Clinical HERBALISM

PLANT WISDOM FROM EAST AND WEST

Rachel Lord, BA, RN

Registered Nurse
Certified Master Herbalist
American Herbalists Guild
Aurora, Colorado

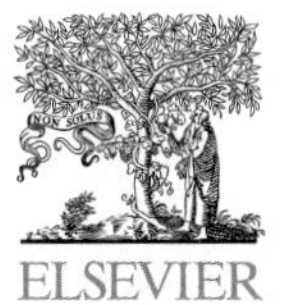

Elsevier
3251 Riverport Lane
St. Louis, Missouri 63043

CLINICAL HERBALISM ISBN: 978-0-323-72176-9

Notice

Practitioners and researchers must always rely on their own experience and knowledge in evaluating and using any information, methods, compounds or experiments described herein. Because of rapid advances in the medical sciences, in particular, independent verification of diagnoses and drug dosages should be made. To the fullest extent of the law, no responsibility is assumed by Elsevier, authors, editors or contributors for any injury and/or damage to persons or property as a matter of products liability, negligence or otherwise, or from any use or operation of any methods, products, instructions, or ideas contained in the material herein.

Disclaimer

This information is for educational purposes only and is not intended as a substitute for professional medical advice, diagnosis, or treatment. Always seek professional medical advice from your physician or other qualified healthcare providers with any questions you may have regarding a medical condition.
Because medical herbalism is an ever-changing field, herbal indications, dosages, and drug interactions may change as new research dictates. What is presented in this text are guidelines – as the relative safety of any substance depends on the quality of product and the health of the consumer. Always check with the latest reliable sources.

International Standard Book Number: 978-0-323-72176-9

Photographs loaned with permission from THE BOTANICAL SERIES are copy-written by Jennifer Anne Tucker and Gerald Lang from the Studio at Hill Crystal Farm. www.jennifer-tucker.com

Joan Zinn, Chief editor, reviewer, photographer, and illustrator, www.medicinehillherbs.com

Senior Content Development Manager: Lisa Newton
Senior Content Strategist: Linda Woodard
Content Development Specialist: Andrew Schubert
Publishing Services Manager: Julie Eddy
Senior Project Manager: Abigail Bradberry
Design Direction: Amy Buxton

Printed in India

Last digit is the print number: 9 8 7 6 5 4 3

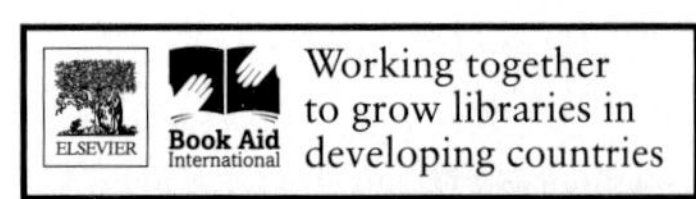

Contents

Herbal Reviewers

Joan Zinn
Western Herbalist, American Herbalists Guild
Original illustrations
Owner, Medicine Hill Herbs
Centennial, Colorado

Matthew Berk, L.Ac.
Eastern Herbalist
Acupuncturist
Pacific College of Oriental Medicine
San Diego, California

Preface

"We do not become healers. We came as healers. We are."
Clarissa Pinkola Estes, from *A Simple Prayer for Remembering the Motherlode*

The Call for More Clinical Herbalists

Herbal healing is one of the oldest practices on the planet, yet one of the newest up-and-coming professions. Reliance on healing botanicals has gone in and out of fashion and acceptance over its long history. The good news for present day herbalists is that there is an increased interest in wellness and willingness to modify lifestyle for the sake of health.

Although *herbalism* is not listed as one of the top ten career paths on popular websites or in the press, health care professions certainly are. There is a reported growing shortage of nurses, doctors, and home health aides as more people, especially the elderly, get sicker and sicker. Modern medicine keeps them alive longer, but quality of life decreases with chronic illnesses, dementias, Alzheimer's disease, and depression. Furthermore, diseases such as diabetes, obesity, and hyperactivity disorders are creeping into our children's lives due to poor dietary and lifestyle choices and peer pressure, among other factors.

An herbalist's intention has historically been to keep people healthy, to use preventative measures, and to be proactive. Maintaining optimum health is our mantra, rather than chasing symptoms and diseases around later. So, who says that herbalism is not, once again, a legitimate up-and-coming profession? If you are trying to become a millionaire, this isn't it. But if looking for a rewarding career, with a chance to heal yourself and others while helping the planet survive, then proceed full speed ahead.

Intentions of the Text

This herbal textbook is the one I always wished for. It is meant to be a practical and understandable user-friendly tool for solo seekers, formal students, educators, herb schools, and colleges. I set out to provide the foundations needed for the modern herbalist and to explain things step by step in a clear and understandable manner. It is meant to help launch into whatever next step appears along the herbal journey. If starting from scratch, welcome. This guide, along with a good teacher or herb school, is a way to go. At the other end, schools will find this a useful text to augment their programs. Perhaps you have already taken herbal classes, gone to a school, found a mentor, or studied on your own. Then this text is aimed at being a good reference to fill in a blank spot or help with memory. Say you forgot the proportions for putting up a tincture or are wondering, "What was that herb, again, for menstrual cramps?" Just flip open this reference to find the answer.

A message to educators: for the all the wonderful herb schools, trainings, and teachers already out there, I know from experience that finding a good text to augment existing curriculums is a challenge. Most herb schools are small, and they typically piece together handouts from their own experience, past classes, and other sources. The volume of herbal information is daunting. A college program, especially, needs a good solid text.

I thought it would be lovely to present what is needed under one tree, so to speak. I certainly would have loved it, had this resource been available for me, way back when. Therefore, I provide what I believe is a beginning and not so beginning guide for school use. In that vein, an *Instructor's Manual* containing suggested lab activities and pop quizzes with answers is available online for instructors. Selections for the hands-on lab sections actually work. I have successfully used those very formulas, gathered from all over, and tested out the activities in my own school. Every class needs some breakout lab time to provide hands-on time—to mix up the medicine and to smell, taste, and experience the plants. Otherwise all you get are a lot of glazed-over eyeballs.

This text is very thorough. My intention is to take nothing for granted and to cover all bases. My hope is that at the end of the day, those with a passion can go out there with enough confidence to carry on as a competent clinical herbalist. This textbook will always be around in a pinch, an old familiar friend. It is a reference to return to for reminders, review, and support when faced with the sometimes scary task of devising a challenging formula and health plan for a complicated client. Nobody is an expert right away, if ever.

Every herbal program or class needs the personal take and touch of its instructor. Exposure to different points of view is enriching, much more interesting, and fun. I believe we all bring our own wisdom and life experiences into the mix of whatever endeavor we embrace. I respect that and you.

The East-West Format

One of the pitfalls of a lot of Western herbal programs and books is that there is really no method provided to make a good assessment of a client's individual condition, nor to determine the best herbal choices from a laundry list of possibilities. It embraces a *take this for that* approach or, one could say, a cookbook mentality.

Other ancient herbal traditions such as Ayurvedic, Unani-Tibb, and Traditional Chinese Medicine have honed assessment skills for patients that are elegant and earth-based. These are incredibly successful in a clinical sense, having evolved over thousands of years. They provide a holistic approach that includes the planet we live on, its elements, the weather, seasons, plants, and animals. These ancient healing traditions appreciated what is referred to as the qualities of a plant, its energetics. They include qualities such as heat, cold, dry, or damp, or some version thereof.

In turn, determinations were made about patients by examining aspects such as the tongue, urine, pulse, personality, or body type, which were then matched up with remedies to heal a given condition. Later, the American Eclectics borrowed from these various systems to develop their unique energetic format.

The modern Western medical approach has pretty much abandoned all this wisdom in favor of a single-minded obsession with science and technology. When this works, it is lifesaving. But it often doesn't work, especially with chronic illness. Throughout history, Western herbalism has always been entangled, often at odds, with the prevailing and dominant medical philosophy of the times. In the modern era, Western herbalists have tended to follow the allopathic lead, perhaps in an attempt to appear more *credible* and respected.

Western herbalism has now come full circle. We are getting back to our roots. It makes for a more successful practice and healing system. Therefore, I have chosen to combine Chinese botanicals with traditional and beloved Western herbs. This is how I learned. I have included Chinese syndromes or disease patterns with a close-as-possible comparison to Western disease names. I am a nurse, after all. I have included Chinese assessment methods of pulse and tongue examination, along with tools that a Westerner might use, such as how to take a blood pressure.

This provides the best of both worlds. It is not the easiest route, because there is a great deal to learn. For a Westerner not trained in Chinese Medicine, it's like learning another language. Even Chinese organs have different meanings than their corresponding Western anatomical parts. But in the end, it's worth it.

Overall Organization

A huge amount of material is organized in what I deem a logical sequence, one that actually makes sense. Any way material is juggled, there is arguably a better order. I placed this material in a sequence that worked for myself and my classes, but as I went along, I would switch things around in real time to fit a unique classroom need. So, I recommend that any school or individual looking to create their own curriculum start here, and then expand, mix or match, and reorganize as needed.

For instance, at first I put the medicine-making segment near the end, but I later discovered that students wanted to get their hands into the nitty gritty of remedy-making much earlier. If it was late spring, a logical time for an herb walk, everyone itching to be in the great outdoors with the baby plants popping up, what good would botany, plant families, and proper identification be tucked in at the end of the program, not yet covered? With these considerations, the text is divided into five parts.

Part I The Basics

This comprises the basics of herbal medicine complete with history, botany, wildcrafting, herbal preparations, and instructions on medicine-making. Chemical constituents come next, providing a scientific segue into traditional plant energetics. Then comes what seems the most challenging topic for Westerners untrained in Chinese Medicine: namely the foundational elements of Western and Chinese Medicine, how they mesh, how they don't, and why this understanding is essential to obtaining good results as an herbalist. For example, a lot of practice time and class labs must be devoted to Chinese pulse and tongue assessment, so it may be used effectively in clinic.

Part II Materia Medica

The all-important Materia Medica, the basic plant information section, is divided into two chapters—the first being a well-rounded selection of individual herbs, and the second comprising groups of similarly acting botanicals, such as a group of cooling demulcents with the nuances between them. Each botanical follows the same format, making the information consistent. I have chosen twenty-five basic herbs that *I think* all herbalists must know. Then come a few important groupings. The Materia Medica includes Western and Chinese botanical selections.

Choosing a good basic Materia Medica always boils down to personal favorites. There are some indisputables, such as the need for Licorice root and at least one berberine, such as Western Oregon Grape root or Chinese Coptis Huang Lian (Goldthread root). But after that, possibilities abound, with what has worked either historically or from personal experience. A beginning Materia Medica should be chosen from common plants that are readily available and not too expensive. There should not be too many. It is best to include a couple of versatile representatives of each body system or energetic quality. For example, a good warming or neutral anti-infective, such as Osha root or Echinacea root, and a cooling antibiotic or antiviral, like Usnea thallus or Andrographis Chuan Xin Lian (Heart-Thread Lotus leaf).

Part III The Herbalist in Action

This is the practical preparation for student clinic. Here we stop being theoretical or intellectual. Instead it's what is needed to know in real time, in a real live clinic setting. A chapter is involved with herbal safety and herb-drug interactions—important information, not necessarily requiring memorization, but still essential. Above all, do no harm. Then comes how to put any given formula together, proportioning out each herb—called *dispensing*. Proper dosing is an essential aspect.

Finally, comes the interview—taking a health history, making an accurate assessment using all described tools, and devising a feasible, effective plan. At the end comes documentation. Health forms are provided to copy and use at will. These appear in the text and in Appendix A.

Part IV Case Histories: Therapeutics and Formulations

This is approached in Western style by body systems. General information is presented about each system. Included are *functional medicine* concepts, with basic understandings that help herbalists get to the root of chronic health problems, including gut health, inflammation, oxidative stress, and liver detoxification. Chinese syndromes or disease patterns with typical pulse and tongue examples are given and are correlated as much as possible with Western diseases.

A small list of important Chinese and Western herbs not previously mentioned in the original Materia Medica section is highlighted here because they are pertinent, a *must* for that body system. Herbal categories are given along with numerous tables to help in creating a personalized formula.

Finally come various case histories showcasing conditions that an herbalist is most likely to encounter, complete with sample formulas and their rationales. The Western disease is explained, and its most likely Chinese syndrome given. The presentation is given in S.O.A.P. format (Subjective, Objective, Assessment, Plan), a standard method of charting and organizing a treatment strategy.

Part V Getting Out There

The final but highly important chapters include current entities and herbal organizations, such as Germany's Commission E, the American Botanical Council, and the American Herbalists Guild. Included are the legal aspects of herbal medicine and herbs. Where do we stand and what are the issues? How are legalities handled in other countries? The debate still rages about herbal standardization, an issue enmeshed in politics, the American Medical Association (AMA), the Federal Drug Administration (FDA), and among herbalists themselves. A discussion is included about Good Manufacturing Practices (GMP) and what that means for us. If being a clinician isn't your bag, mention is made of the various and potentially lucrative other areas an herbalist might explore while still using their skills and love of healing plants.

How to Use This Text

Ground Rules

- *Some knowledge of anatomy and physiology.* The text assumes a basic understanding of each body system. If clarification is desired, obtain a simple beginner's anatomy and physiology reference, such as Cohen and Taylor's *Structure and Function of the Human Body*, listed in the Bibliography.
- *Herbal strengths.* The herbs used in this text are mild and medium strength only. None are very toxic or strong. *Mild* refers to a plant with minimum to no toxicity that is safe with proper use, such as Milk Thistle seed. *Medium*-strength plants have some potential toxicity. A few are listed, like Valerian and Comfrey root. Cautions and contraindications are clearly presented. *Strong* herbs are highly toxic and potentially life-threatening plants that should never be used without a lot of knowledge, experience, and courage, such as Foxglove herb or Henbane herb. None of those appear in our Materia Medica.
- *Commission E.* Refers to Germany's government-sponsored herbal compendium or monograph that enumerates benefits, approved use, dosages, side effects, cautions, and herb-drug interactions. Occasionally, some of that information is included in our Materia Medica, especially the cautions and contraindications. Commission E is considered an authority and is respected by herbalists worldwide. A lot of research and effort went into its creation.
- *Chinese versus Western.* Chinese organs are capitalized—Heart, Lungs, Spleen. Western anatomical organs are small case—heart, lungs, spleen. Chinese syndromes are capitalized, as in Kidney Qi Deficiency.
- *Herb names.* Nomenclature will be explored. Writing plant names follows a recognized form. Botanical names in Latin are italicized with first name (genus) capitalized; second name (species) italicized in small letters—*Taraxacum officinale.* Common names are capitalized, followed by plant part used in lowercase: Dandelion root. Pinyin names, the official romanization system for standard Chinese, is capitalized—Pu Gong Ying for Dandelion root.

Chapter Organization

Chapters begin with *Chapter Review*, a brief, bulleted outline of the contents therein to determine if that is the needed one. *Key Terms* list the important words presented. They are highlighted in the text, appearing again in the *Glossary*. Then come a few introductory paragraphs to further detail contents. The previewed information follows, concluded by a *Summary*. Sometimes just reading the summary alone can help jog the memory. The final section is a *Review* portion to help determine if the material was understood and retained or if reviewing a particular section might be in order. *Fill in the Blanks* follow, with answers in Appendix B. Finally come *Critical Concept Questions*, a group of open-ended queries with answers for the reader to decide.

The Back of the Book Is a Treasure Trove

- *Glossary.* This part gives a quickie guide to important words and concepts used in the text. Think of it as a mini review. Kind of fun to read on its own.
- *Appendix.* This is a vital and quick reference with key information. *Conversions* contain the practical ones I have always used as an herbalist, such as how many drops to a teaspoon or how many milliliters fit in a four-ounce tincture bottle. Then comes average *Doses* to use for tinctures, teas, capsules, and syrups, for both adults and children. The handy *Forms* section follows. These may be reproduced and used if desired.
- *Abbreviations.* A self-explanatory list provides abbreviations used in the text.
- *Cross-referenced Materia Medica.* This is a convenient listing of all herbs I have used, plus others. They are cross-referenced into lists and alphabetized according to botanical name, common name, and pinyin designations.
- *Bibliography.* Listed are the amazing books I referenced, ones that might grace any herbalist's library.

So now with the game plan laid out, the time has come to delve into the specifics of becoming a credible and informed herbalist. Enjoy the ride.

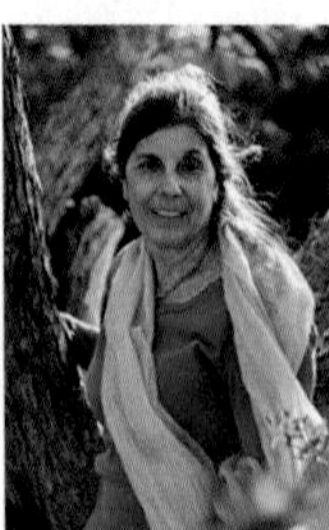

Author Rachel Lord. (Photo courtesy of Sebastian Gorklo, Wolfeyemedia.)

Acknowledgments

It really does take a village. This book could never have existed without my many circles, the herbal community, family, friends, and the star attractions, the plants. At times these circles overlap and intermingle, blurring together into a holistic whole—and at other times, one sphere is singled out, depending on the moment. Thus, my thank you note.

Herbalist Joan Zinn, this text's illustrious illustrator and Western herbal reviewer, has been my faithful backup on Western herbal accuracy, contributing amazing illustrations, photography, computer expertise, copyediting, and attention to detail—endless spelling and punctuation corrections (even when I secretly didn't want to hear it). Her many talents and countless hours glued to the computer go beyond thanks. And, as if her editing expertise wasn't enough, Joan has been my wildcrafting mentor for years, introducing me to plants in the wild through countless herb walks in all kinds of weather, involving plant identification, foraging, and adventuring. She is truly a remarkable teacher and Wise Woman.

Acupuncturist Matthew Berk, Chinese Medicine reviewer, came through brilliantly with his expertise on Chinese herbal medicine and his very gentle corrections to an occasional pulse or tongue *faux pas* on my part.

Photographer and herbalist Jennifer Ann Tucker and husband, professor and photographer Gerald Lang, came along quite serendipitously at the perfect moment. Their magnificent creative collaborations and copyrighted photos, *The Botanical Series*, are loaned with permission from the Studio at Hill Crystal Farm. They are scattered throughout, particularly in the botany chapter.

Herbalist and writer Mary Maruca was there from the start with her encouragement and knowledge about the world of publishing and her valuable advice on approaching that daunting area. Which segues to Elsevier, this text's publisher, having the vision and confidence in me to accept this manuscript. My gratitude is heartfelt.

Technical support has come from my loving husband, Mark Felton, who was always there when I panicked about a computer crisis, not to mention his constant encouragement and patience through a very lengthy process that left us little time to enjoy other activities together.

My children and extended family have always had my back. Their unconditional love, support, and psychic energy (in this and a lifetime of undertakings) has been a constant. Soul sister Andrea Lord was always game, be it helping me wildcraft, hiking anywhere, or doing what she does best—listening.

The herbal community has given me nothing but good vibes and inspiration. I have learned from them all, whether they know it or not. And finally, my herbal allies have been important spiritual teachers and provided countless hours of communion, healing, and joy.

This book is dedicated to my special friend Joan Zinn—chief editor, illustrator, and consultant in all things herbal—who went above and beyond in her help and support. And with love and gratitude to the plant spirits, and all my friends and relations.

1 From the Heart

"It takes SEVEN lifetimes to become an herbalist."

—Herbalist Susun Weed

Your Stories

This textbook is for all those drawn to healing plants. We all have our stories or special people in our lives who opened doors. Perhaps a wise mother or grandmother brewed up a remedy from the garden when you were small. You always remembered the taste and smell of her elderberry honey elixir or her soothing peppermint-licorice tea. If herbal healing runs in the family and you are continuing that legacy, how fortunate.

Perhaps an inspirational teacher or mentor crossed your path at the right time and place. Maybe you apprenticed with a wise old soul, or a dear friend dragged you along on a hike, and in spite of yourself, you found yourself checking out every plant along the trail with her. Some people are gardeners who find joy in watching plants grow and love putting their hands in the dirt. Many grow ornamental flowers first, followed by a more practical vegetable garden. Next, they may add a few cooking herbs that are also medicinal, such as oregano, marjoram, or rosemary. One step leads to another.

Sometimes a nightmarish experience with an insurance company starts an herbal journey. You might have been rejected because of a preexisting condition or not have had the coverage needed to receive an expensive, but life-saving, cancer drug. Maybe you couldn't afford any health insurance at all, leaving no choice but to find an alternative. Did you become disillusioned with the medical establishment because of a bad experience? There sure are plenty of horror stories out there of doctors who do not listen, misdiagnose, prescribe strong drugs with bad side effects, and perform botched or unnecessary surgeries.

There are also the seemingly impossible, too-good-to-be-true, real-life miracles that have changed many lives. Did an herbalist or alternative healer cure you of some serious chronic disease when traditional medicine utterly failed? Some variation of this story is often the inspiration for beginning holistic health studies, whether in herbalism, acupuncture, or massage therapy. The alternative-medicine list is huge. Perhaps you, like me, originally trained as a nurse but eventually sought out other modalities because so few of your patients were truly healed. There are many stories and reasons to turn to plant wisdom. The upshot is that here you are, seeking more.

My Story

It took a long time for me to get to the point where I had the courage to write a textbook that I felt would actually provide useful information and serve as a go-to guide for others. I zigzagged around the signposts pointing me in that direction until finally I arrived.

I live in Colorado where the outdoors and the mountains are a way of life. In the old days, I was a tree checker-outer and a flower-picker. The flower-picking part was done in all innocence with no awareness that, just possibly, I was removing potential seeds that would ensure continuation of next year's blooms. One day, to my embarrassment, I got busted. At Yosemite National Park, I was caught in the act. A park ranger put an end to my wild bouquet creativity.

Then came a July day in 1960s when I drifted by a street fair high up in Telluride, Colorado. One of the booths featured displays of dried herbs lovingly arranged in bundles and tied with natural jute and ribbons. Recycled gallon pickle jars contained mysterious dried plants. It was all very alluring. I asked the wise lady managing the booth about a jar of beautiful red berries. "Rosehips," she replied. "They grow all through the mountains." Wow. And thus it began.

Little did I know then that I would take a slight detour, becoming a nurse and entering the health field in a very conventional way. After nursing school, I worked in an intensive care unit (ICU) for many years, becoming a high-tech adrenaline junky. Working in the ICU is not for easygoing, mellow types. For a while, I found the work challenging and stimulating. I treated a lot of trauma patients, and the heroic saves that followed made me feel proud. Trouble was, very few of my patients with chronic illnesses actually got any better. In fact, they were readmitted multiple times for the exact same problem. We nurses joked that they were the "frequent fliers." Looking back, I think that those comments were not too kind, perhaps, but still true.

During those years, my view of conventional allopathic medicine started to change. For trauma and emergencies, orthodox medicine saved lives, but for the rest, it provided no more than Band-Aid cures. Disillusioned, I reduced my hospital hours, eventually weaning myself out of the ICU and all the while taking courses in holistic health. (This, by the way, is a path many nurses took before me and likely will continue to follow.) After becoming a certified massage therapist and then a national board-certified reflexologist, I opened a private practice. I even taught at my former massage school for a while. Having a nursing background certainly didn't hurt my credentials.

I went to every holistic, alternative medicine workshop I could find and afford, on all kinds of topics. Some were fabulous; some were just ok. My critical test was that the workshop had to be practical. I wanted to be sure I could turn around the next day and really start using what I had learned, both on myself and in my own practice. I had no time for what was intellectual and interesting; I sought the type of workshop that would leave me wondering, "Now what do I actually do with this?"

Later, the same criterion became the standard I aspired to attain in my herb school, Just for Health. I wanted graduating students to be able to take the plunge after attending classes and begin to use the herbs. I wanted them to feel comfortable going out into their communities as practicing herbalists, rather than putting their notes and handouts back on the shelf to collect dust, with the hope they would get back to them someday. So many folks are enthusiastic starters but poor finishers. They don't use their education after shelling out a chunk of cash to learn a subject. I found the key to success for my students was to provide lots of hours of student clinic and practice with actual clients while they still had the safety net of the school and its instructors. A good long clinical experience can make it or break it for a budding herbalist.

So after sampling many holistic classes, I had found my passion and enrolled in a major herbal medicine training with Peter Holmes, licensed acupuncturist, master herbalist, and aromatherapist. I was officially hooked on herbs. Time flew by while I made herbal tinctures; before I knew it, dinner time was long gone. I was so engrossed in herbology that I developed a large apothecary containing both Western and Chinese herbs. Every time I learned about a fabulous new herb, I added it to my must-have list.

My herbal tincture collection grew far beyond the well-known, such as echinacea root and goldenseal root. I remember thinking, "I have to have Salvia Dan Shen" an exemplary Chinese herb for the heart. So I ordered a pound and made it up. Oh, yes, and then I had to gather some Western bilberry leaves in the mountains to help with blood sugar balance. Of course, I hunted out more and more must-have plants. Herbal medicine became an obsession, a dedication, a meditation, a new way of life. I spent my money on whatever next plant I couldn't live without.

In 2003, I opened a Colorado state-approved school called Just for Health School of Reflexology and Healing Arts. When dreaming about how to establish the school and develop the herbal curriculum, I believed it had to include both Western and Chinese philosophies and botanicals to achieve true healing. That's the way I was taught. After I enlisted the help of an acupuncturist to teach the Chinese aspects of the curriculum, we launched ourselves as a cross-cultural East–West herb school. Along the way, as we taught classes, I learned what was needed to help students develop the confidence to really make a go of an herbal practice. I discovered my program's strong points, pitfalls, and holes. Because I could find no textbook in print that covered what I needed, this book organically evolved.

Herbalism Is Community

Now here's a bonus, something wonderful I discovered on my herbal journey. There is a whole tribe of kind-hearted, like-minded people who will embrace and support you on your herbal path and gather together in community with you—if you let them. Your only requirement is to adore and respect plant wisdom. If you do that, you're in. Education or lack of credentials are not the defining criteria. You may have no credentials at all, and you will still be welcome if you love plants. In this community, students of all ages are accepted. Herbalist grandmothers tend to mentor and encourage the newbies. Supporting new herbalists is critical, because all who love plant medicine want the tradition to continue generation after generation—and to raise herbalism's status in the 21st century and beyond.

Communities of supportive herb people are critical, because there always comes a time when the help of a practiced herbalist to save a plant or help with a medicine is needed. One such time came for me when I had the opportunity to acquire fresh *Avena sativa* (milky oat berry), a brain food and nervous system restorative extraordinaire. This is one of the herbs you must have when it is fresh. It is much less effective when dried. The milky stage of the berry is when the young, green immature oat seed is fresh and moist. It is available only about 2 weeks out of the year, so acquiring it at that time is a sensitive, challenging endeavor.

Fortunately, I'm part of an amazing community. So when milky oat berry became available, the Boulder-Denver herbal community pipeline was sent into operation, and a text went out. Pacific Botanicals, an Oregon herb company and farm, had just announced that milky oats would soon be harvested. The community asked if I wanted to go in on an order. Of course, I did! I took a pound.

Fresh herbs need to be sent out via overnight air so that they don't get mildew and moldy in transit. They also have to be tinctured immediately on arrival. Well, time came for the herbal delivery, and just then I had to go out of town. So I asked a dear herbalist friend to pick up my order and tincture it for me right then and there. The oats were safely sitting in alcohol when I returned.

Then there are herbal gatherings. Sometimes we meet at the home of my friend and fellow herbalist Brigitte Mars every summer for a nerdy, annual herbalist potluck. The main topic is some plant or other. We geek out. Brigitte always blends up and serves a fresh Nettle smoothie, along with other veggies and fruits.

Numerous groups have periodic herbal symposia all over the country and abroad. I have found them well worth attending. They offer a wonderful learning, connecting, and joyous herbal ride. If you didn't know anyone before you got there, you could be sure to have a bunch of herbal buddies and connections by the time you leave.

Herbalism Is a Spiritual Journey

For me, botanical medicine is much more than a profession. Herbalism is a spiritual path, a mind-opening experience, an opportunity to explore other realms. Herbal wisdom comes from many sources. Books are one avenue. More esoteric sources of plant wisdom also exist, if you choose to travel there. They involve altered levels of consciousness, meditative and altered states that let you establish a relationship with a plant. Shamans, medicine men and women, curanderos, and the ancient goddess cultures have all known and practiced these forms of connection. Communing and sitting with a plant in the wild can be a mind-opening practice. The plant beings will convey secrets, tell you who they are, let you know who their medicine is for, and give other information—but only if they are treated with respect. And gratitude. And patience.

I have had the great fortune to be gifted with some fresh *Cereus grandiflorus* (Night-blooming cactus flower and stem) (Fig. 1.1)

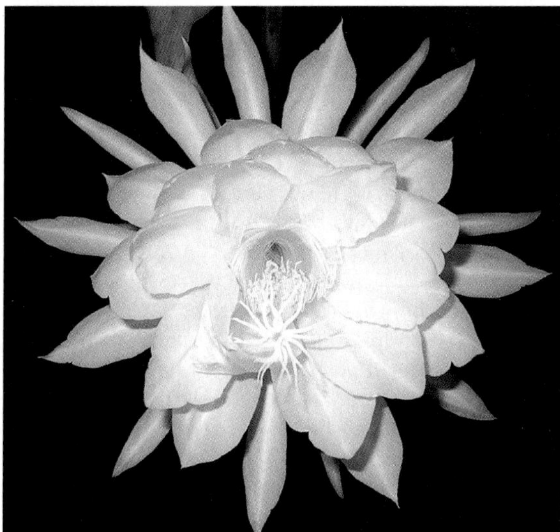

• **Fig. 1.1** Night-blooming *Cereus* flower. (Greenhouse grown and photographed by Joan Zinn.)

grown in a greenhouse. The fleeting cactus blossoms bloom for one night only, giving off a heavenly sweet scent. By morning, the flowers are folded and gone. This cactus flower is strong heart medicine, loved and revered by the famous American Eclectic herbalists of the 19th century.

While tincturing these gorgeously huge white flowers, I drifted into another dimension, complete with visions of a mysterious lady and connection to her spirit. We had never met before, but I now know she is one of my teachers who will instruct me in how to use *Cereus* carefully, with intuition, wisdom, and care. Books say *Cereus* is strong medicine, with a potential for toxicity. But as poet Bob Dylan sang, "You don't need a weatherman to know which way the wind blows." I now know this herb and her personality from a personal space as a powerful and sometimes dangerous ally to be treated with respect.

Caution: *Cereus* is not a plant for beginners and is not recommended for a basic apothecary. Thus I have not detailed its use in our text. I mention it only as part of my own personal medicine journey. Your own allies will appear for you when you are ready—and when the time is right.

Herbalists Are Stewards of the Earth

Being out in nature, going on foraging expeditions known as wildcrafting, or simply walking along and identifying plants up in the mountains is my idea of heaven. I might be alone or with a like-minded friend. Either way, I can think of no other place I'd rather be than in this primal, quiet, peaceful space outdoors. Even when I am not gathering herbs for my apothecary, I am always checking things out, field guide in hand. I'm generally going slowly, looking down, but sometimes up. Or sideways. I don't cover much physical territory, but I do get lost in another world. I return home muddy and rejuvenated (Fig. 1.2).

Digging into the earth for a root or snipping off a flower must be done consciously. To do this, give thanks, ask permission, and if not forthcoming, move on to another spot. Always leave enough in a stand, a group, or plant family, for another day and another year. And then, please cover your tracks. Fill in the hole. Cover the spot with dried grass or branches. Leave no trace. And for heaven's sake, be sure of correct identification.

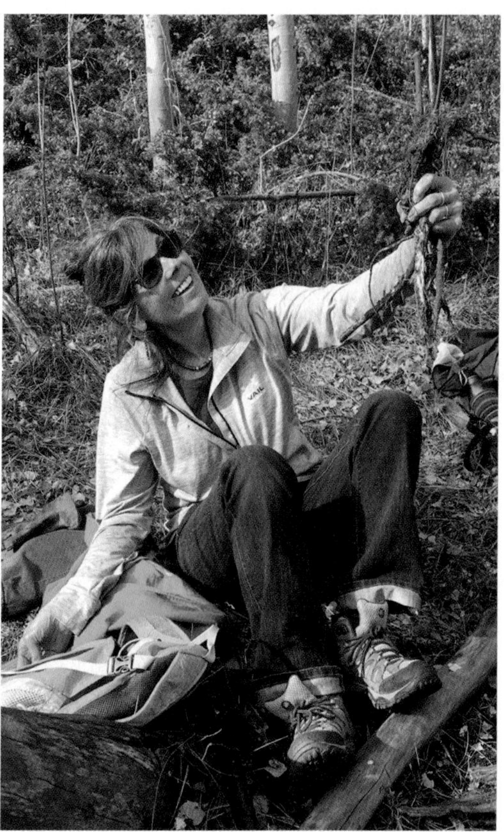

• **Fig. 1.2** Rachel and her hard-won Osha root.

The most obvious thing that draws most people to a new plant is its flower, which is usually seen in summer. A flower's scent and texture are important. Next, we notice the leaves— their pattern, shape, and stem arrangement. Finally, as we become more sophisticated, we know the plant through the other seasons. We recognize her in the fall when she has gone to seed, and in the winter when brown and dry with only a couple of seeds, dried flowers, or crackly leaves still hanging on. Then comes spring, when baby leaves pop up fresh and new through the earth. I am not fully acquainted with a plant until I can recognize her in all guises and seasons. Meeting the botanical all chopped-up in a package bought from a store is never quite as powerful.

Whenever you have the opportunity to check out whole growing plants, wherever you live, seize the moment. I confess that herb walks and outings were the most popular part of my school, more so than any brilliant lecture I had ever prepared. Over the years, I added more and more walks to the program. The students could not get enough. Walking the earth awakens our primal connection to the plants and Earth. We remember who we are, who we were, where we come from.

The most ancient and the latest sources of wisdom say we are all connected. This includes the plants, people, animals, and even the rocks. Native Americans have always known and taught this. Now scientists say that the microflora in our gut and on our skin are similar to the underground fungal mycelium and bacteria connecting the roots of plants. Our bodies and the plants are all really one enormous organism. We are truly a hologram, part of a holistic whole. If this is so, how could we possibly disrespect and tear down nature, the planet, deplete our natural resources, destroy ourselves?

This understanding and consciousness could be one important answer to saving our earth—stopping climate change and healing the planet. Plant people carry with them that grave responsibility for healing at all levels. Herbalists understand this communion with all that lives, and the resulting need to conserve and protect resources, to wildcraft responsibly, to take only what we need and leave enough to grow another day. In this way, acting as true stewards, we gift our children and others with this deep truth.

Herbalism Is a Good Excuse to Travel

Herbalists, medicine men and women, and ethnic healers can be found all over the planet, each practicing their own healing wisdom. Certainly, there are plants indigenous to specific areas of the world that you've never heard of, seen, or met. Think of the Incas of South America who use the healing herbs from the Andes and Amazon rain forest. Daydream about native cultures from Central and North America, including Canada. Don't forget the Hawaiian kahuna shaman, Australian aborigine wisdom, and African medicine women and men. The list is as long as those of plants and humans who love and learn from them.

Opportunities may present for herbal study, apprenticeships, workshops, or expeditions to other countries. Some herb schools offer these experiences as part of their curriculum. If you find one, consider yourself blessed. Dr. Rosita Arvigo knows the healing ways of the Maya in the rain forest of Belize. She offers American herbalists opportunities to study ethnobotany and Maya abdominal massage. I know more than one wise woman who has returned to Belize multiple times to learn and apprentice with beloved Rosita.

Various organizations offer special tours for herbalists also. I was fortunate enough to join a group of healers with Plants and Healers International, based in Asheville, North Carolina. We traveled to Peru's magnificent Sacred Valley and enjoyed a 2-week herb walk, mixed in with visits to Machu Picchu and other spectacular Inca ruins. We learned a lot from our enthusiastic guides, who with much joy, song, and humor dispensed scientific knowledge coupled with deep spiritual understanding of the plants and culture.

Such trips are peak experiences that you'll never forget and cherish forever. They can be enjoyed by visiting another country or by remaining in your own. Wise women and men are everywhere. Look and ask around, and I know yours will be the perfect expedition at the perfect moment.

A Few Words of Wisdom

First. Appreciate the plants and their teachings. Herbalism, in its truest sense, is connecting with the earth and the Earth Mother. We are the stewards of the green. Respectful wildcrafting is very important so that our herbal legacy and our natural medicines will still be available for our children, their children, and future children through the seventh generation. We must protect our resources, learn from nature, and give thanks.

Second. The best way to know a plant is to sit with it where it lives and listen with all the senses. If this is impossible or if a particular herb doesn't grow nearby, no worries. Feel, taste, and smell the bag of herbs you have and say, "Hello." Try sitting with a common plant in your neighborhood. Lady dandelion grows all over the world, so she certainly grows near your house. Countless so-called medicinal weeds are adapted to city environments. Others adapt to specific countries on the map. Granted, you can't find ginseng in a desert in the Southwest desert or osha root at sea level, but you can get to know plenty of plants who grow happily wherever you are. Order the ones that don't grow nearby from a reputable, conscious, Earth-loving herb company.

Third. Herbal knowledge and healing is a health insurance policy. If we know about the healing plants and how to use them, we empower ourselves, our families, and our clients to heal and live up to their health potential under their own steam. What if the modern medical system were to crash? How probable is that scenario? Our backups and saving graces have always been our botanical bounty and the herbalists who know how to use medicinal plants. These gifts from nature grew on Earth before medical doctors, clinics, and hospitals arrived on the scene.

Fourth. Herbs may not do it all, but I for one avoid going to medical doctors as much as possible. Keep in mind that this statement is coming from a former nurse also, or especially, because I was one. I know firsthand how broken the medical system can be. Of course, we respect the modern medical establishment as a part of the whole, to be used when needed, but also to call on wisely. For instance, a few years ago, I had a bout of serious difficulty breathing—pneumonia. Then, 2 years later, I suffered a fractured hip. On those occasions, I wasted no time in getting to the nearest modern emergency room. But choosing a gentler healing method whenever possible and appropriate is what herbalism is about. I always turn to my own herbal formulas first.

And fifth. Positive energy and enthusiasm associated with your personal plant work will rub off on your children, friends, family, and community. So get involved. Pass on our precious legacy. Teach others when possible, and make sure the gifts and teachings from the plants are not lost. And please have fun with this never-ending journey. It's like peeling the onion. Learning and understanding plant wisdom goes on and on. Just when you think, "I've finally got this down," there's more to learn, more to be discovered —as another botanical, a new healing plant emerges from the rain forest, desert, or to our consciousness. Or suddenly a new medical use for an old favorite comes along. Let the excitement shine, because you have a lifetime of adventures ahead. Did you have any idea what you were getting into?

2

The History of Herbalism: A Short History of Medicine

2000 BCE	*Here, eat this root.*
CE 1000	*That root is heathen. Here, say this prayer.*
CE 1850	*That prayer is superstition. Here, drink this potion.*
CE 1940	*That potion is smoke oil. Here, swallow this pill.*
CE 1940	*That pill is ineffective. Here, take this antibiotic.*
CE 2000	*That antibiotic is artificial. Here, eat this root.*

— ***Anonymous***

CHAPTER REVIEW

- Prehistory: Plant healing before written records, Goddess and Wise-Woman traditions.
- Ancient times: Greece and Hippocrates; Rome and Galen; Hygeia, Gaia, and Persephone; spice trading; Materia Medicas.
- Western Europe Middle Ages: Europe, Arab pharmacy, alchemy, chemistry, Black Plague; Hildegard von Bingen; the Inquisition; Doctrine of Signatures.
- Renaissance and The Rise of Science: Scientific method; challengers to Galen, Paracelsus, and Culpeper.
- America: Native Americans. Movements: Thomsonian, Physiomedicalists, Eclectics, Popular Health Movement; Lydia Pinkham and Rene Caisse.
- Merging into the Present: Flexner Report and aftermath; U.S. Pharmacopeia and National Formulary. Progressive Era—Elizabeth Blackwell, Margaret Sanger, Mary Gove Nichols, John Hoxey, and Jethro Kloss.
- Historical timeline.

KEY TERMS

Alchemy
Apothecary
Black Plague
Chemist
Doctrine of Signatures
Eclectic movement
Flexner Report
Four humors
Laudanum
Materia Medica
Physiomedicalism
Simple
Thomsonian movement
Unani-Tibb
United States Pharmacopeia (USP)
Wise-Woman Tradition

This chapter looks at the history of herbalism and its turf wars with the medical establishment. The history of herbalism is interwoven with medicine and the status of women. The use of plants used to be *the* stand-alone healing way. Medicine and herbalism did not diverge until the last few hundred years of the Renaissance, when the scientific method began to dominate. Medical technology began to replace old plant wisdom, a rivalry still not resolved. Colorful individuals, historical events, and movements during these eras led us to our current position on the herb-drug continuum.

Key contributors to the history of herbalism were the Wise-Woman healers, whose status fluctuated from revered healer to witch, as trust in plant medicine gave way to support of what became the medical establishment. Women, originally respected as healers protecting the secrets of life and death, were transformed into evil witches and sorceresses influenced by the devil, as mainstream religious practices and organized medicine grew in Europe. Which version was accepted depended on the dogma of the times and political climate. As medicine became an increasingly male-dominated profession, women as healers were downgraded, dismissed, and sometimes persecuted.

So, in tracing the history of herbalism, we must consider two parallel timelines—one being plant medicine versus allopathic Western medicine, and the other the history of women as healers whose influence fluctuated according to their status in society.

Prehistory

How Did Healing Begin?

Humans and animals have always used plants for food and medicine. Often, human knowledge of plant wisdom came from watching animals select plants for their own healing. Overall, learning was undoubtedly intuitive and based on trial and error, with many of our ancestors discovering the hard way what would help or harm.

Archeological finds testify to this phenomenon. A 60,000-year-old grave site of a Neanderthal man located in a cave in Iraq had been scattered with the flower pollen of many medicinal plants still found and used in the area today. Marshmallow, yarrow, and ephedra were there.[1] In addition, Sumerians left written cuneiform records of plants they used. Ancient Egyptians wrote down herbal remedies on papyri. Jars still retaining the aroma of essential oils have also been found in their tombs, a testament to the reverence the ancients had for healing oils and herbs.

The importance of plant remedies is evident in every civilization for which we have either archeological discoveries or written records. Common threads among these civilizations and fundamental principles indicate that plant discoveries and healing practices evolved simultaneously in many cultures and locations. For instance, dandelion grows just about everywhere on earth, an indication of its benefit to humans as a useful and universal remedy.

Shamans, Witch Doctors, Priestesses, and Priests

Ancient communities invariably had wise, respected, and significant female and male healers. Depending on the culture and its deepest healing practices, people of one gender or the other would be respected as shamanic healers capable of reaching altered states of consciousness and bringing back information from unseen realms. These healers relied heavily on plants to achieve access, approaching healing in a ritualistic/talismanic manner. They treated illness holistically, tapping into the spiritual, emotional, and physical ailments of their clients. Frequently, dream work, trances, or exorcisms were used. Wellness could not occur without addressing all realms.

Although people of many cultures achieve altered states today, these practices, often based in herbology, are not recognized as part of the Western scientific medical model. Nevertheless, those who practice magical uses of plants or employ shamanism offer important contributions to their communities, where such beliefs are essential aspects of a cure. Native American traditional healers, Hispanic *curanderas* and *curanderos*, and modern wiccans are all present-day examples of those who carry on the old ways with much success. Many books include magical uses of herbs, but you will not find this information either in Western medical schools or medical libraries.

Overview of the Wise-Woman Tradition

Once upon a time, as far back as human prehistory, the ***Wise-Woman Tradition*** offered ancient peoples healing. The Wise-Woman Tradition is the oldest type of healing known on our planet, yet one that is rarely identified, and rarely written or talked about.[2] It is an oral tradition in which knowledge and use of local plants is passed down by women from generation to generation.

Archeological evidence suggests ancient health practitioners were likely women. Women have always been healers. It is their natural role, the role of the feminine. The Wise-Woman Tradition goes back through millennia, and women in ancient societies who practiced this intuitive knowledge traditionally tapped into the Divine Feminine, the Goddess. Women have long overseen the human process from birth to death, attempting to make the span of time between these two events as easy and comfortable as possible. But the role of woman as respected healer has cycled back and forth, depending on the time and culture in which she lived. Women have long been caregivers and collectors of healing herbs and plants, particularly in hunter-gatherer societies with a deep connection to the earth.

The Divine Feminine continues to be reflected in our knowledge of plants for healing. More than a thousand years of collective experience has taught us how to use herbs safely and effectively. As caregivers, midwives, wives, and mothers, many women naturally gravitate to the healing art and science of plants.

Unfortunately, hardly any Wise-Woman knowledge was written down, having been communicated orally during those distant eras. Much later, as medicine and writing became the purview of men, women were forbidden to speak and write in Latin, the language of physicians and scholars. If they were educated women and actually managed to record their ideas, authorship generally was attributed to a man.

As a result, women tended to pass on information orally from grandmother to mother to daughter—from woman to woman. This oral tradition produced respected rural herbology, the folk wisdom still practiced in small communities (Fig. 2.1). Sometimes women wrote herbal formulas down, using the form of household recipes, having long considered plants as food and as medicine. Many male counterparts, then and now, supported women in their roles as part of the larger herbal community.

As scientific inquiry advanced in Western societies during the Renaissance, older simpler ways lost popularity and eventually were shunned. Trained male physicians claimed the turf once managed by women. They used violent, dangerous, and dramatically heroic procedures, such as bloodletting, applying blood-sucking leeches to

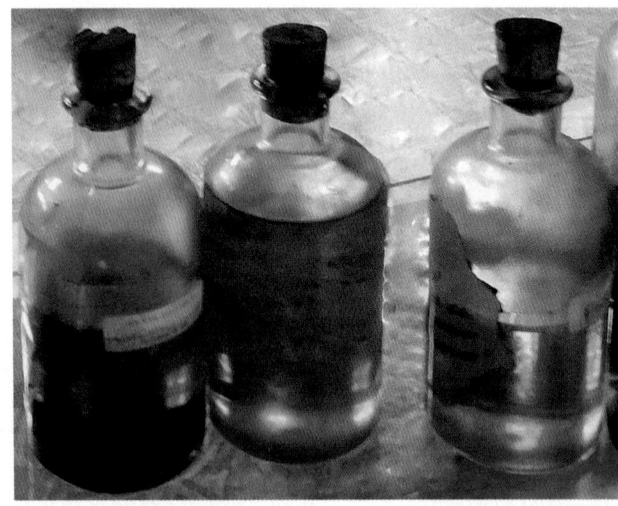

• **Fig. 2.1** Medicine bottles.

the skin, as well as purging, vomiting, and administering mercury. These techniques, so different from the gentler arts of the oral tradition and folk herbalism, led to the diminishment of women's wisdom, which frequently became known as "old wives' tales." Women healers were mocked and given titles like midwives, old wives, crones, green women, nurses, nuns, and, most derisively, simple.

At its most extreme, women were accused of witchcraft. These horrific shameful chapters became part of the Inquisition in Europe and the Salem witch trials in America. Torture and murder were routine. Patriarchal religious doctrine became entangled with medicine. Its persuasive power won out for many centuries, forcing the Wise-Woman way to go underground.

Today Wise-Women and Wise-Men are on the rise. Before most of us venture to consult health care professionals, a large percentage consults a friend or family member with knowledge of herbs. These informal sources of information are overwhelmingly female, though they are joined by more men every day. The feminine principle is beginning to even things out.

Ancient Times

Hippocrates of Greece (460–377 BCE) (Fig. 2.2) is known as the father of Western medicine. He borrowed and expanded on the Perso-Arabic Islamic traditional medicine that was being practiced in India and in Muslim cultures. Known as ***Unani-Tibb,*** it dates from 400 BCE. *Unani* is a Persian word meaning Greek and *Tibb* is an Arabic word meaning medicine.

Hippocrates' medicine was a rational science that used a holistic approach to body type and personality, based on what he referred to as the ***four humors***. Each humor indicated a particular human constitution and had a characteristic personality, temperature, degree of moisture, and a specific pulse and tongue to match—an approach that is similar to the energetics practiced by Ayurvedic and Chinese medicine. For instance, a person with a sanguine (blood) humor was considered happy and optimistic, with a warm and moist quality, an appreciation of the sweet tastes, a strong pulse, and a red tongue.[1] The other humors—yellow bile, black bile, and white phlegm—all had to be in balance with the blood.

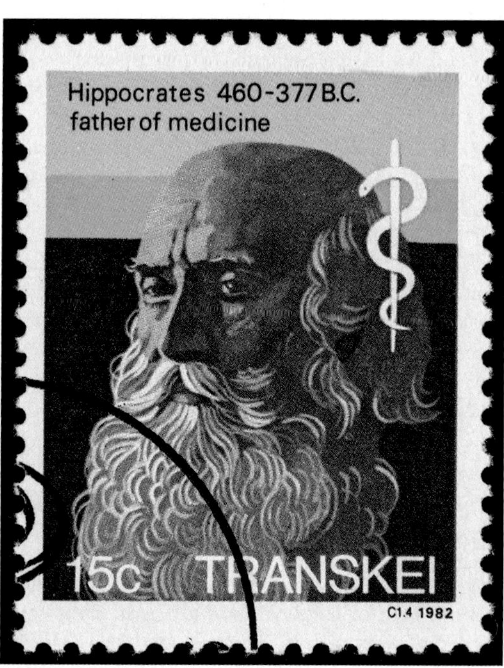

• **Fig. 2.2** Hippocrates stamp (iStock.com/ID#175438227. Credit: PictureLake).

Hippocrates asked questions and conducted physical exams to ascertain which therapy, herbs, and foods patients needed. Signs and symptoms evolved from natural causes and the progression of a disease. Hippocrates was the first to classify illnesses according to their similarities and differences. He encouraged looking into natural causes for illness and restoring balance. Before this approach, at least in the West, and according to the information that has been uncovered to date, the causes of illness and disease were commonly based on superstition or the wrath of angry gods.

Hippocrates, and later Galen of Rome, elaborated on Unani-Tibb Islamic theories. Hippocrates is most remembered today for the Hippocratic Oath, which established high ethical standards for the practice of medicine. A famous and wise quote from one of its many translations is "First, do no harm"—a directive we would all do well to follow.

Another notable Greek physician, pharmacologist, and botanist was Pedianos Dioscorides, who lived c. CE 40–90. Dioscorides wrote *De Materia Medica,* a large encyclopedia of medicinal substances. The text listed and explained approximately 600 herbs and was widely read for the next 1500 years.[3] Among its readers was the famous Islamic physician, Ibn Sina, who lived in the Middle Ages and is discussed later in this chapter.

Dioscorides' *De Materia Medica* was a precursor to modern pharmacopeias. For this reason, Dioscorides is considered the founder of Western herbal medicine. The plant genus *Dioscorea,* which includes the medicinal Wild Yam rhizome, was later named after him by the taxonomist, Carl Linnaeus.

Women Healers in Ancient Greece

Women healers in ancient Greece were few. By that time in history, their role in society had been minimized to that of servant and wife. The study of medicine was punishable by death.[4] However, as hypocritical and contradictory as it sounds, the Greeks still respected women for their healing abilities. A Greek queen and healer named Artemisia discovered the medicinal uses of wormwood, causing the herb now to be included in the genus *Artemisia.* Furthermore, the Olympian goddess, Artemis, ruled the hunt, moon, and chastity and was later associated with childbirth and nature, all interesting connections.

Greek healing goddesses abound. Gaia, goddess of Earth, attests to women's healing powers.[5] The Greeks considered the goddess Hygeia, whose statues include the snake-entwined caduceus, to be one of the children of Asclepius, and today these statues appear in some hospitals (Fig. 2.3). The concept of *hygiene,* so basic to preventative medicine, derives from her name. Demeter, the matriarch who cared for the home, women, and children, made her contribution to the health field through the food she allowed to be raised from the soil, and her daughter, Persephone, cured teeth and eyes. There may well have been many mortal women who made original contributions to Greek medical texts and treatises, but their works have been obscured by centuries of plagiarism and confusion over authorship.[5]

Galen of Rome, c. CE 130–210

Galen, a leading Roman physician, created a system of rules and classifications based on Greek Hippocratic medicine. He too emphasized balancing the four humors (red for blood, black for black bile, yellow for yellow bile, and white for phlegm). Unlike Hippocrates, however, he didn't bother to examine the patient.

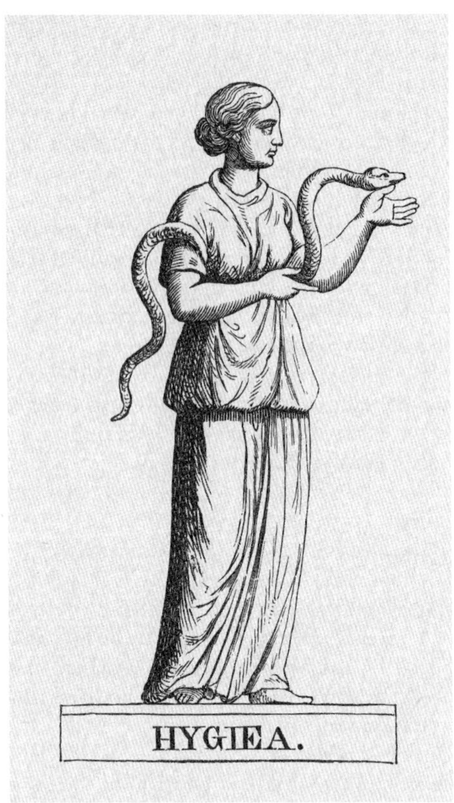

• **Fig. 2.3** The Greek Goddess Hygiea and her snake. (iStock.com/ID:508548651 Credit: ZU_09)

Galen had a rigid system of rules, as well as expensive, complex formulas. His system evaluated plants in terms of the humors and fit them in to a complicated arrangement that was difficult to learn. It ultimately separated the rich and educated from the uneducated and poor, creating an elitist understanding of healing that discounted folk medicine. Right or wrong, this system strictly controlled Western medical philosophy for the next 1500 years, and woe to any brave soul who disagreed, including a Wise-Woman here or there.

Galen's influence managed to paralyze European medical thinking for 1500 years and dominate the doctoring practiced during the Middle Ages.[6] It led to aggressive methods of bloodletting, purging, and use of exotic medications like toad tongues or red ox gall. The more abstruse and awful a remedy, the better. Nothing changed much until the 1860s when Pasteur's scientific germ theory finally supplanted the Galen methods.

Overall, Galen is remembered for disempowering those who practiced individual and community healing. His principles separated and caused the removal of medical practice from the people who had trust in herbs and the healing power of nature. It caused individuals to give up their health care to others, rather than healing themselves. The idea of a single or simple, one-herb cure, as used by common folk, went out of fashion and was scorned. Hence, a simple changed meaning and came to indicate an inferior remedy possessing only one quality, such as heat or moisture, which was used by the uneducated or so-called "simpletons." Instead, the Western medical establishment used the Galenic approach, combining many herbs into complex expensive formulas. Today the word ***simple*** has come full circle and is no longer considered derogatory. The use of a single herb, a simple, is a respected and useful healing protocol in many cases.

Galen and the practitioners of ancient Greece and Rome had such a tremendous influence on modern medicine today that two well-recognized symbols emerged from these traditions—the caduceus and the rod of Asclepius (Box 2.1).

Woman Healers in Ancient Rome

Overall, women's social status in ancient Rome proved better than that of Grecian women. They enjoyed more freedom and prestige, particularly those from aristocratic families. Such women acted as midwives, devised herbal formulas, and functioned as physicians. Octavia, Mark Antony's wife, wrote a book of prescriptions. There was Margareta, an army surgeon, and Fabiola, who founded the first public hospital in history and took advantage of opportunities afforded Roman citizens to help improve human health. As time went on, however, increasing numbers of men became physicians, edging Roman women out of mainstream medicine and delegating them to more peripheral and less lucrative tasks.[5]

Isolated Ancient Cultures Traded Spices: Similar Herbs Used Independently

As the ancients traded spices, exotic plants from foreign lands came into use. Sailors brought cloves and cardamom from the Middle East to Europe. Chocolate from South America was later brought to Europe in the 1500s and transformed from a sacred drink of the Andes into multiple secular uses, ranging from consumption as a delicious beverage to use in candies and liquors. Occasionally, use of similar herbal remedies sprang up independently. Because many of the same plants grow world-wide, their use evolved simultaneously and similarly in many places. Examples of this serendipity include:

- *Angelica archangelica* (Angelica root) and *Glycyrrhiza glabra* (Licorice root). Asians, Europeans, and Native Americans all used these for respiratory ailments.
- *Humulus lupulus* (Hops flower) and *Mentha* spp. (the mints). Many ancient herbal traditions used these to soothe the stomach.
- *Rubus* spp. (Blackberry leaf) *and Rubus idaeus* (Raspberry leaf). These two have a universal history in treating diarrhea.
- *Arctostaphylos uva-ursi* (Uva-ursi leaf). Asians, Europeans, and Native Americans used this as a diuretic.
- *Salix alba* (White Willow bark). The major healing traditions of East Indian Ayurvedic, Chinese, Western European, and native ethnic groups' medicine all used this bark to treat pain and inflammation.

In the 19th century, when science and chemistry became king, chemists homed in on herbal knowledge from around the world. Extracts of the plants in this list became some of the first pharmaceuticals. In fact, 75% of the pharmaceuticals that came to drug companies' attention did so because of their traditional herbal medicine usage.

Historic Ancient Materia Medicas from Around the World

A ***Materia Medica*** is an herbal list, literally meaning the materials of medicine. These collections serve as vehicles for transmitting plant knowledge, written in the language of the day and containing significant information on herbs and their prescriptions. Materia Medicas have been written and recorded throughout written history. They are found in ancient China, Babylon, Egypt, India,

• BOX 2.1 The Caduceus Versus the Rod of Asclepius: A Convoluted History

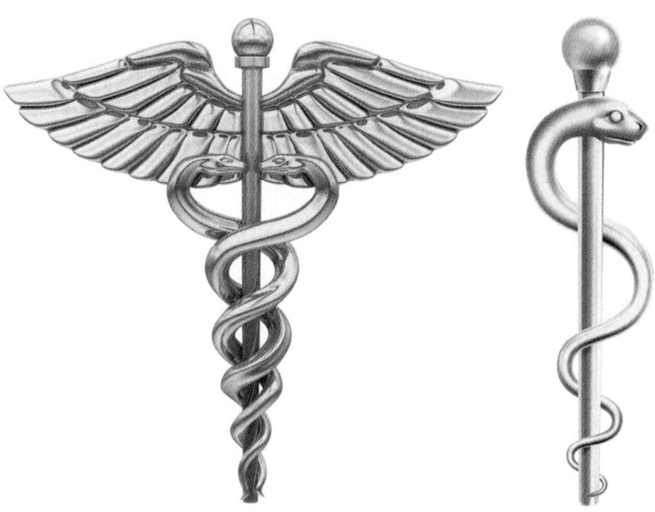

Caduceus (*left*) and Gold rod of Asclepius (*right*) (Left, iStock.com/ ID:1144689533 Credit: Nerthuz. Right, iStock.com/ID:493148816 Credit: Chris Gorgio.)

The caduceus is an ancient symbol representing the staff carried by Hermes, the winged messenger god in Greek mythology. His Roman counterpart was Mercury. The staff is short, entwined by two serpents ending with wings at the top. Sometimes the symbol is shown with one snake and no wings. This version stands for the rod of Asclepius, a famous ancient Greek physician. Historically, the symbols have been used to represent commerce, negotiation, science, mathematics, and medicine.

The symbols are ancient, however, predating Greek and Roman mythologies. They have had both esoteric and mundane meanings. From the 16th century onward, printers used both symbols as printers' marks, particularly as frontispieces for pharmacopoeias in the 17th and 18th centuries. Printers saw themselves as diffusers of knowledge; hence, their choice of images.

Esoterically, the entwined serpents have represented positive and negative kundalini energy moving up through the chakras around the spine (the staff or rod and what is also referred to as the central channel or balancing midline of the body). Serpents have also depicted the evolution of human consciousness and serve as a model for the structure of the universe. When a snake sheds its skin, it symbolically represents a renewal of youth and health. The rod or staff also symbolizes a magical artifact, the wand. The wings are interpreted as swiftness and ascend upwards to the heavens. Both symbols have been used as magical power objects.

The medical link probably came from alchemy. Alchemists were referred to as the sons of Hermes, or Hermetists, practitioners of the hermetic arts. At the end of the 16th century, alchemy included medicine, pharmaceuticals, chemistry and metallurgy. The element called quicksilver was named mercury in honor of the Roman messenger god. Thus the scientific age of medicine has its roots in the mythological and esoteric past. Through these symbols, medicine retains its connection to the old ways, reminding us of the healing process and its work to combat disease.

Over time the caduceus and the rod of Asclepius emerged as symbols of medicine. The World Health Organization and the Medical Council of New Zealand adopted the Asclepius rod and single serpent as their logos.

In the United States the double-snaked caduceus became the insignia of the U.S. Army Medical Corps in 1902 and is the well-known symbol of physicians. The single-snake design appears on ambulance doors and medical products, and it is the American Medical Association insignia.[7]

Greece, and other locations. Today, countless Materia Medicas exist, organizing plants by various categories, traditions, or nationalities. A few famous early ones listed here help us appreciate the cross-cultural influences on these important collections.[1]

- *Pen Ts'ao, China, 2800 BCE.* The *Pen Ts'ao*, written by a Chinese herbalist named Shen Nung, included among other plants, Ephedra Ma Huang (Ephedra stem) still in use today. The *Pen Ts'ao* contained high-quality woodcuts and descriptions of 414 species of plants, of which 276 were described for the first time. This Materia Medica was reprinted and updated many times.
- *Ebers Papyrus, Egypt, 1500 BCE.* The *Ebers Papyrus* listed 500 plants, including the well-known Aloe Leaf, Chamomile herb, Coriander, Fennel and Sesame seed, Thyme herb, Garlic, and Onion bulb. Garlic and Onion of the Lily family were known as the *stinking ones* and rose to fame due to the Egyptian obsession with them to fight disease and strengthen the body. Modern research supports their immune-strengthening properties.
- *The Charaka Samhita, India, 700 BCE.* The *Charaka Samhita* was an early text on traditional Indian medicine, known as Ayurveda. It was the first known major medical encyclopedia, containing 500 herbal formulas. Early versions date from 900 BCE to 600 BCE, and later additions came along as time evolved. This Materia Medica contains eight sections that include areas such as drugs and their uses, preparations, diet, duties of a physician, pathology of eight chief diseases, diagnostics, and anatomy.
- *De Materia Medica, Dioscorides, Greece, CE 77.* Dioscorides is known as the Greek founder of Western herbal medicine and his *De Materia Medica* was the first accurate Western herbal text (Fig. 2.4). A practicing surgeon, he traveled widely with

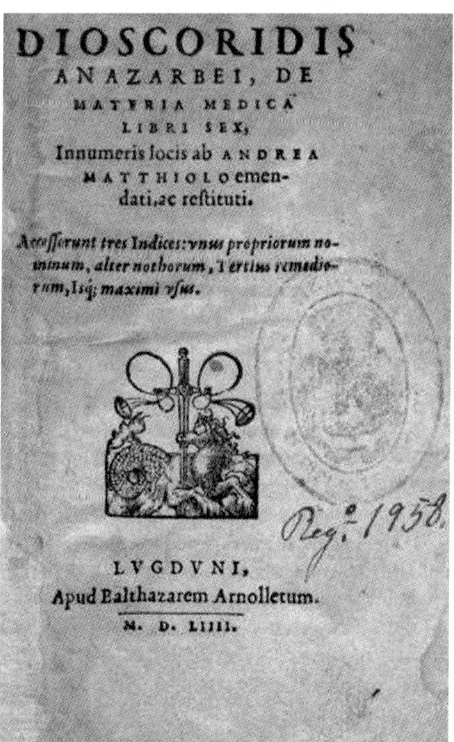

DIOSCORIDIS
ANAZARBEI, DE
MATERIA MEDICA
LIBRI SEX,
Innumeris locis ab ANDREA
MATTHIOLO emendati, ac reſtituti.

Acceſſerunt tres Indices: vnus propriorum nominum, alter nothorum, Tertius remediorum, Isq; maximi vſus.

Reg.º 1958

LVGDVNI,
Apud Balthazarem Arnolletum.
M. D. LIIII.

• **Fig. 2.4** *De Materia Medica*, book 6, 1554, published in Lugdunum [modern-day Lyon, France]. (Pedanius Dioscorides - Self-photographed (Original text: Photo taken from the archives of the History Library of Madrid. 2010. I release the file to public domain. File: 1554Arnoullet.jpg)

the far-ranging Roman armies of Nero. During his travels, he became a skilled pharmacologist and botanist, collecting information from the locals he met while journeying throughout Asia Minor. *De Materia Medica* took the form of a five-volume encyclopedia with precise information about herbs. Entries describe the plants, showing a picture of each. Notes included medicinal properties, preparation methods, dosage, and warnings. Understandably, the book became an indispensable field guide and medical reference. Almost every Western herbal published through the 17th century referred to it. Still quoted today, it is a prototype herbal and pharmacopeia.

- *The Classic of Herbs, China, CE 100.* Sheng Nong's herb guide, *The Classic of Herbs*, listed 237 herbal prescriptions using dozens of herbs, including rhubarb root and opium poppy latex. This work grew over the centuries to contain 11,000 herbal formulas. Today, Chinese medicine uses about 300 individual herbs, 150 of which are considered indispensable by most practitioners.[8]

Western European Middle Ages

From the fall of Rome to about CE 1300 was a bleak time for medicine and women in general. Medicine had not advanced since Galen's time. The Church, the plague, superstition, accusations and convictions of witchcraft, fear, and lack of common sense dominated everywhere. The number of ingredients in remedies grew to outrageous quantities, reaching into the hundreds.

Woman healers who did manage to practice during this period had to exercise extreme caution to remain safe and continue helping people. Regardless of social class, women served as midwives and healers of children, and even though they knew a lot about herbs and cures, they often had to dispense their remedies in secret. These were sane, practical, Wise-Women of the community who carried on the oral herbal traditions they had received from the mothers and grandmothers before them. These simple cures actually promoted health in times of public superstition, fear, and other practitioners' frequent use of sometimes unpleasantly weird, disgusting remedies like the sexual organs of animals, tongue of eagles, saliva, blood, and various toxic minerals. Most prevailing so-called medicines were only remotely connected to simple, sensible botanics.[5]

The European Apothecary of the 1100s, Alchemy, and Chemistry

European apothecaries became an independent profession from the practice of medicine, beginning in the 12th century. Originally an ***apothecary*** was a medical professional who formulated and dispensed herbs and remedies to physicians, patients, and surgeons. The word eventually evolved to denote a physical space that stored wine, spices, and herbs. Allopathic *pharmacists* in America and ***chemists*** in England have taken over the old *apothecary* designation as professionals who dispense drugs. Many modern herbalists have reverted to calling their herbal collections and herbal shops apothecaries.

New exotic herbs coming from Arabia and China turned up in European apothecaries. Apothecaries embraced the profitable new remedies made by Ibn Sina (Avicenna) from Arabia. Included were animal, mineral, and vegetable medicines. The medieval apothecary's shop housed weird animal parts such as viper's flesh, crab's eyes, rhinoceros and unicorn horn, oil of earthworms, scorpions, swallows, moss from a dead man's skull, and urine from a goat, as well as more appetizing items from the Plant Kingdom.

Apothecaries, alchemy, and chemistry have their roots in this period. Modern chemistry actually evolved from the study of alchemy, its medieval forerunner. ***Alchemy*** was a combined physical, metaphysical, and spiritual investigation into the transformation of matter, turning one substance into another. It had many goals, depending on who the practitioner was and how he or she practiced the art. Some aimed to convert ordinary metals into the purest form of matter, which was considered to be gold, to find a universal elixir called the Philosopher's Stone—a way for immortality to be achieved. Others aimed to free and purify the spirit or soul. Alchemy ultimately morphed into the apothecaries and then into the science of chemistry.

Ibn Sina, CE 980–1037, and the Invention of the Arab Pharmacy

The Arabs had a very advanced society, a bright spot in terms of healing. After Rome fell, this part of the world simplified Galen's complicated medicines. Ibn Sina (anglicized as Avicenna) was a leading Islamic physician who developed the world's first pharmacies—professional drug stores—as a field apart from medicine. He excelled in compounding remedies. He used herbs in new ways and developed techniques to produce syrups, ointments, tinctures, elixirs, pills, suppositories, and inhalations. He wrote extensively, leaving behind his encyclopedic five-volume *Canon of Medicine,* which influenced Western medicine throughout the Middle Ages. Some refer to Ibn Sina as the father of modern medicine, whereas Hippocrates holds the title of father of Western medicine. Then, of course, Dioscorides holds the title of founder of Western herbal medicine. Multiple titles, a lot of fathers—no mothers.

Surgeons on active duty during the Crusades used Ibn Sina's new, practical formulations to help the wounded. Ibn Sina influenced European apothecaries, and his work set the standard throughout Europe. New Arabian herbs, such as Nutmeg seed, Clove bud, and Saffron stigma (the part of a flower's ovary that catches the pollen), were introduced to Western practices.

Trotula of Salerno, 11th Century

Trotula of Salerno, Italy, was a rare shining star who is sometimes regarded as the world's first gynecologist. She was a leading physician at the famed Salerno learning center for training medical practitioners. Both men and women attended this center, which attracted Greeks, Arabs, Jews, and Latins among its faculty and students. Known for her wise diagnosis and management of women's problems and diseases, she emphasized the need for hygiene, used opium for pain, and successfully used anesthetic inhalations of the poisonous Hemlock (any part of the plant) and Mandrake root,[5] which could have been disastrous. Trotula's use of these techniques was far ahead of her time and remarkably similar to modern medical practice.

Hildegard von Bingen and the Wise-Woman Tradition, 12th Century

Another bright spot for medieval women healers was a notable German Benedictine nun named Hildegard von Bingen (1098–1179) (Fig. 2.5), remembered today because she was one of the very few known women of her time to record and write down her healing herbs and experiences.[9]

After Rome's domination of the known world ended, the Church dominated European medieval medicine, preaching illness and disease as God's punishment for sinning. Treatment of disease came in the form of prayer and penance. Fortunately, some of the nuns and

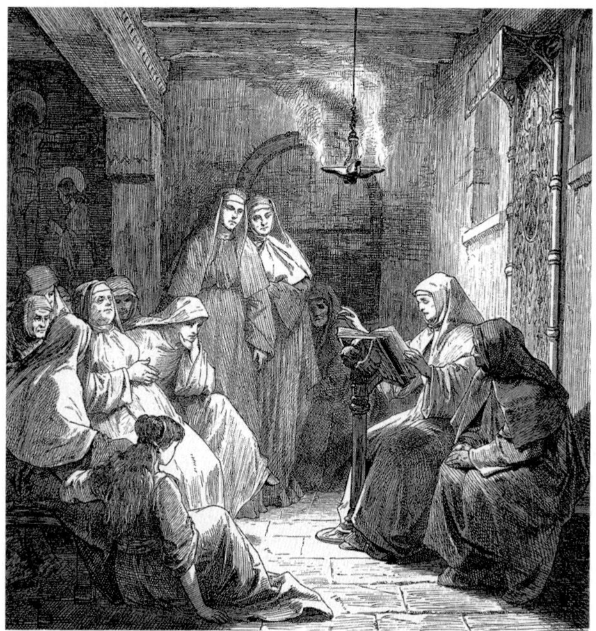

• **Fig. 2.5** Hildegard with her nuns (iStock.com/ID:1092276466 Credit: clu).

monks in the monasteries preserved old Greco-Roman herbal knowledge by planting herb gardens and helping townsfolk in need.

As an herbalist, musical composer, and mystic, Hildegard did more than copy the work of the Greeks and Romans, as others were doing. She was one of the few medieval women to leave a written account of the Wise-Woman Tradition. Her Materia Medica, titled *Physica,* emerged from her own experience. She recorded long lists of herbs, 485 to be exact, still used today. She included Aloe leaf, Basil herb, Bayberry berry, Blackberry leaf, Caraway seed, Celery seed, Clove bud, Dill seed, Fennel seed, Garlic bulb, Hyssop herb, Licorice root, Marjoram herb, Myrrh resin, Nettle herb, Nutmeg seed, Onion bulb, Oregano leaf, Raspberry leaf, Rosemary leaf, Rue herb, Thyme herb, and Watercress leaf (Fig. 2.6). This large array is reminiscent of old European gardens and their nurturing plants. Hildegard von Bingen was a profound scientist of her time.[10]

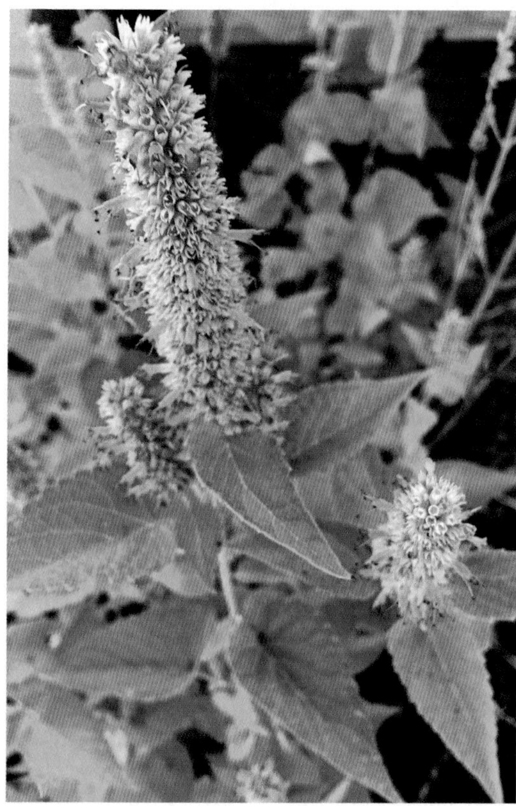

• **Fig. 2.6** *Hyssopus officinalis* (Hyssop herb) appeared in Hildegard von Bingen's garden. The herb is still used today.

Black Plague or Bubonic Plague, 14th Century

The ***Black Plague*** was a horrific pandemic that began in China and eventually spread throughout the Middle East to parts of Africa and Europe, peaking in Europe in 1346–1353. The plague was caused by a bacterium carried by the oriental rat flea, *Yersinia pestis,* living on rats and other rodents.[1] Hygiene, as we know it today, was not practiced until the 19th century. The streets of major cities flowed with raw sewage, dead animals, and garbage, allowing any transmissible disease to spread quickly.

People had no understanding of the cause or treatment for this highly contagious disease. Plague victims suffered from high fevers, sweating, shaking, terrible sores or buboes full of blood and pus, coughing, pneumonia, and pain followed quickly by death. Some blamed the plague on a wrathful, displeased God. Concepts of bacteria and bacterial infections were unknown. Some of the so-called cures involved ingesting mercury or arsenic, bloodletting, hanging pomanders (fragrant balls of flowers or herbs) around the patient's neck, drinking wine, and wrapping the buboes in a live chicken, frog, or leech.

Eventually ships believed to carry the infection were required to stay in port for 40 days, the origin of the word *quarantine.*[11] Terrified people fled the cities. At least one-third of the people in Europe died. Left untreated, 80% of those who contracted the plague succumbed within 8 days.

Because there was no effective treatment, this tragic event eventually necessitated changes in medical thought and discovery. Before an effective cure could be discovered, many useless and dangerous methods were attempted, and countless folks suffered greatly. It was not until 1928, when Alexander Fleming discovered penicillin after observing mold forming in a petri dish, did antibiotics become the recognized treatment for the Black Plague in the present day.

Syphilis: End of the 15th Century

Approximately 150 years after the plague, the sexually transmitted disease syphilis became a major medical problem, with the use of mercury as the biggest medical hoax that promised to cure it. Mercury poisoning leads to tremors, seizures, and death (Fig. 2.7). However, alchemists introduced mercuric quicksilver, and it became the medicine of choice for over 450 years, paving the way for future drugs at the expense of herbal medicines. Today syphilis is cured with the antibiotic penicillin.

In the Americas, healers used the native *Smilax aristolochia* (Sarsaparilla root). Though not a syphilis cure, at least it did no harm. Healers also tried out *Nicotiana tabacum* (Tobacco leaf), *Sassafras albidum* (Sassafras root), and a purging herb called *Ipomoea jalapa* (Jalap root).[1]

Some of the dangerous and useless medieval remedies used by doctors to eradicate the plague, syphilis, and everyday ills caused poisoning—doing more harm than good. One response to this in England was The Herbalist's Charter, an Act of Parliament

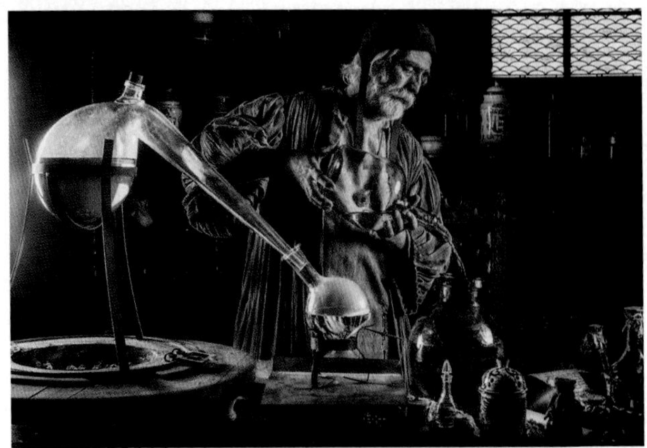

• **Fig. 2.7** The alchemist (iStock.com/ID:1006115078 Credit: aluxum)

• BOX 2.2 The Herbalist's Charter of 1543

King Henry VIII of England (1491–1547) had a keen interest in medicine and dabbled in cures for his well-known painful ulcers and leg sores caused by gout. Many of the remedies he tried were well-known herbal plants and flowers known since the time of Dioscorides, such as plantain, mallow, fenugreek, linseed, and "*Oyle of Roses*" (Rose water).

At that time, doctors used expensive, complicated, and dangerous remedies, and they were outraged that Henry was embracing simple cures. In 1518, as a way to respond to the king, they established the Royal College of Physicians in London (the oldest medical college in England). The College influenced Parliament to pass laws to protect their province of complex medications and mineral cures, and to give them control of both surgeons and apothecaries.

This stratagem backfired, however. Physicians enraged local unlicensed practitioners, one being the brewer, who apparently had friends in high places. He managed to get Parliament to pass a new law allowing laypeople to practice herbal medicine and healing. The final words of the Act warned physicians not to meddle with the newly legalized herbalists.[1]

Outraged doctors called it "the Quack's Charter." But modern herbalists refer to this victory as the "Herbalist's Charter." It ensured the survival of their profession and empowered knowledgeable men and women to administer much needed medical services to the poor.

ordained and implemented by King Henry VIII, making it lawful for any English subject with the "Knowledge and Experience of the Nature of Herbs, Roots, and Waters. . ." to practice their art. This law allowed lay people to use their own herbal cures and folk medicine, despite doctors and the medical establishment who wanted a monopoly on this right. (Box 2.2).

The Inquisition: The Wise-Woman Tradition Hits Bottom

Dark, dark times accompanied by the rise of the witch hunts and revival of the Inquisition occurred in various countries at different times until about 1693, the end of the Salem witch trials in America. After the 1300s, the image of the kindly female folk herbalist changed from helpful Wise-Woman to an evil, devil-possessed witch. Women were accused of conjuring up all kinds of black magic potions with assistance from the devil. Notable witch trials occurred in Germany, France, and, later, in Salem, Massachusetts, in the U.S. Literature and theater reflected fascination with poisonings. Shakespeare's Lady Macbeth threw the roots of mandrake and belladonna into a bubbling cauldron. *Grimm's Fairy Tales* depicted Snow White killed by a poisoned apple prepared by her evil stepmother, whose true identity was a witch. The exact plant was not specified in the original tale.

So what happened? Some of the thinking during this time may have followed traditions from the Greek and Roman days of herbal assassinations. Remember Socrates, the Greek philosopher and teacher who drank the poison hemlock? Many theories and possible reasons have been offered for the witch hunts and the Inquisition. The climate was right for a blame game. Women as healers bore the brunt, especially because they were not allowed to formally study medicine, and any plant knowledge they had was considered to be channeled from the devil. Possible explanations for these twisted thoughts include:

- *Dominant male culture.* The rise of secular medicine to a male-dominated profession turned society against women folk healers and raised fears that they were involved in supernatural shamanic practices.
- *The Church's power.* A suspicious, patriarchal, and powerful Roman Catholic Church wanted to dominate healing and medical practice.
- *The plague.* Women were blamed for the deaths from the Black Plague.
- *Birth control information.* Women were accused of dispensing forbidden information about birth control and how to ease pain in childbirth. The Church found this practice unacceptable, considering women guilty of original sin and thus deserving to suffer and sometimes die in childbirth. As merciful midwives and dispensers of herbs to prevent or enhance pregnancy and childbirth, women were tagged as evil-doers and sinners. Some of the plants they used to create miscarriages were quite effective. Pennyroyal, Artemisia, and Rue were used then and are known today as *morning after* herbs.
- *Judicial use of poisonous plants.* Women were accused of using strong, potentially toxic herbs that could heal when used correctly and knowledgeably but could easily kill in larger amounts. One example was *Aconitum carmichaeli* Fu Zi (Monkshood or Wolfbane root), used for shock and coma. The prepared (less-toxic form) is still used in Chinese and Ayurvedic medicine today. We can't forget that highly schooled, professional male physicians routinely poisoned their patients with horrific, dangerous remedies—mercury and arsenic—and no one ever blamed them for those deaths.
- *Belladonna for beauty.* In Italy, the deadly nightshade, *Belladonna atropa,* meaning *beautiful lady,* cosmetically and topically dilated women's pupils. This was an extremely dangerous practice because Belladonna contains the alkaloid atropine, which can slow a rapid heartbeat. Too much atropine can stop a heart altogether.[12] The likelihood is great that many women died because of this vain habit. Belladonna was also implicated as part of the so-called *flying ointment* that witches supposedly used to fly.
- *Digitalis purpurea* (Fig. 2.8). Foxglove flowers were called *witch's bells* or *witch's gloves*, an accusatory designation for what may be a dangerous, but also useful, plant. All parts of foxglove are lethal in high doses because it can cause cardiac arrest. Therapeutically, it can relieve congestive heart failure and is the source of today's heart drug, digitalis, though exact dosage is critical. Overdoses from foxglove probably occurred at that time, though heroic saves did also, and the Wise-Woman never received credit for those.

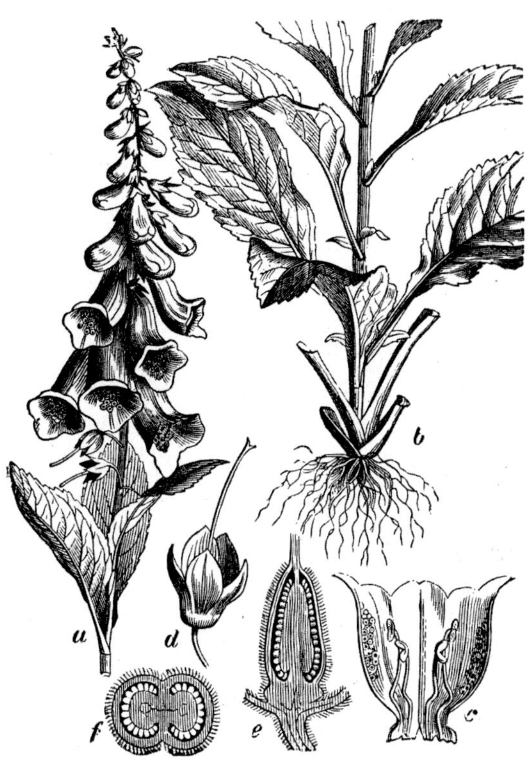

• **Fig. 2.8** Digitalis purpurea (Foxglove, Common Foxglove, Purple Foxglove, Lady's Glove) (iStock.com/ID:651692646 Credit: ilbusca)

These elements forced women's practice of herbology and folk medicine to go quietly under cover. Those who practiced openly would have feared for their lives.

Doctrine of Signatures, 15th Century Italy

In the CE 1st century, Dioscorides described healing plants according to divine intention. It was one of the cultural assumptions of the Galenic era. Dioscorides believed that God marked objects with signs or *signatures* of their purpose. This belief persisted throughout the Middle Ages after the appearance in 1621 of a book by the German mystic, Jakob Boehme, called *The Signature of All Things*, which defined the principle we have come to know as the ***doctrine of signatures***. An herbalist could find in a plant's appearance a clue as to its medicinal use, which had been designed by the creator for this purpose. A plant's overall shape, smell, or characteristic could reveal its healing abilities.[1] Occasionally, this happened to be true but sometimes not.

Examples of plants that do adhere to these observations and support the doctrine of signatures are *Panax ginseng* (Ginseng root), which is shaped like a human male and is a renowned men's tonic; *Caulophyllum thalictroides* (Blue Cohosh root), which branches like contorted limbs and relaxes muscles in muscular spasms; and *Sanguinaria canadensis* (Blood root and sap), which has a beautiful blood-red color is therefore a blood purifier. Another such plant, *Lobelia inflata* (Lobelia herb), has flowers shaped like a stomach (if you have a good imagination) and is a good emetic when taken in large doses. *Hydrastis canadensis* (Goldenseal root) is a yellow-green root that might remind you of the colors of jaundice and pus and is successfully used for infection.

Renaissance and the Rise of Science

Paracelsus—The Rebel Challenges Galenic Medicine, 1493–1541

A Swiss-German alchemist and considered a revolutionary in his time, Paracelsus is credited with being the founder of modern pharmaceutical medicine or chemical pharmacology. He wrote and spoke against the current Galenic practices, which took a lot of courage. He was challenged, ridiculed, and shunned by the medical establishment.

Although he embraced mineral poisons like mercury and antimony, he also appreciated the common folk herbs used in Swiss-German medicine. He tempered his use of poisonous quicksilver for syphilis patients with common healing plants; that approach was possibly why his patients survived.[1] Working in his alchemical lab he developed addictive ***laudanum***—tincture of opium—that later citizens of Victorian England and America abused.

Nicholas Culpeper,1616–1664—Activist and Author of *The English Physician*

Nicholas Culpeper was a reformer who furthered the English tradition of domestic herbal medicine. The son of a rector, Culpeper became an educated English pharmacist, botanist, physician, and astrologer. He also published *The English Physician*, in which he recommended the gentler botanicals growing in one's own backyard, rather than exotic plant medicines that were expensive, hard to obtain, and possibly useless.[1]

He also discouraged using purges and violent remedies, then so in vogue. Culpeper questioned traditional methods and knowledge and explored new solutions for healing, making them more accessible to lay people by educating them about maintaining their own health. The success of *The English Physician* both embarrassed and angered Culpeper's medical contemporaries.

America

Native Americans

Native Americans contributed greatly to herbal knowledge. Compared to Europeans, the native people in the Americas generally enjoyed strong teeth and tremendous physical stamina. Their herbal wisdom was impressive, as was the vast array of native plants they relied on for healing. They appreciated and practiced personal hygiene and isolating the sick. Hot springs and smoke lodges were used for ritualistic and physical cleansing. In these communities, women often maintained knowledge of plant wisdom and practiced it for healing.

Stories exist of European trappers and settlers who had fallen ill being taken in by friendly natives who treated and cured them. Some of a long list of native herbs introduced to the Europeans were *Actaea racemosa* (Black Cohosh root), *Viburnum prunifolium* (Black Haw bark), *Eupatorium perfoliatum* (Boneset herb), *Rhamnus purshiana* (Cascara Sagrada bark), *Echinacea* spp. (Echinacea root), *Larrea divaricata* (Chaparral leaf), *Hydrastis canadensis* (Goldenseal root), *Lobelia inflata* (Lobelia herb), *Mahonia repens* (Oregon Grape root), *Smilax glauca* (Sarsaparilla root), *Ulmus fulva* (Slippery Elm bark), *Prunus serotina* (Wild Cherry bark), and *Hamamelis virginiana* (Witch Hazel herb).

The Shakers, Early 1800s

The Shakers were a religious sect that broke off from the Quakers in the early 1800s and became America's premier medicinal herb growers. They had beautiful herb gardens and prepared and sold herbs and seeds in America—a total of 142 herbs, roots, and barks. They developed a reputation for honesty and herbal purity and supplied the Union Army with its main supply of Opium Poppy latex during the American Civil War. They also sold herbs to hospitals and invented the modern pill form for medicines. When patent medicines became popular after the Civil War, they marketed several. Their biggest seller was Dr. Corbett's Shaker Sarsaparilla Syrup, consisting of Sarsaparilla root, Dandelion root, Black Cohosh root, Yellow Dock root, Juniper berries, and others. The Shaker's herb business died after World War I but has since revived, starting in the 1960s.

Thomsonian Movement, Early 1800s

Samuel Thomson helped return herbal medicine to sanity and place it again in the hands of the people when he started the Popular Health Movement or the ***Thomsonian movement***. Introduced to herbs by an American Wise-Woman named Mrs. Bento, he found himself impressed by her herbal knowledge, writing in 1834, "We cannot deny that women possess superior capacities for the science of medicine."[4] That said, no other credit was given to Mrs. Bento ever again. Thomson rebelled against the regular medicine of the time, such as the practice of bloodletting, use of violent laxatives called cathartics, and use of the toxic minerals like mercury, arsenic, antimony, and sulfur. Over half the population of Ohio adored him, and he was considered throughout the Midwest as a voice of reason.

Thomson was a mixed bag, however, and was part sensible, part extreme in his practices. Although he discounted bloodletting, he advocated harsh treatments, such as purging, vomiting, and sweating. Thomson's two main radical tenets were to raise the body temperature, particularly with *Capsicum annuum* (Cayenne pepper), and to clear it of toxins with high doses of *Lobelia inflata* (Lobelia herb), commonly called Pukeweed (with good reason). For the record, lower doses of Lobelia herb are a good relaxant for stress, anxiety, pain, and seizures without causing vomiting.

To his credit, Thomson often promoted an essential feature of the herbal tradition, supporting the body's own recuperative efforts—everything else being secondary. His more conservative approach prompted scorn, indignation, and resentment in the average North American doctor who was still deep into dramatic, heroic cures like bloodletting. All in all, the Thomsonian approach paved the way for two new important movements—the Physiomedicalists and the Eclectics.

The Physiomedicalists and William Cook's *Physio-Medical Dispensary*, 1869

Physiomedicalism was an offshoot of the Thomsonian movement. A split occurred regarding the issue of medical education and whether licenses should be granted to its physicians. The Physiomedicalists advocated for a formal medical education and a larger Materia Medica, whereas Thomson was opposed to them.

William Cook, the most prominent of the Physiomedicalists, wrote *The Physio-Medical Dispensatory* in 1869, which became famous and is still quoted by herbalists today. It was the primary Materia Medica and pharmacy text for the sect until the last Physiomedicalist school closed in 1915. The book contains more than 440 plants and is considered to have the most complete descriptions of North American herbs in print. Cook was a hands-on clinical herbalist and herbal pharmacist, and the text carries the authority of firsthand knowledge in both arenas.

Physiomedicalism lasted until the early 20th century in North America, when politics intervened. This intervention occurred because of the combined opposition of the Eclectics, homeopaths, and regular establishment physicians. Those groups, along with the American Medical Association (AMA), formed an alliance to demand licensing laws for themselves, denying licensure to the Physiomedicalists who started the furor in the first place.

Fate of the Physiomedicalists and Ties to Britain

Cook's beloved Physiomedicalism survived because some of its followers jumped the Atlantic and traveled to England, strongly influencing British medical herbalism. The Physiomedicalists grouped together against the traditional British Medical Association of the time, whose doctors rarely cured anyone. The Physiomedicalists formed the National Institute of Medical Herbalists in 1864, which is still in existence today. This led to the birth of Anglo-American herbalism, the oldest body of herbalism in the Western world.[13] When people talk about Western Herbalism, these are its roots.

Rise and Fall of King's Eclectic Movement and Medical Schools, 1840s–1939

The ***Eclectic movement***, founded by John King, M.D., emerged as an extension of Native American herbal traditions and a reaction against the purges, bloodletting, and violent treatments being used by the medical establishment of the day. The Eclectics gained popularity because they provided treatments that did not kill their patients. Eclecticism can be defined as borrowing ideas and theories from multiple sources, which they did.

The Eclectics integrated whatever worked, and they borrowed from Native American healers, Samuel Thomson's natural theories, homeopathy, Asian medicine, and African slave herbology. They also promoted scientific herbalism, employing chemical analysis and extraction of active ingredients. This approach greatly influenced the early pharmaceutical industry which, by that time, was extracting drugs from herbal sources. The first pharmaceutical drug developed was morphine, derived from the Opium Poppy in 1805 by a German chemist.

The Eclectic movement is entwined with the turbulent early history of medical schools in the United States, at first extremely influential but ultimately forced to close down. At their high point, Eclectic schools trained nearly one-sixth of the medical students in America, using an all-encompassing curriculum that included herbalism and homeopathy and more orthodox medical training.[14] John King founded the Eclectic Medical Institute, the first medical school to admit women and black students. It opened in 1840 in Cincinnati, Ohio, and graduated more than 4,000 physicians over the next 100 years. Sadly, the school closed its doors in 1939 because of political infighting regarding medical philosophies and a declining quality of teaching.

The U.S. federal government's ***Flexner Report*** of 1920 exposed the alleged shortcomings of the Eclectic Institute. Supported by the powerful AMA and the Carnegie Foundation, it helped shutter the Eclectic schools and led to a new gold standard for the training of physicians. Herbalism's role as part of the medical school curriculum came to an end with the Flexner Report. The Eclectics faded away. All things herbal never again blossomed at such a national level. Notable Eclectic herbalists follow.

- *John King, 1813–1893.* Founder of the Eclectics, and the most prolific and famous of them all, King wrote *The American Dispensary.* The *Dispensary* covered the use of herbs used in American medical practice, particularly those used by the Eclectics. King founded the last herbal medical school, The Eclectic Institute.
- *John Uri Lloyd, 1849–1936.* A visionary pharmacist, Lloyd updated King's *American Dispensary.* The Lloyd Library in Cincinnati, Ohio contains the accumulated libraries of all the Eclectic medical schools. Lloyd wrote the succinct motto adopted by Eclectic physicians, "Sustain the vital forces."
- *Harvey Wicks Felter, M.D., 1865–1936.* Felter revised King's *Dispensary* in 1898 and wrote the *Eclectic Materia Medica, Pharmacology and Therapeutics* in 1922.
- *John Milton Scudder, M.D., 1829–1894.* Scudder was a beloved Materia Medica professor at the Eclectic Medical Institute, who tried, but failed, to reform and save the college as enrollment dropped. He worked to improve common medical practices, spurred on by his own wife's untimely death. Physicians often used mercury chloride, called *calomel,* as a purgative and fungicide. Calomel, combined with bloodletting, created a society of unhealthy women who were weak and bedridden, being slowly poisoned by the medical profession. Women's sickly condition was considered the female norm at the time, not the result of this ill-advised treatment. Scudder's herbal formula, *Alterative Supreme,* was so good it remains on sale today (Box 2.3).
- *Finley Ellingwood, 1852–1920.* Ellingwood wrote *The American Materia Medica,* and its popularity gave him a huge following. He grouped herbs according to modern body systems and also into therapeutic herbal classifications, such as sedatives and depressants, or stimulants and excitants. Most of these categories are still used in Western herbalism.

Women Join the Popular Health Movement in America

During the pioneer push west, women became active community healers by necessity. With male doctors in short supply, pioneer women reemerged with a do-it-yourself attitude. They delivered babies, served as doctors and midwives and did anything that was needed. Some brought herbs and remedies from Europe and planted medicinal gardens. They learned from the Native Americans.

During the Industrial Revolution, a women's place still may have been in the home, but there they ruled. Men were increasingly away working long hours, giving women ample unchallenged authority at home. They extended their talents as caregivers and herbalists. Hydrotherapy, the use of baths and water cures, homeopathy, and Thomson's botanical remedies proved to be the popular practices of the day.[5]

The Thomsonian Popular Health Movement of the 1830s and 1840s gave women new opportunities and empowered them even more. Boston Women's Medical College opened in 1848 and was the first contemporary medical school for the training of female physicians. Restricted from working in male-run hospitals, women founded their own, employing doctors and nurses of both sexes.

Eventually, after her applications to other medical schools had been rejected, Elizabeth Blackwell was accepted into the all-male Geneva Medical College in upstate New York. Blackwell became the first woman to be awarded a medical degree in America. In spite of extreme obstacles, she broke through the barriers established to prevent female medical achievements. She famously noted, "Methods and conclusions formed by half of the race only must necessarily require revision as the other half of humanity rises into conscious responsibility."[5]

Some women educated communities of ladies about their bodies' health and hygiene. They advocated healthy lifestyles, good nutrition, diet, and exercise, and they pushed for elimination of *Gone with the Wind*–style constricting corsets. Mary Gove Nichols was a noted reformer in the Popular Health Movement who contributed to the *Water Cure Journal* and empowered women to take health and healing into their own hands. She wrote about the need for women to embrace their sexuality and not to be repressed or ashamed. She was not afraid to address taboo topics such as birth control, childhood problems, bathing, or teething.[5]

Later, birth control and contraception became an issue during the Progressive Era of the early 1900s. Activist Margaret Sanger's work in New York led to legalization of contraception. Better prenatal care, maternal health care, and childcare increased the health and safety of women and children.

• BOX 2.3 Scudder's Formula Remains for Sale

Gaia Herbs, a present-day herb company, sells a blend called *Scudder's Alterative Supreme.* The Gaia site explains: "This traditional Eclectic formulation encourages healthy removal of cellular wastes and healthy uptake of cellular nutrition. It promotes excretion, detoxification, and healthy skin and appearance. Scudder's Alterative Supreme supports healthy immune system functions, too."[15]

The formula as written on the bottle contains:

Almus serrulata (Alder bark) regulates bowel, liver, and digestive function.

Podophyllum peltatum (Mayapple root) is for detoxification, indigestion, and constipation.

Corydalis Yan Hu Suo (Asian Corydalis corm) regulates bowel, liver, gastrointestinal, and lymphatic function.

Scrophularia nodosa (Figwort root and herb) is a great alterative for the skin.

Rumex crispus (Yellow Dock root) promotes bowel function and iron.

Lydia Pinkham, 1819–1883

Lydia Pinkham was an entrepreneur, a colorful addition to the patent medicine furor of the 1800s. In her home kitchen, she concocted and marketed Lydia E. Pinkham's Vegetable Tonic in 1875 for $1.00 a bottle. It was a wildly popular women's formula that reportedly helped with menstrual symptoms or "female complaints." Her face appeared on medicine bottles everywhere (Box 2.4). Apparently, she derived her formulating information from sources such as Eclectic John King's *American Dispensary,* which she is known to have owned and used.

A pamphlet inside her tonic bottle packaging encouraged women to write to her with their questions. At that time, standards of modesty kept women woefully ignorant about their bodies and how it functioned. Pinkham's work encouraged the ladies to ask uncomfortable questions about menses, menopause, and reproduction. Pinkham answered their queries, dispensing information along with the tonic, and provided forthright talk and advice about women's medical issues.[16] This private and discrete question–answer opportunity empowered women to take charge of their own health, an unheard of and revolutionary concept at that time.

Rene Caisse's *Essiac,* 1888–1978

Caisse was a Canadian nurse-pioneer who challenged the establishment by creating a cancer-curing tea called *Essiac,* her name spelled backward (Box 2.5). Living in Bracebridge, Ontario, she treated people for 60 years, making and using her tea to cure cancer and

• BOX 2.4 Lydia Pinkham's Vegetable Tonic of 1875

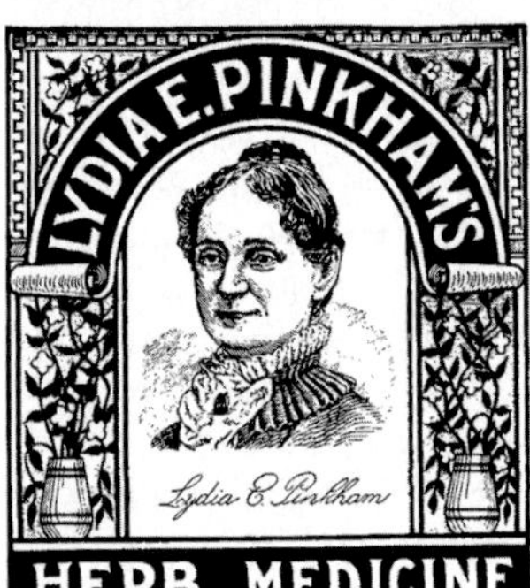

Lydia Pinkham's patent herb medicine label. Her formula remains on the market. (No artist's credit. *This media file is in the* ***public domain*** *in the United States.)*

This tonic is still on sale today at major drugstores and online, although the formula has changed a bit over the years. It was identified for menstrual cramps and other complaints.

- 8 oz. Aletris farinosa (Unicorn root)—Uterine tonic.
- 6 oz. Senecio aureas (Life root)—Uterine and nerve tonic.
- 6 oz. Actaea racemosa (Black Cohosh root)—Hot flashes and cramping.
- 6 oz. Asclepias tuberos a (Pleurisy root)—Prevents prolapse.
- 12 oz Trigonella foenum-graecum (Fenugreek seed)—Digestive aid.
- Alcohol 18% to make 100 U.S. pints.

promote general health. She ran her cancer clinic from 1932 to 1942, taking no money. She once wrote a series of articles titled, "I Was Canada's Cancer Nurse."

Caisse learned about the formula in 1922 from a patient, a prospector's wife, who had breast cancer. The formula had originally come from an Ojibway traditional healer. The patient's cancer never came back.[17] Nurse Caisse wrote down the herbs and began to use them on hopeless cases with much success. No conclusive studies ever proved that the tea worked. Caisse met with resistance from the government and medical associations and spent much of her life in back-and-forth hassles, threat of arrest, and being scammed out of legalizing the cure.

Merging into the Present

Colleges and Medical Schools with New Requirements

The medical schools and the doctors they produced in the late 1800s had terrible reputations; too many poorly trained doctors were graduating from low grade schools. In 1902 the AMA formed a council to investigate medical training in the United States. They found faculty, equipment, and standards lacking. The Eclectic schools fared no better.

As a result, Johns Hopkins Medical School, which opened in 1873, fashioned itself on German-style training and required that applicants have a college degree to qualify for admission. Harvard University put together an undergraduate medical training referred to as *pre-med.* However, some of these improvements backfired on the sound practice of herbalism, and herbal preparations were replaced by drugs. Eclectics Scudder and King, who simply wanted to improve the Eclectic Institute but not close it down, got more than they bargained for.

• BOX 2.5 Essiac Tea Formula by Rene Caisse

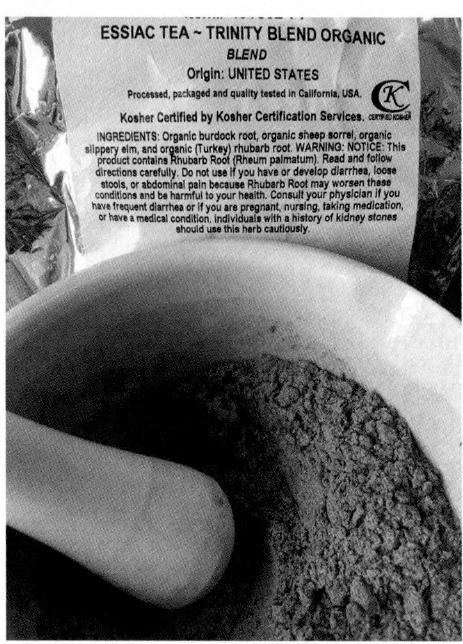

Essiac tea formula herbs are ground and decocted (boiled and steeped), to make the traditional preparation.

The original four herbs in combination actually prevent tumor growth and cancer cell reproduction and cut down on oxidative stress and tissue inflammation. The formula can well be used today as an adjunct supportive tea, along with other therapies for cancer.

- *Rumex acetosella* (Sheep Sorrel herb and root). An antioxidant-rich herb with proven antiproliferative, antineoplastic effects against cancer cells.
- *Arctium lappa* (Burdock root). An alterative, a blood cleanser, and has apoptotic effects on cancer, meaning it stimulates death of malignant cells.
- *Rheum officinale* (Turkey Rhubarb root). Antiinflammatory, antitumoral properties, protects the lungs for those at risk for lung cancer, and is a strong laxative. It is a favorite Eclectic remedy.
- *Ulmus fulva* (Slippery Elm bark). A moisturizing demulcent that soothes and reduces inflammation and supports immune system.

United States Pharmacopeia and National Formulary, 1820

The ***United States Pharmacopeia (USP)*** and National Formulary (NF) was formed in 1820 in response to a lack of uniformity of standards regarding medical practice and the compounding of drugs and herbal formulas. Because of bitter disagreement between establishment doctors and the Thomsonians and Physiomedicalists, the USP was established as a self-sustaining, independent, science-based, nonprofit, public health organization.

By law, all prescription and over-the-counter medicines and herbs available in the United States were to meet USP quality control and public standards, if such exist, for the product being marketed. Then and now, the USP became identified as the official public standards-setting authority for all dietary supplements (including herbs), prescription and over-the-counter medicines, and other health care products manufactured and sold in America. Manufacturers and regulators in more than 140 countries refer to and use USP standards.

Approximately 100 herbs were originally included in the pharmacopeia. Today it publishes countless herbal monographs in the *Herbal Medicines Compendium* that is freely available online. Each monograph contains standards for ingredients used in herbal medicines and follows with specifications for analytical testing to assure quality and lack of contaminants. A large listing of herbs is included, and more are reviewed and added periodically.

Landmark Flexner Report on Medical Education Eliminated Herbal Healing, 1920

In 1920, the wealthy Carnegie Foundation financed and appointed Abraham Flexner to carry out a report on the training of doctors. The report changed the direction of medical practice. It surveyed the quality of the nation's medical schools, praising the Hopkins-Harvard model and condemning all others. The widely circulated Flexner Report, along with the previous AMA recommendations, spelled doom for the Eclectics. Seven of the eight medical schools they ran closed down, as did many others.[18]

In addition, standard medical schools flourished with the help of the Carnegie Foundation. Their scientific, drug-oriented, nonherbal approach promoted the growth of the modern pharmaceutical industry with its now-current near monopoly of the medical profession. By 1940, every surviving U.S. medical school's curriculum was based on the Hopkins-Harvard model. Botany was no longer considered necessary because schools did not provide training in herbal healing. Today, no U.S. medical school can exist without AMA approval[1] and all that approval entails.

A Few Herbal Die-Hards, Despite the Flexner Report

- *Benedict Lust.* In 1895, naturopath Benedict Lust opened the nation's first health food store to promote his water cures. Lust established sanitariums based on healing baths and herbal medicines. His nephew, John Lust, wrote an influential herbal, *The Herb Book,* still in print.
- *John Hoxey.* An herbalist in the mid-1900s, Hoxey proclaimed his herbal formula cured cancer. He sold the formula and opened a cancer center with branches in 17 states. He cured hundreds of people, but not everyone. Hoxey was attacked by the AMA, who won the suit. His clinic was closed down by the U.S. Federal Drug Administration (FDA) for violating drug labeling regulations. His herbs were not FDA-approved cancer treatments. Hoxey's cancer formula is in use today. Most of its herbs have antitumoral action. It consists of *Berberis vulgaris* (Barberry root), *Rhamnus frangula* (Buckthorn bark), *Arctium lappa* (Burdock root), *Cascara sagrada* (Cascara sagrada root), *Trifolium pratense* (Red Clover flower), *Glycyrrhiza glabra* (Licorice root), *Phytolacca americana* (Poke root), *Zanthoxylum americanum* (Prickly Ash bark), and *Sanguinaria canadensis* (Bloodroot).
- *Jethro Kloss* (Fig. 2.9). A health food pioneer, Kloss wrote the American herbal classic, *Back to Eden,* in 1939 (Fig. 2.10). This book is another of the old standbys still in print. I referred to it many times during the early years of my health studies and herbal journey.

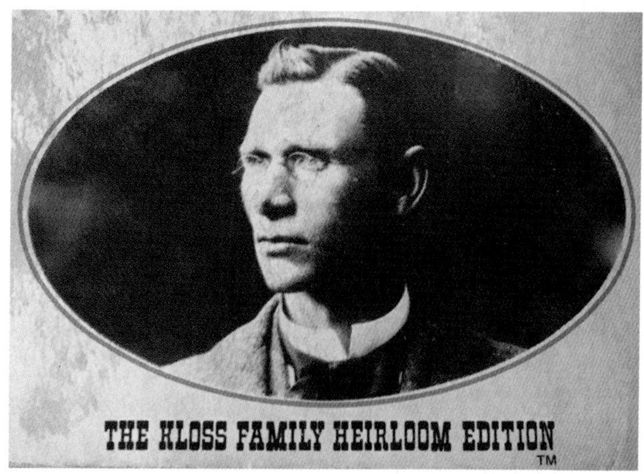

• **Fig. 2.9** Jethro Kloss, author of *Back to Eden*, an American herbal classic.

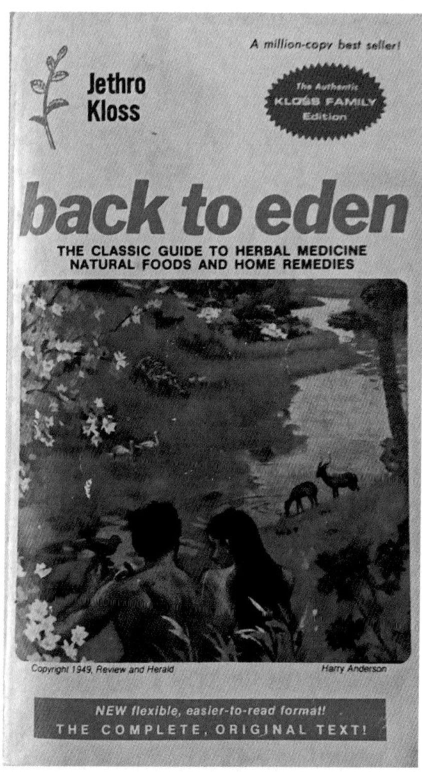

• **Fig. 2.10** *Back to Eden* focuses on herbal home remedies, natural nutrition, and gardening. It helped create the natural foods industry.

We leave off here, with herbalism being abandoned in medical schools and replaced with what is now termed modern medicine (Table 2.1). What goes around comes around. Herbalism has survived many a defeat, only to become a resource for those interested in more natural and often more reliable treatments to promote human health.

The latest evolution of herbalism involves legislation of various sorts, another paradigm shift. This tale will show up later (Chapter 29). There, we sort through the ins and outs of modern legislation and discuss where herbalists stand and what may come next.

TABLE 2.1 Herbal Historical Timeline

Years BCE	
7000–6500	Neolithic, primeval prehistory, shamans, priestesses, priests, beginning of food production, Wise-Woman Tradition begins.
2800	China, *Pen Ts'ao*, Materia Medica.
1500	Egypt, *Ebers Papyrus*, Materia Medica.
700	India, *Charaka Samhita*, herbal encyclopedia.
c. 400	Hippocrates from Greece. Father of Western or modern medicine, four humors. Expanded on Islamic Unani-Tibb tradition.
c. 350	Numerous Greek healing goddesses: Hygiea, Gaia, Persephone, Demeter.
350	Artemisia Greek queen and healer, discovered Wormwood herb as a cure.
Years CE	
c.77	Dioscorides from Greece, founder of Western herbal medicine, wrote *De Materia Medica.* Arabic translations formed basis for future advances in pharmacology and pharmacy.
c.130–210	Galen, Roman physician expanded upon ideas of Hippocrates and influenced medical thought throughout Middle Ages.
c.399	Fabiola of Rome, woman physician who founded first public hospital.
476	Fall of Rome and beginning of the Dark Ages.
980–1037	Ibn Sina invented the professional Islamic pharmacy. Wrote *Canon of Medicine* that became a standard medical text in Islam and Europe up until the 18th century.
c. 1000's	Trotula of Salerno, Italian physician and teacher, world's first gynecologist wrote manuscripts on women's health.
1098–1179	Hildegard von Bingen, first known woman to record her healing knowledge and founder of scientific natural history in Germany.
14th Century	Black or bubonic plague, worldwide.
1478–1600's	Inquisition, witch trials, persecutions on and off in Europe, then America.
1493–1541	Paracelsus challenges Galen. Founder of chemical pharmacology.
1543	The Herbalist's Charter enabled lay practice of herbalism and healing in England.
15th Century	Doctrine of Signatures, Italy.
1616–1664	Nicolas Culpeper's *The English Physician* championed herbs for laypeople.
Early 1800's	The Shakers, America's premier medicinal herb growers.
Early 1800's	Samuel Thomson's Thomsonian Movement in America, responsible for Popular Health Movement. Many women joined in this effort.
1819–1883	Lydia Pinkham's Vegetable Tonic.
1820	U.S. Pharmacopeia and National Formulary formed and set standards for medicines and herbs.
1830's to early 1900's	Physiomedicalist Movement. Basis for Anglo American Western herbalism.
1869	William Cook wrote *Physio-Medical Dispensary,* still loved and used today.
1864	National Institute of Medical Herbalists formed in the United Kingdom, the birth of modern Western herbalism.
1845–1939	Eclectic Movement, King, Lloyd, Felter, Scudder, and Ellingwood.
1847	American Medical Association (AMA) founded.
1849	Eclectic Medical Institute founded by King. First medical school to admit women and black students and last to offer herbology as part of medicine.
1810–1884	Reformer Mary Gove Nichols, part of the Popular Health Movement.
1821–1910	Elizabeth Blackwell, first woman to graduate from all-male medical school.
1879–1966	Margaret Sanger, Progressive Era, advocates birth control.
1910	Flexner Report responsible for closing Eclectic Institute.
1888–1978	Rene Caisse, Canadian nurse famous for herbal formula *Essiac.*

Summary

This chapter showed that the history of herbal medicine and the Wise-Woman way is an integral part of human history. The story is linked with the history of medicine, women's status and is intertwined with politics, religion, medical schools, and the male versus female principle.

In the Middle Ages and beyond, competition ensued between Galen's complex four humors system versus simpler cures. Dangerous practices competed with safer botanicals, compliments of the Wise-Woman way. Benedictine nun, Hildegard von Bingen became the first woman to record herbal knowledge, moving forward from the exclusively oral tradition. The Renaissance and the rise of science brought discoveries in anatomy and chemistry leading to the eventual development of the pharmaceuticals industry. Botanical medicine was scorned as old-fashioned.

America had numerous medical movements. The Thomsonians advocated medical and herbal reform. William Cook's American Physiomedicalists formed the basis for Anglo American Western herbalism. The Eclectics rebelled against the prevailing medical establishment, borrowing from many cultures. The Popular Health Movement included Lydia Pinkham and Rene Caisse. Margaret Sanger pushed for birth control.

The USP of 1820 set standards for herbs and medications. The Flexner Report of 1929 forced the closing of the Eclectic Institute and all U.S. medical schools dropped botanical medicine from their curriculums.

Review

Fill in the Blanks

(Answers in Appendix B.)

1. The Father of Modern or Western medicine was___.
2. A sexually transmitted disease of the Middle Ages was ___.
3. Hildegard von Bingen's Materia Medica was called ___.
4. Three dangerous medical cures of the Middle Ages were___, ___, ___.
5. The symbol of two coiled snakes with wings is called ___.
6. Whose influence halted medical progress from Rome through the Middle Ages? ___
7. The Arab pharmacy was invented by ___.
8. USP stands for___.
9. Name four important Eclectics. ___, ___, ___, ___.
10. The ___movement formed basis for Anglo-American Western herbalism. Its leader was ___ who wrote ___.

Critical Concept Questions

(Answers for you to decide.)

1. How did Galen influence the history of medicine?
2. Explain the Wise-Woman Tradition. How does it fit into the history of herbalism?
3. Is the doctrine of signatures valid?
4. Why is Hildegard von Bingen an important historical figure?
5. What were some reasons for persecution of women during the Inquisition?
6. What was the Thomsonian Movement?
7. Who were the Eclectics? Why are they important?
8. Who was John Cook?
9. How and why did the practice of herbalism disappear from U.S. medical schools?
10. What is the significance of the Flexner Report?

References

1. Griggs, Barbara. Green Pharmacy: The History and Evolution of Western Herbal Medicine (Rochester, Vermont: Healing Arts, 1991).
2. Weed, Susun. Healing Wise (Woodstock, New York: Ash Tree, 2003).
3. "Greek Medicine" History of Medicine Division, National Library. National Institutes of Health https://www.nlm.nih.gov/hmd/greek/greek_dioscorides.html (accessed August 14, 2019).
4. Romm, Aviva. Botanical Medicine for Women's Health. (St. Louis: Elsevier, 2010).
5. Achterberg, Jeanne. Woman as Healer. (Boston: Shambhala Press, 1990).
6. Murray, Michael. The Healing Power of Herbs (Rockville, CA: Prima,1999).
7. Nozedar, Adele. The Illustrated Signs & Symbols Sourcebook. (New York: Metro Books, 2008).
8. Jin, R et al. "Classification of 365 Chinese medicines in Shennong's Materia Medica Classic." PubMed, National Library of Medicine, National Institutes of Health http://www.ncbi.nlm.nih.gov/pubmed/21669172 (accessed August 14, 2029).
9. Flanagan, Sabina. Hildegard of Bingen, a Visionary Life. (London: Routledge, 1989).
10. Strehlow, Wighard and Gottfried Hertzka. Hildegard of Bingen's Medicine (Santa Fe, NM; Bear, 1988).
11. "History of Quarantine." Centers for Disease Control and Prevention https://www.cdc.gov/quarantine/historyquarantine.html (accessed August 14, 2019).
12. Hofmann, Albert, et.al. Plants of the Gods: Origins of Hallucinogenic Use. (New York: Van der Marck, 1987).
13. Bone, Kerry and Mills, Simon. Principles and Practice of Phytotherapy. (London, UK: Elsevier, 2013).
14. Alfs, Matthew. 300 Herbs; Their Indications and Contraindications. (New Brighton, MN: Old Theology Book House).
15. "Gaia Herbs Scudder's Alterative Supreme." Acupuncture Atlanta. https://www.acuatlanta.net/gaia-herbs-scudders-alterative-supreme-2-oz-p-63096.html (accessed August 14, 2019).
16. "Lydia E Pinkham." Encyclopedia Britannica https://www.britannica.com/biography/Lydia-E-Pinkham (accessed August 14, 2019).
17. "Discovering Essiac." Written by Rene Caisse and was published posthumously by the Bracebridge Examiner, January 1979. http://www.essiacinfo.org/caisse_pop_1.htm (accessed August 14, 2019).
18. "The Flexner Report—100 Years Later." U.S. National Library of Medicine, National Institutes of Health. https://www.ncbi.nlm.nih.gov/pmc/articles/PMC3178858/ (accessed August 14, 2019).

3 Philosophical Constructs of Herbology

"There can be no Lotus flower without the mud: No mud, no Lotus."

—from The Art of Transforming Suffering by Thích Nhất Hạnh, Vietnamese Buddhist monk

CHAPTER REVIEW

- Herbal terms.
- The main herbal traditions: Ethnic, Ayurvedic, Western European, and Chinese.
- Vitalistic versus analytic approach to herbalism and medicine.
- The Seven Steps of Healing and how to use them.

KEY TERMS

Analytic/analytical
Ayurveda
Herbalism
Herbology
Herb
Pharmacognosy
Qi
Qigong
Tuina
Unani-tibb
Vitalistic/vitalism

Herbalism is ancient, and it is good to know its roots (Fig. 3.1). Botanical healing knowledge has been passed along since the beginning. The four main herbal traditions are Ethnic, Ayurvedic, Western European, and Chinese Medicine. Others that may seem to be left out are grouped within these four main headings. For instance, Kampo is the Japanese adaptation of Chinese Medicine, so it is included in that tradition. Egyptian and Islamic herbal knowledge evolved into Western European, and Ethnic includes cultures from all over the world.

The *vitalistic* versus the *analytic* approaches to healing are basic. They represent two opposing philosophies. The *Seven Steps of Healing* help us see how people go back and forth between vitalistic and analytic thinking to arrive at personal decisions about their own healing process.

Certain herbal terms appear repeatedly throughout the book. To an herbalist, an ***herb*** is a plant used for medicinal purposes. ***Herbalism*** is the study or practice of the medicinal and therapeutic use of plants, using natural plants or plant extracts that are taken internally or applied to the skin. ***Herbology*** is the study of herbs. ***Pharmacognosy*** is the study of plants as a natural source of drugs and the science of plant chemistry.

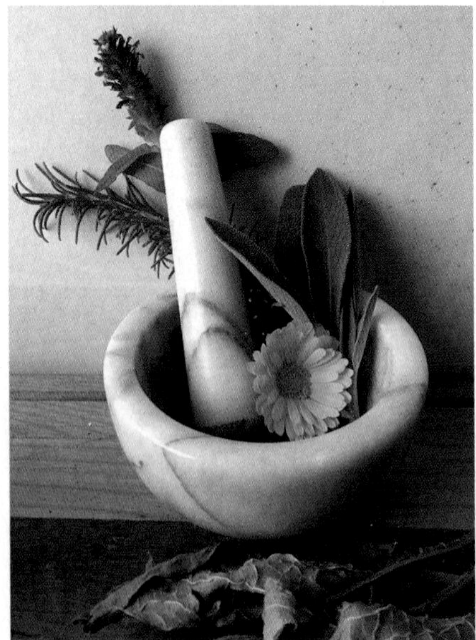

• **Fig. 3.1** Mortar & Pestle.

Main Herbal Traditions

The main herbal traditions—Ethnic, Ayurvedic, Chinese, and Western European—sprung from our worldwide need for healing and represent systems from various continents. As people traveled for trading, exploration, or war, they learned from one another. For instance, the Greek-born botanist and surgeon, Dioscorides, traveled with the Roman army and was introduced to new techniques and plants wherever he went.

During the European Age of Discovery, sailors learned new medicines and healing methods from the Caribbean and the Americas, relaying this often lifesaving information back to France, England, Spain, or their place of origin. Generally, the newer traditions borrowed from the older ones and added to or modified their own systems as years went on. Many are blended combinations. Modern herbalists often use a combination of these traditions for their assessment techniques.

Ethnic, Traditional, or Cultural Healing

One could call this the oldest and most basic form of structured medicine ever practiced, before anything had a name (Fig. 3.2). It is the one from which all later forms of medicine developed, including Chinese, Greco-Arabic, and Western. Traditional healing was part of seminomadic and agricultural tribal societies from prehistoric times, probably predating the last Ice Age.

These healers include traditional healers; shamans; healers from Africa and from North, Central, and South America; Australian aborigines; South Sea Islanders; Nordic healers; and many others. The traditions use tribal herbal wisdom, and sometimes include magic and ceremony, dreams, emotions, prayer, and intention. They comprise knowledge that has been accumulated over thousands of years, based on personal experience and connection with the natural world, using different levels of consciousness within the human psyche.

In most tribal groups, there were usually one or two people who stood out as the *wise ones* or the one most connected to how natural laws influence living things. They became highly respected, sought-out healers of the community. Much of this wisdom has been abandoned and brushed aside in favor of modern medicine.

Today there has been a revival and renewed appreciation of what was lost. Cold, scientific-based Western medicine is, for many, missing something important. In the holistic sense, we must consider more than the physical body. Many modern thinkers and practitioners have written and practiced a more mind-body approach. Examples are found in the works and practices of Deepak Chopra, M.D., Christiane Northrup, M.D., and Louise Hay, medical intuitive. In the West, we are beginning to appreciate and realize that for real healing to occur, we must use the entire human experience.

Ayurveda from India, 5000 Years Old

Ayurveda comes from the Sanskrit words: *ayur* (life) and *veda* (knowledge) (Fig. 3.3). Called "the Science of Life," Tibetan Medicine and Chinese Medicine both have their roots in Ayurveda. Early Greek Medicine also embraced many concepts originally described in the classical Ayurvedic medical texts dating back thousands of years.

Ayurvedic medicine is based on the holistic concept of keeping the body in health and balance first and treating disease second. It provides guidelines on seasonal routines, diet and exercise, behavior, and use of

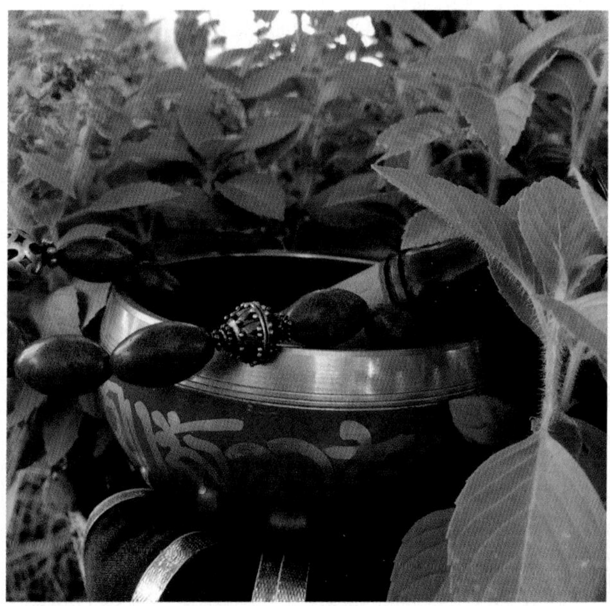

• **Fig. 3.3** Ayurvedic Mala beads, Singing Bowl, and Holy Basil.

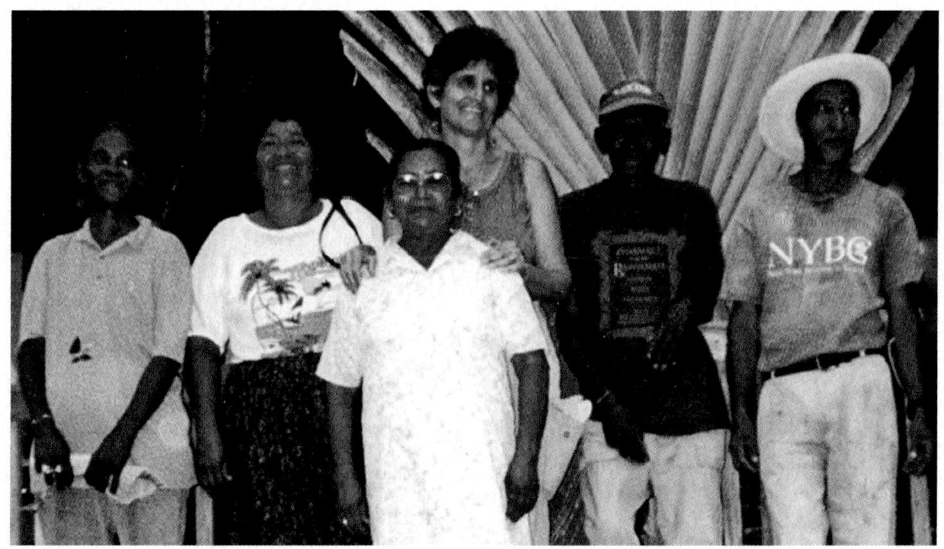

• **Fig. 3.2** Traditional Healers. Pharmacy from the Rainforest Belize Teacher Guides. (Credit Joan Zinn 1995).

our senses. It takes into account body, mind, and spirit and recognizes that, to be in health, we must integrate these three elements.

The tradition recognizes three doshas or body types. These are Vata (wind), Pitta (fire), and Kapha (earth). Each of us has a unique proportion of these three forces that shapes our nature. If Vata is dominant in our system, we tend to be thin, light, enthusiastic, energetic, and changeable. If Pitta predominates, we tend to be intense, intelligent, and goal-oriented, and we have a strong appetite for life. When Kapha prevails, we tend to be easygoing, methodical, and nurturing. Although each of us has all three forces, most people have one or two elements that predominate.[1]

Western European Herbalism with Egyptian and Unani Roots

In ancient Egypt around 525 BCE, medical practice was highly advanced for its time (Fig. 3.4). It included simple noninvasive surgery, bone setting, and an extensive pharmacopeia, titled the *Ebers Papyrus.* Egyptian medical thought influenced later traditions, including that of the Greeks.

Greek ***Unani-tibb*** (tibb means *medicine* in Arabic) is sometimes called Unani. It is a form of traditional medicine practiced in the Middle East and South Asia. It is based on the teachings of Hippocrates and Galen, who had been influenced by the Egyptians.[2] Hippocrates and Galen had a great influence on the medical system of the European Middle Ages that continued to be based on the four humors of phlegm, blood, yellow bile, and black bile (Chapter 2). Unani herbalism eventually evolved into what we now call Western herbalism and medicine from its Greek and Roman roots.

According to Unani medicine, management of any disease depends on the diagnosis. In the diagnosis, clinical features, such as signs, symptoms, laboratory features, and temperament are important. Western European medicine grew from this. It is based on old wisdom, experimentation, and modern use of herbs. Later, pharmaceuticals entered the mix. Because we are Westerners, we are likely most familiar with this method and grew up with it.

Chinese Medicine, 2800 BCE

This ancient tradition uses concepts of qi, yin and yang, plant energetics of taste, moisture, temperature, and conditions such as hot and cold, dry and damp, and strong and weak (Fig. 3.5). Chinese medicine dates back to around 2800 BCE. Its main tenet or objective is to maintain the ***qi*** or life force and energy. Good health depends on the balanced flow of this energy, which circulates through pathways called meridians. Maintaining good *righteous qi* is managed through acupuncture, which is the insertion of hair-thin needles in key points along the meridians and by the use of herbal medicine. Certain classic Chinese herbal formulas have been in use for thousands of years and, when selected properly, are incredibly effective.

The intention of Chinese Medicine is to keep the body in balance, strengthen its defenses, and treat any illness that occurs. It is

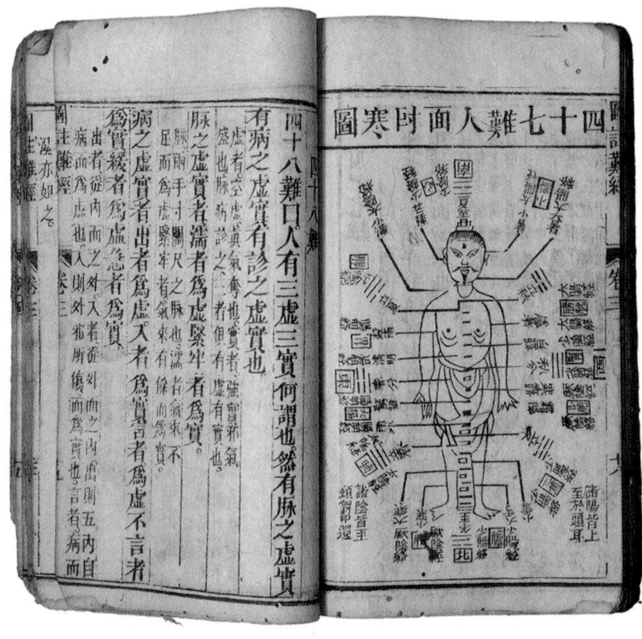

• **Fig. 3.5** Chinese traditional medicine ancient book with Clipping Paths. (iStock.com/ID # 91705422. Credit:4X-image)

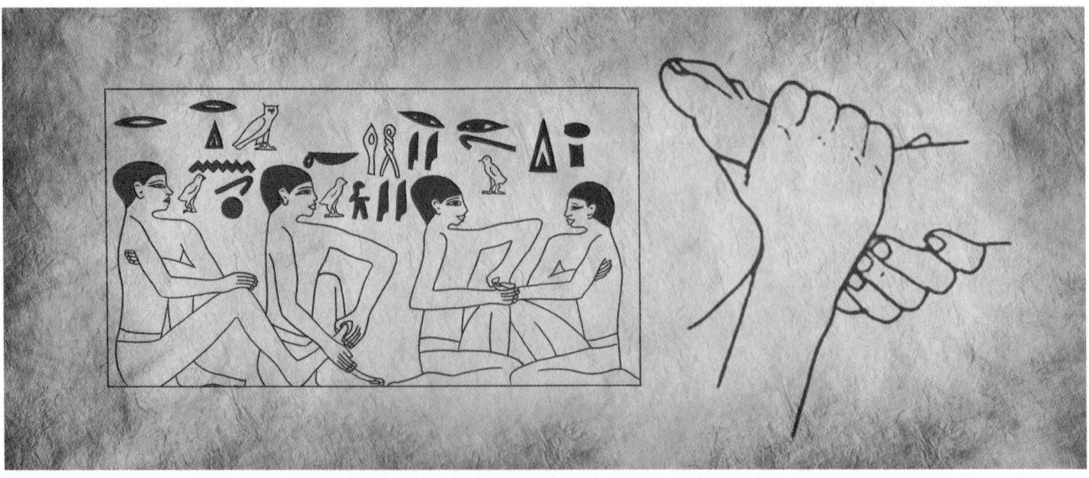

• **Fig. 3.4** The Ancient Practice of Reflexology. (iStock.com/ID:698567840. Credit: NikkiZalewski)

very holistic and takes into account mind, body, and spirit. It is concerned with seasons, weather, time of day when symptoms occur, emotions involved, colors, tastes, and all the senses.

Chinese medicine uses herbs, acupuncture, a type of massage called ***tuina***, and a form of energy movement therapy called ***qigong***. Practice of qigong enhances the flow of *qi* in the body by integrating posture, body movements, breathing, and focused intention. Tuina incorporates many massage techniques, such as kneading, rolling, and range of motion.

Vitalistic Versus Analytic Approaches to Herbalism and Medicine

One of the main differences in the way medicine is practiced allopathically or holistically involves the concepts of vitalism versus analytic. These are two opposing ways of looking at the body and understanding how it heals. ***Vitalism*** means seeing the body as a whole unit that works together. The ***analytic*** approach views the body as a machine made up of various parts—fix or replace the damaged part, and the whole will work again.[3]

Chinese practitioners talk about identifying and treating *the root, not the branch* of a problem, meaning *find the cause, don't just chase symptoms.* Good herbalists do this if they can. For instance, the general fix for a headache could be to stop pain and treat the symptom with aspirin-like Willow bark. The deeper fix for that headache is to find and treat the cause. The headache could arise from liver congestion, in which case you might select Dandelion root; if from a stomach upset, specify Catnip herb; if from tension, choose Valerian root; if from weakness, opt for Cinnamon bark.

Analytic Approach

Conventional Western medicine sees the body in separate boxes *analytically*. Other words to describe this are reductionist, scientific, materialistic, objective, or left-brain linear thinking. This is the way anatomy and physiology are taught in nursing and medical schools. An enormous amount of information is put into boxes to make it more manageable. The body systems and their organs are the parts. There is the digestive system, the respiratory system, and the cardiovascular system, etc. We have gastroenterologists, pulmonologists, and cardiologists, each concentrating in one area. When I worked as a nurse in a modern hospital intensive care unit, these specialists would visit patients and prescribe only for that body system or part. Rarely did they look at the whole person and see more than a heart or a lung with "tunnel vision." It was the nurse's job to look at the whole patient and try to coordinate the treatments to ensure that the whole person's needs were addressed.

Analytic traditions stem from Hippocrates, Aristotle, Newton, and Descartes. They saw the body as a machine made up of organs and chemicals. The whole was understood by reducing things to their parts. This sometimes works well. The periodic table of elements or classifications of body systems are examples. With this reductionist thinking, everyone who has the same diagnosis receives essentially the same treatment.

Herbal medicine can also use the analytic approach. When herbs are classified under categories such as *diuretics*, *demulcents*, *astringents*, or *emmenagogues,* this is analytical thinking. It can be useful information, as long as one does not become trapped into only chasing symptoms and ignoring the cause. A good herbal formula will have components to help symptoms (the branch), but it also needs to contain herbs that treat the cause (the root).

Vitalistic Approach

Vitalism sees the body as a dynamic, ever-changing organism, adapting to its needs and desires. Other words to describe this approach are holistic, energy-based, right-brain, feeling, balancing, restoring, and mind-body. Vitalism assumes that that there is an intelligence and order in the organism that is designed to heal. Body systems coordinate functions with each other. Hearts do not work without lungs. One example of this intelligence is healing after a cut in the skin. The body knows, without any input from the individual, to send certain inflammatory factors to kill off any bacteria, activate clotting factors to stop the bleeding, and initiate tissue growth to heal the wound.[4]

If an herbalist were to use a vitalistic approach, she would look at herbs as energetics. This is the viewpoint taken in books such as Peter Holmes' *Energetics of Western Herbs.* Here, Western herbs are approached from a vitalistic perspective. Is the herb hot or cold, dry or damp, sweet or bitter? What is its overall effect on the individual? Is the person's constitution hot and dry? Then the herbalist cools her down with something cooling and moist. This approach treats the root and considers healing from an energetic level.

Blending the Two Approaches

Of course, the vitalistic and analytic approaches are not mutually exclusive. In reality, herbalists use both. Sometimes one is preferred over the other. If someone comes into a clinic with horrible stomach pain, cramping, and diarrhea, you would best begin by relieving their symptoms (analytic). It would be handy to know that maybe some Peppermint herb to relieve pain and Cranesbill herb to ease diarrhea could be starters. Then, when immediate symptoms are addressed, you would follow with a vitalistic-based gut restorative plan to fix the cause.

Herbalists tend to look at the body as nonlinear. At best, the herbalist's goal is to build up the constitution, strengthen immunity, and maintain health. Medical herbalism is concerned more with overall effects on the individual than with treating symptoms. If you have an irritable bowel, see a vitalistic herbalist for plants and dietary suggestions. But if you fall off a roof or are in a car accident, your best bet is to get to a modern science-based emergency room and see a good trauma doctor.

The majority of diseases affecting Americans today are chronic diseases, such as heart disease, diabetes, dementia, or obesity, often caused by poor health choices. They are governed by lifestyle, diet, and psychological issues, which are better treated with a vitalistic approach. This process is how Chinese, Native American, Ayurvedic, Shamanistic, and Wise-Women and Wise-Men, also called Traditional Healers, approach healing. They see the body as more than the sum of its parts; they see it as a holism. Healing becomes intuitive and spiritually oriented. It requires looking within and finding causes. The practice of herbalism is a juggling act. Sometimes we are on the vitalistic side, sometimes the analytic, and sometimes a little of each (Table 3.1).

Seven Steps of Healing

We all get sick from time to time. Wellness follows a continuum from feeling vibrant and healthy to being deathly ill. Some days are better than other days. These seven steps are adapted from herbalist Susun Weed's *Six Steps of Healing.*[6] They describe the process one might go through to handle a situation and figure out the best approach. The steps can easily be placed into the paradigm of the vitalistic versus analytic approaches just discussed.

TABLE 3.1 Comparison of the Vitalistic and Analytic Approach

Category	Vitalistic	Analytic
Historical	Shamanism, Native American, Ancient Greek Middle Ages, Wise-Woman, Traditional Healing, Ayurvedic.	Aristotle, Hippocrates, Pasteur, Renaissance, Allopathic.
Thinking	Holism, based on perennial wisdom and experience, i.e., Five Element Theory.	Theory-based, linear, logical, reductionist (a stomachache hurts, so treat the pain).
Psychology	Right-brain, feeling, intuition, unconscious.	Left-brain thinking, conscious.
Education	Integration of knowledge from separate disciplines.	Specialization, didactic, based on authority.
Physics	Quantum universe made of vibration, intelligent universe.	Universe and body as a machine made up of atoms.
View of the Body	Self-regulating, self-organizing, seeks homeostasis.	Machine that needs to be fixed.
Healing Approach	Experience, case histories, observation help validate effective remedies.	Scientific double-blind placebo-controlled studies (the gold standard for *truth*).
Diagnostic Approach	Find the syndrome; observe whole person considering mind, body, and spirit. Find disharmony.	Find the disease; analyze body to find diagnosis. Primary consideration is at the physical level.
Treatment Approach	Rebalance energetic disharmony, including physical.	Intervene on physical body to mechanistically alter physical dysfunction.
Treatment Objective	Protect, balance, restore.	Direct, remove, replace.
Side Effects	Hopefully all positive. Life force reengages.	Negative. Life force reacts to invasive treatment.
Symptoms	Relieved. Symptoms not always bad.	Suppressed. May reappear later or new ones occur.
Pharmacology (From *Pharmos,* Greek for plant or remedy)	Natural substances. Nontoxic, energetic-based on qualities such as warming, cooling.	Biochemical. Chemical constituents react with target tissues. Usually strong; sometimes toxic.
Client Interaction	Active. Herbalist in partnership with client. Client responsible for own health.	Passive. Patient acted on. Victim. Responsibility belongs to doctor.
Disease	Multiple causes. Multiple solutions. Not always bad.	External invader to be conquered. One cause; one solution.
Healing	Body heals self. Self-correcting. Has higher innate intelligence.	One cause; one solution.[5]

The steps are guidelines followed by many, but not always in the given order. There is no right way or one way, just as there are many paths to healing. The trick is to choose well and match yourself or your client to the method that fits or resonates. Timing is important. If you wait too long to seek help, things could escalate, and the problem could become more serious.

Knowing whether to approach the problem on the physical, emotional, mental, or vibrational level is helpful. Some people see it one way only. Either it's all vitalistic or all analytic. But if one always goes holistic, shunning Western medicine, or always rushes to a doctor at the first sign of illness, she is cheating herself out of a range of possibilities. It is often a bit frightening to try out an unfamiliar approach. Leaving your comfort zone is not easy, nor is admitting you were wrong.

Sometimes we become fixated at one step and cannot move on to the next. This circumstance could happen from fear or denial. If stuck at a level, it usually helps to go down to the step before for clarity. The healing journey is not always linear. At times we jump around, using the steps out of order, or even take two at a time. Steps one, two, and three are the Wise-Woman or Taoist Way. Four and five are mainstream Chinese, Greek, and Ayurvedic approaches. Steps six and seven refer to the Western, allopathic route.

Step One: Do Nothing

Here we are looking within (Fig. 3.6). This might sound simple, but there is a lot going on. When we don't rush to do or ingest

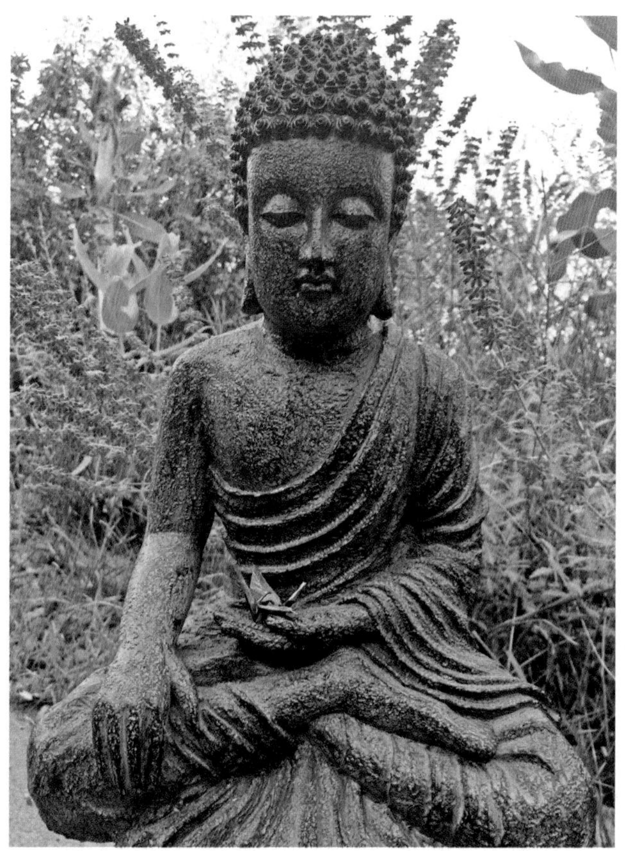

• **Fig. 3.6** Step One: Do Nothing. The Image: Meditation—The Buddha.

something, we are allowing our inner wisdom to give us a clue. It assumes we are taking time out to rest, meditate, sleep, or fast. We are allowing answers to come.

Doing nothing can be empowering and Zen-like and implies we are letting our guides speak. This process, of course, takes time. Patience is a must. Or doing nothing can mean we are in denial and have decided to ignore any messages. We just keep going blindly, hoping it will go away. We decide to tough it out because there is no time to be sick.

Step Two: Collecting Information

At this point, we are not doing anything physically, but we are looking within and also seeking wise council (Fig. 3.7). We want to know what is going on and why. Let's call it "low-tech diagnosis." We are conferring with ourself, our higher self, or other wise men or women we trust. We might fast or dream the answer, channel, or use hypnotherapy. We could consult the internet, use a support group, or look up possibilities in a book, evaluating this information on a psychic level. We may be seeking a message. Why did this happen to me? What is the lesson? We could see illness as an opportunity to slow down, rest, stay home. We might say, "Now I have a good excuse to take a day off."

Step Three: Engaging the Energy

At this point we try mind medicine. We use prayer. We use other energy medicines (Fig. 3.8). These include homeopathy, visualization, ritual, laughter, chakra balancing, therapeutic touch, and Reiki. All are energy based. Homeopathy uses the energetic template of a highly diluted substance with none of its original matter. Reiki and therapeutic touch channel energy. Chakra balancing is from the Hindu tradition and connects the spinning vortexes of energy residing in our bodies.

We could use journaling, qigong, acupuncture, or past-life regression. In some of these, we are not trying to manifest an outcome. Reiki allows the energy to connect and the body to heal. The practitioner is a channel. There is no ego involved and no expectations other than allowing the process to unfold. In other techniques, such as visualization, we are picturing a result through

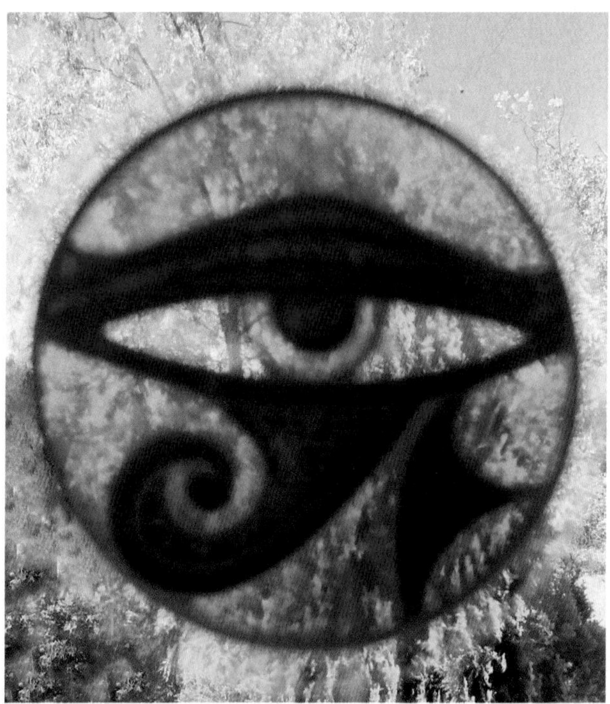

• **Fig. 3.7** Step Two: Collecting Information. The Image: The Third Eye.

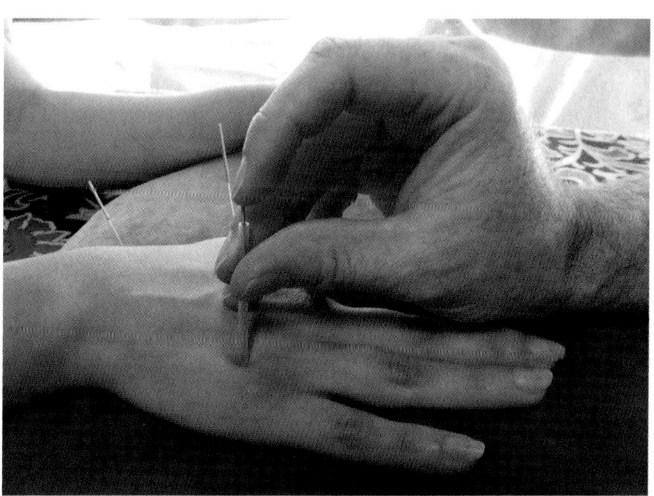

• **Fig. 3.8** Step Three: Engaging the Energy. The Image: Acupuncture–Inserting the needles.

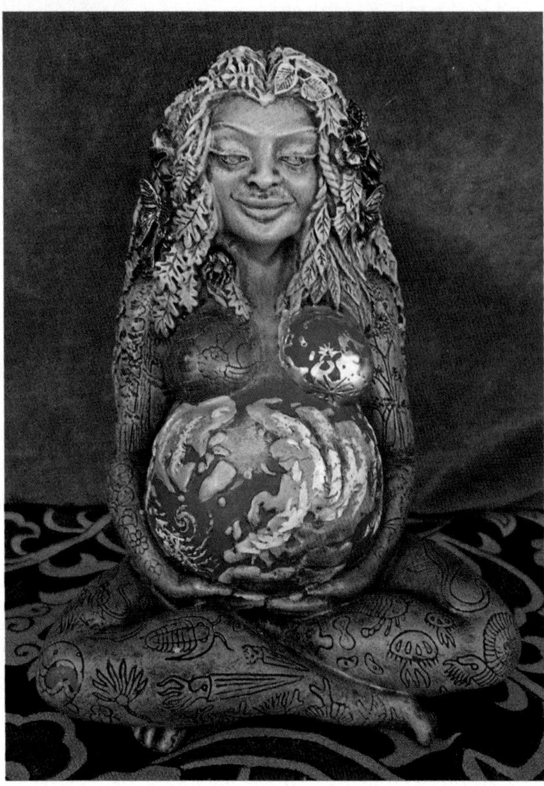

• **Fig. 3.9** Step Four: Supporting and Nourishing. The Image: Earth Goddess.

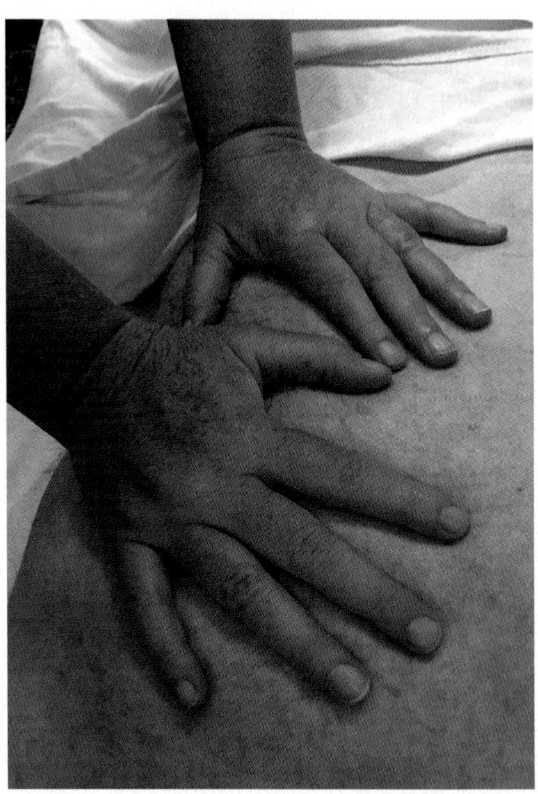

• **Fig. 3.10** Step Five: Altering Energy. The Image: Massage Therapy.

focus and concentration. In acupuncture and qigong, we are opening up energy pathways in the body to allow the smooth flow of qi.

A word of caution here. Energy methods aren't for everybody. They are far over on the vitalistic side. If these methods don't fit into a person's life view and belief system, then leave them alone. As we said earlier, steps can be skipped, and order can be interchanged. If the shoe fits, wear it.

Step Four: Supporting and Nourishing

Now we begin to do something (Fig. 3.9). Call it lifestyle medicine. It's chicken soup time. We try nourishing, tonifying, or strengthening with herbal infusions, hot lemon, and honey or a hot toddy. We choose wild foods like dandelion greens or use mustard plasters on painful muscles. We attempt yoga, tai chi, walking. We take a hot bath containing essential oils and place candles all around. We obtain physical and spiritual nourishment with physical, mental, and emotional support from others.

Spiritual nourishment comes in friendships, family, children, laughter, crying, or playing. We allow someone to bring us a cup of tea. Maybe we watch a silly TV show or movie. We stay at home to heal. We cocoon ourselves and feel loved. We love ourselves.

We do what we need. Maybe we take a little trip to the hot springs, a Turkish bath, steam room, sauna, or sweat lodge. Maybe walk around the block. We pursue a change of scene.

Step Five: Altering Energy

This step is when we try alternative medicine and actually make an appointment (Fig. 3.10). Something is done to someone else. The energy becomes goal oriented with an outcome in mind. The therapy will alter the energy, we hope, for the better. It is getting more specific. Ideally, we have figured out what we need and which modality to try. That is important. There is so much out there. A Wise-Woman friend from the collecting information step may have guided the decision.

We could go natural with herbal medicine or Bach flower remedies. We might try a hands-on type of bodywork such as massage, reflexology, or Rolfing. We could alter our thoughts with the mental approach and consult a psychotherapist. The key is that we are doing something about it—taking action.

Step Six: Going to the Doctor

With this step, we are definitely on the invasive, analytic side (Fig. 3.11). We are going to a doctor and entering pharmaceutical realms. We have given up on the gentler approaches and are hoping for fast action. This is the world of allopathic medicine. It disregards life force or the natural progression of things, but it is quick. It uses active ingredients, supplements, and strong medicine.

The downsides of this route are the side effects of drugs and their interactions with other substances. Drugs are easy to misuse. Dependency or addictions are possible and common. Are the side effects worth the cure? Is chemotherapy or radiation worth it? Sometimes we must be thankful that this aggressive medicine exists. It is lifesaving in the right situations.

Examples of this step are drugs, casts for fractures, dentures, glasses, hearing aids, organ transplants, hip and knee replacements, and blood transfusions. This is hard-core stuff. Addictions to sleeping pills, psychoactive drugs, and pain pills abound. Leading causes of death are through misuse of prescribed drugs, overdoses, hospital drug errors, or addiction from illegal drug use.

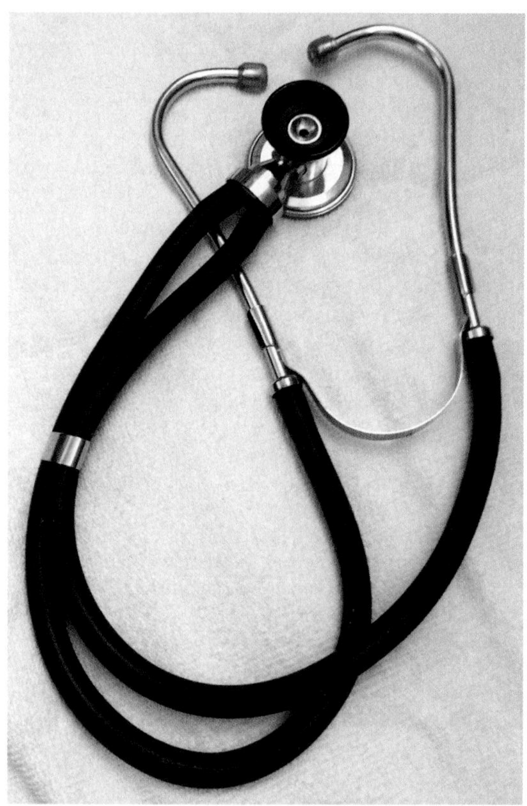

• **Fig. 3.11** Step Six: Going to the Doctor. The Image: Stethoscope.

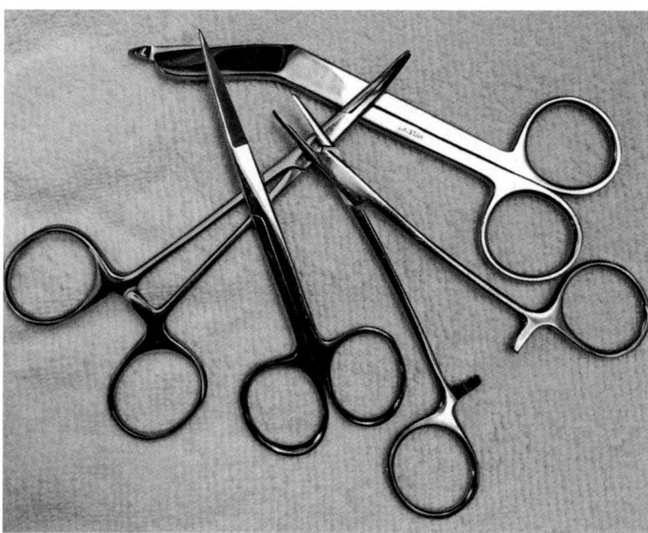

• **Fig. 3.12** Step Seven: Breaking and Entering. The Image: Surgical Instruments.

Step Seven: Breaking and Entering

With Step Seven, we are invading a person's natural barrier or boundary of skin or soul. It disregards natural life force, although the intent is to heal (Fig. 3.12). Here we have high-tech, heroic, Western medicine. This is the world of surgery, MRIs, CAT scans, X-rays, and invasive diagnostic tests like spinal taps. It involves specialized techniques that are done to you. They are goal oriented but have high potential to hurt and harm.

Breaking and entering are acute, intensive, and aggressive approaches. Results can be miraculous or disastrous. As a former intensive care nurse, I've seen real-time side effects of diagnostic tests go bad. For instance, in a cardiac catheterization, a catheter is threaded all the way up from the femoral artery or vein in the groin to a coronary artery surrounding the heart. It is easy to pierce the heart or artery or have a patient bleed to death from this diagnostic procedure. On the positive side, it shows where heart blockages occur so that a stint can be placed to open up the artery, thus saving a life. Quite a range. Don't take it lightly.

Please be very cautious with steps six and seven, *Going to the Doctor* and *Breaking and Entering*. Many folks use these last two as their first resort rather than the last. If you need them, be thankful they're there. But don't abuse them.

How to Use the Seven Steps of Healing

Putting the steps to practical application can be done in three ways. We can take a linear approach, working our way up from steps one to seven systematically. We might take a more global approach, using many steps simultaneously. Or we could skip around.

For instance, if we had undiagnosed back pain, we could do research on the internet, go to the doctor for a pain prescription, and get a massage. If we find a breast lump and are scared, we might get an MRI, see a psychic, and ask for herbs at the health food store, all on the very same day.

Summary

An herbal remedy is a plant or plants used for medicinal purposes. Herbalists practice using these plants for healing. Herbology is the study of plants. Herbalism is a medical model or system that uses natural plants or plant extracts for internal and external use. Pharmacognosy is the study of plants as a natural source of drugs and the science of plant chemistry.

Different cultures have had different approaches to herbalism, medicine, and healing. There are four basic herbal traditions into which most systems fit: Ethnic, Ayurvedic, Western European, and Chinese Medicine. There are two basic approaches to healing: vitalistic and analytic. The vitalistic approach is the holistic method. The analytic approach is more scientific. Vitalism views the body as a dynamic, ever-changing organism, adapting to its needs and desires. The analytic approach can be described as more scientific and objective. The analytic approach is the dominant way medicine is practiced in the West. Both approaches would do well to adopt a little of the other for a more balanced outlook.

The Seven Steps of Healing are the thought processes many use to confront illness. Most people go through some or all of these steps, not necessarily in order. Understanding them is useful for an herbalist who works in a clinical setting.

Review

Fill in the Blanks

(Answers in Appendix B.)

1. In the vitalistic approach, which side of the brain is used? ___.
2. The four herbal traditions are ___, ___, ___, ___.
3. Which is the oldest of the four traditions? ___.
4. What do the Seven Steps of Healing mean? ___.
5. "The *body is a machine* that needs fixing" is which approach? ___.
6. Name the step of healing for getting your appendix removed. ___.
7. Which step of healing may involve choosing qigong? ___.
8. Which step of healing may involve going to bed if your throat hurts? ___.

Critical Concept Questions

(Answers for you to decide.)

1. Of the four herbal traditions, which do you connect with most and why? Which one do you feel most comfortable with?
2. What do we mean by the energetics of herbs?
3. Using the Seven Steps of Healing as a reference, describe what you do personally, should you twist your ankle?
4. Using the Seven Steps of Healing as a reference, describe what you do personally should you find a lump on your breast. This question applies to both men and women.
5. Compare and contrast the vitalistic versus analytic approach to healing.

References

1. Brannigan, Johnny. "The Three Doshas." The Chopra Center. https://chopra.com/articles/what-is-a-dosha (accessed September 20, 2019).
2. "Unani Medicine." Encyclopedia Britannica. http://www.britannica.com/topic/Unani-medicine (accessed September 20, 2019).
3. Mills, Simon. *The Essential Book of Herbal Medicine.* (London: Penguin Books, 1991).
4. "Mechanism versus Vitalism." Wilderness Chirop. http://wildernesschiropractic.com/mechanism-vs-vitalism (accessed September 20, 2019).
5. Holmes, Peter. *Energetics of Western Herbs* (Boulder, CO: Snow Lotus, 2006).
6. Weed, Susun. *Down There: Sexual and Reproductive Health* (Woodstock, NY: Ash Tree, 2011).

4

Taxonomy and Botany for Herbalists

"Sedges have edges, rushes are round, grasses are hollow. What have you found?"

—Anonymous wildcrafting wisdom

CHAPTER REVIEW

- Taxonomy and Linnaeus: Seven-tiered system of plant classification. Phylogeny.
- Naming plants. What's in a name? Common names. The botanical or scientific Latin name: binomial system, International Code of Botanical Nomenclature and basic principles. The pharmaceutical name. The pinyin name.
- Botany: Monocots, dicots, flowers, and leaves.
- Plant families: Lamiaceae (Mint), Apiaceae (Parsley), Brassicaceae (Mustard), Fabaceae (Pea), Liliaceae (Lily), Poaceae (Grass), Rosaceae (Rose), and Asteraceae (Aster).
- Keying out herbs in the field.

KEY TERMS

Angiosperm
Apiaceae
Asteraceae
Binomial system
Botanical name
Botany
Brassicaceae
Carpels
Common name
Dicot
Fabaceae
Family
Genus
Gymnosperm
International Code of Binomial Nomenclature (ICBN)
Keying out
Latin name
Linnaeus
Lamiaceae
Liliaceae
Monocot
Petal (corolla)
Pinyin name
Pharmaceutical name
Phylogeny
Pistil (stigma, style, ovary, carpel)
Poaceae
Rosaceae
Scientific name
Species
Stamen (pollen, anther, filament)
Subfamily
Taxonomy
Tribe

Taxonomy involves the organizing, classifying, and naming of living things. As far as plants are concerned, this process involves a familiarity with the work of renowned naturalist and taxonomist Carl Linnaeus, who lived in Sweden in the 1700s. A degree in botany is not necessary, but some basic information is.

An important aspect of herbalism is the question of plant names. Many plants have more than one common name, and some common names are duplicated for other botanicals. There are also Latin names, pharmaceutical names, and Chinese anglicized pinyin names. This chapter sorts them out. If herbalists know the Latin name of a plant, they are in a safe zone, because Latin is the official designated worldwide naming system. Latin names require an understanding of Linnaeus's binomial system.

To identify plants that are growing in the field with any degree of safety, assurance, and accuracy, we need to have a familiarity with common medicinal plant families and how they fit into the overall scheme. When out wildcrafting, accurate plant identification is vital.

Taxonomy and Carl Linnaeus, 1707–1778

Swedish naturalist ***Carl Linnaeus*** is considered the father of modern taxonomy. ***Taxonomy*** is the science of identifying, naming, and classifying living organisms based on their structure and evolutionary history. Linnaeus focused on the plant kingdom and classified plants based on structure. Taxonomy is a way to categorize extinct and living species. Herbalists would be well-served to know how the plants they use for healing fit into the big picture. Linnaeus organized it into a seven-tiered classification system. Whenever there is a large amount of puzzling information, we tend to arrange it into understandable boxes and categories. The field of taxonomy takes this on.

Before Linnaeus, various systems had been toyed with. Aristotle in ancient Greece was the first to attempt classification of living things 2000 years ago. He divided them into plants or animals based on appearance. The Romans were more specific and added types of organisms, for example, a flower or a dog. As more flora and fauna were discovered, the need arose for further breakdown (e.g., the many types of flowers or dogs). As new organisms were classified, lengthy and cumbersome descriptions were added, such as the plant with the tall yellow flower and pointy leaves or the brown and white, shaggy-haired dog with long legs that could run fast.

As we gain new information about a plant or animal, classifications can and do change. Taxonomy is not static—it's a living, changing entity that is debated and amended. With genetic research now going on, taxonomic reclassifications are occurring at a rapid pace.

The Linnaean Seven-Tiered System of Plant Classification

This system begins with the broadest designation and works its way down to the smallest, most specific, detailed group (Box 4.1). The classification for *Salvia divinorum* (Divine Sage) is shown, but any botanical could have been used as an example. From an herbalist's perspective, pertinent information begins on the last three rungs of the hierarchy: the family, the genus, and the species.

Kingdom

Kingdom is the broadest and top level. Aristotle designated two kingdoms: plant and animal. At this writing, it's up to six kingdoms and will most likely keep climbing as we discover more.

- *Animal.* This is the largest kingdom. One-celled animals are included. Animals can move, reproduce, and respond to stimuli. The animal kingdom includes more than a million species.
- *Plant.* This is the second-largest kingdom. Plants have multicellular complex cells. They have strong cellulose cell walls, contain chlorophyll, and conduct *photosynthesis*, the ability to convert light into energy, from which they give off oxygen. They don't move and don't have real sensory systems. There are about 250,000 species of plants. They range from tiny mosses to giant trees.
- *Fungi.* These are multicell, complex organisms that do not conduct photosynthesis. The largest group is mushrooms. Others are yeasts, molds, and mildews. Fungi do not make their own food but generally live on dead, organic matter and decaying plant parts, such as old logs. There are around 100,000 species of fungi. They are not plants, nor are they animals.
- *Eubacteria.* Complex and one celled, most bacteria fall into this category, for example, *Staphylococci, Streptococci, Escherichia, Salmonella,* and *Acidophilus.* They can have sphere, rod, or spiral forms.
- *Archaebacteria.* This one-celled group is *anaerobic* bacteria, meaning they live without oxygen. They live in extreme, hostile environments, such as salt water, volcanos, acid environments, hot springs, and the human gut. They were first discovered in the thermal waters of Yellowstone National Park.
- *Protist* or *eukarya.* These organisms are the ancestors of the plant, fungi, and animal kingdoms. Most are one-celled and have a nucleus and complex specialized organelles. Some, like seaweed, have many cells. Blue-green algae, diatoms, and protozoa are in this group. There are more than 250,000 species in this kingdom.

• BOX 4.1 Linnaeus's Seven-Tiered Classification System

Salvia divinorum (Divine Sage)

Kingdom: Plant

Division: Angiosperm or Magnoliophyta.

Class: Magnoliopsida (dicotyledons). Class names end in *opsida.*

Subclass: Asteridae. Subclass names end in *idae.*

Order: Lamiales. Order names end in *ales.*

Family: Lamiaceae. Family names end in *aceae.* Sometimes subdivided into Subfamilies and Tribes, which end in *eae.*

Genus: *Salvia.* Genus names are italicized or underlined.

Species: *divinorum.* Follows genus name, lowercase, italicized or underlined.[1]

Division

The next Linnaean plant category is the *division* (Table 4.1). Plants are placed into divisions based on whether they reproduce by seeds or spores, and whether they are vascular. Seed-bearing plants are further divided into *gymnosperms* (naked seeds) and *angiosperms* (seeds enclosed in an ovary).

- *Lycopodiophyta.* The earliest land plants were the nonvascular plants with no seeds and with no inside support system to transport water and nutrients. For that reason, they are small plants that grow close to the ground with green, branched stems, scalelike leaves, and no flowers. Imagine mosses, hornworts, and liverworts.
- *Pteridophyta.* These are spore plants with a vascular system, such as ferns, clubmosses, and horsetails. They have roots and stems but no seeds or flowers. *Pteridophyta* were the first vascular plants, which was significant because it allowed the plant to stand upright. For millions of years, spore plants formed giant forests (that later became our coal deposits) in warm tropical areas. These plants reproduce by dropping spores to the ground and growing a *thallus.* The thallus eventually forms female eggs and male sperm, which fertilize and grow into new plants.
- *Gymnosperms.* ***Gymnosperms*** are vascular and have naked seeds in cones that are exposed to air. They include the conifers, cycads, and one lone Ginkgo. They first appeared in the fossil record about 360 million years ago and were the first plants to evolve beyond spores and have true seeds.
  - *Gymnosperm reproduction.* Gymnosperms produce male and female cones. The large cones produce egg cells, and the smaller cones produce sperm cells. The seeds are naked because their egg cells are exposed to the air and fertilized when pollen lands directly on them.[2] Some species have male and female cones on the same tree; others have them on separate trees. Pollen from the male cone reaches the egg cells in the female cone and fertilizes them. They start to grow briefly, and then the new seeds drop to the ground. These are in the pinecones and other cones you see on the

TABLE 4.1 Land Plant Divisions[2]

Division	Examples	Number of Species	Spores	Seeds
Nonvascular spore plants	Mosses	14,500		
	Hornworts	100	Yes	No
	Liverworts	8500		
Vascular spore plants	Clubmosses	1200		
	Horsetails	20	Yes	No
	Ferns	12,000		
Naked seeds exposed to air (Vascular gymnosperms)	Conifers	550		
	Cycads	100	No	Yes
	Ginkgo	1		
Seeds enclosed in ovary (Vascular angiosperms)	All flowering plants	260,000	No	Yes

ground near their mother tree. If all goes well, such as having good water and soil, the baby seed resumes growth.[2] These seeds have a head start and developmental advantage over spore plants, which simply drop to the ground.

- *Angiosperms* or *Magnoliopsida* (called both). ***Angiosperms*** are all the flowering plants that have their seeds enclosed in a fruit.[3] They were the last to evolve around 100 million years ago and are the most numerous plants on Earth. The flowers evolved into showy petals to attract insects for pollination. The seeds develop inside the flower in an enclosed ovary. Angiosperms also have leaves, stems, and roots. This division includes most crops, trees, shrubs, grasses, and garden plants. Angiosperms are the most common realm of the herbalist.
  - *Angiosperm reproduction*. Seeds have the best chance for survival and propagation of all the plant divisions. Angiosperm seeds are fully enclosed and protected in an ovary which, in turn, is inside a flower. Angiosperms probably coevolved with the insects that were needed to pollinate them, their colorful petals being insect attractors. As the floral parts evolved, they eventually formed a *stamen*, the male part. The pollen is transferred from the stamen to the female ovary by birds and insects, particularly bees. This transfer happens via the *pistil* (top appendage of the ovary). The seeds develop in the ovary. The advantage of angiosperms over gymnosperms is the efficient seed dispersal systems that have developed from the closed ovary. Some seed-containing ovaries become fruits that are eaten and dispersed in animal feces. Other seeds, such as the Maple or Milkweed (Fig. 4.1), are carried by the wind. Dandelions have little wind-borne *umbrellas*, for example.

Class

Class comes next, under division. The two plant classes under the angiosperm division are the monocots and dicots. *Monocots* have one seed leaf and parallel leaf veins; they are vascular and have flower parts in multiples of three (examples are iris, lilies, orchids, and yuccas). *Dicots* have two seed leaves and netted leaf veins; they are vascular and have floral parts in multiples of four or five.[3] More on this topic in the "Botany" section of this chapter.

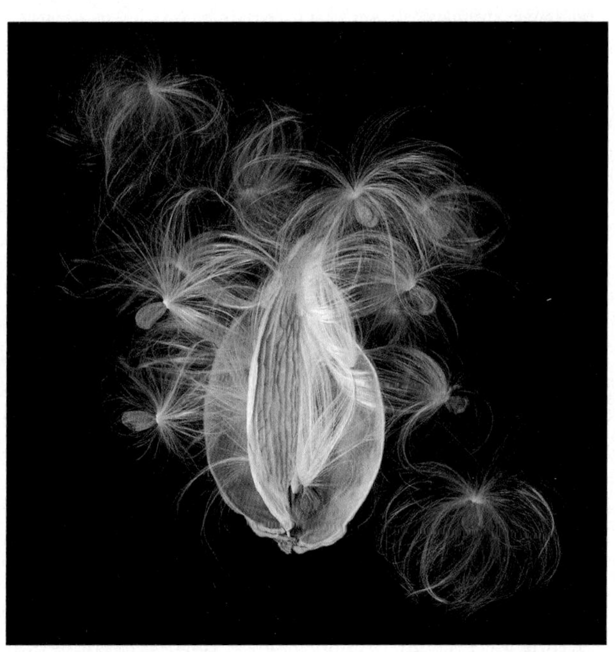

• **Fig. 4.1** Milkweed seedpod. (Copyright Lang/Tucker Photography. Photographs loaned with permission from *The Botanical Series* are copyrighted by Jennifer Anne Tucker and Gerald Lang from the Studio at Hill Crystal Farm. www.jennifer-tucker.com.)

Order

Order is used to group similar families. Various scientific organizations differ regarding where a plant belongs. As far as plant identification goes, the *order* level contains plants that are so varied and different from one another that there are few useful structural patterns to work with. A new taxonomic cataloging system by the Angiosperm Phylogeny Group (APG) uses evolutionary history and genetics, ***phylogeny***, instead of the older structural system used by Linnaeus (Box 4.2).

• BOX 4.2 The Angiosperm Phylogeny Group (APG)

Phylogeny is the use of evolutionary history and genetic relationships to classify plants. Linnaeus didn't know about DNA and based his plant filing system on what was known at the time: structure (morphology) and chemistry.

The Angiosperm Phylogeny Group (APG) is an international team of taxonomists who have been gaining clout and prestige in the world of taxonomy since 1998, when they broke away from the traditional Linnaean system. The APG came together to establish a consensus on the taxonomy of flowering plants (angiosperms) that would reflect new genetic knowledge, rather than relying on the older method of hit-or-miss observation, which had many exceptions to patterns.[4]

Linnaeus divided flowering plants into monocots and dicots. The APG does not support the classification of monocots as a distinct group. It recognizes monocots as a *clade* (a species or group of species) and their most recent common ancestor, the plant's lineage to date. Angiosperm classification begins with the descendants of a particular clade or monocot group, and formal scientific names are not used above that level.

The APG shows this information on a branching diagram or a family tree and depicts a plant's common evolutionary relatives. Common genetic descendants of a particular group branch off on the tree.[5] From order on down the hierarchy, the APG follows Linnaeus's system. Order, family, genus, and species are retained. A limited number of orders (narrowed down to 40 from 232) are considered more useful, and orders containing only a single family are avoided when possible. There are still 25 families of uncertain position. Expect more changes.

The APG is attempting to revamp the Linnaean scheme. Taxonomy is not dead.

Family, Subfamily, and Tribe

Plants with similar flower, fruit, and seed structures are placed into a ***family***.[3] Recognizing plant families is extremely useful for field identification, because if we can learn a distinctive family pattern, we will already narrow down the possibilities for knowing a plant's identity, its genus, and its species. You will automatically know if it is likely poisonous or edible and will know some of its medicinal aspects. Major families for an herbalist to recognize are the Mint, Parsley, Mustard, Pea, Lily, Grass, Rose, and Aster families. There are about 45,000 species in these 8 families alone.[2] That's a lot of plants.

A ***subfamily*** is a designation below a family and a ***tribe*** is a subgroup under a subfamily. Each group has smaller botanical differences than the one above, but each level usually comprises many different plants.

An example of this arrangement is the Pea family name ***Fabaceae***, a subfamily within it being Faboideae (plants with flowers having a banner, wings, and keel structure) and under that, the Clover tribe, Trifolieae with three-parted leaves. Notice that family names end in *ceae*, subfamilies end in *deae*, and tribes end in *eae*. The Pea family (Fabaceae) and the Sunflower family (Asteraceae) have many tribes.

Genus

A ***genus*** is a group of plants within a family that has more traits in common with each other than with any other plants in that family.[3] It is basically the surname of a plant, like *Smith*. Many plants can have the same genus name (the entire related Smith family), but they have to be botanically similar and genetically connected. It is the first listing in the binomial designation.

• BOX 4.3 Herbalists and Linnaeus

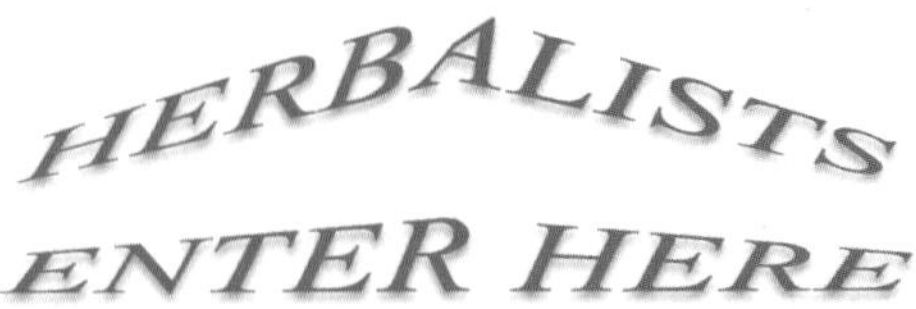

From the perspective of plant identification, the family, genus, and species level is where herbalists join the picture.

Species

The species is the second listing in the binomial designation and the most individual, identifying the specific plant. A ***species*** is a group of organisms that resemble each other more closely than those of any other group and are capable of reproducing with one another to produce fertile offspring.[1] There can only be one plant per species. If the genus is the surname *Smith*, then the species is the first name, *Mary*. These last three groups—family, genus, and species—are the most important for an herbalist to know (Box 4.3).

Naming Plants

What's in a Name?

How do you know which plant is which? How are identifications made and herbs acquired? Will you refer to an herb catalog where herbs are already named, or will you go foraging or wildcrafting? How can a plant that is growing in a field or backyard be accurately identified? This information is pretty basic stuff. The best way to know a plant is to sit with it as it is growing in the ground. Before that, learn her name and something about her.

There are two related aspects and answers to these questions. One involves *taxonomy*, the science of classifying plants into ordered categories and related groups based on some factor common to each, such as structure, embryology, or biochemistry. The other is ***botany***, the science of plants and the branch of biology that deals with plant life and plant structure.

Common Names

When using plants as medicine, it is essential to ensure we have the correct plant and its correct name. This process can be confusing. A single plant often has many nicknames or ***common names***, which may be what it is called in a certain location or region based on common usage. Plantain leaf has been called Ribwort, Lamb's Tongue, Dog's Ribs, Ripple Grass, Leechwort, and Windles, to name a few. *Echinacea* spp. is also known as Purple Coneflower, Red Sunflower, Comb flower, Hedgehog, Scurvy root, and Indian Head.[7] Different countries, towns, and locales have their own preferred names. For good communication, herbalists use the Latin name that is recognized worldwide by all.

If out wildcrafting, where does one start? It is extremely difficult to tell what something is by comparing it to a picture or a sketch in a book. Pictures and the real plant don't always match. Even photos are not always clear. And what if the field guide is organized by flower color and the flowers are long gone, because they died in mid-July, and you are out identifying plants in late August? What if the field guide organizes plants into families, but you haven't a clue which family your plant is in? What if the guide is organized alphabetically? Then you have to rifle through the entire book and hope you are lucky enough to find a picture that remotely matches.

The Botanical Name, Based on the Binomial System

Linnaeus proposed a ***binomial system*** or two-name system of classification for all living things. The first name is the general name, the ***genus***, and the second name is the specific name, the ***species***. This binomial system streamlined and revolutionized botany. The binomial name is considered the ***scientific name***, ***Latin name***, or ***botanical name*** of a plant. There are certain recognized rules to follow when writing botanical names.

- *Proper way to write a binomial:* either *italicize* or underline. The genus is capitalized, and the species begins with a lower case and is italicized or underlined as well. Garden Sage herb is *Salvia officinalis* or Salvia officinalis. Cayenne pepper is *Capsicum annuum* or Capsicum annuum. Although underlining is less often used nowadays, it is useful to understand the convention. Just as medical terms are written in Greek or Latin, plant binomials are also. Ancient Greek and Latin are dead languages. A *dead* language is not spoken anymore, so it does not change. The use of Greek and Latin is very convenient in science because it always remains the same and is standardized all over the world.
- *The plant namer's initials follow a binomial.* A binomial is followed by the name or initials of the botanical authority who named the species. Because Linnaeus named numerous species, his surname initial appears after many plants. For example, *Vaccinium myrtillus* L., *Aloe vera* L., *Marrubium vulgare* L., *Rhodiola rosea* L., were all named by Linnaeus. Others are *Ligusticum porteri* Coulter and Rose, *Carduus benedictus* Bruns, *Nasturtium officinale* R. Brown, and *Ulmus fulva* Michaux.
- *Plural genus notations.* These are used when talking about many different species of the same genus. Perhaps you want to talk about the 11 or so different species of the genus *Artemisia.* They are similar and related plants, so instead of writing out *Artemisia* for each one, the genus name can be abbreviated after writing it the first time: *Artemisia absinthium, A. annua, A. apiacea, A. argyi, A. tridentata,* and *A. vulgaris.* If you want to talk about the whole group at once, you would just write out *Artemisia* spp., in which spp. means *species plural.* The species plural designation (spp.) is not italicized because it is not part of the binomial designation.
- *The binomial name is considered its botanical and its scientific name.* These terms all refer to the same designation.
- *Derivations of botanical names.*[1] This methodology refers to various ways plant names were chosen. Names can incorporate the place a plant grows, its color, or its properties, etc. As we get to know some of these category names and their meanings, the botanical name of a specific herb will make more sense and be easier to remember (Box 4.4). Learning botanical names is part of an herbalist's training. Sometimes botanical names have become the plant's common name as well, such as rhododendron, magnolia, chrysanthemum, and petunia.

• BOX 4.4 Derivations of Botanical Names

- **Mythology**. *Achillea,* from the Greek warrior Achilles, whose bleeding heel was treated with *Achillea millefolium* (Yarrow herb). *Artemisia,* from the Greek goddess of the hunt, as in *Artemisia tridentata* (Sagebrush herb) or *Artemisia annua* (Annual Wormwood herb).
- **Habitat**. *Montana,* meaning growing in mountainous places, such as *Arnica montana* (Arnica flower). *Riparius,* meaning growing by rivers or streams, as in *Elmyrus riparius* (Riverbank Wild Rye).
- **Places**. *Eschscholzia californica* (California Poppy herb), *Dianthus chinensis* (China), *Solidago canadensis* (Canadian Goldenrod herb).
- **Uses or properties**. *Leonurus cardiaca* (Motherwort herb) used for heart palpitations. *Ranunculus repens* (Creeping Buttercup), *repens* means creeping; *Cicuta maculata* (Spotted Hemlock), *maculata* means spotted.
- **Classical names**. The large genus *Ligusticum* (Lovage), derived from the Italian region of Liguria. Narcissus in Greek mythology, known for admiring his own beauty, provides the name for *Narcissus,* a genus that includes Daffodils and Jonquils.
- **Commemorating people:** Chamomile flower, *Matricaria recutita* L. for Linnaeus. Wild Cherry bark, *Prunus serotina* Ehrhart, for a German botanist; Dandelion root, *Taraxacum officinale* Weber, for a French botanist.
- **Anatomical name**. *Chondrus crispus* (Irish Moss), *crispus* means curled. *Achillea millefolium* (Yarrow herb), a thousand-leafed or many cuts.
- **Colors**. *Paeonia lactiflora* (White Peony root), *lactico* means white. *Echinacea purpurea* (Purple coneflower), *purpurea* means purple. *Piper nigrum* (Black Pepper), *nigrum* means black. *Rhodiola rosea* (Rhodiola root), *rosea* means rose. *Rheum* spp. (Rhubarb leaf stalk), *ruber* means dark pink.

The International Code of Botanical Nomenclature for Algae, Fungi, and Plants

The ***International Code of Binomial Nomenclature (ICBN)*** determines and governs the naming of plants. This is a different group from the APG, which deals with phylogeny. The ICBN publishes the set of rules and recommendations that govern the formal botanical names given to algae, fungi, and plants. The International Botanical Congress (IBC) meets every few years in different countries to revise, reclassify, or add names as more is learned or discovered. The original meeting to decide all this was held in Paris in 1867 about a century after Linnaeus. The words *algae, fungi,* and *plants* were in added in July 2011.

As more information is collected on plants, their family, genus, or species may change. Some plants have gone through many name changes and reversals. Roman Chamomile was once in the genus *Anthemis* but is now a member of the genus *Chamaemelum.* Family names have also changed. Major groups have gone from general names to those representing an important genus of the family. The Compositae family is now ***Asteraceae***, named after the common *Aster* genus. The Mint family used to be called Labiatae for its two-lipped upper petals but is now Lamiaceae. The old Cruciferous family is now the Brassicaceae.[2] It's not all that clear cut. The ICBN publishes updates each time it meets and after all the botanists reconsider plants' botanical names, characteristics, and origins.

The Basic Principles of the ICBN

- *It begins with Linnaeus.* Agreement was made to use the works of Linnaeus as a starting point for all scientific names of plants. The formal starting date is May 1, 1753, the publication date of Linnaeus's *Species Plantarum.* His binomials, or the earliest ones published after him, would have priority.

- *New names are declared by original author's publication.* The first published name of a plant is accepted as its correct name and is associated with a particular specimen, declared by the author in her or his original publication. This specimen is usually a dried plant (rarely a photo) that is preserved in an herbarium.
- *All new names use the binomial system.* They are assigned in Latin, and there is only one correct name per plant. Deciding what that name will be is a work in progress, as illustrated by the International Botanical Congress's approved name for Black Cohosh (Box 4.5).

• BOX 4.5 Black Cohosh Botanical Name Reverts Back and Forth

(Make up your mind, already!)

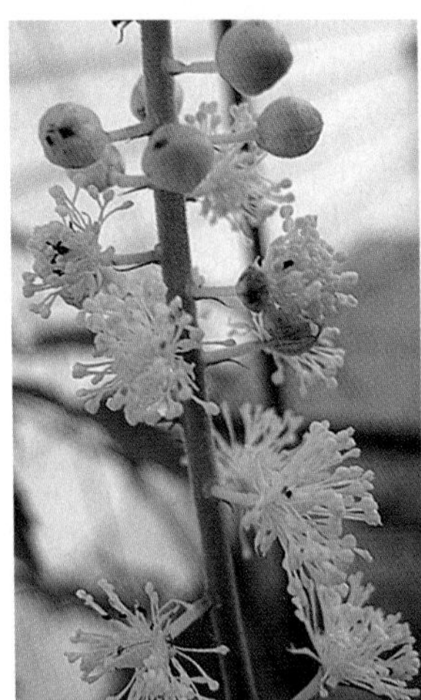
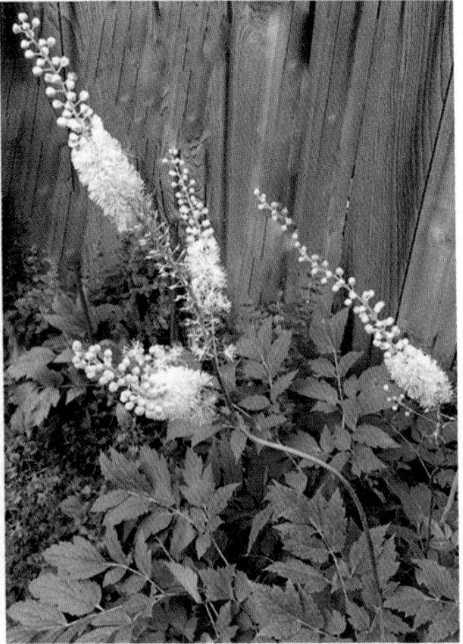

Left, Black Cohosh flower close-up. *Right*, Black Cohosh flowering.

A recent botanical name change was for Black Cohosh. Linnaeus originally listed it in his *Species Plantarum* (1753) under the genus *Actaea (Actaea racemosa*, L.) based on its morphological characteristics of inflorescence (flowers) and seeds. Later, Thomas Nuttall had its genus changed in 1818 because of the dry follicles it produced, typical of the species *Cimicifuga (Cimicifuga racemosa*, Nutt). However, in 1999, based on new morphological and DNA sequence studies by James Compton of the University of Reading, UK, Black Cohosh has been switched back again into Linnaeus's original genus, *Actaea*.[9]

The Pharmaceutical Name

The binomial name of a plant is considered its botanical or scientific name. We have also discussed a plant's common name. To further complicate the name issue, in Chinese Medicine, plants are often named another way, by their ***pharmaceutical name***. The name is composed of the plant part used in Latin, such as *radix* for root, *fructus* for fruit, *flos* for flower (Table 4.2). The plant part is followed by the genus, and occasionally the species. Examples are Licorice root (Radix Glycyrrhizae), Green tea leaf (Folium Camelliae sinensis), Chrysanthemum flower (Flos Chrysanthemi). The advantage of the pharmaceutical name is that you always know the plant part in question; the disadvantage is that you don't always know the species, which is sometimes mentioned and sometimes not.[10]

The Pinyin Name

There is yet another name to be familiar with when considering herbs used in Chinese Medicine. This is the ***pinyin name***, based on a system for transcribing the pronunciation of the Mandarin dialect with its Chinese letters into the Latin alphabet. It was adopted by the People's Republic of China in 1979 and was used to teach standard Chinese and word pronunciation (Table 4.3).

In most books on Chinese herbs and in Chinese herb catalogs, the pinyin name is given along with some combination of the common, botanical, or pharmaceutical name. Pinyin is the Chinese pronunciation of the herb in English. If you shop for herbs in a city's area of predominantly Chinese residents and businesses, the pinyin name is often the only name the Chinese shopkeeper knows. If you can't request your herb and can't pronounce it correctly in pinyin, you may have difficulty buying the herb you seek. If unsure of pronunciation, write down the pinyin name before you go, just in case. For example, Bupleurum root is Chi Hu; Astragalus root is Huang Qi. Examples of the four types of names just discussed are provided (Table 4.4).

Botany

Botany is the study of plant structure: flowers and their parts, leaf structures, and plant families. The ability to name and recognize basic plant structures is needed to identify plants actually growing in the ground. The capacity to pinpoint a few plant families will provide clues about a plant's probable medicinal properties. What follows is basic botanical information for herbalists, but by no means an exhaustive investigation.

TABLE 4.2 Plant Part Names in Latin
(Part of the pharmaceutical name.)

Bulbus = bulb	Fructus = fruit	Rhizoma = rhizome
Cacumen = treetop	Gemma = bud	Semen = seed
Caulis = stalk or stem	Herba = herb, aerial part	Thallus = thallus (same word)
Cortex = bark	Pericarpium = rind or peel	Tuber = tuber (same word)
Flos = flower or blossom	Radix = root	Turio = sprout or shoot
Folium = leaf	Ramulus = twig	Lichen = lichen (same word)

TABLE 4.3 Some Pinyin Meanings, Pronunciations, and Examples

Mandarin Pinyin Word	English Translation	English Pronunciation	Herbal Example
Gen	Root	*G* as in *guy* but less pronounced	Ban Lan Gen Isatis root
Ye	Leaf	*Y* as in *yen* but softer	Da Qing Ye Isatis leaf
Hua	Flower	*Ua* as in *guava*	Jin Yin Hua Honeysuckle flower
Zi	Seed	*Zi* as in *zen* *I* as in *seem*	Zhi Zi Gardenia seed
Pi	Peel	*I* as in *seem*	Chen Pi Ripe Citrus peel or rind
Ren	Kernel	*R* as in ran with tongue curled back on palate, *I* in *Yi* as in *seem*	Yi Ren Coix kernel
Huang	Yellow	*Uang* as in *w* plus *ung* as in *hung; Qi* as in *we*	Huang Qi Astragalus root
Bai	White	*B* as in *mob*	Bai Zhu White Atractylodes root
Hong	Red	*G* as in *gong* *Ao* as in *now*	Hong Zao Red Jujube berry
Xiang	Fragrant	*X* between the *s* in *saw* and the *sh* in shawl; *iang* as the *e* in *seem* and the *ung* in *dung*	Xiang Ru Aromatic Madder herb
Gan	Dry	*G* as in *guy* but less voiced; *iang* as in *hung*	Gan Jiang Ginger rhizome
Zhi	Frying with Liquid	*Zh* as in *jungle* but pronounced more with the teeth; *Cao* as in *sow*	Zhi Gan Cao Honey Fried Licorice root
Sheng	Fresh or Raw	*Sh* as in *wash; aung* as in *hung*	Sheng Di Huang Raw Rehmannia root
Shu	Prepared	*Sh* as in *wash; aung* as in *hung*	Shu Di Huang Prepared Rehmannia root

TABLE 4.4 The Same Plant, All Four Names

Common Name	Botanical Name	Pharmaceutical Name	Pinyin Name
Licorice root	*Glycyrrhiza uralensis*	Radix Glycyrrhizae	Gan Cao
Garden Sage leaf	*Salvia officinalis*	Folium Salviae	None
Alfalfa herb	*Medicago sativa*	Herba Medicaginis	Mu Xu
Hawthorn berry	*Crataegus oxyacantha*	Fructus Crataegi	Shan Sha

Monocotyledons and Dicotyledons

Flowering plants are angiosperms. Their seeds are enclosed in an ovary and are divided into two major groups: the *monocotyledons (monocots)* and the *dicotyledons (dicots)*. A *cotyledon* is a seed leaf, the first leaf that sprouts from the seed. Monocots (one) have one seed leaf because the seed is all once piece (e.g., a corn kernel). Dicots (two) have two seed leaves because one leaf sprouts from each half of the seed (e.g., a bean). Beyond observing seed leaves, there are other ways to recognize them, in case you see the plant long after its seed leaf has died.[3] Recognizing whether a plant is a monocot or a dicot is the first step in its identification.

- *Monocots.* One seed leaf, parallel veins in the leaves, horizontal rootstalks, floral parts mostly in threes. Examples: Grass (Fig. 4.2), Wheat, Lilies, Yucca, Bamboo, Palms, Corn.
- *Dicots.* Two seed leaves, netted veins in the leaves, generally tap roots, complex branching, floral parts mostly in fours and fives. Examples: Rose, Sunflower, Violet, Columbine, Oxeye Daisy (Fig. 4.3).

Be aware that like everything in the plant world, there are exceptions. Some monocots have netted veins. Some dicots have parallel veins. Sometimes the flower parts vary from threes, to fours and fives. To know for sure, one has to key out a plant by using a flow chart technique where characteristics are ruled out one by one through the process of elimination. More on this in the "Keying Out a Plant" section later in this chapter.

Flowers

Flowers have evolved over time as a result of modifications from a structurally simple magnolia flower to the complex flower heads of the Aster family (Fig. 4.4). Leaves transitioned into sepals, then to petals, then to stamens. This change is revealed in the plant's structure. Sometimes it is hard to determine whether the colored part commonly called a flower is a petal, a sepal, or a combination of the two.

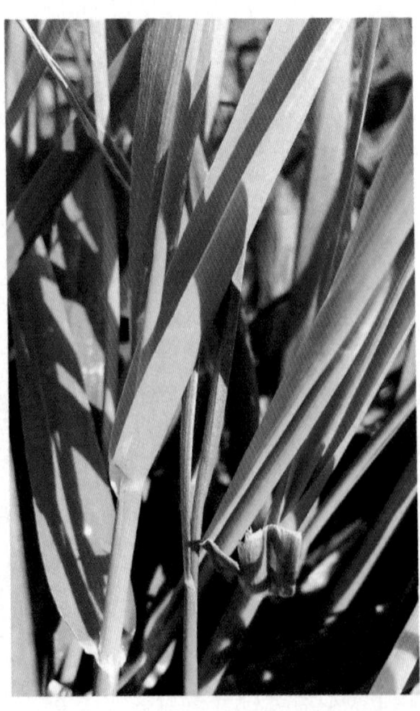

• **Fig. 4.2** Grass, a monocot with parallel veins and nodes.

Flowers vary in shape. Some are symmetrical and regular, with the parts of a set all identical in size; others are irregular, with parts of the set different (Fig. 4.5). Asters have symmetrical daisy-like shapes, and Pea flowers are asymmetrical. Sepals, petals, and stamens can be above, below, or in the middle of the ovary. The parts of a flower follow (see Fig. 4.4).

- *Pistil.* The female part of a flower is the ***pistil***. It consists of the top ***stigma***, the middle ***style***, and the bottom ***ovary***. The ovary contains the *ovules*. After fertilization, an ovule develops into a seed (Fig. 4.6).
- *Stamen.* The male parts of a flower are the ***stamens***. They consist of the ***pollen*** on the tip, the ***anther*** on which the pollen sits, and the ***filament*** or stalk. A useful reminder of the parts is "Stamen *stay men*" (Fig. 4.7).
- *Sepals.* Usually green, leaflike modifications below the petals or under the ovary. The *calyx* is the sum of all the sepals.

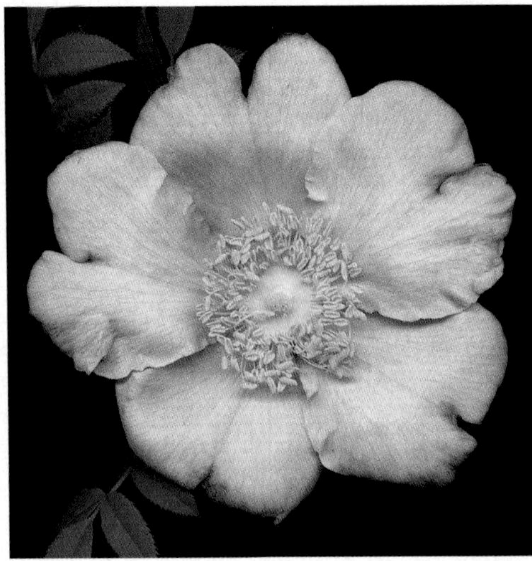

• **Fig. 4.3** Rose flower, a dicot with five petals. (Copyright Lang/Tucker Photography. Photographs loaned with permission from *The Botanical Series* are copyrighted by Jennifer Anne Tucker and Gerald Lang from the Studio at Hill Crystal Farm. www.jennifer-tucker.com.)

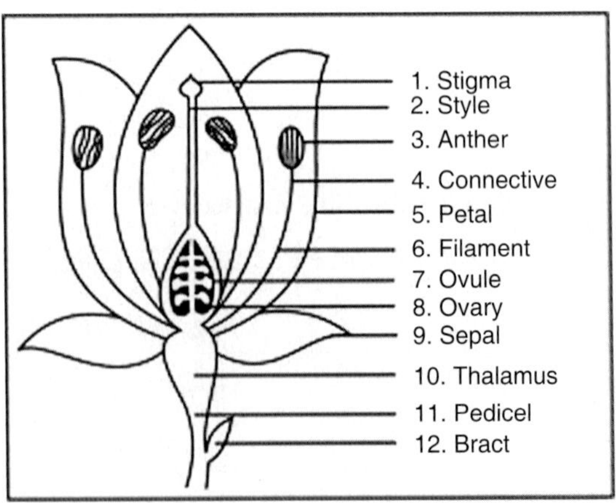

• **Fig. 4.4** Parts of a Generic Flower. (Credit: From Biren N. Shah, A.K. Seth: *Textbook of Pharmacognosy and Phytochemistry*, 1st ed. 2009, Elsevier Ltd.)

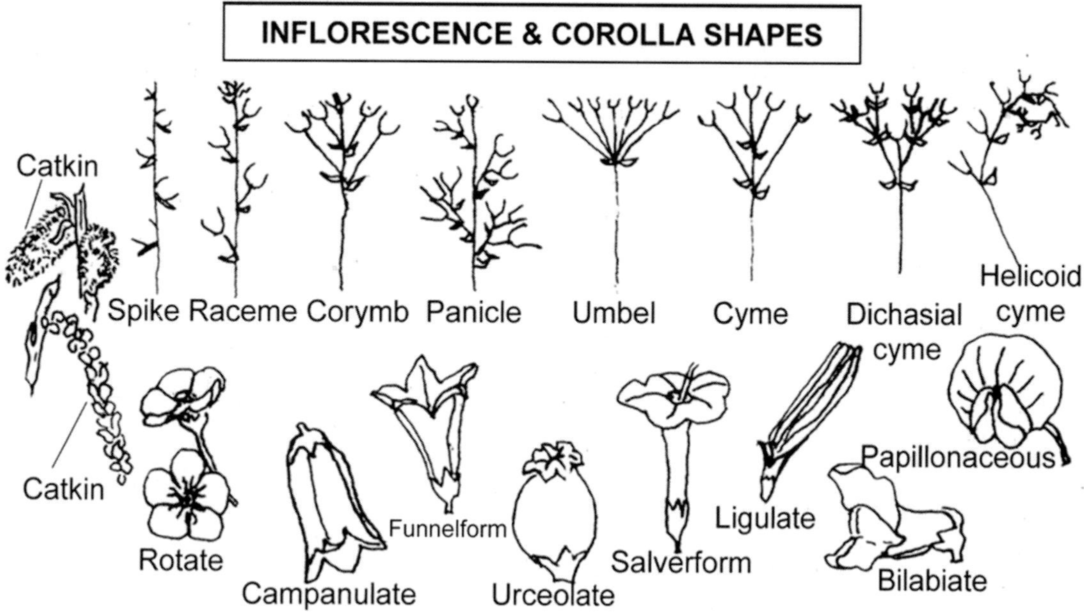

• **Fig. 4.5** Inflorescence and Corolla Shapes. (Illustration by Joan Zinn referenced from *Hortus Third, A Concise Dictionary of Plants Cultivated in the United States and Canada*, by Staff of the L. H. Bailey Hortorium, Cornell University. New York: Macmillan 1976)

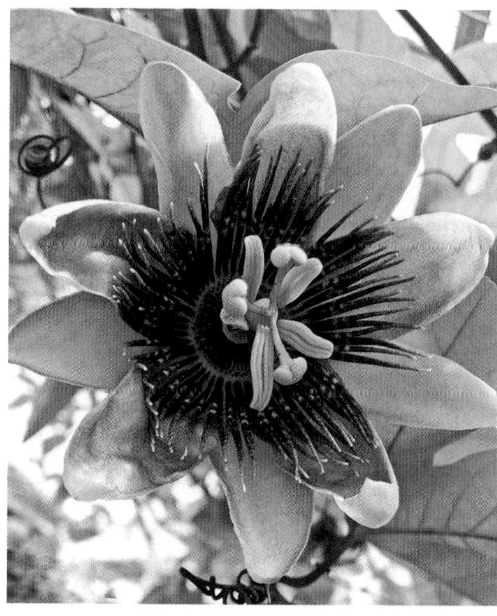

• **Fig. 4.6** Passionflower shows five stamens with yellow anthers; from the ovary arise three widely spreading styles, each ending in a button-like stigma. (Photography Joan Zinn)

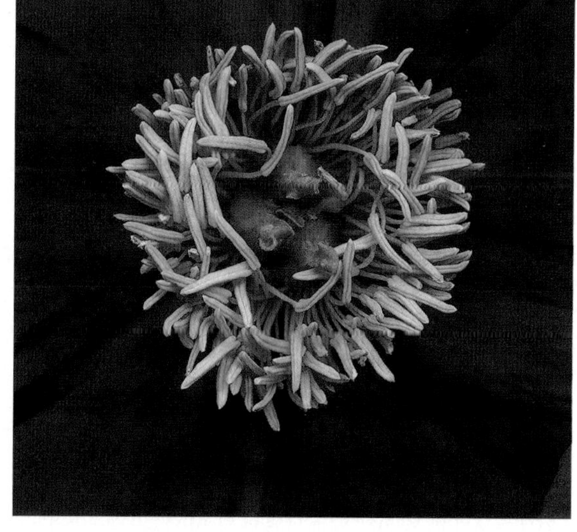

• **Fig. 4.7** Red Peony with numerous yellow stamens and fused ovary with three carpals. Copyright Lang/Tucker Photography. (Photographs loaned with permission from *The Botanical Series* are copyrighted by Jennifer Anne Tucker and Gerald Lang from the Studio at Hill Crystal Farm. www.jennifer-tucker.com)

- *Petals*. The ***corolla*** is the sum of all the ***petals***, sometimes called the inflorescence.
- *Complete flowers* have sepals, petals, stamens, and a pistil.
- *Incomplete flowers* lack one or more of the above flower parts.
- *Bisexual flowers* have both male and female parts.
- *Unisexual flowers* have male and female flowers appearing either separately on the same plant or on separate plants.
- *Ovaries* can be single chambered, many chambered (compound), or fused.
- *Carpal.* A chamber of an ovary. It is common for plants to have a compound ovary consisting of many united/fused carpals.
- *Style and stigma structure*. These parts are easy to see outside the flower and provide a clue about the ovary structure within. A pistil with three separate styles indicates an ovary with three united carpals. If a stigma has four parts, there are probably four carpals in the ovary.[2]

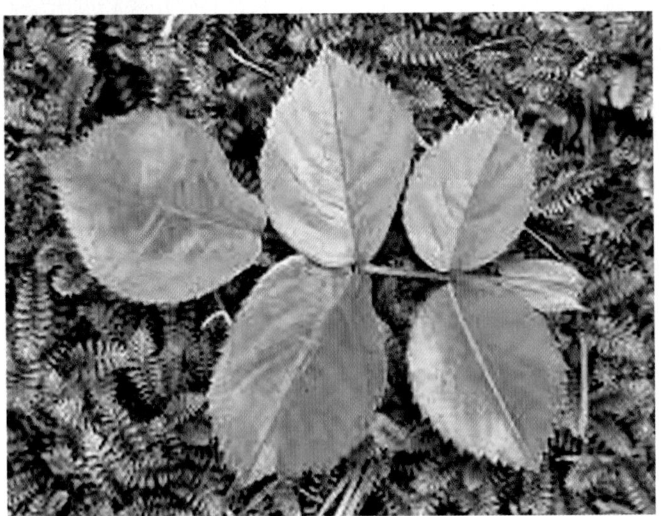

• **Fig. 4.8** Odd-pinnate Rose leaf divided into a group of serrated leaflets.

Leaves

Leaves come in many sizes and shapes. Leaves last much longer than flowers and are a major way to identify plants when sorting out families. Some leaves are actually many leaflets arranged in a group (Fig. 4.8).

- *Margins* or *shapes*. The margins are the edges that give the leaf a shape. Examples are round, oval, lancelike, heart-shaped, arrowhead, pinnately lobed, palmately lobed, serrated, and lobed (Fig. 4.9).
- *Arrangement. Basal* leaves come up in a cluster from the ground with no stem, as seen in a first-year basal Mullein rosette or Green Gentian before flowering (Fig. 4.10). *Alternate* leaves alternate up the stem. *Opposite* leaves grow opposite each other on a stem. *Whorled* leaves grow in a circle around the stem, attached at one node, as seen in Cleavers herb (Fig. 4.11).
- *Divisions*. A simple leaf is one undivided leaf attached to a stalk by its stem or petiole. One leaf can be divided in one, two, three, or many leaflets, making it *compound*. The leaflets can be even or uneven in number. A fern frond is considered a large compound leaf made up of many smaller leaflets. Some leaflets have curly tendrils on the end.
- *Stipule*. A pair of leaflike appendages at the base of a leaf stem.
- *Bract*. Any form of modified leaf.

Plant Families for Herbalists

Now we get into the fun of identifying plant families using our powers of observation, the senses. This skill is essential for any wildcrafter. I can testify that wildcrafting and walking among the plants is one of life's greatest joys. We will consider a few major families that contain many medicinal herbs.

Observing patterns helps place a plant in a family and knowing the characteristics of a family allows us to make an educated guess as to the plant's properties. We use information about leaf structure and flower parts to decide. We count stamens and observe their length. We decide if flowers are symmetrical or irregular and whether the petals are united or separate. We look at the stem to see if it's round, square, rough, or hollow, and if there is juice inside. What shape and pattern do the leaves have, and do they grow on the stem in an alternate, opposite, or whorled position? How does the leaf or flower smell? Are there aromatic oils? Is the texture rough or smooth?

Families are presented with key words to help you remember. Major families are listed here with descriptions, examples, and general characteristics. If you can identify these few families, you already have the potential to know about 45,000 species worldwide![2]

Mint Family (Lamiaceae)

Stems are square (Box 4.6). The leaves are opposite one another on the stem. If you crush or rub a leaf between your fingers, the leaf and your fingers will usually smell strongly aromatic. This scent will quickly distinguish it from other plants. Mint flowers are very tiny and irregular, two-lipped with two lobes above and three lobes below, all united. The flowers have four stamens, two long and two short. You might need a magnifying glass to see them. Other flowers with square stems and opposite leaves are found in the Verbena, Stinging Nettle, and Loosestrife families. Those plants are not aromatic, however. The two-chambered ovary matures into a capsule containing four nutlets. The Mint family has about 3500 species worldwide (Fig. 4.12).[2]

Some Mint family plants are rich in the volatile oil called menthol, which provides the traditional minty smell to Peppermint, Spearmint, Paleo Mint, Wintergreen, Eucalyptus, and Pennyroyal herbs. Rub one of these leaves between your fingers and smell it. Menthol acts medicinally to open the airways, stop pain and inflammation, help digestion, and stop stomachaches. One or two drops of Peppermint essential oil rubbed on the abdomen is a great nausea remedy.

The Mint family tends to be a very safe, nontoxic group and is one of the easiest families to become acquainted with. Many of our seasonings, culinary spices, and aromatic essential oils abound in components of this family, such as the leaves of Marjoram, Oregano, Basil, Garden Sage, Rosemary, and Thyme. Other ***Lamiaceae*** family members are Horehound herb for any kind of cough; Motherwort herb, a woman's ally; Catnip herb for stomachaches; Skullcap and Lemon Balm herbs for sleep and relaxation; and Hyssop herb for opening the airway. *Monarda* spp. (Wild Bergamot, Wild Oregano, Bee Balm) attract bees like crazy, and grow abundantly in the Rocky Mountains. It is a great wild food to spice up camp meals. A little goes a long way.

Parsley or Carrot Family (Apiaceae)

The ***Apiaceae*** family used to be called the Umbelliferae because of its umbel-shaped flowers reminiscent of umbrellas (Box 4.7, Fig. 4.13). The umbels are compound, meaning that the stems of each flower cluster radiate from a single stalk. That stalk in turn meets other stalks at a single point, making it compound or an umbel within an umbel. Each flower is very tiny and has five sepals, five petals, and five stamens that you might need a magnifying glass to see and count (Fig. 4.14). The leaves are usually fernlike, pinnate shaped. Stems are generally hollow. The ovary has two chambers or ***carpels***.[2]

Wild Carrot, commonly known as Queen Anne's Lace, and Parsley are well-known Apiaceae members, as are spicy Fennel, Celery, Dill, and Caraway seed. All of these plants contain volatile oils that are stimulating, warm, and diaphoretic. They are also digestion-helping carminatives. Candy-coated Fennel seeds are often offered in a basket after East Indian meals for that reason. Other medicinal members are the Parsnip, Water Parsnip (roots

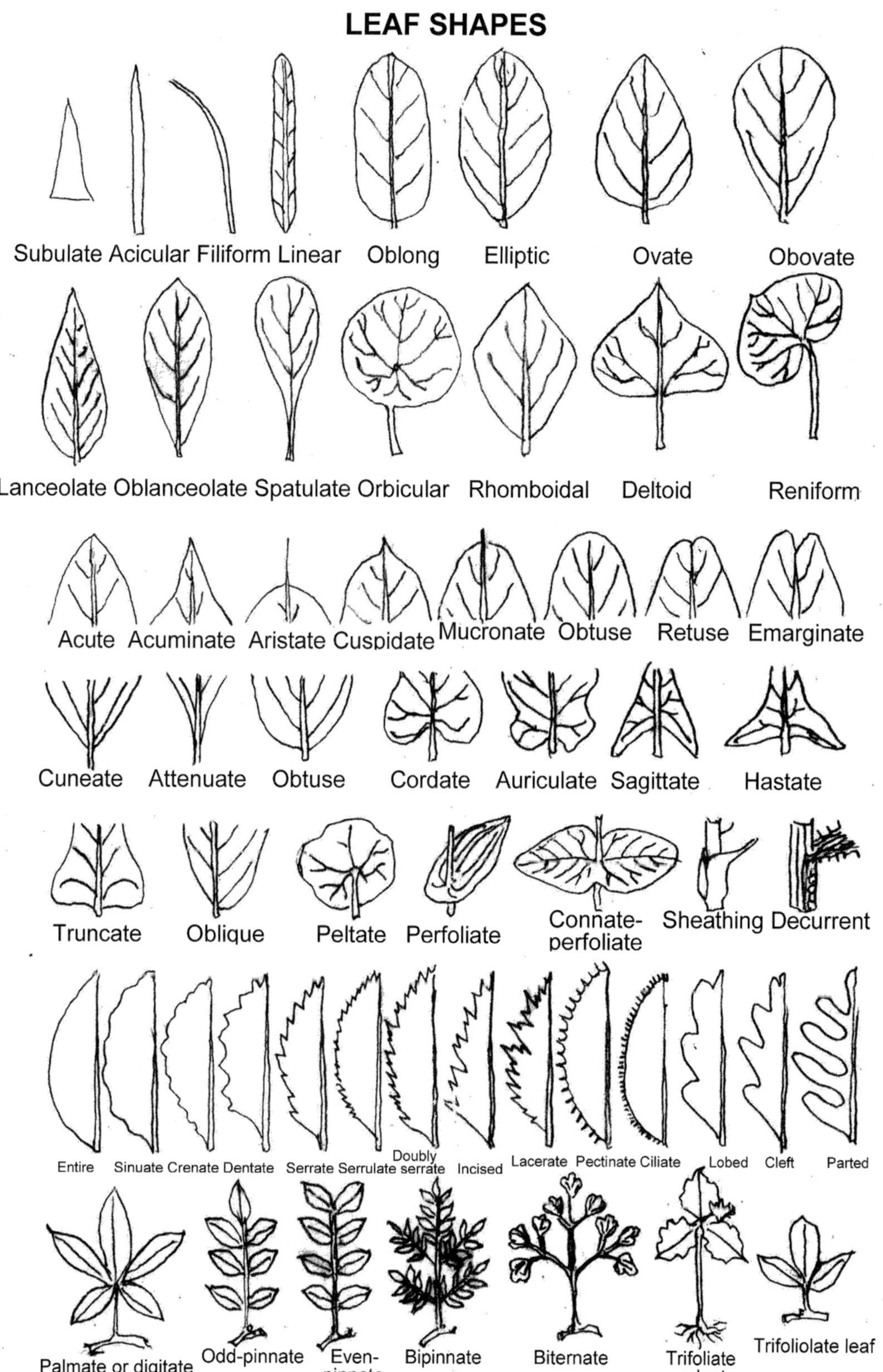

• **Fig. 4.9** Leaf shapes. (Illustration by Joan Zinn referenced from *Hortus Third, A Concise Dictionary of Plants Cultivated in the United States and Canada*, by Staff of the L.H. Bailey Hortorium, Cornell University. New York: Macmillan 1976)

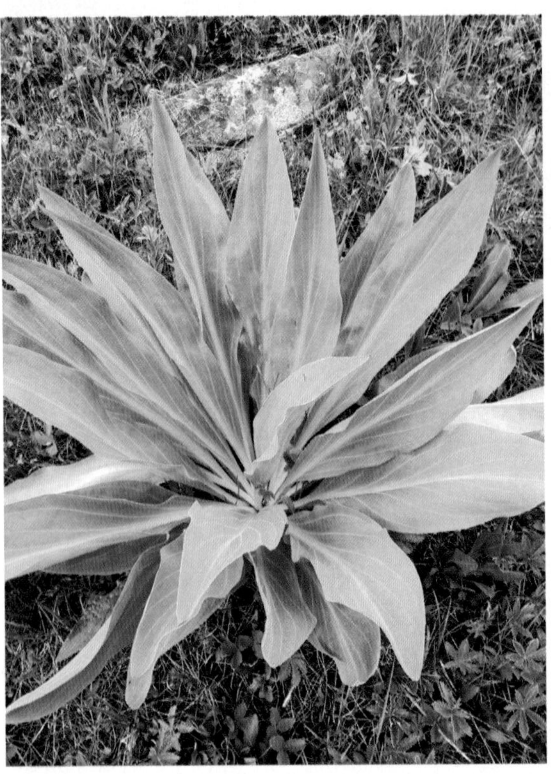

• **Fig. 4.10** Green Gentian rosette showing a basal leaf arrangement.

can be poisonous to livestock), and Cow Parsnip root, whose seeds are carminative and also a tooth and gum analgesic. Then there are the pungent, spicy celery-smelling *Ligusticum* plants, such as *L. porteri* (Osha root) for colds and flu, and the closely related *Levisticum officinale* (Lovage root), a draining diuretic. Also, the *Angelica* genus, such as *A. archangelica* (Angelica root) from the West, for digestion and expectoration, and the famous *A. sinensis* Dang Gui (Dong Quai root) from China, known for helping with women's reproductive problems.

Last but not least are the dangerous and poisonous Apiaceae family members. *Cicuta maculata* (Water Hemlock) is considered the deadliest plant in North America. It can cause seizures and quick death in 15 minutes. *Conium maculatum* (Poison Hemlock), often mistaken for Wild Carrot because of leaf similarity, causes paralysis and death but not seizures, and famously

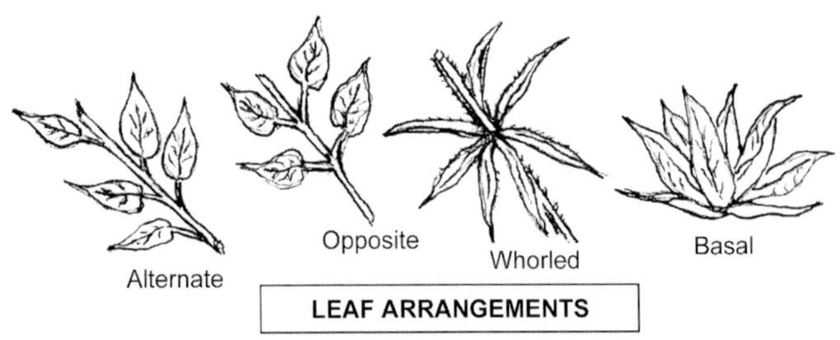

• **Fig. 4.11** Leaf arrangements. (Illustration by Joan Zinn.)

• BOX 4.6 MINT FAMILY. KEY WORDS: * Square stalks * Opposite leaves * Irregular flowers * Usually aromatic *

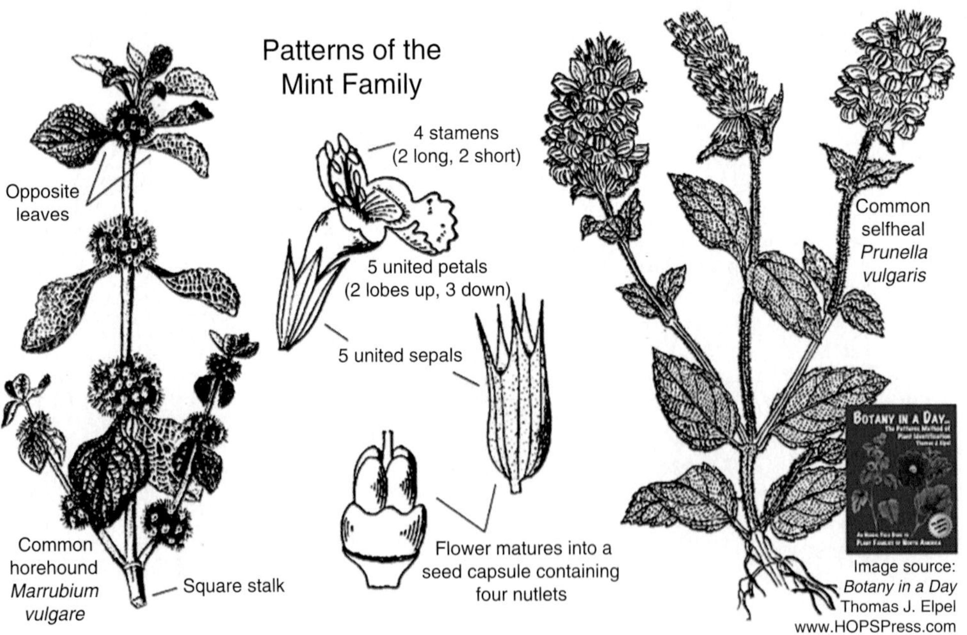

Patterns of the Mint family. (Image Source: *Botany in a Day* Thomas J. Elpel, www.HOPSPress.com.)

was fatal to Socrates in 399 BCE.[11] Both Hemlocks grow in the Rockies, as do Osha and Wild Carrot. Hemlocks have very stinky, mouse-smelling roots and smell nothing like pungent, celery-like Osha root or carroty Wild Carrot. Although Parsley members are very valuable medicinally, it is imperative that you make a positive identification before using. Always go out walking with an expert before any wildcrafting, root chewing, or tasting is attempted.

Mustard Family (Brassicaceae)

The Mustards are numerous, easy to recognize, safe to eat, and they have a spicy flavor. The Radish is the best known. Mustards grow prolifically and bloom early. In early spring, they are visible in fields all over. They like disturbed soil and barren ground (Box 4.8). Mustard family flowers have six stamens, four tall and two short. The flowers grow in an H or X shape (Fig. 4.15). The ovary is superior to the petals, with two united carpels in a single chamber. The seed pods are distinctive and grow in many shapes. They will split open to reveal a clear middle membrane. The pods hang by short stems and spiral up the stem at equal distances in a radial pattern, forming a *raceme* (Fig. 4.16).

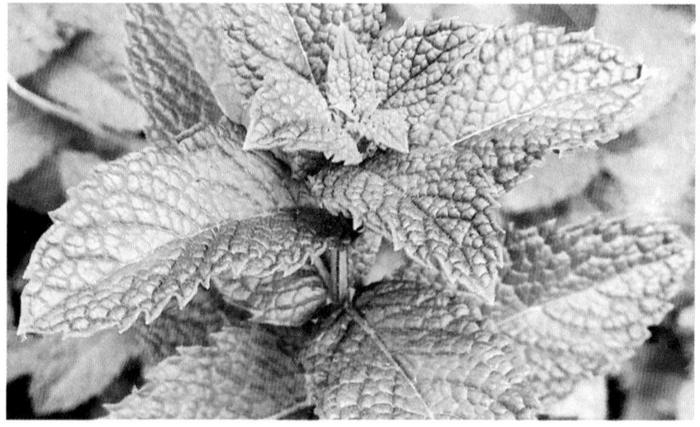

• **Fig. 4.12** The Mint family's Moroccan Mint showing square stem and opposite leaves.

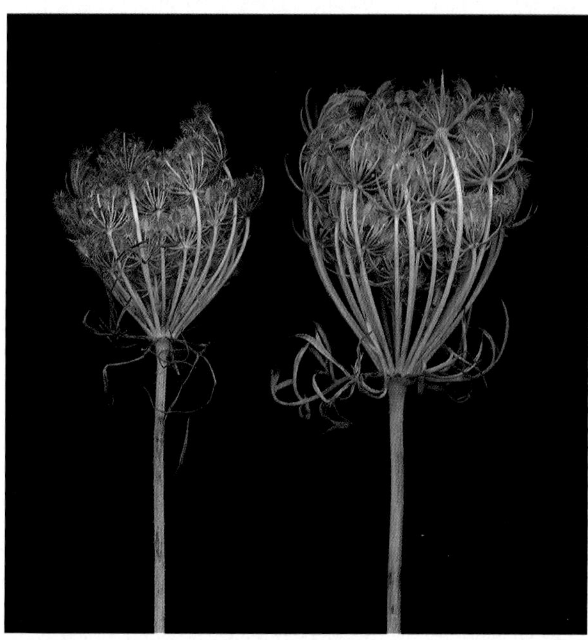

• **Fig. 4.13** The umbel flower formation of *Daucus carota* (Wild Carrot/Queen Anne's Lace seedpods) is characteristic of the Apiaceae (Parsley or Carrot) family. (Copyright Lang/Tucker Photography Photographs loaned with permission from *The Botanical Series* are copywritten by Jennifer Anne Tucker and Gerald Lang from the Studio at Hill Crystal Farm www.jennifer-tucker.com)

• BOX 4.7 PARSLEY FAMILY. KEY WORDS: * Compound umbels * Usually hollow flower stalks *

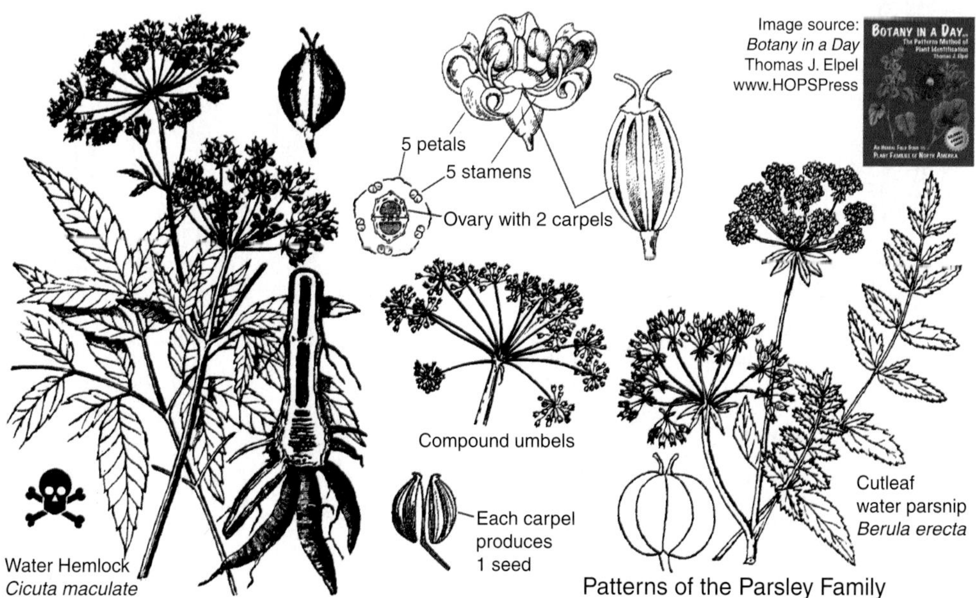

Patterns of the Parsley family. (Image Source: *Botany in a Day* Thomas J. Elpel, www.HOPSPress.com.)

Mustards contain acrid sulfur glycosides, which are irritants. They help digestion in small amounts and cause heartburn in large amounts.[2] A mustard poultice or plaster is very hot and irritating to sensitive skin but can open up the airway and relieve sore muscles. Some well-known medicinal mustards are *Capsella bursa-pastoris* (Shepherd's Purse herb), used as an astringent vasoconstrictor to slow bleeding, and water-loving *Nasturtium officinale* (Water Cress leaf), which is filled with vitamin C and chlorophyll and is a pleasure to munch on in the wild.

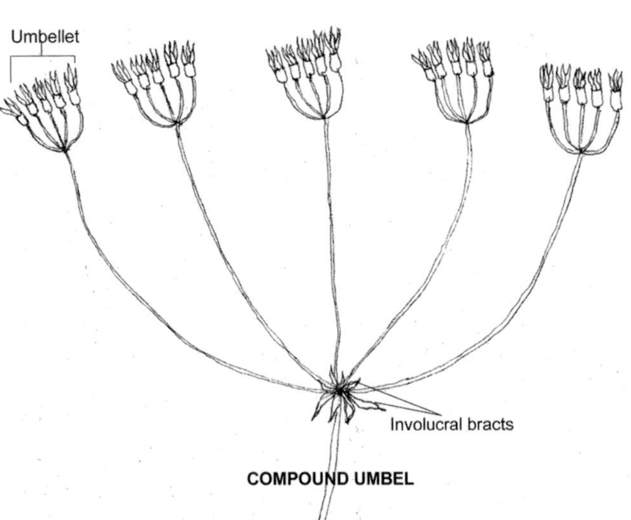

• **Fig. 4.14** Compound umbel. (Illustration by Joan Zinn.)

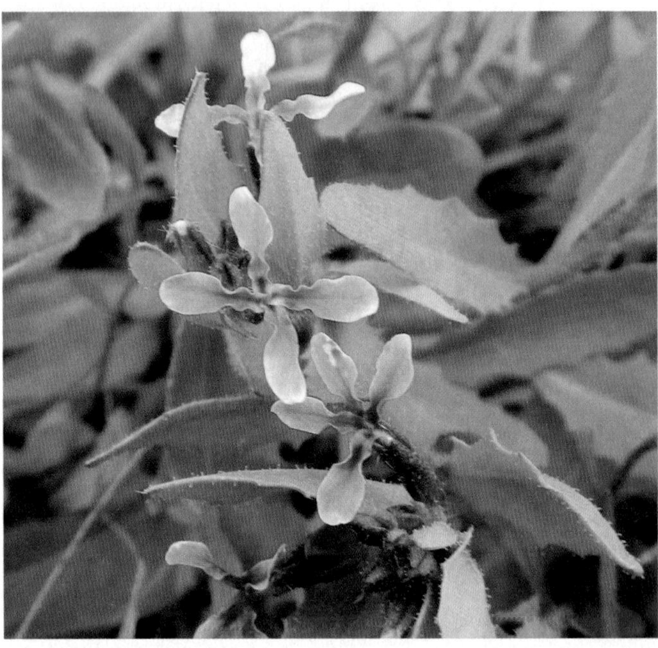

• **Fig. 4.15** Typical four petaled X-shape of the Mustard family. Shown: Purple Mustard.

• BOX 4.8 MUSTARD FAMILY. KEY WORDS: * Four petals * Six stamens, four tall and two short *

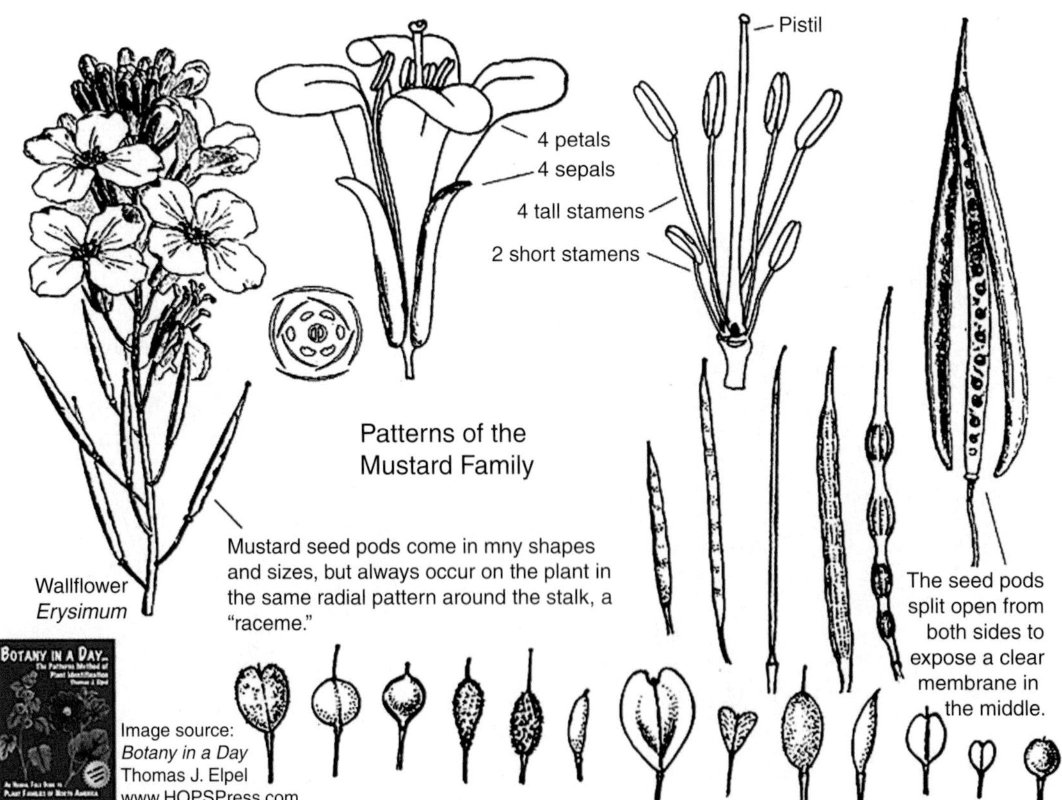

Patterns of the Mustard family. (Image Source: *Botany in a Day* Thomas J. Elpel, www.HOPSPress.com.)

Commercially, the ***Brassicaceae*** family, formerly known as the Cruciferae, gives us many well-known antioxidant-rich *cruciferous* vegetables, such as cauliflower, broccoli, and Brussels sprouts. Other vegetables in the family are cabbage, kohlrabi, and kale. All of these were bred from a single species, *Brassica oleracea*. The condiment called mustard is made from *B. nigra* (Black Mustard seed). Grey Poupon anyone?

Pea Family (Fabaceae)

The entire Pea family is third largest, after the Aster and Orchid families, with 18,000 species worldwide (Box 4.9). The Pea family is divided into many subfamilies, many of which contain individual tribes. Our northern hemisphere U.S. Pea subfamily (*Faboideae*) has a distinctive irregular banner, wings, and keel flower formation, but not all Pea family members have that flower shape. The Mimosa (*Mimosoideae*) subfamily has a five-separate-petaled flower arrangement. The Bird-of-Paradise subfamily (*Caesalpinia*) has showy, irregular flowers. These flowers get bigger and brighter as they work their way south of the U.S. border. Although the flowers of these last two subfamilies do not have the typical banner, wings, and keel shape, they still have pealike pods opening down two seams and pinnate leaves.[2]

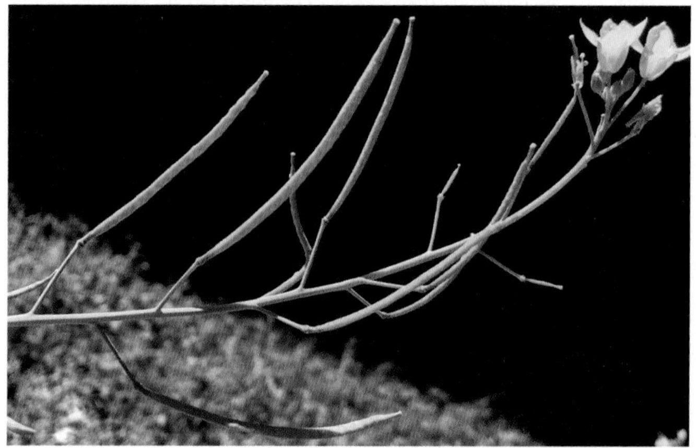

• **Fig. 4.16** A typical radial raceme pattern shown in Arugula seedpods of the Mustard family.

Many Pea family members are also *legumes*. The former name for the entire family was once *Leguminosae*. These tribes include beans, peas, lentils, and peanuts. Legumes have a cooperative, symbiotic relationship with the nitrogen-fixing bacteria in the soil. The bacteria absorb nitrogen from the atmosphere and feed it to the plants. As the plants decompose, they feed the nitrogen back into the soil.

In the Pea subfamily is a variety of *tribes*. The most well-known are the Pea, Licorice, Clover, and Bean tribes.

Pea Subfamily/Pea Tribe (Fabeae)

We are familiar with this subfamily in the northern hemisphere. The flowers have a characteristic five-petal arrangement of a top-lobed and fused banner, two wings, and one bottom keel shape (fused). There is one carpal and five to ten stamens. The carpal becomes a pea pod that opens along two seams with several seeds (peas or beans) inside. A peanut is an underground pod with seeds/legumes inside. They are not actually nuts in the botanical sense but mistakenly have that name. Pea subfamily leaves are pinnately divided and have *tendrils*, specialized curly vinelike stems that react to touch and climb whatever is near.

• BOX 4.9 PEA FAMILY. KEY WORDS: * Banner, wings and keel * Pea-like pods * Often pinnate leaves *

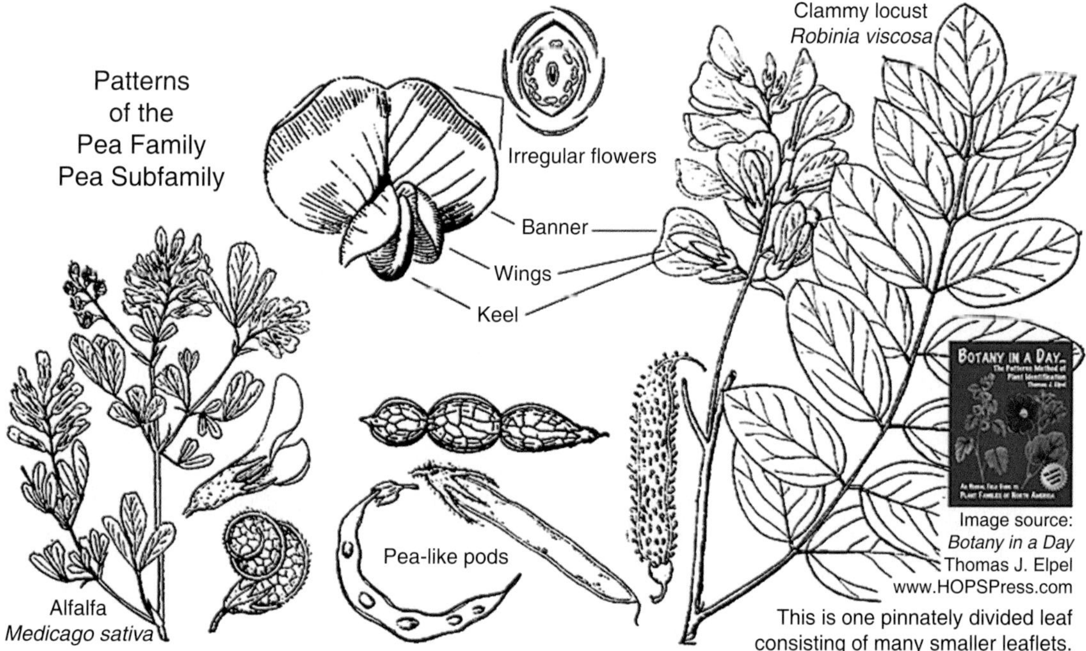

Patterns of the Pea family. (Image Source: *Botany in a Day* Thomas J. Elpel, www.HOPSPress.com.)

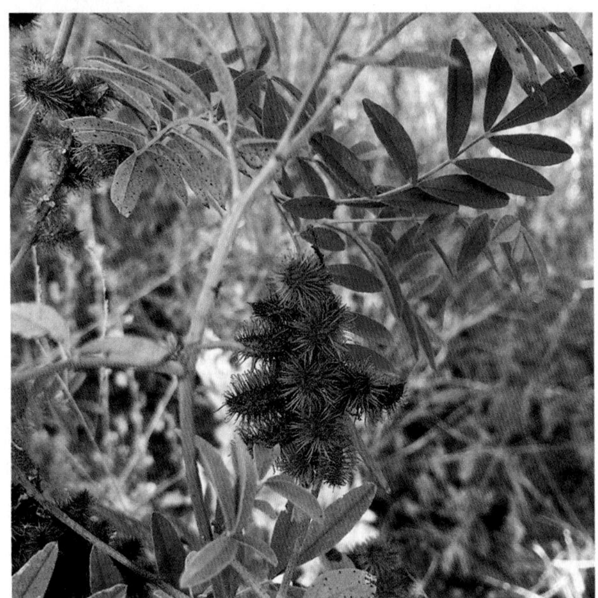

• **Fig. 4.17** *Glycyrrhiza lepidota* (Wild Licorice) from the Pea Subfamily/Licorice Tribe (Galegeae).

Plants in the Pea subfamily/Pea tribe include the familiar *Pisum sativum* (Garden Sweet Peas), *Lens culinaris* (Lentils), and *Vida americana* (American Vetch). Some can be toxic to humans and grazing animals. For instance, common sweet garden peas can cause nervous disorders if eaten in large amounts and over extended periods of time. This effect is particularly true of those growing in hot climates.[2]

Pea Subfamily/Licorice Tribe (Galegeae)

This tribe has pinnately divided leaves, banner, wings, and keel flowers, but no tendrils. The Licorice family contains *Glycyrrhiza lepidota* (Wild Licorice) (Fig. 4.17). It is found in North America west of the Mississippi River and is not as strong or sweet as European *G. glabra* or the Chinese *G. sinensis* Gan Cao. But, in larger amounts, the root can substitute. Sweet-tasting Licorice is a main player in Western and Chinese herbalism. It is used as a demulcent and antiinflammatory in throat and cough formulas, a healer of the gut in ulcers, and an endocrine immune stimulant. It also adds a sweet taste to balance out a bitter formula and lessens any possible toxicity of other herbs.

Another important Licorice herb tribe is the vetches, the *Astragalus* genus. *A.* Huang Qi (Astragalus root) is an important Chinese adaptogen. The dried root is often broken up and added to soups and broths for an immune-boosting tonic, along with some Shitake and Reishi mushroom pieces.

Pea Subfamily/Clover Tribe (Trifolieae)

Clovers have distinctive trifoliate leaves, divided into three leaflets. (If you find one with four leaflets, it's lucky, but unusual.) The flowers have the typical banner, wings, and keel arrangement, but each is quite small. The flower looks like a cluster of many tiny flowers appearing as one large flower ball unless you look closely. Clovers are particularly important in Western herbalism. *Trifolium pratense* (Red Clover flower) is known as a detoxifying herb that is cooling and astringent, and it can dry up wet conditions. *Melilotus officinalis* (Sweet Clover herb) is calming and clears heat, and it is full of sweet-smelling coumarin, which if spoiled and fermented, has a blood-thinning action (Chapter 8). *Medicago sativa* (Alfalfa herb) is a safe, nutritive herb, containing vitamins, minerals, trace minerals, amino acids, and protein. It makes a good tonic for nourishing the liver and relieving fatigue.[7]

Pea Subfamily/Bean Tribe (Phaseoleae)

The familiar bean plants are often seen climbing up a trellis, pole, or fence. They are clinging vines with three-parted leaves. This group includes *Phaseolus* spp. (Common Bean), *Glycine max.* (Soybean), and *Vigna unguiculata* (Black-Eyed Pea).

Pueraria montana (Kudzu vine), which grows all over the southern United States, was introduced in the late 1800s as an ornamental shrub to control erosion. It has taken over and crowds out native species by climbing up and all over them, depriving them of light.[12] In Chinese Medicine, *P. lobata* Ge Gen (Kudzu root) is used to treat symptoms of high blood pressure, such as headache and dizziness, as a moisturizing demulcent for dry coughs, and is taken internally for cold sores, shingles, and genital herpes. The plant has many redeeming qualities as a medicine.

Lily Family (Liliaceae)

Liliaceae plants have three sepals and three petals (Box 4.10) (Fig. 4.18). Although obvious structures in the Mariposa Lily, often these parts are undifferentiated, identical in size and color, and hard to distinguish. The sepal-petal designation has been lumped together into the word *tepal.* There are six stamens. The ovary is superior, with three united carpals with partitioned walls. The pistil is three-parted. Leaf veins are parallel. Many species grow from bulbs (garlic, onions, and tulips); some have rhizomes. Chives, scallions, and leeks are part of this family. Lilies are ancient plants, having evolved approximately 52 million years ago.

Historically, there has been controversy among taxonomists as to how to divide up and assign plants to this family. The Lily family used to be a catch-all group for plants that did not fit elsewhere. Mountain and Meadow Death Camases, often confused with wild onions, are examples (Box 4.11). Now many former Lily plants have been reidentified and reassigned to other homes. (They sound like orphans.) Presently, there are close to 640 species and 16 genera.[2]

Lily Subfamily (Lilioideae)

This Lily subfamily has very showy flowers, more so than others. They grow from bulbs or corms, which are sometimes edible but not always. So, be careful. Tulips belong here and have edible flowers and bulbs, but their bulbs are usually coated commercially with a toxic fungicide to prevent rotting (Fig. 4.19). *Fritillaria thunbergii* Zhe Bei Mu (Fritillaria bulb) from this subfamily is used in Chinese Medicine. It's especially important as a respiratory sedative and mucolytic expectorant for stubborn, sticky sputum-type coughs with yellow phlegm.

The Grass Family (Poaceae, formerly Gramineae)

Grasses are everywhere (Box 4.12). Worldwide, we find 650 genera and nearly 10,000 species in the ***Poaceae*** family. Grasses are monocots, just like the Lily family. They have hollow stems with knee-like nodes or joints and parallel veins on the leaves. The flowers of grasses are contained in modified leaves called *bracts.* Not too impressive looking alone, but they are a beautiful filler in dried

• BOX 4.10 LILY FAMILY. KEY WORDS: * Monocot flowers with parts in threes * Sepals and petals usually identical * Parallel veins *

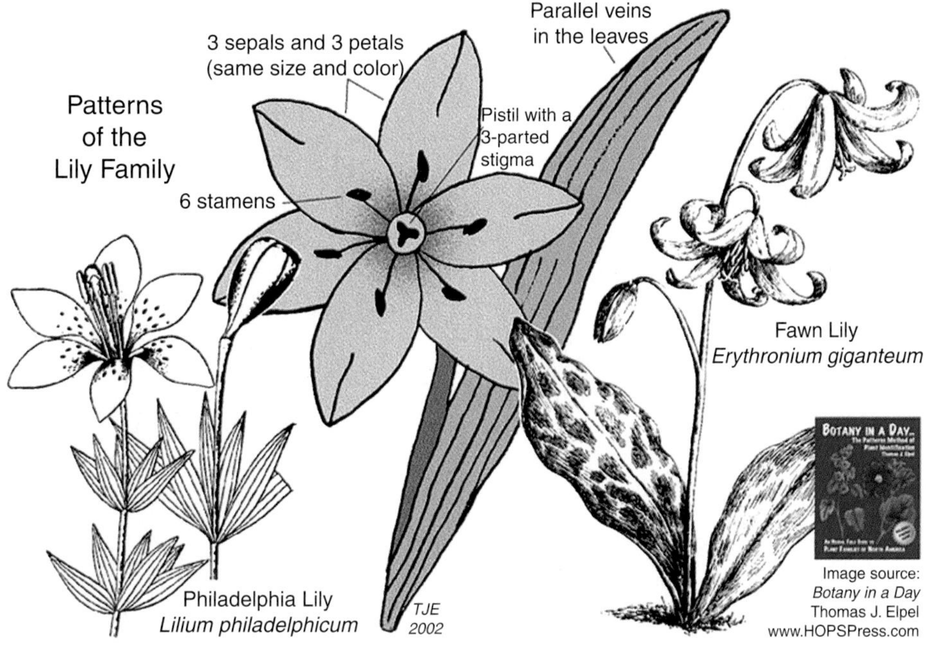

Patterns of the Lily family. (Image Source: *Botany in a Day* Thomas J. Elpel, www.HOPSPress.com.)

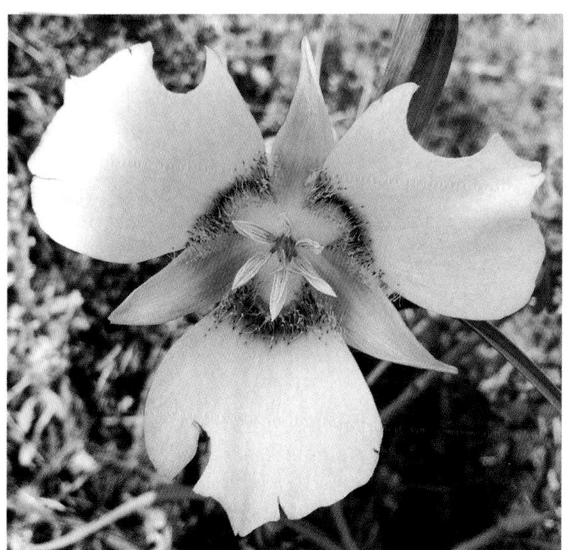

• **Fig. 4.18** Mariposa Lily with three petals and three sepals from the Lily family.

arrangements and winter bouquets, and they are spectacular in fields of grasslands when blowing in the wind. When grass seeds are harvested, the bracts (chaff) must be separated from the seeds (grain). This ancient process is called *winnowing*. It removes the lighter chaff after it is broken away from the grain. Once the seeds are separated, they can be ground into flour for baking or cooked down into a cereal.

Grasses play a large part in our economy and food supply. *Triticum repens* (Couch Grass root) has been used since ancient Greek and Roman times to treat kidney problems. Many grasses are our cereal grains. We have *Secale cereale* (Rye), *Triticum aestivum* (Wheat), *Oryza sativa* (Wild Rice), *Hordeum vulgare* (Barley), *Zia mays* (Corn), *Avena sativa* (Oats), and others (Fig. 4.20). Sugar cane, corn, and sorghum are processed for sugar. High fructose corn syrup is a sweetener in many of our foods, including soda pop, dairy products, and canned fruits, all of which can contribute to type 2 diabetes and insulin resistance, and it is more dangerous than table sugar. Fast-growing Bamboo, with its characteristic grass-family notches, is used for cloth and flooring. Buffalo grass, Fescue grass, and Kentucky blue grass are used for lawns and landscaping. Crab grass is often an unwanted weed dug up by gardeners. Sweet grass is a lovely sugary-smelling grass, made into baskets and often braided and used as a ceremonial smudge by Native Americans.

Grasses are easily confused with rushes and sedges, which are in their own families. (Heed the quotation under this chapter's title.) Grasses have unimpressive wind-pollinated flowers that don't need to be colorful and showy to attract insects. The flowers usually have three stamens. The ovary has three united carpals that form one chamber. The ovary matures as a single seed that we call a *grain*.

Claviceps purpurea or *C. paspali* (Ergot fungus) can form a blackish or purplish powder on most grasses, particularly wheat, rye, barley, and oats. The alkaloid it contains can be very poisonous. Symptoms of ergot poisoning include painful seizures, spasms, diarrhea, mania, psychosis, delirium, hallucinations with effects like those of lysergic acid diethylamide (LSD), and even gangrene. Epidemics have occurred throughout history, and bizarre

• BOX 4.11 Mountain and Meadow Death Camases

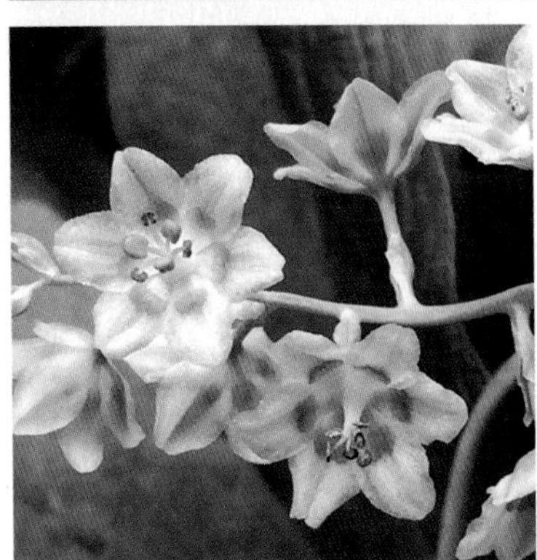

Mountain Death Camas, from the Lily subfamily, Liliodeae.

These two Camases were once classified in the Liliaceae (Lily) family but have been reclassified to the Melanthiaceae (Bunchflower) family. They have been confused with wild onions but don't smell like onions. Their toxic alkaloids are more poisonous than strychnine. The bulbs of both species can be fatal, and people who ingest them present with, dry, burning mouth, nausea, vomiting, headaches, cardiac irregularities, loss of muscle control, coma, and death. The plants are toxic to humans, livestock, and honeybees.

If it looks but doesn't smell like an onion, it isn't an onion!

The two fake onions are *Anticlea elegans* (Mountain Death Camas), formerly *Zigadenus elegans*, and *Toxicoscordion venenosum* (Meadow Death Camas), formerly *Zigadenus venenosus*. They both grow in the Rockies from Canada to Mexico. The mountain variety grows in subalpine and moist tundra areas. The Meadow Death Camas grows in lower meadows and sagebrush areas of the foothills and montane areas. They have narrow grass-shaped, mostly basal leaves with parallel veins, and white flowers arranged in racemes. Mountain Death Camas has nodding buds that are erect when open and stamens in a funnel near the center. Meadow Death Camas flower buds do not nod. The stamens are spread away from the ovary.[11]

behavior observed from poisonings has been blamed as a cause of bewitchment, both by the accusers and the condemned. This played a part in the Salem witch trials.[8]

Ergot has been used historically to induce abortions because it causes strong uterine contractions. The drug ergotamine is now used in controlled doses to induce labor in hospitals. It is also used to treat migraine headaches. Dr. Albert Hofmann, the so-called father of LSD (lysergic acid diethylamide), discovered the mind-altering drug when experimenting with ergot (although there is no LSD in ergot).[13] Today the ergot content of grains is regulated to 0.3% of weight. This regulation has been in effect since 1916. However, if you pick grass in the wild, be sure there is no blackish or purplish powder on it. This fungus is most likely to occur if the climate is wet and damp.

The Rose Family (Rosaceae)

We are surrounded by the Rose family (Box 4.13). Roses are the subject of poetry and symbols of love, friendship, kings, and the Rosicrucians. The ***Rosaceae*** family ranges from plants found in beautiful cultivated rose gardens to all kinds of luscious foods, including strawberries, raspberries, blackberries, cherries, apples, plums, apricots, peaches, pears, and almonds. Many have thorns, which aid in their defense. One of the main chemical constituents of the Rose family is tannic acid, an important astringent used medicinally for discharges, diarrhea, bleeding. This characteristic is good to know about, even if you can't identify the exact plant. You can always make a first-aid tea or poultice to stop those annoying symptoms.

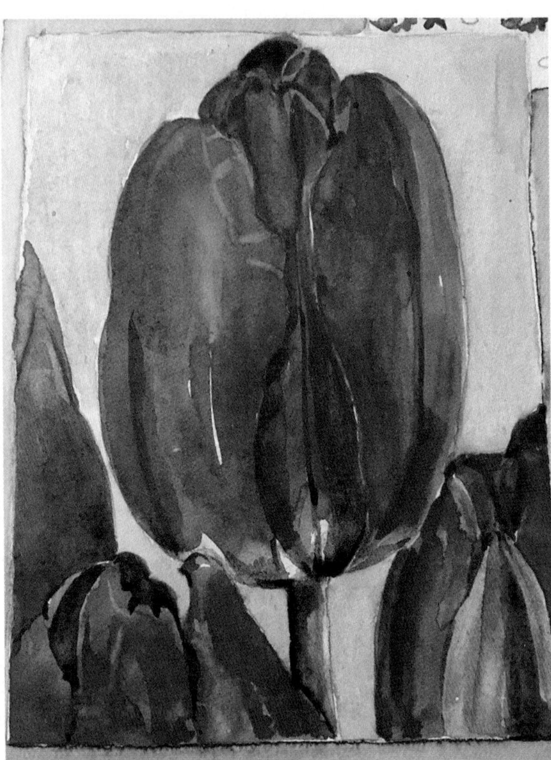

• **Fig. 4.19** Watercolor painting of the Lily family's Red Tulip. (Credit: Collection Joan Zinn. Isolated photo from unsigned watercolor painting by Randy Child.)

The signature of the Rose family is five. There are five petals, five sepals, and a minimum of five stamens, and usually many more in multiples of five. The center of the flower looks fuzzy, with numerous styles surrounded by countless stamen. A wild rose has five lovely petals. Cultivated garden roses with their numerous folded petals have been hybridized for that layered look. Rose family leaves are alternate and can be simple, trifoliate, palmate, or pinnate. The single leaves or leaflets are generally serrated and oval in shape. They have stipules, which are leaflike appendages on the base of the leafstalk (with the exception of the genus *Spiraea*).

Rose Family/Rose Subfamily (Rosideae)

This family is where you find the *Rosa* spp. (Wild Rose) (Fig. 4.21) of high-vitamin C rose hip tea fame, *Agrimonia eupatoria* (Agrimony herb) used for stopping discharges, and *Alchemilla vulgaris* (Lady's Mantle herb), a very important herb for control of heavy menstrual bleeding and cervical discharges. You also find the *Rubus* genus here, with its raspberries, salmonberries, thimbleberries, and blackberries.

Rose subfamily flowers have a domed receptacle beneath the pistils. They also have stipules, which are leaflike growths beneath the leaf stem. They have multiple pistils, each one theoretically or botanically forming its own separate fruit or seed. A raspberry is an example, being an aggregate of many tiny fleshy fruits that cover a domed receptacle. However, the wild rose has many pistils, each producing a seed enclosed in a fleshy fruit known as the hip. This is considered a false fruit. Regardless of name, rose hips are best picked and chewed on after the first frost, when they are the sweetest.

• BOX 4.12 GRASS FAMILY. KEY WORDS: * Grassy hollow flower stems * Knee-like joints or nodes *

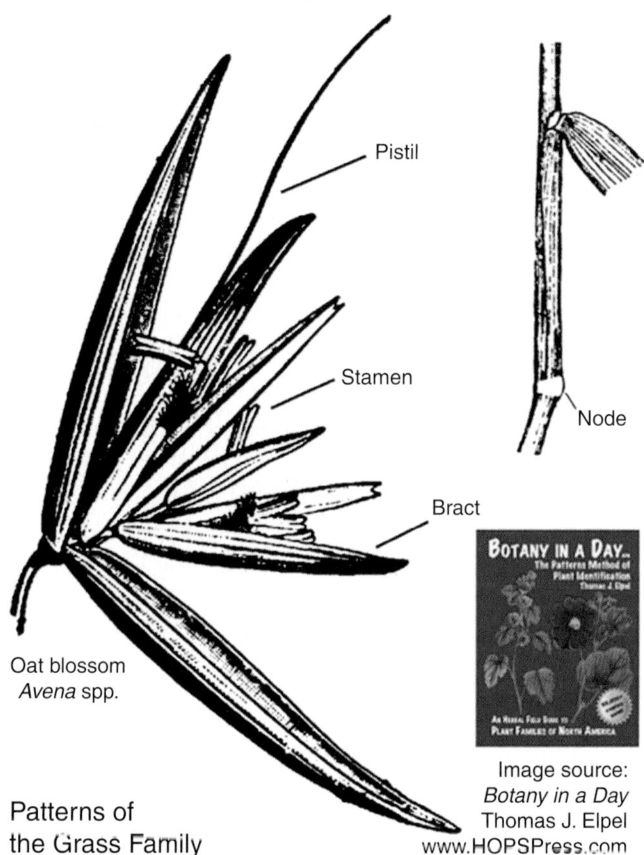

Patterns of the Grass family. (Image Source: *Botany in a Day* Thomas J. Elpel, www.HOPSPress.com.)

Rose Family/Almond Subfamily (Plums–Amygdaloideae)

The Almond subfamily, plums, includes the genus *Prunus*. Most produce luscious fleshy summer fruits with *drupes*, large throwaway pits containing a hard seed. Included are plums, cherries, apricots, peaches, and nectarines. However, the subfamily's namesake, Almond, has a throwaway fleshy fruit and a hard pit, better known as the nut, that we open and eat. All the seeds of drupes have an almond-like shape.

Prunus has two distinguishing characteristics. One is a noticeable seam, evidence of its one chambered carpal, down one side of the fruit. The other is the source of the subfamily's name. Prunus contains amygdalin, which breaks down into benzaldehyde (the bitter almond flavor used in cooking) and cyanide, a poison in large doses. The Sweet Almonds we eat contain very little cyanide, but Bitter Wild Almonds are quite poisonous when raw.[2]

Rose Family/Almond Subfamily (Apples–Amygdaloideae)

Apple subfamily members have a signature five-pointed star on the bottom of the fleshy fruit. (Rose hips have this also.) Apple-type flowers have inferior ovaries. Some are sweet; some are very sour and astringent, making you pucker up. Cultivated members are pears, apples, quinces, and loquats. The most important apple subfamily member for the herbalist to know is *Crataegus* spp. (Hawthorn berry, leaf, and flower), in the form of (usually) thorny bushes and trees. Hawthorn is the most used cardiac tonic herb in the West, being restorative, nourishing, and strengthening. Hawthorn belongs in almost any heart formula and is useful for treating essential hypertension, after heart attacks, reduced circulation, and arrhythmias.[7] The berries are full of Vitamin C and antioxidant bioflavonoids.

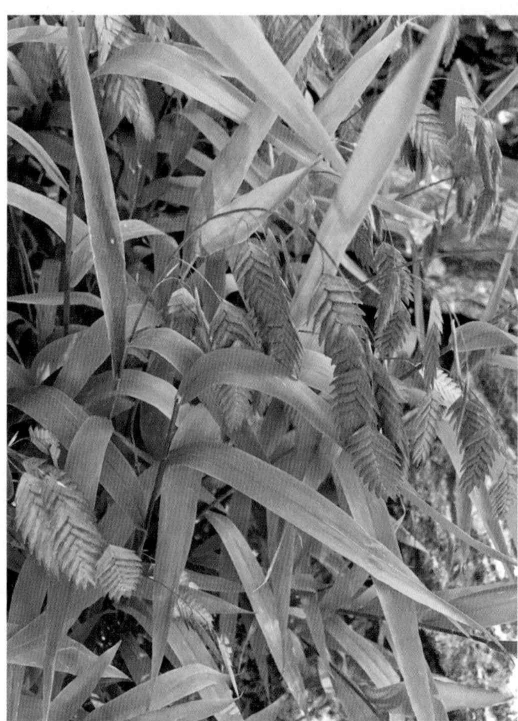

• **Fig. 4.20** *Avena sativa* (Oat grass), a common Poaceae family member.

Aster or Sunflower, Daisy Family (Asteraceae)

Aster means *star* in Greek and is the second largest of the flowering plant families, the Orchid family having the most species of all (Box 4.14). From an evolutionary standpoint, Asters were the most recent family to develop. Worldwide, there are 920 genera and 19,000 species. Because there are so many, there is great variety in their structure. The former name for the Aster family was actually Compositae. Aster plants can be trees, shrubs, vines, or herbaceous plants. They can have tap roots or fibrous roots, be fleshy or woody, and leaves can be alternate, opposite, or whorled.

The flowers are all complex, but these can be deceptive, because they do not all look like your typical daisy. Some have hundreds of flowers in what appears, superficially, to be a single *flower*. It took a long time for this arrangement to evolve. When we identify flowers, we generally proceed from the outside in, going from sepal to petal to stamen to pistil. For Asters, this process of identification doesn't work. What look like normal *sepals* on the outside are actually *bracts* or modified leaves that occur in many layers under the flower heads (Fig. 4.22). These bracts have sometimes been reduced to small scales. The *petals* or outside colorful *rays* are each an entire individual flower with their own stamen and pistil. The multiple disk flowers in the middle (within the flower head) have their own individual petals, stamens, and pistils as well. They are tiny, sometimes requiring magnification to see. The sepals on

• BOX 4.13 ROSE FAMILY. KEY WORDS: * Five sepals * Five petals * Numerous stamens (usually) * * Oval, serrated leaves *

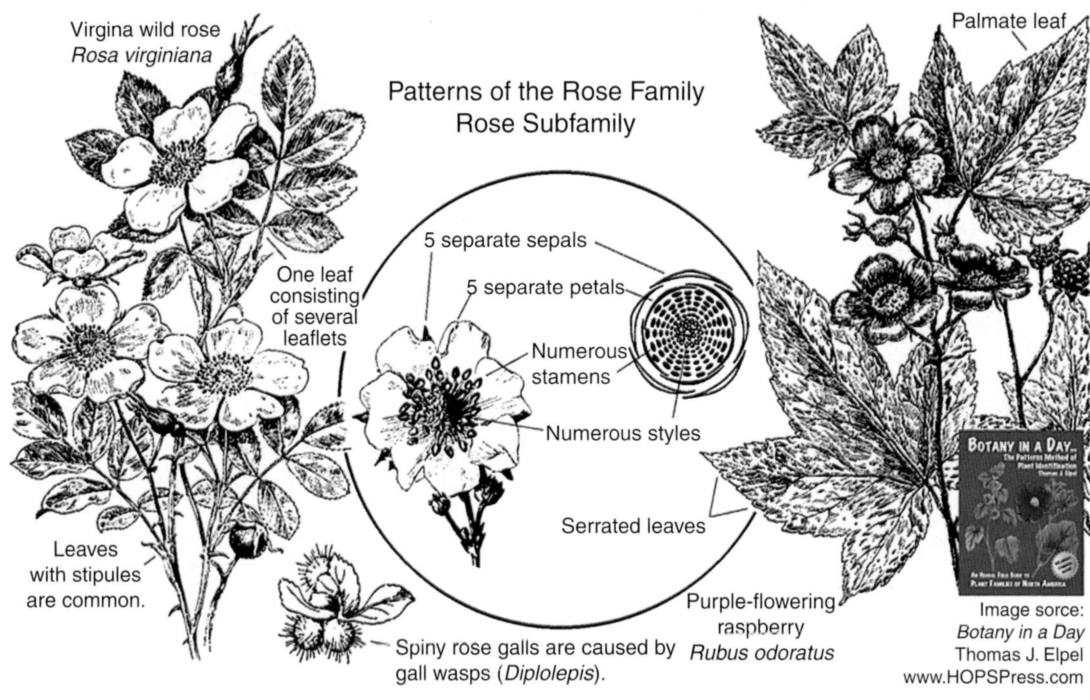

Patterns of the Rose family. (Image Source: *Botany in a Day* Thomas J. Elpel, www.HOPSPress.com.)

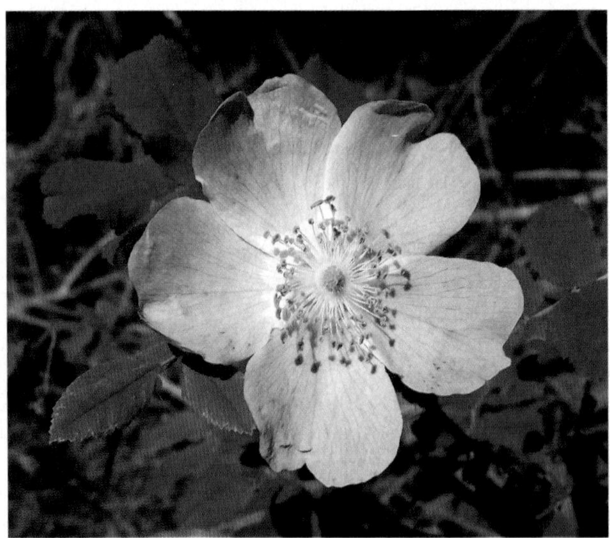

• **Fig. 4.21** *Rosa woodsii* (Wild Woods' Rose) from the Rose subfamily, Rosideae.

these disk flowers have been reduced to a hairy *pappus*. Sometimes they are not even there (Fig. 4.23).

A few important herbal members of this family include *Echinacea* spp., *Calendula officinale* (Calendula flower), *Achillea millefolium* (Yarrow herb), *Taraxacum officinalis* (Dandelion root and leaf), *Grindelia squarrosa* (Gumweed flower), *Silybum marianum* (Milk Thistle seed), *Solidago* spp. (Goldenrod herb), *Matricaria* spp. (Chamomile flower), *Arctium lappa* (Burdock root), and Chrysanthemum Ju Hua (Chrysanthemum flower).[14] Because of its diversity, the Aster family is subdivided into Chicory, Dandelion, Thistle, and Aster subfamilies, among others. Some of the subfamilies are further divided into tribes. We will address a few that are most interesting to herbalists.

Aster Family Chicory/Dandelion Subfamily (Cichorioideae)

This subfamily is characterized by *strap*-shaped ray petals, meaning flat, not pointed or tapered, tips. There are no disk flowers. The ray petals go to the center. The stems contain milky juice that is often bitter but edible. Herbally speaking, this subfamily gifts us with Chicory, Wild Lettuce, and Dandelion.

Cichorium intybus (Chicory root) (Fig. 4.24) is a woody herb that has hairy, alternate, lance-shaped leaves and lovely sky-blue strap-shaped ray flowers (no disks), stalkless along the stem.[2] The roasted and ground roots are best known as a coffee substitute, if you have a good imagination. It is a liver-friendly digestive bitter, and the latex in the stems reputedly destroys warts.

Lactuca serriola (Wild Lettuce leaf) is sometimes called opium lettuce because of the milky white latex from the stems and is found in disturbed ground. It can grow up to 3 feet tall. The undersides of the deeply lobed leaves have a characteristic prickly spine (allowing for a telltale method of identification).[11] The yellow ray flowers are small. Prickly Lettuce is a mild child-friendly sedative and analgesic often used to encourage sleep.

Last is *Taraxacum officinale* (Dandelion root), which is so important herbally that it will be addressed in detail in the basic *Materia Medica* (Chapter 11). As most gardeners will testify, it has a long,

• BOX 4.14 ASTER or SUNFLOWER FAMILY. KEY WORDS: * Composite flowerheads * Ray and disk flowers *

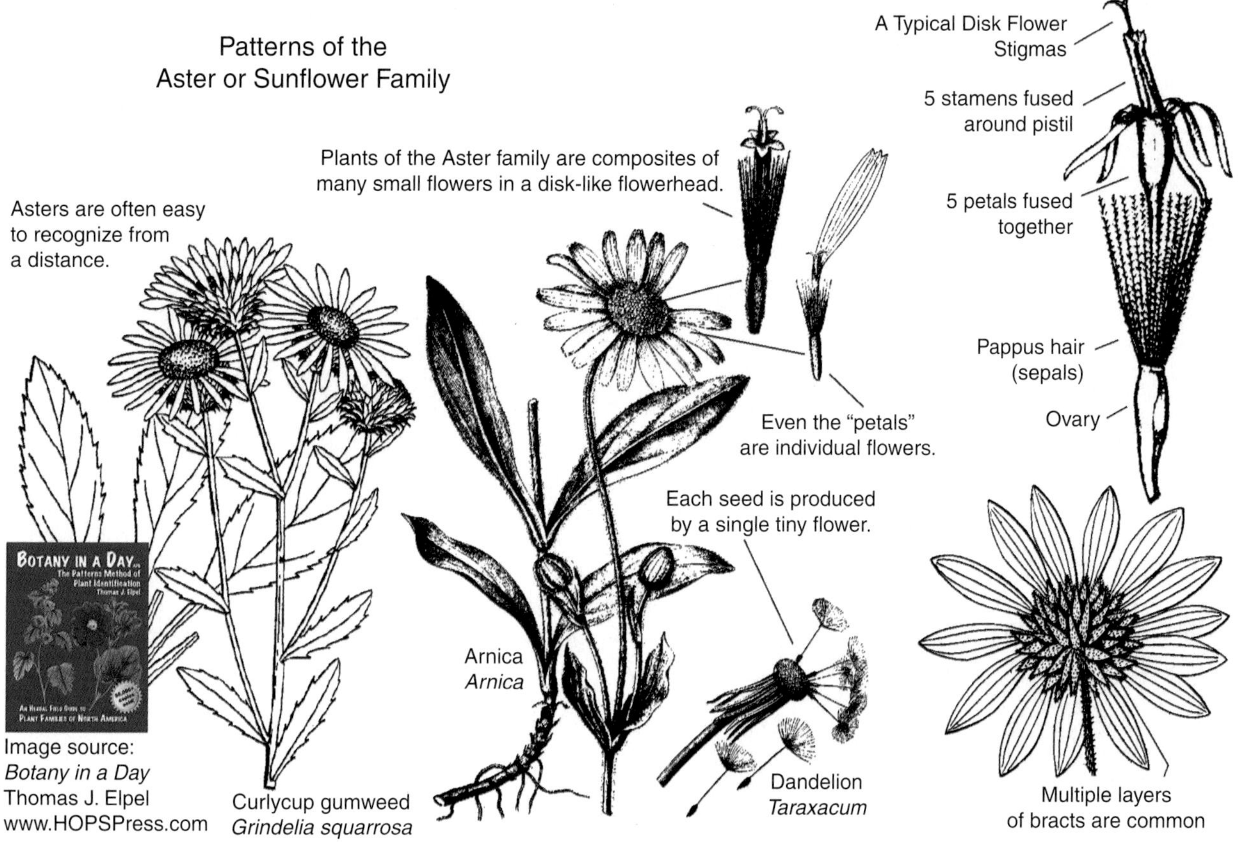

Patterns of the Aster or Sunflower family. (Image Source: *Botany in a Day* Thomas J. Elpel, www.HOPSPress.com.)

stubborn, thick tap root (best to gather in the early spring before flowers come, or in late fall). The root is a great liver stimulant, diuretic, and because it increases bile flow, mildly laxative. The leaves are long and slender, simple, lobed—usually with teeth—and grow in basal rosettes. They are diuretic, make a great spring tonic in tea or salads, are perfect for a liver cleanse, and its bitterness makes it an effective digestive stimulant. Dandelion's signature yellow rays (no disk flowers) eventually become the white wind-carried puff balls/umbrellas we all know and love. The stems are hollow.[2]

Aster Family/Thistle or Artichoke Subfamily (Carduoideae)

This subfamily has plants with the flower heads inside a tight wrapping of bracts. Much of the plant is prickly, especially around the flower heads and bracts. Most are edible. Artichokes are a notable example where the edible portion is the end of the modified leaf (bract) that leads to the delicious fleshy heart inside. Some thistles such as the Musk, Scotch, Bull, and Plumeless are considered invasive species in the American Southwest.[6]

Herbally speaking, Burdock root and seed and Milk Thistle seed are important medicines. *Arctium lappa* (Burdock root) promotes detoxification and is used in the Western sense as a lymphatic mover; for skin problems, such as eczema and psoriasis; and as a kidney diuretic and stone dissolvent. In Chinese Medicine, the seeds of the same plant, Arctium Niu Bang Zi (Burdock seed) are used as an upper respiratory sedative and demulcent. *Silybum marianum* (Milk Thistle seed) is considered a prime liver decongestant and restorative, and a digestive bitter.

Aster Subfamily/Chamomile Tribe (Anthemideae)

This one is an important Aster subfamily tribe for herbalists. The plants here are mostly aromatic, and the bracts surrounding the flower head are thin, dry, and translucent. Herbal medicinals from this group include *Matricaria recutita* (Chamomile flower), *Achillea millefolium* (Yarrow herb), *Artemisia dracunculus* (Tarragon herb), *Artemisia absinthium* (Wormwood herb), *Tanacetum vulgare* (Tansy herb), and *Chrysanthemum* spp.

Matricaria recutita (German Chamomile flower) and *Anthemis nobilis* (Roman Chamomile flower) are used interchangeably. Chamomiles contain a huge list of chemical constituents that provide it with many uses. First and foremost, Chamomile flower is a nervine, a relaxant used in sleep teas for adults and children. It helps stomachaches and seizures and is a muscle relaxant and analgesic, making it good for headaches and muscle pains.

Achillea millefolium (Yarrow herb) looks like an umbel at first glance, so don't be fooled. Its many tiny individual flowers have white rays with a yellowish disk that make up a flat-topped cluster, a composite. Yarrow has been horticulturally bred to have pink or yellow flowers, but those lack the strong aromatic medicinal oils contained the wild, white-flowered variety. Wild Yarrow grows all

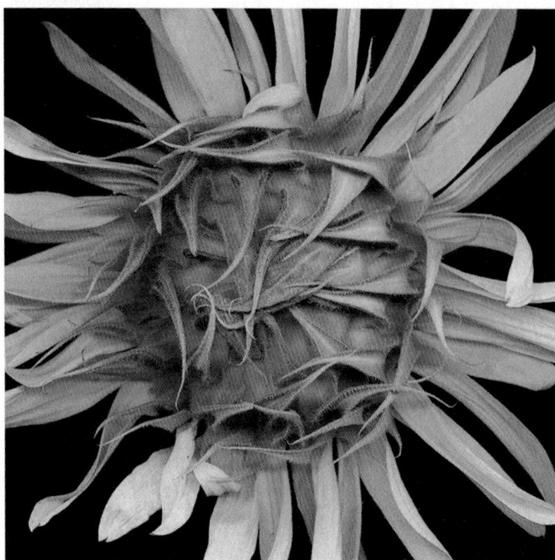

• **Fig. 4.22** Sunflower showing bracts. (Copyright Lang/Tucker Photography. Photographs loaned with permission from *The Botanical Series* are copywritten by Jennifer Anne Tucker and Gerald Lang from the Studio at Hill Crystal Farm. www.jennifer-tucker.com)

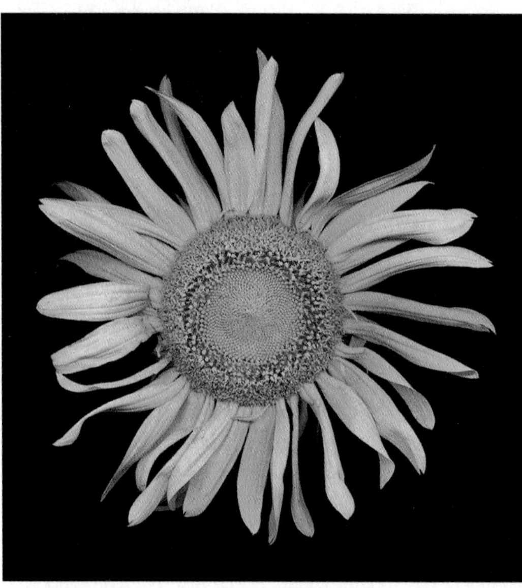

• **Fig. 4.23** Sunflower (*Helianthus giganteus*) from the Aster family, Sunflower subfamily, Heliantheae tribe. (Copyright Lang/Tucker Photography. Photographs loaned with permission from *The Botanical Series* are copywritten by Jennifer Anne Tucker and Gerald Lang from the Studio at Hill Crystal Farm. www.jennifer-tucker.com)

through the Rockies and has many chemical constituents (just like Chamomile), so is extremely versatile from a healing standpoint. Yarrow is foremost an astringent (one of its common names is Nosebleed Plant), but it is also cool, dry, and bitter. Its many uses are as a cold and flu diaphoretic, an antiseptic, and a styptic (it stops bleeding from wounds, bruises, and hemorrhoids).

Artemisia spp. comprise the prairie and mountains sages. (Do not confuse this genus with Garden Sage, which is a *Salvia). Artemisia* spp. are highly aromatic, often burned as a cleansing spiritual smudge and used as an insect repellant. There are many species with gray-green fringelike leaves, including Mugwort,

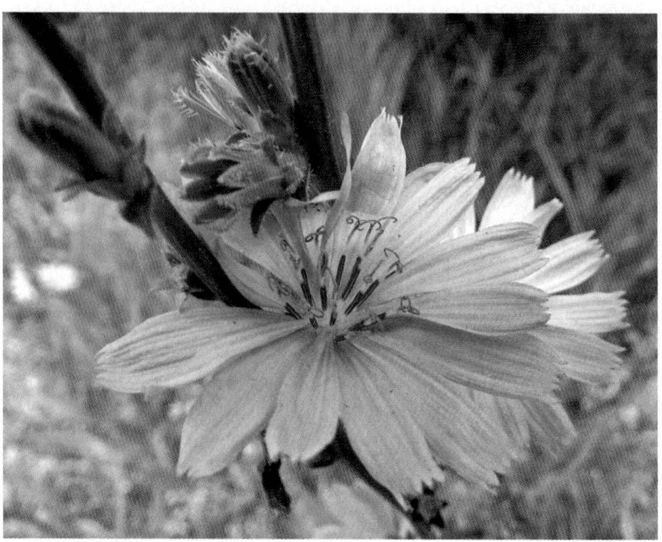

• **Fig. 4.24** Chicory flower with strap-shaped petals, from the Chicory/Dandelion subfamily, Cichorioideae.

Fringed Sage, Prairie Sage, Alpine Sage, and Sweet Annie. Most are antibacterial, antifungal, and antiparasitical, and all are very bitter.

Aster Subfamily/Sunflower Tribe (Heliantheae)

The flowers of this tribe generally have small bracts attached to the base of each disk flower, which you will see if you pull apart a whole disk. They smell and taste resinous. The dramatic huge Sunflower bears the tribal name *Helianthus giganteus*.

Echinacea purpurea (Purple Coneflower), *Rudbeckia hirta* (Black-eyed Susan), *Arnica montana* (Arnica flower), *Ambrosia* spp. (Ragweed herb), and Xanthium Cang Er Zi (Cocklebur) are members. So is the inulin-rich sweet *Helianthus tuberosus* (Jerusalem Artichoke, Sun Choke tuber) of gut-healing fame, which stimulates the growth of a healthy intestinal microbiome. This is a different plant from the common Artichoke of the Aster/Thistle subfamily already discussed.

Echinacea angustifolia, *E. purpurea*, and *E. pallida* roots are so well known, they are now endangered, having been picked almost to death. They are used as an immune stimulant to boost white blood cell count and help treat the common cold and other viral infections. They reduce inflammation and can also give relief from allergies. There are few left in the wild, so it is best to use the cultivated varieties, or substitute with other effective herbs like *Rudbeckia laciniata* or *R. ampla*.[11]

Arnica spp. is a cheerful daisy-looking plant with yellow rays and yellow disks. It has heart-shaped (cordate) basal leaves (*A. cordifolia)* and a few opposite leaves growing on the stem. The leaves are noteworthy because they smell like Juicy Fruit gum. Arnica is classic in first-aid creams. It increases circulation, decreases inflammation, and helps heal injuries. It is best used externally for bruises, strains, and muscle pain, and it is considered poisonous when taken internally. It can cause gastroenteritis unless used in homeopathic doses for shock, trauma, and sprains.[1]

Keying Out Plants

After perusing major medicinal herb families, we are at the stage where we can identify a plant with reasonable certainty. A useful method is to key it out. Keys are sometimes found in field guides, and they help identify a plant. A key is a systematic method of proceeding from general to more detailed observations, using the process of elimination. It is a flow chart method that asks you to follow the dots. If it's not this, then it's that, so go down that path. This chapter has provided the botanical foundation for this skill of ***keying out*** a plant. To use any key (they are not all the same), you must be able to recognize basic botanical structures and make decisions. Is a plant a monocot or a dicot? What type of leaves does it have, and what is their arrangement? What type of stem? What type of flower, and how many petals? How many stamens, and what type of ovary? Knowledge of the basics of botany are necessary for this keying out process.

Different authors have their own ways to key out a plant. One relatively stress-free approach is to use plant family recognition. Narrowing a plant down to its correct family makes sense for beginners. Once a family is determined, almost any field guide can be consulted to arrive at the genus and species. Think of it as a treasure hunt. Sometimes a magnifying glass is helpful. An example of the procedure follows and is explained in greater detail in *Botany in a Day* by Thomas J. Elpel.

A Keying-Out Process for Flowering Plants

- First, determine the major grouping of your specimen. We're assuming it's in the plant kingdom. Is it a nonvascular spore plant like a moss, a vascular spore plant such as a horsetail or fern, a naked seed plant as in a pinecone, or is it a flowering plant with enclosed seeds such as a Rose? If it is anything other than a flowering plant, turn to the appropriate page.
- Is it a flowering monocot or dicot? Monocots have parallel veins and have flower parts in threes, like a Lily. Dicots are usually net-veined and have parts in fours and fives, like a bean. If it is a monocot, go to the key for monocots. If it is a dicot, continue on in the dicot section.
- Is the dicot a member of the Aster family? Because this is the largest family in northern latitudes, if you live there, start with Aster and then eliminate. If it *is* an Aster family member with multiple flowers in the rays or heads or both, you're done. You know the family. It's now time to narrow down the genus and species by referring to a field guide.
- If it's *not* an Aster family member, continue on. Profile your non-Aster-family dicot flower using the dicot flower key. Once you have determined the flower's characteristics, you can then choose the particular dicot key that matches your flower. There are many choices. The flower could have numerous petals (11 or more), as in a Prickly Pear cactus flower. It could be a regular (symmetrical) flower, such as a mustard. The flower could have three, four, five, or six petals. The petals might be irregular, as in Sweet Peas, a united funnel shape, as in a Morning Glory, and so on.
- If it is a tree or shrub, follow that pathway.[2]

Summary

Taxonomy refers to plant organization, Linnaeus's seven-tiered plant classification system. The broadest grouping comes at the top of the hierarchy, and each consecutive category becomes more detailed. For an herbalist, families, genus, and species are the most important. Families are plants with similar physical characteristics. A genus consists of two or more closely related plants. The species is the specific plant name.

Common names vary from place to place, and different plants may have the same name. The Latin/botanical/scientific name is based on the binomial system. Pharmaceutical names are arranged according to anatomical features, such as fruit, leaf, or root. Chinese pinyin names transcribe plant pronunciation of the Mandarin dialect with its Chinese letters into the Latin alphabet.

Botany refers to the structural arrangements of flowers, leaves, and stems. Important plant families were described using Thomas J. Elpel's pattern-recognition method from *Botany in a Day*. This knowledge helps us identify a plant and determine its medicinal characteristics. Keying out is a plant identification technique that uses the process of elimination to narrow down a vast array of plants to the correct one.

Review

Fill in The Blanks

(Answers in Appendix B)

1. What is the binomial system of nomenclature? ___ First name is called the ___ and the second name, the ___.
2. Name Linnaeus's seven tiers of classification. ___, ___, ___, ___, ___, ___, ___.
3. What is the difference between a gymnosperm and an angiosperm? ___.
4. What is the difference between a monocot and a dicot? ___.
5. Name the three parts of a stamen ___, ___, ___.
6. Name the four parts of a pistil ___, ___, ___, ___.
7. Fill in the current Latin family names. Mint___ Parsley ___ Mustard ___ Pea___ Lily___ Grass ___ Rose ___ Sunflower ___.
8. List three major characteristics of the Lamiaceae family. ___, ___, ___.
9. List flower, seed, and leaf characteristics of the Fabaceae family ___, ___, ___.
10. The Apiaceae family has this type of flower ___ and this kind of stalk ___.

Critical Concept Questions

(Answers for you to decide.)

1. What's wrong with using common names for plants?
2. Discuss advantages of naked seeds over spores and enclosed seeds over naked seeds.
3. Name three ways plant field guides can be organized. Which type do think is most useful?
4. Describe the general process of keying out a plant.

5. What does a pinyin name for a plant mean?
6. The Asteraceae family is the most complex. In what way? Why do you think flowering plants evolved to this point?
7. Do you think an ICBN congressional meeting would be interesting to attend? Why?

References

1. Hoffman, David. *Medical Herbalism: The Science and Practice of Herbal Medicine* (Rochester, VT: Healing Arts, 2003).
2. Elpel, Thomas J. *Botany in a Day* (Pony, MT: Hops, 2013).
3. "Classification and Naming of Plants." University of Nebraska Extension. http://extensionpublications.unl.edu/assets/pdf/ec1272.pdf (accessed September 13, 2019).
4. Fay, Michael. "APG—Classification by Consensus." https://www.kew.org/read-and-watch/apg-classification-consensus (accessed September 13, 2019).
5. "Angiosperm Phylogeny Group." Wikipedia. https://en.wikipedia.org/wiki/Angiosperm_Phylogeny_Group (accessed September 13, 2019).
6. "Field Guide for Managing Annual and Biennial Invasive Thistles in the Southwest." U.S. Department of Agriculture. http://www.fs.usda.gov/Internet/FSE_DOCUMENTS/stelprdb5410130.pdf (accessed September 15, 2019).
7. Holmes, Peter. *Energetics of Western Herbs* (Boulder, CO: Snow Lotus, 2006).
8. "The Witches Curse." Secrets of the Dead. http://www.pbs.org/wnet/secrets/witches-curse-clues-evidence/1501/ (accessed September 15, 2019).
9. Foster, Steven. "Black Cohosh, a Literature Review." American Botanical Council. http://cms.herbalgram.org/herbalgram/issue45/article2659.html?ts = 1568487064&signature = 05b8188f9070e626f570216d136e6398 (accessed September 14, 2019).
10. "Latin (Pharmaceutical) Herb Names Explained for Chinese Herbs." Sacred Lotus Chinese Medicine. http://www.sacredlotus.com/go/chinese-herbs/get/latin-herb-names-explained (accessed September 14, 2019).
11. O'Brien, Mary and Karen Vail. *Edible and Medicinal Plants of the Southern Rockies* (Leaning Tree Tales, 2015).
12. "Kudzu." Invasive. http://www.invasive.org/browse/subthumb.cfm?sub = 2425&start = 1 (accessed September 15, 2019).
13. "Bad Rye and the Salem Witches." Damn Interesting. https://www.damninteresting.com/bad-rye-and-the-salem-witches/ (accessed September 15, 2019).
14. "Asteraceae" Encyclopedia Britannica. http://www.britannica.com/plant/Asteraceae (accessed September 15, 2019).

5 Wildcrafting, Preparation, Storage, and Purchasing

"In some mysterious way woods have never seemed to me to be static things. In physical terms, I move through them; yet in metaphysical ones, they seem to move through me."

—John Robert Fowles, Writer and Teacher 1926–2005

CHAPTER REVIEW

- Out in the wild and conscious wildcrafting.
- Harvesting: When to harvest various plant parts, and fresh herbs.
- Preparing and drying: Shelf life, drying methods, garbling, and storage.
- Buying herbs commercially: Discerning quality, herb farms, and cultivation.
- Wildcrafter's information sheet.
- Herb walks, no collecting.

KEY TERMS

Aerial
Garble
Wildcrafting

What does it mean to get out there, search, identify, wildcraft, forage, collect, gather, and procure our own medicinal plants? We will consider the proper attitude for this endeavor, where to go, when to go, and how to go. The tools of the trade, methods, and times of year to collect roots, herbs, and barks are important. We'll look into the drying and storage of herbs and their shelf life. The importance of conserving our resources and conscious gathering is crucial. We'll investigate herbal commerce, ways to procure herbs commercially, and how to judge quality from stores, companies, and growers.

Out in the Wild

It is one thing to know about herbs on an intellectual basis by reading about them in books. It is quite another type of knowing when we get out in nature and meet the plants, take a few home, and do something with them. Preparing a remedy, smelling and tasting the finished product, and having it actually help or cure someone is very exciting, the ultimate herbalist's experience. Both kinds of knowledge are important, and well-rounded herbalists learn with their heads, hands, and hearts.

Before you make any type of herbal preparation, you need to have the herb, of course. Herbs are our allies, our healing friends. Herbs can be bought from herb companies, a sometimes-frustrating endeavor, unless you like going through lists and wondering about the freshness of the Raspberry leaf listed in a catalog. How long has it been sitting in a warehouse? What is the quality? It is much more fun to go out in the wild and meet the plants when you can. Sit with them. Meditate. Ask its name, its song, its healing energies. Is it male or female or both? Ask what it can do for you. What can you do for it? Is this the time to gather? Should I wait till fall? Will midsummer do? Do I have permission? Perhaps not.

We are visitors in the Green House and must enter and leave with respect and gratitude. An offering of tobacco or a prayer of thanks is the respectful way of native cultures. We are the guests of the Green Man, an ancient pagan symbol and nature spirit personified as a man. He is often seen on medieval churches in the British Isles and throughout Europe depicted with sprigs of leaves and acorns forming his hair. His earliest images date back thousands of years, well before the Roman empire (Fig. 5.1).

Conscious Wildcrafting

Wildcrafting is the mindful gathering of wild plants, the ultimate field trip. It implies going out into the backyard, the empty lot, the

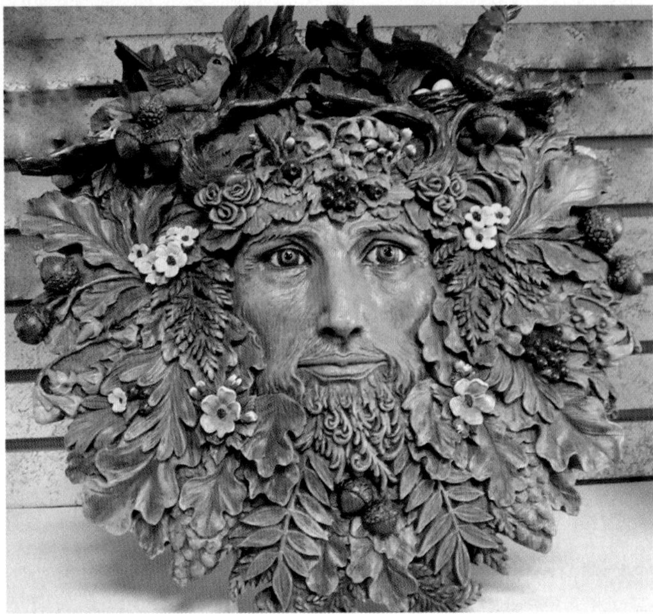

• **Fig. 5.1** The Green Man is an ancient nature spirit.

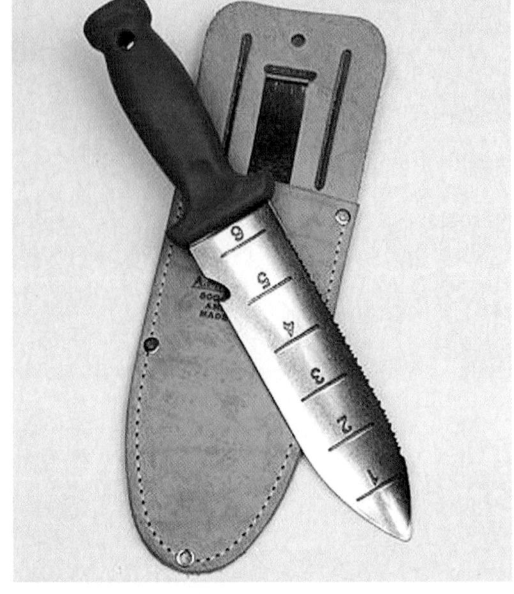

• **Fig. 5.2** This is a hori-hori, a great wildcrafting tool.

woods, the mountains, the fields, the creek-side, or the riverbank with intention.

What to wear and/or bring in your car:

- Clothing in layers
- Extra jacket and rain poncho
- Bottled water and more for car
- Hat
- Work gloves
- Hiking boots and rubber boots, if wet
- Ground cloth or old newspaper
- Collecting basket, paper and cloth bags, zip lock bags
- Pocketknife
- Hand pruner and long-handled pruners
- Little clippers or scissors
- Sturdy trowel or hori-hori
- Small shovel or fold-up army surplus type
- Camera
- Field guides (can't have too many)

You will accumulate your favorite implements as you go along. Mine is a Japanese hori-hori, which means *dig, dig*. It is strong-handled and multipurpose. The handle won't bend, as has happened to many a spade (Fig. 5.2). It is great for digging, cutting, scooping, and measuring dirt depth. It means I don't have to drag along a whole arsenal of tools when one does so many jobs. In addition to these tools, don't forget a camera. Take pictures of the precious plants and label your pictures for later reminders.

Wildcrafting means being conscious and practicing sustainable wild collection. It means gathering only what you need. A year's worth is reasonable. It means leaving the large grandparent plants and the children alone and taking only some of the healthy, mature adults so the stand will propagate and thrive next year. Leave the children to grow and the grandmothers to take care of them. James Green says 10% to 20% of a native plant community is the limit.[1] Michael Moore says one-third.[2] It means going to different places each year and not depleting a stand on your favorite hill, so the plants have a chance to regenerate. It means that after you've finished, all holes are filled in, branches and ground cover are replaced, and your tracks and traces are invisible. Leave a good number of leaves, fruit, or seeds on the plant and ground for next year's growth. It means leaving a site in better condition than when you came. If there is trash, pick it up. Be a steward of the earth. Tread lightly. Wildcrafting consciousness entails looking ahead to the seventh generation to ensure a continuation of our botanical gifts for our children and theirs.

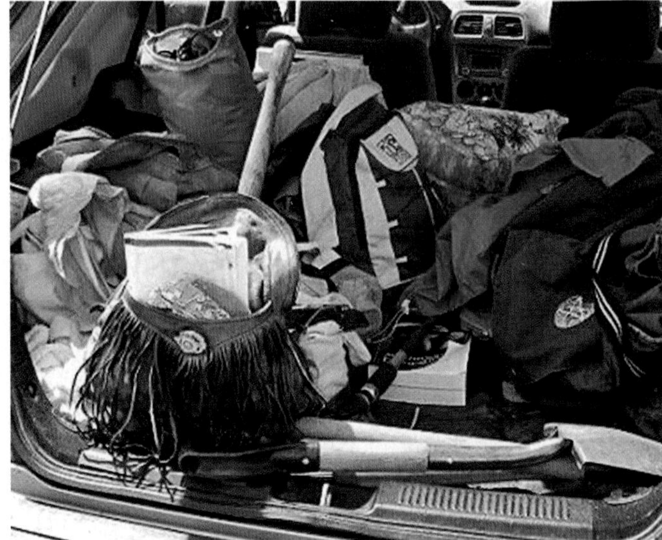

• **Fig. 5.3** A wildcrafter's well-supplied car.

Plant identification (Chapter 4) is of course a must. If you are planning to make medicine, please ensure you actually have what you hope you have. Know your basic plant families. Bring along a field guide, a person who knows, or, preferably, both. (Field guides are listed in the Bibliography.) Put all anticipated tools in your car and carry only what you think you need down the trail (Fig. 5.3). When gathering specimens, paper recycled bags or cloth bags are better than plastic. The plants need to breathe and not sweat and rot before you arrive home. Baskets with handles are lovely.

Harvesting

Be mindful. Harvest in unpolluted areas only, and at least 50 to 100 yards or more away from a road. That's about a football field length. No car fumes allowed. Do not harvest downstream or downwind from polluted areas. Stay clear of areas sprayed with pesticides. Stay away from parking lots, public parks, fertilized lawns, high-tension electric wires, and high-voltage power lines. Those places and structures are bad energy. (Also, avoid putting chemicals on your own lawn.) Always obtain permission before helping yourself to plants on privately owned land. Most owners are more than happy for you to remove so-called noxious, invasive plants, such as St. John's wort or various thistles, but maybe not others. If you want to harvest from Bureau of Land Management (BLM) areas, you are required to obtain a free use permit. The BLM and U.S. Forest Service also prohibit harvesting from campsites, picnic areas, and roadsides. (These areas are probably polluted anyway.)

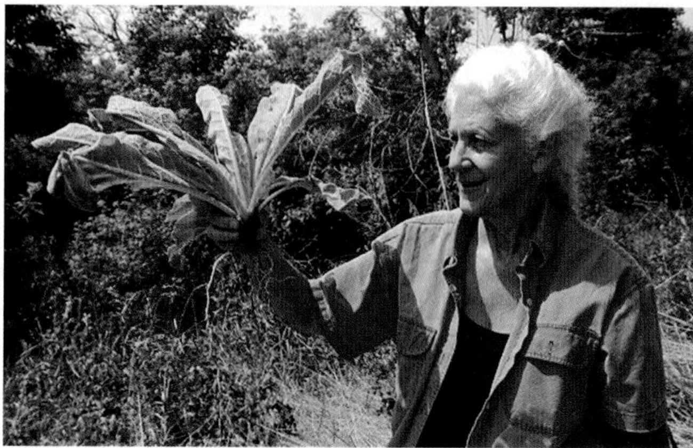

• **Fig. 5.4** Joan Zinn with a Mullein rosette and roots. Joan is our Western review editor and illustrator.

When to Harvest Various Plant Parts

In general, it is best to gather plant medicine when the energy peaks in the part you need. This timing varies. The herb, meaning the upper ***aerial*** aboveground parts like the leaves, stems, and flowers, are best collected in late spring and summer when their plant energy is traveling upward to nourish the upper parts. Roots mature in the fall after the flowers and leaves have died off. The energy is then going downward to nourish the grounding roots, so that's their time. Seeds also are gathered in the fall when they are fully formed and dry.

Moon phases can also be considered. During the waxing moon between new and full, the moon appears larger, tides are high, and the gravitational pull is going up and away from Earth. Plant energy, too, is moving toward the top of the plant. Consequently, this is an ideal time to harvest aboveground aerial parts. Conversely, between the full and new moon as the moon wanes and appears smaller, the tide is low, and the Earth energies are moving downward and inward. This is the time to harvest underground parts, such as roots and rhizomes.[3] *The Old Farmer's Almanac* is published every year and provides extensive detail on the why's, when's, and where's of this type of planning and planting.

- *Annual roots.* These live 1 year only. Dig immediately before they flower. Very few of these are medicinal herbs.
- *Biennial roots.* Biennials live for 2 years. Dig the roots in the fall of the first year or in the early spring of the second year. In the second year, the plant flowers go to seed and the root dies. An example of a biennial is Mullein root. Fig. 5.4 shows Joan Zinn with Mullein rosette and roots. Joan is our Western review editor and illustrator. The first year, Mullein produces a leafy rosette, and the second year, a spike with flowers. So, harvest Mullein root in the fall of the first year when you see a leafy rosette, or early spring of the second year before it starts to form its flower.
- *Perennial roots.* Perennials live more than 2 years. Dig late in the fall after the aerial parts have died down. If you dig them early enough in the spring before the energy rises, roots have had even more time to grow. Later in the spring, the energy has already ascended to the leaves and stem, and so it's too late for roots.
- *Flowers.* These are best gathered in bud or soon after. Early morning is ideal, after the dew has dried. Do not wash flowers or buds. Shake off the bugs and let them dry gently in a shady place. No artificial heat please, or you will dry up the volatile oils. Too much heat when drying takes the color out of the flower. If you have ever seen Red Clover blossoms that have dried brown instead of a lovely pink, that's what happened.
- *Saps.* Pitches and saps are best when gathered in late winter or early spring when the plant is dormant.
- *Fruits.* Gather when they are close to ripe. Fruits make great cordials, syrups, and elixirs. Blackberries, mulberries, raspberries, and strawberries are less glutinous when not totally ripe. Their acids have not yet become sugars, so the aroma is fresher and stronger.[1]
- *Seeds.* Collect when perfectly ripe. They are already quite dry, so they require very little drying. Seeds may be left on stems to dry and then easily rubbed or shaken off. This technique works well with Angelica seed.
- *Stems.* If you plan to use just the stems, harvest before flowering. If you plan to use both stems and flowers, obviously wait until the flowers begin to bud or are just opening.
- *Bark.* First, use small branches or pruned branches, not the fat trunk. Never cut off bark in a ring around the trunk. That will kill the tree. Instead, use longitudinal cuts, no more than one quarter of the branch circumference. Furthermore, most barks herbalists use are from the inner inside, the lighter-colored layer. Wait until after a rain and see if any branches have dropped off on the ground and contain fresh bark. Harvest those. (As for the correct season for bark harvesting, James Green suggests you ask the plant.[1])
- *Leaves.* Gather leaves before the flower has developed and when the leaves are still alive and green. The higher up toward the flower, the more aromatic. An example here are the Mints. If the plant is wilting in the hot noon sun, wait until early morning or evening when the sun is cooler, and the plant perks up and is more hydrated.

Fresh Herbs

Fresh herbs are lovely and vibrant, and they can be potent medicine. St. John's Wort is one of those for which, when tinctured fresh, there's no comparison. It should turn the alcohol or the oil a deep beautiful mahogany red color, which is caused by the hypericin and pseudohypericin content leeching out into the alcohol.[4]

That's how you know its good medicine. If possible, put fresh herbs up for tincture right away out in the field. The famous late herbalist and teacher Michael Moore used to take his students on 2-week camping/wildcrafting excursions. He always kept a supply of alcohol and jars in the back of his truck, so herbs could be prepared and tinctured fresh on the spot. For each of his listed herbs, his field guides have a collecting section that gives explicit, useful gathering tips.

If you're not a Michael Moore type and can't tincture herbs in the field, it's time to get on it as soon as you bring them home. A fresh herb sitting around in a plastic bag, even overnight, starts to spoil. If you can't get to it that same day or evening and want it to stay fresh, put it in the fridge overnight in a paper bag and process the herb the next morning. Fresh herbs are always tinctured in a 1:2 proportion (Chapter 7). This means one-part herb to two-parts 95% to 100% alcohol. No water is added because fresh, undehydrated herbs are already filled with water. In my experience, if you are lucky enough to have a freshly tinctured, wildcrafted herb, it makes superior medicine over the store-bought variety. The plant is bursting with life, and it is imbued with your personal vibes, joy, communion, knowing, and sweat. You know her, and she knows you. That is powerful medicine.

Preparing and Drying

You now know when to go out there and find the plant, but then what? Either you consume it right then or not. Consumables could be a raw nibble or a cooked edible. Possibilities for on the spot consumable wild foods are a salad with Miner's Lettuce leaf, Wild Onion bulb, Wild Oregano, Watercress leaf, and (well-washed) Yucca flowers. Purslane can be cooked as a potherb; berries can be picked or gobbled up. A fresh Peppermint or Nettle leaf tea could be brewed over a fire.

The herb might be used for field first-aid purposes, such as a Plantain leaf poultice to stop an itchy bite or staunch bleeding, or Yarrow herb to disinfect and also stop a bleeding wound. The herb could be tinctured immediately at the back of your car or on a picnic table. Alternatively, you might choose to dry it and prepare it later.

If the plan is to dry the plant for later, the goal is to dry a freshly harvested plant in such a way that it will closely resemble its living component in color, texture, taste, and smell. This implies beginning the process as soon as possible. If they are dried too fast or with too much heat, herbs start to cook and lose potency due to breakdown of enzymes. The leaves turn brown, and flower colors become dull. Sunny yellow Calendula blossoms should still look sunny and yellow when dried. If they stay closed up in a bag for too long, the plant will cook, rot, mold, wilt, or lose its vitamins.

Shelf Life

If dried too slowly, a plant could deteriorate. Even when properly dried and stored, herbs last about a year before the essential oils dissipate, and they lose their potency. Denser roots and barks have a longer shelf life—a year or two, sometimes more—and retain their zest and aroma longer than delicate leaves and flowers do. If you purchase dried herbs commercially from a health-food store or herb shop, open the jar and smell and taste a sample before you buy. You must sort through your own personally dried stash periodically as well, to assess potency, using all your senses and intuition. If the herb has lost its vitality, put it in the compost container. That's why you shouldn't harvest more than needed for about a year. Tossing out those herbs you worked so hard to gather can be wasteful and painful, for you and for the plants and their relatives.

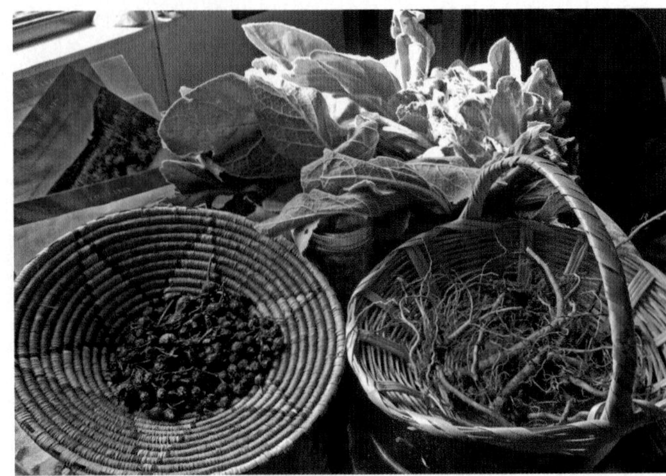

• **Fig. 5.5** Drying Rose hips, Mullein leaves, and Mullein root.

Furthermore, check your herb jars routinely to ascertain freshness, and ensure no moisture has been reabsorbed. The same goes for culinary spices in the kitchen. A rule of thumb for dried herb longevity: leaves, greens, and flowers generally keep for a year; roots, seeds, and barks, 2 to 3 years. Broken, powdered, and crushed herbs lose potency much faster than whole, uncut herbs.

Drying Methods

Drying methods include hanging a small herb bundle upside down, using a flat basket, a drying rack, a dehydrator, an old ladder, a plastic screen, or anything you can dream up that will allow the air to circulate all around the plants. Herbs can look lovely while drying, and it is hard to resist taking a picture or two (Fig. 5.5). The parts shouldn't touch, or the herbs can get mold, bugs, or rot.

- *Aboveground foliage with or without distinct stems.* This category refers to aerial parts, such as those of Nettle herb, Gumweed flower, Plantain leaf, Lemon Balm herb, Vervain herb, Catnip herb, and Dandelion leaf. Handle gently and with care. Don't wash flowers. Brush dust or dirt off leaves only if necessary. No bruising of leaves or delicate flowers, thank you. No leaving in the back of a hot car for hours so that the leaves turn moldy brownish-black. Instead, get them out of the field paper bag, and let them dry out of direct sunlight. If they have stems, you might bundle them in small bunches tied at the woody ends (raffia is attractive for tying) and hang them high and upside down. Or you could spread them out without touching in a flat basket or on a light cloth in a shady spot or indoors. Alternatively, arrange them on an old nylon screen (not metal wire), or use drying racks. It's beneficial to have many baskets. The idea is to allow cool-ish air to circulate above, below, and throughout the plants. Be inventive, and you'll find creative and attractive drying techniques.
- *Roots.* Rinse or scrub off the dirt. If plants are large and aromatic, such as Osha root or Angelica root, split them open once or twice longitudinally, and place in a dry shallow box or basket. Roots must be thoroughly dried before storage, and large hard roots can take a long time. However, the less chopped up or pulverized a root is in storage, the longer it will last. There is less air surface exposure; hence, it retains its good volatile oils and potency. It's best to chop or grind larger pieces just before processing. An exception to this recommendation is

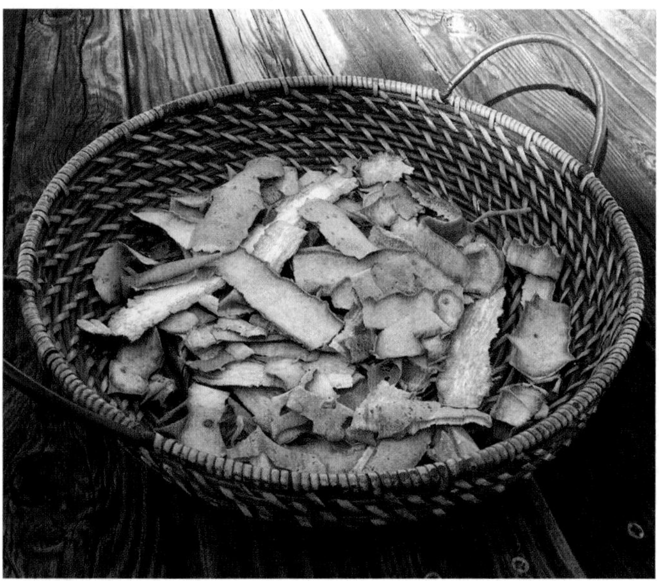

• **Fig. 5.6** Aspen bark drying in basket.

if the plants are very dense, hard, and woody, such as Red root or Oregon Grape root. If such roots aren't chopped or cut up when moist from the ground, you will never be able to do it later without a chain saw. The roots become rock hard, and you probably don't want to break the blades on your grinder!

- *Tree barks*. Pull off the inner bark after collecting (Fig. 5.6). Hang in well-ventilated shade and then chop or break up for storage when dry.

Garbling

Make sure the plant is completely dry. Leaves and flowers should crackle and crumble beneath your fingers; twigs and stems should snap, just as you might have learned in your early fire-building attempts. Roots are dry if you can slice through a thick one and find no moisture. I have been fooled with Rose hips. They seemed shriveled, hard, and dry when I bottled them. Two weeks later, said hips were covered in mold. Obviously, they were not dry enough. Some of this process is trial and error.

Once a plant is dry or during the drying process, the plant is then ***garbled***. This means sorting out and inspecting the dried plant material to remove what shouldn't be there. It includes removing twigs, stray grasses, bugs (dead or alive), and decayed parts of the plant (look for browns, blacks, mold, and moist areas). Everything goes except the beautiful dried plant of the appropriate color.

Storage

Keep herbs out of heat, light, and moisture, because heat and light cause the breakdown of oils and constituents, and moisture can cause mold and rotting. Plastic jars are not the optimal choice; some of the chemicals can leech out into the plant material. So very clean, clear, or better yet, brown glass jars with tight lids are ideal. These containers can be recycled or new. Save canning jars, jelly jars, fancy Italian glass jars, or old mayonnaise jars. Clean coffee cans with plastic lids are ok. If you don't want the herbs on display, keep in a brown bag or zip-lock bag in a dark (not clear), plastic storage bin. I've had dried herbs keep very successfully in the latter, out in a cool, dark garage.

Labeling the jars, bags, or other containers is paramount. Always list the collection date, botanical name, common name, and place of origin. "Place of origin" means, if wildcrafted, include where collected. If purchased commercially, include company name and lot number. It is a good idea to put the label on the jar, not on the lid. This might seem obvious, but it is easy to mix up lids when opening a few jars at a time.

Buying Herbs Commercially

We should be just as picky about the dried herbs we purchase from an herb company or health-food store as we are about our own personally harvested plants. Ideally, they should first look green and fresh in the jar. If that jar of Hyssop herb looks like chopped up little pieces of ancient uniform brown matter, what viability could be left in the plant? If the jars are clear glass sitting on sunlit shelves, I would question the freshness, unless that store has a frequent turnover of products. Check the date on the herb jar. Dated products are ideal. If a flower has been sitting there for a year, it's too old. Ask to see a sample. Rub some leaves together, smell them, and then taste a little. There should be a distinctly herbal scent, and the taste should be distinct and strong—maybe not delicious, but present.

Similarly, follow much of this process if ordering from herb companies. If you do not know the reputation of the company, start with a very small order. Look online for reviews. Ideally, you want to order from a reputable firm, such as Mountain Rose Herbs or Starwest Botanicals, or, for Chinese herbs, the importer Mayway. When you receive the herbs, examine them carefully. The herbs, when received, should have good color, correct taste, and be marked with the date received or harvested and lot number. Obviously, it's best to get the current year's crop, which likely hasn't been sitting around too long. Consider the place of origin. Frontier Herbs, for instance, offers Wormwood from Bulgaria and organic Wormwood from the United States. Which do you think is fresher? Compare notes with other herbalists. Herb companies usually sell by the quarter pound, half pound, pound, or greater. The more you buy, the cheaper it is. Try not to purchase more than you can use up in a year or so, or split a bag with an herbalist friend. Otherwise the unused herbs will lose potency.

Herb Farms and Cultivation

As herbals become more and more popular and the number of herbalists grows, it is increasingly important to obtain plants from herb farms and herb companies that cultivate their own. Our wild plants are not in unlimited supply, and sustainability is important. We must become stewards of the Earth. Frontier Herbs in Iowa cultivates Echinacea root and American ginseng root, among others. Limited availability has already happened with Echinacea, Goldenseal, Ginseng, Black Cohosh, Lady's Slipper, and Pipsissewa. Every year, more plants become endangered. Now, even the common Dandelion (*Taraxacum officinalis)* is being cultivated and coming to market from well-established certified organic farms in Germany, the United Kingdom, and the United States.[5] If you stop using weed killers on your own yard, after 3 years you can count on your own unlimited crop of organic Dandelion.

It is always lovely to support local growers in your area. Perhaps you can visit and inspect their crops! That can become an

TABLE 5.1 Wildcrafting Information Sheet

Herbalist name ________________________
Date gathered __________ Time of day gathered __________
Botanical name ____________________________
Common name(s) ________________________ Batch number ________
Type of plant part(s) gathered ____________________
Weather conditions during harvest ____________________________
Location of area where gathered (map, directions as needed.) ________________
Description of area where gathered (terrain, distance from highway, mountain, prairie, river, open field, backyard) __________
Permit information (Whose land? Permit: Yes, No. From where or whom? Date?) __________________
Cleaning method (shaking, peeling, washing, tools) __________________
Drying method and conditions (tinctured fresh, racks, dehydrator, basket, temperature, ventilation, indoors or outdoors?) __________________
Assessment of process (Did drying, cleaning, gathering methods work? Suggestions.) __________________
Fresh weight (g or oz.) __________ Dried weight (g or oz.) ________
I have gathered these herbs in a manner which is harmonious and respectful to the earth and in an area that was unpolluted and did not disrupt the ecosystem.
Signed ________________________ Date ______________

adventure in itself. Perhaps you would like to become an herb cultivator. What a joy to grow some of your own herbs if that is your bent. Even a little pot of Peppermint for tea and spice is worth having on a balcony or kitchen windowsill. At least you will know where it came from and how it was grown.

The best way to be successful when growing herbs is to duplicate their favorite environments as much as possible. This environmental compatibility includes soil type, climate, shade or sun, water requirements, how and when to plant, and how well the plants take to being cultivated. Obviously, you'll have more success with a plant that grows naturally where you live than trying for a moisture-loving woodland plant if you live in Arizona. *Ligusticum porterii* (Osha root), for instance, likes to grow in the Rockies at around 8,000 feet in montane to subalpine elevations. Attempts to grow it in Denver are most often unsuccessful. On the other hand, endangered American ginseng root, which grows naturally in moist Eastern forests, has been cultivated successfully by Frontier Co-Op, a Midwestern herbal company in Norway, Iowa. If you are not experienced, start with a candidate that enjoys your home conditions.

Horizon Herbs is a seed catalog company that sells non-GMO organic medicinal seeds and plants, including hard-to-find Chinese Ephedra Ma Huang (Ephedra stem), *Arnica montana* (Arnica flower), *Sambucus nigra* (Elderberry berry), and *Actaea racemosa* (Black Cohosh root). The company has a catalog with very cheerful and helpful growing tips, phone support, and an extensive website.[6] Common and very unusual Western, Chinese, and Ayurveda herbal seeds are available. Not hybrids, but the real thing. Just looking through the catalog will make you dream of spring.

If you must have a fresh herb and it's not in your backyard or the back forty, there are herb companies that will ship fresh herbs overnight from their own farms. One such company is Pacific Botanicals in Oregon. You have to order in advance, well before planting and when their crop is harvested (a variable date). They immediately notify you and ship it out. Just don't be out of town and return to find a carton on your porch containing a bunch of melted ice, rotting plants, and soggy plastic! There are many possibilities. The quest for high-quality herbs can get very interesting.

Wildcrafter's Information Sheet

Table 5.1 shows a sample sheet that you are free to copy and use for your wildcrafting records. This form may be modified in any way to accommodate need. It is very good to keep track of where you found plants. It is surprisingly easy to forget which trail, Arnica hill, or Aspen grove you visited or become confused about where the Hops or the Vervain that you saw last month (not to mention last year) originated. Occasionally, give an area a rest and find a new place to go the next time, so one spot is not wildcrafted and loved to death. Keeping records helps you to remember these details. It is also helpful to go back in your notes to see how you processed a given herb and whether it worked out well. No use reinventing the wheel. In addition, if last time was not very successful, you won't repeat the process. Do some research. Try something new.

But do keep records. When you actually process your herbs, be they fresh or dried, that medicine-making information will require a separate sheet (Chapter 7). Sample forms to copy, (Appendix A).

Herb Walks, No Collecting

There is great joy in walking, exploring, and being, with no taking involved. A walk through the fields or woods with your trusty camera or herb pal is uplifting and educational. A pocket guide for your area, or a good herb plant identification app is a plus. Recall your basic herb families and how to key out a plant (Chapter 4). If you're not sure of a plant, take a picture, and look it up later. Label the picture as soon as you know. I personally have certain plants that I see again and again and just draw a blank every time. Sometimes your friends can jog your memory and you theirs. Another tactic is to visit a local botanical garden if you are lucky enough to have one close by. The plants there are often labeled with common and botanical names, so you can quiz and check yourself. It is a wonderful way to conduct a self-guided tour. Also, check out the same plants at different times of the year, and learn to recognize their early spring leaves, summer flowers, and fall seeds or pods.

Summary

Gathering herbs in the wild is called wildcrafting. Proper attitude and respect must be given to the plant, the environment, and the ecosystem. Collect only what you will use, doing so consciously. Tools needed in a seasoned herbalist's car could include a small shovel, hori-hori, collecting bags, and a good knife. Keep what you need in the car because you never know when you may find herbs, but don't carry all your tools down the trail. A few good field identification guides should always be handy, to make sure you have what you intend.

Knowing the proper time of year and season to collect assures good quality. Generally, herbs and flowers are gathered in early spring and summer; root and seeds are gathered in the fall. The moon phases and time of day are factors. There are pros and cons of fresh versus dried plant preparations. Fresh is generally best. Always follow recommended methods for drying and safekeeping.

Purchasing our herbs is perfectly acceptable and becoming more and more necessary as availability of wild stands decline along with our other natural resources. How do we judge quality when purchasing botanicals? Consider their source, when, where, and how collected, any cultivation methods, and the reputation of the company. The best judge is your senses. Smell and taste a sample, if possible, to evaluate freshness and vitality. Herbs should be stored in cool, dark places for best shelf life. A quality product will result in a good remedy. Have fun discovering new and reputable herb sources and support your local growers.

Review

Fill in the Blanks

(Answers in Appendix B)

1. The best time to gather roots is when the energy of the plant is ___. Season of the year would be ___.
2. The best time to gather leaves is when the energy of the plant is ___. Season of the year would be ___.
3. Name five useful tools to take wildcrafting. ___, ___, ___, ___, ___.
4. How long do perennials live? ___.
5. Name three techniques for drying herbs. ___, ___, ___.
6. For best storage, keep herbs out of ___, ___, ___.
7. For best drying results, the air must ___.
8. Shelf life of greens and flowers is ___. Shelf life of roots, seeds, and barks is ___.
9. Name four items to include on a dry-herb label. ___, ___, ___, ___.
10. How is bark correctly stripped from a live tree? ___.

Critical Concept Questions

(Answers for you to decide.)

1. List the pros and cons of wildcrafting.
2. Do you think you will wildcraft? Reasons?
3. Why are fresh herbs preferred by many herbalists?
4. How do you judge the quality of an herb?
5. What are some garbling techniques?
6. How do you tincture a fresh herb? What are the recommended proportions?
7. What are some considerations in cultivating an herb?
8. What does conscious wildcrafting mean?
9. Why is use of a Wildcrafter's Information Sheet a good idea?
10. You are harvesting Burdock root. When would you go? Which tools would you take?

References

1. Green, James. *The Herbal Medicine-Maker's Handbook* (New York: Crossing, 2002).
2. Moore, Michael. *Medicinal Plants of the Mountain West* (Santa Fe, NM: Museum of New Mexico Press, 2003).
3. Burgess, Stephanie. "Harvesting and Preparing Herbs by the Lunar Phases." AltNature Menu. https://altnature.com/library/lunarphases.htm (accessed September 16, 2019).
4. Ganora, Lisa. *Herbal Constituents: Foundations of Phytochemistry* (Louisville, CO: Herbalchem, 2009).
5. Engles, Gayle and Josef Brinckmann. "Herb Profile: "Dandelion, *Taraxacum officinale*." *Herbalgram, Journal of the American Botanical Council,* Feb-April 2016.
6. Horizon Herbs Catalog. P.O. Box 69, Williams OR 97544. Request catalog online: www.horizonherbs.com.

6 Types of Herbal Remedies

"This large and expensive stock of drugs will be unnecessary . . . the common resources of the lancet, a garden, a kitchen, fresh air, cool water, exercise, will be sufficient to cure all the diseases that are at present under the power of medicine."

***—Dr. Benjamin Rush (1745-1813) American physician, Continental Congress member, and a signer of the* Declaration of Independence.**

CHAPTER REVIEW

- Types and uses of herbal preparations and considerations for choice.
- Infusions: Hot and cold, discussion and preparation.
- Decoctions: Discussion and preparation.
- Mouthwashes and gargles: Discussion and preparation.
- Steams, smokes, and baths: Discussion and preparation.
- Capsules and suppositories: Discussion and preparation.
- External plasters, poultices, and compresses: Discussion and preparation.
- External salves, creams, and lotions differentiated.
- Tinctures: Discussion of menstruum types, extracts, percolations, and liniments.
- Essential oils: General information and quality control. Hydrosols.
- Syrups: Simple syrups, cordials, oxymels, electuaries, and honeys discussed.

KEY TERMS

Aromatherapy
Baths
Capsules
Compress
Cordial
Cream
Decoction
Electuary
Essential oils
Extract
Fixed oils
Fomentation
Glycerin/glycerite
Hydrosol
Infusion
Liniment
Lotion
Maceration
Marc
Menstruum
Neat
Oxymel
Percolation
Plaster
Poultice
Salve
Smokes
Spirits
Steams
Suppository
Syrup
Tincture
Vinegar

The numerous and varied herbal preparations are identified and explained with their pros and cons, along with guidance for how to choose among them. Some types, like vinegars or electuaries, have gone in and out of fashion, but tinctures and creams are very important for the modern herbalist.

The hope is that experimentation with basic herbal medicinal teas will begin early on in your studies. Teas should first be made as simples (one plant only), and then in blends. Teas are a good way discover a plant's properties and to discover how it tastes and reacts in the body.

It is also hoped that other easy preparations will be tried—external applications like poultices, compresses, steams, baths, and gargles. Complex herbal medicine-making appears in Chapter 7.

Types and Uses of Various Herbal Preparations

Countless types of preparations can be made with any given plant. Proper choices depend on therapeutic intention, what a client is willing or able to actually ingest, and the extraction method appropriate for a specific plant. For example, very mucilaginous plants, such as Marshmallow root or Slippery Elm bark, are best extracted by cold water. A plant high in volatile oils might also do best in a cool oil extraction form, because heat breaks down the aromatic quality. Plant proteins (albumen) also like cold water better because heat makes them coagulate, just like an egg white. Hot water preparations are best for herbs containing starch. Others do better with alcohol, and some need both. Gums and sugars do well in either.[1]

Types of preparations might include a sweet syrup for a child, a syrup to soothe a cough, a strong alcoholic tincture for a bad infection, a hot tea to sip (infusion or decoction), a topical first aid cream, a ***glycerite*** (a sweet viscous fat extracted from plant oils) for someone who cannot ingest alcohol, or an herbal vinegar to give away at the holidays. Herbs can be dispensed to be used topically, internally as tinctures, in glycerites or capsules, in baths as hand or foot soaks, as an anal suppository, or for inhalation as steams. It is very useful for herbalists to learn the art of herbal preparations and to recognize situations where one particular type of remedy is appropriate over another. Ready-mades can be quite expensive, and the quality could be, perhaps, lacking. It all depends on your time, desire, and budget.

Considerations for Preparation Choice

- *Condition of client.* One or two forms might work. If client has a sinus infection, the herbalist might choose an internal tincture directed at the sinuses and an external aromatic steam to open the airway. If a client has had a burn, an external salve that's cooling and healing and an internal antibiotic-type tincture would be appropriate. If a health-promoting tonic is required, you might make a pleasant tasting tea to sip daily and a yuckier-tasting tincture to quickly take 3 times a day.
- *Same herb, fresh versus dried.* Sometimes, a fresh versus a dried preparation of the same botanical will change its therapeutic effect. For example, Chinese and Ayurvedic traditions consider the fresh and dried forms of Ginger rhizome to be different medicines with distinct therapeutic actions. A tea made from fresh *Zingiber officinale* (Ginger rhizome) is preferred if sweating is desired, but dried Ginger, in tincture form, is best for nausea or stomach aches.
- *Chemical constituents.* Information about a plant's chemistry can determine choices. Saponins are water-soluble chemicals extractable in cold water. Plants containing alkaloids and amino acids require alcohol for best extraction results. Some plants, such as Ganoderma Ling Zhi (Reishi mushroom), require both hot water and alcohol to extract both its water-soluble and alcohol-soluble ingredients.
- *Age of client.* Children do well with preparations containing vegetable *glycerin* or *glycerol* or with alcoholic preparations in hot water with lots of sweetener added. Elders may benefit from the same types of preparations.
- *Intention.* The different forms in which an herb is administered may influence your choice of preparation of the herb. Rosemary essential oil can be stimulating, warming, or relaxing. White Horehound leaves taken as a hot infusion promote sweating; when taken cool they stop sweating and promote urination.[2] A hot Burdock root infusion tastes different and feels different in the body from a Burdock root tincture of alcohol and water.
- *Route of administration.* People with absorption problems may do better using a rectal suppository than taking a preparation by mouth. Elderly people often have greater body fat over lean muscle and water mass.[3] For them, a fat-soluble glycerin form of administration may work best. Tinctures often absorb more quickly and are more bioavailable than a ground-up herb in a capsule, because the stomach does not have to break the whole thing down by digestion and process the plant fiber. Essential oils work well when applied topically, inhaled directly, or used in a diffuser or steam inhalation. (See later section for a full discussion of essential oils.)
- *Compliance.* Always find out what a person can and is willing to do. Is the remedy practical for the situation? Can they handle the taste? It does no good to prepare an elaborate dried tea mix if the person isn't willing to drink it 3 times a day. Compresses for sore muscles are time-consuming to prepare if they have to be made up each time. A liniment is quicker, easier, less messy, and more portable. If a person works 5 days a week, their remedy should be easy to transport. Often a tincture in a little brown bottle is the easiest.

Infusions and Preparation Instructions

An ***infusion*** is a preparation of a plant part steeped in hot water and the most basic way of brewing a tea. It is standard for preparing *lightweight* plant parts, such as dried leaves, seeds, flowers, and stems, by letting them stand in hot water for 10 to 20 minutes. A ready-made tea bag immersed in a cup of boiling water creates an infusion. The United States Pharmacopeia (USP) has its own particular proportions and infusion methods, and the British Pharmacopeia (BP) has its own versions. There are various folk ways and variations among them, including the elaborate tea-making rituals in Japanese tea ceremonies. Learn to prepare teas first as simples, then in blends. It's a good way to discover a plant's properties and how it tastes and reacts in the body.

Infusions are used for water-soluble herbs. The plant material can be dry or fresh. If dry, less herb is needed by weight because its dehydration makes it stronger. If fresh, more plant is required by weight because of its higher water content. For fresh herbs, generally use twice the weight of the dried form of the same plant. Medicinal teas are stronger-tasting than a standard commercial tea bag because more plant material is required for a therapeutic effect. If an herb (like Goldenseal root) is very bitter, use less. If strong and intense, like Cayenne fruit, use only a pinch. Mild-tasting, light, and fluffy plants, like Raspberry leaves, require more plant material.

Hot Infusion Directions

- *Hot infusions.* The herbal portion is added to just boiled water, removed from stove, covered, and left to steep for 10 to 20 minutes.[1] Covering while steeping preserves important healing essential oils of aromatic plants such as Chamomile flower,

Fennel seed, or Peppermint herb. Other herbal examples for infusions include light plant parts such as Chrysanthemum flower, Cleavers herb, Comfrey leaf, Dandelion leaf, Elder flower, Ginkgo leaf, Mugwort herb, Mullein leaf, and Nettle herb.

- *Containers.* The best containers for infusions are previously warmed glass, glazed earthenware or porcelain pots with a lid, so when the water is poured in to steep, it is not cooled by the pot. The herb should sit in the top portion or section of the water (solvent) so that the most efficient circulatory displacement (diffusion) occurs. That is why some teapots have little ceramic baskets at the top for the plant material. I personally love the French press, which allows plenty of water for the herbs to float around in and steep, and the pressing or straining step is handily taken care of when you push down the plunger.
- *The metric system.* The metric system of measurements is practically universal and is used by most professional herbalists today. Metric measurements are used in all U.S. hospitals and pharmacies. The only countries in the whole world not on the metric system for all their measurements are the United States, Burma (Myanmar), and Liberia. Therefore, getting into the habit of using the metric system and investing in a metric scale makes sense. Grams (g) refer to dry weight and milliliters (mL) refer to volume (either liquid or packed dry herb).
  - When making tea, herbs are usually (but not every time) measured out in *weight* rather than volume. This practice is because a gram or ounce of fluffy flowers takes up much more space (volume) than a gram or ounce of dense root (weight). Another way to express this is that 1 ounce of feathers takes up a lot more space (volume) than 1 ounce of lead (weight). For general purposes, 1 oz equals approximately 30 g dry weight or 30 mL liquid volume. One pint equals 500 mL equals 16 oz equals 2 cups. (Appendix A, see Conversions.)
- *Standard infusion proportions.* When making herbal teas, a proportion refers to a given amount of dried or fresh herb to a given amount of water. One ounce of dried herb is generally added to 1-pint boiling water. This ratio translates by metric to approximately 30 g dried herb to 500 mL boiled water. (If the herbs are fresh, chop coarsely and double the weight, because so much of it is from water in the plant.) These standard infusion proportions make *very strong* medicinal teas and will have a robust taste.
- *Milder proportions and dose.* Today, many herbalists use a little less herb than that indicated in the previous section, making their infusions a little milder and more dilute, and obtain better compliance because so many herbal medicinal-strength teas are not that pleasant tasting. The milder proportion is still effective and curative. A milder proportion is 3 to 5 g herb in 250 mL (about 1 cup water).
  - Some sources express this proportion by volume by recommending 2 to 3 tablespoons of dried herb per cup of water.
- *Use common sense when measuring out herbs for teas.* The take-away from this discussion is that there is really no equivalent of weight-to-volume when measuring out herbs for teas. Deciding which measurement to use really comes down to experience and consideration of the nature and density of the plant part used. Sometimes one way works, sometimes the other. The quantities given above are merely guidelines to get you started.
  - *Dose for standard and mild infusion proportions.* One cup 3 times a day. It's easier to make up one day's supply (3 cups) to keep in the refrigerator in a glass jar between doses and gently heat each time. Don't make up more than this at one time because it can spoil.
- *Boil water.* Pour measured boiling water over the herbs.
- *Steep.* Remove boiling water from heat. Cover and let stand 10 to 20 minutes in a warm place.
- *Strain.* If possible, press out the ***marc***, the plant material. One way is to press it down through a strainer with a spoon. Bulky herbs will absorb water, and if not pressed, you won't end up with sufficient liquid. Add extra hot water if necessary to make infusion measure 500 mL (1 pint).

Cold Infusion Directions

- *Cold infusions.* These infusions are not heated. Instead, the herb is soaked overnight in water.
- *Use and examples for cold infusions.* Cold Infusions are used for plants high in mucilage and for those high in essential oils that would dissipate if heated. Examples are Burdock root, Chamomile flower, Cleavers herb, Comfrey root, Cramp bark, Marshmallow root, Mugwort herb, Nettle root or whole herb, Peppermint herb, Uva ursi leaf, and Slippery Elm bark.[1] Notice that some of these plants are also in the hot-infusion list and can be infused either hot or cold.
- *Proportions.* One part herb to 20 parts water or 30 g (1 oz) coarsely ground herb to 500 mL water. Use less herb if very mucilaginous, like Marshmallow root or Slippery Elm bark, or you will have a slippery, gooey mess.[1]
- *Soak overnight.* Place loose herb into water or put herb in cotton pouch or tea bag and submerge in water overnight. Place herb into water and let remain overnight at room temperature.
- *Strain the herbs.* Squeeze out the pouch and press the marc.
- *Add cold water if necessary.* Do this to insure finished infusion measures 500 mL (1 pint).

Decoctions and Preparation Instructions

A ***decoction*** is a standard method for preparing hard plant parts, such as dried roots, barks, twigs, and some seeds, using prolonged simmering for 10 to 20 minutes. This method is good for the tougher constituents found in roots, such as resins and tannins.[2] Rather than steeping, the herb is simmered in water to draw out constituents that would not be coaxed out by infusion.

To decoct means to boil down or boil away, so it is the chosen method used for extracting herbals that are then used in fomentations, syrups, and enemas. Decoctions would *not* be used for mucilaginous herbs, such as Slippery Elm bark and Marshmallow root, or for herbs with delicate volatile oils, such as Mint herb, Hyssop herb, or Fennel seed. Decoctions are not for resinous plants, such as Gumweed flower or Yerba Santa herb, or for delicate flowers like Rose buds or Elder flowers.[1] Save decoctions for plants not easily injured by heat, like Wild Cherry bark, Fenugreek seed, Licorice root, Astragalus Huang Qin (Astragalus root), or Sarsaparilla root.

Decoctions are traditional preparations in Chinese Medicine. Oriental medical doctors give their patients strong raw and dried herbal mixtures in paper bags so they can prepare them at home. The instructions are very specific, often complicated. One should use enamel, crockery, or glass pots, not metal; metal can adversely affect the herbal ingredients. Decoction time and methods used are important. Patients can spend an hour or so cooking up a tea, smelling it, and then sipping it, all part of the healing experience. Decoctions are often prescribed for long-term therapy for chronic illnesses lasting a few months.[4] In many Chinese hospitals, a daily decoction is prepared each morning and delivered to the patient's bedside in a thermos.

Decoction Directions

- *Slice roots*. Diagonal slices provide better surface coverage. Alternately, chop or grind finely if the root is very hard.
- *Fresh roots and seeds*. Slice thinly or shave down to small pieces. Lightly crush seeds.
- *Container*. Use glazed earthenware, porcelain, or glass pot with lid. Do not use iron because root tannins react with the iron, causing discoloration, and never use aluminum pots because the hot water can leach out the metal.
- *Proportions*. 30 g of herb (1 oz) to 1 pint of cold water. If you want it milder, use less herb; for example, 1/4 less. If herb is fresh, double the weight.
- *Macerate herb*. It helps to soak or macerate dense herbs in water for a few hours or overnight to soften them. Place herbs in the pot.
- *Add measured cold water*. Begin with cold water to ensure complete extraction of all soluble constituents by slow heating.
- *Cover and bring to a slow boil.*
- *Decrease heat to a simmer* for 10-15 minutes. The harder the material, the longer it takes. Use clinical, herbal judgment.
- *Press herb* and discard marc.
- *Cool and strain*. Cool to below 104°F and strain once or twice with a fine strainer or filter paper.
- *Add more hot water*, if necessary, to replenish lost water volume back to 500 mL.
- *Dose and storage*. Make a 24-hour supply—3 cups. Refrigerate extra in a glass jar and reheat. Make a fresh batch each day. Dose: 1/2 to 1 cup 3 times per day, depending on situation and body weight.[1]
- *Dosage interpretation*. The weight of the herb used in each cup is the herbal dose.
- *Examples for decoctions*. Blackberry root bark, Black Cohosh root, Burdock seed, Comfrey root, Cramp bark, Dandelion root, Echinacea root, fresh or dried Ginger rhizome, Mullein root, Ganoderma Ling Zhi (Reishi mushroom) decocted 45 minutes, Eleutherococcus Ci Wu Jia (Siberian Ginseng root), Willow bark, and Yellow Dock root.

All the above tea preparations—hot herbal drinks infused in just boiled or boiling water in one way or another—are classic ways to make medicine, probably the most ancient herbal delivery system of them all. For more information on tea, refer to Box 6.1.

• BOX 6.1 Tips for Herbal Teatime

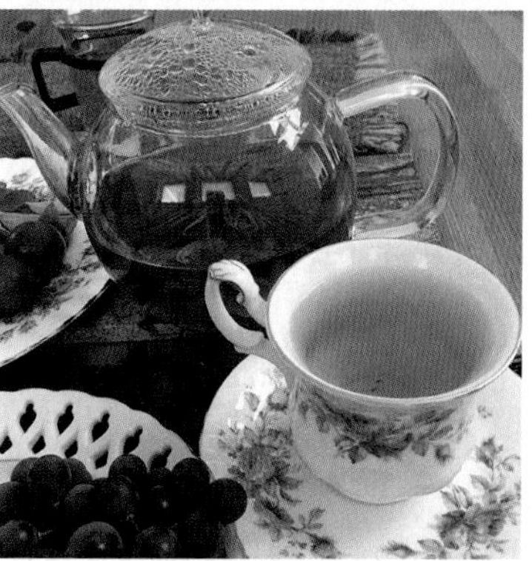

Charming herbal tea presentation using a glass pot.

If you are making a tea with roots and flowers, do you infuse or decoct? Do both. First simmer the roots separately for 10–15 minutes, remove from heat, cover, and then add the leaves to steep for about 10 minutes more. At the end, strain it all.

- The longer you simmer, the stronger it becomes.
- The longer it stands before straining, the more bitter it becomes.
- Be flexible. Experiment and adjust amounts of herb to taste. This takes experimentation. The proportions given are only guidelines.
- Glass French presses are your friends. Steeping and straining is done in one container. Don't use the same French press that you use for coffee when making herbal teas, or the tastes will mingle.
- Sun teas and moon teas give celestial energy to the brew. Put herbs and water in a lidded glass jar and let it stand, covered, in the hot sunlight for a few hours. Overnight cold infusions could sit outdoors in the moonlight.
- Doses: Acute problems like a cold, a headache, or a toothache: 1/4 cup every 2 hours. For chronic problems such as hay fever, arthritis, or insomnia:
  3-4 cups daily for several weeks.[5]
- For children, make teas into herbal popsicles or blend with fruit juice. Add sweetener appropriate for their age.

Tea and Honey

The World Health Organization and the American Academy of Pediatrics say not to give raw or unpasteurized honey to children under 1 year old because of rarely occurring infant botulism toxicity. Botulism is caused by *botulinum* toxin, a natural poison produced by *Clostridium botulinum* bacteria. Honey is almost always raw and seldom, if ever, heated or pasteurized. Doing so would destroy all its healthy vitamins and enzymes. The reason for caution is the concern about botulism spores being present in some soils in which bee-attracting plants grow. If the bee pollinates those infected flowers, they could carry the botulism spores to their hives, thus contaminating their honey.[6]

Older children and adults can tolerate the small amount that may be present due to having more mature, acidic stomachs that counteract the botulinum toxins. Babies haven't matured to this point, so for them, botulism toxicity could be serious. Signs of botulism in babies include lethargy, poor feeding, constipation, weak cry, floppy muscle tone, facial weakness, and impaired gag reflex. Therefore, it is best to err on safety's side. Substitute sweeteners for the little ones are maple syrup, rice syrup, or vegetable glycerin. Of course, many cultures past and present have fed and do feed their babies honey from birth with no ill effects. Perhaps this toxicity is a result of our more polluted soils.

Mouthwashes, Gargles, and Preparation

For mouthwashes and gargles, use double-strength herbal infusions or decoctions and rinse mouth and/or gargle the back of the throat. Sometimes a gargle is used for bad breath caused by eating garlic or onions, but if a person has persistent, chronic halitosis, she or he should see a dentist or doctor. Reasons for bad breath include local tooth or gum infections, dry mouth, poor oral hygiene, or systemic problems, such as kidney or liver problems, acid reflux, or chronic respiratory conditions, like bronchitis, pneumonia, and postnasal drip. Many excellent uses for gargles are listed below and are mainly used for acute conditions.[2]

- *Disinfect and astringe local tissues.* This technique is therapeutic for loose teeth, inflamed, bleeding gums (*gingivitis*), and mouth and tongue sores. Astringents and antiseptics to use for these purposes are Garden Sage leaf, Calendula flower, Myrrh resin, or Echinacea root. Myrrh is often added to toothpaste.
- *Decongest mucous.* When needed for conditions such as chronic laryngitis, sore throat, sticky or stuck mucous, or sinus infection, warming and stimulating gargles are called for, made with herbs such as Cayenne fruit, Mustard seed, Garden Sage leaf, Ginger root. Sinus infection and congestion respond to Tea Tree and Lemon Myrtle essential oils.
- *Acute inflammation/irritation of mouth and throat.* Sore throats require moist, demulcent, cooling, analgesic herbs, such as Plantain leaf, Marshmallow root, and Rose petal for mouthwashes and gargles, plus internal, systemic preparations.
- *Tooth cavities and gingivitis prevention.* Bitter and strong Creosote or Chaparral leaf work well. Clove essential oil is analgesic, antimicrobial, and numbing.

Steams, Smokes, Baths, and Preparation

Steams

A ***steam*** refers to breathing in the vapors of an herbal infusion high in essential oils. As the medicated steam is inhaled, it coats the mucous membranes of the upper and lower respiratory passages. Steams are simple to make. Boil water in a small stainless-steel saucepan and remove from heat. Then add 4 to 6 drops of essential oil. Alternately, make an infusion with the herbs. Set the pan on table with a hotplate underneath, sit down, and cover your head and the pan with a towel and inhale the volatile oils for 10 to 15 minutes, 2 to 3 times daily or more, as needed.

A *vaginal steam* is a partner of the steam inhalation. Here a bowl of relatively hot, steamy, medicated water is placed on the floor, and the client squats over it for a few minutes, allowing the volatile oils to medicate the perineum. This treatment can soften and relax the pelvis and cervix during the last 2 or 3 weeks of pregnancy, relieve spasms from kidney stones, or relax and relieve menstrual cramping.

There are many situations and signs and symptoms in which steams would be a wise remedy choice. This list provides a few ideas to add to your arsenal with appropriate herbs and essential oils for each case:

- *Sinus infections and congestion.* Use steams to loosen sinus mucus, disinfect the tissues, and relieve pain and pressure. Suggested herbs are Eucalyptus, Camphor, Lavender, Chamomile, Rosemary, Ravensara, and Peppermint essential oils or herbs.
- *Middle ear infections.* Let steam envelop one ear at a time to disinfect and relieve congestion and inflammation. Suggested herbs are Eucalyptus, Chamomile, Thyme, Ravensara, Rosemary, and Magnolia bud essential oils or herbs.
- *Lung mucus congestion.* This type of congestions is caused by bronchitis, with coughing and chest pain. Here the herbalist needs to stimulate and decongest the chest with steams containing expectorating, stimulating, and decongesting herbs and essential oils, such as Eucalyptus, Pine, Fir, Spruce, and Hyssop.
- *Chest wheezing and tightness.* Especially for asthma, use respiratory relaxants such as Hyssop, Thyme, Aniseed, and Cypress essential oils and herbs.
- *Tension and stress.* Use calming essential oils such as Lavender, Marjoram, Bergamot, Chamomile, and Clary Sage.
- *Woman's issues.* Vaginal steams, the counterpart to the upper airway steam, are used for childbirth preparation, menstrual cramps, and kidney stones. Relaxing essential oils to use are Clary Sage, Marjoram, Laurel, and Garden Sage.[2]

Smokes

Smokes are the therapeutic smoking of dried, relaxing herbs and blends. They can provide immediate temporary relief from tight respiratory conditions. Indulging in herbal smokes every day can be hot and irritating to the lungs, but occasionally, about 6 to 10 puffs from a pipe will relieve tightness. Although smoking may seem counterintuitive to lung relief, the herbs used here have a relaxing effect.

Make a blend. Mix chopped herbs with some honey and water, lay out to dry, and then store in a beautiful airtight tin. Adding at least 10% Coltsfoot herb ensures a good burn.[2] Herbs that work well for coughs, bronchial congestion, and asthmatic breathing are Coltsfoot herb, Mullein leaf, Lobelia herb, Nettle herb, Lavender herb, and Elecampane flower. For wheezing, try Catnip herb, Mullein leaf, Hyssop herb, and Lavender herb.

Baths

Therapeutic ***baths*** are the immersion of the body or a body part in hot, warm, tepid, or cold water with or without the addition of herbs. Therapeutic use of water is called *hydrotherapy* and has been used for centuries. Hot mineral springs were considered sacred sites, where American Indian tribes would gather in peace, regardless of politics or states of war. The Baths of Caracalla were public baths used in ancient Rome. Scandinavian saunas employ moist or dry heat followed by plunges into cold water. Simple baths are, first of all, cleansing and relaxing. A plain un-medicated bath following a long, stressful day is therapeutic in itself. Other functions of bathing are to draw out toxins; restore and revive; relieve tension from the head, the emotions, and the muscles; reduce fever; and relieve skin burns, bites, and itches. Essential oils may be added to a medium such as Epsom salt, dry milk, or unscented bath gel before being added to the water. Otherwise, the oil will just float on the surface of the water.

Bathing in various water temperatures have different therapeutic effects, ranging from invigorating and cooling to hot and relaxing soaks.[1]

- *Cool.* Water 65° to 75° F. Cool means slightly warmer than the cold, shocking plunge after a hot sauna, which can be a physiological tonic and invigorating in healthy people. Cool baths are reviving and stimulating and should only last 1 to 2 minutes.
- *Tepid.* Water 75° to 85° F. Tepid is approaching normal body temperature, so the effect is mild. This temperature is used most often for skin cleansing.
- *Warm.* 85° to 98° F. This is just below or at normal body temperature but gives a sensation of warmth because it is hotter than our surface skin. This is your standard bubble-bath temperature. Recommended here would be full immersion in a large, comfortable, claw-foot tub (if available) left over from the days when people took their time bathing.
    - If fever is present, warm baths feel even warmer because the skin surface is cooler than the elevated core temperature. Warm baths can cause therapeutic sweating when we get out and dry off, another way that body

temperature is lowered. Such baths are relaxing, help with sleep, relax muscles, and help decongest the chest and throat mucous.

- *Hot.* Water 98° to 104° F. Initially it excites the nerves, and then depresses or relaxes them. It relaxes smooth and skeletal muscles. That's why people feel mellow and relaxed after a hot soak. Hot water dilates the capillaries, brings blood to the surface, and increases circulation. It can relieve dysmenorrhea (menstrual cramps) and bring on menses, relieve chronic arthritis and sore muscles, relieve colic, and prepare the skin for cold applications. Very hot baths are not recommended in cases of cardiac weakness, brain or spinal cord inflammation, atherosclerosis, and the treatment of debilitated people, the elderly, infants, or those affected by sunstroke.

Baths can be used for various therapeutic outcomes and do not always refer to submersion of the whole body. Specialized types are hand and foot soaks, eye washes, and douches. Whole herbs and essential oils (or both) can be added for different therapeutic outcomes.[1]

- *Detoxifying bath.* Detoxifying baths draw out toxins accumulated from poor diet, smoking, chemical exposure, and drug use or chemotherapy. The toxins pass out through the skin into the bath water. You can accomplish this detoxification with the additions of large amounts of remedies such as Epsom salt, baking soda and salt, trace minerals, seaweed, and Lemon or Grapefruit essential oils.
- *Essential oil bath.* To enhance bathing pleasure, help relaxation, reduce anxiety, and aid sleep, essential oils are recommended. Try Chamomile, Lavender, Rose, Geranium, Neroli, or Ylang-Ylang. If the intention is to relax sore muscles, try a few drops of Birch, Camphor, Lavender, Lemon Grass, Wintergreen, Peppermint, Basil, or Cypress. Because oil and water don't mix, combine the oils in Epsom salt, dry milk, or unscented bath gel. Dissolve the essential oil mixture under running water.
- *Dried or fresh herbal bath.* Make a strong herbal tea from any selection of plants and pour into bath water. Alternately, make an herbal tea bag. Wrap fresh or dried herbs up in a sock, stocking, or scarf, or place in a muslin tea bag. Toss into the water or tie bundle to the faucet under running water. This is an infusion. Use 2 to 3 oz of herb per tub.[2]
- *Restoring, reviving bath.* For conditions of weakness, such as severe stress, recovery from long illnesses, sickness, childbirth, or after surgery, restoratives are needed. Milky Oats, Seaweeds or minerals, and essential oils of Sage, Pine, Spruce, Basil, Thyme, or Ravensara are helpful.
- *Stimulating, warming bath.* For cold conditions, use warming herbs, such as Black Peppercorns, Prickly Ash bark, Cinnamon bark, Horseradish root, or Mustard seed.
- *Baths to clear heat and reduce fever.* For onset of fever and if chilled, use sweat-inducing, stimulating diaphoretics such as Cayenne fruit, Ginger root, Horseradish root, or Peppermint herb. Later, if fever becomes too high and the person feels very hot, use cooling herbs or essential oils like Lemon Balm, Lavender, Borage, or Chickweed.
- *Hand and foot baths.* Hands or feet are soaked to warm, cool, or relax. Either the feet are soaked up to the ankles in a tub, or the hands are submerged up to the wrists in a basin. Other than for manicures and pedicures, these baths are good for warming or cooling the body. The radial artery in the wrist and the pedal pulses in the foot are close to the surface and rapid carriers of warmth. Use the same herbs for warming and cooling as given in earlier sections. These extremity soaks are furthermore useful for spasms, cramps, arthritis, dysmenorrhea, dry skin, and eczema. If alternating hot and warm water is used, pain is relieved.
- *Sitz baths.* Sitz baths are also known as hip baths. *Sitzen* means "to sit" in German; thus one sits in hot or cold water up to the waist, covering the hips. These can be used with various combinations of hot and cold water. Sitz baths are useful for conditions of the urinary, genital, and lower gastrointestinal (GI) systems. Cool Sitz baths are used for heavy menses, intermenstrual bleeding, and bleeding hemorrhoids. Hot Sitz baths are used for delayed menses, dysmenorrhea, post-childbirth episiotomies, lumbar pain, gout, constipation, and urinary disorders.[1]
- *Eye baths.* (These are technically called *washes.*) You can wash out an eye with a sterile eye cup or a bulb syringe. Start with a well-strained lukewarm infusion or decoction. Eye washes are used for inflammations, infections, and allergy symptoms, so require antiinflammatory, cool antiseptic herbs such as Chamomile flower, Eyebright herb, Goldenrod herb, Fennel seed, Meadowsweet herb, Goldenseal root, or Elder flower. Make sure the wash is completely free of herb particles because those can irritate the eyes. Essential oils are contraindicated in eye baths.
- *Douches.* These are a vaginal wash using herbal tea preparations, diluted tinctures, or essential oils in water. Douching is useful for acute infections, itching, and soothing irritation but use it for no longer than a week, once a day. Excessive douching disrupts the normal healthy vaginal flora and the pH, which can cause further infection. Douche bags can be purchased in drug stores. FYI: Vinegar douches, once popular as a post-sex birth control method, are extremely unreliable.
    - *For cervicitis or yeast infections,* use Goldenseal root, Oregon Grape root, *Phellodendron* Huang Bai, or *Coptis* Huang Lian (Goldthread root). Powdered acidophilus may be dissolved in a tea. Essential oils of Myrrh, Tea Tree, Cinnamon, or Savory work nicely.
    - *For bacterial vaginal discharges and itching,* use astringents and disinfectants such as Plantain leaf, Yarrow flower, Cranesbill root, Stone root, essential oils of Lavender, Sage, or Sandalwood.

Capsules and Suppositories

Capsules

Capsules or *gelcaps* are containers for filling and administration of dry, powdered herbs. They are usually made of vegetable gelatin. They come in two sizes: small 0 caps and larger double 00 caps. Small 0 caps are good for children if they will or can swallow one and for administering strong herbs when you need only small amounts, such as Goldenseal root, Lobelia herb, Wormwood herb, or Cayenne pepper. Large double 00 caps are better for use by adults. For amounts of dried powered herb needed for a 1- or 2-week supply of capsules, see Box 6.2.

Capsules can be filled by hand. First, powder the herb finely. Mix the simple herb or the various powdered herbs of the formula together well. Take apart the capsule. Fill the bottom portion and push top half down over bottom. Alternately, there are little capsule-making machines available from herb catalogs, which are basically two flat pieces with 12 to 24 holes (see Figs. 6.1 and 6.2).

• BOX 6.2 Capsule Making Machine and Amount of Dried Herb Needed to Fit in Capsules

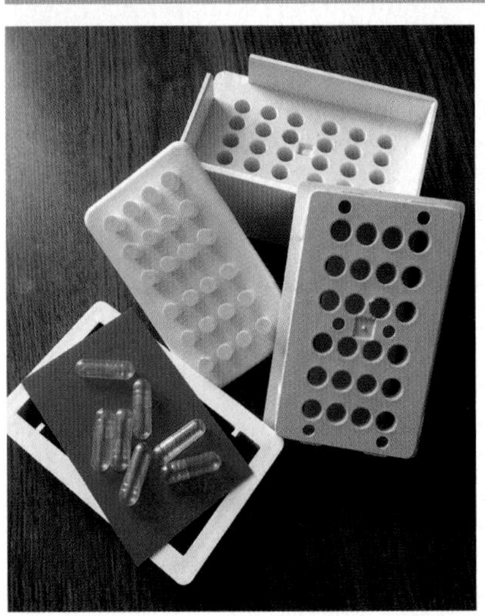

Capsule making machine showing upper and lower halves with capsule holes, tamping tool, green spreader, and empty capsules on the stand.

- Two small 0 size caps equals 1 large double 00 size cap.
- 1 oz finely ground herb fills about 60 single 0 caps.
- 1 oz finely ground herb fills about 30 double 00 caps.
- One double 00 cap holds about 1/4 teaspoon or 0.5 g of dried finely powdered herb.

Dose: Average adult dose is 2 double 00 caps 2-3 times daily. For children: one double 00 cap, or 2 single 0 caps 2-3 times daily. Take with juice or water, as you would any pill.

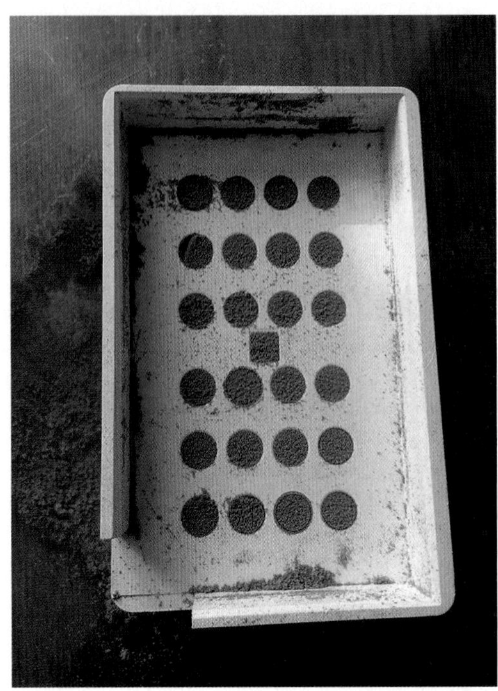

• **Fig. 6.1** Making capsules. Lower half of capsule filled with Turmeric powder.

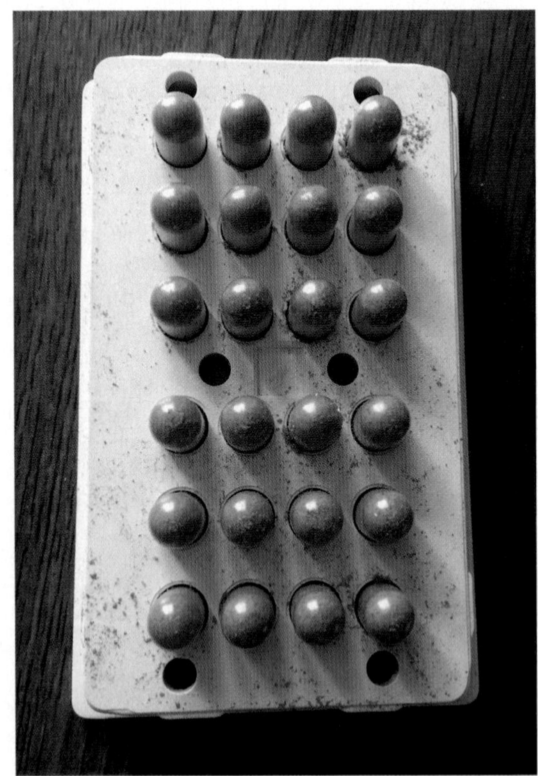

• **Fig. 6.2** Turmeric capsules assembled in capsule making machine.

Place bottom half of the capsules in the holes of one piece and the top half of the capsule in the holes of the other flat piece. After filling, the top and bottom pieces are tamped down, fitted together, and voilà, you have many filled capsules (Fig. 6.3).

Like anything else, there are benefits and drawbacks with capsule administration. From an apothecary standpoint, capsule-making can be rather time-consuming. If the adult dose is 2 capsules 3 times daily, that's 6 a day, or 84 capsules needed for a 2-week supply.

- *Capsule benefit.* Good for small amounts of herb, such as 1/2 to 3 g (a minuscule amount).
- *Capsule benefit.* Hides nasty and bitter tastes, as in Chinese antibacterials that clear heat, like Andrographis Chuan Xin Lian (Heart-thread Lotus leaf) or Coptis Huang Lian (Goldthread root), Western Goldenseal root, Creosote/Chaparral leaf, or intensely bitter Ayurvedic *Boswellia serrata* (Frankincense resin). Halitosis-producing Garlic bulb would be another good herb to encapsulate.
- *Capsule benefit.* Capsules are convenient to take, and they travel well. No broken bottles. Herbalists may have better compliance with clients' taking them over long periods of time. Taking some herb is better than taking no herb.
- *Capsule benefit.* Capsules are an option for people who cannot ingest alcohol.
- *Capsule drawback.* Capsules are bit of trouble for the herbalists to make.
- *Capsule drawback.* Capsules have a short shelf life. Dried herbs dry out quickly and lose their potency. Make sure the herbs you use are fresh to begin with. Purchased powdered herbs off the shelf or from an herb company can be old before you start. Capsules made with potent herbs should last a year if kept in a cool, dark place.
- *Capsule drawback.* Absorption (in my experience) is not as good as with tinctures. The body has to first dissolve the

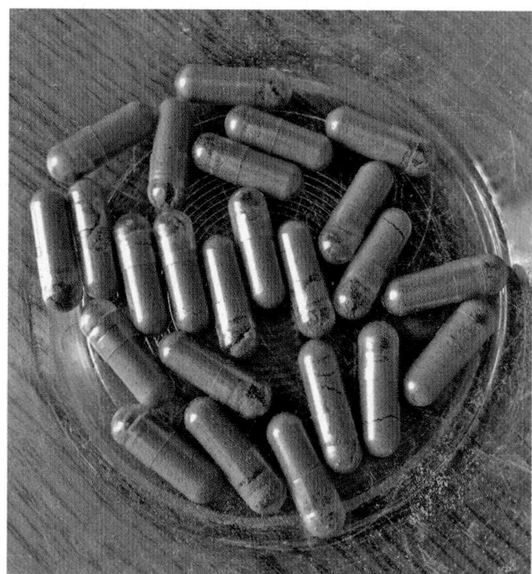

• **Fig. 6.3** Turmeric capsules, 24 made at once.

capsule, and then the plant material needs to be broken down and digested. This process is especially difficult if the herb is not finely and evenly ground up or if there are little bits of stem or root left in small chunks.

Suppositories

A ***suppository***, or a *bolus*, is a single-dose preparation inserted into the rectum or vagina. Suppositories can be effectively used locally for rectal hemorrhoids or for vaginal infections. Because these orifices are quite vascular, the herb will affect the tissues it touches and also enter the systemic circulation through the capillaries to affect related parts. This is the principle of the allopathic rectal suppository Phenergan, which is used for nausea when a pill taken by mouth would cause emesis. Rectal suppositories, the best route for systemic relief from pain or fever, are easy to administer to infants and children.

To make suppositories, ground herbal material is mixed in a melted cocoa butter base to form a paste and then molded into the appropriate shape. Molds can be purchased or made from a simple foil tube. Store suppositories in the refrigerator because cocoa butter easily melts when inserted. They're messy, but effective. Have clients wear old underwear or have them apply menstrual pads to recover leakage and protect bedding and clothing. Put a towel on the sheet. For hemorrhoids, use tightening astringent herbs, such as White Oak bark or Witch Hazel leaf. For vaginal yeast infections, use antifungals, like Pau d'arco bark, Oregon Grape root, or Creosote herb. Saw Palmetto berry and Echinacea root work for prostatitis.

External Plasters, Poultices, Compresses, and Preparation

Plasters

A ***plaster*** is a long-lasting oil-based or wax-based medication applied topically. It allows for continuous, slow absorption through the skin and is combined with internal remedies. The end product is supposed to be thick, soft, and waxy, so it will adhere to the skin. In general, a plaster base is made of beeswax, paraffin, lanolin, or castor oil that is melted together and cooled while being mixed constantly. Essential oils or powdered herbs are then added. If the herbs in the plaster are hot and irritating, oil should be rubbed on the skin before applying. A famous hot plaster is the Mustard seed plaster. Mustard is very hot and irritates the skin, acting as a counterirritant. It must be mixed with cool (not hot) water, so the enzymes stay activated. It is then diluted with cornmeal, flaxseed, or flour, so it does not blister the skin.

Poultices

A ***poultice*** is a relative of the plaster. It is a soft, mushy, external application of herbs made into a paste using hot water, spread thickly on or in a cloth and applied hot to the skin. For a cooling poultice, use cool water. A poultice must be changed often and can be used repeatedly if reheated each time. Moist heat drives the medicinal properties into the skin, so they must be kept warm and damp. Herbs (best fresh) are chopped, mashed, or bruised, mixed with hot water or hot apple cider vinegar (ACV). Once it has become soft, warm, and moist, the poultice is applied to the skin. The major three herbs for poultices are Calendula flower, Comfrey root and leaf, and Plantain leaf.[1] *Calendula officinalis* is for cleansing and healing wounds, and it is antibacterial and antiinflammatory. *Symphytum officinale* (Comfrey root and leaf) is the ultimate healer for wounds, ligaments, tendons, and bones. *Plantago* spp. (Plantain leaf) removes pain, draws out toxins from stings, and staunches bleeding.

Other than water or ACV, bentonite clay can be added to a poultice for thickening. Two parts tincture to one-part water are added to the clay to make a paste of a peanut butter consistency. Poultices may be used on the mouth, teeth, and gums to reduce inflammation, for drawing out splinters, to bring pimples to a head, and for infected sores (Box 6.3).

Compresses

A ***compress*** or ***fomentation*** is composed of hot or cold water-soaked herbs applied externally with a cloth. Make a strong or double-strength tea and soak a piece of white flannel, absorbent sock, or cloth into the hot or cold-water solution. Wring out and apply lightly over the body part. Air must be allowed to circulate through the cloth, which helps retain heat. Keep moist. You may cover it with a heating pad or ice pack as indicated. Keep compress moist and change often, just like a poultice. Cold compresses clear heat, edema, and inflammation. Arnica flower would be a good choice. Warm compresses restore heat in cold conditions, such as weakness, fatigue, cramps, muscles spasms, or pain. Alternating hot and cold compresses helps bruising, sprains, edema, menstrual cramps (pelvic congestion), engorged breasts, and tumors.[2]

External Salves, Creams, and Lotions Differentiated

Salves

Salves are also called *ointments and unguents*. Salves are a semisolid, fatty herbal mixture prepared for external use and made from a wax

• BOX 6.3 Poultice Ideas

TO AVOID THE "MESSY POULTICE" PROBLEM, USE TWO TUBE SOCKS

Put powdered or chopped fresh herbal materials into two clean, white, cotton socks tied shut at the top. Alternate use. Place sock in bowl and pour hot water over prefilled sock to soak the dry herb or heat up the fresh herb. Knead sock until herbs are mixed and hot. Apply to affected area until poultice is cool. Repeat with the other sock, back and forth. Maintain hot applications.

EYE POULTICE

The above sock method is used, substituting two small muslin tea bags. (These are available in herbal catalogs and health food stores.) Chamomile herb, Eyebright herb, Fennel seed, and Red Raspberry leaf are some eye disinfectants. Good for styes, pink eye, and irritations.

PLANTAIN POULTICE

The ultimate first aid poultice when out on the land. Boil water. Wet some broad- or narrow-leaf Plantain leaves (*Plantago* spp.). They grow all over the planet in wet areas. Apply and tie with bandanna or Ace wrap or gauze pad or plastic bag and tape. Plantain draws out splinters, toxins from wounds and bites. Stops pain from stings, bug bites, spider bites, dog bites, and snake bites; and soothes inflammation; and staunches bleeding. If you don't have tape or gauze available, crush the leaves with a tiny bit of water until wet and plop on area. Messy, but it works. In the case of tick bites, pull tick straight out first. For bee stings, remove stinger by sliding edge of credit card or equivalent along skin up to stinger and nudging it out.

HONEY POULTICE

Put honey on a minor burn after the burn has been rinsed with cold water. Honey soothes, cools, and moistens; is antiseptic; pulls water from a wound (hygroscopic); and seals off burns from air. Alternately for burns, apply a split-open Aloe Vera leaf, gel side down, if you have one.

and oil base. They are prepared over low heat and then poured into individual containers to cool (Chapter 7). The average herbal salve uses a fixed oil, such as sesame, olive, or almond, in combination with a wax, such as beeswax, which is responsible for the thickening, hardening element. The herbal component comes from essential oils or previously prepared fresh or dried macerated oils like Arnica flower, Calendula flower, or Chickweed herb.[1] A ***balm*** is a salve that contains a lot of volatile oils. Examples are various lip balms that use Peppermint, Camphor, or Tea Tree essential oils for their refreshing and stimulating effects.

Body heat melts the wax in a salve, and the oil provides quick absorption through the skin. Salves melt quickly in hot cars and keep best in cooler locations. Salves do not appreciate constant alternating cooling and reheating. Medicinally, salves can cool and soothe skin inflammations such as sores, cuts, and fungal infections. Marshmallow root, Slippery Elm bark, Selfheal herb, and Chickweed herb do well for these purposes. For damp heat skin conditions, such as eczema or boils, use Calendula flower, Mugwort herb, Chickweed, and Comfrey leaf. For psoriasis, use Nettle herb or Cleavers herb. To protect and heal wounds from cuts, sprains, or abrasions, use Calendula flower, Arnica flower, and Selfheal herb. For varicose veins, use astringents, such as Calendula flower, Horse Chestnut seed, or Witch Hazel leaf.

Creams and Lotions

Creams and ***lotions*** are both moisturizers that are combinations of fat and water, which will separate, so consequently need to be stabilized or emulsified. This can be done by carefully pouring the oil into the water in a thin constant stream while agitating (Chapter 7). A cream is a light oil preparation emulsified with a medicated liquid. A lotion is just a thinner, more liquid cream. In comparison with salves, lotions and creams are a bit more challenging to make because you are combining oil and water. Salves do not contain water, just fat.

Creams and lotions are used extensively in the cosmetics industry but can be herbally medicated for healthier skin care. Herbwise, the same medicinals for salves are used in creams and lotions. Herbs can be added in tincture, hydrosol, or essential oil form. Emulsifiers may be lanolin derived from sheep's wool, vegetable glycerin, or lecithin—fatty substances in plants and animals. Beeswax used alone is not a true emulsifier and may be used as a thickener and hardener that holds the oil-water emulsion in suspension (unless it's left in the sun and melts in the heat).

Tinctures

A ***tincture*** is an alcohol or alcohol and water preparation suitable for roots, seeds, fruits, or herbs. They are ***macerations*** (soaks) that are then strained or pressed. Like capsules or teas, there are always advantages and disadvantages. When deciding whether a tincture is the best delivery system for a client, consider the following points.

- *Tinctures have a long shelf life.* Alcohol is the best-ever preservative and kills bacteria. Therefore, alcoholic tinctures last in the apothecary for years to decades. A dried herb in a jar has about a year of viability for aerial parts and about 3 years for roots stored in tight-fitting containers, out of direct exposure to light, air, and heat.
- *Tinctures provide fast delivery.* Tinctures require very little digestion and move quickly into the bloodstream.
- *Tinctures are concentrated.* Tinctures, percolations, and extracts are very strong medicine. A little goes a long way. Average dose of a standard tincture is 3 to 4 mL 3 times per day. That's about three squeezes of the dropper per dose, which is much quicker and easier than dealing with teas.
- *Tinctures and compliance.* Tinctures are easy to take. You can carry around your tincture in a pocket, pack, or purse with ease. A client typically gets a little 1-, 2-, or 4-oz bottle with a dropper top. Very convenient and beneficial for folks who have no time to work with teas. One swallow in a little water, and your dose has been taken.
- *Tinctures are consistent medicine.* Properly made, tinctures are very reliable as to potency.
- *Tinctures are not for alcohol intolerance.* Tinctures are not appropriate for alcoholics, those on Antabuse, and anyone with alcohol intolerance. For children, you can dilute a little in tea or juice. The amount of alcohol in a dose is minimal and won't hurt them, but if the parents are concerned, most of the alcohol can be evaporated off in hot water. If that's not an option, the child can be given teas or glycerites (Chapter 7).
- *Concentrated.* Tinctures are very strong-tasting. It's best to dilute when taking with a little water or juice. If people are expecting candy-coated pills, they may not tolerate a tincture.

Types of Menstruum Used as Tincture Solvents

In a tincture, the liquid solvent is called the ***menstruum***, and the solid plant part is the ***marc***. The word *marc* comes from the

French *marcher* (to trample, as on grapes). After the marc is trampled or pressed, the final result is a tincture. Tinctures have to macerate (soak) for about 2 weeks to 1 month and be shaken daily before pressing. They are very easy and foolproof to make and turn out consistently well (Chapter 7).

A tincture's solvent breaks down the plant cell wall by varying degrees, allowing its medicinal constituents to be released into the menstruum. Another solvent function is to act as a preservative. Solvents can be water, pure alcohol, vinegar, wine, brandy, vodka, gin, rum, or glycerin. Various solvents are discussed.

- *Water.* Known as the universal solvent. Water dissolves more substances than any other known liquid. Cold water dissolves sugars, proteins, mucilages, pectins, tannins, and mineral salts. Hot water causes tough plant tissues to swell and bursts open their tough, fibrous cells.[1] Hot or cold, water is the menstruum used for infusions and decoctions. In a tincture, water is part of the menstruum; the remainder will be some type of alcohol that extracts substances that water cannot and also acts as a preservative. Water does not preserve anything. A refrigerated water extract (tea) lasts only 1 to 2 days unless frozen.
- *Alcohol.* Alcohol is the best microbe destroyer and preservative available. Pure ingestible 95% to 100% medicinal-grade ethyl alcohol, also called ethanol, grain alcohol, and EtOH, may be obtained from a grain company. It contains ethane and will preserve a well-made tincture for up to 10 years or more, even with water added. Noningestible isopropyl alcohol (rubbing alcohol) contains propane, a cheap and poisonous cousin that can only be used externally.
  - Alcohol is a selective extractor and will extract non-water-soluble resins, alkaloids, and volatile oils. Unlike a water solvent, it will not extract gums, starches, mucilages, albumins, or some minerals. Alcohol will also inactivate enzymes that destroy alkaloids and glycosides and control chemical decomposition of glycosides and saponins, due to the presence of water.[1] When using alcohol, use the highest percentage possible. Vodka, for instance, is only 40% alcohol or 80-proof. Water plus alcohol, and water plus glycerin combine very well for use as a menstruum in any proportion.
- *Water plus alcohol.* This duo is used in tincture making extensively. They are combined in various proportions, determined by the chemical components of the particular herb in question (Chapter 7).
- ***Glycerin.*** This is the sweet faction of a fixed oil found in fats of plants and animals. In herbal preparations, we use vegetable glycerin (also spelled glycerine, as on the label shown in Fig. 6.4). Most commercial glycerin is derived from coconut oil. It is really a class of alcohol, and thus, a good preservative. It is not a carbohydrate and therefore contains no sugar. Glycerin is slowly metabolized by the liver and does not cause blood sugar imbalances.[1] Therefore, this is a possible solvent for diabetics because it does not raise glucose levels. Glycerin can be used alone or mixed with pure ethyl alcohol. It is syrupy, sweet, colorless, odorless, and antibacterial. It is a very good substitute for people who cannot tolerate or ingest alcohol and a great answer to the *yuck factor* for kids and adults. Glycerin extracts tannins very well but not alkaloids. Glycerol extractions are neither as strong as those containing alcohol, nor do they preserve as well.
- *Vinegar.* A ***vinegar*** is a sour-tasting liquid containing acetic acid obtained by fermenting dilute alcoholic liquids, such as wine, cider, or beer. Commonly used vinegars are apple cider, plum, rice, wine, or balsamic. Vinegars are sour because of their acetic acid content. They are chemically classed as an alcohol derivative due to being fermented. They make a good solvent and a fair preservative and can be substituted for alcohol in extract preparations. Vinegars can extract some alkaloids and water-soluble compounds. In comparison with alcohol, their preservative action is much weaker, and vinegars can decompose quickly due to their inherent vegetable matter.[1] Vinegars were once popular in the late 1800s but fell out of favor, only to enjoy a small revival among modern herbalists.
- *Wine.* Wines are lovely, tasty menstruums. The alcoholic content of wine is naturally low, about 14%, so they are weak in terms of extraction and preservative action. Sometimes adding a little extra alcohol to a wine or adding some brandy can improve preservative qualities. Historically, white wines were used as menstruums because of their smaller proportion of tannins.[1]

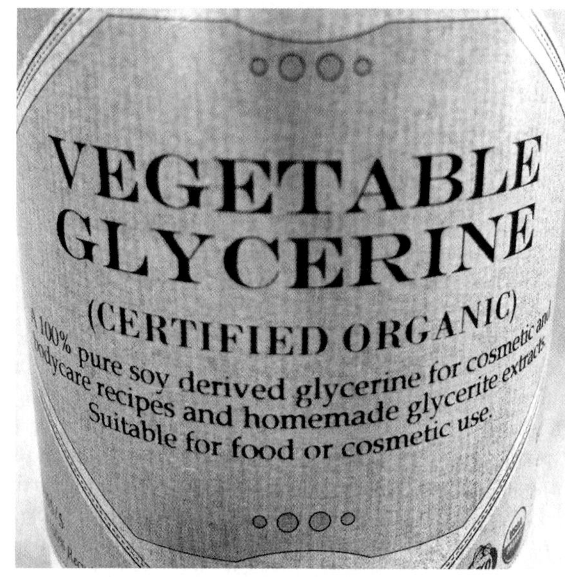

• **Fig. 6.4** Vegetable Glycerine solvent, a sweet, non-alcoholic menstruum.

Fixed oils are nonvolatile oils of plant or animal origin. They do not contain alcohol. They are not used in tinctures but appear in *medicated oils*. Herbalists commonly use olive, almond, avocado, and grapeseed fixed oils to extract ingredients from a plant. The plant material is eventually pressed out, leaving behind a medicated oil that can be used by itself for compresses, dropped warm into the ears, or added to other ingredients in lotions, salves, and creams.

- *Emulsification.* Oil and water don't mix, unless we force them to do so. Emulsification happens by vigorously beating the oil and liquid by hand or using an electric mixer until the oil breaks down into smaller droplets and forms a stable blend. Emulsifying substances added to herbal preparations include vegetable glycerin, lecithin, and lanolin. Chefs use egg yolk to emulsify the oil and the water when making mayonnaise.
- *Common herbs used in medicated oils.* Calendula flower, Comfrey root, Arnica flower, and St. John's wort herb are commonly used. Oils can spoil and become rancid without the addition of antioxidants and use of refrigeration. Essential oils are often added to salves and creams made with medicated oils to provide additional medicinal value and some antioxidant preservative action.

Other Types of Tinctures

An ***extract*** or *concentrate* is a very strong tincture. An extract can be twice as strong as a tincture. An equivalent dose would be smaller, so less alcohol would be ingested. An extract is a very efficient way to administer herbs. One problem with an extract is that it is hard to make with very fluffy or high-volume herbs. Some plants, like Red Clover flower or White Horehound herb, are extremely light and absorbent and will soak up menstruum like a sponge, requiring much more liquid than would be used for an extract. The proportions sound good on paper, but don't work in a practical herb-making setting for all herbs.

A ***percolation*** is another type of tincture. In the percolation method, the soluble constituents of an herb are extracted by slow passage of the solvent through a column or cone of dried, powdered plant that has been packed in a percolator. A favorite low tech, low investment percolator cone is an upside-down Perrier or sparkling water glass bottle with the bottom cut off. Expensive, more impressive-looking glass cones are also available from scientific supply stores. The menstruum flows down by gravity through the herb in the cone and into a collecting jar (Chapter 7). *Percs*, as they're affectionately called, make very concentrated, strong medicine. They can be made quickly in 24 hours or less, whereas the standard macerated tincture needs to sit for 2 weeks to a month. Percolations do not work with resinous plants such as Gumweed flower or Myrrh resin or with fresh plants that are gummy or mucilaginous. Resins clog the cone, and the menstruum will not flow through them. Fresh plants have too much water and volume. Percs work best with finely and evenly ground, dried plant material that doesn't expand much when moistened.

A ***liniment*** is an external, thin, medicated tincture that is rubbed or massaged into the skin. The menstruum, the liquid portion, can be vinegar, ethyl alcohol, or isopropyl alcohol. Liniments used for muscular-skeletal pain usually have a warming effect and are used for myalgia, neuralgia, numbness, soreness, sciatic pain, or muscle spasm (Box 24.4). Likely muscle pain herbal candidates are Panax San Qi (Notoginseng root), Cayenne fruit, Prickly Ash bark, Ginger root, and essential oils of Marjoram, Peppermint, Birch, Wintergreen, or Ginger. For closed injuries, swelling, and contusions, use Arnica flower, St. John's Wort, Tansy herb, or Marigold flower. For insect repellents, use Pennyroyal or Citronella essential oil.

Essential Oils

Essential oils are steam or water distillations of aromatic plants that are extremely concentrated and strong. *Distillation* refers to converting a liquid into a vapor and then condensing it back into a liquid form. Examples of plants used for steam or water distillations or cold pressing of peels include aromatic Peppermint and Eucalyptus leaf, Lemon and Tangerine peel, Hyssop herb, Rose petal, Lavender herb, Cinnamon bark, and Myrrh and Frankincense resins. ***Aromatherapy*** is the use of essential oils for healing and is a subspecialty of clinical herbalism. It can constitute an entire study on its own. An excellent reference is by Australian aromatherapist, Salvatore Battaglia.[7]

The distillation process for essential oils requires a lot of expensive equipment, time, and skill and is not in the realm of simple homemade tinctures and ointments. Medicated oils made in the kitchen by most herbalists are different and were described earlier. They are macerations, not distillations. Do not confuse the two. Most herbalists and aromatherapists purchase essential oils from suppliers or distilleries that do the actual production and have all the equipment for production and quality testing. Essential oils are very strong medicinally and may be used externally or topically—even internally, as long as they're of high food-grade quality. They are also added to creams and salves in drop-by-drop amounts.

Essential oils contain potent constituents of the plants and can be highly effective physiologically as antiinfectives, antiseptics, and relaxants and for healing skin conditions. They have powerful psychological and emotional effects and are used to treat depression, anxiety, memory issues, and emotional issues. The nose leads to the olfactory bulb and the limbic system in the brain, which houses the amygdala where emotional memories are stored. When we inhale an aroma through the nose, these brain areas are stimulated.

Because essential oils are so strong, only tiny doses are needed: 1 to 2 drops at a time is a approximate amount. This dosage of course varies, depending on the particular oil, its potency, and its recommended use. For instance, Lavender is a mild one, generally safe for babies, whereas Oregano is much stronger and could burn the skin unless mixed and diluted with an inert vegetable carrier oil, such as olive oil or grape-seed oil. No matter which is chosen, it is always recommended to test a drop in a small spot (as on the back of the hand) to determine whether there are any reactions like redness, burning, or allergy. Redheads, fair-skinned individuals, babies, and elders tend to be more sensitive than others. It is best to dilute essential oils for use on babies, children younger than 12 years old, our elders, and those on heavy medication. Controversy exists on safe usage by pregnant women.

Quality Control of Essential Oils

Quality control is an important factor when using essential oils. The cheap versions are just that, often adulterated and of bad quality, filled with artificial additives, common in the fragrance industry. This is notoriously true of Lavender, which is not always what it seems. Lavender essential oil must contain a certain percentage of the terpene linalool to be of good quality. Reliable and effective therapeutic results can be obtained only if essential oils are pure and contain the correct chemical substances in proper amounts to provide healing results. These pure varieties are often much more expensive than cheaper, contaminated versions. You get what you pay for.

The most reliable standards of essential oil quality have either an Association French Normalization Organization Regulation (AFNOR) certification from the French Standardization Association or an International Organization for Standardization (ISO) designation. These entities perform chemical analysis of essential oils and report what a given batch contains. If an oil passes AFNOR or ISO standards, it contains the correct chemical constituents at therapeutic levels. The best we have in the United States is a Generally Regarded as Safe (GRAS) status that comes from the U.S. Food and Drug Administration (FDA) (Chapter 29). It issues a long list of oils considered safe as food additives and that can thus be ingested without harm.[8] However, GRAS does not provide chemical breakdowns, whereas companies that use AFNOR or IOS standards can provide certificates of analysis (Box 6.4).

Other Essential Oil Facts

- *External use.* Essential oils are fat soluble and therefore absorb quickly through the fatty subcutaneous skin layer into the bloodstream. A drop applied ***neat*** (undiluted) absorbs quickly. Traditionally, external applications were and still are used in the

• BOX 6.4 Criteria and Methods to Assure Quality Essential Oils

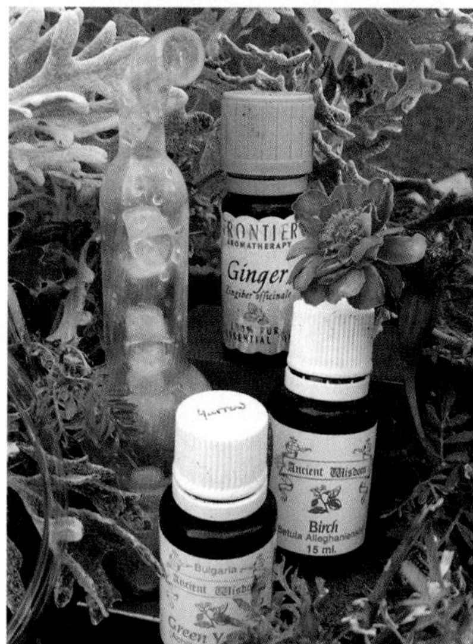

Assorted essentail oils and a glass diffuser.

TO ASSURE QUALITY ESSENTIAL OILS:

- Determine evidence of chemical analysis from AFNOR or IOS.
- Buy from companies owned by certified aromatherapists or essential oil specialists, who have relations with distillers and can supply a batch-specific specification report for each oil it sells and can also provide material safety data sheets.
- Determine longevity of supplier. If the company has been around a long time and is known and used by other aromatherapy practitioners and educators, it's a safe bet.
- Assess the price. The essential oil should be within expected price range. For instance, If it's much cheaper than any other normally expensive Frankincense brands you can find, it's probably a bad quality, adulterated oil.
- Trust your intuition. Always smell and experience a company's oils yourself. Lemon Balm from one source can smell quite different from that of another company.
- Frequent health food stores to sniff and compare. This is fun and educational.

United Kingdom. Most remedies discussed in essential oil texts are for external use only in the form of skin applications, steams, sprays, air diffusers, in baths, lotions, creams, or cosmetics.

- *Application.* Apply to the forehead or temples for a headache, or to the abdomen for a stomachache, etc. Essential oils are effective when rubbed over acupuncture or acupressure points. The soles of the feet are one of the safest areas because the skin there is thicker and the fat pads on the ball of the foot allow quick penetration.[9] For this reason, reflexologists frequently apply them on the foot reflexes. Herbalists can rarely go wrong or do harm with external applications, as long as skin sensitivity is tested with a drop or two.
- *External dosage.* (See Appendix A for essential oil doses.) Essential oils can be used as swabs, as compresses, in baths, or as direct applications to a wound or bug bite with a cotton applicator. One to three drops mixed with 1/2 teaspoon pure vegetable oil is a good starting point.[9] If used for massage, add 10 to 25 drops per ounce of almond or avocado carrier oil. Suggestions for use are stimulating Peppermint, relaxing Lavender, or anxiety-reducing Lemon Balm.
- *Internal use.* Internal use is traditional in France but is discouraged by many practitioners in the United States. Since it is more controversial than external usage, more care is required because essential oils are such strong substances. Make sure any oils used internally are pure and of the highest medicinal quality, as explained above. The GRAS status list has at least 100 essential oils deemed safe for internal use. Examples include three species of Chamomile flower; Rose family members like Rose petals, Citrus peel, and Almond; six species of Cinnamon bark; Ginger; Licorice; and Mint family associates like Hyssop, Horehound, Thyme, Basil, Lavender, Garden Sage, and, of course, Peppermint and Spearmint.
- *Internal dosage.* Two or three drops per 8-hour period. Dilute in a fat, milk, or honey base.[9] For use in tinctures, my experience has been that 1 drop of a mild GRAS-approved essential oil per 1 oz of tincture is a safe and effective ballpark amount. This helps with flavor and is a nice way to add a good dose of medicine and aroma and still leaves room in the bottle for other botanicals. I have never had a problem with this regimen. Some of my favorite and safe choices for use in tinctures are relaxing Lavender, anxiety-relieving Lemon Balm, carminative Tangerine or Fennel, airway-opening Peppermint or Hyssop, and female balancing Clary Sage or Geranium.
- *Douche* dosage. Twenty drops of essential oil to 1 pint warm water plus 1 tablespoon of ACV to maintain acid pH if indicated, once per day for 1 week.

Hydrosols

Hydrosols are an offspring of steam distillations of aromatic plants, the essential oils. They are an aromatic water and volatile oil combination. In a hydrosol, the process of distillation is used to separate the liquid parts (the water and volatile oils) from the solid parts of the plant. The result is a gentle aromatic water combined with a volatile oil. The smell is fragrant and delectable. Because it has a water base, it is not nearly as strong as an essential oil.

The method of making a hydrosol involves the setting up a primitive home still (Figs. 6.5 and 6.6).[1] The still consists of an enameled canning pot into which the plant material is simmered; the condenser is the lid of the canning pot placed upside-down on the pot with ice on top; the receiver is a bowl placed inside the pot on a stainless-steel folding steamer-basket insert with the handle removed. This ingenious setup is easily created at home.

Hydrosols are safe to drink and may be taken internally. Incidentally, they are the best choice for use on animals; pure essential oils are too strong. They also make excellent water bases for making creams, lotions, syrups, and fomentations. Store hydrosols in the refrigerator in tightly sealed sterilized bottles. A Lavender hydrosol in a pretty spray bottle would make a glorious gift.

Syrups

A ***syrup*** is a thick, sweet liquid that is a saturated solution of sugar in pure water or other aqueous liquid. The sugar (sucrose) acts as a preservative but must be used in adequate concentrations. If not enough is used in the syrup, the mixture attracts bacteria. If used near saturation point, the sugar in a water solution acts as a preservative, stopping the growth of microorganisms, especially yeasts and molds.[1] If the sugar content reaches concentration, the sugar can crystallize as it cools, which is then very difficult to redissolve. In the days before refrigeration, this preservative quality of sugar was greatly valued. If a syrup is refrigerated, it will last longer, maybe 1 to 2 years. Syrups can

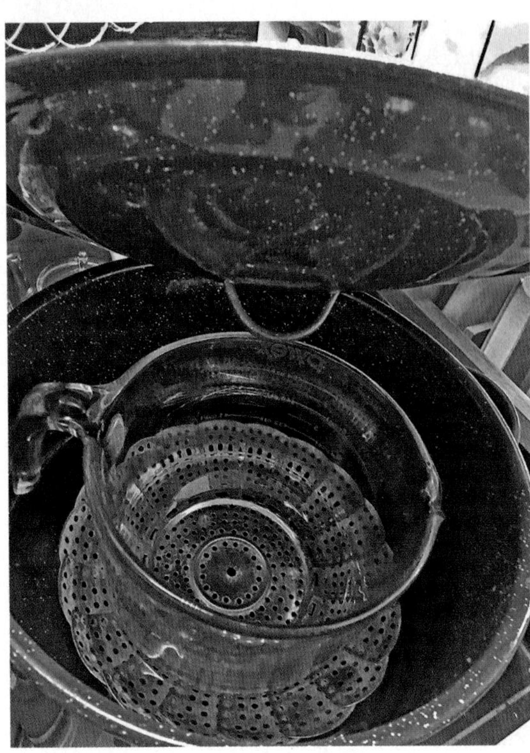

• **Fig. 6.5** Homemade still for making hydrosols. Set-up involves a large enamel pot and a tempered glass measuring cup placed on adjustable steamer basket.

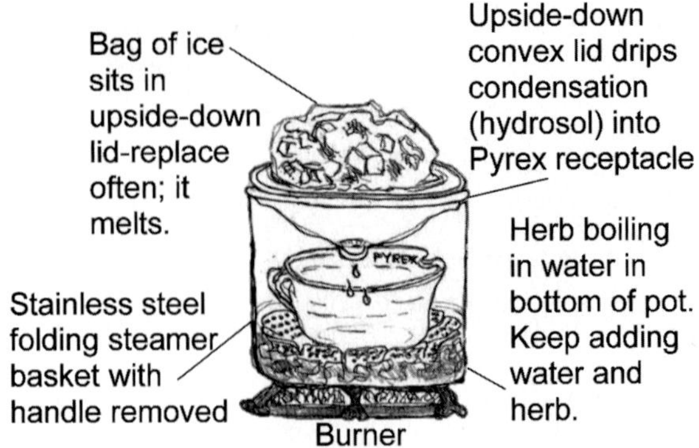

• **Fig. 6.6** Homemade hydrosol still diagram.

ferment and spoil if the glass containers used are not perfectly clean, preferably sterilized by boiling.

Syrups are used for soothing irritated lungs, throats, stomachs, and intestines. Their absorption is gentle and gradual—good for children, elders, and individuals who are weak. They are beneficial for any inflamed conditions that reflect as dryness—dry coughs, constipation, and sore throats. Common types are herbal cough syrups (often with brandy) with wild cherry concentrate added. Elderberry syrup is classic for early-onset colds and fever. Garlic syrup is good for coughs and lung congestion. The herbs chosen for a syrup should reflect the therapeutic intention. Dose is typically 1 teaspoon as needed.

- *Simple syrup*. An unmedicated syrup made with water and sugar, honey, glycerin, or combinations thereof. Think of it as the base for the other types.
- *Medicated syrups*. A simple syrup with a medicinal herb added.
- *Dried herb syrup*. This method uses dried herbs. An herbal infusion or decoction is simmered down to one-half the original quantity. This is then added to and simmered with the basic syrup.
- *Cordial*. A syrup with one part tincture to three parts simple syrup is a ***cordial***.
- *Oxymel*. A specialized sweet and sour herbal honey. In an ***oxymel***, a sweet honey is mixed with a little sour vinegar. This mixture becomes the carrier for infusions, decoctions, and tinctures.
- *Electuary*. An ***electuary*** is also known as a confection or conserve. Nasty tasting, finely ground herbs are disguised by adding honey or fruit pulp and shaped into marble sized bites. Modern examples of an ***electuary*** are edibles known as *Brain Balls* and *Love Balls*, made with herbs good for each body area, plus the addition of some yummy carob, chocolate chips, coconut flakes, nuts and nut butters, seeds, and/or dried fruit. You can have fun with this one. Trick or treat?
- *Spirits or essences*. Combinations of food-grade essential oils and grain alcohol are ***spirits***. These preparations may be added to syrups, used alone as a flavoring agent, or diluted into syrups, tinctures, honeys, and elixirs.
- *Honeys*. Thick honey is used as a base with herbs added. Glycerin can be added, as can essential oils such as Cinnamon, Ginger, or Peppermint. Use 1 to 2 drops essential oil to 1/4 cup honey. If too strong, add more honey.

Summary

The more you try out various types of herbal preparations, the more comfortable you will become at making them for yourself and others. The best way to fully understand a preparation method is to make it yourself a few times and then to teach someone else. If you recommend that your client prepare a decoction at home, be able to provide clear directions.

Determining the type of remedy to use is based on the condition and age of your client, route of administration, intention, and degree of compliance. Often a combination of remedies works best. The most basic ones are water-based teas—infusions and decoctions.

Essential oils are highly concentrated steam or water distillations that require specialized equipment to produce. Safe usage and the need for unadulterated, high-quality products are important. Essential oils are different from simple medicated oils that are macerated at home by most herbalists. A tincture is an herb that is soaked in some type of menstruum (various solvents) and then pressed to obtain the liquid remedy. Menstruums may be alcohol, water, glycerin, wine, brandy, vinegar, fixed oil, or combinations. They extract different constituents and have varying preservative abilities. A syrup is a thick, sweet, saturated solution of sugar in pure water or other aqueous liquid. Sweet syrup bases can be made into medicated syrups, oxymels, cordials, and electuaries.

Review

Fill in the Blanks

(Answers in Appendix B.)

1. Name five different menstruums. ___, ___, ___, ___, ___.
2. Name five kinds of baths. ___, ___, ___, ___, ___.
3. Name two preparations for which double strength decoctions could be used. ___, ___.
4. Tincture proportions are ___. Extract or concentrate proportions are ___.
5. Ethyl alcohol is for ___ use. It is used to make ___ and contains the chemical ___.
6. Isopropyl alcohol is for ___ use. It is used to make ___ and contains the chemical ___.
7. Name three uses for a base syrup. ___, ___, ___.
8. Arrange the following menstruums from most preservative to least. Water, glycerin, vinegar, alcohol.
9. A salve has a ___ base. A cream has a ___ and ___ base and requires ___ to mix the two.
10. When using alcohol and water to make a tincture, the process involved is called a ___. The solvent is called the ___ and the pressed-out plant material is the ___.

Critical Concept Questions

(Answers for you to decide.)

1. Give client instructions for how to prepare a fresh Dandelion leaf tea.
2. Give client instructions for preparation of a fresh Dandelion leaf and Red Clover blossom tea.
3. Ms. Jones asked if she should give her 6-month-old daughter any honey. You say?
4. Explain the difference between a poultice, a compress, a plaster, and a fomentation.
5. In what situations would you choose a tea over a tincture?
6. Discuss the benefits and drawbacks of an herbal capsule. Contrast the two sizes.
7. A client has a cold but cannot ingest any alcohol. What are your options?
8. Your client has pinkeye. Explain how to prepare and administer an eye wash.
9. How can an herbalist use essential oils? Are they herbs? How is quality assessed?

References

1. Green, James. *The Herbal Medicine-Maker's Handbook* (New York: Crossing Press, 2002).
2. Holmes, Peter. *Energetics of Western Herbs* (Boulder CO: Snow Lotus, 2006).
3. Hoffman, David. *Medical Herbalism: The Science and Practice of Herbal Medicine* (Rochester, VT: Healing Arts, 2003).
4. Dharmananda, Subhuti. Institute for Traditional Medicine. "Dosage and Form of Herbs." http://www.itmonline.org/arts/dosage.htm (accessed September 17, 2019).
5. Gladstar, Rosemary. *Herbal Recipes for Vibrant Health* (North Adams, Maine: Storey, 2008).
6. "Infant Botulism—Why Babies Should Not Eat Honey." Wholesome Baby Food. http://wholesomebabyfood.momtastic.com/infantbotulismhoney.htm (accessed September 17, 2019).
7. Battaglia, Salvatore. *The Complete Guide to Aromatherapy* (Australia: Black Pepper Creative, 2018).
8. "How to Determine the Quality of Essential Oils." *Mother Earth News*. https://www.motherearthnews.com/natural-health/determine-the-quality-of-essential-oils-part-2-zbcz1509 (accessed September 19, 2019).
9. *People's Desk Reference for Essential Oils* (Essential Oil Publishing Company, 1999).

7

Preparation of Tinctures, Infused Oils, Salves, Lotions, Creams, and Syrups

"Herbs ought to be distilled when they are in their greatest vigor, and so ought Flowers also."

—Nicholas Culpeper, English herbalist, botanist, and physician.

CHAPTER REVIEW

- Apothecary equipment: Jar assortments, other tools, and labels.
- Folk method and weight-to-volume tincture discussion and preparation. Alcohol. Solubility, determining alcohol to water percentages in a menstruum and plant to menstruum ratios.
- Directions for weight-to-volume tincture making: Practice calculations for custom weight-to-volume menstruums.
- Directions for preparing percolations, dual extractions, and glycerites.
- Worksheets for internal preparations.
- Infused oil preparations: low heat, accelerated blender version, and sun oil.
- Directions for preparing salves, lotions, creams, and syrups.

KEY TERMS

Cream
Dual extraction
Ethyl alcohol
Fixed oil
Folk method
Glycerin
Isopropol alcohol
Lotion
Maceration
Marc
Menstruum
Percolation
Polar
Polarity
Precipitation
Proof
Rancidity
Salve
Sandcastle
Solubility
Syrup
Tincture
Weight-to-volume method (w/v)

This chapter covers the basics, the nitty-gritty how-to of making advanced herbal preparations. The list includes various types of tinctures, glycerites, infused oil preparations, salves, creams, lotions, and syrups—a large project. Try them little by little, and you'll soon have your own apothecary in the works. Refer further to *The Herbal Medicine-Maker's Handbook* by James Green, a classic, practical reference for the ins and outs and pitfalls of making herbal remedies.[1]

Before beginning, please review the definitions and general information already covered. (Chapter 6). The steps in the present chapter can be viewed as a practical, hands-on lab. The content provides the benefits of my practical experience and that of others, complete with worksheets and record-keeping methods, so you can always refer to it and look back to see how a remedy turned out and what might be done next time to improve results.

Apothecary Equipment

Most herbalists begin their medicine-making experiences in their school labs or at home in their kitchens, where we have traditionally worked. Eventually, this endeavor could extend into an industrial kitchen that meets health department regulations for food

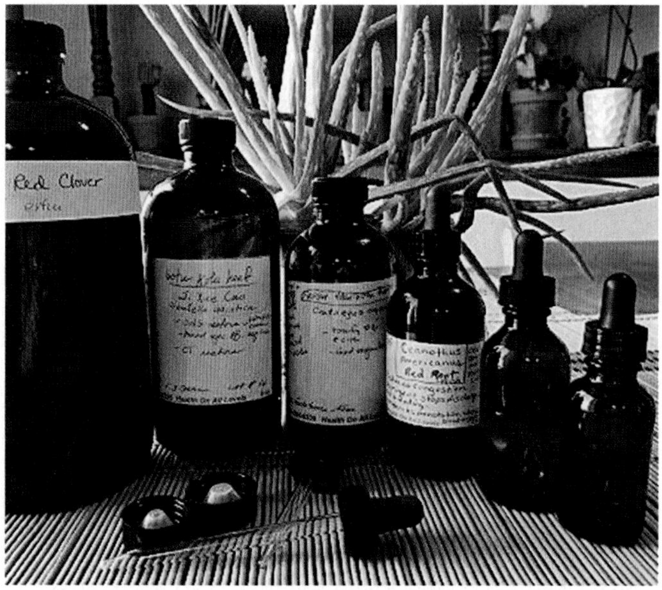

• **Fig. 7.1** Boston rounds in various sizes with caps and droppers.

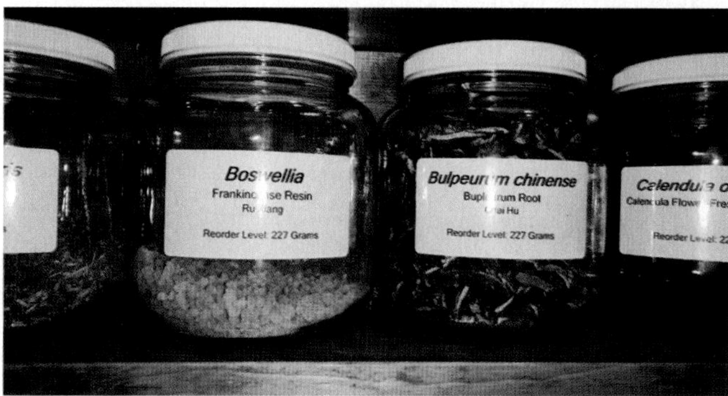

• **Fig. 7.2** Wide mouth half gallon jars holding dried herbs.

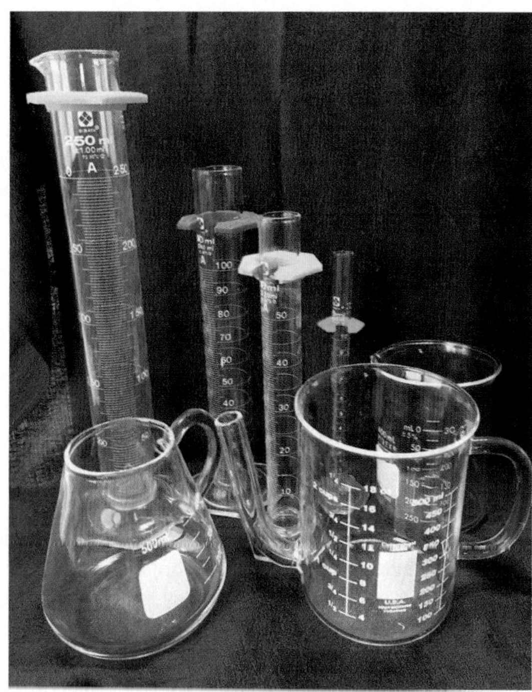

• **Fig. 7.3** Graduated cylinders and assorted beakers.

preparation. But first things first. Begin low tech with a few well-chosen utensils; many are already in most kitchens. If possible, reserve a separate cabinet or area dedicated to medicine-making equipment. Choose natural materials of glass and stainless steel, ceramic, unchipped enamel, and wood—no plastic. Plastic stains can leech into the herbs. As you proceed, you will accumulate a variety of favorite utensils to make your processes fun and easier.

Jar Assortments

Jars and bottles are basic. They are needed to store tinctures, put up macerations, dispense remedies to clients, and hold herbs. A good place to start is the hardware store for the purchase of various sizes of wide-mouth Mason or Ball canning jars with two-part lids that have seals. Most useful are pint, quart, and half-gallon sizes. Get a case of pints (12), a case of quarts (12), and a case of half gallons (4). All canning jars can handle boiling water. To obtain half-gallon sizes with extremely wide mouths that are useful for tincture maceration, access a commercial bottling company and order a case of six. Save and recycle other jars. Collect them in all shapes and sizes, which look very artsy, eclectic, and fun on a shelf. Just be sure they're made of glass.

When you are ready to get a little more professional, turn to container companies. Amber glass Boston rounds that keep out light are the best options (Fig. 7.1). These come in 1- to 32-oz sizes. The 1-, 2-, and 4-oz bottles have matching droppers and are good for dispensing. The other sizes only come with lids.

Wide-mouth half-gallons with plastic lids are perfect for macerating and shaking tinctures and for storing and displaying dried herbs (Fig. 7.2). (Metal lids tend to rust.) They are generally available commercially in cases of six. Sometimes lids cost extra.

Other Tools

Measuring items are necessary. Glass Pyrex measuring cups with lips come in 1-, 2-, 4-, and 8-cup sizes. Get used to metric conversions (Appendix A). The measuring cups have a side showing measurements in ounces and the other side in milliliters. This design is helpful to get a sense of equivalents. Graduated milliliter cylinders from scientific supply companies are necessary for measuring out formulas. They come in a large range of sizes and are available in glass and plastic (Fig. 7.3). The glass ones are very esthetic but break easily. While you're still at the scientific supply store, purchase a 500-mL beaker, which comes in very handy. Add a set of stainless-steel measuring spoons.

Other practical tools are mixing spoons, choppers, strainers, stainless-steel funnels, graters, knives, cutting boards, bowls of many sizes, saucepans for salves and oils, a turkey baster, muslin cloth, rags, sponges, a box of latex or vinyl gloves, and a nice supply of zip-lock plastic bags and aluminum foil. In addition, an assortment of long-handled wooden stirring spoons is useful, and they feel good in the hands and work well (Fig. 7.4). Also helpful are large and small metal spoons. A fun place to visit is a restaurant supply store for ideas and good-quality utensils. Get a large

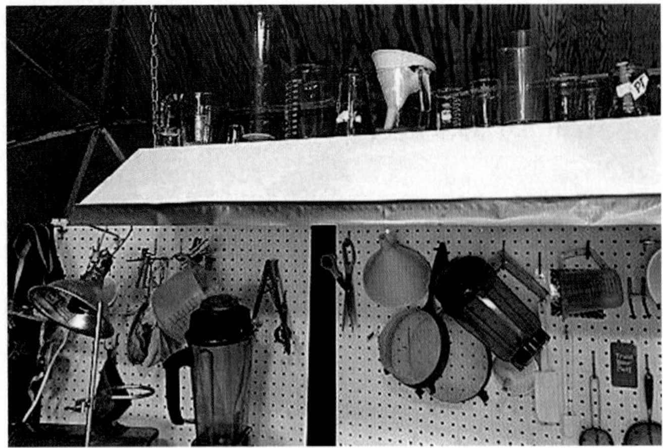

• **Fig. 7.4** Tools of the trade hanging on pegboard.

package of a dozen chopsticks. I love chopsticks. These are invaluable for poking, coaxing, and stirring. Strainers of many sizes and meshes, from fine to large holes are invaluable. A few decent knives are important. Get a set of nested stainless funnels, small to large.

You can't have too many stainless-steel mixing bowls of many sizes. Unbleached, natural muslin from the fabric store that you can cut to size, or white unbleached cotton dish rags, are necessary for wrapping herbs and pressing out the marc in an herb press or for twisting them out by hand. Wash the muslin or any new cloth before using to eliminate any starch or chemicals. Consider acquiring nut milk bags, which are easy to clean and nifty for pressing herbs.

Finally, purchase a sensitive scale that will accurately weigh small to large amounts. Small means a few grams. Large is 1 pound or 2. One ounce is equal to about 30 g. It is helpful to get a metric scale that converts alternately from ounces to g, and avoirdupois to metric. Make sure the scale has a container large enough to keep a pound of fluffy Calendula flowers from spilling or overflowing. That way the plant material will not fall all over the counter and floor, necessitating multiple steps of weighing, clean up, and waste.

Another necessity is a grinder. Blenders can be used to grind and blend herbs. Regular commercial blenders are marginal: the blades break, and the motor burns out with rough use and repeated attempts to grind hard roots or blend herbal oils. The recommended grinder is the tried-and-true, sturdy and unbreakable Vitamix 3600 or Vitamix Maxi 4000 commercial juicer, preferably with a stainless-steel container. The company has now replaced its stainless container with a new and improved plastic one. That's progress. However, if you are lucky, you might locate an older gently used stainless model. If not, get a new one with the plastic container. Herb grinding may scar the plastic over time, but these plastic containers are replaceable and of food-grade quality. Also available are some grinders from China, which are available from Mayway Herbs and other Chinese companies. They are very durable and pulverize hard roots into fine powder. However, the motor has gone out on one of mine with continual use.

The largest apothecary item is the herb press. After you have laboriously hand-squeezed out a few dozen tinctures, you'll be ready to invest. Most presses are a few hundred dollars but well worth it. There are electric ones, cheesemaker types, and other models. The one I love is pictured here and was specially designed and fabricated for making herbal medicines (Fig. 7.5).[2] It is basically an indestructible hydraulic car jack that is cranked up against a stainless-steel plate until it presses out the menstruum, which then flows down a tube into a waiting half-gallon jar. This press squeezes out every last drop and works well. It also provides a little exercise.

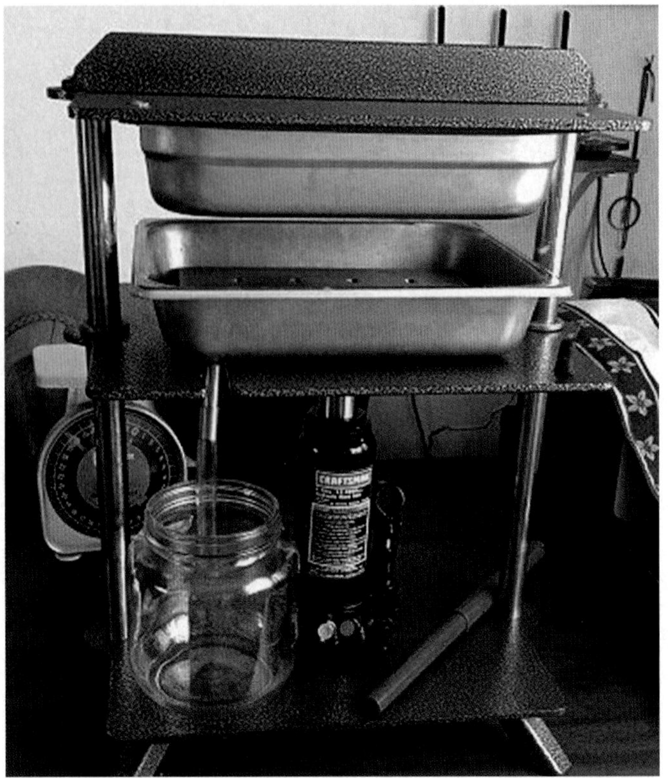

• **Fig. 7.5** Hydraulic herb press.

More and more companies now offer presses. Make sure the press you purchase will hold the quantity of menstruum you generally use so you won't have to go through repeated pressings due to small capacity. The yield of my personal home tinctures average about 750 to 1000 mL per batch (a little over 4 cups, or 1 liter). This amount fits nicely into the half gallon collecting jar.

Labels

Don't forget labels. They are a challenging project. Labels can be store-bought stick-ons, computer generated, or hand printed and cut. Some herbalists have labels made up by outside companies with pretty pictures and their logos. Whatever your source, make sure indelible ink is used, unless you think smeared writing increases the esthetic value.

Paper labels that get wet are a useless mess. When any labeled concoction is used up, the bottles and jars must be washed. The catch is that before this happens, the label must be removed. It can be a true hassle and sometimes impossible to wash and scrape off any glue that invariably sticks to the glass. One solution is not to use any glue in the first place. After much trial and error, I now center a paper label on the jar and adhere a strip of clear, heavy-duty shipping tape over it and the bottle. This makes a waterproof label that is easy to peel off when done, and no glue is involved.

When you need a temporary label during production, masking tape and a felt-tip indelible marker are very convenient options. All herb jars must be labeled (even if only used temporarily), or you will soon forget what you have in which jar.

Tincture Preparation: Folk and Weight-to-Volume

A ***tincture*** is an alcohol or alcohol and water preparation suitable for roots, seeds, fruits, or herbs. Technically, a tincture is an alcoholic ***maceration***. The medicinal plant is macerated, (slowly soaked or steeped) in a liquid solvent, the ***menstruum***, for a few weeks, and then pressed out. The leftover plant material is the ***marc***, and the tincture is the finished product. Various types of menstruums and their extraction and preservative qualities were previously discussed (Chapter 6). Menstruums are usually a combination of alcohol and water, but glycerin, vinegar, or wine may also be used. In a tincture, the job of a menstruum is to break down the cell walls of a whole plant. It then extracts, coaxes, and conjures out the chemical constituents.

Wise Woman/Folk Method to Prepare a Tincture

The Wise Woman or ***folk method*** is ancient and requires no weighing and measuring. It involves putting your dried or fresh herb in a jar and covering it with menstruum so that about 1/4 inch of menstruum comes above the top of the herb. The maceration sits for 2 weeks or so, and the liquid menstruum is then pressed out. The resulting folk tincture makes good medicine, and this technique has been used quite successfully for hundreds of years.

The downside is that you really don't know what your proportions are. If vodka containing 40% alcohol was used as the total menstruum, it implies that the tincture (if made from a totally dried herb) contains 40% alcohol: no more, no less. The remaining 60% of menstruum out of that bottle of vodka is water. You know you have a menstruum containing 40% alcohol, but there is no way to know the proportion of herb to alcohol, because nothing was weighed or measured.

Because the proportion of menstruum to herbal material in the folk method is so vague, or hit or miss, it is difficult if not impossible to duplicate or control the tincture from one batch to another. The strength of the tincture or the proportion of herb to menstruum is unknown. In these days of the FDA-mandated Good Manufacturing Process (GMP) requirements (Chapter 30), which is an attempt towards herbal standardization, the folk method is not accurate enough. When we enter into commerce, the picture changes, the plot thickens, and more accuracy is required. But for home use or in situations where precision doesn't matter—the folk method will suffice.

Instructions for Making Tinctures Using the Folk Method

- *Grind dry herb.* Make a moderately coarse powder.
- *Place the ground herb into glass jar.* Use a tight-fitting lid.
- *Add prepared menstruum.* Use commercial vodka, if possible, 80 to 100 proof. ***Proof*** means twice the percentage of the alcohol content. One hundred proof means the vodka is 50% alcohol, and 80 proof means it is 40% alcohol. Both strengths are more than sufficient to preserve the tincture. This is possibly not a high enough proof to extract all the ingredients, but this is the folk method, so you've made the decision that precision is not required.
- *Cover the herb with menstruum.* Make sure it's at least 1/4 inch above the surface of the herb, so the herb will not be exposed to air and become moldy. If a lot of the menstruum is absorbed overnight and the plant material pokes out above the menstruum, add more vodka to cover it up. Another option is to weigh the herb down into the menstruum with a rock or crystal or other heavy object.
- *Cap jar tightly.* A good seal is necessary. Canning jars have excellent sealing lids.
- *Shake daily.* The container should be shaken daily for 2 weeks, minimum. It never hurts to leave it macerating longer. After a few weeks, all that's ever going to extract out into the menstruum will have done so, but leaving it longer does no harm.
- *Press.* Pour off the clear menstruum from the top, and press the marc. Wrap the herb in an unbleached muslin cloth or a nut-milk bag and hand squeeze it out. An herb press is easier on the hands and will squeeze out much more of your precious tincture.
- *Bottle.* Pour the tincture into a bottle, and cap and label the bottle.[1]
- *Fresh plant folk tincture.* A fresh (not dried) plant already contains about 50% water and therefore dilutes the menstruum. For that reason, you need a high percentage (proof) of alcohol. Vodka won't do. The product with the highest percentage obtainable in a liquor store in most states is a bottle of Everclear containing 95% alcohol, which is 190 proof. This is strong enough to macerate and preserve fresh herbs. Chop the herb and pack it down tightly into jar. Add Everclear to 1/4 inch above the marc. If plant material is too fluffy and pops up above the menstruum, pour the entire contents into Vitamix or other blender to create a denser slush. Pour the mushy menstruum back into the jar. Close tightly. Shake daily for 2 weeks. Strain, bottle, and label. Date the label and make sure it reads *Fresh Mullein leaf in 95% alcohol.*

The Weight-to-Volume Method

The ***weight-to-volume method (w/v)*** is where precise amounts of herb, alcohol, and water are calculated and measured out to produce a specific tincture strength. Weight-to-volume implies that 1 cubic centimeter (cc) of water weighs 1 g. This is a 1-to-1 equality between the weight or mass of a solid (the marc) and the volume of a liquid (the menstruum). When making tinctures, this convenient fact applies to any menstruum or combination thereof, including water, alcohol, wine, vinegar, or glycerin (Fig. 7.6). The w/v method is preferred over the folk method because a precise ratio of herb to menstruum can be calculated, as can the percentage of alcohol within the menstruum.

The relationship, proportion, or ratio of the plant material to the menstruum is expressed as the weight of the herb to the volume of menstruum.[1] Common ratios are 1 part dried herb to 5 parts menstruum written as 1:5 (pronounced "one to five"); or 1 part herb to 3 parts menstruum, written as 1:3 (pronounced "one to three"); or as in fresh herbs, 1 part herb to 2 parts menstruum written as 1:2. There can be other ratios. Determining the correct ratios for a given tincture depends on convention, the plant constituents, and the ratio necessary to extract the active ingredients out of the plant. The smaller the second number (volume or part of menstruum), the stronger the tincture. Generally speaking, denser plants and roots require larger percentages of alcohol.

Alcohol

For tincture making, use alcohol that is 95% to 99% pure ingestible ***ethyl alcohol***. Ethyl alcohol is also referred to as ethanol, grain

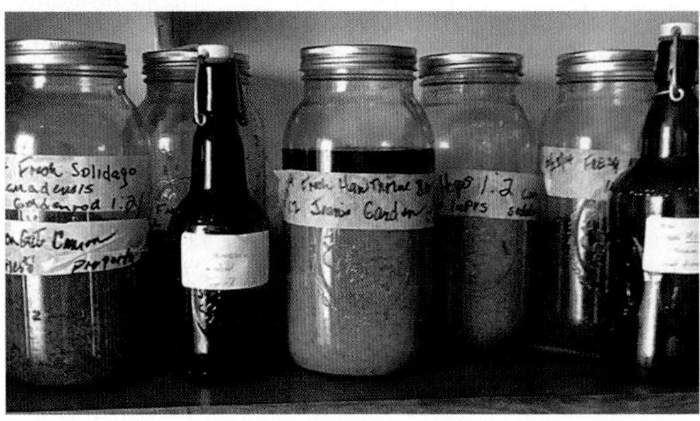

• **Fig. 7.6** Weight-to-volume tinctures macerating.

alcohol, or EtOH. It is not chemically possible to get every drop, all 100% of the water out of the alcohol, but distilleries come close. If pure alcohol is exposed to the air, it will absorb moisture from the atmosphere and self-dilute down to about 95%. Herbalists use 95% to 99% alcohol but round it up to 100% for calculation's sake.

Always use the highest alcohol percent possible—that way there is no water content to worry about or factor in. Less than 95% alcohol literally waters down or dilutes the menstruum. Commercial Everclear (grain alcohol), in states where this concentration is available, is 95% alcohol—190 proof. Most vodkas are about 50% alcohol, or 100 proof. When you get into tincture making in any quantity, it is most economical to purchase 95% to 100% ethyl alcohol or ethanol directly from a distillery in a 5-gallon container. This quantity of alcohol is more than enough to get started. Don't worry, it won't spoil if it isn't used up right away. Alcohol is the best preservative known.

Isopropol alcohol, known as rubbing alcohol, contains propane and is highly toxic and *not* ingestible. It is a good disinfectant and will extract alcohol-soluble constituents. Use this type only for external remedies.

Solubility: Determining Alcohol to Water Percentages in a Menstruum

Solubility refers to the ability of a given substance to dissolve in a particular solvent. From a practical standpoint, plants with predominately water-soluble constituents need a higher percentage of water; plants with predominantly alcohol-soluble constituents need more alcohol in the maceration. For instance, plants high in tannins and mucilages do better with a lot of water, and plants high in alkaloids and resins require higher alcohol concentrations.

Solubility is influenced by heat, pH, concentration, and presence of various constituents. In general, solubility runs on a continuum.[3] No plant is all water or all alcohol soluble. Plants contain many different chemical constituents, so sometimes decisions must be made as to which chemical needs to be extracted the most.

A molecule that has an uneven distribution of electrical charges is ***polar***. It has areas of partial positive charge and areas of partial negative charge. As far as herbal menstruums are concerned, water is the most polar and is known as the universal solvent. Then comes vinegar, glycerol, and finally, ethanol, the least polar.

Substances of similar polarities will dissolve in one another. Plant constituents that are very polar dissolve well in water.

• BOX 7.1 Solubility of Various Constituents

More Water Soluble (Require smaller alcohol proportions.)	**More Alcohol Soluble** (Require higher alcohol proportions.)
Carbohydrates, polysaccharides	Alkaloids
Tannins	Volatile oils (terpenoids)
Mucilages	Lipids
Some flavonoids	Resins, oleoresins
Saponins	Gums
PA alkaloids, as in Comfrey root	Steroids[4]

Carbohydrates are highly polar and hence are very water soluble. Plant constituents that are least polar dissolve in solvents that are also least polar, in our case ethanol. Turmeric root and Ginger root have low ***polarity*** and therefore dissolve well in high-percentage ethanol mixtures (Box 7.1).

Obviously, a plant contains more than one biochemical. To obtain the synergy of all the chemicals working together, it's wise to extract as many chemicals as possible. For this reason, we generalize as to proportions of solvents. Alcohol and water together will extract quite a few. Therefore, we need to use both to cover our bases. The proportion of alcohol to water depends on what needs to be extracted the most and on what is needed to break down plant cell walls. Sometimes water temperature is an additional factor. Hot water or prolonged simmering heats dried plants and breaks down tough cell walls of certain plants that room temperature water cannot. Other considerations as to how much alcohol versus amount of water to use in w/v tinctures follow.

- *Minimum amount of alcohol.* The percentage of alcohol in any tincture regardless of solubility should be at the very least 35% grain alcohol to ensure preservation and safety, although some sources specify as little as 20%.
- *Determining biochemical constituents.* One way to find out which chemical constituents a plant contains is to consult a Materia Medica that lists them. These days, many do. Peter Holmes's *Jade Remedies* on Chinese herbs[5] and *Energetics of Western Herbs*[6] contain fine lists.
- *Grinding well.* A finely ground plant will ensure that more of any kind of solvent will reach a greater surface area, resulting in more constituents extracted.
- *Density of the herb material.* Very generally speaking, soft herbal or leafy materials need less alcohol, approximately 30% to 35%. Soft seeds, fruits, and roots of medium density require more, approximately 40% to 60% alcohol. Hard roots and seeds could require 60% to 80% alcohol. Use these percentage ranges as a safe guide.
- ***Precipitation*** means falling out of solution. Precipitation occurs when two different previously clear tinctures are mixed together and suddenly result in murky, milky-looking solid particles leaking out. This is a little startling and unattractive but not harmful. It happens when a high-alcohol and highly alcohol-soluble component are mixed together with a high water and highly water-soluble component, such as resinous Myrrh and water. The polarities are incompatible; thus, precipitation occurs. Best to shake these types thoroughly before using, so all components will be temporarily mixed before ingestion. This is why labels should state *shake well before using*. A few minutes later, precipitation will reoccur.
- *Tradition, experience, and observation.* Old texts and new ones have various recommendations for plant-to-menstruum ratios

and for alcohol-to-water percentages, based on time and experience. They do not always agree. Honor this, as well as your own observations. Keep records of your proportions and alcohol percentages and always taste and smell a tincture to decide for yourself. Observe how a remedy works for you and your clients. If you're not happy, try another proportion.

Determining Plant to Menstruum Ratios

- *Fresh herb ratios.* Fresh herb ratios. Fresh herb ratios are easy. The International Protocol adopted in Brussels in 1902 says that a fresh plant ordinarily requires a metric 1:2 w/v 50% tincture using 190-proof undiluted ethyl alcohol. This assumes that a fresh plant contains a large amount of water. If 95% or 190-proof or greater grain alcohol is used as the menstruum, it will conform to the International Protocol standards. The results will be a near perfect 1:2 w/v tincture (also called a ½ or 50% w/v tincture). Note that metric weight to volume (w/v) refers to the weight of the original plant material and the volume of the original alcohol. Because there is no such thing as exactly 100% or 200-proof alcohol and fresh plants vary in water content the calculations will never be precise, but experience demonstrates these proportions will produce effective herbal remedies.
- *Dried herb ratios.* Varied information abounds. Different sources provide conflicting ratios. The gold standard for most herbs used to be a 1:5 ratio of w/v plant material to total menstruum. Herbalist Michael Moore pretty consistently recommended 1:5 for most herbs.[8] He followed in the Eclectic's footsteps. Peter Holmes reports that the current norm is 1:2 or 1:3.[7] These last two are concentrations stronger than 1:5.
  - *Author's preference.* I personally use a 1:3 ratio in most cases. This provides stronger, more concentrated medicine than a 1:5 would provide. There is less volume involved, so less tincture is needed for an equivalent dose. The bottle lasts longer. Dosage can then be adjusted up or down depending on the person, their size, condition, and tolerance. Start small; you can always go up. Another factor is that as micro-organisms have become more virulent and the environment more toxic, we need larger or stronger doses these days than in the past, when the 1:5 proportion was the standard ratio.
- *Volume of plant material versus amount of menstruum.* Sometimes the plant decides this question for you. Botanicals such as Mullein leaf, White Horehound herb, or Artichoke leaf soak up menstruum like sponges. Therefore, you have to use more liquid to ensure the top of the herbal material is covered. If the plant is a closely packed nonporous root, less menstruum is needed to cover it. There has to be at least enough menstruum to do this to avoid spoilage.
- *Bottom line.* Plant-to-menstruum ratios are really a judgment call, based on your sense of the finished product. If unsure, pick a good source or go middle of the road, and experiment. Table 7.1 gives suggestions for the percentages of alcohol to water to use for selected herbs.

TABLE 7.1 Average Weight-to-Volume Ethanol Percentages and Proportions for Dried Plant Tinctures

Lower Ethanol 20%-40%	Medium Ethanol 40%-60%	Higher Ethanol 60%-90%
Bladderwrack thallus 1:4 20%-30%	*Artemisia annua* (Sweet Annie herb) 1:4 50%-60%	*Angelica archangelica* root 1:3 70%-75%
Cascara sagrada bark 1:4 20%-30%	Astragalus Huang Qi (Astragalus root) 1:3 40%-50%	Angelica Dang Gui (Dong Quai root) 1:3 60%-70%
Cleavers herb 1:4 30%-35%	Black Walnut hull 1:3 40%-55%	Arnica flower 1:4 65%-70%
Dandelion root 1:4 30%-45%	Bloodroot 1:3 50%-60 %	Ashwagandha root 1:3 60%-65%
Eleutherococcus Ci Wu Jia (Siberian ginseng) 1:3 30%-40%	Blue Cohosh root 1:3 55%-65%	Black Cohosh root 1:3 60%-80%
Eyebright herb 1:4 25%-40%	Blue Vervain herb 1:4 40%-45%	Buchu leaf 1:4 75%-85%
Ganoderma Ling Zhi (Reishi mushroom) 1:5 20%-25%	Boneset herb 1:4 40%-45%	Cayenne pepper 1:4 70%-85%
Gotu Kola herb 1:3 25%-40%	Bugleweed herb 1:4 40%-60%	Chamomile flower 1:3 60%-70%
Green Tea leaves 1:5 25%-40%	Burdock root 1:4 40%-60%	Chickweed herb 1:3 65%-70%
Horsetail herb 1:4 30%-40%	California Poppy herb 1:4 55%-60%	Cinnamon bark 1:3 60%-70%

(*Continued*)

TABLE 7.1 Average Weight-to-Volume Ethanol Percentages and Proportions for Dried Plant Tinctures—cont'd

Lower Ethanol 20%-40%	Medium Ethanol 40%-60%	Higher Ethanol 60%-90%
Licorice root 1:3 25%-35%	Cat's Claw bark 1:3 50%-65%	Devil's Claw root 1:3 60%-65%
Marshmallow root 1:4 20%-30%	Celandine herb 1:4 50%-55%	Elecampane root 1:4 65%-70%
Milky Oat berry 1:4 30%-50%	Chamomile flower 1:4 50%-60%	Fennel seed 1:3 60%-65%
Panax spp. (Ginseng root) 1:3 20%-40%	Cilantro leaf 1:4 50%-60%	Ginger root 1:3 60%-80%
Pau d'Arco bark 1:3 25%-40%	Coleus root 1:4 40%-60%	Ginkgo leaf 1:3 55%-65%
Raspberry leaf 1:4 35%-65%	Coptis Huang Lian (Goldthread root) 1:3 50%-60%	Goldenseal root 1:3 55%-65%
Red root 1:3 30%-40%	Cornsilk style 1:4 50%-55%	Gumweed flower buds 1:4 65%-70%
Sarsaparilla root 1:3 20%-30%	Cramp bark 1:3 50%-65%	Holy Basil herb 1:3 65%-80%
Uva-ursi leaf 1:4 35%-60%	Damiana leaf 1:4 55%-65%	Jamaican Dogwood root bark 1:3 70%-80%
Willow bark 1:3 20%-40%	Dandelion root 1:4 35%-45 %	Kava root 1:3 65%-90%
	Devil's Club root 1:3 50%-55%	*Larrea divaricata* (Creosote bush) 1:3 60%-75%
	Echinacea root 1:3 45%-60%	Lavender flower 1:4 80%-85%
	Elderberry berry 1:4 40%-50%	Milk Thistle seed 1:3 65%-75%
	Fenugreek seed 1:3 50%-60%	Myrrh resin 1:3 70%-90%
	Feverfew herb 1:3 50%-65%	Olive leaf 1:4 85%-95%
	Ginkgo leaf 1:3 55%-65%	Oregano herb 1:4 65%-75%
	Goldenrod herb 1:4 50%-55%	Osha root 1:3 65%-70%
	Gotu Kola herb 1:4 40%-50%	Passionflower 1:3 65%-75%
	Hawthorn berry 1:3 40%-45%	Peppermint herb 1:4 60%-90%

(Continued)

TABLE 7.1 Average Weight-to-Volume Ethanol Percentages and Proportions for Dried Plant Tinctures—cont'd

Lower Ethanol 20%-40%	Medium Ethanol 40%-60%	Higher Ethanol 60%-90%
	Helonias root 1:4 40%-45%	Propolis 1:3 75%-90%
	Hyssop herb 1:4 50%-55%	Rosemary leaf 1:4 65%-70%
	Lemon Balm leaf 1:4 45%-60%	St. John's Wort 1:4 50%-75%
	Lobelia herb 1:4 40%-45%	Sage leaf, Garden 1:3 70%-75%
	Maca root 1:3 50%-60%	Saw Palmetto berry 1:3 60%-80%
	Mistletoe herb 1:3 45%-50%	Schisandra Wu Wei Zi berry 1:3 70%-80%
	Motherwort herb 1:4 40%-60%	Thyme herb 1:3 70%-75%
	Mullein leaf 1:5 40%-50%	Turmeric root 1:3 60%-70%
	Nettle herb 1:5 40%-55%	Usnea thallus 1:4 60%-95%
	Olive leaf 1:4 55%-65%	Vitex berry 1:3 60%-75%
	Oregano herb 1:4 55%-65%	Wormwood herb (*Artemisia annua*, Sweet Annie) 1:4 50%-75%
	Oregon Grape root 1:3 40%-65%	Yarrow herb 1:4 55%-70%
	Passionflower 1:3 50%-60%	Yerba Mansa root 1:4 70% 75%
	Pau d'arco bark 1:3 40%-50%	Yerba Santa leaf 1:4 70%-75%
	Plantago spp. (Plantain leaf) 1:3 45%-55%	
	Raspberry leaf 1:4 40%-60%	
	Red Clover flower 1:4 40%-50%	
	Red root 1:3 45%-55%	
	Rhodiola root 1:3 40%-60%	
	St John's Wort 1:4 50%-75 %	

(*Continued*)

TABLE 7.1 Average Weight-to-Volume Ethanol Percentages and Proportions for Dried Plant Tinctures—cont'd

Lower Ethanol 20%-40%	Medium Ethanol 40%-60%	Higher Ethanol 60%-90%
	Sarsaparilla root 1:3 40%-50%	
	Schisandra Wu Wei Zi (Five Taste berry) 1:3 55%-65%	
	Skullcap herb 1:4 40%-50%	
	Shepherd's Purse herb 1:3 40%-45%	
	Stoneroot 1:3 35%-50%	
	Uva-ursi leaf 1:3 35%-60%	
	Valerian root 1:4 50%-60%	
	Wild Geranium root 1:4 50%-55%	
	Wild Yam root 1:3 45%-60%	
	Wood Betony herb 1:4 55%-60%	
	Wormwood herb 1:4 50%-75%	
	Yellow Dock root 1:3 40%-55%	

Ethanol percentages courtesy of Lisa Ganora, director of Colorado School of Clinical Herbalism and author of *Herbal Constituents*; proportions from James Green[1] and Rachel Lord. Based on old pharmacopoeias and general contemporary practice.

Directions for Weight-to-Volume Tincture Making

- *Weigh plant.* Weigh dry plant material, preferably in grams.
- *Grind plant.* Grind plant finely and reweigh. Some can mysteriously disappear.
- *Herb in jar.* Place dried plant material into a glass jar with tight lid.
- *Prepare custom menstruum.* Decide on ratio of herb-to-menstruum and alcohol percentage of menstruum. Then calculate amount of alcohol and water to use (Box 7.2).
- *Label jar.* Include date; botanical and common names; proportions, such as 1:3 50% or 1:5 60%; and type of preparation, in this case a maceration. Include the mL of alcohol and the mL of water used. This temporary label can be made with a piece of masking tape and permanent ink felt-tip marker.
- *Combine menstruum and herb.* Pour measured menstruum into a separate jar. Mix the alcohol and water together. Pour mixed menstruum into the jar with the ground herb and close lid tightly.
- *Shake it up.* You might have to retighten lid to allow for air loosening it. Make sure that all dried plant material is thoroughly wetted down and that nothing dry is left at bottom of jar.
- *Shake daily for 2 to 4 weeks.* Watch the miracle of the maceration changing color and becoming darker day by day. Faithful shaking is important.
- *Decant clear liquid.* Pour out the clear tincture portion that rises to the top through a funnel or strainer into a clean glass jar. Amber glass Boston round jars keep out the light, and lids with inverted plastic cones inside (called polycones) keep the jar tightly closed.
- *Press plant and measure yield.* Press the rest in an herb press or squeeze through twisted muslin cloth or nut-milk bag, using lots of elbow grease, until every last drop of tincture is extracted. Measure the *yield*, the amount of extracted menstruum in milliliters. Compare yield, or what was actually extracted, to the original total menstruum amount. If the difference is over 100 mL, too much extra menstruum, which was not pressed

• BOX 7.2 Practice Calculations for Custom Weight-to-Volume Tinctures

Directions

1. Figure out total weight of herb in grams. (1 oz = 30 g)
2. Figure out amount of total menstruum (TM). Multiply total grams times proportion of menstruum.
3. Figure out amount of alcohol. Multiply percentage of alcohol times total menstruum.
4. Figure out amount of water. Multiply percentage of water times total menstruum.

EXAMPLE: Calculate a 1:4 45% menstruum for 8 ounces dried Dandelion root.
8 oz = 240 g dried herb (1 oz = 30 g, 8 oz × 30 g = 240 g)
4 × 240 g = 960 mL total menstruum (TM) (4 × more menstruum than herb, because it's a 1:4)
45% of TM = 432 mL of alcohol (0.45 × 960 = 432 mL).
55% of TM = 528 mL of water (0.55 × 960 = 528 mL).

EXAMPLE: Calculate a 1:3 75% menstruum for 230 g dried Licorice root.
3 × 230 g = 690 mL of TM (3 × more menstruum than herb because it's a 1:3).
75% of TM = 517.5 mL of alcohol (round up to 518 mL).
25% of TM = 172.5 mL of water (round up to 173 mL).

EXAMPLE: Calculate a 1:5 50% tincture for 5½ oz of dried Burdock root. Use metric.
5.5 oz herb = 165 g (5.5 oz × 30 g)
5 × 165 = 825 mL of TM (5 times more menstruum than herb because it's a 1:5).
50% of TM = 412.5 mL of alcohol, round up to 413. mL
50% of total menstruum = 412.5 mL of water, round up to 413. mL

EXAMPLE: Calculate menstruum for 6 oz of fresh St. John's Wort—always 1:2 50%
6 oz = 180 g
2 × 180 = 360 mL of TM which is 95% ethanol, no water.

out, was absorbed in the marc. Some loss is normal, and dense plants tend to press out more efficiently than spongy flowers.

- *Bottle and label.* On finished label: Put the date, botanical name, and proportions, such as *Echinacea purpurea* root, 1:3 60% tincture. Give it a lot number and a batch number. Perhaps include an informational cheat sheet on the label to jog your memory about use of the plant.

Percolation Preparation

A ***percolation*** (perc) is another type of tincture. It is a method in which the soluble constituents of an herb are extracted by the slow passage of a solvent through a column of dried, powdered plant.[1] This happens mostly by the pull of gravity. The plant is packed in a special apparatus known as a percolator (cone). A percolator can be made from an upside-down glass sparkling water bottle with the bottom cut off, or a fancy readymade cone can be purchased from a scientific supply store (Fig. 7.7).

There is debate in the herbal community as to which is better, a macerated tincture or a percolation. In my experience, percolations taste stronger, and the menstruum appears darker in comparison with the same weight of plant material in a w/v maceration. They can be made quickly in 24 hours or less, whereas the standard tincture needs to sit for 2 weeks to a month.

Percs work best with finely and evenly ground plant material that neither swells much when moistened, nor takes up too much

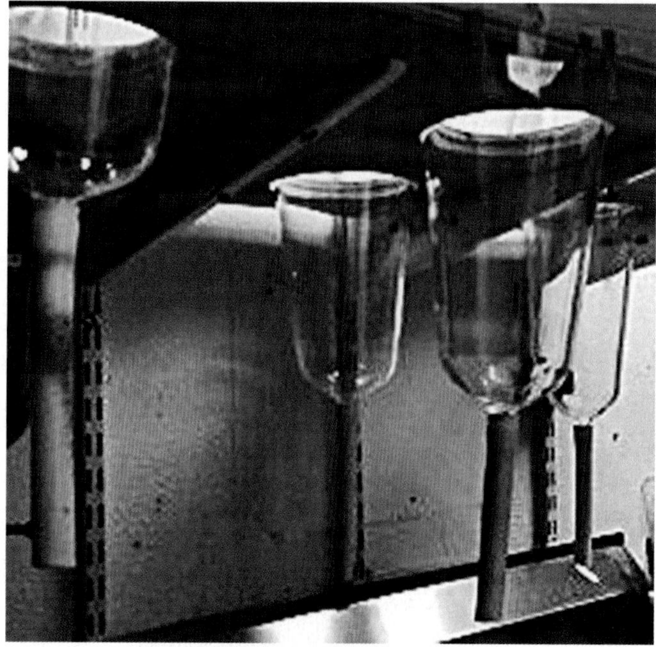

• **Fig. 7.7** Professional percolation cones.

cone room. That's a lot of plants. Percolations sometimes require no pressing, and the marc that's left in the cone can be discarded or composted.

Percolations do *not* work with resinous plants, such as Gumweed flower or Myrrh resin, because resins clog the cone, and the menstruum will not flow through. They do *not* work with glycerites because sticky glycerin can prevent the flow of menstruum through the cone. Fresh plants contain too much water and have a volume too large for the cone. In the end, percolations work better for certain plants, and old-fashioned macerations are better for others. Know both methods. The trend in tincture concentrations among present-day herbalists seems to be calling for stronger and stronger extracts, such as 1:3 or 1:2. Percs certainly work better for those kinds of preparations.

At first, percolation making is ideally done with a mentor or in a class setting. It is a delicate, tricky process. If the cone or upside-down bottle is packed too tightly with herb, nothing will drip through. If it is too loose, the menstruum will flow through too quickly. If there are holes or air pockets or uneven packing, the menstruum can redistribute itself, creating little streaks or rivulets without soaking through the entire herbal material. Proper and even cone packing is key. Some herbalists put a paper coffee filter inside the bottle. I prefer not. Either way, the intent is to get the menstruum to drip slowly through the plant material, dissolving out and taking the constituents along for the ride, just like a coffee percolator. The bottle is placed neck-down into a gallon or half-gallon jar (Fig. 7.8). The screw top can be adjusted tighter or looser to control drip rate. They say about 1 drip per 3 seconds is about right, to the tune and rhythm of the American song "Battle Hymn of the Republic." Sing it slowly.

Directions for Percolations

- *Weigh herb.* Use dry finely ground herb and put in a half-gallon jar. Label.

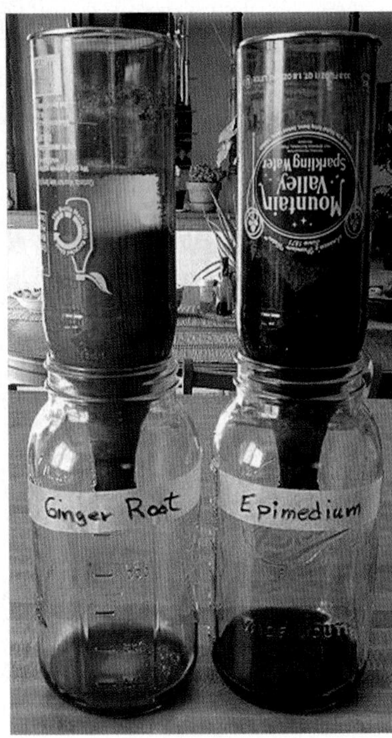

• **Fig. 7.8** Percolations in progress, using cut-off upside-down bottles with adjustable screw-top lids.

• BOX 7.3 Menstruum Abbreviations

Original Menstruum (OM)
Added Menstruum (AM)
Total Menstruum (TM)

- *Calculate the original menstruum.* Menstruum for a perc is calculated just as for a tincture (Box 7.2). Then there is an additional step—calculating a little more menstruum.
- *Calculate amount of additional menstruum—30% rule.* Some additional menstruum must be added to the original menstruum just calculated to account for the liquid loss that invariably occurs in the cone. Thirty percent extra is an average amount that works in most cases. This means the *added menstruum* (AM) will be 30% more than was in the *original menstruum* (OM).
- *Mix up alcohol and water menstruum.* The total mixture includes the OM that reflects the chosen proportion, plus whatever extra you are adding for cone loss (AM). The two added together become the *total menstruum* (TM) that will be used. Put the TM aside in a separate closed half-gallon jar that is labeled with date, herb name, menstruum proportions, and milliliters of alcohol and water.
  - *Alternate way to calculate additional menstruum.* If you didn't resonate with the above 30% rule, another way to determine AM is to pack a measuring cup or beaker with the ground dried herb. That *volume* is the AM. If the packed cup measures 100 mL, the AM is 100 mL. The calculated OM and the AM is combined to equal the TM. The TM is put aside in a closed half-gallon jar and labeled. See menstruum abbreviations in Box 7.3 and practice percolation calculations (Box 7.4).

• BOX 7.4 Practice Calculations for Custom Weight-to-Volume Percolations

Directions

1. Figure out amount of OM as was done for a tincture.
2. Figure out amount of AM to account for cone loss. (Thirty percent is written as 0.30 or 30%.) Alternately, use amount of dried herb in packed measuring cup for amount of AM. If packed cup of dried powdered herb reaches the 40-mL mark, this means to add 40 mL of additional menstruum.
3. Figure out TM by adding original menstruum plus added amounts together.
4. Figure out amount of alcohol and water needed for the TM as was done for a tincture.

EXAMPLE: Ginger root 1:3 65% percolation using 250 g of dried root.
3 × 250 g = 750 mL OM (3 × more menstruum than herb because it's a 1:3).
Add 30% more to original menstruum to get total menstruum.
750 mL × 30% = 225 mL = AM (750 mL × 0.30 = 225 mL = AM).
750 + 225 = 975 mL TM.
Calculate Amount of alcohol and water.
65% of TM = 633.75 mL alcohol (0.65 × 975 = 633.75, round up to 634 mL)
35% of TM = 341.25 mL water (0.35 × 975 = 341.25; no rounding up when it's less than half).

EXAMPLE: Lobelia 1:4 45% percolation using 6½ oz of herb.
6.5 oz × 30 = 195 g dried herb
195 × 4 = 780 mL OM (4 × more menstruum than herb because it's a 1:4).
Add 30% more to original menstruum to get total menstruum.
780 mL × 30% = 234 mL AM (780 mL × 0.30 = 234 mL)
780 + 234 = 1014 mL TM
Calculate amount of alcohol and water.
45% of total menstruum = 456.3 mL alcohol (0.45 × 1014 = 456.3 round down to 456 mL)
55% of total menstruum = 557.7 mL water (0.55 × 1014 = 557.7 round up to 558 mL)

EXAMPLE: Garden Sage herb 1:3 75 % using 300 g dried herb.
300 × 3 = 900 mL OM (3 × more menstruum than herb because it's a 1:3)
Add packed dried herb amount to original menstruum amount.
Packed herb was 300 g or 10 oz = 300 g per w/v (300 g divided by 30 = 10 oz).
300 g + 900 mL OM = 1200 mL TM (total menstruum)
Calculate amount of alcohol and water.
75% of TM = 900 mL alcohol (0.75 × 1200 = 900 mL).
25% of total menstruum = 300 mL water (0.25 × 1200 = 300 mL).

- *Moisten the dried herb (sandcastle).* The dried ground herb needs to be slightly moistened (not soaked) with some of the TM, so it can expand a bit and begin to break down or digest. The AM was added to allow for this step, as well as the cone loss during the percolation process.
  - The easiest way to do this process is to put the herb into a bowl, add a bit of menstruum and stir with wooden spoon or gloved hands until all the herb is damp, with no dry patches. Add a little TM at a time. If the herb gets too wet, it won't perc, and the only alternative is to change plans and make a normal maceration. So, go slowly. The idea is to build baby ***sandcastles*** between your fingers so that when the herb is pinched, it holds the shape and stands up in little peaks like meringue. That's how you know you have it right.
- *Return moistened herb to jar.* Pack herb back into jar and close lid. This sandcastled herb, moistened with alcohol and water, needs to sit for 2 to 24 hours. This process begins the breaking down of its constituents.

- *Packing the cone.* We will use the low-tech, sparkling-water bottle version with the loosely screwed-on cap. Turn it upside-down and begin to pack the cone part carefully, layer by layer, so the menstruum will pass through all the plant material and not get stuck or divide up into little streams. Keep the top surface flat and level. This is an art, not a science. Place a crystal or small rock on top to weigh down the herb if necessary.
- *Pour in menstruum. Slowly.* Set the cone in a wide-mouthed half-gallon Mason jar. Loosen bottle cap on the percolator bottle for now. Very slowly pour in a little menstruum, trying not to disturb the herb. The menstruum should gradually and evenly progress down through the cone. When it reaches the bottom, it will begin to drip out into the jar. Pick up the bottle and adjust the cap as best you can until menstruum is dripping 1 drip or drop every 3 seconds or more. As the menstruum flows down into the herb, continually keep jar topped off, so an inch or more of menstruum covers the top of the herb. This prevents air getting in and disturbing the process. When dripping at proper rate, cover the top with the Mason jar's flat lid. Its diameter usually fits perfectly on a sparkling-water jar percolator.[1]
- *Be patient.* Sometimes it takes a long time for the menstruum to start dripping through, even an hour or longer. But if it's just not happening, if it's too gummy and thick, don't waste your precious herb and menstruum. Make a simple macerated tincture instead. Pour the whole works into a jar. If there is any menstruum not yet added to the cone, remove the calculated added amount. That way, the finished tincture will be relatively close to the same proportions and alcohol percentage that you hoped the perc would have had.
- *Finishing touches.* Measure the menstruum yield and compare to original calculations to see whether yield is close to original menstruum amount. How much was lost? Record your results so you can adjust added menstruum (AM) next time you put up that herb. Individual herbs have different absorptive properties. Bottle and label the completed percolation.
- *Practice percs.* Until you get the hang of percolation production, it is wise to begin with inexpensive materials. Recommended less-expensive herbs to perc are Fennel seed, Peppermint herb, and Nettle herb.

Dual Extraction Preparation

A ***dual extraction***, also called a *double extraction*, is an advanced method of making a tincture, in which a simmered *water* decoction and *ethanol* are both used as solvents. This is done because certain herbs are chemically complex and require both extraction methods to release a full-spectrum of their precious water-soluble *and* alcohol-soluble ingredients.

One notable herbal category that provides exemplary therapeutic results when the dual extraction method is used are the immunomodulating adaptogens that help the body deal with stressors that make us sick. Examples are *Ganoderma* Ling Zhi (Reishi mushroom) and other medicinal mushrooms, *Echinacea angustifolia* (Echinacea root), *Glycyrrhiza* spp (Licorice root), *Withania somnifera* (Ashwagandha root), Schisandra Wu Wei Zi (Five Taste berry), Astragalus Huang Qi (Astragalus root), and others.

- *The hot-water decoction.* Hot simmered water does a particularly good job of extracting immunomodulating, hepatoprotective, and cancer-fighting beta glucans (polysaccharides) present in adaptogens. To do this, the herb requires simmering in very hot water for a length of time to break down the cell walls and extract the water soluble beneficial constituents—a bit more than simply macerating in room temperature water, as is done in a basic w/v tincture method.
- *The ethanol maceration.* Alcohol excels in the extraction of immune-stimulating, antiinflammatory terpenes, alkaloids, and essential oils. Adaptogens are particularly rich in alkaloids and so require this step as well.

In the herbal world, there is a bit of controversy over which step is done first—the decoction or the maceration. Recommended decoction time varies from an hour to a few days in a slow cooker. One method described by herbalist Stephen Harrod Buhner for Reishi mushroom is to make the water decoction first; next, press, reserve, and then soak the marc in an alcohol maceration. The alcoholic tincture and the water decoction are eventually combined.[9]

Another method recommends the reverse: first making the alcoholic maceration, pressing and reserving the tincture, and then decocting the pressed marc, which had been previously soaked in alcohol.[10] Some research suggests that having a little alcohol left in the marc may partially break down the water-soluble polysaccharides that are being extracted from the decoction.

A method given by herbalist Guido Masé for Ganoderma Ling Zhi (Reishi mushroom) is a compromise. Masé suggests dividing the plant material in half. One half is decocted, the other half is macerated, and then the two are combined.[13]

A fourth even more complicated method is a percolating-steeping-decocting procedure that herbalist Michael Moore described for an Echinacea dual extraction. The plant is first percolated with alcohol and a portion of the total water. The pressed marc and water are then steeped for 2 hours, the marc pressed and removed, and the decoction (minus the plant) simmered down until it evaporates to the calculated amount. The completed decoction and percolation are combined.[16]

To determine which method is best, a chemical analysis would be required for the same herb batch with the same proportions prepared in all the various ways. In lieu of this, the subjective inspection, taste, and smell test (*organoleptics*) should be used so you can reach your own conclusions. In my experience, the decoction-first and the maceration-first techniques work equally well and make excellent medicine. The only drawback to either is a rather large buildup of precipitation, herbal material that sinks to the bottom of the jar of completed extraction, despite repeated straining. I have chosen to present the version in which the alcoholic maceration is done first, and decoction method is second.

Directions for Dual Extraction

Part One: The Maceration (Use only the Ethanol Fraction)

- *Weigh and grind herb. Astragalus membranaceus* (Astragalus root) 350 g using 95% ethanol.
- *Determine proportions and percentages of alcohol to water.* We will use 1:3 50%. Calculate for a usual w/v alcohol/water menstruum. 350 g times 3 equals 1050 mL TM. Ethanol and water are 50% each. Menstruum will consist of 525 mL water and 525 mL ethanol. Check your math. Add menstruum and water amounts together, and you get 1050 mL.
- *Place ground herb in jar.* Macerate by adding the 535 mL of 95% ethanol (not the water). Using masking tape and marker, temporarily label as *dual extraction, ethanol fraction, 535 mL EtOH.*

- The finished dual extraction will be: Astragalus Huang Qi 1:3 50%. The separate water decoction will be added to this later. If the temporary labeling is done very explicitly, there won't be any mix-ups later.
- *Shake* alcohol-only maceration daily for 2 weeks, minimum.
- *Press and reserve menstruum* in the rinsed out and labeled jar. Save the marc; set aside for decoction, part two.

Part Two: The Decoction

- *Chopstick trick.* Place pressed marc from the maceration with the water (525 mL) into a double boiler. Place your trusty chopstick into it and mark or tape it at the top level of the water. This way you have created a measuring stick to use later that will tell you how far down you need to simmer. After water level of 525 mL is marked on the chopstick, more water is added—another 525 mL to simmer and evaporate down to original amount.
- *Decoct marc.* Add the additional water, 525 mL or even a little more. Bring to a simmer with lid off and *very* slowly evaporate down to original 525 mL. The chopstick measuring tool placed vertically along the outside of the pot is the guide. When the menstruum is decocted by half, it should be very thick and rich smelling because the heat pulls out the water-soluble constituents.
- *Strain and press.* Strain out decoction. You should have 525 mL of a thick syrup mixture. If amount is a little short, press on the marc to push out more water, which is inevitably absorbed within. Let the decoction cool. To end up with a 50% solution, the measuring needs to be precise. If a little extra decoction is left over, go ahead and drink it—to give yourself an immune boost.
- *Combine alcoholic menstruum into cooled-off decoction.* Very slowly pour the alcoholic menstruum into the cooled, strained, and pressed water decoction, not the other way around. This is to avoid excess precipitation.
- *Re-label.* The mixture now contains both the alcohol and the water decoction. A new label should reflect this: *Astragalus membranaceus* Huang Qi (Astragalus root) 1:3 50% dual extraction. The dual extraction is now completed.

Glycerite Preparation

Glycerin is the sweet faction of a fixed oil. (***Fixed oils*** are nonvolatile, nonevaporating fats found in plants and animals, such as olive, almond, or fish oil.) Glycerin is a class of alcohol, but nonalcoholic. Even though it tastes sweet, it is *not* a carbohydrate and contains no sugar. It is slowly absorbed into the bloodstream and slowly metabolized by the liver without causing any blood sugar imbalances.[1] Therefore a glycerin maceration, called a *glycerite*, is an alternative for diabetics who cannot tolerate sugar and a treat for those who prefer it sweet. Glycerites are also good options for children's health care, because compliance with this sweet substance is high. Sounds too good to be true.

Glycerites mix with both water and alcohol, so they may be added to finished water/alcohol extractions. Glycerin can be used in a menstruum containing water, alcohol, vinegar, or any combination of the three. If alcohol is added, less glycerin is required, because it is a weaker preservative and extractor. It does not extract volatile oils very well, as with those present in Peppermint herb or Lavender flower, and preserves them for only a short time. In such a case, more alcohol is required. Vinegar can be used in a glycerite if alcohol is not a good option. Vinegar extracts some alkaloids and water-soluble compounds, has some antiseptic properties, but is a weak preservative.

Glycerin also binds to or absorbs tannins really well. This information is useful because when a plant high in tannins (such as White Oak bark and other barks, or Rose family herbs, such as Raspberry leaf or Hawthorn berry) is combined with any alkaloid (present in countless plants), precipitation occurs, and the alkaloid is rendered inactive. A bit of glycerin included in small proportions in any formula containing tannic acid allows the alkaloids and tannins to separately do their medicinal duties.[1]

The downside of glycerin is that it is only a fair preservative and does better with refrigeration. When kept cool, a glycerin tincture without alcohol has a shelf life of about 2 years. (An alcoholic w/v tincture lasts for many years.) As a solvent, it works best for primarily water-soluble compounds and does not generally dissolve alkaloids. It is slightly antiseptic but less so than alcohol.[1] Call it "a middle of the roader."

Glycerin absorbs water readily from the air. Because of this, commercial glycerin already contains 5% water by volume before the bottle is ever opened. If using glycerin as the sole preservative in a menstruum, use 60% glycerin by volume to account for this.[1] Remember that at least 30% alcohol (190 proof) alone is needed to preserve a tincture. So, if you use less than 60% glycerin, there needs to be some preservative-acting alcohol added to make up the difference. If alcohol isn't an issue, some herbalists make a traditional w/v alcohol and water maceration with a little glycerin added for the flavor factor. I have noticed this combination appearing in health food stores.

Glycerite/water menstruums for fresh plants do not work very well and are a special consideration. Fresh plants already contain 50% water, and they are made in a 1:2 ratio of plant material to ethyl alcohol. Therefore, a *lot* of glycerin, 80% to 90% by volume, is needed to preserve the menstruum with only 10% to 20% water. That will taste sickeningly sweet for most people. It is probably best to make glycerites out of dried plants for this reason. However, an exception is a fresh Ginger glycerite mixed up in a Vitamix. It is excellent, a beneficial and delicious remedy for digestion and respiratory problems.

Directions for w/v Glycerites

Vegetable glycerin already contains about 5% water by volume. To allow for the 5% of water already in the glycerin, we need to use a minimum of 60% glycerin by volume. This provides the right amount of pure glycerin for the menstruum to maintain proper shelf life/stability and is necessary if glycerin is the only preservative solvent. If 95%-100% grain alcohol is also added to the glycerite, the total volume of glycerin can be less, since the grain alcohol makes up the difference in preservative action required.

Definitions.

Vegetable glycerin. The commercial product purchased that contains pure glycerin with 5% water.

Glycerite. The finished preparation that includes glycerin as a solvent. This is also called the *yield* or *menstruum*. It is expressed as the percentage of glycerin used: such as a 40% or a 60% glycerite.

Ratio (1:4). The weight of herb (grams) to the volume of total fluid or menstruum (mL).

Percent glycerin. The percentage of commercial glycerin to glycerite (for example 60% glycerin and 40% added water).

- *Weigh and grind herb.* Place in labeled jar with tight lid.
- *Prepare custom menstruum.* Calculate amounts (Box 7.5). Menstruums may be water/glycerin, water/glycerin/alcohol, or water/glycerin/vinegar. Whatever the menstruum combo, make

• BOX 7.5 Practice Calculations for Vegetable Glycerin Menstruums

Directions

1. Figure out amount of total menstruum (TM) as was done for a regular w/v tincture.
2. Figure out amount of vegetable glycerin needed, keeping in mind that there must be enough to preserve the menstruum.
3. Figure out menstruum amounts of remaining solvents (water, vinegar and/or ethanol).

EXAMPLE: Calculate a 1:4 60% glycerite with 300 grams dried Ginger root.
Glycerin must be 60% by volume of menstruum to maintain shelf life, since there is no other preservative.

Total Menstruum	**1200 mL TM**	**300 g × 4 = 1200 mL**
Glycerin	720 mL	TM 1200 mL × .60 = 720 mL needed glycerin
Water	+ 480 mL	TM 1200 mL × .40 = 480 mL needed water
	1200 mL TM	

EXAMPLE: Calculate a 1:5 60% glycerite that includes 5% vinegar with 250 grams dried Skullcap herb.
Glycerin must be 60% by volume of menstruum to assure stability, even though a little vinegar is added. Apple cider vinegar has very little to no alcohol and is a poor preservative, so we calculate as if glycerin were the only preservative.

Total Menstruum	**1250 mL TM**	**TM 250 g × 5 = 1250 mL**
Glycerin	750 mL	TM 1250 mL × 0.60 = 750 mL needed glycerin
Vinegar	+ 63 mL	TM 1250 mL × 0.05 = 62.5 mL rounded up = 63 mL needed vinegar
	813 mL	
Water	+ 437 mL	TM 1250 mL−813 mL (glycerin + vinegar) = 437 mL needed water
	1250 mL TM	

EXAMPLE: Calculate a 1:3 40% glycerite that includes 20% ethanol with 6 ounces dried Chamomile flower.
Ninety-five to one hundred percent grain alcohol provides 20% of total menstruum's alcohol requirement. Glycerin must provide the remaining 40% to total the 60% required preservative. The rest of the menstruum is water.
Herb 6 ounces of dried Chamomile flower: 6 oz × 30 grams = 180 grams

Total Menstruum	**540 mL TM**	**180 g × 3 = 540 mL**
Ethanol	108 mL	TM 540 mL × 0.20 = 108 mL needed alcohol
Glycerin	+ 216 mL	TM 540 mL × 0.40 = 216 mL needed glycerin
	324 mL	
Water	+ 216 mL	TM 540 mL−324 mL (glycerin + ethanol) = 216 mL needed water
	540 mL TM	

sure to mix it all together first in a separate jar *before* adding to the dried plant.

- *Add thoroughly combined menstruum to powdered herb.* Stir all the sticky stuff together with your chopstick.
- *Shake daily* for at least two weeks.
- *Decant, press, and filter.* Again, sticky glycerin filters very slowly.
- *Bottle, cap, and label.*[1]

Worksheets for Internal Preparations

The following worksheets are very useful guides for calculating and recording the internal preparations presented in this chapter. Please make copies (Appendix A). They can be placed in a three-ring binder to keep records of your tinctures, percolations, dual extractions, and glycerites. Taking notes is also useful, so each succeeding preparation can either be made the same or modified and improved on as to taste, strength, proportions, and technique. It is helpful to refer later to these sheets to see which company the herbs were obtained from and your impression of the quality and freshness. If and when you undertake GMP certification (Chapter 30), these worksheets will provide invaluable information and give you a head start recording lot and batch numbers (Tables 7.2–7.6).

Preparing Infused Oils: Solar, Double Boiler, Accelerated Blender

These three approaches for preparing an infused oil are done by macerating or steeping fresh or dried herbs in a fixed oil menstruum, where the oil is the solvent. They are folk methods requiring no measuring. Preparation of infused oils is the first step in making many other remedies. Infused oils can be prepared into salves with a thickening element such as beeswax or be used in creams and lotions with the aid of an emulsifier such as lanolin, glycerin, or lecithin. They may be used topically as a massage oil, wound/scar healer, or moisturizer. Infused oils are not essential oils. They are much simpler to prepare. All that is needed is the sun, an herb, a jar, and a previously prepared fixed oil.

Common fixed oils used for macerations include olive, almond, grape-seed, sunflower seed, or combinations. Oils can become rancid if not stored properly. ***Rancidity*** means that the oil or fat has become spoiled or degraded due to combining with oxygen in the atmosphere, causing oxidation.[11] Rancidity produces a distinctively nasty odor and taste, making it unfit for consumption. To avoid this, oils should be stored in tightly sealed amber bottles away from air, heat, light, and moisture. In other words, keep the macerated oil in the refrigerator or freezer with the jar filled to the top to eliminate contact with oxygen in the air and to minimize

TABLE 7.2 Dried Plant Tincture Worksheet

General Information
Herb botanical name ______________________________
Common name ______________ Pinyin name ______________
Company or location of collection ______________________
Date received/wildcrafted __________ Company lot number __________
Apothecary production lot number__________ Batch number __________
Herbalist's name______________________________

W/V: Weight-to-Volume **TM: Total Menstruum**
TOM: Total Original Menstruum **OE: Original Ethanol**
AM: Added Menstruum **AE: Added Ethanol**

W/V Ratio ☐ 1:2 ☐ 1:3 ☐ 1:4 ☐ 1:5 ☐ Other __________
Ethanol % _______
Weight of herb ________ g
W/V ratio ______ g x ______ = TM mL ________
Ethanol needed % ethanol _______ x TM = _______ = mL of needed ethanol ______
Water needed % water ________ x TM = ________ = mL of needed water _______
Maceration date ______ Date pressed ______TM ______mL Yield ____ mL Loss ____mL
Initials _____
Notes: Taste; Energy; Changes for next time?

TABLE 7.3 Fresh Plant Tincture Worksheet

General Information
Herb botanical name ______________________________
Common name ______________ Pinyin name ______________
Company or location of collection ______________________
Date received/wildcrafted __________ Company lot number __________
Apothecary production lot number__________ Batch number __________
Herbalist's name______________________________
W/V ratio ☑ 1:2
Ethanol 95%-100%
Weight of fresh herb ________ g
W/V ratio ______ g × 2 = TM ________ mL
Ethanol needed ________ TM mL
Water needed None
Maceration date ______ Date pressed ______TM mL ______ mL Yield ____ mL Loss ____mL
Initials _____
Notes: Taste; Energy; Changes for next time?

any condensation in the bottle. As the oil is used and the level goes down, switch to a smaller container.

There are three basic ways to macerate an oil, and all utilize a very low heat.[12]

- *Sun or solar oil.* This is a pack-and-cover approach where a jar is tightly packed to the top with plant, covered with fixed oil and set in the summer sun for 4 to 6 weeks.
- *Double boiler digestion.* In this method, the herb and oil are slowly heated in a double boiler or slow cooker for a few hours over very low heat.
- *Accelerated blender.* For this version, the herb is moistened in a little alcohol for about an hour and then blended until warm. A regular blender or Vitamix is used.

All three work. I prefer the sun oil method, if time is not an issue, because it looks beautiful sitting on a windowsill or outside in the summer taking its jolly time. All of the methods utilize low heat for maceration. It is essential that the heat stays low and does not cook the herbs. Natural solar heat will be just right; the double-boiler method must be carefully monitored so as not to become too hot; the blending method warms it slightly but takes a while to build up heat. The challenge with a blender is to get the oil heated before the motor overheats or blows out. For this reason, an old sturdy Vitamix is your best bet. Heat must be present, or the oil will not macerate.

Directions for Pack-and-Cover Sun Oil

- *Pack the plant.* Stuff an absolutely dry, preferably sterilized glass jar full to the top with dried or fresh herbs. If fresh herbs are used, let them wilt for 2 to 24 hours to evaporate off a

TABLE 7.4 **Percolation Worksheet**

General Information
Herb botanical name ______
Common name ______ Pinyin name ______
Company or location of collection ______
Date received/wildcrafted ______ Company lot number ______
Apothecary production lot number______ Batch number ______
Herbalist's name______
W/V ratio ☐ 1:2 ☐ 1:3 ☐ 1:4 ☐ 1:5 ☐ Other ______
Ethanol % ______
Weight of herb ______ g
W/V ratio ______ g × ______ = TOM ______ mL
Add to cone TOM ______ × 30% or mL of dry herb pressed in cup = AM ______mL
Total menstruum TOM ______mL + AM ______ mL = TM ______mL
Ethanol needed % EtOH______ × TM = ______mL = mL of needed ethanol ______
Water needed % water ______ × TM = ______ = mL of needed water ______
Sandcastle date ______ Initial ______
Perc date ______ Date bottled ______ TM ______ mL Yield ______ mL Loss mL ______
Initials ______
Notes: Taste; Energy; Adjustment for cone addition; Did herb perc well? Changes next time?

TABLE 7.5 **Dual Extraction Worksheet**

General Information
Herb Botanical Name ______
Common Name ______Pinyin Name ______
Company or Location of Collection ______
Date Received/Wildcrafted ______ Company Lot Number ______
Apothecary Production Lot Number______ Batch Number ______
Herbalist's Name______
W/V Ratio ☐ 1:2 ☐ 1:3 ☐ 1:4 ☐ 1.5 ☐ Other______
Ethanol % ______
Weight of Herb ______ g
Method: Maceration and Decoction
W/V Ratio ______ g × ______ = TM ______ mL
Ethanol Needed % EtOH______ × TM = ______ = mL of needed ethanol ______
Water Needed % water ______ × TM = ______ = mL of needed water ______
Alcohol to Macerate = ______ mL
Water to Decoct = Needed water mL ______ × 2 = ______mL. Decoct down to ½ = ______mL
Date completed ______ OM ______mL Yield______ mL Loss ______mL
Initials ______
Notes: Taste, Energy; Changes next time?, Did more water need to be added to decoction?

little water. Fresh herbs may be chopped, ground, or left whole. If dried, grind coarsely.

- *Pour in fixed carrier oil.* Choose your oil and pour it in up to the top. Extra virgin olive oil is a good, heat-stable oil. Oil should cover herb totally with no air space between it and the inside of the lid. If herbs try to float to the top and peek out over the oil, weigh them down with cheesecloth and a rock. This eliminates condensation, mold, and air.
- *Macerate, steep, infuse.* Let stand for 4 to 6 weeks. Keep in sun, warm shade, or in brown paper bag in a warm place, placing the jar on a dish or old pie plate to catch spills that invariably occur. Keep an eye on it. If a little oil leaks out over top as the plant soaks it up and expands, add more oil, so there is no space at the top for condensation to form. You will notice the oil taking on the color and aroma of the plant as it macerates, a signal that it's ready.
- *Strain.* Use a fine strainer, cheesecloth, or knee-high nylon stocking and press oil out of the pulp. Can also wrap it in a muslin cloth or nut-milk bag and press with an herb press. This last method does a good job but makes a mess to clean up. Wear gloves and apron, unless you want a greasy moisturizing treatment for your hands and clothes. Also be aware of touching the oil, because bacteria from your fingers can develop in the closed container and spoil the oil.

TABLE 7.6 Vegetable Glycerite Worksheet

General Information
Herb Botanical Name ____
Common Name ____________________ Pinyin Name ________________
Company or Location of Collection ________________________________
Date Received/Wildcrafted ____________ Company Lot Number ______________
Apothecary Production Lot Number____________ Batch Number __________
Herbalist's Name____________________________
W/V ratio ☐ 1:2 ☐ 1:3 ☐ 1:4 ☐ 1:5 ☐ Other __________
Glycerin percentage of menstruum (If only using glycerin, it has to be at least 60% by volume to maintain shelf life/stability, a 60% glycerite.)
Glycerite includes what percent ethanol? _____%. Glycerin %______
Glycerite includes what percent vinegar? _____% Weight of herb _____ g
W/V ratio _______ g × ________ = TM _______ mL
Glycerin needed % glycerin ______ × TM _______ = _______mL glycerin
Ethanol needed % ethanol_________ × TM = ______ = _______ mL ethanol
Vinegar needed % vinegar ______ × TM = ______ = ______mL vinegar
Water needed Glycerin mL _____ + EtOH mL_____ + Vinegar mL____ = ______mL
TM _______mL − sum of glycerin + ethanol + vinegar = _____mL water
Date completed ______ TM ______mL Yield_______ mL Loss _______mL
Initials _____
Notes: Taste, energy, changes next time, how did it taste? Need more or less glycerin?

- *Storage.* Keep in a dark, cool place in a sterilized amber bottle. Label.
- *Tips for preparing sun oils* (Box 7.6).

Directions for Double Boiler Digestion: Slow, Low-Heat Method

- *Place herbs in receptacle.* A double boiler, slow cooker, or electric yogurt maker is fine.
- *Fill container with carrier oil.* Pour oil at least 1 to 2 inches above the herbs. Again, extra virgin olive is recommended. It has some preservative value itself, slowing down the possibility of rancidity.
- *Heat gently.* Heating must be done very slowly and carefully over a very low heat (100°F to 140°F.) for 1 to 5 hours until the oil takes on the color and scent of the herb. Do not deep fry.
- *Allow to cool.* Turn off heat and be patient.[1]
- *Strain.* Use a wet and wrung-out cheesecloth, fine strainer, or knee-high stocking. You may add few drops of vitamin E to serve as antioxidant.
- *Storage.* A sterilized amber bottle in a cool, dark place is best. Label.

Directions for Accelerated Blended Version

- *Prepare herb.* Coarsely grind and place herb in a bowl. (We are not measuring anything.)
- *Moisten with alcohol.* Use 95% EtOH. Just get it moist, not soaked. This begins the breaking-down process, because a head start is needed for this quick version. Let it stand for 1/2 to 1 hour.
- *Return herb to Vitamix or blender.* Add fixed oil to cover top of herb.
- *Blend until warm.* This step is the important part; otherwise the oil, which is the solvent, will not macerate the constituents. The outside of the blender will feel warm; the oil will feel warm also.
- *Strain.* Use a knee-high stocking, nut-milk bag, cheesecloth, or strainer. Press and recycle the marc.
- *Storage.* Choose a cool, dark place. Store oil in sterilized amber bottle with label.

• BOX 7.6 Clinical Pearls for Macerated Sun Oil Preparations

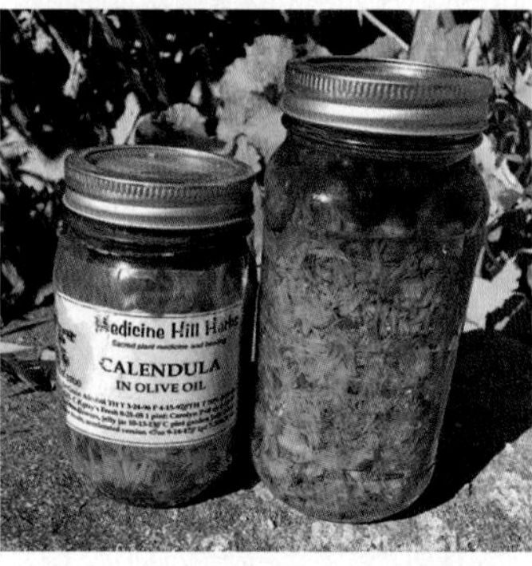

Macerating Calendula flower sun oil sitting outside.

Avoid rancidity. Store in amber containers out of heat, light, moisture and air. Use natural antioxidants: Because rancidity is caused partially by oxidation, use natural antioxidants to avoid this. Suggestions are Rosemary essential oil, vitamin E, or citric acid (vitamin C).

Use vitamin E for preserving. Prick a capsule on either end with a needle and squeeze out capsule contents into the oil, salve, lotion, or cream.

Easy straining method. A good no-hassle, easy clean-up technique is to strain through a clean knee-high nylon stocking. Wet and squeeze dry. Pull stocking top over top of jar. It will be nice and snug. Strain oil through and then wring medicated oil out of the stocking. Best to use gloves so as not to transfer bacteria to the oil from your hands. Then discard stocking. No washing up involved, and area remains relatively clean.

Preparing a Salve

Salves are semisolid fatty preparations applied externally. They are also known as *ointments, unguents, or balms*. They can vary in consistency from thick and hard to greasy and soft, depending on the amount of thickener used. Salves are combinations of a medicated fixed oil and a wax to make them thick. The most common wax is beeswax. Often volatile essential oils are added, which contribute further medicinal action and have preservative value.

Salves can be made starting with a previously made herbal oil infusion or with a dried herb and plain unmedicated fixed oil. Oils and wax are both measured out and heated. The correct amount of beeswax must be added to a set quantity of oil to obtain desired thickness as it cools and hardens. The more wax, the harder it will be. One method to test hardening is to dip a metal spoon into the warm oil and place the spoon in a freezer. When it hardens, test consistency. If too soft, add a little more wax; if too hard, add a little more oil infusion. Basic proportions are 1 cup of infused oil to 1/2 to 1 oz of beeswax.

Directions for "Joint Ease" Salve Using Previously Infused Herbal Oils

- *Assemble ingredients and equipment* (Table 7.7). You'll be glad the containers are all laid out and ready when your hands are holding a pot of hot liquid salve.
- *Prepare a double boiler and heat water.* Either use a commercial double boiler or hook handle of a 2-cup Pyrex measuring cup over the side of the saucepan filled with water. Heat water. Cup must be large enough to prevent boiling water splashing into the oil and beeswax.
- *Heat infused oils slowly.* Place combined oils in top of double boiler or Pyrex measuring cup. Water should come to boil slowly. Do not let it splash up into the oil. Do not stir. (Water and oil don't mix.)
- *Add beeswax to oils.* Beeswax beads are easier to measure and melt faster than a chunk of beeswax that you shave off. Either way, heat until completely melted. Keep temperature very low. Again, don't let any water in.
- *Remove oil from heat.* Dry off outside of oil container with a clean towel. No water.

TABLE 7.7 "Joint-Ease" Salve Assembly

Ingredients	Equipment
• 4 oz. Arnica infused olive oil. • 4 oz. St. John's wort infused olive oil. • ½ oz. beeswax, shaved or beads. • Scant tablespoon Wintergreen essential oil. • Vitamin E oil (100%)—use small amount as a preservative, i.e., prick and empty a capsule.	• Double boiler or 2-cup Pyrex measuring cup and saucepan. Set-up described in instructions. • Measuring spoons. • Stainless steel spoon. • Rubber spatula to clean out oil. • Clean dish towel. • Chopstick. • Salve containers and lids. Set up in row with lids off and face up.

- *Add Wintergreen essential oil.* Stir constantly with a chopstick until it smells good and strong.
- *Add vitamin E oil, stirring constantly.* You don't want it to harden too quickly.
- *Line up salve containers* in good positions for pouring. Stir as you pour to keep essential oils mixed in. Or add a couple of drops of essential oil into each container first, just prior to pouring in the warm salve mixture.
- *Let filled containers cool.* Keep lids off. If you cover them, the salve will sink down in the middle.
- *Label.* Include name of salve, ingredients, ounces, and date made.
- *Storage.* Choose a cool location where salve will remain semisolid and not continue to remelt and resolidify, which can happen in a hot backpack or car. If stored correctly, salves will last for 1 to 3 years. Refrigerate for best longevity (Fig. 7.9).[13]

Directions for Salve Starting with Dried Herbs, Fixed Oil, and Beeswax

- *Prepare infused oil.* Because the herb-infused oil was not made in advance, it has to be done now. To 1 cup of olive or almond oil, add 1 to 2 oz of powdered herb or herbal combination. The volume of dried herb depends on density. There has to be enough oil to make the herbs wet and oily.
- *Slowly heat the oil.* Use the double boiler method described under infused oils. Heat under low heat 100°F to 140°F slowly for 3 to 5 hours.
- *Strain.* Line strainer with a cotton muslin cloth, unbleached coffee filter, or nut-milk bag. Pour the warm oil mixture through strainer. Let this sit until well-drained. Press out remaining oil and recycle marc.
- *Return 1 cup infused oil to double boiler.* Use low heat and warm slowly.
- *Add beeswax.* Use shaved or beads. One-half to 1 oz of wax per cup of oil, approximately.
- *Complete process.* Proceed from here as for a salve with previously infused oils.

Preparing Lotions and Creams

Lotions and ***creams*** are moisturizers that are combinations of water and fat. A cream is simply a thicker lotion. Because water and fat don't mix, they must be emulsified with substances that can combine them, such as lecithin, glycerin, or lanolin, or blended together properly so they stabilize. Beeswax can be added to thicken and harden a properly emulsified cream made without an

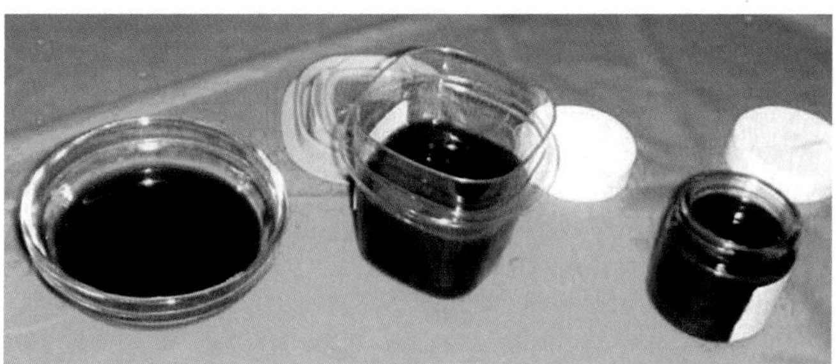

• **Fig. 7.9** Freshly poured salves beginning to harden. Lids ready and waiting.

emulsifier. Making a nice lotion takes a little practice, as does making a fine mayonnaise. The water content of a lotion may be in the form of distilled water, an infusion, decoction, tincture, vinegar, hydrosol, or witch hazel. The oil or fat content may be a plain fixed oil such as olive, almond, jojoba, avocado, or grape; an infused medicated oil; a butter such as cocoa or shea; or any combination of oils or butters. A preservative is frequently added.

Lotions and creams allow the skin to breathe and don't clog the pores. Lotions penetrate the skin faster than creams, but they need to be applied more frequently. Lotions, because of their soft, easy spread are nice for the delicate, sensitive skin of elders, infants, and children. Creams and lotions can be cleansing, softening, soothing, astringing, toning, or pain relieving.[7] In general, the same herbs used for salves are also used in creams and lotions. The choice depends on the therapeutic intention.

You can preserve creams and lotions for about 4 to 6 weeks to 6 months without refrigeration, by using clean utensils, by keeping fingers out of jars, and by taking advantage of the naturally occurring bacterial and mold- and fungus-fighting qualities of the ingredients. Jojoba, avocado, and olive fixed oils, Aloe Vera gel, Tea tree essential oil, vitamin E oil, and honey already have these attributes. Other preservatives include citric acid powder, Geranium and Rosemary essential oils, Grapefruit seed extract, and Green Tea extract.

The proportions of water, oil, and emulsifier vary in lotions, depending on the specific ingredients chosen. Follow a proven recipe for starters. Then branch out. General proportions are as follows:

- *Water base.* About 60% to 80% of the whole consists of distilled water, infusion, decoction, tincture, hydrosol, or prepared witch hazel.[14]
- *Oil base.* About 12% to 14% of the whole consists of fixed or herb-infused oils of cocoa butter, apricot kernel oil, coconut, and others.
- *Emulsifiers.* If any are used, they most often consist of vegetable glycerin, deodorized hydrous lanolin extracted from sheep wool, or *lecithin,*[1] a yellow-brown fatty substance occurring in animal and plant tissues that is amphiphilic (attracting both water and fat). Emulsification can be also be accomplished by careful blending, and no additional emulsifier being necessary. To do this, the oily portion is trickled slowly in a thin stream into a churning blender that contains the watery portion until the oil and water are combined into a creamy mixture that does not separate, and not a single unincorporated drop of liquid can be seen.[15]
- *Preservative 0.5% to 1%.* Choose vitamin E oil or Rosemary essential oil.
- *Creams.* Technically, if the water drops below 50%, the lotion is considered a cream.
- *Extra special lotion-making tips* (Box 7.7).

Very Specific Fail-Safe Directions for a Generic Cream

- *Assemble ingredients and equipment* (Table 7.8). Life is easier when organized.
- *Set up* blender *with water base.* Pour 8 oz of water base (hydrosol or distilled water or decoction or tincture combo) into clean Vitamix or blender. Set aside.
- *Measure out oil.* Pour fixed oil into the top of the double boiler and water in bottom. Or improvise by using a 1- or 2-cup Pyrex measuring cup and hooking it over a saucepan with water in the pan. Put enough water in the saucepan to come to top level of the oil when a Pyrex cup is in the pan. Be careful not to splash water into the oil.
- *Heat oil.* Do this slowly, so water does not boil and splash up into the oil.
- *Add beeswax.* Put 1/2 oz beeswax into the oil and heat until wax is melted.
- *Remove oil from heat.* Remove double boiler or Pyrex cup with oils, wipe outside dry, and set aside.
- *Cool oil.* Wait until a thin rim of hardened wax encircles the inside of oil container (check often).
- *Turn on blender with water covering blades.* Turn blender with water base on to medium speed, lid secured.
- *Add oil slowly.* Very, very gently and gradually and with a steady hand, pour a thin stream of oil/beeswax mixture into top of blender spout using plastic or rubber spatula for scraping the side of the cup occasionally to get all the hardened wax from sides, and then clean the spatula with the chopstick. Do not touch cream with your fingers.

• BOX 7.7 Cream- and Lotion-Making Clinical Pearls

- ***The oil and water mixing must be perfect.*** To properly emulsify, be precise. The mixing/emulsification process is magical and entails the use of a medium or high-speed blender into which the oils are *s-l-o-w-l-y* added until the mixture gradually thickens into a creamy cream or lotion; no water droplets allowed. This might involve banging the blender bottom against the counter a few times and tipping the container to release and pop any water bubbles that appear on the surface or are contained in the air bubbles. If you still see even 1 droplet, emulsify a bit longer and make sure they are all gone.
- ***Keep fingers out.*** Lotions and creams must be stored in perfectly dry and clean (sterile, if possible) containers and lids. No fingers are allowed in any container (including the blender) or you will be introducing microorganisms, mold, and spoilage. This has been the downfall of many a lotion. Although some preservative essential oils and vitamin E might be added, these are not guarantees and are often not enough to counteract inadvertently introduced bacteria.
- ***Herbal tincture suggestions for lotions.*** For chapped, inflamed skin use 1 oz Calendula flower and 1 oz Burdock root. For eczema and chronic skin problems, use 2 oz Oregon Grape root, but know that the berberine content can color skin yellow temporarily. For bruises and sore muscles and joints with no open sores, use 2 oz Arnica flower.

GOOD LUCK and PRACTICE MAKES PERFECT

TABLE 7.8 Generic Cream Assembly

Ingredients	Equipment
• 6 oz olive oil (or other fixed oil) • 8 oz Lavender hydrosol or other hydrosol, distilled water, decoction, combo, or tincture. • 1/2 oz Beeswax shaved or beads (beads are better at melting evenly). • Few drops Lavender or other essential oil. (Start with few drops and add more if needed.) • Few drops pure vitamin E oil.[13]	• Vitamix or blender. • Plastic or rubber spatula. • Chopstick. 1- or 2-cup Pyrex measuring cup. • Stainless steel saucepan large enough to bathe the measuring cup; alternately, use a double boiler. • Containers for cream. • Paper towels.

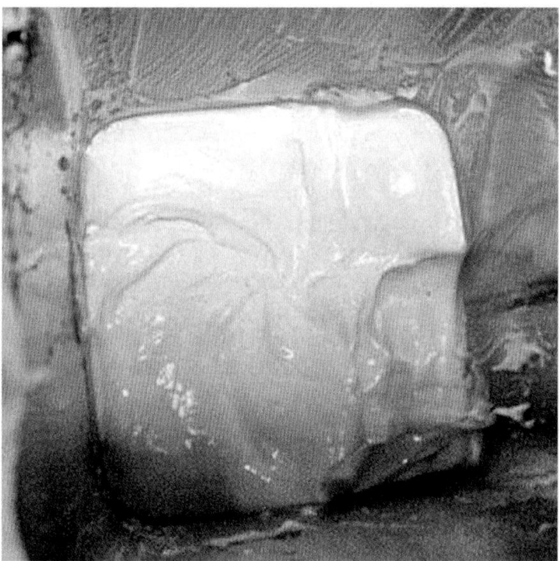

• **Fig. 7.10** Peeking inside a Vitamix holding a cream with no bubbles.

- *When all oil is in blender, turn to high.* Stop machine occasionally to remove lid and scrape sides and lid with the plastic spatula.
- *Listen for cream.* Blend until you hear the cream slap side of the blender. Running the blender too long will heat the cream, so stop in regular intervals to check and scrape. Allow to cool if needed. Rosemary Gladstar says that it "coughs and chokes" and has a buttercream-frosting consistency (Fig. 7.10).
- *Check for water droplets.* Open the blender lid and check for any water droplets. Scrape side again and blend until there are absolutely no droplets of water. Turn off, bang blender bottom against counter, and tilt to let cream run against the side of the container to release air bubbles. Repeat the blending, tilting, and banging until all bubbles are free of water and all water droplets are visibly gone.
- *Add preservative.* Drip in a few drops of vitamin E oil. Sparingly add a few drops of essential oil a little at a time. If too much gets in, you can't take it out.
- *Pulse blender.* Replace the lid and pulse a few times just to mix. Don't overmix.
- *Smell and adjust the cream.* Remove the lid and breathe in the scent. If needed, add only a few more drops of essential oil at a time. Put on the lid and pulse to mix. Then, smell the mixture again. Repeat until just right.
- *Line up clean cream jars.* Place in easy pouring position, setting lids aside.
- *Pour cream into clean waiting jars.* Use a spatula to clean sides of blender. Use a chopstick to guide cream into the jars.
- *Wipe.* Clean the edges of jar with paper towels, *not fingers.*
- *Put on lids.* Then label with the name of cream, ingredients, ounces, and date made.
- *Finishing touches.* Smear remaining cream from blender all over yourself. Wipe utensils with paper towel before cleaning with hot soapy water.

Making Syrups

A ***syrup*** is a thick, sweet liquid that is a saturated solution of sugar in pure water or other aqueous liquid. It is traditionally used for sore throats and in cough mixtures, and it tastes good. Hiding the medicinal taste in a syrup helps the medicine go down. Kids love them. Syrups act as a preservative and can take the place of alcohol or refrigeration in that regard. Only permanent simple syrups can remain unrefrigerated. Syrups containing vinegar, honey, etc., are *not* permanent and require refrigeration.

Syrups may also contain vinegar, honey, glycerin, or small amounts of alcohol or brandy. A *simple syrup* is a saturated sugar solution. A *flavored syrup* contains pleasant, aromatic substances, such as cherry, peppermint, or blackberry. A *medicated syrup* contains soluble principles from various medicinal plants, such as Marshmallow root, Garlic bulb, Elderberry berry, Horehound herb, Black Cohosh root, and many others. Some syrups start from a simple syrup and are further flavored and medicated. In medicated syrups, a decoction is concentrated, simmered down to a half or a third of its original volume, and used as the aqueous element, replacing the pure water. Essential oils may also be added for therapeutic effect.[1]

A little sugar diluted in water spoils quickly and is a magnet for yeasts, molds, and other microorganisms. However, as the saturation of sucrose increases, the chance for these growths decreases. Simple sugars need to approach saturation but not quite reach it. If a syrup is fully saturated, meaning no more sugar can enter solution, chances for crystallization increase as it cools. The resulting crystals or precipitates are difficult to redissolve, and what's left is a solution with insufficient sugar. This again encourages microorganism growth. Vicious circle. To avoid these pitfalls, check Box 7.8.

Syrups can be made with sweeteners other than sugar. Honey, brown sugar, vegetable glycerin, maple syrup, or rice syrup may be used. Honey has antibiotic and enzymatic properties that will break down under high heat. It is a preservative as well. Generally, syrups made with these other sweeteners require refrigeration after a short time.

• BOX 7.8 Syrup-Making Clinical Pearls

- ***Type of water.*** Use recently boiled, distilled water, which is free from mineral matter and spores that might cause fermentation in the presence of sugar.
- ***Type of sugar.*** Use very dry, refined white sugar in crushed, powdered, or granulated form, which is uncontaminated, chemically pure sucrose. These syrups require no refrigeration for storage and are good for traveling, camping, or off-the-grid lifestyles—if in exact proportion of sugar to water to make a permanent simple syrup.
- ***Correct proportion of sugar to water.*** Eighty-five grams of pure sugar to 47 mL of pure water is the ideal proportion for a self-preserving, perfectly concentrated solution.[1] But know there are other proportions out there.
- ***Be sure to strain finished syrup.*** After syrup is prepared, strain through a wet, wrung-out, clean muslin cloth before bottling. This removes any inadvertent dust and dirt that may have crept in.
- ***Sterilized or immaculate containers are important.*** Use very clean, if not sterilized, dry, glass bottles. Store out of air, sun, heat, and light in cool place with uniform temperature. Use small containers so that a large quantity of syrup is not exposed to air every time container is opened.

Directions for Making Cough/Sore Throat Syrup

- *Assemble ingredients.* These can be dried herbs and others (Table 7.9).
- *Weigh dried herbs.* Approximate parts to equal 60 g (2 oz).
- *Soak herbs in water.* Soak herbs in 1 l (1 quart) distilled water for a few hours to soften.

TABLE 7.9 Ingredients Assembly for Cough/Sore Throat Syrup

Parts	Dried Herbs 60 g/2 oz	Other Ingredients
4 parts	Fennel seed	1 l (quart) distilled water.
2 parts	Licorice root	1 cup honey, more or less as desired.
2 parts	Osha root	4 tablespoons Wild Cherry concentrate.
2 parts	Horehound herb	4-8 tablespoons brandy.
2 parts	Wild Cherry bark	
2 parts	Valerian root	
1 part	Slippery Elm bark	
1 part	Cinnamon bark	
1 part	Ginger root	
1/8 part	Orange peel	

- *Decoct herbs.* Simmer until liquid is reduced to half of original volume (500 mL or 1 pint). Use chopstick measuring method described in dual extraction section.
- *Strain and press herbs.* Remove from heat, and then strain and press. Measure decoction.
- *Return decoction to pot.* Measure it to make sure there is 1 pint. Add a little water, if necessary.
- *Add desired sweetener.* Add to decoction at 2:1 ratio (two parts herb to one part sweetener). Approximately 1 cup sweetener to 2 cups or 1-pint decoction. Sweetener can be honey, white or brown sugar, maple syrup, rice syrup, vegetable glycerin, or any combination. It will be sweet. Always start with less and then add sweetener to taste if refrigeration is used, and storage not an issue.
- *Warm up sweetener.* Use low heat and mix decoction and sweetener together until fully dissolved.
- *For thicker syrup.* Simmer for 20 to 30 minutes more. Remember, if honey is used, heat will destroy the enzymes. It's a tradeoff. (To thicken this more, increase Slippery Elm proportion.)
- *Add brandy and wild cherry syrup.* Brandy relaxes smooth muscles and suppresses cough. Wild Cherry is a cough suppressant and adds flavor. This step could make the syrup a little diluted.
- *Allow to cool.* Although not in above formula, this is when essential oils would be added. Add only 1 drop at a time and test flavors. Essential oils are strong and could overpower the whole thing. Peppermint, Ginger, or Anise are possibilities.
- *Bottles.* Use clean small bottles and label.

Summary

Advanced herbal remedy making was presented in the form of a hands-on lab. Materials and equipment needed to equip an apothecary were described.

Making tinctures includes the folk method that does not require calculations and more precise w/v techniques that do. Weight-to-volume is based on the fact that 1 cubic centimeter (cc) of water weighs 1 g. Precise amounts of herb, alcohol, and water are calculated to produce a specific tincture strength. Instructions and worksheets were provided for simple macerations, percolations, dual extractions, and glycerites. A factor in determining alcohol percentages requires knowledge of which plant constituents are water soluble and which are ethanol soluble. A handy table for this is provided.

There are three kinds of infused oils: the slow solar method, double boiler, and blender methods. They all require heat. Directions and pitfalls of making salves, lotions, creams, and syrups were provided in detail with tips for successful results.

Review

Fill in the Blanks

(Answers in Appendix B.)

1. W/V method assumes ___.
2. Ingestible alcohol is called ___ and external use alcohol is called ___ .
3. Four water-soluble chemical constituents include ___, ___, ___.
4. Four alcohol-soluble constituents include ___, ___, ___, ___.
5. Plants high in ___ require very high ethanol around ___ to ___ percent. Two herbal examples are ___ and ___.
6. We are using 8 oz of dry Uva ursi. Need a 1:4 60% alcohol to water menstruum. Herb weight = ___ g. TM = ___ mL. Water = ___ mL. Alcohol = ___ mL.
7. We want a 50% 1:3 percolation of 200 g of dry Xanthium Cang Er Zi. Calculate OM, AM, and TM. OM = ___ mL. Added menstruum = ___ mL. TM = ___ mL. Total water = ___ mL. Total alcohol = ___ mL.
8. A dual extraction is a combination of two methods. What are they? ___, ___.
9. Name three types of oil infusions and how long to make each. ___, ___, ___, ___, ___, ___.
10. Three important points for successful lotion and creams are to ___, ___, ___.

Critical Concept Questions

(Answers for you to decide.)

1. What equipment will you purchase initially for your herb remedy-making set-up?
2. What are the advantages/disadvantages of the w/v method versus the folk method?

3. A tincture label says it contains 1:4 65%. What does that mean?
4. Which is stronger: 1:6 50% or 1:2 50%? Why?
5. You have 5 oz of Burdock root and want a 1:4 45% tincture. How much water and how much alcohol are needed? Next time you try a percolation with same amount of plant and above proportions. How much water and how much alcohol this time?
6. Name some instances where a glycerite would be indicated.
7. Why must the sugar content in a good syrup approach saturation?
8. Explain how you make a dried herb into a syrup?
9. What is a dual extraction? Why would you choose this method? What kind of herbs should be dual extracted for best results?

References

1. Green, James. *The Herbal Medicine-Maker's Handbook* (New York: Crossing, 2002).
2. Made by Isaiah Scott of ISCO Limited. Listed for sale on herbalist Joan Zinn's website: http://www.medicinehillherbs.com/products/products.htm
3. Romm, Aviva. *Botanical Medicine for Woman's Health* (St. Louis, MO: Elsevier, 2020) (Section written by Lisa Ganora).
4. Ganora, Lisa. *Herbal Constituents: Foundations of Phytochemistry* (Louisville, CO: Herbalchem Press, 2009).
5. Holmes, Peter. *Jade Remedies: A Chinese Herbal Reference for the West* (Boulder, CO: Snow Lotus, 1996).
6. Holmes, Peter. *Energetics of Western Herbs* (Boulder, CO: Snow Lotus, 2006).
7. Green, James. *The Herbal Medicine-Maker's Handbook* (New York: Crossing Press, 2002).
8. Moore, Michael. *Medicinal Plants of the Mountain West* (Santa Fe, NM: (Museum of New Mexico Press, 2003).
9. Buhner, Stephen. *Herbal Antibiotics* (North Adams Maine: Storey, 2012).
10. "How to Make a Medicinal Mushroom Double-Extraction Tincture". Herbal Academy. https://theherbalacademy.com/make-medicinal-mushroom-double-extraction-tincture/ (accessed September 23, 2019).
11. "What is Rancidity?" The World's Healthiest Foods. http://whfoods.org/genpage.php?tname = dailytip&dbid = 356 (accessed September 26, 2019).
12. "How to Infuse Oil with Herbs (3 Methods)". Mountain Rose Herbs. https://blog.mountainroseherbs.com/making-herbal-oils (accessed September 26, 2019).
13. Zinn, Joan. http://www.medicinehillherbs.com/
14. "Make Your Own Lotions". Glenbrook Farms. http://www.glenbrookfarm.com/make-your-own-lotions.htmL (accessed September 26, 2019).
15. "How to Create Handmade Lotion Recipes". Soap Queen. https://www.soapqueen.com/bath-and-body-tutorials/lotion/how-to-create-homemade-lotion-recipes/ (accessed September 26, 2019).
16. Moore, Michael. *Medicinal Plants of the Desert and Canyon West* (Sante Fe, New Mexico: Museum of New Mexico Press, 1989).

8 Chemical Constituents For Herbalists

"The molecular world is far more mystical, fluid and dynamic than your college chemistry classes might have suggested."

***— Lisa Ganora, director, Colorado School of Clinical Herbalism, author of* Herbal Constituents**

CHAPTER REVIEW

- Overview: Pharmacognosy, primary and secondary metabolites.
- Synergy: The whole herb is greater than the sum of its parts.
- Phytochemistry basics. Elements.
- Carbohydrates: Monosaccharides, disaccharides, oligosaccharides, polysaccharides, immunomodulating polysaccharides (IPs), gums, mucilages, pectins, inulin, and organic acids.
- Amino acid derivatives: Amines, sulfur compounds (allium plants), and glucosinolates.
- Lipids: Saturated fatty acids, unsaturated fatty acids, essential fatty acids, omegas, triglycerides, and alkamides.
- Phenolic compounds: Salicylic acid, coumarins, lignins, flavonoids, and phytoestrogens.
- Terpenes: Monoterpenes, sesquiterpenes, diterpenes, triterpene saponins and steroidal saponins, cardiac glycosides, and tetraterpenoids.
- Alkaloids, Allantoins, pyrrolizidine alkaloids (PAs), protoberberines, purines, piperidines, and sanguinarines.

KEY TERMS

Alkaloids
Alkamides
Amino acids
Carbohydrates
Cardiac glycosides
CB receptors
Coumarin
Drug
Endocannabinoids
Endocannabinoid system
Essential amino acids
Free radicals
Gum
Immunomodulating polysaccharides (IPs)
Inulin
Lignins
Lipids
Pectin
Pharmacodynamics
Pharmacokinetics
Pharmacology
Pharmacognosy
Phenolic compounds
Photosynthesis
Phytochemistry
Phytoestrogens
Salicylic acid
Saturated fatty acids
Synergy
Terpenes
Trans fatty acids
Unsaturated fatty acids

The archetypal constituents consist of the *primary metabolites* that keep a plant alive. These are carbohydrates, proteins, lipids, enzymes, and chlorophyll. A plant's *secondary metabolites* are not necessary to sustain plant life, but they increase its survival in the natural environment. Examples are alkaloids, which play a defensive role against pathogens and herbivores (plant eating animals), and tannins, which protect the wood in living trees from microbial decomposition and insects. Understanding the properties of these metabolites provide us with clues as to how a plant affects the body and its medicinal characteristics.

The intention is to introduce the herbalist to ***phytochemistry***, the study of the major substances found in plants and the therapeutic properties that result. The six major categories for this understanding are carbohydrates, amino acid derivatives, lipids, phenolic compounds, terpenes, and alkaloids. Basic nutritional information becomes a natural part of the discussion.

Chemicals in plants affect the energetics of taste (Chapter 10). Carbohydrates are sweet. Tannins are astringent. Organic acids are sour. Glucosinolates are pungent. Alkaloids are bitter. Plant chemical constituents also affect the therapeutic actions a plant has on the body. Included here are the major herbal phytochemicals.

Plant Chemistry Overview

Plants are chemically complex. There can be hundreds of constituents in a single one. *Phyto* means related to plants. Close to 45% of modern pharmaceuticals contain chemicals originally found in herbs. Herbs can be active medicine for the body. By understanding the basic plant chemicals, we can see how a given herb affects the body without having to memorize what does what.

Phytochemicals are compounds that occur naturally in plants (Table 8.1). They can be thought of as the active ingredients. They have specific tastes and other properties. They are responsible for plants having a mild gentle tonic effect (e.g., Nettle herb), strong therapeutic properties (Lily of the Valley herb), or deadly poisonous elements (Water Hemlock root).

Synergy

Any given plant has numerous components, not all of which are considered active ingredients. Some work in harmony in a single plant or even in a formula to balance and modulate one another for a particular therapeutic effect. This characteristic explains why a whole herb can be safer or more effective than an isolated constituent or a single-molecule pharmaceutical or drug. There is *synergy*, implying that the whole herb is greater than the sum of the parts. It explains why a very mild constituent can be enhanced by other ingredients or why a strong, toxic substance is safer in the context of the whole plant than when in isolation.

Synergy is the interrelationship between constituents of a plant or formula. This coaction results in an altered therapeutic effect that we would not have had with a single substance. An example of this is the famous antidepressant herb, *Hypericum perforatum* (St. John's Wort). The first ingredients ever isolated from this plant were hypericin and pseudohypericin. Later in other studies, hyperforin, hyperin, and melatonin were found to work synergistically with hypericin.[1] They work better together than by themselves. Early extracts of *H. perforatum* had historically been standardized to a certain percentage of its assumed *active ingredient* hypericin—with much hype and little regard for the other ingredients. Now, the other coactive components are also included and standardized to provide a more effective antidepressant extract.

However, you can rest assured that a weight-to-volume tincture of St. John's Wort made with the fresh flowering tops and no chemical alteration or standardization will also provide the active synergy to treat mild to moderate depression. And there may be many other substances in St. John's Wort not yet analyzed that also add to its synergy. Many plants are far from having a complete chemical analysis of constituents.

Definitions

- ***Pharmacology***. The study of the interaction of biologically active agents in a living system. *Plant pharmacology* is the study of the key chemical constituents in a plant.
- ***Pharmacognosy*** is the study and science of phytochemistry or plant chemistry and potential drugs that may result.
- ***Pharmacodynamics***. The effect of a chemical at active sites in the body. This is the therapeutic effect.
- ***Pharmacokinetics***. The study of what happens to a constituent from the time it enters the body to when it exits. It involves *absorption* and how well the constituent reaches where it needs to go (bioavailability); *distribution*, how and to what organ it tends to go (tropism); *metabolism*, how it breaks down (biotransforms) into something the body can use, which is generally done in the liver; and *excretion*, the avenue and time taken to eliminate a substance (usually through the kidneys). This knowledge provides information about correct and safe dosing, dosing intervals, and how long the drug lasts and works in the body before it is metabolized and excreted.
- ***Drug***. Usually one or two pure chemicals, considered the active ingredient and dispensed as a remedy. Many drugs or their precursors were derived from plants. Drugs are dispensed as a single pure chemical, rather than in a plant matrix. They are also patented and usually synthesized (Chapter 29).

Phytochemistry

The elements common to all living things are carbon, hydrogen, oxygen, nitrogen, sulfur, and phosphorus. Some plants have other elements too, such as calcium, magnesium, iron, copper, or selenium.

TABLE 8.1 Summary of Phytochemical Organization

Carbohydrates	Amino Acid Derivatives	Lipids (Fatty acids or FAs)	Phenolic Compounds	Terpenes	Alkaloids
Monosaccharides	Amines	Saturated	Salicylic acid	Monoterpenes	Allantoins
Disaccharides	Sulfur compounds and allium plants	Unsaturated	Coumarins	Sesquiterpenes	Pyrrolizidine alkaloids (PAs)
Oligosaccharides	Glucosinolates	Essential FAs	Lignins	Diterpenes	Protoberberines
Polysaccharides		Omega-3, -6, -9	Flavonoids	Triterpenes	Purines
Immuno-modulating polysaccharides (IPs)		Triglycerides	Phytoestrogens	Triterpene saponins	Piperidines
Gums		Alkamides		Triterpene steroidal saponins	Sanguinarines
Mucilages				Cardiac glycosides	
Pectins				Tetraterpenoids	
Inulin					
Organic acids					

- *Carbon* (C) occurs in all phytochemicals and living things. It forms the backbone or the so-called skeleton of organic molecules.
- *Hydrogen (H).* Hydrogen gas is the smallest and lightest element. It is a fundamental component of water and all life.
- *Oxygen (O).* Oxygen gas, the most abundant element in all living things, is an odd one, because we can't live without it, but it can also do damage to cells and even be lethal when out of check. This happens when oxygen forms one or more unpaired electrons called ***free radicals*** (reactive oxygen species, ROS), which are highly unstable atoms that damage cells, proteins, and DNA by altering their chemical structure.
  - Plants (and humans, thanks to our awesome livers) naturally inhibit these free radicals and guard against ROS, which cause cellular damage (Chapter 19). When various antioxidant-rich foods and herbs are ingested, they help toxin-overloaded livers quench free radicals and thus protect us from oxidative stress.[2] Plant antioxidants give a plant its color. The blues and purples in elderberry, bilberry, and blueberries are notoriously healthy foods due to their antioxidants. Consuming a variety of colorful foods assures a well-rounded antioxidant supply.
- *Nitrogen* (N). Nitrogen occurs in 78% of the atmosphere but is not absorbed directly by plants. Instead, many Fabaceae/Pea family members have root nodules on which nitrogen-fixing bacteria (*Rhizobia* and others) live symbiotically. Beans, peas, clover, soy, and alfalfa depend on the bacteria to convert nitrogen into soil nitrates, which are usable forms and necessary nutrients for healthy soil, plants, and the animals who eat them.
- *Sulfur* (S) gives some plants their hot, pungent taste as evidenced in garlic, onions, and wasabi.
- *Phosphorus* (P) can glow in the dark in some forms. It occurs in adenosine triphosphate (ATP), the cell's energy source, and is a part of the double helix of genetic DNA.

Single elements are *atoms*. These do not occur by themselves but are held together in *molecules* by various types of bonds. There are also functional groups, which are specific small groups of atoms that are the parts of a larger molecule. The groups are chemically active, and this is where most reactions and changes occur. Examples of these are an ester group, an amino group, or an ethanol group.

Furthermore, some or a series of atoms in a compound can be connected to form a *ring*. This happens most often with carbon. Carbon can form a frame or ring to which other groups of atoms are attached. Although these various molecules are really three dimensional, they are often represented graphically by two-dimensional lines or a line formula, with symbols of the atoms included. The phytochemical groups in this chapter's figures are drawn in the two-dimensional fashion.

Carbohydrates

Carbohydrates are present in all living beings on the planet. Carbohydrates, a major phyto molecule, are any type of *sugar* made from carbon, hydrogen, and oxygen (CHO). If you chew any carbohydrate long enough, you will taste the sweetness. Carbohydrates are the product of photosynthesis in plants and the building blocks of all other phytochemicals.[3] In ***photosynthesis***, plants use their light-absorbing green pigment—*chlorophyll*—to convert carbon dioxide and water into glucose for their food. In the process, plants give off oxygen as a byproduct and thus are crucial in maintaining our atmosphere.

As herbalists, we are interested in the nutritional value of carbs and the types that pop up in herbal remedies. Humans use glucose, a simple sugar, to create ATP. This energy source keeps the heart beating, the muscles working, and the brain functioning. An adequate intake of carbs also spares proteins and helps with fat metabolism. Carbohydrates are generally water soluble—sugars and starches being examples. Dietary carbohydrates include *glucose*, *fructose*, *starch*, and *cellulose*.

Carbohydrates are classified into the number of sugars they contain. As they proceed from one sugar to many sugars, they get more and more complex and take longer for the body to break down and digest. From a nutritional standpoint, the more complex a carbohydrate, the slower the spikes in blood sugar and the healthier that carbohydrate is. Hyperglycemia, insulin and leptin resistance, metabolic syndrome, and type II diabetes can result from excess carbohydrate intake, particularly from simple monosaccharides with one sugar, and disaccharides with two sugars (Chapter 27).

- *Monosaccharides* are single, simple sugars: *glucose*, the form the body uses to make energy and present in ripe fruits and some onions; *fructose*, found in fruits and honey; and *galactose*, mammals' milks. These provide energy, some vitamins and roughage, and immune protection through mother's milk.
- *Disaccharides* have two simple sugars combined, such as 1 glucose plus 1 fructose equals *sucrose* (table sugar and sugar beets) or 1 glucose plus 1 galactose equals *lactose* (dairy) or 1 glucose plus 1 glucose equals *maltose* (barley or malt) (Fig. 8.1).
  - Many people are lactose intolerant. Lactose intolerance results from lack of the enzyme *lactase* that digests lactose. Populations where this intolerance is prevalent are people of African and Asian ancestry. But adults and even kids of any descent with chronic ear infections may have this problem.
- *Oligosaccharides. Oligo* means *a few.* These sugar units range between 2 and 10. One important type is the *fructooligosaccharides* (FOS). These are prebiotics—foods and herbs that stimulate the growth of healthy bacterial intestinal flora and are present in Jerusalem artichokes (sunchokes), asparagus, onion, Burdock root, Dandelion root, Chicory root, and Garlic bulb.[1]
- *Polysaccharides*, also known as *glycans*, have from 10 to thousands of sugar units. They are the long-chain *complex carbohydrates* found in starchy root vegetables, such as potatoes and whole grains, that take a while to digest, providing nutrition and energy with less stress on the pancreas than simple carbs. Polysaccharides include immunomodulating medicinal mushrooms, inulins, pectins, mucilages, and gums. These are so important herbally, they will be addressed separately.

Immunomodulating Polysaccharides (IPs)

Polysaccharides that modulate and balance the immune system—***immunomodulating polysaccharides (IPs)***—are a very important group of carbohydrates. These are present in most adaptogenic herbs and the medicinal mushrooms, such as Ganoderma Ling Zhi (Reishi mushroom) (Fig. 8.2). They are phytochemically complex and contain both water- and ethanol-soluble constituents, requiring dual extraction (Chapter 7) for best results.

Adaptogenic IPs

IPs help the body maintain vitality, health, and resistance to infection. Adaptogens occur all over the planet. *Echinacea angustifolia* is the most notable Western adaptogenic polysaccharide, Eleutherococcus Ci Wu Jia (Siberian ginseng root) is from Russia, and *Withania somnifera* (Ashwagandha root) is from India. Notable Chinese

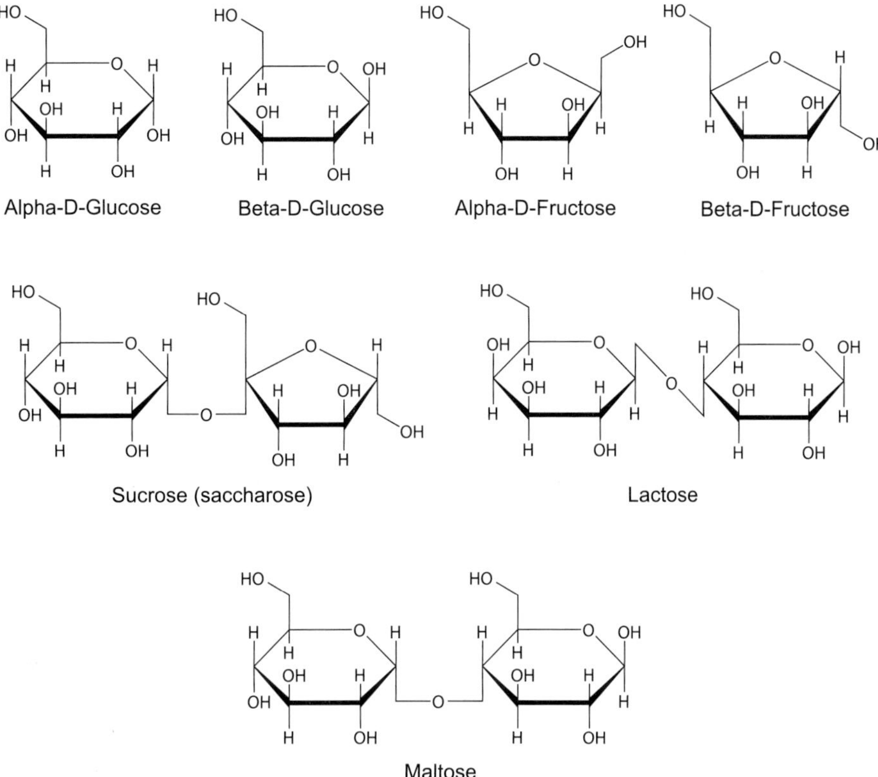

• **Fig. 8.1** Chemical structures of main sugars showing monosaccharides with one simple sugar and slightly more complex disaccharides with two simple sugars. (iStock.com/Credit: chromatos.)

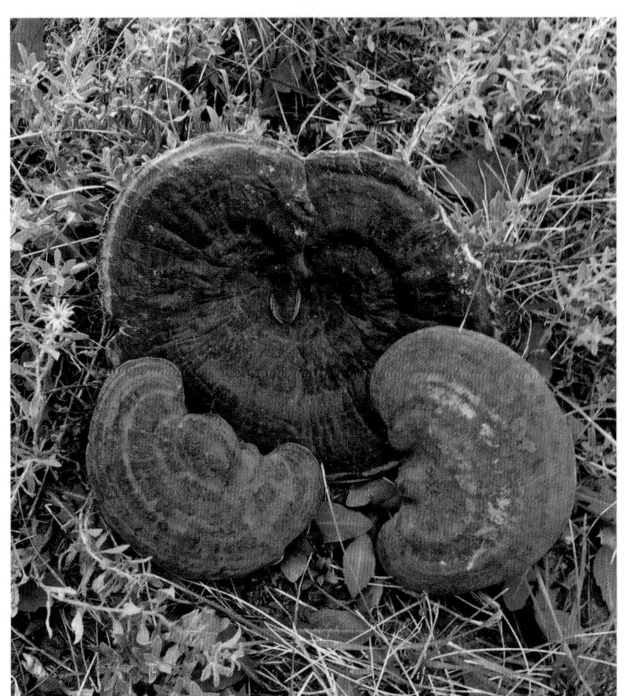

• **Fig. 8.2** Ganoderma Ling Zhi (Reishi mushroom), rich in immunomodulating polysaccharides.

adaptogens, other than the mushrooms, are Lycium Gou Qi Zi (Goji berry or Wolfberry), Panax Ren Shen (Asian ginseng root) and Panax Xi Yang Shen (American ginseng root). IPs do the following in the body:

- *Slow down aging.* IPs have antiaging properties, and some inhibit cancer cells.
- *Decrease oxidative stress.* Many IPs inhibit oxidation of lipids (lipid peroxidation). Lipid peroxidation causes oxidative stress and tissue breakdown.
- *Increase immunity.* Some IPs stimulate function of plasma proteins and antibodies, boosting resistance.
- *Decrease stress.* Other IPs affect the neuroendocrine system and decrease stress by normalizing the hypothalamus–pituitary–adrenal axis (HPA axis), which releases the stress hormones cortisol and adrenaline (Chapter 27).[4]

Gums

A ***gum*** is a water-soluble polysaccharide secretion produced by algae and plants in response to trauma, insect attack, or infection.[1] Gums are often found on the woody parts of a tree or on seed coatings in response to damage. They are thicker and stickier than a mucilage. Gums attract water molecules and become hydrated, viscous hydrocolloids. They stop other ingredients from separating out of a mixture and are therefore used as stabilizers in the cosmetic industry. Agar and carrageenan are seaweed gums used for these purposes. Gums are soluble dietary fiber that can bind to bile acids and help lower cholesterol, thereby lowering risk of colon cancer, coronary artery disease, and diabetes.

Mucilages

Mucilages are polysaccharides that form viscous solutions with water. The key action of mucilages occur on the surfaces with which they come in contact.[5] They produce a slimy, cooling yin-generating effect that is soothing, cooling, and itch reducing. Mucilages are the *demulcents* of herbal fame. They act as emollients for the mucous membranes of the urinary, respiratory, reproductive, and digestive systems. They calm irritating coughs, help with urinary tract infections, and soothe stomach cramps, lesions, and ulcers. Demulcent herbs extract best in cold water. Examples are Marshmallow root and leaf, Flax seed, Purslane herb, Plantain herb, Slippery Elm bark, Comfrey root and leaf. Mucilaginous Psyllium seed husk is very fibrous and gelatinous and has a pulling and bulking action on the bowel.

Pectins

Pectins are water-trapping colloidal polysaccharides found in the primary walls of most plant cells, especially fruit tissue. In solution, they create a gel and are used as a setting or thickening agent in jams and jellies. Pectins are usually found in the white material inside the rind of the fruit, notably apples, oranges, and grapefruits. Apple pectin and organic unfiltered apple juice are often used in bowel cleanses because they pull water and toxins into the bowel for elimination. Pectin has been used to lower high cholesterol and high triglyceride levels and for colon and prostate cancer prevention. It is also used in the treatment of diabetes and gastroesophageal reflux disease (GERD) and to prevent poisoning caused by lead, strontium, and other heavy metals.[6] These uses are all because of pectin's pulling action in the gut that helps with detoxification.

Inulin

Inulin is an indigestible oligosaccharide. It is *not* insulin, so don't confuse the two. Inulin provides soluble fiber for humans, although we lack the enzyme to digest it. However, our important intestinal microflora can and do metabolize it and use it for food. Inulin-rich gut foods are known as *prebiotics*. Healthy food for the gut microbiome translates into numerous happy gut flora. Maintaining gut flora is crucial in managing and/or eliminating irritable bowel disease (IBS), Crohn's disease, and ulcerative colitis. Many prebiotics are Lily family members, such as onion, garlic, leeks, scallions, and Blue Camus bulb.

Inulin has numerous other functions. It helps stabilize blood sugar by decreasing glucose absorption. It lowers fatty triglycerides in blood plasma by reducing synthesis in the liver, and it aids the gut-associated lymphoid tissue (GALT) by increasing immunoglobulins that boost the immune system (Chapter 18). *Inula helenium* (Elecampane root) is named after inulin. One of the best-known herbs containing inulin is Dandelion root.[1] It helps absorption of calcium and magnesium and has anticancer properties.

Organic Acids

Organic acids are derived from monosaccharides. There are many types, including the fruit acids of *citric, malic, tartaric,* and others such as *formic acid, oxalic acid,* and *ascorbic acid* (vitamin C). Organic acids supply the sour taste.

- *Fruit acids. Citric acid* occurs in citrus fruits and gooseberries, black currants, and strawberries. It tastes tart and sour. Although it is an acid, it (counterintuitively) breaks down or metabolizes into alkaline bicarbonates. Citric acid is thus good for acid conditions, such as arthritis and degenerative diseases, and also helps stop acid-dependent tooth decay. Being sour, citric acid increases bile flow from the liver.
  - *Malic acid* occurs in apples, grapes, cherries, and plums. These fruits contain antioxidants and have sour, tart flavors, and like citric acid, do not increase the body's acidity. Lemons contain both citric and malic acids and have long been considered liver stimulants. In Chinese medicine, the taste for the liver is sour.
  - *Tartaric acid.* Although citric and malic acids do *not* increase the body's acidity, tartaric acid *does* because it is *not* broken down by metabolism.[5] Tartaric acid is found in tamarinds, cranberries, Prickly Pear Cactus fruit, and other plants.
- *Oxalic acid (oxalates).* This acid occurs in plants in the form of insoluble calcium salts or water-soluble sodium or potassium salts. Oxalic acid might be an issue if a person has kidney problems (Chapter 26). It can be the source of kidney stones formed by precipitation of excessive oxalates in acid urine. Many common foods and herbs contain oxalates, such as Rhubarb family plants, Yellow Dock root, Chickweed herb, Lamb's Quarters herb, spinach, beet greens and roots, Swiss chard, and parsley. The oxalate content of these foods can be reduced 30% to 90% by boiling in water, if necessary.[1] If a client has a problem with kidney stones, refer to a longer list of oxalate-rich foods and herbs.
- *Formic acid* and *nettle. Urtica dioica* (Nettle herb) is covered in stinging, painful hairs (Fig. 8.3), which contain a mixture of formic, oxalic, malic, acetic, and tartaric acids and inflammatory modulators, including histamine, serotonin, and acetylcholine.[1] Consequently, fresh Nettle herb—with its stinging hairs—is used as a local irritant for treating chronic joint inflammation and arthritis and is often rubbed against the skin for this therapeutic purpose. It creates itchy, stinging, red welts (the sting) that disappear in about 10 to 15 minutes

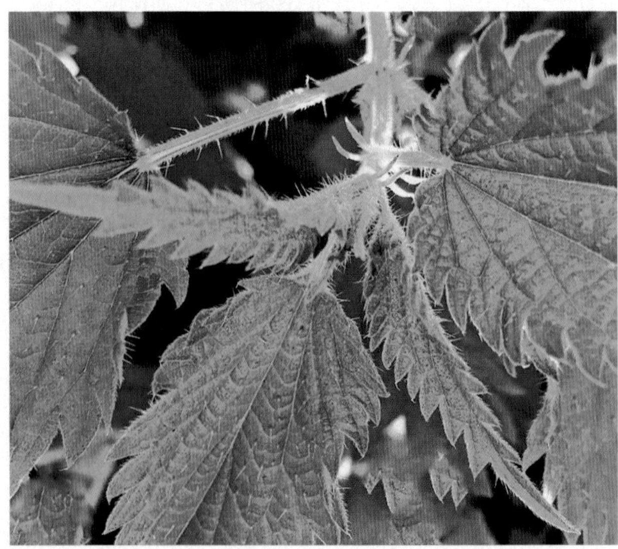

• **Fig. 8.3** Nettle herb showing stinging hairs containing formic acid.

as pain relief begins. When Nettle is heated, cooked, or tinctured, formic acid is inactivated. If wildcrafting the plant, use gloves unless you seek the stinging effect.

Amino Acids

Proteins are made up of ***amino acids*** (AAs), which are one of the three *macronutrients* the body requires along with carbohydrates and fats. Amino acids are organic compounds that contain various numbers of amine and carboxylic acid functional groups. They are the building blocks of plant and animal proteins. In plants, amino acids are precursors, used and combined to form proteins, peptides, enzymes, amines, the sulfur allium compounds, and cyanogenic glycosides, which are alkaloids.[1] In humans, proteins are needed primarily for tissue growth and repair. When proteins are digested, they are broken down into amino acids. There are 20 to 22 biogenic amino acids (*biogenic* means brought about by living organisms) (Fig. 8.4). The exact number is up for debate.

Essential amino acids cannot be made by the body yet are indispensable for health. As a result, they must come from food. There are nine essential amino acids: histidine, isoleucine, leucine, lysine, methionine, phenylalanine, threonine, tryptophan, and valine. The other amino acids that the body does make are alanine, asparagine, aspartic acid, glutamic acid, arginine, cysteine, glutamine, tyrosine, glycine, ornithine, proline, and serine. AAs are water soluble, except the aromatic ones (phenylalanine, tryptophan, and tyrosine). Insufficient protein dietary intake leads to muscle wasting, weakness, fatigue, decreased immunity, and anxiety.

Animal sources of protein are numerous and include meats, eggs, dairy, and fish. An egg, considered a perfect food, contains all nine essential amino acids. For people on vegetarian or vegan diets, obtaining balanced protein sources is a little more challenging, particularly if no dairy is consumed. Plant sources of amino acids include whole grains, legumes, seeds, and nuts. Excellent high protein foods are soybeans, spirulina algae, and yogurt. The hulled seeds of *Cannabis sativa* (Hemp seed) contain all the essential amino acids and essential fatty acids (FAs) that our bodies need, making it a perfect protein supplement. Kelp contains over 12 vitamins, 20 major amino acids, and 60 chelated trace minerals.[7]

Amines

Amines are small structures with one phenolic group or more. *Histamine* is an amine. It causes allergic symptoms and is found in Nettle herb stingers, discussed earlier. Another amine is *ephedrine*, similar to the human sympathetic hormone, adrenaline.[1] Chinese *Ephedra* Ma Huang (Ephedra stem) is a fabulous herb that is warm, dry, and relaxing and has been used in Chinese Medicine for thousands of years to dry up mucous and to treat asthma, bronchitis, and hay fever.

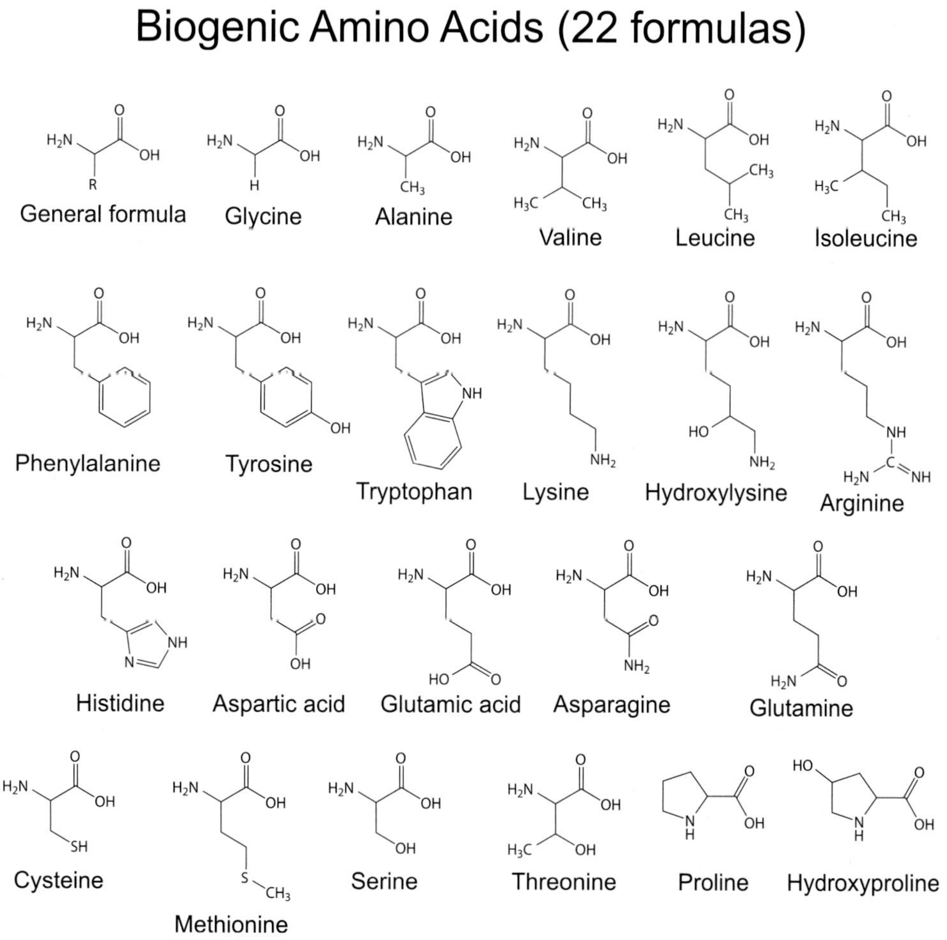

• **Fig. 8.4** Amino acids are the building blocks of plant and animal proteins. There are 20 to 22 amino acids made by living organisms. (iStock.com/ Credit: chromatos.)

Sulfur Compounds and Allium Plants

Lily family plants of the *Allium* genus contain bioactive sulfur compounds derived from the amino acid, cysteine. We are speaking of *Allium sativum* (Garlic bulb), onions, and leeks. Fresh Garlic bulb contains alliin, a derivative of the amino acid cysteine. When a clove is crushed or chopped, the enzyme alliinase is released. The two interact to form allicin.[1] *Allicin* is the pungent-smelling component in Garlic bulb that kills bacteria and fungus, and has cardiovascular and anticancer benefits. It will stay active at room temperature for about 12 to 16 hours. Most sources report that Garlic bulb is more beneficial raw than cooked; the reason is that when heated or microwaved, alliinase and its subsequent conversion into allicin cannot take place. It tastes good, but it is not as therapeutic. When using Garlic bulb in cooking, it is best to add it near the end.

Glucosinolates

Glucosinolates are highly pungent-tasting compounds synthesized from amino acids, especially the sulfur-containing cysteine and methionine.[1] Examples are the Mustards: Japanese *Wasabi japonica* and Horseradish root (Fig. 8.5). All are strong sinus openers that cause tearing and other extreme reactions. Sulfurous Mustard family foods like broccoli, cauliflower, cabbage, and Brussels sprouts contain chemoprotective glucosinolates.

Lipids

This is a complex group. ***Lipids*** are fatty, oily substances that are usually not water soluble. Some are liquid and some are solid. There are many subgroups in the lipid category: fats, triglycerides, phospholipids, steroids, and fatty acids.

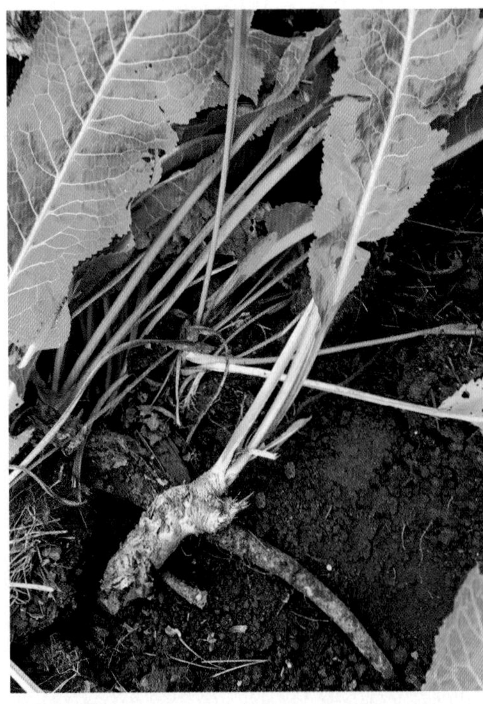

• **Fig. 8.5** Exposed Horseradish tap root containing pungent sinus-opening glucosinolates.

Lipids provide energy, provide the building blocks for phospholipid cell membranes in plants and animals, and act as raw materials that can be converted to other substances, such as hormones. Examples of lipids include fats, oils, waxes, fat-soluble vitamins (A, D, E, K), cholesterol, steroids, and hormones. Olives, avocados, and palm berries are fatty fruits. Nuts and seeds, like flax, walnuts, and almonds, have a fatty component that provides energy storage for the plant and are healthy for humans. Note that essential oils are not lipids; they are terpenes (explained later in this chapter), but most of them will dissolve with plant oils.

Fatty Acids (FAs)

The properties of fats and FAs depend on their degree of hydrogen saturation and the length of their molecules, or *chain length*. Chemically, a fatty acid is a chain of carbon atoms with pairs of hydrogen atoms attached and with an *acid group* attached to one end of the molecule (Fig. 8.6).

FAs have hydrocarbon tails that terminate with a carboxylic acid group. They are made up of carbon, hydrogen, and oxygen. There are many kinds of FAs. Some are healthy; some not. Research is constantly providing new information about good fats and bad fats (Table 8.2). The previously reviled saturated fats from animals and tropical oils have come back into favor with the Paleo diet (mainly meat and vegetables) and with information that coconut oil is the oil of choice for cooking, as it remains stable and does not oxidize and turn rancid under high temperatures. Olive oil is a smart fat to include in the diet in nonheated forms, such as for salad dressing; but it is not very stable when heated.

- ***Saturated fatty acids*** (SFA). These are *saturated* with hydrogen atoms, and the tail is bonded to as many hydrogen atoms as possible. The tail is straight. They are solid at room temperature. Coconut oil, palm oil, cocoa butter, and animal lard are examples. Human breast milk, which contains 54% saturated fat, is the food of choice for infants. Fats that are universally implicated in heart disease are *hydrogenated* synthetic *trans fats*, like margarine.

```
        H   H   H   H   H   H
        |   |   |   |   |   |
COOH — C — C — C — C — C — C—H
        |   |   |   |   |   |
        H   H   H   H   H   H
```

Saturated Fatty Acid

```
        H   H   H   H    H
        |   |   |   |    /   H
COOH — C — C — C — C = C   /
        |   |   |         \C
        H   H   H        /   \H
                        H
```

Unsaturated Fatty Acid

• **Fig. 8.6** Saturated fatty acid with H atoms totally filling the straight tail, and an unsaturated fatty acid with an empty space causing the tail to bend or kink. (Courtesy Joan Zinn.)

TABLE 8.2 Dietary Examples of Fatty Acids
(Body needs fats in small amounts. An asterisk (*) indicates an excellent choice)

Saturated Fats (Animal and tropical plant oils)	Unsaturated Fats (Monos are the best; the polys are okay in small amounts.)	Trans Fats (Artificially made solid; undisputedly unhealthy.)	Omega-3 Fatty Acids (Unsaturated, omega-3 FAs are highly recommended.)	Omega-6 Fatty Acids (Unsaturated. Eat less omega-6 and more omega-3.)
*Coconut oil (cook with this)	**Monounsaturated**	Margarine	*Tuna	**Seeds**
Cocoa butter	*Olive oil/olives	Cookies	*Herring	Sunflower seeds
Butter	*Avocados	Crackers	*Sardines	Hempseed
Palm oil		Cakes	*Mackerel	
Tallow	**Polyunsaturated**	French fries	*Salmon	**Oils**
Suet	Peanut oil	Onion rings	*Krill oil	*Flax seed and oil
Lard	Canola oil	Donuts	*Black Currant seed oil	Chia oil
Processed meats	Sesame oil	Snack chips	*Evening Primrose seed oil	Corn oil
Fatty meats	Sunflower oil	Many deep-fried foods	*Walnuts	Soybean oil
		(Read labels)	*Pumpkin seeds	Cottonseed oil
	Nuts		*Egg yolks	Peanut oil
Dairy	Almonds			Canola oil (this one is overly processed)
Cheese	Peanuts			
Whole milk	Cashews			
Ice cream	Brazil			
Cream	Hazelnuts			
	Macadamia			
	Pecans			
	Pistachios			

- ***Unsaturated fatty acids*** (UFAs). These have at least one double bond, and the hydrogen atoms do not fill up the tail, so the tail kinks. They are liquid at room temperature. There are two kinds: monounsaturated FAs (MUFAs) and polyunsaturated FAs (PUFAs). Monos are missing one pair of hydrogens. Polys contain more than one double bond and are missing more than one pair of hydrogens. Olive oil and avocados are very healthy MUFAs. Walnut oil and canola oil are PUFAs.
- *Essential fatty acids* (EFAs). The designation *essential* in nutrition means that the substance must be obtained from the diet, because it is not manufactured by the body. (The same goes for essential amino acids/proteins.) The two EFAs we are concerned with here are omega-3 alpha linoleic acid (ALA), and omega-6 linoleic acid (LA).[1] There are also other omegas. The end of the fatty-acid chain opposite the acid end is the *omega end.* The location of the first double bond from the omega end dictates whether a fatty acid is an omega-3, omega-6, omega-9 (oleic acid), or another member of the omega family.
  - *The ratio of omega-3 to omega-6 is important.* Humans require both omega-3 fatty acids and omega-6 FAs in the diet. But for good health, the antiinflammatory omega-3 fatty acids need to be in higher amounts. Unfortunately, most Westerners consume just the opposite—more omega-6 FAs than omega-3 FAs. Recommended ratios are 1:3, 1:4, or 1:5 (omega-6 to omega-3 FAs), depending on a person's health and condition. Larger amounts of omega-3 fatty acids are important to combat all kinds of inflammatory conditions such as metabolic syndrome, high serum cholesterol, heart disease, macular degeneration, osteoporosis, decreased mental acuity, dementias, depression, anxiety, inflammatory bowel disease, cancer, and autoimmune diseases.[8]
  - Pregnant and breast-feeding mothers also need larger amounts of omega-3 FAs. Animal forms of the omega-3 FAs are eicosapentaenoic acid and docosahexaenoic acids, called EPA and DHA for short. Although fats should be eaten in moderation, EPA and DHA from cold water marine fish, shellfish, and krill are important nutrients.
- ***Trans Fatty Acids*** (TFA's). These are the notoriously unhealthy, artificially made fats. Trans fats were originally produced in the form of margarine during World War II but are now prevalent in many so-called junk foods. They are chemically altered by overheating, oxidation, and partial *hydrogenation*, the forced addition of hydrogen in the form of omega-6 polyunsaturated oils, making them semihard at room temperature. They are artificially (*trans*) formed. Hydrogenation of unsaturated liquid fats produces a saturated solid fat that is worse to consume than the natural saturated fats. Some of their detrimental effects include increased LDL (so-called *bad cholesterol*) levels; elevated markers of inflammation, such as C-reactive protein; and increased risk of sudden cardiac arrest, coronary artery disease, and insulin resistance with resulting type II diabetes.
- *Triglycerides*. These are the main constituents of natural fats and oils. They consist of three molecules of fatty acid combined with a molecule of the alcohol glycerol. Triglycerides are the major form of fat stored by the body. They come from the diet and are also produced in the body. Elevated serum triglycerides can be a risk factor for stroke and heart disease. Plants store triglycerides in seeds and oily fruits like olives and avocados, and in palm berries such as Dwarf Palm and Saw Palmetto berries.

Alkamides

Alkamides are a class of lipophilic (dissolving in fats) polyunsaturated fatty acid molecules found in Echinacea root, Prickly Ash bark, and several peppers, including Black Pepper and Long Peppercorns, among others. Some have a pungent taste and cause numbing and salivation. Notable herbs containing alkamides appear in the following list.

- *Isobutylamides in Echinacea. Echinacea* spp. contain at least 14 different isobutylamides, which are types of alkamides. They are responsible for the immunomodulating and antiinflammatory actions of the plant, and for the herb's numbness and tingly effect on the tongue. The alkamides in Echinacea bind to cannabinoid (CB) receptors of various white blood cells, adding to its immune-enhancing action.
- *Sanshools in Xanthoxylum americanum* (Prickly Ash bark). This plant contains the alkamide group called the *sanshools*. Warm, dry, and pungent, Prickly Ash bark is used for Wind Damp Cold Invasion, a syndrome or condition described in Chinese Medicine. It also promotes sweating and opens the sinuses, stimulates the GI tract, and is good for toothache. It is a circulatory stimulant (blood mover) and useful for acute and chronic arthritis.
- *The Peppers*. The pepper species, *Piper longum, P. nigrum* (table Peppercorns) and *P. tuberculatum* are pungent, dry, and warming, and they resolve cold and damp conditions due to the alkamides found in the leaf, root, and fruit.

Alkamides and the Endocannabinoid System

Discovery and research on the ***endocannabinoid system*** (ECS) began in the 1960s and is ongoing. The ECS is a system in our body, which naturally produces compounds or *lignins* that activate specific cell receptors and have numerous health benefits. Various alkamides interact with cannabinoid (CB) receptors. ***CB receptors*** were named after the plant that led to their discovery, *Cannabis sativa* (Marijuana). These receptor sites are located in cell membranes, particularly the brain, spinal cord, and peripheral nervous system, but also occur throughout the body in the organs, tissues, glands, and immune system cells.

CB receptors are ancient and evolved in primitive animals. The most well-known receptors are CB1 and CB2 found in mammals, birds, reptiles, and fish. ***Endocannabinoids***, made in fat cells, are the substances our bodies naturally make to stimulate these receptors. *Phytocannabinoids* are plant substances that stimulate human CB receptors. Delta-9-tetrahydrocannabinol (THC) is present in *Cannabis* spp. and is the most psychoactive and well-known of these substances, but other nonpsychoactive cannabinoids in the plant, such as cannabidiol (CBD) and cannabinol (CBN), are constantly undergoing research due to a variety of healing properties, notably treatment for cancer and seizures (Chapter 24).

Dravet syndrome is a rare and severe type of epilepsy in children that is *retractable* or especially resistant to standard medications. An instance of the benefits of CBD treatment involved a little girl named Charlotte Figi, who was having up to 50 brain-damaging seizures a day (Fig. 8.7). At age 5 she was suffering severe cognitive decline, multiple cardiac arrests, and could no longer walk, talk, or eat (she had a feeding tube). Eventually her family heard of a particular hemp cultivar of *Cannabis sativa*, high in CBD and low in THC, that quiets the excessive electrical and chemical activity in the brain that causes seizures and had been found to work for Dravet syndrome.[9]

The family moved to Colorado, where CBD oil was legal, and she was admitted to the University of Colorado Children's Hospital. Charlotte began taking the CBD oil there, in conjunction with some of her existing medications. Eventually (at age 6), the seizures decreased to two or three a month, mostly in her sleep, and she was weaned off the antiepileptic drugs.[10] The strain was named Charlotte's Web, after the little girl. To end this story, sadly

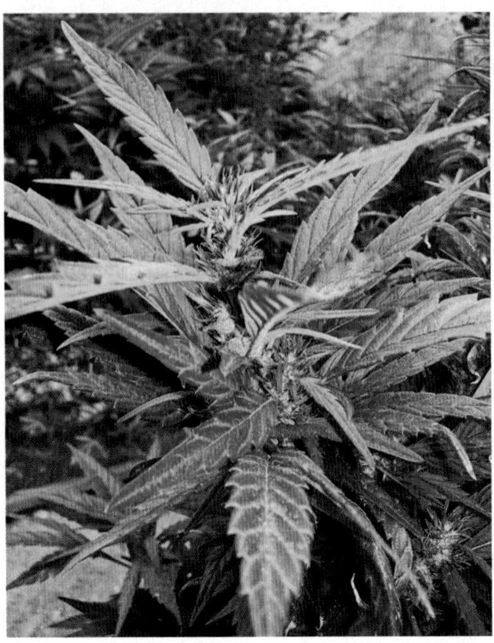

• **Fig. 8.7** *Antiepileptic strain, Cannabis sativa* 'Charlotte's Web'.

Charlotte died in April 2020 at age 13 due to complications of the novel coronavirus (COVID-19), as the pandemic was beginning to sweep the world.

Cannabis is not the only plant or substance that binds to CB receptors. *Echinacea purpura* has been found to contain nonpsychoactive cannabinoids. As more phytocannabinoids are identified and added to the list, the designation *cannabinoid*, referring to *Cannabis* spp., will probably create confusion. Additional suspected cannabinoids occur in broccoli of the Mustard family, *Ruta graveolens* (Rue herb) from the Rutaceae/Citrus family, and the substance *falcarinol* in carrots of the Apiaceae family.[11] It would not be surprising if many more healthy fruits and vegetables join the phytocannabinoid group.

Phenolic Compounds or Polyphenols

These are a huge and diverse group. There are close to 8000 naturally occurring plant phenolics, and about half of them are in the grouping of flavonoids. All ***phenolic compounds*** (polyphenols) have an aromatic benzene ring structure with two or more hydroxyl groups.[1] They include coumarins, salicylic acids, flavonoids, lignins, and phytoestrogens (Fig. 8.8).

Polyphenols provide the flavors and colors of many herbs. Tastes can be bitter or sweet. Flavonoids provide yellows, blues, reds, golds of fruits and flowers, depending on the chemical makeup. Pharmacologically, polyphenols may be antiinflammatory, as in *quercetin*, liver-protecting as in *silybin*, or phytoestrogenic as in *genistein* and *daidzein*. Many are antioxidants that quench free radicals and guard against oxidative stress, as in *resveratrol*, found in the reddish-blue skins of grapes, blueberries, and raspberries. In general, many phenols are bactericidal, antiseptic, anthelmintic (eliminates or destroys gut parasites), and anesthetic.

Salicylic Acid and Coagulation

Salicylic acid is a phenolic acid derived from the naturally occurring salicylic glycosides found in plants.[1] In nature, it is the form

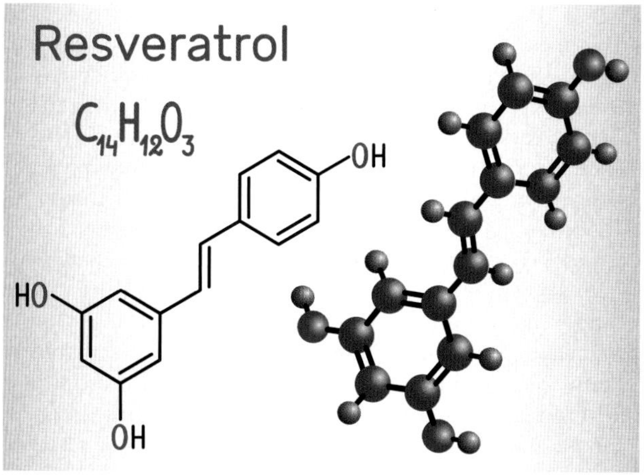

• **Fig. 8.8** Resveratrol, a powerful antioxidant in red grape skins, is a polyphenol with 2 benzene rings and 3 hydroxol groups. (iStock.com/ Credit: Bacsica).

called *methyl salicylate*. It is antiinflammatory, antipyretic (decreases fever), analgesic, and externally, a skin irritant/rubefacient, which can ease painful joints and even remove warts. The drug version known as acetylsalicylic acid (ASA) or aspirin, has an extra acetyl group added, which gives it its anticoagulant properties and consequent side effect of gastric or other types of bleeding in susceptible individuals. Its anticoagulant effect is used therapeutically to help prevent heart attacks and strokes.

Plants containing salicylic acid *do not* inhibit platelet aggregation, clotting, or blood thinning or cause gastric bleeds. This is an important distinction and one that creates much confusion, particularly in the medical community.

Naturally occurring methyl salicylic containing herbs are White Willow bark, Meadowsweet herb, Wintergreen leaf, Sweet Birch bark, Cramp bark, Black Haw bark, and the Poplars, including Aspen bark. Oil of Wintergreen is absorbed through the skin and is useful for arthritis. All are antiinflammatory, analgesic, and antipyretic. They may be taken internally in tinctures and applied externally in ointment or liniments. Internal and external remedies used in tandem are effective for arthritic, joint, and muscle pain. Methyl salicylate is an ingredient in the external Chinese patents White Flower Analgesic Balm and Kwan Loong oil.

Salicylic acid in the form of aspirin is the basis for the enormous group of drugs that are used internally and externally, over the counter (OTC), and by prescription, some as additions to narcotic drugs. There are countless brands of plain aspirin. Other drugs in combination with aspirin include Aleve, Excedrin, Aspergum, Alka Seltzer, Percodan, Darvon, and many more. Aspirin has been in use for more than 100 years, and its exact mechanism of action is still not fully understood.

Coumarins and the Clotting Issue

Coumarins are phenolic compounds that generally exist in the form of glycosides. Coumarins are found in the legume plants of the Fabaceae/Pea family, particularly *Melilotus officinalis* (Sweet Clover herb) and in the Poaceae/Grass family. When coumarin ferments, it becomes *dicoumarol*. Dicoumarol provides the sweetly fermented mowed-hay smell of cut grasses and is responsible for a strong anticoagulant effect.[5] But unspoiled coumarin is *not* anticoagulant.

The drug Coumadin (generic name warfarin) is an anticoagulant/blood thinner used in the treatment of strokes, heart attacks, or deep vein thrombosis, conditions where blood clots are the issue. Dosage must be titrated and monitored to therapeutic levels and can cause dangerous hemorrhage in those with a history of bleeding ulcers, hemorrhagic stroke, or easy bruising. This has led to confusion among the medical establishment and herbalists. Coumadin thins the blood; but fresh, unspoiled, unfermented herbs containing *coumarin* are not blood thinners.

Newly mown grass or hay that has fermented in the field—and is no longer fresh—is sometimes eaten in large quantities by grazing animals. Veterinarians have reported delayed clotting times and even hemorrhaging in animals foraging large amounts of fresh legume plants and moldy Red Clover and grasses.[1] Hence, the "bad rap," overreaction, and fear associated with coumarin-containing herbs in the literature. This issue presents an excellent opportunity for herbalists to educate the public and medical establishment.

In general, herbs and plants containing derivatives of coumarin are antioxidant, antiinflammatory, and tonic to venous and lymphatic vessel walls. They are traditionally used for edema, varicose veins, and hemorrhoids. *Aesculus hippocastanum* (Horse Chestnut seed) is a classic treatment for varicose veins. Meadowsweet herb, Sweet Grass, Sweet Woodruff, Sweet Clover herb, and Tonka bean are other examples of plants containing coumarin.

Lignins

Lignins are a class of polyphenols. They are a diverse group, high in fiber, which can contribute many actions. Various kinds of lignins are part of the active constituents in adaptogens, phytoestrogens, anticarcinogenics, and hepatoprotective herbs.[1] Some big players are in the following list of herbs.

- *Flax seed.* Whole or ground, antioxidant rich flax seeds are extremely high in fibrous lignins, ALA, and mucilage. They can be considered a wonder food. Some of the benefits, according to recent research, are antibacterial, antifungal, anticarcinogenic, antiinflammatory, phytoestrogenic and heart healthy. Flax seed and especially the pressed oil provide good sources of ALA, a plant-based form of healthy animal-based omega-3 FAs that benefit the heart. This is considered an EFA and must be obtained from the diet. The high mucilage content of Flax seed helps the digestive tract and nutrient absorption.
  - *Flax seed and estrogen.* The seeds can lower breast cancer risk by decreasing estradiol and estrone sulfate (forms of estrogen) levels in postmenopausal women (Box 8.1). They are phytoestrogenic and displace so-called *bad* estrogen *16-hydroxy* and *4-hydroxy* pathways on binding sites.[12] This lowering of bad estrogen can help relieve PMS symptoms in women with estrogen dominance (Chapter 28).
- *Silybum marianum* (Milk Thistle seed). The plant is called Milk Thistle because of the milky whitish veins in its leaves. Because of its superb hepatoprotective and hepatogenerative qualities, Milk Thistle seed shines as the premier liver restorative herb in Western herbalism. The lignin it contains is actually a *flavonolignan*, a combination of flavonoids and lignins called *silymarin*.[1] Milk Thistle seed can be ground up and eaten daily, just like Flax seed, and used as a liver tonic, antioxidant, and restorative.
- *Schisandra berry.* Schisandra Wu Wei Zi contains a number of lignins, giving it its antioxidant, hepatoprotective, and adaptogenic properties. It is a valuable and complex herb. Schisandra is also

• BOX 8.1 Flax Seeds and Oil, an Herbalist's Ally

Whole Flax seeds can be freshly ground in a coffee bean grinder and sprinkled over foods. They're good on cereal, salads, and casseroles.

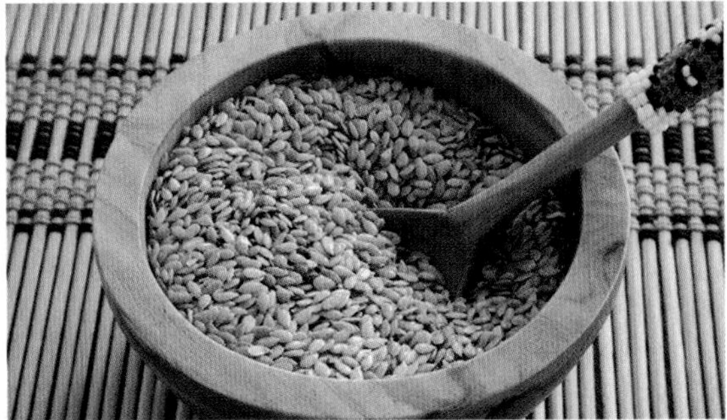

Flax seeds in bowl.

- Store the ground seeds or oil in the refrigerator to stop rancidity. Once the seed is cracked open by grinding or pressed into oil, this happens quickly.
- Flax oil should not be used for cooking because it breaks down at very low temperatures.
- Flax seeds are part of the herbalist's arsenal and require no processing, only grinding. Just instruct your clients to purchase inexpensive, plump golden Flax seeds from the health food store.

called Five Taste berry. The varied chemicals creating those tastes make it a versatile and useful Chinese adaptogen to have in an apothecary.

Flavonoids

Flavonoids are a large subclass of polyphenols that occur in plants as flavonoid glycosides. Flavonoids are powerful antioxidants known to be cancer preventing and health promoting. Being antioxidant, they protect plants against free-radical damage and oxidative stress. When we consume them, they do the same for us. Antioxidants are billed as major contributors to keeping us healthy and cancer free. Flavonoids are prevalent in flowers, fruits, and leaves. They appear in many fruits, vegetables, coffee, and even chocolate, and they provide the famous healthy rainbow diet of many colors that is rich in antioxidants of all kinds. *Flavus* means yellow, the first plant color where the chemical was discovered. Later flavonoids were found in reds, blues, purples, and colorless varieties. Flavonoid concentration is high in citrus fruits, buckwheat, and white and yellow flowers.

Many types of flavonoids sound alike with slightly different spellings because of their various molecular structures and substituents. Here is a list of a few flavonoids:

- *Anthocyanidins*. A subclass of flavonoids that provide the blue, red, and purple antioxidant pigments found in blueberry, blackberry, elderberry, currants, raspberries, blood oranges, cabbage, eggplant, and purple potatoes.[5]
- *Flavanols*. These are found especially in green tea under the flavanol names *catechin* and *epicatechin*. Green tea is known for its antioxidant, anticarcinogenic, and antihypertensive properties.
- *Flavanones/bioflavonoids/vitamin P*. This flavonoid subclass is found in citrus fruits, concentrated in the inner spongy white layer of the peel. They have been called bioflavonoids and sometimes vitamin P. The *P* stands for *permeability factor*. Consequently, this subclass is famous for regulating capillary permeability and fragility, toning blood vessels, and thus stopping easy bruising, bleeding, and varicose veins.
  - *Naringenin and the liver*. This is a flavonoid present in grapefruit that inhibits the cytochrome P450 detoxification pathway in the liver (Chapter 19). In plain English, ingesting grapefruit slows down and alters metabolism/breakdown of certain drugs. Hence, those drugs are not supposed to be taken with grapefruit or grapefruit juice—because grapefruit increases the drug's bioavailability. This can lead to increased serum blood levels, resulting in overdose.[13] A *caution* is included on the drug insert and sometimes put on the offending bottle by the pharmacy. On the other hand, a *smaller* drug dose might be needed if taken *with* Grapefruit, which is perhaps not such a bad thing.
- *Isoflavones*. This is another large subgrouping of flavonoids. Of great interest to herbalists are the ***phytoestrogens***, plants with estrogen-like activity or plant estrogens. They are not identical to human estrogens but have structural similarities allowing them to bind to estrogen receptor sites in human cells and block other harmful *exogenous* estrogens from the environment and *endogenous* estrogens produced in the body. They have been found to help menopausal women with hot flashes and vaginal dryness, and reduce risk of stroke, osteoporosis, and breast cancer. Herbal and food examples are *Trifolium pratense* (Red Clover flower), lignin-rich flax seeds, soybeans, walnuts, other seed nuts, and whole grains (Chapter 28).

Terpenoids or Terpenes

The first terpene to be isolated was turpentine, distilled from Pine oleoresin. ***Terpenes*** are the largest group of secondary plant metabolites. Their basic structure is a five-carbon precursor isoprene. These units can be assembled chemically in many different ways, accounting for their diversity. They differ in their functional groups and in their basic carbon skeletons. They are classified by molecular weight, increasing from light molecules with 5 carbon units to heavy molecules with 40 carbons. For example, monoterpenes have 10 carbon units, sesquiterpenes have 15 carbon units, diterpenes have 20, triterpenes have 30, and so on. Terpenes include essential oils, resins, steroids, carotenoids, and rubber.[3]

- *Some terpenes are fragrant volatile oils*. These are mainly the monoterpenes and sesquiterpenes. *Linalool* in Lavender essential oil (Fig. 8.9) excites the parasympathetic nervous system (PNS) and has a calming influence. *Menthol* gives Peppermint its aromatic smell; *thujone* provides the strong smell of Garden Sage leaf and Yarrow herb; *limonene* gives citrus its outer rind's zesty quality; *oleoresins* provide conifers with their Christmas-tree aroma.
- *Terpenes provide many therapeutic qualities. Sesquiterpene lactones* impart a bitter principle and give Dandelion and Wild Lettuce their milky-white, latex-like sap. *Thymol* provides Thyme herb and Oregano herb antiseptic and antifungal qualities. *Artemisinin* in *Artemisia annua* (Sweet Annie herb) treats malaria and skin diseases. *Cineol* provides antimicrobial and antiseptic properties against *E. coli* and is toxic to gram-positive bacteria. *Cineol* is found in *Melaleuca alternifolia* (Tea Tree) and *Eucalyptus globulus* essential oils.[1]

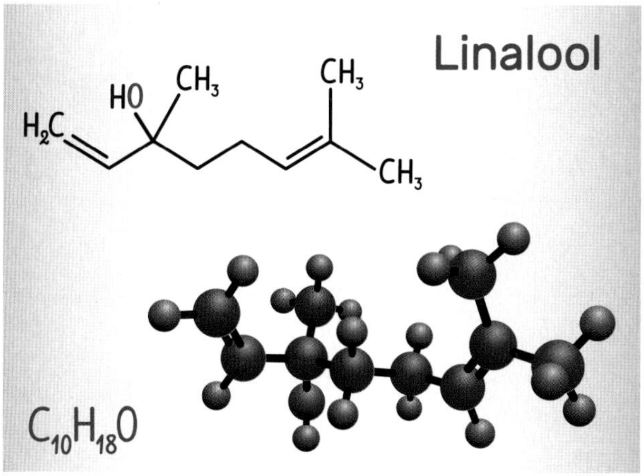

• **Fig. 8.9** Linalool, a fragrant volatile monoterpene in Lavender essential oil that is calming to the nervous system. (iStock/Bacsica).

Monoterpenes

Monoterpenes have 10 carbons. They are responsible for many diverse therapeutic actions of essential oils and whole herbs. *Camphor*, a local rubefacient, occurs naturally in Camphor Tree wood and is also in Rosemary leaf, *Artemisia* spp., and Chrysanthemum Ju Hua (Chrysanthemum flower). Camphor and menthol are paired in many external liniments and creams. *Thujone* from *Salvia officinalis* (Garden Sage) essential oil is antiseptic and carminative. *Thymol* in Thyme herb is fungicidal. *Iridoids* are a subclass of monoterpenes that give us the bitter principle. At least 500 various terpenes have been identified.[1] They are responsible for the herbal category of digestive bitters, including *Gentiana lutea* (Yellow Gentian root). They also provide the cat psychotropic in *Nepeta cataria* (Catnip herb).[5] *Pulegone* in *Mentha poeciloides* (Pennyroyal essential oil) repels mosquitoes and fleas.

Sesquiterpenes

Sesquiterpenes have 15 carbons. Sesquiterpenes provide the volatile aspect of many essential oils. *Chamazulene* is found in Chamomile essential oil and Yarrow herb, *humulene* is found in Hops flower, and *zingiberene* is a carminative in Ginger and Turmeric root. A subclass called the *sesquiterpene lactones* are antiinflammatory, anticancer, antibacterial, antiparasitic, and antispasmodic; they also stimulate digestion.[1]

Diterpenes

Diterpenes have 20 carbons. These molecules are too large to be volatile and many are oleoresins and resins. They require high percentages of alcohol as solvents. Diterpenes include *grindelic acid* in *Grindelia squarrosa* (Gumweed flower), *carnosol* in Rosemary leaf, and *ginkgolides* in Ginkgo leaf. Some diterpenes are toxic, notably a group called the *grayanotoxins*, which are present in *Rhododendron* spp. (the Mountain Laurels).[1]

Triterpenes

Triterpenes have 30 carbons. This is the largest terpene subgroup. *Ursolic acid* appears in Olive leaf and essential oil, Privet berry, Agrimony herb, Rosemary leaf, Oregano herb, Thyme herb, Lavender flower, Peppermint herb, Pomegranate fruit and seed,

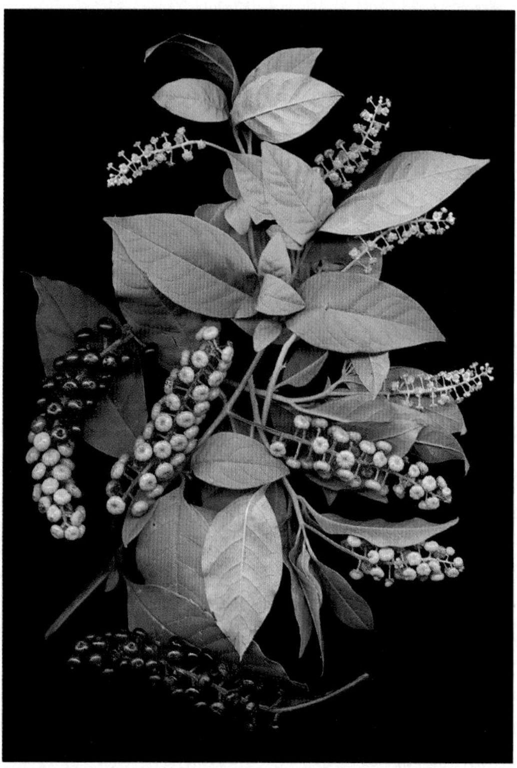

• **Fig. 8.10** *Phytolacca americana* (Poke root) a medium-strength saponin. (Copyright Lang/Tucker Photography. Photographs loaned with permission from *The Botanical Series* are copywritten by Jennifer Anne Tucker and Gerald Lang from the Studio at Hill Crystal Farm. www.jennifer-tucker.com.)

and Hawthorn berry. Triterpenes are anticarcinogenic, chemoprotective, hepato-protective and antiinflammatory.[1]

- *Triterpene saponins.* Saponins are soap-like; *sapo* means soap. They taste bitter and alter the surface tension of water to form stable foam when shaken in water, hence being water soluble. Soapwort herb Yucca root, Pokeberry, and Sarsaparilla root contain saponins. *Glycyrrhizin glabra* (Licorice root) contains *glycyrrhizin*, which inhibits stomach acid and heals the gut lining. Eleutherococcus Ci Wu Jia (Siberian ginseng root) contains *eleutherosides*, which provide its adaptogenic action.
- *Some saponins are poisonous.* The valuable herb *Phytolacca americana* (Poke root) (Fig. 8.10) can irritate gastrointestinal mucosa and cause symptoms like bleeding, nausea, and diarrhea when uncooked mature leaves and roots are eaten in large quantities. Therapeutically, this plant is a medium-strength remedy but safe if used wisely. It is an important detoxifying ally for dissolving hard lumps, tumors, and moving lymph.
- *Triterpene steroidal saponins* have 27 carbons. *Diosgenin* was isolated in Wild Yam rhizome. This can be bought over the counter in a weak cream form, which is a useful phytoestrogen. Other steroidal saponins occur in Soybean, Sarsaparilla root, Fenugreek seed, and Beth root. *Ginsenosides* are a group found in *Panax* spp. (Korean, Chinese, and American ginseng root) providing tonic/restorative effects on the nervous system that enhance energy, stamina, and longevity.

Cardiac Glycosides

Cardiac glycosides are terpenes, which can be toxic. One of them, *digitalis*, has been synthesized into a powerful heart drug used for congestive heart failure (CHF) and other cardiac problems. Cardiac glycosides are steroidal saponins with an additional lactone ring. The three herbal cardioactive herbs in order of toxicity from most to least are the famous *Digitalis purpurea* (Foxglove herb), *Convallaria majalis* (Lily of the Valley herb), and *Drimia maritima* (Squill bulb). Foxglove is toxic and dangerous for herbalists to use because the exact dose is critical and must be controlled precisely. All parts of the plant, sap, seeds, flowers, nectar, and especially the dried leaves contain poisonous *digitoxin* and other cardiac glycosides.

Cardiac glycosides are used allopathically in the form of digoxin, synthesized from Foxglove herb, for treating CHF and atrial fibrillation. Therapeutically, they increase cardiac output by making the heart pump harder and lowering heart rate. The downside of this is that serum blood levels must be carefully monitored to maintain therapeutic range and prevent a dangerously low heart rate and/or digitalis toxicity and possible death.

Foxglove's cardiac affect has been known for centuries. In 1785, the English doctor William Withering studied Foxglove and published a paper on its properties. Its subsequent use in medicine is regarded as the beginning of modern pharmacology. *Convallaria majalis* (Lily of the Valley herb) is a safer and less powerful alternative to Foxglove and can be used for CHF, as a neurocardiac restorative and for treating arrhythmias and palpitations. If using Lily of the Valley as a simple, take a 10-day break after 10 days of continuous use.[14] Be sure not to combine the herb with the drug Digoxin (digitalis). Leave at least four days between the two, with no overlap because the herb and the drug combined can lead to digitalis toxicity and cardiac arrest.

Tetraterpenoids (Carotenoids)

This group of terpenoids are lipid-soluble antioxidants. There are over 600 types of carotenoids. Rich sources are yellow, orange, and red vegetables, fruits, and flowers. *Lycopene* occurs in tomatoes, watermelon, pink grapefruit, papaya, Calendula, Dandelion, and Nasturtium flower. *Beta carotene*, a precursor of vitamin A, helps maintain visual acuity, immunity and is cancer protective. It is present in Rose hip, carrot, oats, yams, and sweet red peppers. *Lutein* is in all green leaves and is also found in yellow-orange plants such as carrots, tomatoes, corn, and Calendula flower. Lutein is an important antioxidant that guards against macular degeneration.[1]

Alkaloids

Bitter ***alkaloids*** are the "drama queens" of herbalism. They are the most potent of all the herbal constituents. Many have strong physiological, psychological, and therapeutic effects. Of all the categories, alkaloids have been the most investigated by modern science. This huge group displays much structural diversity, but all have at least one nitrogen atom in a heterocyclic ring, and classification is based on the type of ring system present.[3] The pH of alkaloids is alkaline. It has been surmised that alkaloids play a protective function in plants by protecting them against insects. Alkaloid-containing plants are more common in hot climates than in cold ones. Many are named after the plant from which they were discovered. Alkaloids are mainly alcohol-soluble, not water-soluble, and require high ethanol percentages in tincture.

Alkaloids can cure or kill, depending on which plant is chosen. In herbology, this is not a tremendous problem because the synergy of plant chemicals tones down toxicity. Furthermore, vomiting and diarrhea tend to be warning signs that a therapeutic dose has been exceeded. This is not true in allopathic medicine, where plant alkaloids have been isolated and synthesized into potent and dangerous drugs. Often the drugs need to be titrated by microgram increments so as not to exceed therapeutic doses.

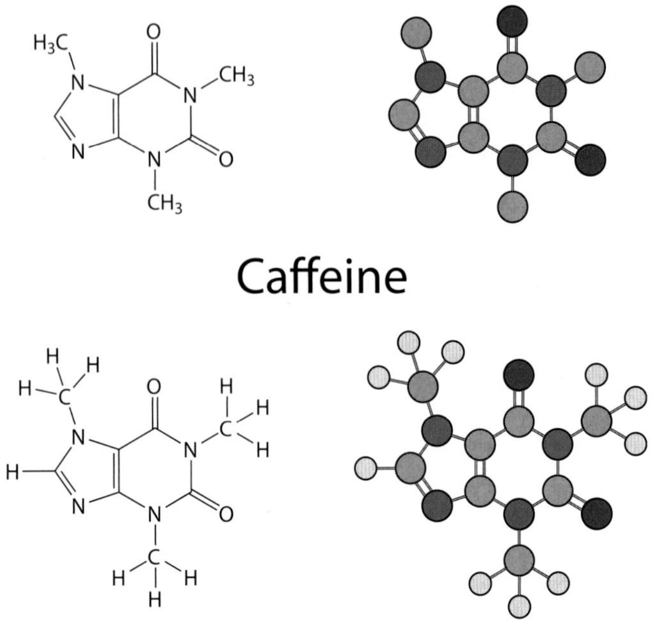

• **Fig. 8.11** Caffeine, a stimulating and addictive methylated purine alkaloid (iStock.com/Credit: Chromatos.)

Plants containing alkaloids range from common foods and herbals in the Solanaceae/Nightshade family such as Ashwagandha root, the peppers, tomatoes, and potatoes, to the poisonous nightshades, *Atropa belladonna* (Deadly Nightshade herb), *Hyoscyamus niger* (Henbane herb), and *Datura stramonium* (Jimson Weed herb). Garlic bulb is another common and edible alkaloid from the Lily family.

Some alkaloids are addictive, such as *nicotine* from *Nicotiana tabacum* (Tobacco leaf). Others are both addictive and analgesic: *heroin* from *Papaver somniferum* (Opium Poppy seed pod) and *cocaine* from *Erythroxylum coca* (Coca leaf). Some alkaloids are psychoactive: *mescaline* from *Lophophora williamsii* (Peyote Cactus button) and *psilocybin* from many types of *Psilocybe* spp. (Psilocybin mushroom). The stimulating alkaloid, *caffeine* (Fig. 8.11), is found in coffee, black and green tea, maté, kola nut (the fruit/seed of *Cola acuminata*), and cocoa beans (chocolate). New alkaloids are constantly being discovered.

From a medicinal standpoint, the pharmacological actions of alkaloids are extensive. Therapeutic actions can be narcotic, analgesic, vasoconstricting, muscle relaxing, and antineoplastic, and they can provide local anesthesia, be hyper- or hypotensive, and function as cardiac and respiratory stimulants or relaxants.[3] No wonder so many alkaloid pharmaceuticals are on the market. Many profitable drugs have been derived from these powerful substances.

Allantoin, Pyrrolizidine Alkaloids (PAs), and Comfrey

The alkaloid *allantoin* is a constituent of *Symphytum officinale* (Comfrey leaf and root), which is known to stimulate wound healing, stop scarring, slough off dead skin cells, and enhance growth of healthy tissue. Comfrey is famous in healing salves and was used during the Civil War in poultices to wrap wounds and fractures because of healing allantoin.

Pyrrolizidine alkaloids (PAs) are a group of alkaloids that are *negatively* associated with Comfrey root and leaf. Herbalists should be aware of the PAs because some forms can be toxic because of their metabolites that accumulate in the liver. There have been reports of livestock poisonings and problems with contaminated food crops from PAs. However, not all PAs have similar toxicity, nor are they all toxic.

Comfrey is sometimes cited as being hepatotoxic when taken internally because of the presence of PAs. This attribution is controversial. Nevertheless, caution should be taken when giving Comfrey in pregnancy, in individuals with liver disease and with elevated liver enzymes, or as a simple. Some herbalists recommend Comfrey for external use only, although it has been used safely internally in formula by many herbalists, including me. *Symphytum officinale*, found in most gardens, is much less toxic than other varieties. At any rate, to remain on the safe side, do not give for long-term internal use.

Other herbs containing PAs are *Tussilago farfara* (Coltsfoot herb), *Petasites* spp. (Butterbur root), *Senecio* spp. (Ragwort herb), and *Agrimonia eupatoria* (Agrimony herb). Remember that a plant's toxicity is greatly lessened due to the synergy of many constituents. It is best for the herbalist to use judgment and caution with dosage in PA-containing botanicals.

Protoberberines

Herbs that contain protoberberine alkaloids and their derivatives are extremely important to have in any herbal apothecary. *Berberines* are found in seven plant families and are a bright yellow, very bitter, water-soluble substance appearing on the inner bark. It is antibacterial, antifungal, antimalarial, antitumor, cytotoxic, and hepato-protective.[3] Berberines serve as digestive stimulants and antidiabetics because of their bitter quality, as astringents for mucous membranes of the stomach and respiratory mucosa, as antiseptics in eyewashes, as wound creams and poultices, and as cholagogues that stimulate bile flow in the liver.

Berberine-containing herbs are dry, bitter, astringent, and cooling. *Hydrastis canadensis* (Goldenseal root), which contains *hydrastis*, is the best known, but it is also endangered and very expensive. A better choice is to use *Mahonia aquifolium* (Oregon Grape root) or *Berberis vulgaris* (Barberry root), both of which contain berberine, among other alkaloids. Chinese berberine-containing herbs are relatively inexpensive and include heat-clearing Coptis Huang Qi (Goldthread root) and Phellodendron Huang Bai (Siberian Cork Tree bark). *Huang* means *yellow* in pinyin.

Purines

This alkaloid class is also designated as methylated purines. The chief alkaloids in this group are *caffeine*, *theophylline*, and *theobromine*.[3] *Caffeine*-containing purines include black and green tea and kola nuts. Caffeine is a CNS, cardiac, and respiratory stimulant, a diuretic, and vasoconstrictor. *Theophylline* is used most as a bronchial smooth muscle relaxant in asthma, chronic bronchitis, and emphysema. Its drug form is Aminophylline.

Theobromine is found in *Theobroma cacao* (Cacao seed or bean). Cacao (or the chopped-up nibs) is the purest, most healthy form of chocolate, as long as no sugars, fats, or milk have been added. Pure, unprocessed dark chocolate is a CNS stimulant and contains the antioxidant *flavanol*. Consumption of 1 oz per day may lower bad LDL cholesterol, reduce blood clots, increase coronary artery blood flow, and lower blood pressure. It also enhances mood by increasing serotonin and endorphin levels in the brain.[15] Did we really need an excuse to enjoy chocolate?

Piperidines

This group of alkaloids, *piperidines*, is found in deadly *Conium maculatum* (Poison Hemlock) but more usably in *Lobelia inflata* (Lobelia herb) in the form of *lobeline*. In moderate dosage, Lobelia herb is famously used as an antispasmodic bronchodilator for asthma and bronchitis. Large doses are highly emetic and were used for purges by the Eclectics. *Piperine* is the main pungent constituent of Black Peppercorn.

Sanguinarines

It is one of many alkaloids in the Papaveraceae/Poppy family, which includes *Papaver somniferum* (Opium Poppy) and medium-strength *Sanguinaria canadensis* (Bloodroot) (Fig. 8.12). Though pungent, hot, and dispersing, Bloodroot is also antibacterial, antiviral, and antifungal. It has been used topically for cold, damp congestion and for removing warts, reducing tumors in breast cancer, and treating nasal polyps.

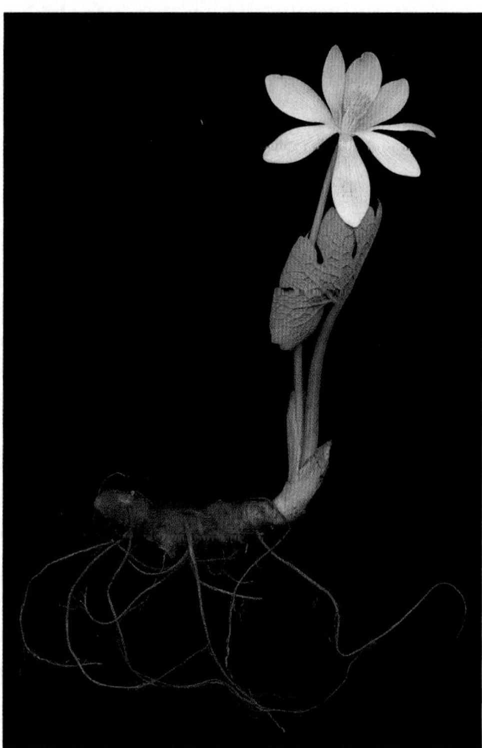

• **Fig. 8.12** *Sanguinaria canadensis* (Bloodroot) gets its botanical name from the alkaloid sanguinarine and is a member of the Poppy family. (Copyright Lang/Tucker Photography. Photographs loaned with permission from *The Botanical Series* are copywritten by Jennifer Anne Tucker and Gerald Lang from the Studio at Hill Crystal Farm. www.jennifer-tucker.com.)

Summary

The six key chemical groups in plants, known as archetypal plant constituents, include carbohydrates, amino acid derivatives, lipids, phenolic compounds, terpenes, and alkaloids. Understanding these major categories helps the herbalist appreciate therapeutic actions, tastes, energetics, and which solvent proportions work best in tincture.

Dietary macronutrients include carbohydrates (sugars), lipids (fats), and amino acids (proteins). Important carbohydrates are the adaptogenic immunomodulating polysaccharides (IPs) present in *Echinacea* spp. and medicinal mushrooms. Another is inulin, present in prebiotic plants that feed gut flora. Healthy fats include olive fruit and oil, coconut oil, monounsaturated avocados, and omega-3 flax seed. Amino acids are the building blocks of plant and animal proteins.

Phenolic compounds can be bitter or sweet, antiinflammatory, phytoestrogenic, and antioxidant. Terpenes are a diverse phytochemical category, which includes volatile essential oils such as thymol in Thyme and humulene in Hops, the cardiac glycosides, and steroidal saponins.

Alkaloids are the most potent and diverse group of all the herbal constituents. Herbalists should be aware of the pyrrolizidine class of alkaloids (PAs), which are present in some plants, including Comfrey, and may be toxic to the liver. The antimicrobial, bitter protoberberines are important medicinally, and the purines are types of alkaloids that include caffeine, theobromine (found in chocolate), and bronchodilating theophylline.

Review

Fill in The Blanks

(Answers in Appendix B.)

1. ___ is the study of plant chemistry.
2. The major six herbal constituent categories are ___, ___, ___, ___, ___, ___.
3. The three macronutrients are ___, ___, ___.
4. Name six herbs that contain salicylic acid. ___, ___, ___, ___, ___, ___.
5. The active ingredient in Garlic bulb is ___.
6. Three plants with fibrous lignans are ___, ___, ___.
7. ___ provide a rainbow diet of many colors. These are in the main constituent category of ___.
8. Three phytoestrogenic herbs are ___, ___, ___.
9. Essential oils are all in the large chemical group called ___. Antibacterial, antifungal Thyme and Eucalyptus essential oils contain ___. Citrus zest contains ___. Gentian root is bitter because of ___. The sinus opening quality of Peppermint is from ___. Licorice heals the gut because of ___.
10. The ___ are a class of bright yellow, bitter alkaloids, which have an ___ effect on the body. Three examples are ___, ___, ___.

Critical Concept Questions

(Answers for you to decide.)

1. What makes something a drug?
2. Why is the drug digitalis much more dangerous than a Lily of the Valley percolation?
3. You have put Red Clover flower in a tea. Your client is worried that it will cause bleeding. How do you answer?
4. What is the difference between inulin and insulin? What is each one used for? Which plants contain inulin?
5. Explain why we need omega-3 and omega-6 FAs in our diet. In what ratio? What is the difference between a saturated fat and an unsaturated fat? Give examples of each.
6. Why can pharmaceutical alkaloids be toxic but herbal ones not as toxic? Give examples of some drug alkaloids and plant alkaloids.
7. Which alkaloid is in chocolate? Is chocolate a healthy choice? Name benefits and disadvantages.
8. What are cannabinoid (CB) receptors and the endocannabinoid system? What does Echinacea have to do with this?
9. What is the difference between Coumadin and coumarin?
10. Explain the best way to use Garlic clove and why.

References

1. Ganora, Lisa. *Herbal Constituents: Foundations of Phytochemistry* (Louisville, CO: Herbalchem, 2009).
2. Lobo, V. et al. "Free Radicals, Antioxidants and Functional Foods." Pharmacognosy Review, US National Library of Medicine, National Institutes of Health. http://www.ncbi.nlm.nih.gov/pmc/articles/PMC3249911/ (accessed September 27, 2019).
3. Hoffman, David. *Medical Herbalism: The Science and Practice of Herbal Medicine* (Rochester, Vermont: Healing Arts, 2003).
4. Yance, Donald R. *Adaptogens in Medical Herbalism* (Rochester, VT: Healing Arts, 2013).
5. Mills, Simon Y. *The Essential Book of Herbal Medicine* (London, UK: Penguin, 1991).
6. "Pectin." WebMD. http://www.webmd.com/vitamins-supplements/ingredientmono-500-ctin.aspx?activeingredientid = 500&activeingredient name = pectin (accessed September 27, 2019).
7. "Seaweed, Raw, Kelp." https://www.nutritionvalue.org/Seaweed,_raw,_kelp_nutritional_value.html (accessed September 27, 2019).
8. Jacob, Aglaee. Today's Dietician. https://www.todaysdietitian.com/newarchives/040113p38.shtml (accessed September 28, 2019).
9. Saundra, Young. "Marijuana Stops Girl's Severe Seizures." *CNN Health*, 2019 https://www.cnn.com/2013/08/07/health/charlotte-child-medical-marijuana/index.html (accessed December 20, 2019).
10. Maa, Edward and Paige Figi. "The Case for Medical Marijuana in Epilepsy." *Epilepsia*, 2019 https://www.theroc.us/images/Maa%20The%20case%20for%20medical%20marijuana%20in%20epilepsy%20Epilepsia%202014.pdf (accessed December 20, 2019).
11. "Scientists Find New Sources of Plant Cannabinoids Other Than Medical Marijuana?" https://montanabiotech.com/2011/03/26/scientists-find-new-sources-of-plant-cannabinoids-other-than-medical-marijuana/ (accessed September 29, 2019).
12. "Nine Causes of Estrogen Dominance and What to Do About It." Amy Meyers MD. https://www.amymyersmd.com/2019/03/9-causes-estrogen-dominance/ (accessed September 2, 2019).
13. Shalansky, Karen. "Grapefruit Juice-Medication Interactions." Pharmaceutical Sciences, 2019 http://www.vhpharmsci.com/Newsletters/1990s-NEWS/Article22.htm (accessed September 29, 2019).
14. Holmes, Peter L. *Energetics of Western Herbs* (Boulder, CO: Snow Lotus Press, 2007).
15. Martinez-Pinilla, Eva, et al. "The relevance of theobromine for the beneficial effects of cocoa consumption." *Frontiers in Pharmacology*. https://www.ncbi.nlm.nih.gov/pmc/articles/PMC4335269/ (accessed September 30, 2019).

9

The Basics of Chinese Medicine

"One disease, many treatments; one herb many diseases."

—***Old Chinese adage***

CHAPTER REVIEW

- Five main branches of Chinese Medicine: Qigong, massage, nutrition, herbal therapy, and acupuncture.
- Yin and Yang.
- The Fundamental Substances: Qi, blood, jing, shen, and fluids.
- The Five Element Theory: Correspondences, the Five Organ Network, and the Five Element Cycles.
- The five yin organs and their yang partners: liver/gallbladder, heart/small intestine, spleen/stomach, lung/large intestine, and kidney/bladder.
- The External Pernicious Influences: wind, cold, heat, damp, dry, and summer heat.
- Physical assessment: reading the pulse and tongue.
- Eight Principle Patterns of Assessment: cold/heat, deficiency/excess, interior/exterior, yin/yang.

KEY TERMS

Acupuncture
Blood
Correspondences
Disharmonies or syndromes
Eight Principle Patterns of Assessment
Five Element Cycles
Five Element Theory
Five Organ Network
Fluids
Jing
Palpate
Pulse (Chinese)
Qi
Qi gong
Shen
Six External Pernicious Influences
Tongue (Chinese)
Tuina
Yang
Yin

The basic premises of Chinese Medicine will be examined from an herbal therapy perspective. The assumption is that you are primarily a Western herbalist with no or little background in Chinese Medicine. It is a beginning. If you have training already, please be tolerant. Important concepts include the principles of yin and yang; the Fundamental Substances of qi, blood, jing, shen, and fluids; the Five Element Theory and Correspondences; the Five Organ Network; the Five Element Cycles; the External Pernicious Influences; and the Eight Principle Patterns of Assessment. These concepts are so critical that they are traditionally capitalized.

From this basic theory emerges a diagnostic tool, namely pulse and tongue assessment, which will prove invaluable to the Western herbalist. If these assessment techniques are practiced and appreciated, and the theoretical principles and basics understood, we will be gifted with an important way to assess our clients and to choose superb herbal combinations to facilitate healing. This chapter is an overview and introduction and in no way goes into the detailed methods required of a skilled Chinese Medicine practitioner. It is meant to be a tool in our pocket, along with many others, to help us become expert herbalists.

The Five Main Branches of Chinese Medicine

- *Medical qi gong*. The oldest of the five and the least invasive. ***Qi gong*** is a mind-body practice and an energetic form of movement used to enhance the flow of qi through the body. It uses body movements, breathing, and focused intention to improve mental and physical health.
- *Nutrition*. In addition to its therapeutic value, food is considered in terms of its energetics: its taste, temperature, and how it affects different organ systems.

- *Chinese massage therapy*. A specific type of body work called **Tuina**.
- *Herbal therapy*. This therapy is the use of Chinese herbs based, in part, on the concepts of yin and yang; qi, blood, and essence; and the Five Element System and Correspondences. Its diagnostic system includes pulse and tongue diagnosis and the Eight Diagnostic Principles of body illness.
- *Acupuncture therapy*. **Acupuncture** is a hands-on therapy that involves placement of thin needles on specific points of the skin along energy lines called meridians. In this way, qi is accessed, and proper flow of energy is restored throughout the body. Harmonious energy flow is necessary for good health.

The Principle of Yin and Yang

Yin and yang are a key concept in Chinese medicine. The principle represents the idea of dualism, or how forces that appear to be opposites actually complement one another. All is one in the universe. We are all one. Out of the one is the connected, intertwined opposites, or polarities of ***yin*** and ***yang*** (Fig. 9.1). Yin and yang encompass everything. The universe is always in motion, so yin and yang are always in motion, changing, and complementing one other. If you check out the yin-yang symbol, you will see that the dark, yin blends into the light yang. In the dark yin is a dot of light yang; in the light yang is a dot of dark yin. The feminine and masculine principles intertwine. A woman has female yin in her, but within that woman is a little yang maleness. A man has masculine in him, but within that man is bit of the feminine.[1]

Yin-yang is an interwoven relationship, never static. Yin and yang are in everything. Sometimes a thing is more yin; sometimes more yang. For there to be hot, there is cold; for heaven, there is earth; for masculine, there is feminine; for the light is the dark. Sometimes the very same thing is yang, and sometimes it is yin. Or it could be more yin than yang or more yang than yin. It depends on the point of view of the observer. Yin and yang are always in flux, cyclic, and a circle. As Donovan once sang in the song "Circular Motion," "Everybody is a part of everything anyway. . ."

In general, yin is cool, dark, and moist. Yang is warm, light, and dry. Yin is female; yang is male. Yin is the moon; yang is the sun. Yin is the receptive; yang is the creative. As above, so below. Yin and yang are part of the conditions of human illness and wellness. We have the dualities of dry and damp, hot and cold, internal and external, weak and strong, and excess and deficient. When we investigate herbal qualities and human conditions, the concept of yin and yang are paramount.

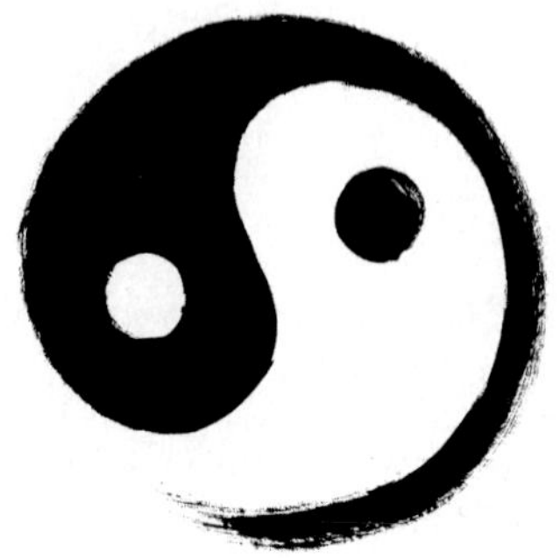

• **Fig. 9.1** The yin-yang symbol holds its roots in Taoism, a Chinese religion and philosophy. (iStock.com/ Credit DKsamco.)

Yin and Yang in a Nutshell

- Yin and yang are relative (Box 9.1).
- Yin and yang result from the infinite movement of the universe.
- Yin attracts yang, and yang attracts yin. The greater the difference, the greater the attraction.
- Yin repels yin, and yang repels yang. The greater the similarity, the greater the repulsion.
- Everything has a yin and yang aspect.
- All things are constantly changing their yin-yang proportion.
- Yin is not better than yang; yang is not better than yin. Both are beautiful and perfect. They need each other to exist.
- Yin and yang control each other.
- Yin and yang transform each other. One is always changing into the other (Table 9.1).[2]

The Fundamental Substances: Qi, Blood, Jing, Shen, and Fluids

Qi is energy, the life force. It is the active principle that forms part of living things. Think of it as breath, air, gas, and energy. Qi is also the energy that flows through the body along pathways called meridians. When we think of an herbal *qi tonic*, we have an herbal mixture that helps us regain or maintain our energy. If qi is deficient, we are weak or tired.[3]

Functions of Qi

- *Qi maintains our defenses*. It protects us from what is called the *External Pernicious Influences*, or pathogens outside the body. If the qi is deficient, our immune system suffers, and we get sick. Our qi also helps to fight off germs if they do get inside. Death is the absence of qi.

• BOX 9.1 A Taoist Poem

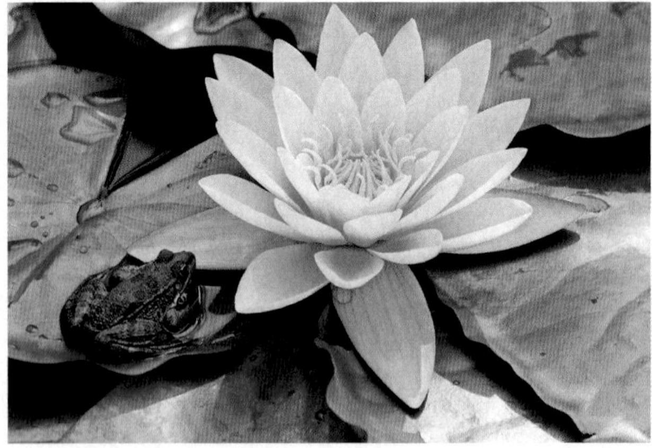

Yin and yang depend on the observer's point of view. (iStock.com/Credit Alexandrite.)

The Lotus and the Frog

To the frogs in a temple pool
The lotus stems are tall.
To the gods of Mount Everest
An elephant is small.

TABLE 9.1 **Comparison of Yin and Yang**

Yin	Yang	Yin Body	Yang Body
Damp	Dry	Female	Male
Night	Day	Internal	External
Cold	Hot	Cold and cool	Hot and warm
Interior	Exterior	Damp or moist	Dry
Deficiency	Excess	Weak	Strong
Descending	Ascending	Forming blood	Metabolism
Chronic	Acute	Weak voice	Loud voice
Small	Large	Hypotensive	Hypertensive
Moon	Sun	Depleted qi	Congested qi

- *Qi transforms substances* in the body. This transformation happens in ways other than those we perceive in the West. When food is ingested, it transforms into substances such as blood, qi, tears, sweat, or urine. It supports metabolism. All these changes and transformations depend on qi.
- *Qi holds things in and together*. It keeps blood in its vessels and organs in place, and it prevents loss of body fluids, such as saliva and sweat.
- *Qi keeps us warm*. It maintains body heat.
- *Qi has proper directions*. It moves upward, downward, inward, and outward. To be alive, qi must travel in all four directions in the body. It must move evenly through the meridians. Too slow and it's sluggish, slow, or stuck, causing pain or clots; too fast and we're hyper, and it can cause bleeding, tremors, or seizures. Qi must also move in the proper direction in each organ. ***Disharmonies or syndromes*** are functional disturbances, or illnesses within the body, and can occur from qi moving in the wrong direction. If stomach qi moves upward instead of downward, we have nausea and vomiting. Insufficient downward movement of Lung qi causes a cough.
- *Qi circulates fluids*. It moves blood and lymph and supports metabolism.

Primary Types of Qi

- *Original or ancestral qi*. This qi is the foundation of all the yin and yang in the body. It keeps the lungs breathing in air and the heart beating and circulating. It keeps us alive.
- *Organ qi*. Each organ has its own qi, such as Lung qi, Heart qi, or Kidney qi. When we refer to Chinese organs, they will be capitalized to distinguish them from Western organs.
- *Meridian qi*. This refers to the qi that circulates throughout the meridians or channel network and flows to each organ.
- *Nutritive qi*. Qi moves nutrients obtained from food through the blood and moves the blood through the vessels.
- *Protective qi*. Qi resists the External Pernicious Influences that come from the exterior environment and guards against pathogens. Protective qi keeps us healthy.

When Qi Goes Badly, There Are Qi Disharmonies or Patterns

- *Deficient qi*. Qi is deficient when there is not enough energy available for it to perform any of its functions. Qi deficiency can occur in a malfunctioning organ, such as the Heart. It could be systemic, meaning throughout the entire body, resulting in general fatigue. It could also apply to specific type of qi, such as deficient protective qi, resulting in an infection, a cold, or cough.
- *Collapsed qi*. Because qi holds things in place in the body, occurrences like a prolapsed uterus, hemorrhoids, or varicose veins, where tissue is thin and weak, would be collapsed qi.
- *Stagnant qi*. If qi circulation slows down or does not flow smoothly, it can affect an organ or body part, depending on where the blockage occurs. Stagnant qi in the legs or knees causes pain there; stagnant Lung qi could cause coughing or wheezing. Stagnant Liver qi causes abdominal distention.
- *Rebellious qi*. In this case, qi is going in the wrong direction. Nausea and vomiting are cases in point. That would be called (you guessed it) Rebellious Stomach Qi.

Blood

The concept of *blood* in Chinese Medicine is different from the Western idea of blood. In the West, blood is a red liquid filled with cells, made in the marrow, that circulates throughout the body in definite anatomical pathways, the blood vessels. In Chinese Medicine, ***blood*** travels through the physical blood vessels but also goes through the energy meridians. In the Western sense, the vessel pathway is important; in the Chinese version, not so much. Blood's *function* is more important, namely to nourish, maintain, and repair the entire body. Because it's a liquid, blood is considered a yin substance.[3]

Chinese blood arises from food that has been transformed through digestion. Food goes to the Stomach and then *ripens* in the Spleen into a pure *essence*. The essence rises to the Lungs and becomes clear. Then nutritive qi turns it into blood. From there, the Heart circulates it, the Liver stores it, when necessary, and the Spleen keeps it in the blood vessels, its correct place. As the saying goes, "The Heart rules the blood; the Liver stores the blood; the Spleen governs the blood." If something goes wrong, the blood has disharmonies.

The Two Main Categories of Blood Disharmonies

- *Deficient blood*. If blood does not nourish the entire body, we become pale, dizzy, and perhaps dry. If it does not nourish a particular organ, such as the Heart, we might develop particular symptoms, like palpitations.
- *Congealed blood*. If blood does not flow smoothly, it becomes obstructed. This obstruction creates sharp stabbing pain and tumors, cysts, or swelling of an organ. It usually affects the Liver.

Jing

Jing is the substance that underlies life from birth to death. Jing is the basis of reproduction and development and part of our DNA. It is supportive and nutritive. We receive prenatal, original jing at conception. At birth, we acquire postnatal jing from our parents. As we grow and mature, our jing is dependent on our lifestyle choices, and it changes accordingly. All life cycles are considered jing. The triad of the *Maiden, Mother*, and *Wise Woman* (Chapter 28) is jing. Jing is the inner essence of growth, decline, and death. If there is disharmony with these life passages, we might have trouble conceiving a child, have sexual dysfunction, experience delayed puberty, or encounter premature aging. A Western concept of a jing disharmony might be a congenital defect.[3]

In Chinese Medicine, the Kidney holds the jing. The Kidney, being the most yin organ, holds our essence and the root of life. The Kidney is deep and watery and the source of life and development. Every part of the body needs Kidney jing to thrive and survive. From a Western perspective, the endocrine system, which manages hormonal growth and development, is part of Kidney jing. The adrenal glands, which anatomically sit atop the kidneys, are major players in Kidney jing.

Shen or Spirit

Shen is spirit or essence. It is associated with the human personality and the ability to live life fully and happily. Healthy shen translates into a sparkle in the eyes. In Chinese Medicine, the Heart stores the shen. This action makes sense if we consider how often we describe our feelings in terms of the heart, as in, "My heart is soaring, My heart is broken, I am sick at heart, My heart aches for you." Shen disharmonies can lead to anxiety, depression, and other mental illnesses. From a Western perspective, we may see insomnia, excessive dreaming, forgetfulness, dementia, or irrational behavior. If the Heart's blood and qi are in harmony, then all is well. We are content.[3]

Fluids

The ***fluids*** consist of all bodily fluids, other than blood. Fluids include semen, urine, lymph, sweat, gastric juices, and mucous membrane linings. They moisten and sometimes nourish hair, skin, membranes, orifices, flesh, muscles, joints, marrow, and bones. Fluids come from ingested food and are absorbed and regulated by the qi of various organs. Fluids are yin. Therefore it is reasonable that a fluid disharmony is a yin disharmony and would result in dryness.[3]

The Five Element Theory

The ***Five Element Theory*** is a world view in Chinese medicine, which includes our relationship with the earth and its natural cycles. It takes into account the five yin-yang organ pairs and their association with the five seasons, five elements, five tastes, five colors, five emotions, and the five sense organs. To this day, Chinese Medicine describes and defines the world and medicine using the influence of day and night, the seasons, and the elements—all circular.

Correspondences

Five Element Theory is a tremendously holistic idea that takes into account the five yin-yang organ pairs and their associations or ***correspondences*** with the natural world. Collectively, this information is organized in a *Table of Correspondences*. It is a way to look at reality and organize what we see. The Five Element Theory includes our life cycle from birth to death, the cycle of a day from morning to night, the 24-hour clock, and the circulation of qi from hour to hour as it passes through each organ (Chapter 15). The five yin elements and their correspondences are the same for their partners, the yang elements (Table 9.2).

The Five Organ Network

Within the Five Element Theory is the ***Five Organ Network***. In Chinese Medicine, the organs do not necessarily have the same functions that they have in the West. They are appreciated in reference to their given functions (physiological and psychological) and to their relationship to the substances and other parts of the body, a network. They occur in pairs; there are five yin organs and five yang organs. The yin organs are more internal and hollower, and the yang organs are more external and more solid. In terms of importance, the yin organs are more essential to life (Table 9.3).[1]

In the Five Organ Network system, there are 5 paired yin-yang organs, equaling 10. In the Chinese *acupuncture* system, there are 6 paired yin-yang meridians, equaling 12. The two extra paired meridian organs are not actual visceral organs. They are concepts, called the *Pericardium* and the *Triple Burner*. The Triple Burner encompasses three areas: the upper (chest), middle (abdomen), and lower part (pelvis) of the torso, and their collective function is to tie together and harmonize the five organs of the network system. The Pericardium protects the heart and the active mechanism of the Heart.[1] The protective Pericardium is yin, and the active, harmonizing Triple Burner is yang.

The Five Element Cycles

The ***Five Element Cycles*** show how organs and their corresponding element interact and work with each other and/or against each other, resulting in health or disease. When in balance, they are drawn as an outside circle with arrows going clockwise. This image indicates them working together in harmony and is called the *creation* or *supporting sequence*. One organ gives birth to the next. Water nourishes wood by moistening it. Wood generates or feeds fire. Fire creates ash that covers earth to form soil. Earth supports metal by forming minerals and bringing them to the surface. Metal revitalizes water by giving it minerals, so it can nourish wood.

The five-pointed star inside the circle is a *destruction or restraining sequence* or cycle. It illustrates how organs can work against each other, causing illness or syndromes. Additionally, they work as a check-and-balance relationship, showing how one organ can stop another from getting out of hand, such as Kidney water cooling and preventing Heart fire from overheating the heart. Metaphorically, Wood inhibits earth by covering it, but also its roots help Earth by moving it around and preventing stagnation. Wood controls water by damming it up and absorbing it. Water controls fire by extinguishing it. Fire melts down metal. Metal chops wood and destroys it (Fig. 9.2).

We live on this earth in connection with the plants, the sky, the earth, the elements, the weather, the seasons, and the animals. The Chinese Five Element Cycle is reminiscent of the Native American Medicine Wheel, which is also circular and also includes an entire cosmology. The Medicine Wheel includes people, animals, plants, rocks, stars, seasons, and the life cycle. A main difference between the two is that the Chinese Five Element Theory includes a system of wellness and sickness in the human body and offers an intricate system of healing.

TABLE 9.2 Five Elements and the Primary Correspondences

Yin Organ	Yang Organ	Environmental factor	Season	Element	Taste	Color	Sense Organ	Tissue	Emotion and Sound
Liver	Gallbladder	Wind	Spring	Wood	Sour	Green	Eyes	Joints, Tendons, Ligaments, Nails	Anger/Frustration-Flow. Shouting
Heart	Small Intestine	Heat	Summer	Fire	Bitter	Red	Tongue	Heart, Vessels	Joy-Sorow. Laughter
Spleen	Stomach	Damp	Late Summer	Earth	Sweet	Yellow	Mouth or Lips	Muscles	Worry-Spaced-out. Singing
Lung	Large Intestine	Dryness	Fall	Metal	Pungent	White	Nose	Skin, Body Hair	Grief/Mourning-Recovery. Crying
Kidney	Bladder	Cold	Winter	Water	Salty	Black or Blue	Ears	Bones, Marrow, Head Hair	Fear-Courage. Groaning[2]

TABLE 9.3 The Five Paired Organs

Yin Organs (More Internal, Hollow)	Yang Organs (More External and Solid)
Liver	Gallbladder
Heart	Small Intestine
Spleen/Pancreas	Stomach
Lung	Large Intestine
Kidney	Urinary Bladder

The Five Yin Organs and Their Yang Partners

Wood: The Liver (Yin) and Paired Organ, The Gallbladder (Yang)

The miraculous liver does so much, having over 100 functions. Almost everyone in the West would benefit from some liver herbals, because the liver is responsible for detoxification. From that standpoint alone, it is vital for health. The liver breaks down chemicals or *deconjugates* them. It takes apart used estrogen and other hormones, drugs, and toxins, so they can be excreted from the body through the bile and urine. The liver also stores glucose in the form of glycogen and regulates glucose metabolism. All diabetics need a nod from the Liver.[1]

Chinese Liver Functions

- *The Liver stores the blood.* The Liver directs the blood around the body with the help of qi. Therefore the Liver maintains the smooth flow of qi and blood. If this is slowed down or blocked, causing pain or cramping, it's a Liver problem.
- *Poor Liver function can lead to blood and qi stagnation.* In qi stagnation, the person complains of stabbing pains, fullness, suppressed emotion, or frustration. If the qi becomes slow enough or stops altogether, PMS, masses, or tumors can develop.
- *The Liver governs the sinews.* This principle means that the Liver is associated with, in charge of, the sinews—the tendons, ligaments, small muscles, and the voluntary motor nerves. Therefore it regulates body movement, which should be fluid and smooth. If blocked, muscle spasms, aches, and cramping occur.
- *The Liver's sense organ is the eyes.* The Liver, therefore, is said to "open to the eyes." The Liver's paired meridians actually pass upward internally through the center of the eyes. Therefore the Liver affects vision and other eye problems.
- *The Liver affects the nails.* The fingernails and toenails are considered a byproduct of the sinews, which are under the control of the Liver. Therefore Liver health is related to the nails.
- *The Liver meridian circles the external genitalia.* If blood slows down and becomes congested in that area, there will be uterine cramping (dysmenorrhea) and reproductive problems.
- *The Liver's emotion is anger.* Unhealthy or excessive anger harms the Liver. If the flow of qi or blood is erratic, emotions rise. The head becomes hot, and a migraine could occur. If blood and qi flow smoothly, so goes our life. If we go with the flow, we have a happy Liver.

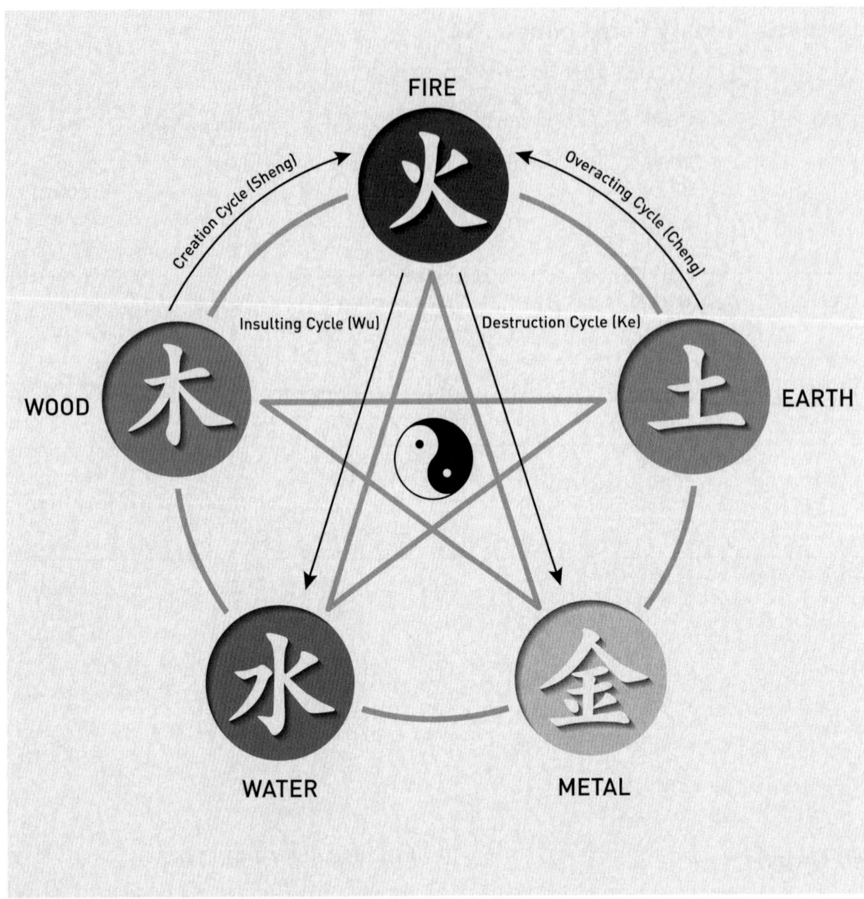

• **Fig. 9.2 The Five Element Cycles**. The outside circle is the creation or supporting sequence and the inside star is the destruction or restraining sequence. (iStock.com/Credit Thoth Adan.)

- *The Liver element is Wood, and the color is green.* Bile is dark green, and leaves turn green in the *spring*, the Liver's season. The taste is sour. Eat lemons for a healthy liver.

Chinese Gallbladder Functions

The yang Gallbladder is the organ paired with the yin Liver, making it part of the Liver network. Most of the correspondences of the yang organs match their partners. The Gallbladder makes and secretes bile (which used to be called *gall*). Bile stimulates peristalsis, breaks down fats, and helps assimilation and elimination. Many liver remedies, called *cholagogues*, stimulate the production and flow of bile and act as a laxative. The Gallbladder is associated with the powers of *decision making, judgment, and clarity*. If we make the wrong decision, or have trouble deciding, the universe often does it for us by default. If we can't see (first, second, and third eye), our vision and understanding are cloudy, and action is not taken.

Fire: The Heart (Yin) and Paired Organ, The Small Intestine (Yang)

Love resides in the heart. The heart is the place of healing, unconditional love, and compassion. It contains the shen, the spirit, the life force, and the personality. If shen is strong, there is mental balance, a healthy outlook, and a positive self-image. Life's problems and dark moments still occur but can be dealt with. A carefree Heart equals a peaceful shen.

Chinese Heart Functions

- *The Heart stores the shen and maintains awareness.* The Heart creates consciousness and feeling. It keeps us mentally healthy. If not, there may be nightmares, sleep disturbances, unclear thoughts, confusion, depression, schizophrenia, or psychosis.
- *The Heart propels the blood through the body.* It brings nourishment and oxygen to the cells and removes waste. The Heart communicates with the cells. Cardiovascular diseases are syndromes of the Heart, along with arrhythmias, chest pain, sweating, restlessness, heart attacks, or congestive heart failure.
- *The Heart's body parts are the blood vessels and the complexion.* The red hemoglobin molecule in red blood cells brings a blush to the skin and gives it a glow.
- *The Heart's emotion is joy.* This ties in with the shen. Damaged spirit can create depression and sadness. If we wall in emotions or avoid relationships, a heart attack could manifest. Overwhelming sorrow, shock, and surprise are all attacks on the Heart. These experiences are affairs of the heart, the mind-body connection.

- *The Heart's sense organ is the tongue.* Humans form words with our tongues. Speech is a Heart function. A clear, strong voice denotes a healthy heart. If we stutter or have speech impediments, it's the Heart trying to speak.
- *The Heart's element is Fire,* the color is *red* like fire, the season is *summer*, and the taste is *bitter*.

Chinese Small Intestine Functions

The yang Small Intestine is the paired with the yin Heart, so it is part of the Heart network. The Small Intestine receives digestive enzymes from the pancreas and liver and separates out solids to the colon and liquid to the kidneys. The Small Intestine is paired with the Heart in communication, because it assists in sending purified food (absorption) to the Blood. The Small Intestine assists the Heart in caring for the spirit by filtering out negativity and what is not needed.

Heart illnesses can manifest as inflammatory (fire or heat) conditions in the Small Intestine. If we are anxious or stressed out from a shen disturbance of the Heart, we can talk too much, develop ulcers, inflammatory and irritable bowel diseases of the Small Intestine, or cystitis. Stress is a major player in many diseases, particularly of the gut. This manifestation is a perfect example of the mind-body or gut-to-brain connection.

Earth: The Spleen (Yin) and Paired Organ, The Stomach (Yang)

The Spleen is like Mother Earth. The Earth holds, houses, and nourishes us, as does the Spleen. It holds us together, keeps us safe, and provides nourishment. The Chinese Spleen is similar to the Western stomach. It supplies nourishment, called *nutritive essence*, which is converted into qi and blood.

Chinese Spleen Functions

- *The Spleen regulates metabolism.* By regulating qi and blood, the Spleen directs our fuel and energy supply. If this supply is weak, we have fatigue. If there is too little blood, we get anemia, pale lips and nails, and fatigue. Further depletion of blood can lead to digestive Spleen qi problems, such as abdominal distention, flatulence, loose bowels, malabsorption, malnutrition. Irritable bowel syndrome may be a Spleen Qi Deficiency.
- *The Spleen is the source of and distributor of body fluids.* It adjusts the thickness of our blood, lymph, and other fluids. It has a tendency to allow accumulation of dampness anywhere in the body. Spleen damp is a significant issue in Chinese Medicine. Excess fluids can build up in the stomach, lymph nodes, joints, or extracellular fluid, causing edema, swollen breasts, and discharges. If there is heat involved, it's damp heat; if cold is involved, it's damp cold.
- *The Spleen holds tissues together and keeps them upright.* The Spleen prevents prolapses when it works correctly. It regulates and makes sure blood flows in the correct places. It maintains tone and elasticity in the blood vessel walls. If they become thin or fragile, we could develop varicosities, bruising, or hemorrhoids.
- *The tissue associated with the Spleen is the flesh.* The modern term for the flesh is *muscle.* This association accounts for Spleen-associated muscle strains and soreness.
- *The Spleen, which deals with food, opens to the mouth and manifests on the lips.* The Spleen's sense organs are the mouth or lips. Mouth sores are Spleen issues.
- *The Spleen governs thought.* Excessive thought and perseveration are associated with *worry or overthinking.* On the other hand, being blank, spaced-out, and unfocused is under-thinking, and also the Spleen's doing.
- *The Spleen color is yellow,* associated with the warmth and fruits of its element, the *yellow Earth.* The Spleen's season is the harvest time of late summer (an extra season in addition to the traditional four seasons). The taste is *sweet.*

Chinese Stomach Function

The yang Stomach is paired with the yin Spleen, so it is part of the Spleen network. It holds and "ripens" or digests food. The Stomach is yang and dry and needs the moisture of the yin Spleen. The Spleen and Stomach work in opposite directions. Stomach qi is supposed to move food downward to the intestines. If it rebels and moves upward, we belch, hiccup, or have nausea and vomiting. Conversely, the Spleen should have upward energy. If its qi is deficient, we have downward prolapses of organs and veins.

Metal: The Lungs (Yin) and Paired Organ, The Large Intestine (Yang)

Chinese Lung Functions

The Lung governs the relationship between the outside (exterior) and inside (interior) of the body. It puts up limits and boundaries and determines what comes in through the qi of heaven (breath) to join with the qi of earth (nutrition).[1] This barrier protects us from the External Pernicious Influences of microorganisms. It sets up the rhythm of the organism through air exchange. Slow, measured breathing can be quieting, conscious, and meditative. The Lungs do this. Qi gong is a discipline that uses this truth for disease prevention.

- *The Lungs provide an interface between the interior and the exterior.* They are the connection between the outer world and the body. They are the portal through which gases are exchanged. Oxygen is inhaled into the body, and carbon dioxide is exhaled.
- *The Lungs maintain defenses and boundaries* by providing the connection between external organisms and the inside of our bodies. This protection is known as *wei qi* or defensive qi, a huge part of our immune system. *Mucous membranes* line and secrete mucus that protects us from organisms entering through the respiratory tract. Mucous membranes are tissues associated with the Lungs and are also part of the immune system.
- *The Lungs connect with the skin, which provides defense.* The skin can be considered the third Lung. Skin is our immune system's first line of defense against outside organisms in the Western sense; the lungs are a close second. It is no surprise that the skin and Lungs are related. If the Lungs are healthy, the skin is smooth, supple, and vibrant.
- *The Lungs maintain balance and rhythm.* Slow, even respirations calm us down and help us relax. Controlled, slow breathing is a key part of meditation and yoga. It elicits the parasympathetic nervous system, decreases stress, and increases immune defenses.
- *The Lungs disperse moisture* to our body. Lungs collect fluid essence from the Spleen, moisture from the air, and send it downward to the Kidney and Bladder. For this reason, the Lungs regulate urine output. If Lung qi does not descend as it should, moisture could build up in the upper body as facial edema or as decreased urine output in the lower body. If Lung

qi is weakened, we experience excessive sweating (perspiration at rest) and incontinence because the body is too weak to hold in water.

- *The Lungs are related to sweating and sweat glands.* They release moisture through sweat glands on the skin. This action explains the tissue connection between the lungs and the skin, sweat glands, and body hair. Sweating, plus wei qi, helps to maintain body temperature and fluid balance.
- *The Lungs open to the nose*, part of the respiratory tract. Problems with the sense of smell are Lung problems.
- *Lung-related tissues* are the respiratory tract structures of the nose, sinuses, nasopharynx, bronchi, skin, and mucous membranes. The other related tissues are the skin, body hair, and sclera of the eye (the skin of the eye).
- *The Lung's emotion is grief, loss, or letting go.* The color is *white*, the season is *fall*, the element is *Metal* or structure, and the taste is *pungent*. Pungent herbs like Garlic bulb, Onion, and Ginger rhizome are used to break up and move out mucous and help us to sweat when a respiratory infection sets in.

Chinese Large Intestine Function

The yin Lung is paired with the yang Large Intestine, so it is part of the Lung network. The lungs filter out stale and unneeded air, and the Large Intestine separates food particles that are unneeded and could make us toxic if allowed to build up. This letting-go of what no longer serves relates to the Lung network's emotion of grief. Appropriate grieving requires release of the old to keep us whole and let in the new. If the Lung and Large Intestine become stressed and restrained, tension arises and leads to stiff, tight muscles, constipation, spastic colon, or asthma. Asthma is when we cannot exhale, release, or let go of stale air.

Water: The Kidneys (Yin) and Paired Organ, The Bladder (Yang)

The Kidney is the most yin organ because it generates, stores, and governs our deep essence, our genetic DNA information called *jing*. Kidney yin is moist and nourishing. It supports reproductive functions. But like all other organs, the Kidney has an active yang side. The Kidneys *rule water* and circulate fluids. This characteristic is an action-oriented yang function. All other organs are dependent on the yin and yang of the Kidneys. The Kidney has a long list of functions and is a very important organ.

Chinese Kidney Function

- *The Kidneys rule the jing* and preserve the essence of human life. The more jing, the longer the reproductive and life span. This factor is determined from our genes at birth and increasingly from healthy choices as we grow and age. Gene expression may be altered for better or worse by healthy or unhealthy lifestyle options, which is crucial information for herbalists to impart to clients. We can all take an active role in staying healthy. Helping our clients to follow the basics of maintaining good diet, exercise, sleep patterns, and attitudes is our job.
- *The Kidney supports reproductive organs and regeneration.* This sphere of influence includes the uterus, ovaries, vagina, testicles, prostate, penis, and their functions. Reproduction is tied up with jing (the life force). If Kidney qi is vigorous, we have a healthy sexual and reproductive life. This influence involves transitions, such as beginning and leaving puberty, libido, healthy menstrual cycles, pregnancy, and menopause. For men it involves libido, sperm count, and a healthy outlook regarding sexuality.
- *The Kidney regulates growth and development.* Loss of Kidney essence includes premature aging, graying and thinning hair, dimming vision, tooth loss, weak and fragile bones, stiff spine, impotence and infertility, foggy thinking, and loss of stamina. We are all aging, of course, but conscious aging helps us with spiritual, emotional, and psychological growth. Developmental errors include central nervous system (CNS) developmental diseases, such as multiple sclerosis, cerebral palsy, and muscular dystrophy.
- *Kidney yin regulates fluid metabolism and balance.* Kidney yin is the basis of all liquid substances, including tears, saliva, mucous, urine, sweat, cerebral spinal fluid, synovial fluid, plasma, and semen. The syndrome called Kidney Yin Deficiency makes us dry and weak.[1] Kidney yang circulates the fluids. If there is fluid retention, we see evidence, such as edema of the ankles and knees, baggy eyes, or swelling of the skin, hands, or tongue.
- *Kidney yang is responsible for basal metabolic issues*, our body's heat. Kidney yang warms the body. If it is high, we are robust and resistant to cold and have good digestion and potency. If Kidney yang is deficient, we are cold or hard of hearing, or may have loose stools, incontinence, dizziness, weakness, and low back pain.
- *The Kidney's emotion is fear*, the opposite of courage, bravery, and facing life confidently.
- *The Kidney opens to the ear.* The ear is the Kidney's sense organ. Deafness and tinnitus reflect this connection and are considered Kidney issues.
- *Tissues related to Kidney.* These tissues include all the reproductive organs, the head and pubic hair, the bones and bone marrow. (In Chinese medicine, the bone marrow is equivalent to the brain and spinal cord.)
- *The Kidney color is midnight blue or black*, the season is *winter*, the taste is *salty*, and the element is *Water*.

Chinese Bladder Functions

The yin Kidney is paired with the yang Bladder, so it is part of the Kidney network. The bladder holds and releases the urine. Because the paired Bladder meridian extends down the midback, back issues and spinal cord problems are related to this network. The Bladder controls the release of urine along with the lower sphincters.

The Six External Pernicious Influences

The ***Six External Pernicious Influences*** that cause disease are wind, cold, heat, damp, dry, and summer heat. They are sometimes called *The Six Evils*. They are climatic influences that enter the environment externally and can penetrate the body.[4]

- *External Wind* is the most important Pernicious Influence. *Wind* implies movement, unpredictability, and sudden onset. Spring, a time of rapid change and a season of wind, is associated with the Liver. The concept of wind implies not only the movement of air, but also a condition of rapid changes shifting movement internally and externally. Wind may penetrate the body's defenses and enter it, accompanied by dampness, dryness, cold, or heat. Examples are *Wind Cold* and *Wind Heat*, which blow in microorganisms from the outside in the form of a common cold or flu. Common colds caused by Wind invasion can be either cold with chills and no fever and/or hot with fever and other symptoms. Cold common colds can turn into hot common colds if not treated promptly. *Wind Damp Cold* and *Wind Damp Heat*, called *Bi Syndromes*, refer to arthritis or nerve pain of either an acute hot or chronic cold type. Bi Syndrome indicates a moving, windy pain in the muscles and joints.[2]

- *Internal Wind.* Internal wind is mentioned here, because the concept of *wind* is so important. When wind affects the skin surface, it can cause sores and itching. When wind gets inside the body, it is then internal and manifests as jerky movement, dizziness, vertigo, labile emotions, incoordination, seizures, strokes, tremors, or moving or migratory pain in the joints and muscles or head. Internal and external wind are both associated with the Liver.

- *External Cold.* This type can attack the body, and acute illness may develop, along with chills, fever, and body aches. If external cold moves inward, it can become chronic. A client would have a pale face, lethargy, and would crave heat and sleep for long periods of time. In the West, this condition might be termed *hypothermia*.
- *External Heat.* This type can invade the body on a hot day, causing overactive yang functions or insufficient yin functions. A person could have a red face, boils, hyperactivity and talkativeness, fever, dry mouth or thirst for cold liquids, and a rapid pulse. Westerners might call it *hyperthermia* or *heat exhaustion*.
- *External Damp.* Dampness can get inside the body and cause various symptoms, depending on its location. It could cause stiff joints (arthritis). If it goes to the Lungs, we are stuffy and have a damp cough. If it goes to the Spleen, it can cause upset stomach, nausea, lack of appetite, a swollen abdomen, or diarrhea. Once dampness is internal, it is hard to eradicate. It produces a heaviness.
- *External Dryness.* Dryness is often accompanied by heat. Heat causes water to evaporate and could create dehydration. If dryness invades the body, we have respiratory problems, such as asthmatic breathing, a dry cough, acute pain, and fever.
- *External Summer Heat.* This type comes from the very hot days of late summer, also called Indian summer. Extreme summer heat can bring on a sudden high fever and lethargy. It often is accompanied by damp.

Assessment: Tongue and Pulse

There are many ways to determine what is wrong. A Western doctor or nurse practitioner would take a verbal health history. They would also conduct a physical exam by listening to the heart, lungs, and bowel sounds with a stethoscope; take blood pressure with a sphygmomanometer; look in the ears with an otoscope; and look in the eyes with an ophthalmoscope. They would run a battery of lab tests of the blood, urine, and sputum. They might take an EKG or X-ray or order an MRI. They would then come up with a *diagnosis* or a name for that disease or problem, such as bronchitis, myocardial infarction, or pneumonia. The process is dependent on machines and technology and, in some cases, can be life-saving.

In Chinese Medicine, doctors depend on their senses, judgment, intuition, and experience, not technology. They begin with questions, obtain a very detailed health history regarding family and personal health, sleep patterns, elimination, menses, weight, food preferences, diet, and stress. They make observations regarding complexion, posture, gait, and nails. They use the senses: smelling for body odor, listening for the sound of voice, and using touch to determine muscle tone, flexibility, temperature, and texture.

Chinese Medicine doctors also use touch for a detailed method of *pulse* P *and tongue* T diagnosis or evaluations, which help arrive at a diagnosis, a *syndrome*, a *disharmony*, or pattern of disease. Examples of syndrome names could be Wind Damp Heat, Spleen Qi Deficiency, Excess Kidney Yang, or Yin Deficiency. A cough comes in many forms and could result from heat, cold, dry, damp, deficiency, or excess. These individual coughs are all different, and each would be treated differently, depending on the results of the pulse and tongue analysis, and other assessments. One universal bottle of cough syrup from the local drugstore does not fit and cure every kind of cough. An aspirin does not treat every kind of headache.

As herbalists, we understand that our assessments will include some of the Western techniques and some of the Chinese. What is optimal is that we begin to learn and use Eastern and some Western methods of assessment. Notice the word *assessment* was used. In the United States, herbalists are not legally allowed to diagnose, treat, or prescribe, *and* they are not allowed to use those words verbally or in writing. By using the Chinese methods, we can make assessments and come up with suggested remedies without making a formal Western diagnosis.

Assessment of pulse and tongue are skills which take time to develop; ideally with an experienced practitioner standing by, to provide a read or reality check for your findings. Just begin. Start to use pulse and tongue assessment and see if they match up with your other assessment modalities. The more tools pointing in one particular direction, the more likely you are to be on the correct assessment track.

Tongue Assessment (Looking)

In Chinese Medicine, the ***tongue*** reflects the condition of the body (Fig. 9.3). We observe it for color, texture, moisture, size, and shape. A healthy tongue is smooth, moist, pale red, and firm. The tongue fits comfortably into the mouth and has a thin white *coating*, also called the *fur* or *moss*, on its upper surface. The *body* of the tongue underneath the fur is sometimes called the tongue material. Changes in the body of the tongue show long-term dysfunctions. Changes in the fur show short-term problems, such as changes in digestion, fluid balance, and heat regulation.[1]

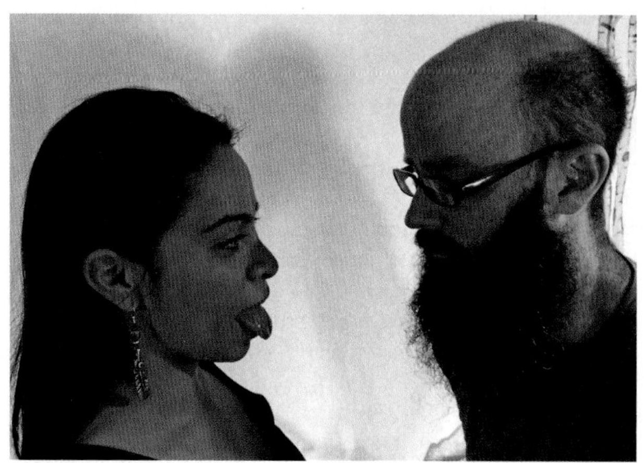

• **Fig. 9.3** Tongue assessment.

Tongue Body Color

- *Normal tongue.* Pale red indicates blood is carried to the tongue by a smooth flow of qi.
- *Paler.* Less red than normal indicates *deficient blood* or *deficient qi* or excess cold.
- *Red.* Redder than normal indicates *heat.*
- *Scarlet.* Darker purplish-red, rather than a red tongue indicates *extreme heat* or heat that has gone internal.
- *Purple.* Purple indicates that qi and blood are not moving, and there is stagnant or congealed qi. Pale purple indicates *cold*, and reddish-purple indicates *heat.*[3]

Tongue Coating, Fur

- *Normal coat.* Normal coat is a thin, white, moist layer, mostly uniform all over the tongue, with uniform thickness or slightly thicker texture in the center or back of the tongue. The tongue body can be seen through it.
- *Coat puddled with moisture.* Indicates excess fluids because of deficient yang or fire, the body's internal heat.
- *Dry coat.* If it looks like dry sandpaper, it's from deficient fluids or excess yang fire and external wind heat attack.
- *Firmly attached coat.* If it looks firmly planted, it indicates good, strong Spleen and Stomach qi.
- *Coat floating on surface.* If it appears to float, the Spleen and Stomach qi are weak.
- *Greasy coat.* An oily film indicates mucus or damp. The pastier the coat, the more extreme the damp.
- *Coat patchy or uneven.* If it looks peeled off in sections, it's called a *peeled tongue*, indicating deficient yin, fluids, or Spleen qi.
- *White coat.* Indicates either normal or a cold illness. If it's white and cottage-cheesy, it's Stomach heat.
- *Yellow coat.* Indicates heat; the deeper the yellow, the greater the heat.
- *Black or gray coat.* Indicates extreme heat or extreme cold. It's heat if the tongue body is red; it's cold if the tongue body is pale.

Tongue Shape

- *Normal shape.* Tongue is normal if it fits in mouth easily and is not too big or too small and neither swollen nor shriveled. Movement should be flexible, with no slant in any direction. There should be no cracks or pimples, but there may be raised papillae.
- *Swollen tongue.* Tongue is swollen if it is puffy with scalloped edges or has teeth imprints. Swollen tongue indicates excess fluids or deficient qi.
- *Thin tongue.* Smaller than normal and indicates deficient blood or fluids.
- *Stiff tongue.* If tongue lacks flexibility, it indicates a windy Pernicious Influence, or mucous obstructing the Heart qi.
- *Trembling tongue.* If it wiggles around or shakes, and body is pale, the qi is deficient and can't regulate movement; if body is red, the internal wind is moving the tongue.
- *Lolls like a panting dog.* A sign of heat.
- *Contracted tongue.* If it won't stretch out, it's serious. If body is pale or purple, it's from cold. If body is swollen, it's from mucous or damp. If body is red, it's heat.
- *Cracks.* These are normal if from birth. If they develop from illness, it's chronic and severe.
- *Red eruptions.* Occasional papillae are normal. Pimples or thorn-like protrusions are signs of heat or congealed blood.
- *Red tip of tongue.* This condition is often a clue to emotional issues of the Heart shen that shows heat—a good diagnostic tip.

If a tongue cannot be analyzed from the parameters in this list of tongue shape conditions, it helps to look at a five organ-tongue correspondence map. Sometimes these characteristics listed here are only seen in one portion of the tongue (Box 9.2). For instance, only the tip may be red; purple coloration might be present only on the edges. If either is the case, the map can be useful to identify the affected organ. This is helpful but not definitive.

Pulse Assessment (Palpation)

Palpating (feeling) the pulse is partnered with a tongue assessment. In Chinese Medicine, a ***pulse*** reflects the blood and qi circulating through the vessels and tells the practitioner about the condition of each organ. Skilled practitioners can make amazingly correct assessments of current body imbalances, past diseases, and future predictions by taking a pulse. This ability is the result of information gathered over centuries of experimentation and effort, a true art that is not quickly mastered.

Each wrist has three positions to palpate along the radial artery. The three positions indicate a metabolic zone known as the Triple Burner or *Jiao* (rhymes with cow). The upper position, closest to the wrist, corresponds to the chest and upper body. The middle position corresponds to the middle body or upper abdomen, and the lower position corresponds to the lower abdomen or pelvis. The rate of speed, depth, degree of strength, and fullness of these pulses give important information about the integrity of the qi and blood and organs.[2]

• BOX 9.2 The Tongue Reflects a Reliable Assessment of the Body

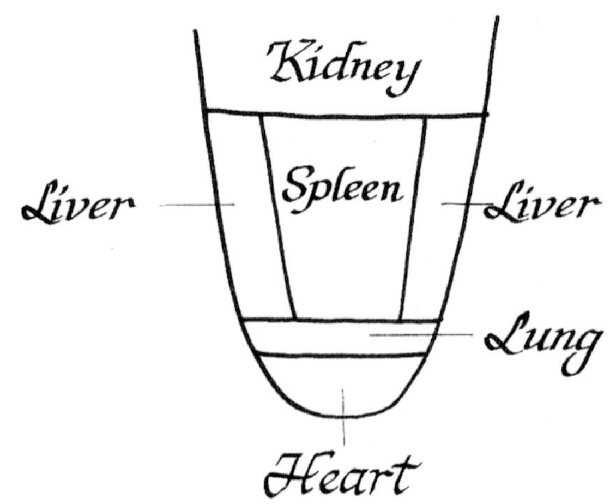

Tongue map showing areas of influence of each yin organ. (Illustration by Matthew Berk, L.Ac.)

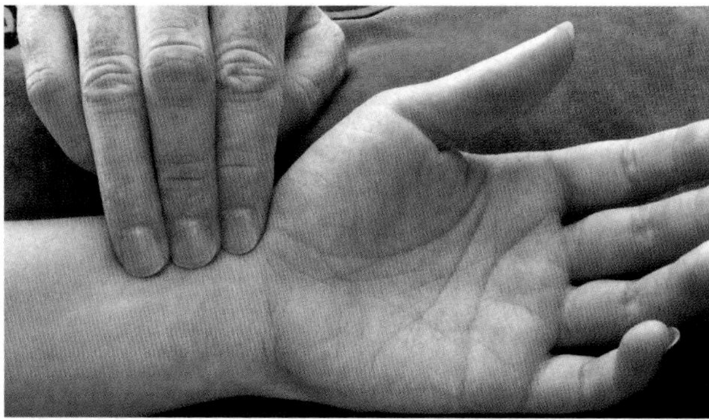

• **Fig. 9.4** Palpating pulses.

How to Palpate Pulses

- *Body position.* Pulses are taken along the radial artery on the thumb side of the inner wrist (Fig. 9.4). You and the client are relaxed. Allow client to rest wrists on a pillow, palms up. Face client or sit to their side and lightly curl your fingers around client's wrist.
- *Finger position.* Practitioner places second finger (index finger) at wrist crease and third finger medial to radial eminence just off the bone; fourth finger will naturally fall next to the middle finger (Box 9.3). The index finger is now on the first point, middle finger on second point, and ring finger on third point. These three points represent the yin organs of each wrist.
- *First, feel for three depth positions: superficial, middle, and deep.* Press deeply against the bone until you have occluded it and can hardly feel the pulse. Then lighten up a little. This second depth indicates strength of the internal, deep yin organs and emotions. Next release pressure to feel the superficial surface pulse just under the skin. This is the external yang pulse that indicates body's strength to overcome external colds, flus, skin problems, and arthritic pains. Do the same for the other wrist and then do them both together to compare.
- *Feel for rate.* Time the beats per minute (bpm) with a second hand for a minute. The average adult rate is 60 to 80 bpm. Less than 60 indicates yin coldness. Greater than 80 indicates yang heat.
- *Now feel for empty or fullness.* Emptiness is a small, yin pulse from a generally thin, timid person. It is soft, like a balloon filled with water. A robust, full pulse is a generally from a more outgoing, yang person. It pounds hard against the fingers at all three depths. Feel for empty or full on both wrists.
- *Normal pulse.* It is felt mainly at the middle level. It should be alive and feels elastic and spirited: not too thin; not too full; not too weak; not too strong; normal rate. Just right. Normal pulses vary. Athletes may have very slow normal pulses; some women may have softer, faster pulses; men can have slower pulses than women; children have faster pulses than adults; heavier people have deeper pulses; thinner folks have more superficial pulses. All are normal.
- *First practice feeling for rate, depth, and fullness.* This practice is the best place to begin. Do this before you get into the individual pulse types and positions.
- *Now feel for each individual organ position and pulse type* (Box 9.3). Use one finger at a time, as when learning to play the piano. Don't start feeling for the type of pulse without first getting a sense of the basics just described, namely depth, rate, and fullness.
- *Each wrist has three positions that denote a yin organ.* The Kidney position on the left hand is Kidney yin. The Kidney position on the right hand is Kidney yang. Added together, 26 basic pulse types can technically be felt in each of three pulse levels (superficial, middle, and deep) in the three positions on each wrist![5] Table 9.4 presents the most common types. Palpating and assessing these possibilities in a systematic manner will and should take a long time. It takes years to master this expertly, but there is no time like the present to begin.[3]

• BOX 9.3 Pulse Positions and Palpation Basics

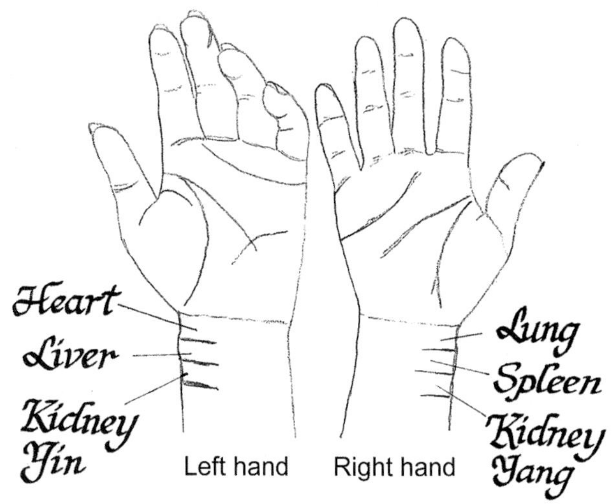

Pulse positions and palpation basics. (Illustration by Matthew Berk, L.Ac.)

To obtain a global analysis of the overall pulse, feel under the middle finger on both wrists. These may also be palpated at each individual pulse position.

FAST PULSE = Heat
SLOW PULSE = Cold
SUPERFICIAL PULSE = External Acute Condition
DEEP PULSE = Internal Chronic Condition
EMPTY OR THIN PULSE = Deficient
FULL PULSE = Excess

The Eight Principle Patterns of Assessment: Cold-Heat, Deficiency-Excess, Interior-Exterior, and Yin-Yang

What does all the information just obtained through taking the patient's health history, observation, and tongue and pulse assessment mean? How will you use it? What herbs should be chosen? The ***Eight Principle Patterns of Assessment*** refer to four sets of opposites that help interpret the data gathered through examination: *cold-heat, deficiency-excess, interior-exterior, and yin-yang* (Table 9.5). They reflect the overall quality and the location of the qi, moisture, and blood in the body and in the organs.

The information helps to figure out the therapeutic principles or objectives, according to the style of Chinese Medicine. Basically, a therapy that is the opposite of the assessment is used. If

TABLE 9.4 **Common Pulse Types**
(These may be felt at each position on each wrist)

Pulse type	Description	Interpretation
Floating Depth	Higher than normal, easier felt with light pressure. Felt at superficial level.	Disharmony in superficial part of body. Combating external influences.
Sinking Depth	Felt at third, deepest depth with heavy pressure.	Internal with obstruction. Yin.
Slow Speed	Fewer than four beats per breath (in and out). Felt at middle depth.	Insufficient qi to cause movement of blood. Yin.
Rapid Speed	More than five beats per breath (in and out). Felt at middle depth.	Heat is moving blood. Yang.
Thin Width	Fine thread, but distinct and clear. Middle depth.	Deficient blood and qi. Yin.
Big Width	Broad and distinct. Middle depth.	Excess and yang. Usually with heat.
Empty Width	Big without strength. Soft like balloon filled with water. Superficial level and slow.	Deficient qi and blood. Yin.
Full Width	Strong, pounding, hard against fingers at all three depths.	Excess and yang.
Slippery Shape	Fluid, smooth, slithers like a fish jumping out of your hand. Middle depth.	Excess, damp, or mucous, pregnancy (when extra blood is needed for fetus).
Choppy Shape	Opposite of slippery. Uneven, rough, and sometimes irregular. Middle depth.	Deficient blood, jing, or congealed blood. Yin.
Wiry Shape	Taut like guitar string. Rebounds against pressure evenly at all depths.	Stagnation against flow of Liver or Gallbladder. Yang.
Tight Shape	Strong and bounces from side to side. Fuller, urgent and more elastic than the wiry pulse. Middle depth.	Excess cold and stagnation. Considered both yin and yang.[3]
Short Length	Does not fill space under the three fingers. Generally felt in only one finger position in middle depth.	Deficient qi. Yin.
Long Length	Goes beyond first and third positions. Felt closer to hand or up to elbow in middle depth.	Excess is yang. May be tight and wiry or normal.
Knotted Rhythm	Slow and irregular that skips beats irregularly. Middle depth.	Cold obstructing qi and blood. Deficient qi, blood, or jing. Yin.
Hurried Rhythm	Rapid and skips beats irregularly. Middle depth.	Heat agitating qi and blood. Yang.
Intermittent Rhythm	Skips more beats than previous two beats. Has regular pattern. Middle depth.	Serious, exhausted state of all the Organs. Yin.
Moderate Rhythm	Normal in depth, speed, length, and width. Middle depth.	The healthy pulse. No one is perfectly normal, but one could come close. This is the ideal.

a person is already too warm, it would make no sense to add more warmth in the remedy; the person needs to be cooled down. Furthermore, this Chinese Medicine style of assessment will later be combined with the Western-type information that is also gathered (Chapter 15).

- *If a person is mainly cold*, the body needs warming with warming herbs. If one is predominantly warm, cooling herbs are needed.
- *If excess exists*, it must be dispersed or spread out. If *deficiency* predominates, it must be strengthened or tonified. Deficiency patterns are often chronic in nature. Excess patterns are more acute and often come from a Pernicious Influence attacking the body.
- *If the disease is internal*, remedies are used that go deep into the body, so the organs can be reached. If *external*, more superficially acting herbs are needed.
- *If yin predominates*, in general, it implies a cold, deficient, and internal condition. If *yang predominates*, it usually implies a warm, excess, and external condition. These are combinations of the earlier three.[1]

TABLE 9.5 **The Eight Principle Patterns of Assessment**

Principle	Body Process	Signs & Symptoms	Pulse (P) Tongue (T)[3]
Cold	Slow metabolic activity.	Decreased measured body temperature, feels chilled, pale skin or mucous membranes, slow, withdrawn, watery stool.	P Slow or tense. T White fur; pale or purple or blue body.
Heat	Rapid metabolic activity.	Feels warm generally or locally, increased measured temperature, flushed or red skin or mucous membranes, constipation, outgoing, fast, thirst.	P Rapid or bounding. T Yellow fur; red body.
Deficiency	Hypofunctioning organs or body processes; decreased resistance to stress or infection. Low immunity.	Systemic or local fatigue, weakness, dull pain relieved by pressure, passive.	P Weak or thin. T Scanty or absent fur; pale, flabby, or scalloped body.
Excess	Hyperfunction or obstruction of organ or process; increased reactivity to stress or infection.	Local or systemic feeling of fullness, tension, agitation, or intense pain, worse with pressure.	P Strong, large or tense, wiry, slippery. T Thickened fur; red, swollen, stiff, or quivering body.
Internal	Affects deeper tissue layers and function, i.e., organs, brain, spinal cord, bones, vessels, nerves, or reproductive organs.	Conditions originating from the inside, caused by improper diet, lack of exercise, emotions, traumatic injury.	P Changes at deep level. Can be excess or deficient. T Changes in tongue body, but also in the fur.
External	Affects superficial layers and function, i.e. skin, hair, nails, muscles, tendons, ligaments, joints, genitals, eyes, ears, mouth, teeth, breasts, or anus.	Conditions occurring from the outside, such as sunburn, itching, bites, wind, injuries. OR conditions which move from the inside out, showing up as visible symptoms of an internal problem—like a pimple.	P Superficial or deep level, depending on the condition. T Changes in fur. Color and shape may also be affected.
Yin	Includes cold, deficient, excess damp, and internal processes.	Contracted, sleeps curled up, tired, withdrawn, weak, quiet, cold, seeks warmth.	P Frail, thin, weak. T Pale, puffy, moist, thin. Coat is white.
Yang	Includes hot, excess, and external processes. Can also be deficient yang, which indicates cold, damp conditions.	In excess, shows heat conditions, such as red face, agitation, high blood pressure, talkative, constipation. When deficient is cold, diarrhea, bloated, edema, often tired.	P Signs of excess, full, rapid, wiry, slippery. T Red, yellow coat, if excess. Swollen, white coat, if yang deficient.

Summary

The basics of Chinese Medicine provide a time-tested, accurate way for us to categorize herbs, assess our clients, and devise herbal formulas. Grasping these fundamentals will help achieve successful clinical results and eliminate guesswork. The West really has no counterpart or organized system to accomplish this.

Yin and yang encompass everything and are relative to any situation. Generally, yin is cool, moist, inward, and feminine. Yang is hot, dry, outward, and male. However, within all yang is some yin; and within all yin is some yang. Bodily disharmonies (syndromes) or pathologies are excesses or deficiencies—too much of one over the other.

The Fundamental Substances are qi, blood, jing, shen, and fluids—and all can have disharmonies. Qi refers to the energy or life force in all living things. Blood arises from transformed food and nourishes the body. Jing is the basis of the life force from birth to death. Shen is the spirit and affects the psyche. Fluids refer to all liquids in the body.

The Five Element Theory is a world view that explains our relationship with natural cycles. External Pernicious Influences are conditions that arise from outside the body, causing imbalance. Two important Chinese Medicine assessment techniques are pulse and tongue analysis. These skills can be practiced and used to assess our clients. There are Eight Principle Patterns of Assessment organized into four opposite pairs: cold-heat, deficiency-excess, interior-exterior, and yin-yang. Once an assessment is made based on health history and analysis of pulse and tongue, a proper herbal remedy can be formulated.

Review

Fill in the Blanks

(Answers in Appendix B.)

1. What are the five divisions of Chinese Medicine? ___, ___, ___, ___, ___.
2. Name three characteristics of yin. ___, ___, ___.
3. What is *protective qi* in Western terms? ___.
4. The Five Elements are ___, ___, ___, ___, ___.
5. Name the yin organs and their yang pairs. ___, ___, ___, ___, ___.

6. Which organ would you associate with mental depression? ___.
7. Which organ would you associate with pink eye? ___.
8. A deficient pulse and tongue would look like: P___ T___.
9. A person is too moist and wet. Describe their pulse and tongue. P ___ T ___.
10. A tongue coat is yellow and very moist and greasy in the center. Body is red. Can you name the syndrome? ___.

Critical Concept Questions

(Answers for you to decide.)

1. Why is Chinese Medicine worth understanding for the Western herbalist?
2. Contrast and describe basic yin-yang concepts.
3. What is the function of the Chinese Liver?
4. A stressed-out person with a fever has an unproductive, painful cough. Give a guess as to the pulse and tongue.
5. Explain the Chinese concept of wind.
6. What is the Five Element Theory? Is it vitalistic or analytic?
7. How can knowing a person's emotional state help one develop a treatment plan?
8. What are the Eight Principle Patterns of Assessment?
9. How do the Eight Principle Patterns of Assessment give you clues as to herbal treatment?
10. How does the Chinese Spleen differ from the Western anatomical spleen?

References

1. Beinfield, Harriet and Efrem Korngold. *Between Heaven and Earth: A Guide to Chinese Medicine* (New York: Ballantine, 1991).
2 Tierra, Michael. *The Way of Chinese Herbs* (New York: Pocket Books, 1998).
3. Kaptchuk, Ted J. *The Web That Has No Weaver* (New York: Congdon and Weed, 1983).
4. "Causes of Illness: 6 Evils or 6 Pernicious Influences." Sacred Lotus Chinese Medicine. http://www.sacredlotus.com/go/foundations-chinese-medicine/get/causes-illness-6-evils (accessed October 5, 2019).
5. Dharmananda, Subuhuti "Institute for Traditional Medicine. The Significance of Traditional Pulse Diagnosis in the Modern Practice of Chinese Medicine. http://www.itmonline.org/arts/pulse.htm (accessed October 5, 2019).

10

Energetics Related to Western Herbology

"We live in a world of energy. An important task at this time is to learn to sense or see the energy of everyone and everything—people, plants, animals. . . . Go to the sacred places of the Earth to pray for peace and have respect for the Earth which gives us our food, clothing, and shelter. We need to reactivate the energy of these sacred places. That is our work."

—Carlos Barrios (Australian artist, born Carlos Manuel Barrios Rosa in 1966 in San Salvador, El Salvador, Central America)

CHAPTER REVIEW

- The why and what of energetics in Western herbalism and its relationship to Chinese Medicine.
- The Three Primary Qualities: Taste (with energy directions), warmth, and moisture.
- The Six Secondary Qualities: Stimulate-sedate, restore-relax, and moisten-decongest.
- Tissue level qualities or descriptions: Astringe-eliminate, solidify-dissolve, thicken-dilute. These qualities appear in Western herbalism.
- Descriptive terms in Western herbalism: Diuretics, laxatives, dissolvents, antibacterials, alteratives, and so many more.
- Organoleptics, evaluating herbal energetics using the senses.

KEY TERMS

Anhidrotics
Antilipemics
Antidiarrheals
Antilithics
Astringents
Bland
Counterirritants
Decongestants
Demulcents
Diaphoretics
Dissolvents
Diuretics
Emmenagogues
Energetics
Expectorants
Hemostatics
Laxatives
Litholytics
Mucolytics/mucostatics
Nervines
Oily
Organoleptics
Primary Qualities
Purgatives
Quality
Relaxants
Restoratives
Secondary Qualities
Sedate
Stimulate
Tonics
Trophorestoratives
Vulneraries
Warmth

This chapter organizes, classifies, categorizes, and arranges herbs based on their energetics from Chinese and Western standpoints, providing the best of both worlds. The terms are found in numerous herb books worldwide and give information about how herbs work.

The Three Primary Qualities or characteristics are taste, warmth, and moisture. These qualities give data about a plant's effect on the body in relation to the senses, a plant's energy, and the direction it moves the qi. The Six Secondary Qualities are specific actions arranged as opposites—stimulate-sedate, restore-relax, and moisten-decongest—indicating what an herb does to the body in very broad terms.

Descriptive qualities are categories traditionally used in Western herbalism. They tell us what an herb does on a tissue level. These groups are also opposites: astringe-eliminate, solidify-dissolve, and thicken-dilute.

Further breakdowns involve the countless descriptive terms used in Western herbalism. They are action words, such as *diaphoretics* that cause sweating, *emmenagogues* that bring on menses, or *anxiolytics* that curb anxiety. Many come from Western allopathic medicine and are intertwined with Western herbalism.

Organoleptics refers to judging the potency, quality, and phytochemical composition of an herb or preparation by using the senses. By attentively tasting, smelling, or feeling, we experience and reach our own conclusions about how an herb acts in the body.

Energetics in Western Herbalism

Rationale for the Energetic Approach

There are countless books about Western herbs with various organizational principles, some more useful than others. One type assigns a descriptive term to a plant that tells about one of its actions, such as *demulcent* or *astringent*, a method typically done in the West. Raspberry leaf is astringent, meaning it pulls in and tightens—therefore a good choice for diarrhea. But if Raspberry leaf were considered only as astringent, another important use is omitted: its nutritive quality. For pregnant women, Raspberry leaf is a prime reproductive nutritive tonic with an affinity for the uterus.

Some books give long laundry lists of actions, but they might leave you wondering which herb to choose. Say there are 20 different antimicrobials listed. Are they all equally effective? Popular magazines often extol the wonders of a popular "herb of the year," such as Echinacea root. Pictures of *Echinacea purpurea* with its purple rays and yellow center appear all over the media. It is supposedly *the* herb to take for colds and infections. But is Echinacea the best selection for every single viral and bacterial illness that comes along?

Herbalism is complex. How do we know which remedies to choose? In my experience, the best way to choose is to use a combination of Western categories of action, *property-based* concepts (actions), combined with Chinese methods that consider *energetics*. Western labels tell you very quickly at least one action for an herb: diuretic, antiinflammatory, or demulcent. Chinese energetics take into account diagnostics, helping to fit the correct herb to the correct condition.

Chinese Energetics in Western Herbalism

Energetics is a system used to organize herbs referring to its qualities, its nature or sensory characteristics, and the broad actions they have on the body. ***Quality*** refers to how an herb acts on contact with tissues like the mouth, skin, stomach, or sense organs. When we eat a lemon, its sour taste causes the lips to pucker and constrict, producing an energy that pulls inward. This is a very different action and direction from that of sweet-tasting Licorice root, which restores or builds up mucous membranes and moves energy outward in gentle waves. Hot and pungent Cayenne pepper moves energy forcefully outward to the extremities, working differently from cold, bitter Gentian root, which pulls energy inward and downward. Chinese Medicine often refers to this directional pull of plants.

Another category of energetics refers to actions, the properties of an herb and its potential for achieving a particular outcome. Ginger root is a *stimulating* herb that warms the body and helps blood circulate outward to the extremities. Lobelia is *relaxing*—it calms down the nervous system. Corn Silk *restores*, or builds up, the urinary system. White Horehound herb *decongests*, or breaks up mucus, in the lungs. Dandelion root does two seemingly contradictory things but they are actually not. It is both *sedating* and *stimulating*, in that it decreases heat (sedates warmth) and encourages the liver to work harder (stimulates).

Western and Chinese traditions both have their place. Use them both in describing, categorizing, and selecting herbs—and end up with an excellent system and great tools. It is beneficial to appreciate the two ways of thinking. Cross-cultural healing deepens our understanding and ability to assess conditions in a patient and to formulate wisely and effectively. Ayurvedic medicine from India also uses energetics, being an important part of that system, as well.

The Three Primary Qualities: Taste, Warmth, Moisture

The three ***Primary Qualities*** of taste, warmth, and moisture provide information about a plant, helping us to choose wisely. They all have local and global effects on the body. We will go through the various tastes, the gradations of hot to cold, and the concept of moisture, ranging from dry to damp.

Taste: Sweet, Sour, Bitter, Salty, Pungent

There are four types of taste buds or chemoreceptors mapped out on the tongue in anatomy and physiology texts. Those receptors are for sweet, sour, bitter, and salty. In Chinese Medicine, five tastes are described: sweet, sour, bitter, salty, and pungent (sometimes called acrid or spicy).[1] In Ayurveda, they speak of six tastes: sweet, sour, bitter, salty, pungent, and astringent. Ayurvedic has added astringent to the mix (Box 10.1).

We will select the five tastes of Chinese Medicine for the discussion of the energetics of taste. In Chinese Medicine, tastes are also

• BOX 10.1 Tastes from Different Traditions

The Four Western Textbook Tastes	Sweet, sour, bitter, salty
The Five Chinese Tastes	Sweet, sour, bitter, salty, pungent (sometimes called acrid or spicy)
The Six Ayurvedic Tastes	Sweet, sour, bitter, salty, pungent, astringent
Extra Qualities	Oily and bland (neutral, pure, or no taste)

assigned *directions*, part of the desired action in a formula, indicating where those herbs will travel in the body.

Herbs usually have two or more tastes in combination, although one generally predominates and is considered the main taste. If you put an herb on your tongue, there will be a taste that you become aware of first, but in a few seconds, you'll probably detect others. Tastes derive from chemical properties in a substance (Chapter 8). Taste buds receive the chemicals, and the brain interprets them.

- *Sweet* comes from carbohydrates, fats, and proteins.
- *Sour* comes from ascorbic acid, citric acid, and acetic acid.
- *Bitter* comes from alkaloids or glycosides.
- *Salty* comes from mineral salts.
- *Pungent* comes from essential oils.
- *Astringent* comes from tannins. (In Chinese Medicine, astringent is considered a subcategory of the sour taste; in Ayurvedic, it's a separate taste.)

Sweet

- *Constituent:* Carbohydrates.
- *Direction:* Moves qi in calming waves, flowing outward.
- *Actions:* Nourishing, moistening, cooling, restorative, harmonizing, and tonifying.

The sweet taste is universally loved and pleasing to all people, regardless of age or culture. It is the first one babies experience with mother's milk. The other tastes, particularly bitter, take some getting used to. Very few children like bitter foods. When experimenting with new plants, ancient tribes found that sweet tastes were generally not poisonous. The macronutrients—carbohydrates, proteins, and fats—are the major food groups necessary for good nutrition. Carbohydrates and proteins contain sweet tastes, and fats enhance the flavor of sugar.

Sugar is a water-soluble carbohydrate, has a crystalline shape, and tastes sweet. The more complex the sugar molecule, the longer it takes the body to digest and the less stress it puts on the pancreas. Simple sugars, such as found in donuts and bagels, cause frequent fluctuations in insulin production, whereas complex carbohydrates in whole grains and vegetables take longer to digest, causing fewer insulin swings. An interesting sweet tasting herb that is not a carbohydrate and that does not cause blood sugar swings is Glycyrrhiza Gan Cao (Licorice root; Box 10.2).

In Chinese Medicine the sweet taste is calming and moist. One often sees honey or sugar being used as the base of cough syrups and other medicines. It is harmonizing. It soothes, coats, and calms irritated throat mucous membranes. It blends together all the herbs in the syrup. In the West, we are so accustomed to eating simple sugars in the form of candies, cakes, and ice cream, that sometimes we don't appreciate the incredible sweetness of a carrot, a sweet potato, or a slice of bread (Fig. 10.1). The Chinese also consider grains, meats, beans, and nuts to be sweet.

Refined sugars in small amounts can be calming. However, if children overconsume sweets, they may become anything but. If sugar were an occasional treat, rather than a major part of the diet, the sugar would be in balance and thus not lead to hyperactivity. The energy of the sweet taste is comforting, with a smooth, soft, wavy feeling and direction. Think of how good an amazing chocolate bar or your favorite sweet makes you feel.

In Chinese Medicine, the sweet taste is considered tonic. ***Tonics*** build, nourish, energize. and treat deficiencies. If one is nourished, the body can make energy. If one has energy, the immune system benefits. If one is calm, there is balance and freedom from detrimental stress, a road toward optimal health. A class of herbs called *adaptogens* has these properties. They are building tonic herbs such as Astragalus Huang Qi (Astragalus root), or Ashwagandha root. These herbs *tonify* the Chinese Spleen, the organ of digestion and assimilation. According to the Five Element Theory of Correspondences, the sweet taste is attributed to the Spleen (Chapter 9). Examples of sweet herbs and foods appear in Table 10.1.

• BOX 10.2 Licorice: An Exception to Sweet

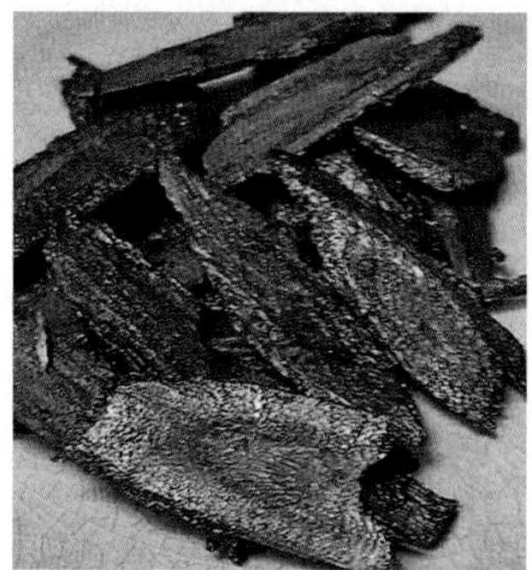

Glycyrrhiza Zhi Gan Cao (Honey fried Licorice root) is warm and nutritive with a calming outward energy.

The glycyrrhizin in *Glycyrrhiza glabra* Gan Cao (Licorice root) is not a sugar or carbohydrate at all (it's a saponin in the terpene category), although if you chew on the yellow insides of its root or rhizome, it tastes 50 times as sweet as cane sugar. Licorice has many tastes, the dominant one being the taste of Anise. But it is also bitter. Raw Licorice root tastes sweet, but to make Licorice into a truly sweet tonic, the Chinese bake it with honey and sugar to neutralize some of the bitter, cooling, and antiinflammatory actions. It then becomes more tonifying.

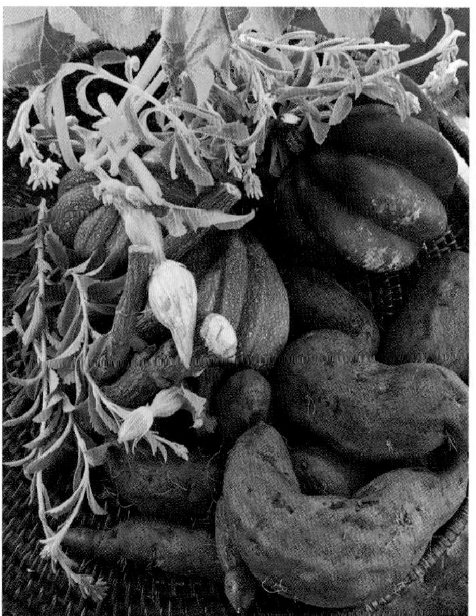

• **Fig. 10.1** Sweet acorn squash, purple sweet potatoes, *Stevia rebaudiana*, and Licorice root sticks.

TABLE 10.1 Examples of Sweet

Sweet Herbs and Some Properties	Foods
Astragalus membranaceus Huang Qi Astragalus root Its polysaccharides proven to help immunity.	Most carbohydrates, honey, molasses
Codonopsis pilosula Dang Shen Downy Bellflower root Restores the GI system. Tonic.	Grains, pasta, rice, bread
Matricaria recutita Chamomile flower Calming and harmonizes digestion.	Carrots
Cinnamomum cassia Rou Gui Cinnamon bark Helps glucose metabolism.	Potatoes
Glycyrrhiza glabra or *G. sinensis* Gan Cao Licorice root. Much sweeter tasting than sugar. Often used to blend, moisten, and to harmonize other herbs in a formula. Tonic.	Meat, fish Winter squashes and pumpkins
Althea officinalis Marshmallow root Moistening.	Nuts
Ophiopogon japonicus Mai Men Dong Dwarf Lilyturf root Moistening.	Yams
Symphytum officinale Comfrey root Moistening and tissue nourishing.	Dates
Ulmus fulva Slippery Elm root Moistening and nourishing to the gut.	Dairy

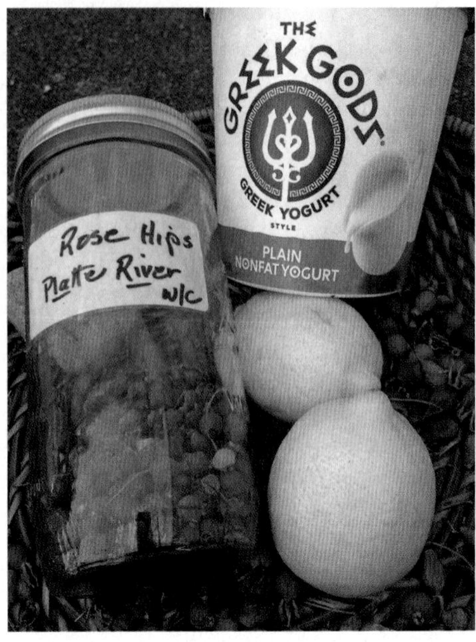

• **Fig. 10.2** Rosehips fruit/seed pods, lemons, and yogurt are all examples of the sour taste.

Sour

- *Constituents:* Organic acids such as citric, malic, ascorbic, and ascetic. Tannins are often present.
- *Direction*: Spiraling inward, sour foods pull in and pucker the lips (Fig. 10.2).
- *Actions*: Cooling, drying, astringent, refreshing, coagulating, and decongesting.

The sour taste is very common in foods, particularly fruits such as lemons, limes, and papayas. Because the sour taste is astringent in quality, it pulls tissue together and spirals energy inward. These actions translate into a tightening, astringent effect that reabsorbs escaping fluids, stopping discharges such as sputum, semen, vaginal fluids, and blood. It is drying to mucous membranes. It is *anhidrotic* (decreases sweating). It is cooling, so it can lower fevers. It is stimulating, meaning it increases the digestive enzymes of the liver, gallbladder, and small and large intestines.

Ayurvedic medicine uses sour tastes to stimulate digestion with foods such as tamarind or sour pickles. As part of the Five Element Correspondences, the sour taste is associated with the Liver. Wine (with tartaric acid) and vinegar (mainly acetic acid) are sometimes used to process herbs that are to be used as liver and blood tonics because of their herbal properties that are similar to those of other sour materials (Table 10.2).[1]

Bitter

- *Constituents:* Monoterpenes, sesquiterpenes, iridoids, alkaloids, and glycosides.
- *Direction:* Moves qi downward toward the feet.
- *Actions:* Grounding, cooling, stimulating, drying, detoxifying, antiinflammatory, antibacterial, and antiviral.

Bitter is widely prevalent in medicinal plants, probably more so than any other taste. Although the sweet taste is universally loved, bitter takes some getting used to for the uninitiated. Do most kids like kale? Many poisonous, toxic plants have a bitter, unpleasant taste, and the tastes were probably warnings to the ancients to spit out or beware. For the same reason some plants are dangerous, they also make strong valuable medicine when used judiciously. Bitter herbs range from the mildly bitter tastes of Chamomile and Yarrow flower to the intensely bitter tastes of *Gentian lutea* Long Dan Cao (Gentian root) and *Artemisia annua* Qing Hao (Sweet Annie herb) used in the treatment of drug-resistant malaria (Box 10.3).

Essential oils contain various kinds of volatile substances found in monoterpenes and sesquiterpenes (Chapter 8). They are found in the conifers, in Thyme leaf, Oregano herb, the Mints, Eucalyptus, White Sage leaf, and others. Citrus monoterpenes are bitter substances found in orange peels, especially the limonene component found in the white and the zest of the peels. They are rich in bioflavonoids, which fight cancer. Next time you eat an orange, be sure to eat some of the bitter peel and white membrane (Fig. 10.3).

The bitter taste has many uses and appears in healing plants used in most body systems. Because bitter is cold, it cools hot conditions and decreases fever, inflammation, and hot anger. Bitter is detoxifying and cleansing and works below the waist to pull off

TABLE 10.2 Examples of Sour

Herbs	Fermented Foods Produced by Microorganisms	Pickled Foods Made with Brine, Lemons, and Vinegar (Some could also be fermented.)	Foods
Rumex acetosella Sheep Sorrel herb	Yogurt, cheeses, kefir	Pickles	Lemons Limes
Oxalis acetosella Wood Sorrel herb	Wine	Pickled ginger	Blackberries
Rosa spp. Rosehips fruit	Vinegar	Pickled plums	Tamarind
Rhus glabra Sumac berry *Sambucus nigra* Elderberry *Crataegus oxyacantha* Hawthorn berry	Sauerkraut, Kombucha	Pickled cucumbers, beets, and other vegetables	Papaya Pomegranates Orange peels
Schisandra chinensis Wu Wei Zi Five Taste berry	Miso, soy sauce, Tempeh	Pickled herring	Greek lemon soup
Paeonia suffruticosa Mu Dan Pi Tree Peony root bark	Kimchi	Pickled olives and peppers	Raspberries

fluids, especially in the gut, kidney, and bladder, which is testament to their downward, grounding direction. They can help clear cholesterol from the liver, and some are laxative.

Because bitter is stimulating, it can decrease water retention and bloating, contributing to a drying action. An entire category of plants is called *digestive bitters* (Chapter 18). Examples are Gentian root, Yarrow herb, Dandelion root, Chicory root, Burdock root, and Chamomile flower. They stimulate the digestive system to secrete digestive enzymes and hormones, increase appetite, decrease sugar cravings, and aid the liver to increase its bile flow and detoxification.[3] Because gastrointestinal (GI) bitters are so wonderful for digestion and glucose regulation, they play a major role in holistic herbal treatment and preventative medicine.

Bitter-tasting pyrrolizidine alkaloids (PAs) are found in Comfrey root, Coltsfoot leaf, and Echinacea root. Comfrey is a renowned wound healer, Coltsfoot an expectorant, and Echinacea an antimicrobial. Examples of antiinfectives and antiinflammatory bitter herbs are yellow-rooted, berberine-containing plants. These bitter alkaloids are found in Goldenseal, Oregon Grape, and Barberry root. Berberines are effective for deep, hot infections. Some notoriously poisonous plants, such as *Datura stramonium* (Jimsonweed), Conium maculatum (Poison Hemlock), *Hyoscyamus niger* (Henbane), and *Atropa belladonna* (Deadly Nightshade), contain strong bitter alkaloids.[2] In Chinese Medicine, the bitter taste affects the Heart in the Correspondences. This is no coincidence, because many bitter heart herbs and allopathic drugs contain alkaloids. The Chinese Heart organ system corresponds to the nervous and circulatory systems of Western medicine, both strongly affected by the bitter taste. Bitter herbs and foods are listed in Table 10.3.

Salty

- *Constituent:* Trace minerals, sodium, and electrolytes.
- *Direction:* Sinking, downward effect.
- *Actions:* Softening, dissolving, sinking, moistening, and antilithic.

The salty taste improves flavors of food, lubricates and moistens body tissues, helps retain body fluids, and stimulates digestion by promoting salivation. Salt can also act as a laxative as in Epsom Salts (magnesium sulfate). The ocean is salty, and some of our salty herbs come from the sea. Seaweeds or sea vegetables are great sources of trace minerals, especially iodine. Kelp thallus is type of red algae, or seaweed, that moistens the mucosa and relieves dryness. It contains macro minerals and trace minerals of iodine, potassium, magnesium, calcium, iron, manganese, germanium, zinc, and bromium.[4] Irish Moss, Kelp thallus, and Dulse are other examples of sea veggies. Nori is type of seaweed that is used to wrap sushi (Fig. 10.4).

Salt is dissolving and softening. Salty ocean water corrodes metals. Taking this further, substances that stick and harden in the body can be broken down by salt. Salty herbs soften tumors, stones, and chronic lymph gland hardness. Salt can break down calcium deposits in atherosclerosis, keeping vessels soft. Echinacea root is primarily considered a pungent herb but is also salty and can reduce tumors and prostate enlargement. Because of salt's sinking, pulling-down action, it is diuretic and can decrease edema. This diuretic action is true of salty herbs, but not true of excess table salt, which can create an osmotic pull on water, causing fluid retention and edema.

A classification of herbs known as ***antilithics*** break down mineral deposits in kidney stones and gall stones. Examples of antilithic remedies include Gravel root, Horsetail herb, Cleavers herb,

• BOX 10.3 Very Bitter *Artemisia Annua* and Malaria

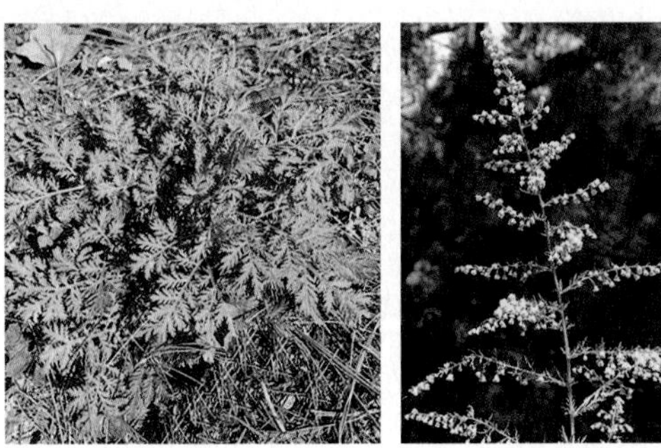

Artemisia annua Qing Hao (Sweet Annie herb), young plant showing it's fern-like leaves (*left*). Fragrant Sweet Annie herb showing its flowering top (*right*). It contains the sesquiterpene artemisinin. (Credit Mary Maruca.)

Artemisia annua Qing Hao, commonly called Annual Wormwood or Sweet Annie, is one of the most bitter plants known. It has been used in Chinese Medicine for more than a thousand years to treat low-grade fevers, skin diseases, parasites, fungus, bacteria, protozoa, and infections of all types, including malaria.

The World Health Organization endorses *A. annua* as a first-line treatment for drug-resistant malaria. Malaria is caused by *Plasmodium* parasites carried by the *Anopheles* mosquito. If bitten, the parasites invade human red blood cells, causing fever and, in severe cases, brain damage and death, especially in children. It is a huge problem in developing countries.

Sweet Annie contains artemisinin. This component, and its derivatives, are powerful medicines known for their ability to swiftly reduce the number of *Plasmodium* parasites in malaria patients. Artemisinin-based combination therapies (ACTs) are recommended for first-line treatment for uncomplicated *P. falciparum* malaria. Chemically, it releases "deadly free radicals once it enters the plasmodia."[4] In 2015 the Nobel Prize in Physiology was awarded to a Chinese woman, Tu Youyou, who revisited the ancient literature and discovered clues that guided her to successfully extract the active component from *A. annua*. Her discovery resulted in the drug artemisinin.

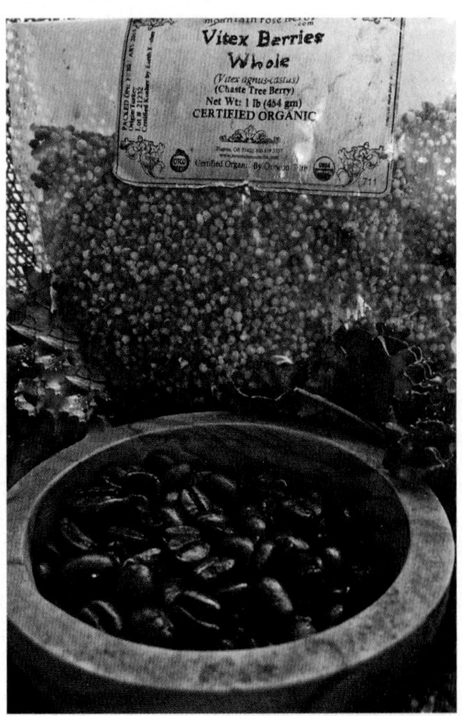

• **Fig. 10.3** Bitter Vitex berries, Coffee beans, and dark greens.

TABLE 10.3 Examples of Bitter

Herbs	Foods
Artemisia annua Qing Hao (Wormwood herb). Very strong.	Kale
Gentian spp. (Gentian root). Very strong.	Brussel Sprouts
Carduus benedictus (Blessed Thistle root).	Tomatillos
Anemopsis californica (Yerba Mansa root).	Water Cress
Arctium lappa Niu Bang Zi (Burdock seed) and *Cichorium intybus* (Chicory root). Mild.	Endive
Taraxacum officinalis Pu Gong Ying (Dandelion root and greens).	Coffee
Achillea millefolium (Yarrow herb).	Bitter Melon
Humulus lupulus (Hops flower).	Arugula
Vitex Agnus-Castus (Chaste Tree berry).	Broccoli

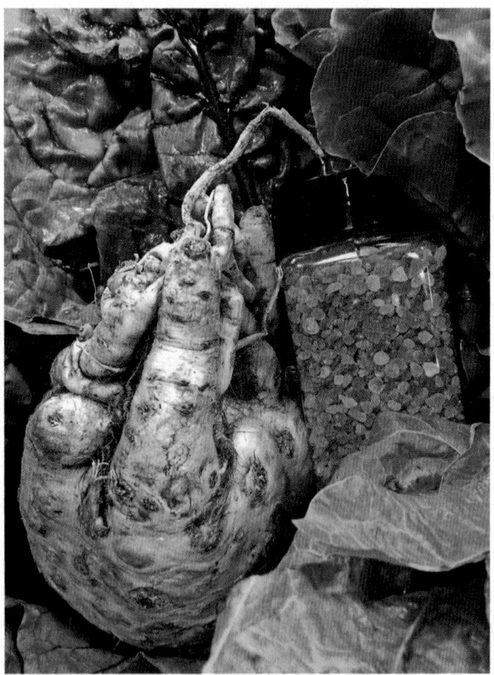

• **Fig. 10.4** Salty Swiss chard, Celery root, and pink Himalayan salt.

and Celery seed or root. They contain significant amounts of trace minerals or organic acids and have a salty taste.

In the Chinese correspondences, the salty taste is associated with the Kidneys and the Bladder. This association makes sense if you think about the organ's relationship with water. The kidney's physiological function is to balance out electrolytes in the blood.

TABLE 10.4 Examples of Salty

Herbs	Foods
Echinacea spp. (Purple Coneflower root)	Dark greens
Apium graveolens (Celery root)	Celery, Fennel
Portulaca oleracea Ma Chi Xian (Purslane herb)	Mineral and sea salt
Stellaria medica (Chickweed herb)	Dandelion greens
Chondrus crispus (Irish Moss thallus)	Lamb's Quarter
Fucus vesiculosus (Bladderwrack thallus)	Soy sauce, tamari, miso
Laminaria spp. (Kelp thallus)	Black olives
Urtica dioica (Nettle herb)	Lox, Gravlax

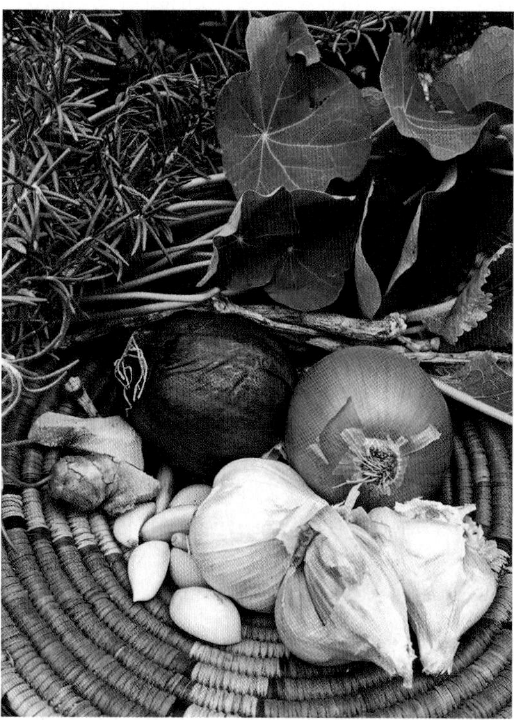

• **Fig. 10.5** Pungent onion, garlic, ginger, rosemary, nasturtium, and horseradish.

Chinese Medicine speaks of kidney essence, life force (*jing*) tonics with a salty taste. Examples here are animal products: deer antler, gecko, placenta, sea horse, turtle shell, tortoise shell, and mantis. The frequently used sour fruits of Cornus Shan Zhu Yu (Japanese Dogwood berry) and the adaptogen Schisandra Wu Wei Zi (Schisandra berry) also have a salty taste. They are used to nourish and astringe the essence.[1] Examples of salty herbs and foods are listed in Table 10.4.

Pungent (Acrid or Spicy)

- *Constituent:* Glycosides and essential oils, i.e., monoterpenes and sesquiterpenes.
- *Direction:* Pushes outward and disperses energy.
- *Actions:* Warming, stimulating, and relaxing.

The chemical constituents in pungent or acrid herbs are mainly glycosides and essential oils. Have you ever sniffed strong Tea Tree essential oil or put a Peppermint or Ginger Altoid candy on your tongue? These are pungent and very spicy. How about eating a bowl of hot chili or Japanese wasabi to open the sinuses? They can make your nose run. Essential oils are highly volatile, giving them a notable fragrance and a dispersing quality. They might feel warming and tingly. Other examples are Thyme, White Sage, and Lavender, which contain monoterpenes, and Chamomile, Ginger, and Turmeric, which contain sesquiterpenes.[2]

Pungent pushes outward. When energy pushes out to the extremities and the skin, it is not stuck or bound up inside the body. In the Chinese arena, energy or qi is supposed to flow easily and evenly throughout the 12 paired meridians, not too quickly and not too slowly. If qi becomes stopped up or blocked, pain results. So it makes perfect sense that an herb that pushes outward would relax and ease pain in the tissues, opening the qi. The Chinese refer to pungent herbs as those that regulate the qi and relieve pain. These pungent herbs tend to be warming and stimulating, like Juniper berry or Rosemary leaf (Fig. 10.5).

From a Western perspective, outward, dispersing energy increases and stimulates circulation. Healthy blood circulation removes toxins and brings nutrients into a sore muscle so that the muscle fibers can heal. It removes waste products produced from an inflammatory response, driving them out and away from an edematous injury and thereby relieving pressure and pain. Stimulating circulation enhances lymphatic flow. Lymph and blood circulation are connected and related. Improved lymphatic flow helps the body detoxify and enhances immunity.

Further, increased blood circulation causes the surface capillaries under the skin to dilate, resulting in sweating and warming of the hands and feet. Consequently, a pungent, acrid-tasting herb increases sweating (*diaphoretic*), becoming a major remedy for early-onset respiratory infections, such as colds and flu. Fresh Ginger root tea accomplishes this, as does a Mustard bath. Sweating removes toxins and cools down a fever. Some lovely immune soups include pungent Onion and Garlic for this reason. Try stimulating the airway with acrid, pungent herbs such as Eucalyptus or Peppermint herb, and feel the sinuses open, creating mucus flow from the lungs. If the sinuses are open and flowing, head pressure is relieved, headaches disappear, and you can relax. Pain causes stress; when pain is relieved, stress dissipates, and you can calm down.

According to the Chinese correspondences, the pungent taste relates to the Lungs (Chapter 9). This relationship exists because the body parts associated with the Chinese Lungs are the skin and sweat glands. Sweat glands are anatomically located in the skin and pungent diaphoretics that help us sweat are frequently used in treating early-onset respiratory infections. A caution using this type of remedy is that sweating can also lead to water loss and dryness. For this reason, a pungent tasting herb should not be used as a simple with someone who is already dry because it could make the dryness worse. Such a client might be dehydrated, elderly, or experiencing an already dry condition, such as eczema. In these cases, the formula should be balanced out with an appropriate

TABLE 10.5 **Examples of Pungent**

Herbs	Foods
Juniperus communis (Juniper berry)	Cinnamon, Clove
Rosmarinus officinalis (Rosemary leaf)	Garlic, Onions
Capsicum annuum (Cayenne fruit)	Chili Pepper
Menthe x piperita (Peppermint herb)	Horseradish
Eucalyptus spp. (Eucalyptus leaf)	Ginger
Melaleuca alternifolia (Tea Tree leaf and essential oil)	Mustard
Asarum canadense Xi Xin (Wild Ginger rhizome)	Black Pepper

cooling, moist herb, such as Marshmallow root, Comfrey root, Asparagus root, Chickweed herb, Iceland moss, or Slippery Elm bark. See Table 10.5 for pungent herbs and foods.

Description of Oily

In addition to the previously described tastes, sometimes the herbal literature mentions *bland* and ***oily***. I believe these are not really tastes but descriptions. They seldom appear in medicinal herbal plants or in foods.

- *Constituent*: Oils.
- *Action*: Slows things down, thickens, and moistens and is nutritive.

Oily is nutritive. It nourishes glands. Fats are needed for energy storage and hormone production. The human body uses fats to absorb and transport vitamins A, D, E, K, and carotenoids. Fat is the slowest burning but most energy-dense macronutrient, supplying nine calories per gram. In contrast, each gram of carbohydrate or protein yields only four calories of energy. As a result, fats represent the body's largest form of energy storage. It also forms the important lipid bilayer of cell membranes and is necessary for growth and development.

Fats move slowly. They are moistening to the skin. Very few herbs can be called fatty. Examples are Saw Palmetto berry, which is useful for underweight or depleted people; Heart of Palm; and Rehmannia Shu Di Huang (prepared Rehmannia root cooked in wine). Among the five tastes, sweet is the one closest to being oily. Fatty foods take a long time to digest, so they would not be recommended for weak digestion or overweight conditions.

However, some fats are necessary for good health. Examples are the *monounsaturated* fats in olives, almonds, peanuts, macadamias, hazelnuts, pecans, cashews, and avocados; the *polyunsaturated* fats in walnuts, sunflower, sesame and pumpkin seeds; and in cold-water marine fish, such as salmon, tuna, mackerel, herring, trout, and sardines (Chapter 8). These healthy fats are necessary for everyone in moderate amounts, and especially for individuals with weight problems.

Description of Bland

Bland is considered the absence of taste. The most important bland herbs are the medicinal mushrooms. Examples, such as Chinese Ganoderma Ling Zhi (Reishi mushroom) and Poria Fu Ling (Hoelen fungus), are described as bland with a slightly sweet taste. Other examples are Couch Grass root, Slippery Elm bark, Pearl Barley seed, and Water Plantain root. These foods and herbs are generally neutral, calming, and restorative.

Warmth: Hot to Cold

When we speak of the ***warmth*** of an herb, we are considering the entire spectrum of gradations from hot to warm, to neutral, to cool, and to cold.[5] Herbs are placed on this continuum for different reasons. Some herb books list temperature in their Materia Medicas; some don't. It is helpful to understand what is meant by this designation. Warmth may be described by the following criteria:

- *Topically*. Effect on the skin surface.
- *Environment*. Effect on the surroundings and air temperature.
- *Subjective taste*. A person's individual reaction to the plant.
- *Ability to alter subjective feelings of warmth*. Includes external and internal.

The quality of warmth or cold on the skin occurs locally as a topical application. Have you ever used Bengay? This common over-the-counter ointment is used as an analgesic rub for muscle and joint pain, sprains, and strains. A commercial preparation called Muscle Pain/Ultra Strength contains 30% methyl salicylate, 10% menthol, and 4% camphor. At first it makes the skin feel warm and tingly, followed by a cooling effect. Similar qualities are found in the Chinese liniment Tiger Balm.

Peppermint and Camphor are warming, and then cooling. Menthol is an organic compound found naturally in Peppermint. Camphor comes from the resin of the Camphor tree. They both initially warm us up and then cause sweating, which cools us down. They are ***counterirritants***. Counterirritants create reddening of the skin caused by vasodilation, raise body temperature, cause sweating, and produce a mild irritation to the skin that reduces hot inflammation deeper in the body.[6] The addition of methyl salicylate, the active ingredient in Aspirin, decreases pain.

We can also think of warmth in relation to the environment. In a hot country such as Mexico, hot herbs and spices like Chili pepper are routinely eaten to cool one down. Chilies and Cinnamon increase blood circulation to the skin surface, creating sweating and subsequent cooling. However, in cold countries, hot drinks may be used to warm one up. Some hot drinks have cold energetics, such as coffee, which in Chinese Medicine is considered to scatter qi.

Another way to consider temperature is from the subjective taste of an herb. Pungent tastes feel warm on the tongue. Think of warm cooking spices like Oregano herb, Rosemary leaf, or Thyme herb. When we swallow a pungent spice, we can feel the warmth as it travels down to the stomach. Choosing Ginger tea on a cold winter's day is warming. Conversely, a cucumber or watermelon eaten in the heat of summer is cooling. Salads are cooling. Spicy turkey stuffing with Sage and Pepper is warming.

We can further consider the hot-to-cold continuum based on a person's condition or what is happening inside. When out of balance, heat leads to irritability, fever, and inflammatory conditions. By its nature, heat rises, appearing as a red face and eyes, sore throat, or dizziness. In Chinese Medicine, if heat affects Heart or Liver, anger may result. Excess heat dries out body fluids. Excess cold can create copious fluids: frequent urination, too much mucus, slow pulse, and pale face. In general, warm conditions are treated with cooling herbs, and cold conditions are treated with warming herbs. It makes sense. Herbs that give energy and strength and activate circulation are warming. Herbs that make us sweat, urinate, or feel calm are cooling (Table 10.6).

TABLE 10.6 Ranges of Warmth

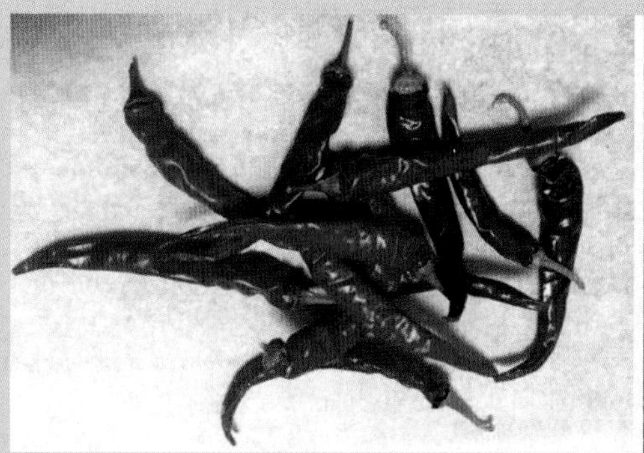
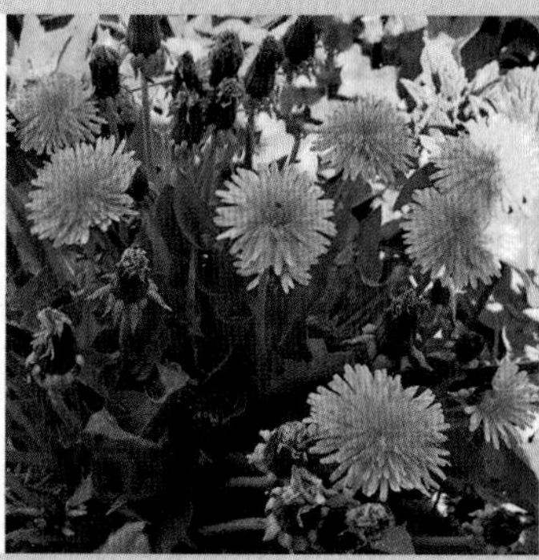

Hot Cayenne pepper and cold Dandelion leaf and root.

Quality	Taste	Warmth	Foods	Herbs
	Pungent	**HOT**	**Spices** Cinnamon Ginger	Cayenne pepper
Stimulants	Pungent		Pepper, Clove, Horseradish, Garlic	Snake root
	Pungent	**WARM**	**Cooking Herbs** Fennel Rosemary Thyme Basil Tarragon Oregano Marjoram	Calamus root Valerian root Osha root
Restoratives	Sweet, Bland, Oily, or Sour	**NEUTRAL**	**Grains** Millet, Barley, Buckwheat	Yarrow herb Lemon sorrel leaf Tamarind fruit
Relaxants	Sweet or Bland		Rice, Wheat	Slippery Elm bark
Sedatives	Sweet Bitter Astringent Salty	**COOL**	**Wild Greens** *(Spring blood cleansers)* Borage Chickweed Dandelion Cucumber Docks	Chickweed herb Nettle leaf Mullein leaf
Sedatives	Bitter	**COLD** (Absence of warmth)		**Medium/Strong** Goldenseal root Goldthread root Isatis root
	Bitter	**VERY COLD** (Nerve Death)		**Poison** Water Hemlock plant Henbane plant Yellow Jasmine plant

Based on class notes from Peter Holmes, L.Ac., M.H.

Moisture: Wet to Dry

In the human body, the degree of moisture or dryness affects the tissues and our health. We contain about 60% water. How many times have you been told to drink more water? Water is held in the body in two main compartments: our intracellular fluids (ICF) within the cell and extracellular fluids (ECF) in fluid compartments outside the cells. The balance of ICF to ECF is very important in physiology. Normally, the kidneys do a brilliant and miraculous job of balancing fluids. When dehydrated, water is retained, urine becomes concentrated and dark, and there is thirst. As we hydrate, our urine becomes lighter and less concentrated, and there is less thirst. Lymphatic circulation, which begins at the capillary level, brings excess ECF back to the heart for recycling.

It is easy to get out of fluid balance. The external environment, weather, and humidity take its toll. We experience dry skin in the low humidity of Colorado or moist dewy skin in wet, humid New Jersey. Stress can make us dry. Infections, such as a flu virus, can make the mucous membranes secrete more than their share. The inflammatory cascade brings fluids to places of injury, causing painful ECF swelling as the blood receives toxins it must remove and replace with nutrients. Dryness can make us constipated. Damp can cause diarrhea. Menopause and aging cause drying when mucous membranes have fewer secretions. Infection with fluid build-up makes us damp. Intestinal permeability causes dampness in the gut, which is called *Spleen damp*.

Fortunately, we have an arsenal of herbs in various categories to regulate damp and dry conditions. For *drier-uppers* in the astringent or cell-tightening category, there are *anhidrotics*, like Garden Sage, which stop excess sweating; there are antidiarrheals like Oak bark for loose stools; stiptics like Cranesbill Geranium herb for excess bleeding; there are *mucostatics* like Goldenrod herb to dry respiratory secretions. *Diuretics* like Dandelion root and leaf help with edema by stimulating urination.

In the *moistening* category for dry conditions, an array of *demulcents* are sweet, moist, and nutritive. The classic Western moisturizer for all organ systems is Marshmallow root. There is also Iceland moss thallus or Slippery Elm bark for the respiratory and gastrointestinal tract, Chickweed herb for reproductive dryness, or Comfrey root for wounds and wound healing.

If something is damp or wet, it gets soaked. If something is soaked, it gets heavy and bogged down and can take a long time to dry out. In Chinese Medicine, this dampness leads to a blockage called *stagnation*. Signs of dampness in the body are phlegm, edema, bloating, and discharges. Skin can ooze or crust, as in eczema. A person feels heavy and may become dizzy. As things become heavy, gravity pulls downward. If damp combines with heat, there is damp heat, indicated by dark, burning urine; thick, foul-smelling stools; yellow vaginal discharges; or jaundice. These symptoms occur in the lower part of the body. Causes can be cold, uncooked or greasy foods, and large amounts of dairy and ice cream, which can cause excess mucus.

If damp combines with cold, there is damp cold. In damp cold, we see pale, scanty urine; hard constipation with mucus; and clear discharges. Damp can also combine with external forces from outside the body, such as *wind*. If wind and damp affect the joints, there is wind damp joint pain, as in arthritis affected by barometric pressure. If wind and damp affect the respiratory system, there could be wind damp cold or even wind damp heat, as in a common cold.

One remedy for damp conditions in Chinese Medicine is to use *bitter*-tasting foods which have a draining property. Leafy green vegetables like kale, mustard greens, dandelion greens, parsley, and celery are good examples of bitter foods that drain damp. Citrus peels are bitter, so if they are added to meat dishes, they can help reduce dampness. Turnips, radish, kohlrabi, asparagus, and broccoli do this also. The Chinese also use pungent, stimulating, and aromatic herbs and diuretics, a favorite being the fungus Poria Fu Ling (Hoelen fungus), to dry up damp.

The Six Secondary Energetic Qualities: Stimulate-Sedate, Restore-Relax, Moisten-Decongest

The six ***Secondary Qualities*** give the key to choosing herbs to treat basic conditions or problems in the body. This group gives a specific clue as to which remedy to use. Herbs with these secondary herbal qualities are used to treat a person having the *opposite* condition.

- *Stimulating herbs*. Stimulants are warm and therefore treat cold conditions.
- *Sedating or cooling herbs*. Sedatives are cold and therefore treat hot conditions.
- *Restoring herbs*. Restoratives or *tonics* build up and therefore treat weak conditions.
- *Relaxing herbs*. Relaxants calm the nervous system and therefore treat tense conditions.
- *Moistening herbs*. Demulcents are wet and therefore treat dry conditions.
- *Decongesting herbs*. Decongestants break things up and therefore treat damp, thickened conditions.[6]

Energetics of Stimulating: Dispersing, Circulating

To ***stimulate or disperse*** in herbalism means to create movement in the body because of cold conditions. As things become cold, they slow down, causing stagnation and lack of flow. We need to move things along. If blood needs moving, we would use arterial *stimulants*. If lymphatic fluid were sluggish, we would use lymph *circulators*. A person might feel sleepy or sluggish because of deficient qi and so would require nerve *stimulation*. An organ might slow down, becoming sluggish and deficient, as can occur when the liver's detoxification processes need a boost, so liver *stimulants* would be used. The small intestine might require digestive enzyme *stimulation*. A muscle could slow down, be in spasm, and need a relaxant to *disperse* the tightness. A cough might be unproductive, requiring a *stimulating* decongestant. All of these examples require stimulating herbs.

Stimulants are warm and pungent. They have an outward energy. They loosen what is stuck, creating movement. The result is a warming effect as they relax, invigorate, and loosen what was sluggish and tight.[7] From the Chinese Medicine standpoint, to stimulate is to tonify yang: warm the interior, transform damp, drain damp, and restore the Liver and Kidney.[5]

Example: Signs and symptoms of a person who needs blood stimulated because of a cold condition: has cold hands and feet, displays inactivity, and has low metabolism; feels cold all the time; and prefers summer and warm clothes. Such a client may like warm foods but might be addicted to cold foods and possibly shows signs of depression. **Pulse (P)** Slow, tight, and deep. **Tongue (T)** Pale and white coat, possibly excessively moist.

Herbs: Warm, pungent arterial circulators to warm and increase blood flow, such as: Prickly Ash bark, Western Angelica root, or Chinese Angelica Dang Gui (Dong Quai root), Ginger root, Rosemary leaf, Juniper berry, Cayenne pepper, Garlic bulb, and Horsetail herb.

Example: Signs and symptoms of person who needs nerves stimulated because of a cold condition: numbness and tingling in the extremities, sleepiness, sluggishness, inability to focus, dizziness, or fainting episodes. **P** Weak, deep, and slow. **T** Pale.

Herbs: Warm nerve stimulators in moderation, such as: caffeine-containing Chinese Ephedra Ma Huang (Ephedra stem), coffee, chocolate, black tea, green tea, and non-caffeinated Rosemary leaf, Prickly Ash bark, Black Peppercorn, Cardamom pod, or Camphor resin.

Energetics of Sedating: Reduce Infection, Heat, or Hyperactivity

To ***sedate*** means to treat excessively hot conditions or hyperactivity. We want to reduce heat in the body and slow things down. We could cool down a very hot infection or calm a hyperactive person. For these purposes, we use cool or cold herbs. Please don't get the quality of *sedating* mixed up with the quality of *relaxing*. In allopathic medicine, sedatives calm down the nervous system, but not here. Herbs that sedate are always cooling or cold. *Relaxants* treat tense conditions of the nervous system and can be either warming or cooling.

In Chinese Medicine, hot conditions are considered excess yang. Sedative herbs clear heat, damp heat, and toxic heat, and they calm the spirit.[5]

Example: Excess yang or heat. Signs and symptoms of people with heat or hyperactivity of the blood: fever, infection, inflammation, red face, anger, dislike of summer, preference for or addiction to hot, spicy foods. **P** Fast. **T** Red.

Herbs: Those that reduce heat are numerous. We use cooling, bitter ones, such as Goldenseal root, Barberry bark, Wild Indigo root, Dandelion root, Gentian root, or Coptis Huang Lian (Goldthread root).

Example: Hyperactivity of nerves. Signs and symptoms of person with hyperactivity: excited, wired, hyperactive, insomnia, ringing in the ears (tinnitus), spasms, unexplained aches, cramps, and smooth muscle spasms of GI or bladder. **T** Varied. **P** Full, wiry.

Herbs: Those that cool and sedate the nervous system are many: Hops flower, Passionflower herb, California Poppy herb, Jamaican Dogwood root, Wild Lettuce leaf, essential oils of Chamomile, Lavender, or Clary Sage are a few examples.

Energetics of Restoring: Tonifying, Nourishing, Building

Restoratives are sweet. They build tissue bulk, nourish, strengthen, and treat weak conditions. This concept is paramount in all herbal medicine traditions. It sustains health and preserves life. All other therapies are dependent on this. Restoratives can treat cells in general, or they can be directed to specific organs for nutritional deficiencies.

The physio-medicalists, like William Cooke, called the nutritive remedies ***trophorestoratives***, which are superlative remedies with an affinity for particular organs and tissues and targets them specifically. Burdock root and Horsetail herb have a tropism to the skin. The liver attracts Dandelion root and Milk Thistle seed. The nervous system leans toward Schisandra Wu Wei Zi (Five Taste berry) or Milky Oat berry. Kidneys go for Goldenrod or Parsley herb. The heart likes Hawthorn berry. Trophorestoratives help the body function and increase metabolism, absorption, and the body's resistance to organisms. They help one overcome conditions that are weakening, such as anemia, chronic illness, malnutrition, dehydration, and fatigue.

Western herbalism claims countless restorative herbs (Tables 10.7 and 10.8). Some of these are general *superfoods* that nourish the entire body rather than having a particular tropism, such as Blue Green algae or Bee Pollen.

In Chinese Medicine, these restoratives are known as *tonics* that treat deficient conditions. One can augment or *tonify* the qi, nourish the blood, and enrich yin or yang.[5] They tend to be warming and nourishing. They can be used over long periods of time, and rather than treat an illness, they strengthen the body to keep us healthy. They are known as the imperial herbs, revered over the centuries and highly valued.

Example: Deficiency signs and symptoms of a person who could benefit from tonics or restoratives: generalized weakness, fatigue, decreased resistance to stress or infection, hypofunction of any organ or physiological process. **P** Weak or thin. **T** Coat pale or absent. Body: thin, flabby, or scalloped; red and cracked in yin deficiency; pale in qi or blood deficiency.

Herbs. Choose an appropriate qi, blood, yin or yang tonic or combination (Tables 10.7 and 10.9).

Qi tonics are energy tonics that increase physiological energy production, but they are not stimulants. Qi tonics help the body function optimally, increase vitality, help nutrient absorption, and oxygenate through the lungs. Energy in the form of oxygen then circulates through the meridian system, providing the basic energy needed to live well.[7]

Blood tonics nourish the blood, so the blood can bring nutrients to the cells. They help with anemia, particularly in menstruating women who lose blood monthly. Some blood tonics increase circulation.

Yin tonics nourish fluids and soft tissues, keeping them moist. Moisture is associated with the Chinese Kidney, and yin tonics are related to jing (essence), the energy stored in the Kidney. These tonics are important antiaging and longevity herbs, especially for women in menopause who need more moisture.

Yang tonics provide power and energy. They use the stored *yin* energy of the Chinese Kidneys and employ it to build will power and creativity, stimulate metabolism, and strengthen muscles and bones of the back, knees, and joints. Yang tonics are used by athletes. Some yang tonics are aphrodisiacs, and energetically they are considered warm or hot.

Energetics of Relaxing: Relax Nervous System, Circulate Qi or Blood

Relaxants treat tense, restrained conditions in the body. Herbs that are *spasmolytics, anticonvulsants*, and muscle relaxants all have a relaxing action. Tense can manifest as pain caused by tight skeletal muscles, high blood pressure caused by smooth muscle constriction in arterial linings, menstrual cramps caused by smooth muscle constriction of the uterine linings, coughing caused by spasms of the bronchi, stomach aches from smooth muscle constriction of the gut, a tension headache from constricted blood flow to the head, or seizures. A person could be tense from stress, anxiety, fear, or worry, which could cause insomnia.

In the Chinese sense, by relaxing, we circulate the qi, subdue Liver yang, release the exterior, and extinguish internal wind.[5] We

TABLE 10.7 Restoratives for Body Systems

Nervous	Heart and Blood Vessels	Kidney	Lungs	Reproductive	Muscular-Skeletal	Skin
Rosmarinus officinalis Rosemary leaf	*Crataegus oxyacantha* Hawthorn berry	*Triticum repens* Couch grass	*Avena sativa* Oat straw and berry	*Avena sativa* Oat straw and berry	*Symphytum officinale* Comfrey Leaf and root For bone.	*Juglans regia* Hu Tao Ren Walnut leaf and hull
Avena sativa Oat straw and berry	*Cereus grandiflorus* Night Blooming Cactus	*Zea mays* Yu Mi Xu Cornsilk	*Equisetum arvense* Horsetail herb	*Serenoa serrulata* Saw Palmetto berry	*Equisetum arvense* Horsetail herb For bone and connective tissue.	*Equisetum arvense* Horsetail herb
Panax spp. Ginseng root	*Santalum album* Sandalwood essential oil	*Asparagus officinalis* Asparagus root	*Cordyceps sinensis* Dong Chong Chinese Caterpillar mushroom	*Rubus idaeus* Raspberry leaf	*Acorus calamus* Calamus root For bone.	*Avena sativa* Oat straw and berry
Pollen Flower pollen	*Citrus vulgaris* Neroli essential oil	*Taraxacum officinale* Dandelion root	*Verbascum thapsus* Mullein leaf	*Fragaria vesca* Strawberry leaf	*Avena sativa* Oat straw and berry For bone and connective tissue.	*Astragalus membranaceus* Huang Qi Astragalus root
Spirulina spp. Microalgae	*Rosmarinus officinalis* Rosemary herb	*Foeniculum vulgare* Fennel seed	*Ophiopogon japonicus* Mai Men Dong Dwarf Lilyturf root	*Rubus fruticosus* Blackberry leaf	*Eucommia ulmoides* Du Zhong Ye Eucommia bark For connective tissue.	Symphytum officinale Comfrey root and leaf
Sesamum indicum Sesame seeds	*Panax quinquefolius* Xi Yang Shen American ginseng root	*Equisetum arvense* Horsetail herb	*Ulmus fulva* Slippery Elm bark	*Angelica sinensis* Dang Gui Chinese angelica root, Dong Quai	*Juglans regia* Walnut hull and leaf For muscles, bones, mineral deficiencies.	*Calendula officinalis* Marigold flower

This table based on information from Institute for Traditional Medicine. (http://www.itmonline.org/articles/taste_action/taste_action_herbs.htm. Accessed October 10. 2019.)

treat excess conditions characterized by hyper-functioning and tension.

Example: Signs or symptoms of a tense condition: tension headaches or migraines; muscle spasms; pain; rough, dry skin; nervousness; agitation; sweating; dribbling; sleep disorders; or hypertension. **P** Wiry and tight. **T** Possible red tip; longitudinal lines.

Herbs: Lily of the Valley herb for the heart; Catnip herb for the stomach; Wild Cherry bark for the lungs.

From the Western perspective, we might use the category of pungent spasmolytics to stop a cough or bronchodilators to relax the respiratory tree in a cough. A general Western classification, *relaxing* ***nervines*** refer to herbs that relax the nervous system. These herbs could be hot or cold in quality. If one were picking a good relaxing nervine, it would be best to choose a cooling one for a hot condition and vice versa. In general, nervines are a broad class of herbs that affect the nervous system in many ways: relaxing it, cooling it down, warming it up, strengthening, and harmonizing (Table 10.10).

Energetics of Moistening: Soothing, Tonify Yin

In Western herbalism, herbs that moisturize and create wetness and lubrication treat dry conditions. They are known as ***demulcents***; they taste sweet or bland; their warmth is neutral to cooling; and they are harmonizing, soothing, and antiinflammatory.[5] A urinary tract infection is usually accompanied by pain on urination (dysuria). The formula would include a demulcent to relieve redness and burning, such as Marshmallow root or Slippery Elm bark. A dry cough makes the throat raw, dry, and sore. That cough formula needs herbs such as Comfrey root, Iceland Moss thallus, or Licorice root, all specific to relieving lung dryness and moistening the mucosa. For irritable bowel disease and inflammatory bowel diseases such as ulcerative colitis and Crohn's disease, a GI demulcent would be in order. General considerations for demulcent usage are:

- *Demulcents do not combine well with astringents high in tannins*. If you think about this, it makes sense. They work at odds with each other: one moistening, and the other tightening and drying up.
- *Demulcents are not usually used on their own in simples*. When used topically in a salve for immediate symptom relief, they are combined with other remedies to address specific imbalances. If dryness accompanies a hot, infectious sore throat, one would combine with an antiinfective or sedating herb that treats hot conditions. If a client had dry hard stools, we would use something for constipation and a moistener.

Often, demulcents are nourishing (or nutritive) and moistening. *Nutritive demulcents* promote secretion of fluids, moisten and nourish mucus membranes, and reduce low-level inflammation and fever. Iceland Moss and Irish Moss thallus nourish the lungs and gut and help heal damaged tissue. Licorice root restores the

TABLE 10.8 **Restoratives for Specific Tissues**

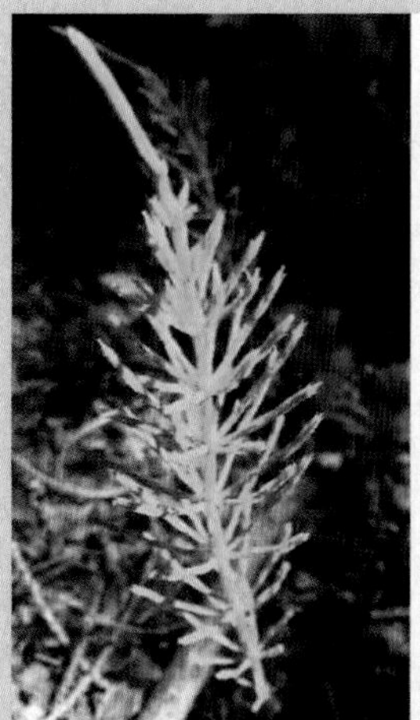
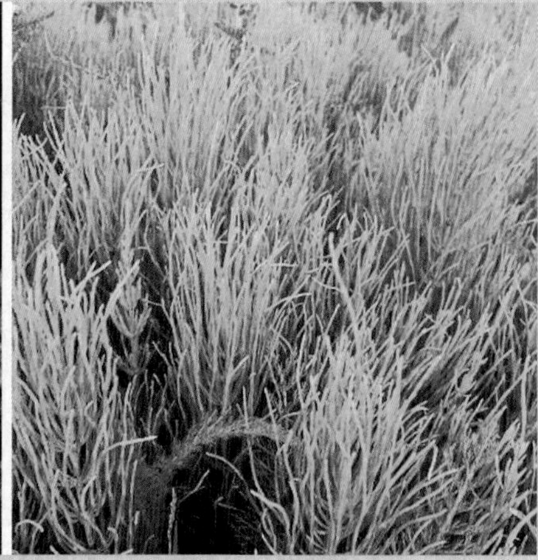

Horsetail sprouting (sterile) and habit. *Equisetum arvense* is a trophrorestorative to the bones, skin, lungs, and kidneys.

Pituitary Gland	Thyroid Gland	Adrenal Gland	Liver	Blood	Connective Tissue
Panax quinquefolius Xi Yang Shen American ginseng root	*Laminaria* spp. Kelp seaweed	*Glycyrrhiza glabra* Licorice root	*Cynara scolymus* Artichoke leaf	*Rosmarinus officinalis* Rosemary leaf	*Equisetum arvense* Horsetail herb
Panax ginseng Ren Shen Asian ginseng root	*Fucus vesiculosus* Bladderwrack seaweed	*Panax quinquefolius* Xi Yang Shen American ginseng root	*Silybum marianum* Milk Thistle seed	*Medicago sativa* Alfalfa herb	*Eucommia ulmoides* Du Zhong Ye Eucommia bark
Eleutherococcus senticosus Ci Wu Jia Siberian ginseng root	Other seaweeds	*Panax ginseng* Ren Shen Asian ginseng root	*Taraxacum officinale* Dandelion root	*Urtica dioica* Nettle herb	*Urtica dioica* Nettle herb
Avena sativa Oat straw and berry	*Withania somnifera* Ashwagandha root	*Urtica dioica* Nettle herb	*Lycium chinense* Gou Qi Zi Wolfberry/Goji berry	*Angelica sinensis* Dang Gui Dong Quai root	*Symphytum officinalis* Comfrey root
Serenoa serrulata Saw Palmetto berry	*Eleutherococcus senticosus* Ci Wu Jia Siberian ginseng root	*Withania somnifera* Ashwagandha root	*Ziziphus jujuba* Da Zao and Hong Zao Black and Red dates	*Trifolium pratense* Red Clover flower	*Juglans regia* Walnut hull and leaf

mucosal lining of the intestines and restores respiratory tract lining. Comfrey root and leaf restores lung tissue and is famous for wound repair, frequently found in first-aid creams.

In Chinese Medicine, moisturizing, demulcent herbs are said to tonify the yin and relieve dryness. The body's fluids and moisture are part of the yin, so dry conditions are considered a yin deficiency. Demulcent lubricating herbs are used, such as Prunus Xing Ren (Apricot seed) or Perilla Zi Su Zi (Perilla seed) for the lungs, or Flax seed and Psyllium seed for the intestines. Western herbs that nourish the yin and moisten dryness are found chiefly in the Plantain family (Plantaginaceae), the Mallow family (Malvaceae), and the Grass family (Poaceae).

Example: Signs and symptoms of person with dryness who needs moistening: dry skin; dry stools; thick, sticky mucus and mucous membranes; concentrated urine; vaginal dryness; and thirst. **T** Dry, sticky, parched. **P** Tight, thin, and possibly wiry.

Herbs: Choose moistening herbs from Table 10.11.

Energetics of Decongesting: Breaking Up, Removing Stagnation

Decongestants break things up; therefore, they treat damp conditions where excessive fluid has built up in the body. Taste-wise, they tend to be pungent, bitter, or bland.[5] Damp (either damp heat or damp cold) is resolved by using herbs that decongest wherever excess fluid has accumulated. This fluid can be in the form of blood and lymph, mucus, or discharges occurring in many body systems. It can occur in any system where mucous membranes exist: respiratory, gastrointestinal, urinary, or reproductive. In general, decongestants cover a range of herbal actions and cover an array of phytochemicals.

Astringent mucus decongestants work on loosening and diminishing lung or GI secretions, like Goldenrod herb, Thyme herb, and Sage leaf. Some are nonastringent plants high in essential oil glycosides, like Cayenne fruit and Yerba Mansa herb. Others are herbs with high polysaccharide content, such as Iceland Moss

TABLE 10.9 Examples of Chinese Tonics

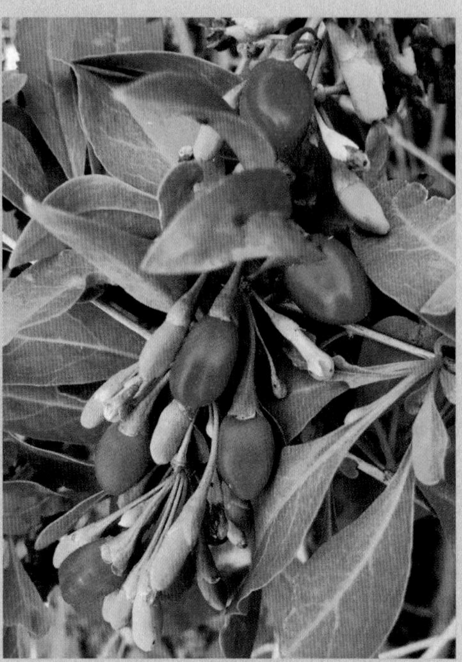

Lycium chinense Gou Qi Zi (Goji or Wolfberry) is an antioxidant blood and yin tonic.

Qi Tonics	Blood Tonics	Yang Tonics	Yin Tonics
Astragalus membranaceus Huang Qi Astragalus root	*Equus asinus* E Jiao Ass hide glue/gelatin	*Astragalus chinensis* Sha Yuan Zi Astragalus seed	*Anemarrhena asphodeloides* Zhi Mu Know Mother root
Dioscorea opposita Shan Yao Chinese Yam	*Euphoria longan* Long Yan Rou Longan berry	*Cervus nippon* Lu Jiao Mature Deer Antler gelatin	*Dendrobium nobile* Shi Hu Stonebushel stem
Codonopsis pilosula Dang Shen Downy bellflower root	*Lycium chinense* Gou Qi Zi Wolfberry, Goji berry	*Cordyceps sinensis* Dong Chong Xia Cao Chinese caterpillar mushroom	*Sesamum indicum* Hei Zhi Ma Black Sesame seed
Ginseng spp American and Asian ginseng root	*Rehmannia glutinosa* Shu Di Huang Prepared Rehmannia root	*Cynomorium songaricum* Suo Yang Lock Yang stem	*Ophiopogon japonicus* Mai Men Dong Ophiopogon root
Glycyrrhiza uralensis Gan Cao Licorice root	*Paeonia lactiflora* Bai Shao Yao White Peony root	*Juglans regia* Hu Tao Ren Walnuts	*Lilium brownii* Bai He Lily bulb
Oryza sativa Gu Ya Rice sprout	*Angelica sinensis* Dang Qui Dong Quai root	*Eucommia ulmoides* Du Zhong Eucommia bark	*Rehmannia glutinosa* Sheng Di Huang Raw, uncooked root
Polygonatum sibiricum Huang Jing Siberian Solomon's Seal root	*Ziziphus jujuba* Hong Zao Red Dates	*Panax ginseng* Ren Shen Asian ginseng root	*Polygonatum odoratum* Yu Zhu Fragrant Solomon's Seal root
Ziziphus jujuba Da Zao Black Dates	*Polygonum multiflorum* He Shu Wu Flowery Knotweed root	**Foods**: Wheat germ, mustard greens, radish, scallions, turnips, leeks, watercress.	**Foods**: Tofu, zucchini, millet, coconut milk, watermelon, string beans.

This chart based on "Taste and Action of Chinese Herbs" by Subhuti Dharmananda, Ph.D. Institute of Traditional Medicine. (http://www.itmonline.org/articles/taste_action/taste_action_herbs.htm.)

TABLE 10.10 **Relaxants per Body System**

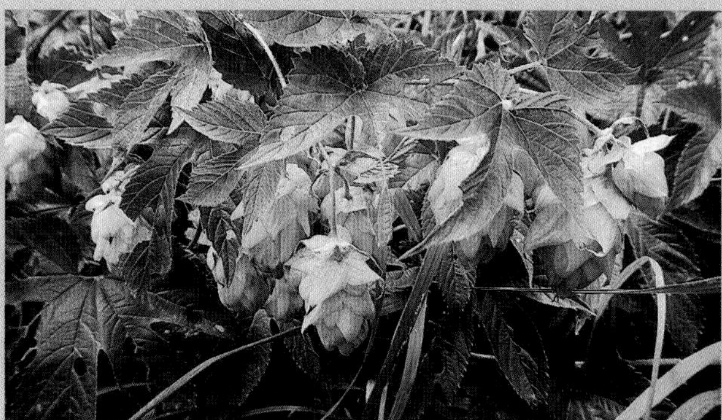

Humulus lupulus (Hops strobile/flower) is bitter, cold, and pungent, a general multi-purpose relaxant.

General	Lung	Heart	Urinary	Gastrointestinal
Lobelia inflata Lobelia herb Major all-system relaxant.	*Verbascum thapsus* Mullein flower and leaf	*Crataegus* spp. Hawthorn berry	*Piper methysticum* Kava root	*Nepeta cataria* Catnip herb
Matricaria recutita Chamomile flower Gentle.	*Prunus serotina* Wild Cherry bark	*Carthamus* Hong Hua Safflower	*Daucus carota* Wild Carrot seed	*Mentha x piperita* Peppermint herb
Humulus lupulus Hops strobile/flower	*Grindelia robusta* Gumweed flower	*Ligusticum* Chuan Xiong Sichuan Lovage root	*Hydrangea arborescens* Hydrangea root	*Viburnum opulus* Cramp bark
Lavandula angustifolia Lavender flower	*Pimpinella anisum* Aniseed	*Scutellaria lateriflora* Skullcap herb	*Petroselinum crispum* Parsley seed	*Humulus lupulus* Hops strobile/flower
Scutellaria lateriflora Skullcap herb	*Actaea racemosa* Black Cohosh root	*Melissa officinalis* Lemon balm leaf	*Hypericum perforatum* St. John's Wort	*Dioscorea villosa* Wild Yam root

thallus or Lungwort lichen. *Circulatory stimulants* move blood away from the affected area, as in Prickly Ash bark or Tangerine peel. *Intestinal mucus* overproduction might occur in the stool, in abdominal distention, and in indigestion, possibly from enteritis, irritable bowel, colitis, ulcers, or the yeast infection *Candida albicans*.

Respiratory decongestants are used when mucus is seen in the respiratory tree and sinuses, as a result of inflammation and irritation from an infection or allergy, excess dairy consumption, drugs, stress, chronic illness, chronic bronchitis, emphysema, and dysbiosis. The membranes lose normal tone and oversecrete sputum. In the old days it was called *catarrh*. Westerners call the condition *congestion*, and Chinese Medicine calls it *phlegm damp*.

Example: Chinese Medicine signs and symptoms of phlegm damp include increased mucus in stools or urine, sinus congestion, chronic sore throat or bronchitis, irregular stools, rheumatoid arthritis, pelvic inflammatory disease, *Candida albicans* yeast, and other vaginal infections. **T** Teeth marks, thick greasy with oily coat. **P** Slippery and/or floating.

Herbs: Primary herbs as suggested earlier in this section, plus various decongestants.

Excess *mucus in the urine or reproductive system* could be from urinary tract infection, vaginal infections, and discharges. In these cases, primary herbs would be used to resolve the cause/root of the problem, such as antimicrobials or gut restoratives. Decongestants, diuretics, astringents, and lymphatic circulators would be added as secondary herbs to dry damp and heal and tighten tissue. An herb of particular interest is *Ceanothus* spp. (Red Root). It is a cooling astringent filled with alkaloids and acids that clears damp heat by tightening veins, capillaries, and lymphatics, particularly in the uterus and liver.[4] By this action, lymph is moved (decongested) and returned to blood circulation, so excess dampness can be ultimately eliminated through the kidneys. In the same manner, Red Root can reduce nonfibrous ovarian and breast cysts by clearing lymphatic stagnation. It takes work to wildcraft, as evidenced in Table 10.12.

Blood decongestants are used when blood pools in the lower extremities, slows down, and eventually clots, causing varicose veins or deep vein thrombosis (phlebitis) in the legs or in the rectal area causing hemorrhoids. Blood can also pool in the pelvic basin from deficient venous flow or decreased lymph circulation, causing cramps. Blood decongestants are generally astringent, cool, and dry. They contain many tissue-tightening tannins, organic acids, and flavonoids and work in three ways:

TABLE 10.11 Some Moistening Herbs with Different Tropisms

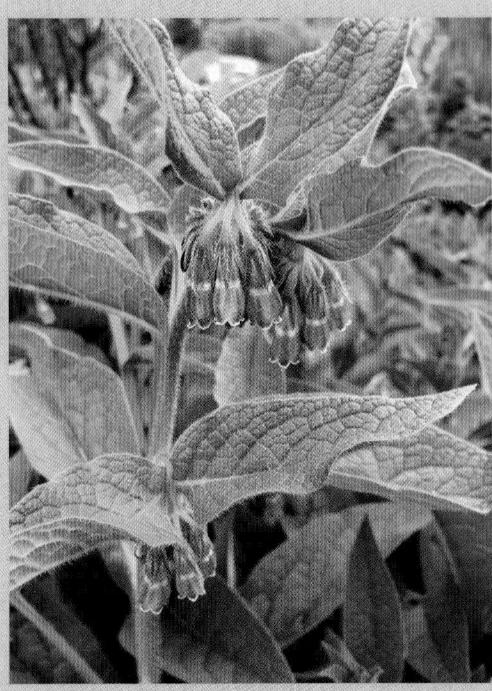

Comfrey flower and leaf. *Symphytum officinale* is cool, moist and healing to the skin, bones, gut, and lungs. A yin tonic.

General	Topical	Lungs	Gut	Urinary
Symphytum officinale Comfrey root and leaf	*Symphytum officinale* Comfrey root and leaf	*Cetraria islandica* Iceland moss thallus	*Ulmus fulva* Slippery Elm bark	*Cetraria islandica* Iceland moss
Stellaria media Chickweed herb	*Aloe* spp. Gel	*Chondrus crispus* Irish Moss thallus	*Cetraria islandica* Iceland moss	*Chondrus crispus* Irish moss thallus
Polygonatum multiflorum He Shou Wu Solomon's Seal rhizome	Honey	*Pulmonaria officinalis* Lungwort lichen	*Althea officinalis* Marshmallow root	*Althea officinalis* Marshmallow root
Althaea officinalis Marshmallow root	*Calendula officinalis* Marigold flower	*Ulmus fulva* Slippery Elm bark	*Glycyrrhiza glabra* Licorice root	*Zea mays* Yu Mi Xu Cornsilk
Ulmus fulva Slippery Elm bark	*Verbascum thapsus* Mullein leaf	*Glycyrrhiza glabra* Gan Cao Licorice root	*Symphytum officinale* Comfrey root	*Plantago major* Plantain seed

- *By tightening dilated vessels.* The astringency tones capillaries and veins.
- *By increasing venous circulation.* This shunts the blood away from the stagnated area, encouraging return into systemic circulation.
- *By strengthening smooth muscle tone.* Smooth muscles line the veins. Herbs that tone (tighten) those muscles contain antioxidant bioflavonoids; examples are Bilberry fruit or Green Tea leaf.

Blood decongestants are called for when blood pools in the extremely vascular uterus, resulting in dysmenorrhea or menstrual pain. Bleeding increases, but if it moves slowly enough, clots form (stagnation). If the situation continues, there is danger of fibroid tumors, endometriosis, and pelvic inflammatory disease (Chapter 28). There are five herbal approaches in cases of menstrual pain that cover many of the herbal categories we have been discussing (Box 10.4).

Note: If blood were to become very thick or stagnate to the point of a clot, anticoagulant herbs would be required. Melilot herb, Cleavers herb, Ginger root, and Ligusticum Chuan Xiong (Sichuan Lovage root) are all anticoagulants, but none are decongestants.

Example: Stagnation. Signs and symptoms of those needing decongestants: Clots, thrombus, excess mucus, discharges, menstrual cramps. **P** Tense or erratic. **T** Purplish body indicates blood stagnation.

Herbs: Pick appropriately from the previous paragraphs in this section and Table 10.12.

TABLE 10.12 Herbs for Damp Congested Conditions

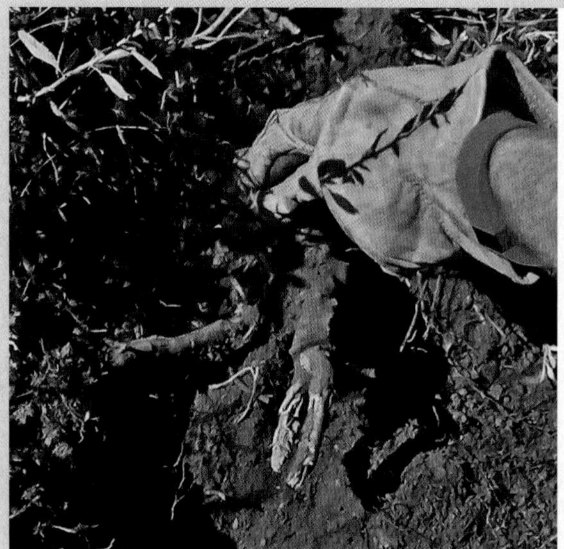

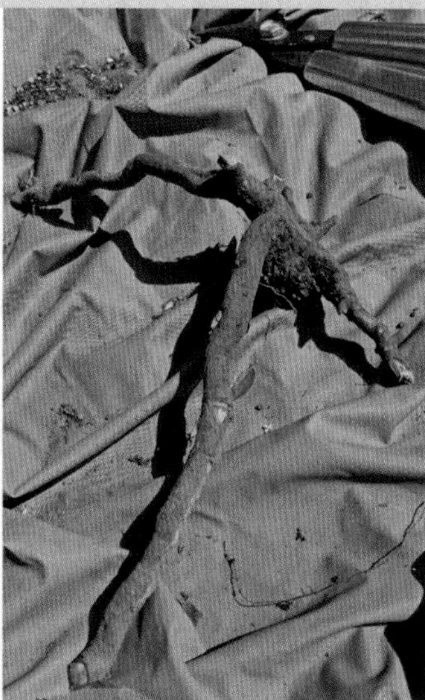

Ceanothus spp. (Red Root), freshly dug, must be split and cut up with pruners in the field. Known as a lymph gland drainer, it is cooling and astringent, a fine uterine and venous decongestant for menstrual cramps and varicose veins, respectively.

Blood (Uterine decongestants)	**Venous Decongestants** (Lower body)	**Phlegm Damp** (Lungs)	**Diuretics** (Urinary and general usage)
Alchemilla vulgaris Lady's Mantle herb	*Aesculus hippocastanum* Horse Chestnut seed	*Eucalyptus* spp. Eucalyptus leaf and essential oil	*Triticum repens* Couch grass root
Capsella bursa-pastoris Shepherd's Purse herb	*Calendula officinalis* Marigold flower	*Angelica archangelica* Angelica root	*Solidago* spp. Goldenrod herb
Mitchella repens Partridge Berry herb	*Hamamelis virginiana* Witch Hazel leaf	*Marrubium vulgare* White Horehound herb	*Taraxacum officinale* Dandelion leaf
Ceanothus spp. Red Root	*Ceanothus* spp. Red Root	*Anemopsis californica* Yerba Mansa root	*Poria cocoa* Fu Ling Hoelen fungus
Anemone pulsatilla Pasque flower	*Achillea millefolium* Yarrow herb	*Salvia officinalis* Garden Sage leaf	Arctium lappa Burdock root

Tissue-Level Qualities or Descriptions: Astringing, Eliminating, Solidifying, Dissolving, Thickening, Diluting

The group of tissue-level *qualities* are Western descriptions of what herbs actually do to the tissues. In fact, these action words were used by the 19th-century Western physiomedicalists. Tissue-level qualities are really subdivisions of the Six Secondary Qualities, discussed earlier. Many Western herb books categorize in this manner, using allopathic-type expressions such as *laxative* or *expectorant*. These are helpful terms when choosing an herb needed for one specific action—and handy concepts to understand. Much of this material is presented in convenient herb chart format that can be referred to later when making up formulas. It will aid in finding a proper herb in the correct category.

In real life, most conditions require more than one category of herbs. Just because clients have a dry condition doesn't mean they require only a moistener like Slippery Elm bark. Herbalists don't just chase symptoms. The whole person must be considered, and the formula should include other herbs to balance it out and get to the root or cause. One might ask, "Why are they dry? Is it interior or exterior? What organ or tissue is dry?" A little detective work helps determine what else is needed in a formula.

Some herbs fit more than one quality. This versatility is because a plant contains many chemicals, each responsible for something different. Yarrow herb is a famous example, containing countless constituents and actions. The chemical listing takes up eight full

• BOX 10.4 Five Herbal Actions for Treating Dysmenorrhea

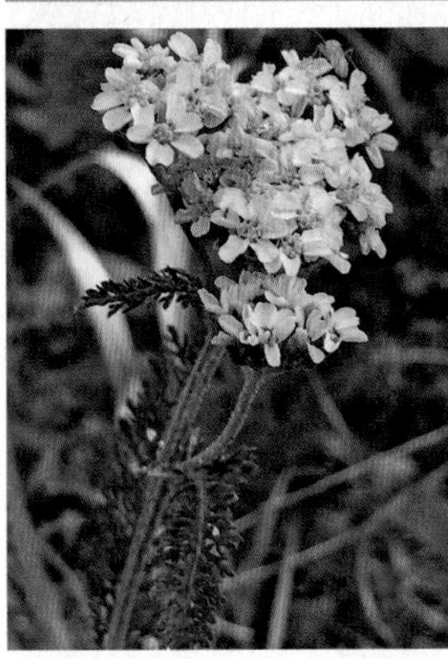

Yarrow flowering. *Achillea millefolium* would be a fine herb to include in a menstrual cramp formula.

When treating menstrual cramps, uterus blood congestion, and/or dysmenorrhea (all the same thing), five herbal actions that include three types of blood movers could be used. And all these for only one symptom.

- *Venous decongestants.* To move excess blood away from the uterus with something like Yarrow herb.
- *Uterine decongestants.* To circulate blood away from the pelvic floor with Yarrow herb, Lady's Mantle herb, or Red Root.
- *Arterial circulatory stimulants.* To move blood from the pelvis through arterial stimulation with Ginger root or Prickly Ash bark.

Additionally, two more actions might be called upon:

- *Spasmolytics.* To ease smooth muscle spasms and pain with Pasque flower or Cramp bark.
- *Hemostatics.* To reduce bleeding with Shepherd's Purse herb or Plantain leaf.[4]

lines in Holmes' *Energetics of Western Herbs*[4] and 46 lines, three columns for each line, in Stephen Buhner's *The Lost language of Plants.*[9] Buhner was referencing another renown herbalist, James Duke. All this was as of 1992! The qualities or actions of Yarrow are stimulating, decongesting, astringing, restoring, and relaxing. It dries mucus, stops discharges, restores kidneys, stops urinary incontinence, promotes sweating, and stops bleeding. This versatile herb can obviously be used for many functions. In terms of space, it is economical to select herbs in a formula that can address more than one need. Tissue-level qualities or actions are:

- *Astringing.* Tightens up tissues to stop discharges, sweating, or bleeding. Includes descriptions like anhidrotics, antidiarrheals, hemostatics, and mucostatics.
- *Eliminating.* Moves fluids or mucus up or down and out. Western descriptions include expectorants, diaphoretics, emmenagogues, diuretics, laxatives, etc.
- *Solidifying.* Strengthens weak or flabby tissues by making them firmer and healthier. Nutritive herbs and tonics are used.
- *Dissolving.* Softens hard deposits. Western descriptions are litholytics or antilipemics.
- *Thickening.* Restores, builds up and heals thin, weak tissues. Descriptive Western terms are nutritive restoratives and tonics.
- *Diluting.* Thins out hyperviscous, dense fluids. Western examples are anticoagulants and mucostatics.

Astringing

Astringents tighten tissue and mucous membranes and stop discharges, ultimately strengthening the tissue (Table 10.13). For this reason, they are drying. ***Anhidrotics*** limit sweating; ***antidiarrheals*** slow excess stool; *mucostatics* reduce mucous secretion; ***hemostatics*** stop bleeding (Table 10.14).

Many astringents also decrease inflammation and infection, making them ideal wound healers in the case of tissue trauma and injury. These types are the ***vulneraries*** or ciscatrizants. Vulneraries should be used internally and externally. A wonderful, classic vulnerary is the Chinese herb *Panax notoginseng* San Qi (Pseudoginseng root) (Chapter 25).

Eliminating: Includes Expectorants, Diaphoretics, Emmenagogues, Diuretics, Laxatives

Herbs that *eliminate* work to break up, move, and remove several things. They are generally pungent and stimulating. They break up stasis of fluids causing edema, sweat, skin rashes, stasis of stool, bronchial sputum, and lack of menses.[5] ***Mucolytics/mucostatics*** break up thick mucus. *Expectorants* move mucus up and out. *Diaphoretics* create sweating, thus removing water and wastes from the skin. *Emmenagogues* increase menstrual flow. *Diuretics* increase urine flow. *Laxatives* increase and move stool down.

- *Expectorants.* Move out thick mucus. (Mucolytics break up the mucus. *Lytic* means to destroy or break up.)
- *Diaphoretics.* Create sweating.
- *Emmenagogues.* Increase menstrual flow.
- *Diuretics.* Increase urine flow.
- *Laxatives.* Move stool down and out.

Expectorants

Expectorants break up mucus and stimulate it to be expelled from the lungs. They are used to treat congestion. Infectious mucus, containing toxins from bacteria and viruses, can make us septic if it remains in the lungs. We need to cough it up and get it out. Expectorants come in warm, cold, and mucolytic varieties (Table 10.15).

Warm, stimulating expectorants are pungent and spicy, with large essential oil content. They are used for cold conditions when there is no hot infection present, as in the early stages of a cold or flu. Sometimes the essential oils of Hyssop or Thyme and others are mixed with a neutral carrier oil, such as Olive or Almond oil, and rubbed onto the chest. Elecampane root, Horseradish root, or Fennel seed are other possibilities.

Cooling, stimulating expectorants are pungent, cool, and sedating. They are used for sputum with infection. They are used when heat is present, with fever, yellow-green sputum, chills, and muscle aches. Cooling expectorants disinfect and clear infection, stop inflammation, and break up mucus. Eucalyptus leaf, White Horehound herb, or Thyme herb are examples.

Mucolytic expectorants break up thick, viscous, and scanty sputum. In respiratory infections, the lungs naturally produce extra sputum because there is irritation on the membranes that creates coughing. This extra sputum must be eliminated. Mucolytic expectorants change a dry, hacky, unproductive cough into one that is wet and productive. They get out the gunk. This effect is because of their saponin content. Saponins act as emulsifiers,

TABLE 10.13 Categories of Astringent Herbs

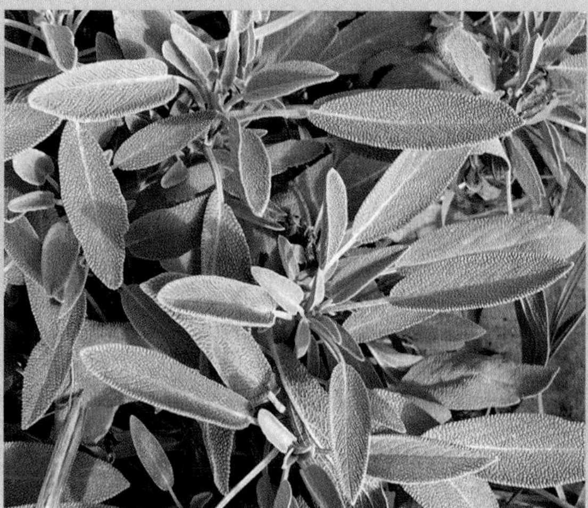

Salvia officinalis (Garden Sage leaf) is an astringent herb that helps stop excessive sweating and heals tissue.

Anhidrotics	Antidiarrheals	Mucostatics	Restrains Urinary System	Vulneraries
Geranium maculatum Cranesbill herb and root	**Children** Rose Family: weaker ones, use leaves; stronger ones, use bark	**Upper Respiratory** *Euphrasia rostkoviana* Eyebright herb	**Dribbling, Enuresis, Involuntary Sperm Loss** *Verbascum thapsus* Mullein root	*Salvia officinalis* Garden Sage leaf
Salvia officinalis Garden Sage leaf	*Rubus idaeus* Raspberry	*Pulmonaria officinalis* Lungwort lichen	*Piper methysticum* Kava root	*Berberis vulgaris* Barberry root
Rhus glabra Sumac bark	*Rubus villosus* Blackberry	*Hydrastis canadensis* Goldenseal herb	*Eupatorium purpureum* Gravel root	*Panax notoginseng* San Qi Pseudoginseng root
Juglans regia Hu Tao Ren Walnut hull	*Fragaria vesca* Strawberry leaf	*Xanthium sibiricum* Cang Er Zi Siberian cocklebur	*Rhus glabra* Sumac root	*Myrtus communis* Myrrh resin
Quercus spp. White Oak bark	**Adults** *Quercus* spp. White Oak bark	**Vaginal** *Trillium pendulum* Birth or Beth root	*Cornus* spp. Dogwood berry	*Euphrasia rostkoviana* Eyebright herb
Astragalus membranaceus Huang Qi Astragalus root	*Berberis vulgaris* Barberry root bark	*Agrimonia eupatoria* Agrimony herb	*Equisetum arvense* Horsetail herb	*Hydrastis canadensis* Goldenseal root
Schisandra chinensis Five Taste berry	*Phellodendron amurense* Huang Bai Siberian Cork Tree bark	**Urinary** *Piper methysticum* Kava root	*Populus* spp. Poplar bark	*Calendula officinalis* Marigold flower

helping oily constituents dissolve in water, like soap. Soapwort root is named for this quality and contains both saponins and mucilage. It bubbles up and lathers when mixed in water, breaking up stubborn, thick mucus.[2]

Diaphoretics to Dispel External Wind

Diaphoretics make us sweat, cool us down, and treat external wind conditions. They are spicy, pungent, stimulating, and vasodilating.[4] Sudoriferous or sweat glands are located in the dermis and subcutaneous layers of the skin. Sweating occurs when the internal temperature becomes too hot. Blood vessels dilate, bringing more warm blood to the surface, causing the release of moisture. As heat is drawn from the skin, we are cooled down (Table 10.16).

Sweating has been used therapeutically in many cultures. Hydrotherapy (water) with the use of either dry or damp heat makes us sweat. The Native American tradition of a dry sweat lodge, Finnish and Swedish dry heat saunas, Turkish hot steam baths, mineral baths, and hot springs from many countries are all examples. The ancient Roman baths of Caracalla are famous.

TABLE 10.14 Astringent Hemostatics
(Constrict vessels and/or coagulate blood.)

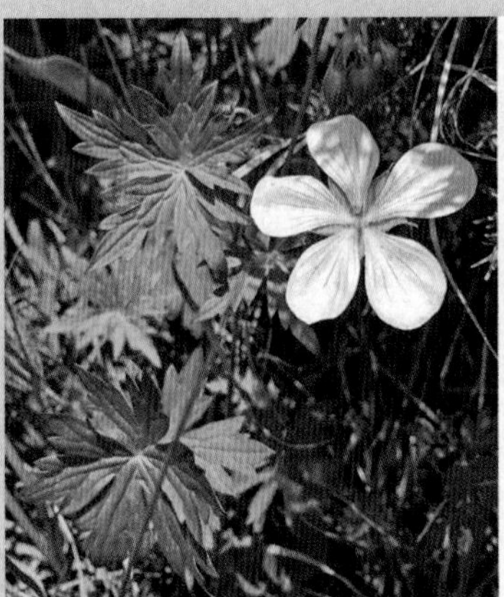
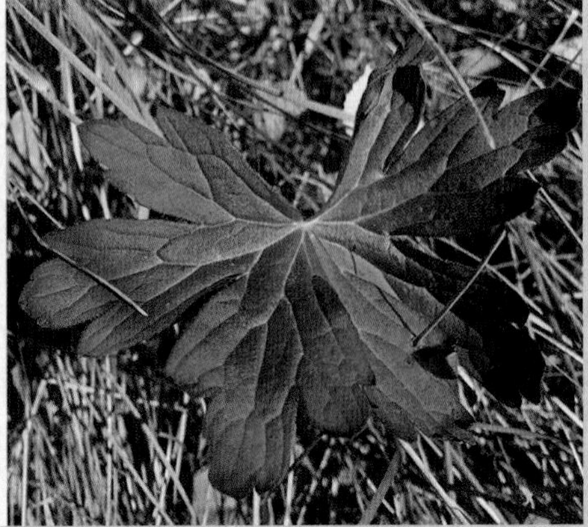

Richardson's geranium in summer and Cranesbill geranium leaf in fall. *Geranium* spp. is a mucostatic and hemostatic astringent.

Menorrhagia (Excess menstrual bleeding from congestion)	**Hematuria** (Blood in urine)	**Blood in Stool**	**Hemoptysis** (Coughing up blood in lungs)
Gossypium spp. Cotton root bark Constricts and coagulates.	*Piper methysticum* Kava root	*Geranium maculatum* Cranesbill herb and root	*Plantago* spp. Plantain leaf
Agrimonia eupatoria Agrimony herb	*Agrimonia eupatoria* Agrimony herb	*Quercus* spp. White Oak bark	*Agrimonia eupatoria* Agrimony herb
Capsella bursa-pastoris Shepherd's Purse herb Constricts and coagulates.	*Rubia tinctorum* Madder root	*Phellodendron amurense* Huang Bai Siberian Cork Tree bark	*Quercus* spp. Oak bark
Trillium pendulum Birth or Beth root	*Arctostaphylos uva-ursi* Uva Ursi leaf	*Hydrastis canadensis* Goldenseal root	*Geranium maculatum* Cranesbill herb and root
Chamaelirium luteum Helonias root	*Eupatorium purpureum* Gravel root	*Plantago* spp. Plantain leaf	*Achillea millefolium* Yarrow herb

Sweating cools us down and drives out toxins, and it is very healing. Think of colds, flus, sinusitis, laryngitis, and other respiratory conditions accompanied by chills, sneezing, sore throat, headache, and possibly a fever. Onset of these ills are initially treated by sweating it out, either by hydrotherapy or by herbs that do the trick (Chapter 20).

Pungent warm stimulating diaphoretics treat or dispel external wind cold conditions. As discussed earlier, external wind comes from the environment (exogenous) and invades our body. External wind cold comes in the form of acute infections, usually from bacteria or viruses. Wind cold produces no fever, very little inflammation, clear or white discharges, and little sweating. **P** is floating and tight, and **T** is normal or pale. For this cold situation, we need pungent, warm arterial stimulant diaphoretics like Garlic Bulb or Zingiber Sheng Jiang (Fresh Ginger rhizome) decocted in tea.

Pungent, cool relaxant diaphoretics treat external wind heat conditions. Wind heat has fever, sweating, inflammation, and yellow or greenish discharges, all indicating infection. These symptoms indicate inflammation. The suffix "itis" means "inflammation of" – examples being bronchitis, laryngitis, and sinusitis. **P** Fast, wiry. **T** Red. For this hot condition, we need cool, peripheral vasodilating diaphoretics to help us sweat, such as Catnip herb, Field Mint herb, Elder flower, or Yarrow herb.[4]

Fevers are not necessarily bad. They actually help the immune system fight infection by stimulating the production of leukocytes (a white blood cell), antibodies, cytokines (inflammation fighters), and a virus-fighting protein called *interferon*, all of which work to protect the body against harmful microorganisms. Germs have a hard time surviving with high core temperatures. As a fever increases, the body naturally sweats to cool us down. That natural process is augmented with herbs.

Emmenagogues

Emmenagogues are uterine stimulants that increase uterine contractions and increase menstrual flow. They can bring on a period that is a few days late because of disruptions in lifestyle or travel. Emmenagogues come in varying strengths (Table 10.17). Some work through bitter stimulation, and others work through localized irritation.[3] If a woman is pregnant, emmenagogues do not work. They will not cause miscarriages.

TABLE 10.15 **Various Types of Expectorants**

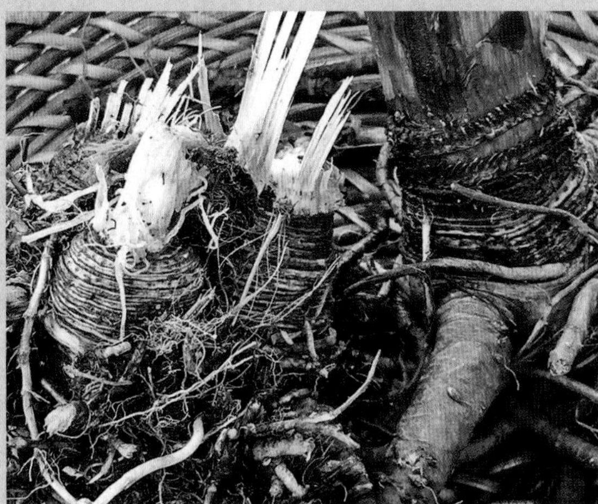

Angelica archangelica (Angelica root) is a warm, dry and pungent expectorant that opens the sinuses and can help a tight cough.

Warm Stimulant Expectorants	Cool Stimulant Expectorants	Mucolytic Expectorants (With saponins)
Angelica archangelica Angelica root	*Asclepias tuberosa* Pleurisy root	*Verbascum thapsus* Mullein leaf
Platycodon grandiflorum Ji Geng Balloonflower root	*Symphytum officinale* Comfrey root	*Grindelia robusta* Gumweed flower
Ligusticum porteri Osha root	*Plantago lanceolata* Ribwort Plantain leaf	*Trillium pendulum* Birth or Beth root
Thymus vulgaris Thyme herb	*Marrubium vulgare* White Horehound herb	*Platycodon grandiflorum* Ji Geng Balloonflower root
Pinus spp. Scotch Pine needle	*Sambucus nigra* Elderberry and flower	*Polygonatum multiflorum* Solomon's Seal root
Ocimum basilicum Basil herb	*Tussilago farfara* Coltsfoot herb	*Saponaria officinalis* Soapwort root

Diuretics

The kidneys are amazing. They maintain proper fluid balance, which is essential for good health. Urine becomes dark and concentrated when the body is dehydrated. With more hydration, the urine becomes lighter and dilute. The kidneys maintain proper internal fluid balance without conscious thought. They work with the liver, lungs, skin, and bowels to maintain a nontoxic internal environment. The kidneys dispose of excess waste through the urine and help maintain the acid-base balance of the blood.

Herbs that promote urination are the ***diuretics***. Whenever there is too much fluid in the body, the Chinese Medicine condition is damp. **P** Slippery. **T** Wet, scalloped or thick and greasy. Diuretics increase the flow and elimination of fluids through urination and therefore are one way to reduce watery damp. In general, the criteria listed here all are indications for the use of diuretics:

- *Damp, edematous conditions.* These concern the face and limbs.
- *Edema with liver weakness.* This condition is edema from the waist down. Here choose diuretics that work directly on the liver, such as Dandelion root, Artichoke leaf, Blessed Thistle herb, Elecampane root, Wormwood herb, and Blue Flag root.
- *Congestive heart failure (CHF) and hypertension.* A chief symptom is bilateral ankle edema. Choose Broom herb, Squill bulb, Lily of the Valley herb, or Cereus stem.
- *Metabolic toxicosis with edema.* Use saponin diuretics such as Goldenrod flower tops or Cleavers herb.
- *Acute urinary tract and kidney infections.* Examples are bladder infections (cystitis) and kidney infections (nephritis). A cooling, refrigerant diuretic is needed that also has a restorative quality, such as Goldenrod herb or Horsetail herb.
- *Acute urinary retention.* This condition assumes existing adequate hydration with scanty urination (oliguria) or stopped urination (anuria). If either of these potentially dangerous situations go on for long, a referral to a physician is urgent. (The nurse in me speaking.)

TABLE 10.16 Diaphoretics

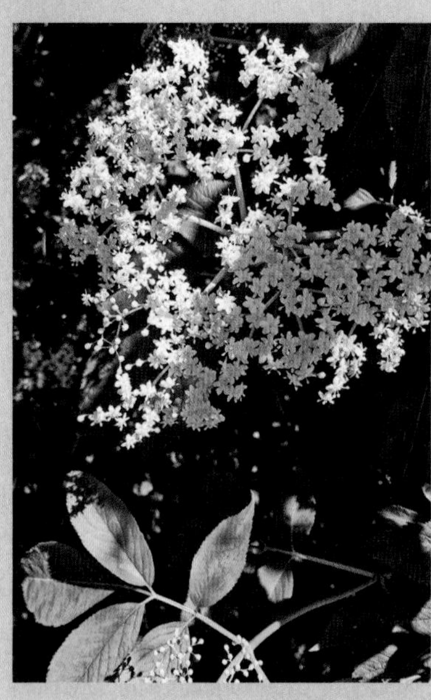

Sambucus nigra (Elder flower, leaf, and berry) are diaphoretic, help us sweat, and can reduce a fever.

Stimulating Diaphoretics (Scatters wind cold)	Vasodilating Diaphoretics (Scatters wind heat)
Cinnamomum cassia Gui Zhi Cinnamon twig	*Achillea millefolium* Yarrow herb
Sambucus nigra Elderberry and flower	*Tilia cordata* Linden flower
Allium sativum Garlic bulb	*Eucalyptus* spp. Eucalyptus leaf
Zingiber officinalis Shen Jiang Fresh Ginger root	*Nepeta cataria* Catnip herb
Brassica spp Mustard seed	*Sambucus nigra* Elderberry and flower
Ligusticum porteri Osha root	*Matricaria recutita* Chamomile flower
Mentha piperita Peppermint herb	*Lavandula angustifolia* Lavender flower
Zanthoxylum americanum Prickly Ash bark	*Chrysanthemum x morifolium* Ju Hua Chrysanthemum flower

TABLE 10.17 Emmenagogues Based on Strength

Mild[3]	Moderate	Strong
Achillea millefolium Yarrow herb	*Actaea racemosa* Black Cohosh root	*Zingiber officinalis* Gan Jiang Dried Ginger root
Calendula officinalis Pot Marigold herb	*Caulophyllum thalictroides* Blue Cohosh root	*Hydrastis canadensis* Goldenseal root
Hyssopus officinalis Hyssop herb	*Mitchella repens* Partridge berry	*Gentiana lutea* Long Dan Cao Yellow Gentian root
Salvia officinalis Garden Sage leaf	*Rubus idaeus* Raspberry leaf	*Ruta graveolens* Rue herb
Thymus vulgaris Thyme herb	*Vitex agnus-castus* Chastetree berry	*Tanacetum vulgare* Tansy herb *Artemisia absinthium* Wormwood herb
		Both Tansy and Wormwood: CAUTION in essential oil form could cause miscarriage

Diuretics may be put into various categories, depending on action desired (Table 10.18). Sometimes it is useful to combine diuretic herbs in a given formula from more than one category to assure that the bases are covered.

- *Dry, pungent diuretics.* These contain essential oils and help when edema begins around the ankles and moves upwards in the body. We may see puffy eyes in the morning, lumbar pain, heavy knees. We might even see chronic kidney diseases, such as nephritis or glomerulonephritis, or salt cravings.
- *Saponin diuretics.* Mucilaginous saponin diuretics stimulate the urinary tract mucosa by a reflex action. They treat urinary water congestion caused from *metabolic toxicosis*, indicated by chronic malaise, headaches, and skin eruptions. (The skin is considered the third kidney.) If kidney function is subpar, the kidneys will not filter toxins out of the blood efficiently, and toxins build up in the body. In this instance, kidney function is encouraged by a diuretic with a detoxifying effect.
- *Saluretics.* Saluretics increase renal excretion of salt. Where salt goes, water follows. This action is useful with edema or hypertension.
- *Osmotic diuretics.* This class contains sugar alcohols, such as mannitol and sorbitol. They draw water from the blood and interstitial fluids into the microcirculation of the kidney glomerulus, enhancing diuresis.
- *Cardio-renal diuretics.* These have cardioactive constituents, such as glycosides and alkaloids. They are go-to diuretics when a person has congestive heart failure (CHF) from cardiac edema or swelling of the ankles and/or hypertension.[4]

Laxatives

Mild herbs that promote bowel movements are known as ***laxatives***, whereas the very strong ones are known as ***purgatives***. Galenic physicians misused purgatives in ancient Greece. Eclectic physicians such as Scudder and Webster of the 19th century followed suit and were known for heavy, dramatic purges and the use of calomel, the highly toxic mercurous chloride.

Herbalists today are much more careful and conservative. Stronger purgatives are only used in extreme cases, for short duration. Before *any* laxative is given, make sure clients are consuming adequate fluids, exercising, and eating a fiber-rich diet. Strong

TABLE 10.18 Diuretic Categories

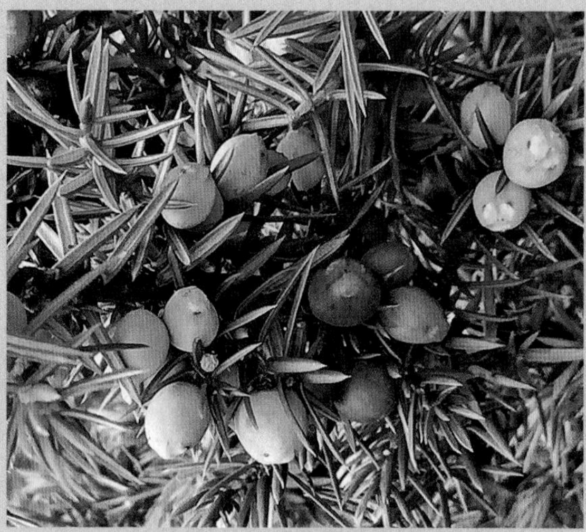

Juniperus communis (Juniper berry), a is a dry, pungent diuretic.

Pungent, Dry	Saponins	Saluretics	Osmotic	Cardio-Renal
Ligusticum levisticum Gao Ren Garden Lovage herb	*Solidago* spp. Goldenrod herb	*Taraxacum officinal* Pu Gong Ying Dandelion leaf	*Triticum repens* Couch Grass root	*Cytisus scoparius* Broom herb
Cochlearia armoracia Horseradish root	*Asparagus officinalis* Asparagus root	*Solidago* spp. Goldenrod herb	*Zea mays* Cornsilk style	*Scilla maritima* Squill herb
Juniperus communis Junipor bcrry	*Galium aparine* Cleavers herb		*Taraxacum officinale* Dandelion leaf	*Convallaria majalis* Lily of the Valley herb
Petroselinum crispum Parsley seed	*Eupatorium purpureum* Gravel root		*Eryngium maritimum* Sea Holly root	*Selenicereus grandiflorus* Night Blooming Cactus stem and flower
Daucus carota Wild Carrot seed and root	*Betula* spp. Birch leaf			*Coffea arabica* Coffee bean
Foeniculum vulgare Fennel seed	*Primula veris* Cowslip root			

stimulant laxatives, like Senna leaf and pod, can be habit-forming and should be given only for short periods, in the lowest dose possible, for stubborn unresponsive cases. Laxative dependency is all too common. Laxatives work to increase peristalsis in a variety of ways (Table 10.19).[4] Further details on laxatives are discussed in Chapter 18.

- *Bulk laxatives.* These mild herbs swell up when mixed with warm water and stimulate peristalsis by enlarging and softening the feces. Bulking agents are normal components of food in the form of indigestible carbohydrate fiber in grains, seed husks, bran, fruits, and vegetables.
- *Sweet stimulant laxatives.* These are mild and sweet and gently stimulate peristalsis. They are used occasionally for children and elders. Licorice root is an example.
- *Demulcent laxatives.* These are mild, sweet, cool, and moist, and they are useful for intestinal dryness with dry, hard stools and straining. Their oily mucilage lubes up the bowel, so contents can slide out. They help prevent hemorrhoids. Examples are Flax seeds and Seaweeds.
- *Saline dissolvent laxatives.* These are mineral salts such as Epsom Salts (magnesium sulfate). They work by osmosis, pulling water into the bowel and dissolving accumulations. The extra water increases intestinal wall pressure, stimulating movements. They work quickly, may cause dehydration, and should not be used continually.
- *Cholagogue laxatives.* This large group of bitter, cold, and stimulating herbs increase bile flow in the liver, gastric, and pancreatic secretions, thus helping the body break down food and evacuate the bowel. There are many yellow bile stimulants, such as the berberine-containing Goldenseal, Oregon Grape and Barberry roots, bitter Artichoke leaf, and Celandine herb.
- *Purgative stimulant laxatives.* These strongly irritate the intestinal wall to create peristalsis. Anthraquinone compounds present in these plants can damage epithelial cells, leading to

TABLE 10.19 Laxative Categories

Bulk (Mild)	Mild Sweet Stimulants (Sugars)	Demulcent (Wet)	Saline Dissolvent (Salty)	Cholagogue (Increase bile)	Stimulant Purgatives (Very strong)
Ulmus fulva Slippery Elm bark	*Glycyrrhiza glabra* Gan Cao Licorice root	*Plantago psyllium* Psyllium husk	Epsom and Glauber's Salts	*Menthe x piperita* Peppermint herb	*Rhamnus catharticus* Buckthorn bark
Linum usitatissimum Ground Flax seed	*Ziziphus jujube* Da Zao Jujube berry	*Linum usitatissimum* Flax seed	**Sea Veggies** *Laminaria* spp. Kelp seaweed	*Carduus benedictus* Blessed Thistle seed	*Rhamnus purshiana* Cascara Sagrada bark
Plantago psyllium Psyllium husk	*Tamarindus indica* Tamarind pulp	*Cannabis sativa* Hemp seed	*Porphyra* spp. Nori seaweed	*Silybum marianus* Milk Thistle seed	*Cassia acutifolia* Senna leaf/pod
Sea Veggies *Laminaria* spp. Kelp thallus		**Kernels** *Prunus domestica* Plum kernel	*Palmaria palmata* Dulse seaweed	*Taraxacum officinalis* Dandelion root	*Rheum officinale* Da Huang Rhubarb root
Porphyra spp. Zi Cai Nori seaweed		*Amygdalus persica* Tao Ren Peach kernel	*Undaria pinnatifida* Wakame seaweed	*Berberis vulgaris* Barberry root	*Menyanthes trifoliata* Bogbean leaf
Palmaria palmata Dulse seaweed		*Prunus armeniaca* Xing Ren Apricot kernel		*Arctium lappa* Burdock root	*Aloe vera* Aloe resin
Undaria pinnatifida Wakame seaweed		**Sea Veggies** *Laminaria* spp. Kelp seaweed		*Cynara scolymus* Artichoke leaf	*Scrophularia ningpoensis* Figwort herb
Grains *Oryza sativa* Rice bran *Triticum aestivum* Wheat bran		*Porphyra* spp. Zi Cai Nori seaweed			*Podophyllum peltatum* Mayapple root—the strongest of all. Caution in high doses.

changes in absorption, secretion, and motility. They can be habit-forming when taken over long periods, causing abdominal pain and gas. They are highly effective for very short-term use. Cascara Sagrada bark, Rhubarb root, and Senna leaf and pod fall into this category.

- *Lubricant laxatives.* Cod Liver or Flax seed oils taken by mouth encourage bowel movements by coating the bowel and the stool with a waterproof film. This action keeps moisture in the stool. The stool remains soft, and passage is made easier.

Solidifying

Tissue that is weak or poorly toned needs to be more dense, solid, and strong. Solidifying herbs work primarily on all types of connective tissue, where many weaknesses can occur. The bones may become soft in the form of osteopenia and osteoporosis, gums may soften, and teeth loosen or fall out. Weak veins cause hemorrhoids or varicosities. The mitral valve in the heart can prolapse. Subluxations, misalignments of the vertebrae, occur because of ligament weakness. A weak anterior cruciate ligament (ACL) is one of the four main ligaments in the knee that connect the femur to the tibia; if it tears, it pushes the knee painfully out of alignment.

The uterus or bladder can prolapse, fall downward, and protrude into the vagina. It sags because of stretched-out ligaments that are normally tight and elastic. Western medicine attributes uterine prolapse to excessive pushing in labor, a history of having large babies, or being overweight. Allopathic treatment surgically tightens supporting ligaments. In Chinese Medicine, the Spleen holds tissues and organs in their correct place and is the organ responsible for giving strength and power to connective tissue. Therefore treatment for prolapse is to strengthen or tonify the Spleen. The syndrome is known as Spleen Qi Deficiency.

Other approaches to solidify tissue are with the use of nutritive herbs that provide the vitamins, minerals, and trace minerals needed to build connective tissue. The list in Table 10.20 divides herbs into categories for solidifying and strengthening various tissues of the body.

Dissolving

Dissolvents soften hardened deposits or tissue. Many contain trace minerals to help this along. Gallstones require dissolvents that have an affinity for the liver. Kidney stones require those with a tropism to the kidneys. Some dissolvents work on fibrosis, which is scarring and thickening that can affect nerves, bones, or blood vessels. This condition could manifest as a thickening of the nerves in a

TABLE 10.20 **Solidifying Weak Tissue**

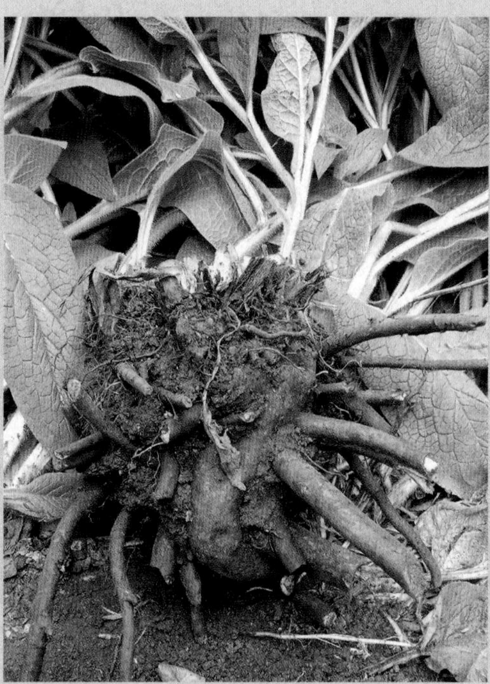

Symphytum officinale (Comfrey leaf and root) strengthens and builds connective tissue of all kinds, especially in the muscles, ligaments, bones, and gut.

Soft Teeth and Bones (Tones and restores with Ca^+ and minerals)	**Prolapses and Subluxations** (Uterus, intestines, bladder, and mitral valve)	**Weak, Flabby Muscles** (Includes arthritic conditions)
Equisetum arvense Horsetail herb	*Equisetum arvense* Horsetail herb	*Medicago sativa* Alfalfa herb
Urtica dioica Nettle herb	*Urtica dioica* Nettle herb	*Taraxacum officinale* Dandelion root
Juglans regia Walnut leaf and hull	*Juglans regia* Walnut leaf and hull	Symphytum officinale Comfrey leaf and root
Medicago sativa Alfalfa herb	*Symphytum officinale* Comfrey leaf and root	*Urtica dioica* Nettle herb
Taraxacum officinale Dandelion root		*Eucommia ulmoides* Du Zhong Eucommia bark
		Liquid Trace Minerals

Morton's neuroma between the third and fourth metatarsal. Bones can fibrose and thicken into extra calcifications called *bone spurs*. Arterial walls can fibrose, becoming hard and nonelastic. Other conditions where dissolvents are important are fibroid tumors, cysts, and polyps. Mucolytic expectorants that break up mucus are actually dissolvents. Types of dissolvents are listed here, and herbs in those categories include (Table 10.21):

- *Litholytics*. Herbs that break up and dissolve kidney stones and gallstones, made up of calcium and other mineral deposits, are called ***litholytics***.
- *Antiatherosclerotics*. They break up fats, cholesterol, and other substances in and on artery walls (*plaques*) that can restrict blood flow. Also, antiatherosclerotic can refer to the vessels becoming thick, stiff, nonflexible, and hardened, causing restricted blood flow.
- *Antilipemics*. Herbs that soften and break up fatty cholesterol deposits in blood and on blood vessels, particularly the coronary arteries, are ***antilipemics***. If a coronary artery, which feeds oxygen to the heart muscle, becomes blocked from blood, cholesterol, or mineral deposits, a heart attack occurs.

TABLE 10.21 **Dissolvents**

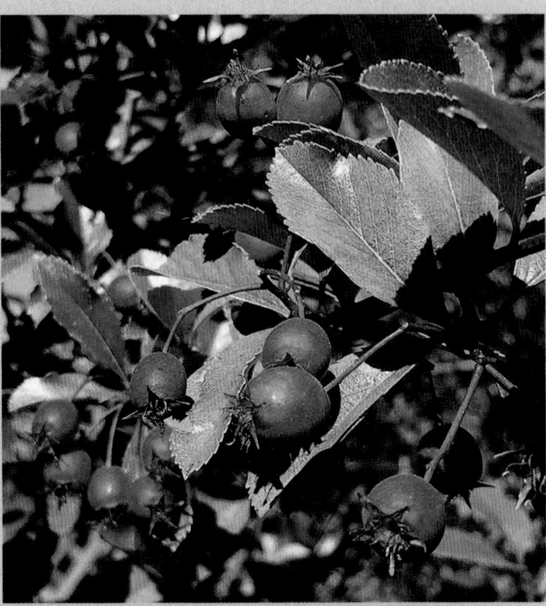

Crataegus spp. (Hawthorn berry) dissolves fatty and mineral deposits in the coronary arteries.

Kidney Litholytics (Kidney stones)	Gallbladder Litholytics (Gallstones)	Antiatherosclerotics (Mineral deposits)	Antilipemics (Fatty deposits)
Zea mays Yu Mi Xu Cornsilk style	*Cynara scolymus* Artichoke leaf	*Equisetum arvense* Horsetail herb	*Cynara scolymus* Artichoke leaf
Hydrangea arborescens Hydrangea root	*Berberis vulgaris* Barberry bark	*Urtica dioica* Nettle herb	*Crataegus* spp. Hawthorn berry
Rubia tinctorum Madder root	*Chelidonium majus* Celandine herb	*Cynara scolymus* Artichoke leaf	*Allium sativum* Garlic bulb
Galium aparine Cleavers herb	*Taraxacum officinale* Dandelion root	*Ginkgo biloba* Ginkgo leaf	*Ligusticum wallichii* Chuan Xiong Sichuan Lovage root
Desmodium styracifolium Jin Qian Cao Coin grass	*Equisetum arvense* Horsetail herb	*Galium aparine* Cleavers herb	*Taraxacum officinale* Dandelion root
Apium graveolens Celery seed	*Urtica dioica* Nettle herb	*Taraxacum officinale* Dandelion root	*Cichorium intybus* Chicory root
Chimaphila umbellata Pipsissewa herb	*Zea mays* Yu Mi Xu Cornsilk style	*Gardenia jasminoides* Zhi Zi Gardenia pod	*Urtica dioica* Nettle herb

Thickening

Nutritive restoratives *thicken* tissues and build them up by nourishing deficiencies. They are for conditions of malnutrition, malabsorption, degenerative diseases, alcohol abuse with malnutrition, chronic illness, and deficient dry conditions. Most of these herbs are sweet and healing and build up tissue.[5] They were addressed earlier under the sweet taste and tonics but can be broken down into more specific tropisms (Table 10.22).

Diluting

The *diluting* quality treats fluid hyperviscosity. Herbs that are ***diluting*** are used for thinning out thick, congealed, or fatty blood, or for lymph node swellings. They help Western maladies such as hyperlipidemia, atherosclerosis, thrombosis, swollen lymph glands, viscous sputum, menstrual clots, and intestinal mucus. They decrease blood clotting factors. Many of these herbs have a detoxifying effect as well and would be useful as a detoxicant assist in treating tumors (Table 10.23).

TABLE 10.22 Nutritive Restoratives/Thickeners

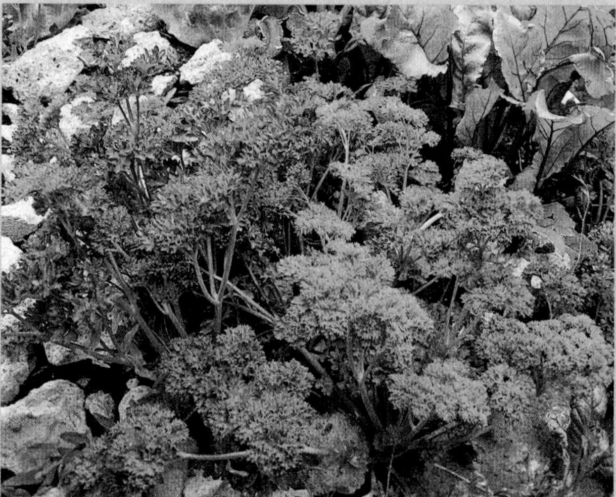

Petroselinum crispum (Parsley herb) is rich in Vitamin C and other antioxidants.

General Deficiencies	Blood Restoratives	Respiratory Demulcents
Pollen Flower pollen	*Petroselinum crispum* Parsley herb	*Stellaria media* Chickweed herb
Chlorella spp. *or Spirulina* spp. Microalgae	*Rumex crispus* Yellow Dock root	*Borago officinalis* Borage leaf
Urtica dioica Nettle herb	*Trifolium pratense* Red Clover blossom	*Symphytum officinale* Comfrey root
Medicago sativa Alfalfa herb	*Smilax officinalis* Sarsaparilla herb	*Althea officinalis* Marshmallow root
Nasturtium officinale Watercress herb	*Codonopsis pilosula* Dang Shen Downy bellflower root	**Insatiable thirst** *Asparagus officinalis* Asparagus root
Triticum aestivum Wheatgrass	*Lycium chinense* Gou Qi Zi Wolfberry or Goji berry	*Ophiopogon japonicus* Mai Men Dong Dwarf Lilyturf root
	Angelica sinensis Dong Quai Angelica root	

An Experiment in Energetics: Organoleptic Evaluations

Have you ever wondered how herbalists over the centuries came up with the energetics of a plant? How did they figure this out long before we knew anything about chemistry and constituents? The fancy word for doing this is ***organoleptics***, which means judging the potency, quality, and phytochemical composition of an herb or preparation by using the senses.

Obviously, energetic information had to come from frequent investigation and experimentation. Herbalists use their senses and instincts, just as animals do. It is a conscious act that takes learning and practice. A quiet, darkened room, with other sensory stimuli kept at a minimum, helps one focus in on the herb being evaluated. It is interesting to do this in a group and then compare notes on what each person determined.

Organoleptics is about our own experience with a plant or herb. If you truly sit with an herb, feel it, taste it, and learn its energy, you will know and understand that herb. When that happens, you will never forget the personality and properties of said plant and will not have to memorize anything. Over time, we have lost this ability but can regain the skill by relearning and training ourselves. Doing so can also help evaluate the quality of our own homemade remedies—or anyone else's. Always give your product the smell and taste test.

TABLE 10.23 **Diluting/Thinning Herbs**

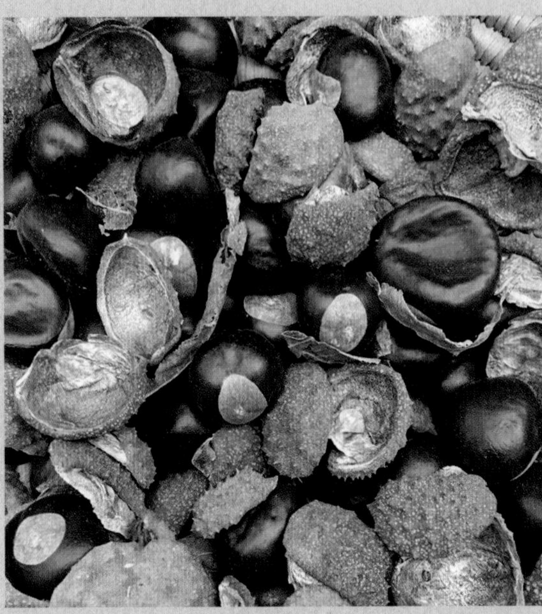

Aesculus hippocastanum (Horse Chestnut seed) thins the blood and breaks up deposits/clots in varicose veins, hemorrhoids, and congestive dysmenorrhea.

Anticoagulants	Antitumoral Detoxicants	Mucostatics
Aesculus hippocastanum Horse Chestnut seed	*Phytolacca decandra* Poke root—Strong.	**Upper Respiratory** *Euphrasia rostkoviana* Eyebright herb
Allium sativum Garlic bulb	*Larrea divaricata* Chaparral herb	*Sticta pulmonaria* Lungwort thallus
Salvia miltiorrhiza Dan Shen Cinnabar Sage root	*Scrophularia ningpoensis* Figwort root	*Solidago* spp. Goldenrod herb
Angelica archangelica Angelica root	*Chimaphila umbellata* Pipsissewa herb	*Xanthium sibiricum* Cang Er Zi Siberian cocklebur
Panax notoginseng San Qi Pseudoginseng root	*Iris versicolor* Blue Flag rhizome	**Uterus/Vagina** *Trillium pendulum* Birth or Beth root
Ligusticum wallichii Chuan Xiong Sichuan Lovage root	*Galium aparine* Cleavers herb	*Agrimonia eupatoria* Agrimony herb
Convallaria majalis Lily of the Valley herb	*Rumex crispus* Yellow Dock root	**Urinary** *Piper methysticum* Kava root
Carthamus tinctorius Hong Hua Safflower herb	Seaweeds	*Commiphora myrrha* Myrrh gum

It is very interesting to practice detecting an herb's energetics before you are told what it is. Don't read the label. Don't check out your plant identification book. Don't worry what the experts say. Above all, don't be concerned if your evaluation doesn't match the official opinion. Try putting a couple of drops of a tincture or tea on your tongue and sit and meditate with it in a quiet space. Give it some time. Allow the sensations to come to you. Herbalist Lisa Ganora suggests using the "wolf snort." Ganora writes, "Rather than politely and delicately sniffing a plant or extract, smell it as a wolf or dog would: repeatedly puff air out of your nose (to vaporize the compounds with warmth) and draw the vapor cloud deeply back inside. . . ."[2] Similarly, when you taste a plant, chew the material thoroughly, moving it around in your mouth until you have fully experienced its character. Then just spit it out if you don't want to ingest it.

Note: If you do taste testing in the field, please rule out anything poisonous first, such as: Poison Ivy, Poison Oak, all plant parts of *Datura stramonium* (Jimson Weed), *Conium maculatum* (Poison Hemlock), or *Cicuta maculata* (Water Hemlock). In fact, no taste testing allowed whatsoever unless you are positive of identification or if you are with a pal who is in the know. Always work with an accurately identified and safe plant.

By doing these taste and smell exercises, you are learning to feel and detect the energetics for yourself before any book or authority tells you the answer.

- Smell: Do this first. Does it have a smell? What kind? Is it pleasant, neutral, or unpleasant? The perfumery industry calls fragrance notes the top, middle (heart), and base notes, referring to which scent is smelled first, second, and third. The top note is the first impression, the middle is the heart of the fragrance, and the base notes linger on.
- Taste: Is it sweet, sour, bitter, pungent, or salty? Is there more than one taste? Which predominates? What do you taste first, second, and last? What taste remains on the tongue?
- Temperature: Is it hot, warm, or cold? How does your body feel? Does it warm your core or make you shiver?
- Moisture: Is it wet, neutral, or dry? Is your tongue getting sticky and dry, or are you salivating?
- Direction: Does it go inward to your organs or disperse outward to your arms and legs? Does it go up or down?
- Qualities: Is it relaxing or energizing? Is it making you sleepy? Does it wake you up? Did it stop your cough? Lower or increase your pulse or breathing?

Summary

The way we classify, categorize, and arrange herbs is by their energetics. The Chinese speak of hot-cold, dry-damp, strong-weak, and their qualities, such as stimulating or relaxing. Westerners think more about actions—what an herb does. Understanding both will be helpful when building herbal formulas and making herbal choices.

The Three Primary Qualities or characteristics are taste, warmth, and moisture—basic concepts in Chinese and Ayurvedic systems. Sweet builds and restores. Sour draws inward and tightens. Bitter is cold, pulls down, and fights microorganisms. Salty dissolves lumps and drains downward. Pungent is warm, pushes outward, and can help circulation. A warm herb is used for cold; a cooling herb for warmth. Drying herbs dry damp conditions, and moisteners cool and lubricate a dry, hot condition.

The Six Secondary Qualities are stimulate-sedate, restore relax, and moisten-decongest. They denote actions. Stimulating makes an organ work harder. Sedating herbs are cooling. Restoring herbs are nutritive. Relaxants calm the nervous system. Moisteners add wetness, and decongestants break up thicknesses.

Tissue-Level Qualities are subdivisions of the Secondary Qualities: astringing-eliminating, solidifying-dissolving, and thickening-diluting. These are active and descriptive terms, categories discussed in Western herbalism. Astringents tighten and slow discharges or bleeding. Eliminating herbs remove substances from the body, such as stool (laxatives), urine (diuretics), or mucus (mucolytic expectorants). Solidifiers strengthen and make something harder. Dissolvents soften deposits and break up stones (litholytics). Thickeners restore (nourish). Dilutants thin blood (anticoagulants) or mucus (mucolytics).

Organoleptics refers to judging the potency, quality, and phytochemical composition of an herb or preparation by using the senses. It is the primary way herbs were understood over the centuries. If we can learn to do this for ourselves, our understanding and true ownership of a plant will increase.

Review

Fill in the Blanks

(Answers in Appendix B.)

1. The Three Primary Qualities are ___, ___, ___.
2. Fill in the taste. Cinnamon bark is ___. Kelp is ___. Goldenseal root is ___. Garlic bulb is ___. Tamarind is ___.
3. What are the Six Secondary Qualities? ___, ___, ___, ___, ___, and ___.
4. Name five superfoods ___, ___, ___, ___, ___.
5. Arrange these herbs in order from hot to cold. The Docks, Oregano, Goldenseal, Ginger, Water Hemlock, Barley.
6. What do dissolvents do? ___. For what would you use them? ___.
7. Name three types of dissolvents. ___, ___, ___.
8. Stimulating herbs treat ___conditions. Sedating herbs treat ___ conditions. Restoring herbs treat ___ conditions. Relaxing herbs treat ___conditions. Moistening herbs treat ___ conditions. Decongesting herbs treat ___ conditions.
9. Name a good laxative herb for a child. ___.
10. Give four conditions when a diuretic would be indicated. ___.

Critical Concept Questions

(Answers for you to decide.)

1. Why does the Western herbal tradition tend not to use energetics?
2. Give advantages and disadvantages of categorizing herbs by energetics versus symptoms.
3. Herbalists value restoratives and tonics. Why?
4. Why would having hot flashes be a yin deficiency?
5. What is the difference between wind heat and wind cold?
6. What is the difference between sedating and relaxing?

7. Why would a blood decongestant help dysmenorrhea?
8. When and why would an herbalist use a diaphoretic?
9. What are some conditions where a person would require solidifying herbs?

References

1. Dharmananda, Subhuti. *Taste and Action of Chinese Herbs: Traditional and Modern Viewpoints*. Institute for Traditional Medicine. http://www.itmonline.org/articles/taste_action/taste_action_herbs.htm (accessed October 7, 2019).
2. Ganora, Lisa. *Herbal Constituents: Foundations of Phytochemistry* (Louisville, CO: Herbalchem, 2009).
3. Hoffman, David. *Medical Herbalism: The Science and Practice of Herbal Medicine* (Rochester, Vermont: Healing Arts, 2003).
4. Holmes, Peter. *Energetics of Western Herbs* (Boulder, CO: Snow Lotus, 2007).
5. Holmes, Peter. *Jade Remedies: A Chinese Herbal Reference for the West* (Boulder, CO: Snow Lotus, 1996).
6. Mills, Simon. *The Essential Book of Herbal Medicine* (London, UK: Arkana, Penguin, 1991).
7. Beinfield, Harriet and Efrem Korngold. *Between Heaven and Earth: A Guide to Chinese Medicine* (New York: Ballantine, 1991).
8. Teeguarden, Ron. *Chinese Herbal Tonics* (Venice, CA: Cha Yuan, 1991).
9. Buhner, Stephen Harrod. *The Lost Language of Plants* (Chelsea, VT: Chelsea Green, 2002).

11 Basic Materia Medica

"The art of healing comes from nature and not from the physician. Therefore, the physician must start from nature with an open mind."

—Paracelsus

CHAPTER REVIEW

- Considerations for choosing herbs for a beginning apothecary.
- Materia Medica format.
- Basic monographs: includes all names, trigger words, family, part used, energetics, strength, key constituents, actions, indications, preparations and dose, side effects, contraindications, Commission E, and author's editorial.

KEY TERMS

5-Alpha reductase (5-AR)
Alterative
Anticoagulant
Antiemetics
Antilipemic
Antilithic
Antipruritic
Anxiolytic
Carminative
Cholagogue
Galactagogue
Hypnotic
Hypotensive
Materia Medica
Monographs
Mucolytic expectorant
Nervine
Paradoxical effect
Potentiation
Pruritus
Styptic
Vulnerary
Wort

A ***Materia Medica*** is an herbal list of medicinal plants that literally means the materials of medicine. This chapter provides a minimal Materia Medica, a collection of plants important to have in any apothecary. Most are Western, and some come from the Chinese and Ayurvedic traditions. All are easily obtainable commercially. Some, like Ginger root and Licorice root, are cultural crossovers used all over the world. Others are specific to a certain place, probably because the plant originally grew and was used there. A precise format is followed, providing thorough information for each botanical. These formats are called ***monographs*** and reflect current herbal usage. Because medical herbalism is an ever-changing field, herbal indications, dosages, and drug interactions may change as new research dictates. Always check with the latest reliable sources.

Who are *your* herbal allies? Choosing a Materia Medica is very personal. It's hard to leave favorites behind. Ask any herbalist, and you'll get a different list, because we all have our go-to herbs and complain bitterly if a beloved plant is left out. In the school I ran, lively discussions arose on which to choose.

You can't have them all. Through time and experience, you will begin to use certain herbs constantly, requiring frequent replacement, whereas others languish, forlorn and forgotten. That's when your true allies reveal themselves. It is best to begin with a classic variety that can cover all body systems and treat many common conditions. We can get esoteric and fancy, but perhaps 50 or so tinctures with their dry herbal counterparts are a decent starting point. You can always expand later on.

Considerations for Choosing a Materia Medica

- *Availability*. What can you purchase on the market or wildcraft? *Ephedra* Ma Huang is very hard to locate and purchase at this writing. Although still a fabulous herb, we will eliminate that one unless we can grow it ourselves.

- *Economics.* The *Ginseng* spp. are wonderful, precious herbs, but last time I checked, cultivated American ginseng root was over $100 for a quarter of a pound, which could price you right out of business. Fortunately, there are substitutes.
- *What grows where you live?* If you are wildcrafting, location is a factor. I love and use *Anemone pulsatilla* (Pasque flower) because it grows near my home in the Rockies. But there are many other herbs with similar therapeutic actions. If I lived in the East, I might choose *Betonica officinalis* (Wood Betony herb).
- *What is endangered?* I refuse to use Goldenseal root or Echinacea root, unless they have been properly and sustainably cultivated. Many other similarly used plants that are not endangered can fill in: Coptis Huang Lian (Goldthread root) could replace Goldenseal root, and perhaps Calendula flower or Lonicera Jin Yin Hua (Japanese Honeysuckle flower) could serve as substitutes for Echinacea root.
- *What is your personal favorite?* It goes without saying that if something calls to you, it is your medicine.

Tips for Learning Herbs

When learning about herbs, always give the part used along with its name. This information is important. Magnolia Xin Yi Hua, (Magnolia *bud)* is an upper respiratory nasal decongestant, whereas Magnolia Hou Po (Magnolia *root)* reduces colic and relaxes the middle burner in gastrointestinal (GI) conditions. Ginger is always used in root or root peel form, not leaf or flower. Also, say the botanical Latin name out loud, along with a plant's common name to help jog the memory. In the case of Chinese herbs, speak and practice the pinyin name and its pronunciation.

Materia Medica Format and Descriptions

The following provides an outline with their explanations of each aspect of our monographs.

- *Names, family, part used, growth, and harvest.* These are the demographics, which are the essentials for accurate plant identification, whether from a catalog or in the field.
- *Trigger words.* You will notice a section at the top of each monograph that lists *trigger words*, a few key phrases to jog your memory about that particular botanical. Examples of trigger words could be *broad-spectrum antibiotic*, or *phytoestrogen*, or for *liver qi stagnation*, or *clears heat*, or *antidepressant*. A trigger word is whatever helps you to remember the main uses for that herb. You can always add your own. Just keep them brief, or they won't trigger anything except confusion.
- *Energetics.* This aspect is important so that you can match the herbal energetics to the Chinese syndrome, Western medical diagnosis, or assessment findings (see Chapter 10). If an herb is moist and cool, it is used for a dry, hot condition, and so on.
- *Strength. Mild* means similar to a food with minimum toxicity. *Medium*-strength plants have some potential toxicity but are nothing to worry about if contraindications are followed. *Strong* herbs are toxic. There are *no* toxic herbs in this Materia Medica.
- *Key constituents.* A few are listed. Some herbal chemicals have not yet been identified. Constituents give important clues to a plant's action and solvent percentages to use in tincturing (see Chapter 7).
- *Actions.* These elements explain the mechanisms of action, how the herb works in the body, based on research or traditional usage. Actions are presented four ways: in Western herbal style, such as being a nervine or a vulnerary; in Western allopathic terms, such as antioxidant, antiinflammatory, or muscle relaxing; as Chinese Medicine actions, such as to dry damp, clear heat, or move blood; and as energetics, such as taste, temperature, or moisture.
- *Indications, syndromes, and disorders.* For what is an herb used? This may be presented by common Western signs and symptoms, such as to use for rhinitis, colic, pain, fatigue, or hypertension. Another is by actual diagnosis/disease names, as provided by a licensed medical doctor, doctor of osteopathic medicine, or chiropractor, such as diabetes, hypothyroidism, or multiple sclerosis. Another indication is by Chinese Medicine syndromes, such as External Wind Heat or Wind Damp Heat. Another is by Chinese herbal categories, as fire toxins, yin tonics, or blood tonics.
  - Alternating between traditions and various descriptions provides a multicultural understanding of the indications for each herb. It helps to match the right herb to the right person, based on findings from pulse and tongue assessment, history, and Western physical assessment (Chapter 15), so the best herbal choices can be made.
- *Dose.* Dosage is stated as either a single dose or a daily dose. It reflects the common amounts used per United States Pharmacopeia (USP), in Chinese Medicine, historical practice, or in contemporary practice. The dose assumes the herb is used as a simple. When botanicals are combined in formula, the dose could change. Dosage determination can take the synergy of herbs into account. When herbs work together, the toxicity of the plant is reduced, so more could be used. The combination of many herbs in a formula could, conversely, potentiate or enhance the effectiveness of a given plant, making a smaller dose necessary to do the same job.
- *Side effects.* Possible adverse reactions described in the literature, usually rare or mild. Anyone can be affected by any substance, including food. If an herbal combination is used in a formula, it's hard to know which is the culprit. In that case, elimination or an educated guess is necessary.
- *Contraindications.* These are the *absolute no-no's.* Don't use this for that.
- *Commission E.* Germany's Commission E publishes herbal indications, side effects, and contraindications, based on research studies. If a plant has not been studied, it is not mentioned by Commission E. When available, it can be useful information.
- *Editorial.* Author's tidbits, opinions, and comments.

Monographs

Actaea racemosa L. Sheng Ma (Black Cohosh root)

Trigger words. * **Muscle/nervous relaxant** * **PMS** * **Estrogenic** *
Botanical name. Actaea racemosa L. (formerly *Cimicifuga racemosa* L. Nutt) (Fig. 11.1)
Common name. Black Cohosh
Less common names. Black Snakeroot, Bugbane, Squawroot
Pinyin name. Sheng Ma
Family. Ranunculaceae (Buttercup)
Part used. Fresh or dried rhizome with attached roots

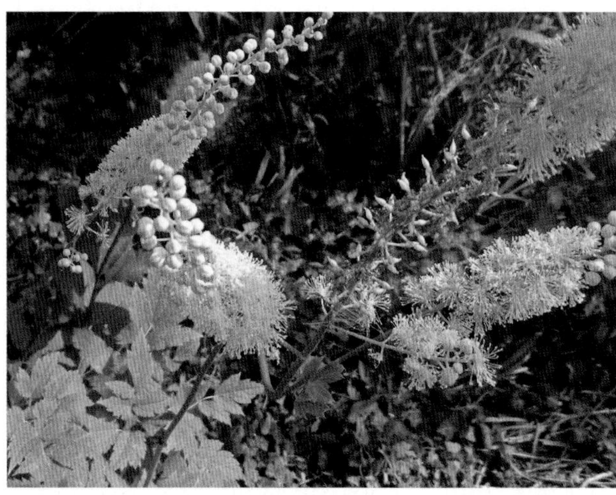

• **Fig. 11.1** *Actaea racemosa* (Black Cohosh root) is used as a muscle and nervous relaxant and for women's reproductive issues.

- *Growth and harvest.* White blossoms, feathery drooping racemes, and dry fruit with numerous seeds. Rhizome is a creeping underground stem with dark brown roots. Native to eastern North America, it is found in rich, shady woods ranging from Maine to Ontario and from Wisconsin south to Georgia and Missouri.
- *Energetics.* Bitter, slightly pungent, cool, dry, calming, and relaxing; uterine restorative.[1–5]
- *Strength.* Mild with minimum toxicity.
- *Key constituents.* Nearly 20 triterpene glycosides including cimicifugoside, aromatic acids, resins.[1–5] (Tincture with a high ethanol percentage of 65% to 85%, due to non–water-soluble triterpenes and resins.)
- *Actions.* (1) General muscle relaxant, spasmolytic, analgesic. (2) General nervous relaxant. (2) Reproduction: used historically and by Eclectics for women's health. Has been considered estrogenic. There are recent conflicting studies as to whether it actually binds to estrogen receptors. It may lower luteinizing hormone (LH) levels at the pituitary level, meaning it lowers progesteronic surges at ovulation, relatively increasing estrogen (a different mechanism of action accomplishing the same effect). (3) Protects against menopausal bone loss somewhat. (4) Improves menopausal mood swings. Does not enhance tumor growth in estrogen-dependent breast tumors, but high doses should be avoided in such cases to be safe.[4] (5) Antiinflammatory, antioxidant.
- *Indications, syndromes, and disorders.* (1) Muscles: menstrual cramps, dull muscle aches, as in arthritis (Wind Damp Heat), myalgia, sciatica. (2) Relaxant: for nervous tension, tinnitus, hypertension, palpitations, seizures. (3) Gynecological problems: irregular cycles, dysmenorrhea, PMS, and menopause. For empty heat (hot flashes).[2] (4) Psychological and physiological symptoms of perimenopause and menopause.
- *Dose.* Decoction: 6 to 12 g per dose. Tincture: 2 to 4 mL (1:5 60%) per dose.[1–5]
  Side effects. Gastric discomfort, frontal headache.
- *Contraindications.* (1) Preexisting liver disease, pregnancy (except to induce labor), and lactation.

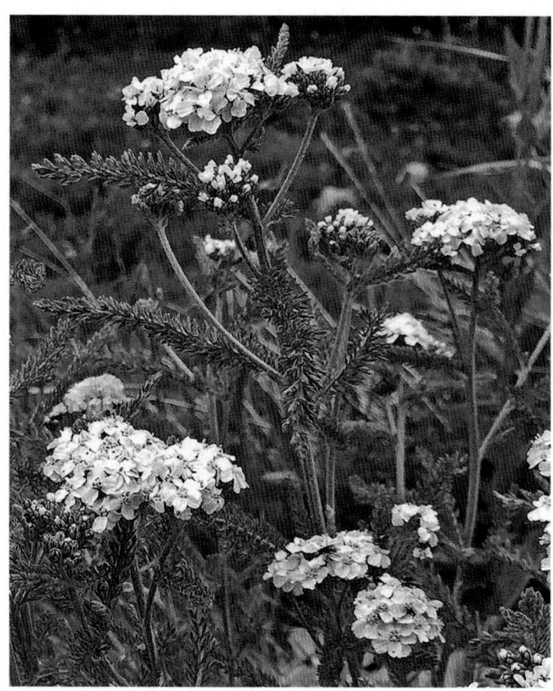

• **Fig. 11.2** Yarrow flowering. Highly aromatic *Achillea millefolium* herb is astringent, diaphoretic, and antiseptic.

- *Commission E.* PMS, dysmenorrhea, and menopausal vegetative ailments. Acteina, a constituent in Black Cohosh, has been studied for use in treating peripheral arterial disease.[6]

Editorial. Do not confuse Black Cohosh with *Caulophyllum thalictroides* (Blue Cohosh root), which is chiefly used for labor and delivery. Blue Cohosh is an indispensable go-to remedy for many women's conditions, sometimes used to induce labor, if begun 2 to 3 weeks before due date. Black Cohosh has become one of the largest-selling herbal dietary supplements in the United States (and in Germany under the name *Remifemin*) for reducing menopausal symptoms. It's especially nice for women who have accompanying cramps, muscle aches, and pains. Black Cohosh also combines well with St. John's Wort in PMS, when accompanied by anxiety and depression.

Native American women used it for menstrual problems, pregnancy, and childbirth; Eclectic John King lauded its properties in the 1840s when it was used routinely among nurses, midwives, and doctors for women's complaints and arthritic pain. The Eclectics also used it as a uterine tonic in the last few weeks of pregnancy, and it even turned up in Lydia Pinkham's famous *Vegetable Compound* of the era for menstrual stress. In Chinese Medicine, it is used completely differently than in the West. Here, Actaea Sheng Ma is used to vent rashes, especially in measles (being cooling and drying), to help with head pain (analgesic property), and to help raise spleen qi (improve digestion) when combined with Astragalus Huang Qi.

Achillea millefolium L. (Yarrow herb)

Trigger words. * **Astringent** * **Diaphoretic** * **Antiseptic** *
Botanical name. Achillea millefolium L. (Fig. 11.2)
Common name. Yarrow
Less common names. Milfoil, Thousand leaf, Nosebleed

Pinyin name. None.
Family. Asteraceae/Compositae/Daisy
Part used. Herb

- *Growth and harvest.* Highly aromatic perennial. Leaves alternate, gray-green, fernlike (*millefolium* means thousand-leafed). Many tiny flowers with white rays and yellowish disc in dense, flat-topped cluster. Habit: not picky. Grows from dry to moist soils, sun to shade, and montane to alpine. Yarrow is bred with yellow or pink flowers for gardeners, but it's not as good as the wild variety, having fewer essential oils. Use the good stuff.
- *Energetics.* Somewhat bitter, astringent, cool, dry, decongesting, restoring, stimulating, and relaxing.[4]
- *Strength.* Mild with minimal chronic toxicity.
- *Key constituents.* Many essential oils, including pinenes, ketones, azulene, eugenol; many alkaloids, 3% to 5% tannins, resins, flavonoids, phytosterols, phenolic acids (caffeic and salicylic among others), amino acids, fatty acids, coumarins, polysaccharides, saponins, sterols, sugars, chlorophyll, many minerals, and vitamin C. (Tincture in 55% to 70% ethanol due to vast array of ethanol soluble constituents, many not listed here.)
- *Actions.* Because of its enormous range of constituents, Yarrow does a lot. The list of descriptive terms: Diaphoretic, astringent, antispasmodic (gentle smooth-muscle relaxant), ***hypotensive*** (reduces blood pressure), antimicrobial, antiseptic, digestive bitter, hemostatic, hepatic stimulant; balances women's hormones and progesteronic.
- *Indications, syndromes and disorders.* (1) Wind Heat/Wind Cold, as a diaphoretic in a tea, for early-onset flu and colds, and for fevers. (2) Women: ally for hormonal imbalances (due to phytosterols). For progesterone deficiency, PMS with dysmenorrhea (it's spasmolytic), menopausal syndrome with flooding/bleeding (astringent), varicose veins, and hot flashes. (3) ***Vulnerary***. Tissue repair/wound healing: due to antiseptic, astringent nature for cuts, bruises, burns, scrapes, and pinkeye. (4) *Hemostatic/astringency* action for nose bleeds, menorrhagia, bleeding wounds, fibroid bleeding, varicose veins, diarrhea, discharges, and urinary incontinence. (5) *GI* as a digestive bitter, appetite stimulant, and for colitis, gastroenteritis, and irritable bowel syndrome.
- *Dose.* Tincture: 2 to 4 mL per dose. Infusion: 1 to 2 teaspoons dried herb per cup (best preparation to induce sweating). Swabs and compresses used for wounds or hemorrhage, along with frequent internal tincture use. Use in sitz baths. May juice fresh.
- *Side effects.* Might cause photosensitivity in prolonged high doses. Possible skin rashes due to sesquiterpene lactone content. Safe in lactation.
- *Contraindications.* Pregnancy; uterine stimulant.
- *Commission E.* Internally for loss of appetite and dyspeptic ailments, such as mild, spastic discomforts of the GI tract. Externally, as a sitz bath for painful, cramplike conditions of psychosomatic origin in the lower part of the female pelvis.[7]

Editorial. Yarrow is chemically rich with many uses. It got its name from the Greek hero, Achilles, who used it to treat his soldiers' wounds in battle because it conveniently grows everywhere. Its astringency, because of the alkaloid achilleine, shortens bleeding time.[8] Yarrow is a great addition to first-aid kits or to pick in the wild for use as a poultice. (If you can't find Yarrow, you might find some Plantain leaves for the same purpose.) Yarrow leaves can be rubbed on the skin as an insect repellent or diffused in a tea to rinse your hair.

Bupleurum chinensis de Candolle Chai Hu (Asian Buplever root)

Trigger words. * **Liver Protective/Tonic** * **Muscle relaxant** * **Chills/fever** * **Antiviral** *
Botanical name. *Bupleurum chinensis* de Candolle, *B. falcatum* L. (Fig. 11.3)
Common name. Asian Buplever root
Less Common name. Hare's ear
Pinyin name. Chai Hu
Family. Umbelliferae
Part used. Root

- *Growth and harvest.* Carrot family with compound umbels of small yellow flowers; leaves are alternate; leaf shape is long and thin, sometimes with parallel veins; grows up to 3 feet high.
- *Energetics.* Bitter, a bit pungent and astringent, cool, very dry, calming, relaxing, solidifying, and stabilizing.[4]
- *Strength.* Medium strength with some chronic toxicity.
- *Key constituents.* Triterpenoid saponins (many saikosaponins), phytosterols, pectin-like polysaccharides (bupleurans).
- *Actions.* (1) Liver antimicrobial, protector. (2) Nervous sedative, analgesic, and spasmolytic. (3) Clears heat: antipyretic, antiinfective, antiviral. (4) Pituitary/adrenocortical stimulant (helping the body to increase cortisol), making it antiinflammatory. (5) Immune stimulator and regulator. (6) Astringent.
- *Indications, syndromes, and disorders.* (1) Liver protector for acute and chronic infections (antiviral, antibacterial), fever, jaundice. (2) Other viral infections: colds and flu; to reduce fever; cooling, clears heat. (3) Nerve and muscle pain: because of its antiinflammatory, spasmolytic, sedative qualities. (4) GI and lung relaxant: dyspepsia, colic, irritable bowel syndrome, spasmodic coughing because of spasmolytic aspect. (5) Immediate allergies, urticaria, otitis media, immune regulation.

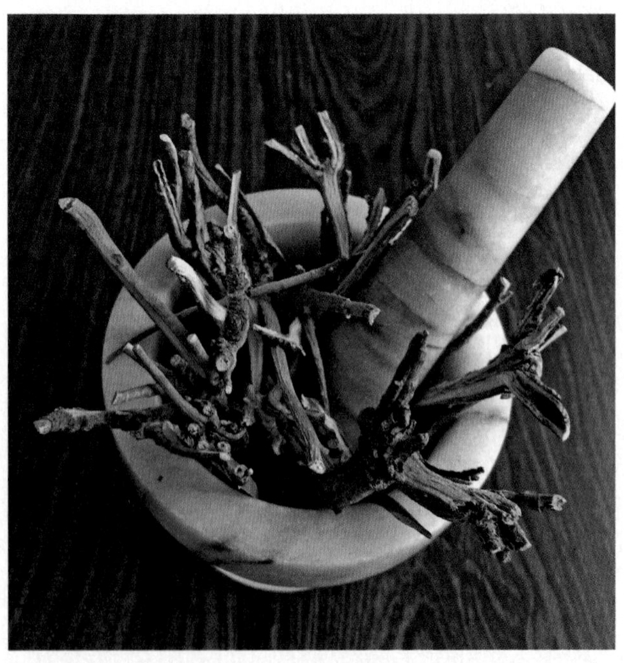

• **Fig. 11.3** *Bupleurum chinensis* Chai Hu (Asian Buplever root) is well-known as a liver tonic, antiviral, and a muscle relaxant.

(6) As an astringent for hemorrhoids, rectal or uterine prolapse, diarrhea.

- *Dose.* Decoction: 3 to 10 g. Tincture: 1 to 3.5 mL.
- *Side effects.* Infrequent nausea/vomiting. Safe in pregnancy and breastfeeding.
- *Contraindications.* None
- *Commission E.* Not listed.

Editorial. Bupleurum has many uses. A good go-to liver protective herb that nicely combines with Milk Thistle seed and Dandelion root. With regard to the liver, it can also be used as a protectant and antiviral in hepatitis. In that case, combine with Scutellaria Huang Qin (Baikal Skullcap root) and Turmeric root. For colds and flu, it not only fights infection and lowers fever but stimulates immune function. Last, it has the advantage of being a sedative-relaxant, helping muscle pain, spasms, inflammation, menstrual cramps, and headaches, and it is a nice choice in PMS for the woman who could always use some liver protection along with relief from her aches and pains.

One of the most widely researched Chinese herbal formulas is *Minor Bupleurum*, known in Japanese Kampo tradition as Sho-Saiko-To. This herbal combination has been used for over a thousand years and is probably the most popular herbal formula in Japan today. Although it contains herbs other than Bupleurum, it is used for many Chai Hu-sounding indications such as immune stimulation, treating acute and chronic hepatitis C, protection against radiation therapy, as an antiallergenic, for prolonged flu and colds, and for chronic digestive problems.

Crataegus spp. L. Shan Zha (Hawthorn berry)

Trigger words. * **Number one Western heart tonic** *
Botanical name. Crataegus oxyacantha L., *Crataegus pinnatifida* Bunge and others (Fig. 11.4).
Common names. Hawthorn berry, Asian Hawthorn berry
Less common names. Hedgethorn, Maybush, Haw, Redhaw
Pinyin name. Shan Zha
Family. Rosaceae (Rose)
Part used. The berry, flower, and leaf

- *Growth and harvest.* Deciduous, and usually thorny shrub or small tree up to 30 feet tall. Often grows as a hedge, especially in Germany, to divide plots of land. Native to Europe. Leaves are serrated or lobed. White flowers. Oval, dark red false fruits contain a small kernel, the true fruit.
- *Energetics.* Sweet/sour, astringent, neutral, dry, nourishing, restorative, dissolving.[4]
- *Strength.* Mild with minimum chronic toxicity
- *Key constituents.* Flavonoids, vitamin C, oligomeric procyanidins (OPCs), and crataegus acid, especially in the berries. Leaves contain the most OPCs, flowers the most flavonoids. (Tincture with medium ethanol percentages of 40%–45%.)
- *Actions.* (1) Cardiac: ***Antilipemic*** (reduces lipid levels), ***antilithic*** (breaks down mineral deposits), and ***anticoagulant*** (decreases blood clots). (2) Tonifies heart and blood qi. Increases force of heart contractions, decreases heart rate, increases coronary artery blood flow, reduces oxygen demand, mild hypotensive (reduces blood pressure), protects against heart damage and arrhythmias. (3) Digestion: improves digestion of fats and proteins, due to the sweet/sour taste.[4]
- *Indications, syndromes, and disorders.* (1) Cardiovascular: congestive heart failure, angina, tachycardia, atherosclerosis, Buerger's disease. (2) Chinese syndromes: Heart, Blood, and Qi Stagnation, Kidney Yin Deficiency with nerve excess. (3) GI: food stagnation.
- *Dose.* Infusion/decoction: 1.5 to 3.5 g per day. Tincture: (1:5) 7.5 to 15 mL per day.
- Extract: (1:2) 3 to 7 mL per day. Needs to be taken for at least 2 months for effect on heart conditions.
- *Side effects.* None, safely used continuously.
- *Contraindications.* None known. Not recommended during pregnancy and lactation due to potential uterine activity.
- *Commission E.* Indicated for weak heart, coronary artery circulatory disturbances, hypotension, and arteriosclerosis.[9]

Editorial. Hawthorn is *the* Western heart tonic. Hawthorn berry's actions, which increase force of heart contractions and decrease heart rate, are exactly what is needed for the treatment of congestive heart failure (CHF). This is the exact action of the drug digitalis, but in a milder and safer form. Combine Hawthorn with the stronger medium-strength Lily of the Valley herb, and you have an excellent early-onset CHF remedy.

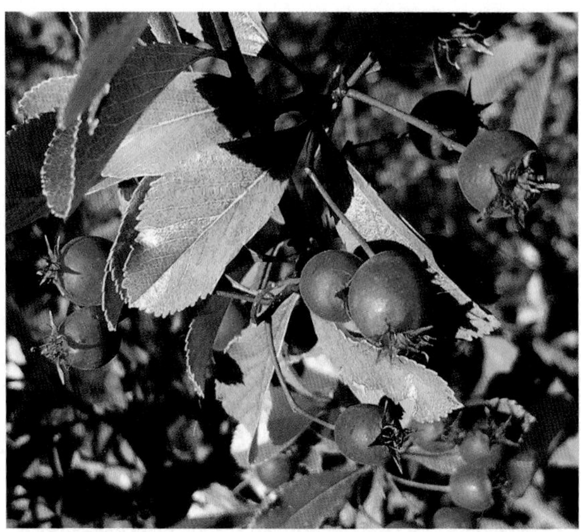

• **Fig. 11.4** *Crataegus* spp. (Hawthorn berry) is a superlative Western heart tonic.

Curcuma longa L. Jiang Huang (Turmeric root)

Trigger words. * **Antiinflammatory** * **Digestion** * **Alzheimer's** * **Insulin resistance** * **Bitter** *
Botanical name. Curcuma longa L. (Fig. 11.5)
Common Name. Turmeric root
Less common names. Wild Zedoary, Constrained Gold, Indian Saffron
Pinyin name. Jiang Huang
Family. Zingiberaceae
Part used. Root

- *Growth and harvest.* Perennial with tufted leaves, flowers trumpet-shaped, dull yellow and close to ground. Oblong rhizome yellow to yellow-orange in two parts; primary part egg-shaped, and many cylindrical secondary rhizomes.
- *Energetics.* Bitter, pungent, aromatic, warming and cooling potential. Stimulating, decongesting, calming, and dissolving.[1]
- *Strength.* Mild with minimal toxicity.
- *Key constituents.* Essential oils including cucumene, camphor, turmerol), and cucuminoids, the yellow pigments. (Tincture at 1:3 with 60%–70% ethanol.)
- *Actions.* (1) Supremely antiinflammatory, antioxidant. (2) Hypolipidemic: dissolves fatty deposits and tumors, and

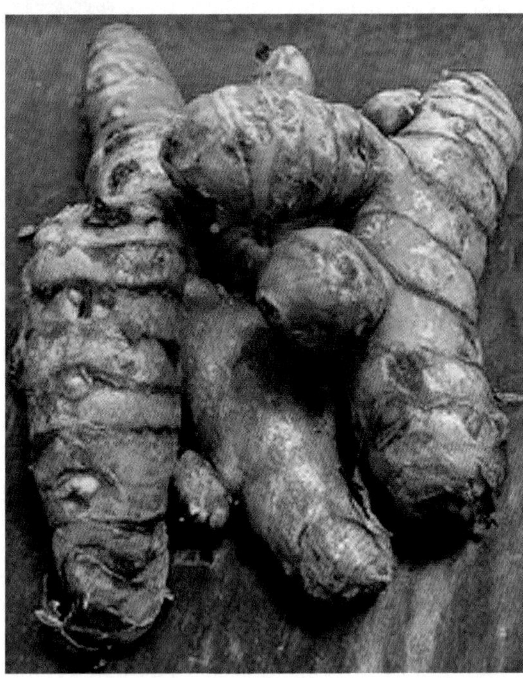

• **Fig. 11.5** *Curcuma longa* (Tumeric root) is warm, bitter, and pungent, often used for dementias and inflammatory conditions.

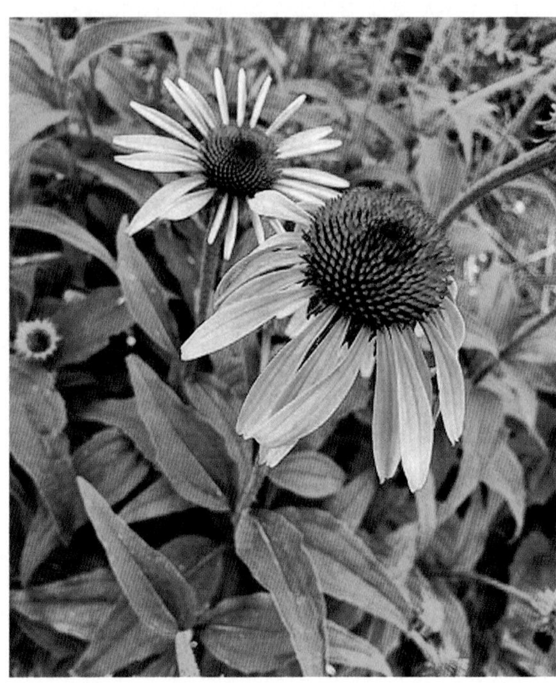

• **Fig. 11.6** *Echinacea purpurea* (Purple Coneflower) with its distinct purple rays and protruding orange-tipped brown flower cone is the species most people identify with Echinacea and the one most easily grown in the garden.

hemostatic. (3) ***Cholagogue***: stimulates bile flow from the liver. (4) Antifungal, antiviral. (5) ***Carminative***: stops nausea, helps digestion. (6) Vulnerary: protects many body tissues, i.e., neurological, cardiac, hepatic, blood vessels. (7) Radioprotective.

- *Indications, syndromes, and disorders*. (1) Neuro: protective and preventative for dementia and Alzheimer's, sedative for seizures. (2) GI: bitter taste helps digestion, bile flow, and constipation, IBS, insulin resistance. (3) Liver: valuable viral hepatitis remedy (Damp Heat), jaundice, gallstones, and Gallbladder and Stomach Qi Stagnation. (4) Cardiac: hyperlipidemia, angina, atherosclerosis. (5) Muscular-skeletal: arthritis, pain, inflammation. (6) Skin: chronic sores, ulcers, wounds, contusions, trauma (especially locally). (7) Bleeding: nose bleeds, coughing up blood, postpartum bleeding, and hematuria.
- *Dose*. Tincture: 2 to 5 mL per dose. Decoction: 5 to 15 g. Powdered: heaping teaspoon mixed with milk to form a slurry 2 times per day for good antiinflammatory effect.
- *Absorption*. Turmeric does not absorb well by itself. Take with *Piper nigrum* (Black Peppercorn). The piperine content increases absorption by 2000%.[10] Because Turmeric is fat soluble, it also needs a fat base. In Ayurvedic, it is traditionally taken in antiinflammatory Golden Milk (Chapter 18).
- *Side effects*. None if taken within dose. High doses may cause diarrhea because it stimulates bile flow. Safe in pregnancy and lactation. Used in India for morning sickness.[1–5] Caution in people with very hot constitutions because it may be too warm.
- *Contraindications*. Biliary tract obstruction.
- *Commission E*. Dyspepsia.

Editorial. Turmeric has long been used in Ayurvedic and Chinese Medicine, and it is now very popular in the West. It is classic in China for liver and gallbladder congestion and inflammation. Research has been done for its preventative action in Alzheimer's and other dementias, as well as for insulin resistance, due to its bitter taste. It was shown to suppress inflammation and beta amyloid plaque accumulation in the brain, which builds up in Alzheimer's.[11] In India, incidence of that disease is low because of the prevalence of Turmeric in curry dishes, a dietary staple. Eat more curry.

Echinacea spp. de Candolle (Echinacea root)

Trigger words. * **Antiinfective/clears toxic heat** * **Immunostimulant** * **Vulnerary** *

Botanical name. *Echinacea angustifolia* de Candolle, *E. Purpurea* Moench, *E. pallida* Nuttall (Figs. 11.6 and 11.7)

Common name. Purple Coneflower

Less common names. Comb Flower, Kansas Snake Root

Pinyin name. None.

Family. Asteraceae (Compositae or Daisy)

Part used. Usually the root, also the flower. (Root most common and considered stronger by many herbalists.)

- *Growth and harvest*. Thick hairy leaves, 1 to 3 feet tall. Seed head cone shaped. White, rose, or purple (*E. purpurea*), drooping ray florets.
- *Energetics*. Pungent, salty, cool, dry, stimulating, dissolving.[4]
- *Strength*. Mild with minimal chronic toxicity.
- *Key constituents*. Phytochemistry varies between species and plant parts. Roots: alkylamides, mostly isobutylamides (creates tingles in the mouth), mainly absent in *E. palladia*; Caffeic acid esters (not in *E. purpurea*). Cynarin (*E. angustifolia* only). Aerial parts: alkylamides, caffeic acid esters, flavonoids, and polysaccharides.[1–5] (Tincture with medium ethanol percentage of 45%–60%.)

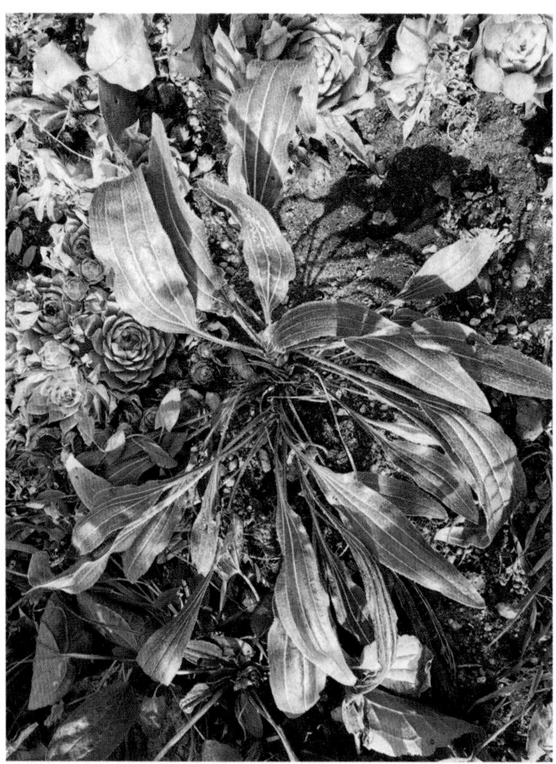

• **Fig. 11.7** *Echinacea angustifolia*, first-year plant in fall has narrow leaves with prominent veining.

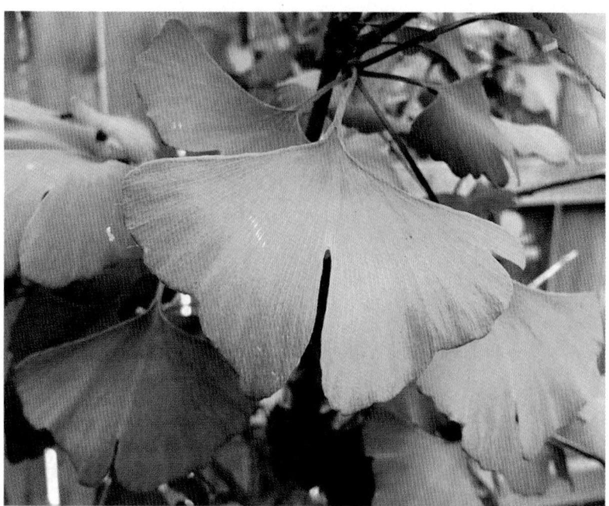

• **Fig. 11.8** *Ginkgo biloba* (Ginkgo leaf) is known for increasing brain microcirculation, repairing veins and capillaries, and decreasing venous clots in blood stagnation.

Tincturing is best done as a dual extraction to draw out all constituents.

- *Actions.* (1) Clears toxic heat, wind heat, damp heat. Antiviral, antibacterial. (2) Regulates immunity short-term, reduces allergy. Increases WBCs, T lymphocytes, and interferon production. (3) ***Alterative***: improves cellular nutrition and lymphatic drainage through detoxification, thereby helping skin conditions. (4) Vulnerary: excels in tissue repair, dissolves tumors. (5) Diaphoretic, causing fever reduction. (5) Binds to cannabinoid receptors.
- *Indications, syndromes, and disorders.* (1) Antimicrobial. For common cold, flu, and upper respiratory tract infections, if used immediately at onset, and for vaginal candidiasis. *E. angustifolia* species clears Streptococcal pharyngitis (Strep throat) when applied directly to infected area. (2) Adaptogenic-like. Immunomodulation. There is controversy regarding its use as a long-term adaptogenic. (3) Skin: damp heat of purulent wounds, abscesses, furuncles, indolent leg ulcers, and herpes simplex.
- *Dose.* Decoction: 1 g cut root several times daily. Tincture: 1:5 45% ethanol: 2 to 5 mL 3 times per day. Extract: 1:2 50% 2 to 4 mL per dose. My opinion is that Echinacea is not effective for long-term prevention of colds or flu and best for early onset of symptoms.
- *Side effects.* Rarely may cause dizziness, nausea, mild throat irritation, joint pain, or gastric upsets, because of its stimulating nature. (Add a little Peppermint or Ginger root in the formula to protect against nausea.)
- *Contraindications.* In principle: systemic diseases such as tuberculosis, leucosis, multiple sclerosis, AIDS, HIV infection, and other autoimmune diseases, and for those taking immunosuppressant medication. No restrictions known for pregnancy and lactation.
- *Caution.* May rarely cause contact dermatitis for those sensitized to plants from Compositae family.
- *Commission E.* Of the four *Echinacea* monographs published by Commission E, two are approved (*E. pallida* root and *E. purpurea* herb) and two are not yet approved because of lack of data.

Editorial. Echinacea was the most popular plant sold in the United States from 1995 to 1998. It is native to the Americas and was used by Native Americans and by Eclectic physicians in the late 1800s and early 1900s. There has been much debate in herbal circles as to which species, plant part, and preparation type does what, and which variety is best. The American Botanical Council (ABC) says there's enough research to support the safety and effectiveness of preparations made from both the aerial parts of *E. purpurea* and the roots of *E. pallida* and *E. purpurea*, and possibly, *E. angustifolia.*[12] The commercial price of *E. angustifolia* root far exceeds the cost of *E. purpurea* root. *E. pallida* is rarely offered in catalogs. Our precious *Echinacea* spp. is an endangered plant. Please use only cultivated varieties.

Ginkgo biloba L. Yin Xing Ye (Ginkgo leaf)

Trigger words. * **Neuroprotective** * **Enhances microcirculation** * **Alzheimer's/dementia** *

Botanical name. Ginkgo biloba L.

Common name. Ginkgo (Figs. 11.8 and 11.9)

Less common names. Maidenhair tree

Pinyin name. Yin Xing Ye (leaf), Yin Gao (nut)

Family. Ginkgoaceae (Ginkgo)

Part used. The leaf. In Chinese Medicine, the leaf and nut.

- *Growth and harvest.* Ginkgo is a gymnosperm (naked seeds like conifers and cycads) and has male and female flowers on separate trees. Tree grows to 100 m and can live for 1000 years. It is planted along many city streets. Leaves have fanlike shape with two distinct lobes (*biloba*). The naked seed or nut is oily and edible. Seed coat is bitter.
- *Energetics.* Sweet, bitter, astringent, neutral, dry, restoring, decongesting, relaxing, diluting, and astringing.[9]
- *Strength.* Medium strength with minimal chronic toxicity.

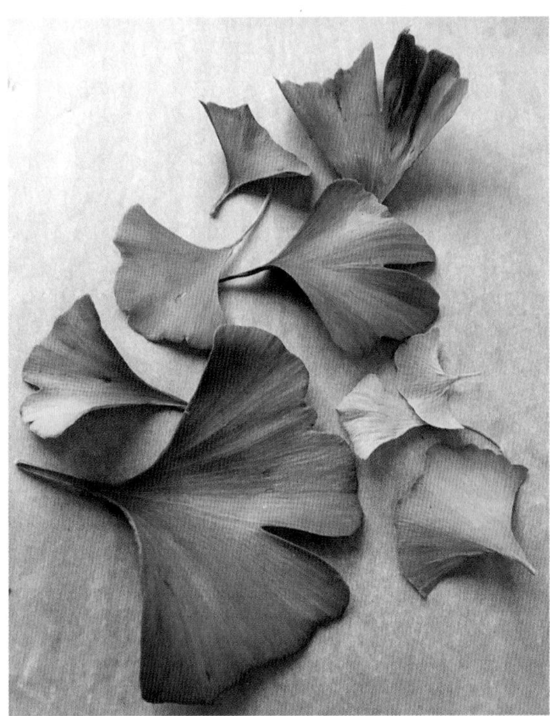

• **Fig. 11.9** Ginkgo leaves are collected for medicine when they start to turn in the fall.

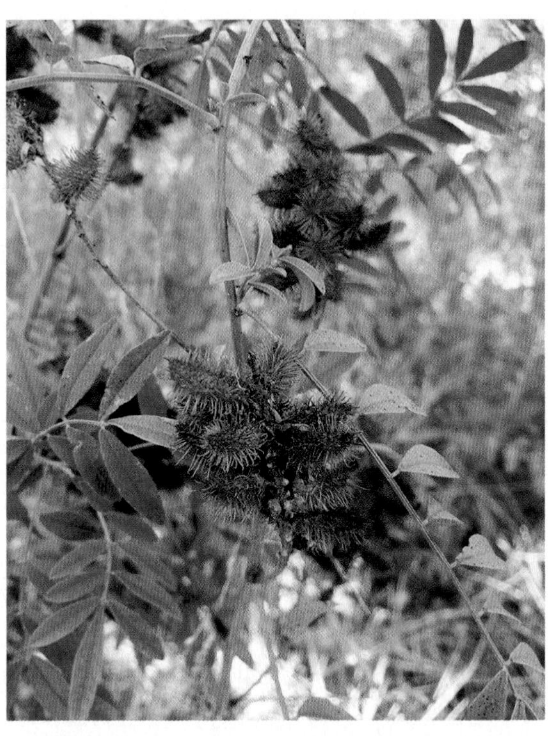

• **Fig. 11.10** *Glycyrrhiza lepidota* (Licorice root) grows in wet areas in Colorado. It is a native species, weaker medicinally than Chinese *G. uralensis* and European/Mediterranean *G. glabra*.

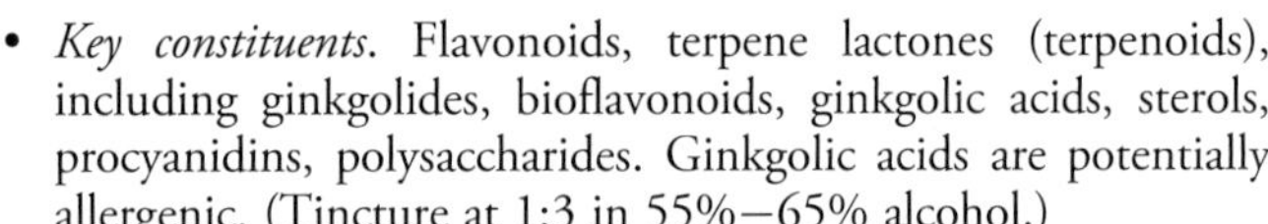

- *Key constituents.* Flavonoids, terpene lactones (terpenoids), including ginkgolides, bioflavonoids, ginkgolic acids, sterols, procyanidins, polysaccharides. Ginkgolic acids are potentially allergenic. (Tincture at 1:3 in 55%–65% alcohol.)
- *Actions.* (1) Antioxidant, and increases microcirculation, blood flow, and oxygenation, from any cause, at any site. Prevents free radical damage to cell mitochondria. (2) Strengthens veins and capillaries. (3) Enhances cognition and memory, due to platelet activating inhibiting factor (PAF) that decreases inflammation, helping in allergies, asthma, and migraines. (4) Neuroprotective. (5) ***Anxiolytic*** (action that reduces anxiety).
- *Indications, syndromes, and disorders.* (1) For any type of vascular disorder, mainly of the head, heart, eyes, and veins. (2) For restricted cerebral blood flow (Kidney Essence Deficiency), resulting in strokes, memory loss, decreased cognition, anxiety, depression, dizziness, tinnitus, vertigo, early stage dementia, Alzheimer's. (3) Eyes: macular degeneration, diabetic retinopathy. (4) For heart, to increase coronary and capillary circulation. (5) For Venous Blood Stagnation, as in varicose veins, phlebitis, and thrombosis. (6) High altitude sickness and radiation damage.
- *Dose.* Standardized extract: Leaf 120 to 240 mg containing 24% ginkgo flavone glycosides and about 6% terpenoids. Tincture: 2 to 5 mL per dose. Takes at least 6 weeks to kick in. Not to be used as a single herb (a simple) for longer than 2 to 3 months due to potential side effects of the ginkgolic acids. Best to use in formula.
- *Side effects.* ***Potentiation*** (creating a stronger effect when combined with the drug) of allopathic blood thinners seems to be overstated and not supported by clinical trials.[1–5] Some folks get mild side effects such as dizziness, headache, fatigue, chest discomfort, and GI nausea/vomiting. Leaves are safe during pregnancy and lactation.
- *Contraindications.* (1) Known hypersensitivity. (2) Ginkgo nuts: a uterine stimulant, not to be used in pregnancy.
- *Commission E.* For symptomatic dementia syndromes, including memory deficits, disturbances in concentration, depressive emotional condition, dizziness, tinnitus, and headache.[3]

Editorial. Ginkgo is an ancient 150-million-year-old tree that thrived with the dinosaurs. It hasn't changed much. Darwin called it a living fossil. The Chinese revered the tree and planted it around their temples and tombs to honor their ancestors. Traditionally in Chinese Medicine, the nuts were used. (The nuts have a cumulative toxicity.) Now they use the leaves as well. The green leaf, or yellow fall leaf, not the odiferous nut, is used today by most herbalists. It's an extremely versatile and useful plant in the modern Materia Medica.

Glycyrrhiza glabra or *G. uralensis* L. Gan Cao (Licorice root)

Trigger words. * **Ulcers** * **Adrenal/qi tonic** * **Expectorant** * **Hepatoprotective** * **Antiviral** *

Botanical names. Glycyrrhiza glabra L. (Western), *G. uralensis* (Chinese), and *G. inflata* (All three medicinally interchangeable) (Figs. 11.10 and 11.11).

Common name. Licorice

Less common names. Sweet Root, Black Sugar, Grandfather herb, Great harmonizer

Pinyin name. Gan Cao

Family. Fabaceae (Pea, formerly Leguminosae)

Part used. Root

- *Growth and harvest.* Perennial grows up to 150 cm tall. Thick rhizome with outside hard reddish-brown and inside yellowish.

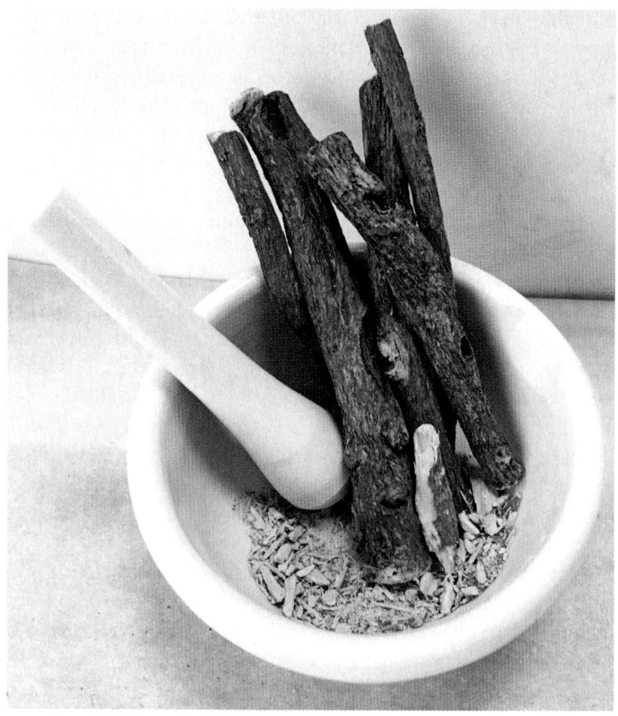

• **Fig. 11.11** *Glycyrrhiza uralensis* Gan Cao (Chinese Licorice root sticks) can be simmered to soften and suckled like a lollipop to relieve an inflamed throat.

Compound leaves; purple flowers have typical banner, wings and keel of pea family.

- *Energetics.* Very sweet, neutral, moist, restoring, calming, relaxing, and softening.[9]
- *Strength.* Mild with minimum chronic toxicity.
- *Key constituents.* Flavonoids, steroids, saponins including glycyrrhizin (the sweet taste), glucose, starch. (Most constituents are water soluble, so tincture at 1:3 proportion, with only 35%–40% ethanol.)
- *Actions.* (1) Antiinflammatory by potentiating the glucocorticoids and inhibiting production of the inflammatory prostaglandin E2. (2) ***Mucolytic expectorant*** (breaks up mucous and helps to cough it out). (3) Hepatoprotective. Chinese Medicine: Tonifies the Spleen (digestive qi), moistens the Lungs, benefits the qi, clears heat, and detoxifies fire poison.[1–5] (4) Supports adrenals and the hypothalamic-pituitary-adrenal axis (HPA axis). A qi tonic. (5) Phytoestrogenic. (6) Antiinfective and supports immunity. Inhibits viruses from creating pores to enter host cells.[13] (7) Anticarcinogenic.
- *Indications, syndromes, and disorders.* (1) GI: dyspepsia and duodenal and gastric ulcers, using the deglycyrrhizinated (DGL) form available as sublingual lozenges. (2) Liver: for chronic viral hepatitis and support. (3) Lungs: for dry coughing, wheezing, helps expectoration. (4) Adrenals: for adrenal fatigue, Addison's disease, tonifying qi. (5) Estrogen deficiency with PMS, menopause, dry skin, depression. (6) Infection: chronic hepatitis. (7) Inflammation: for arthritis, skin problems (dermatitis, eczema, ***Pruritus*** or itchy skin, cysts). (8) Allergies: for both immediate and autoimmune.
- *Dose.* Tincture: 1 to 3 mL of 1:2 per dose. Decoction: 2 to 4 g in 150 mL water, after meals 3 times daily. Deglycyrrhizinated (DGL) tablets: 380 mg DGL 4:1. For acute cases (gastric or duodenal ulcers): chew 2 to 4 tablets before each meal; for chronic cases: chew 1 to 2 tablets before meals.[14] Topical: Mouth ulcers. Washes: as a compress for local inflammations.
- *Side effects.* With very high continued dosage, possible mineralocorticoid excess syndrome with sodium and water retention, and potassium loss. (Therefore, have client supplement with potassium and have low sodium intake.) Possible hypertension with salt-sensitive individuals. Has estrogenic properties and excessive use as a simple can cause gynecomastia (enlarged breasts) in men. Not recommended during pregnancy; no known restrictions during lactation.
- *Contraindications.* (1) Hypertension: related to fluid retention, as in CHF, and edema or kidney-related high blood pressure. (This alludes to Licorice's aldosterone-like effect, which draws sodium and fluids into the bloodstream and pushes out potassium in the urine.) (2) Hyperglycemia: not for diabetics. (It's sweet; however, it will support pancreas and glucose metabolism in hypoglycemia.)
- *Commission E.* Indicated for catarrhs of the upper respiratory tract and gastric or duodenal ulcers.[14]

Editorial. The word *Licorice* is derived from the Greek, meaning *sweet root*, and is widely used in the West, Chinese Medicine, Ayurvedic, and Kampo traditions. In Chinese Medicine, Licorice enters all 12 meridians and is frequently used in formula for nutrient assimilation, sweetening, and harmonizing all the other herbs.

There has been extensive research into Licorice in the treatment of gastric and duodenal ulcers, especially in a concentrated extract with the constituent glycyrrhizin (GL) removed to 3%, because it was found to cause unwanted side effects. This modified form is known as DGL. It inhibits acid secretion and protects the mucosa against damage from gastric acid and bile. In addition, Licorice was found to inhibit 29 strains of *H. pylori*, the bacteria found to be the cause of 90% of duodenal and 80% of gastric ulcers.[1–5]

Most so-called Licorice candy in the United States is made with Anise essential oil, which smells and tastes like genuine Licorice extract. There is no therapeutic effect of Licorice candy in this form, just a lot of sugar. The genuine stuff comes from China and other countries. Licorice is a must-have in cough syrups and for laryngitis, because it moistens dry throat and bronchi.

Hydrastis canadensis L. (Goldenseal root) and *Coptis chinensis* Franchet Huang Lian (Goldthread root)

Trigger words. * **Antifungal** ***Antibacterial** * **Antiviral** * **Damp Heat** * **Cholagogue** *

Botanical name. Hydrastis canadensis L., *Coptis chinensis* Franchet (Fig. 11.12).

Common name. Goldenseal and Coptis

Less common names. Yellow Root, Indian Dye (Hydrastis), Goldthread (Coptis)

Pinyin name. Huang Lian (Coptis)

Family. Ranunculaceae (Buttercup)

Part used. Root and rhizome

- *Growth and harvest.* Goldenseal is native to eastern North America and cultivated in Washington, Oregon, and the Midwest. It favors rich, moist soil of shady woods. Perennial plant with a knotty yellow rhizome that arises from a single leaf with an erect, hairy stem. In spring it bears two five- to nine-lobed rounded leaves near the top, which is terminated

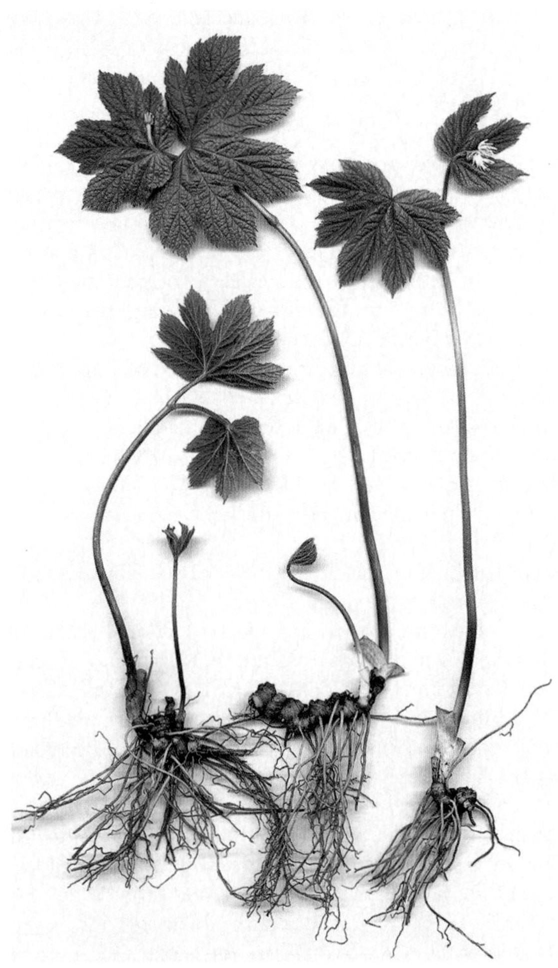

• **Fig. 11.12** *Hydrastis canadensis* (Goldenseal root) is an endangered plant. Substitute with other berberines such as *Coptis chinensis* Huang Lian or Oregon Grape root. (Copyright Lang/Tucker Photography. Photographs loaned with permission from *The Botanical Series* are copywritten by Jennifer Anne Tucker and Gerald Lang from the Studio at Hill Crystal Farm. www.jennifer-tucker.com.)

by a single greenish-white flower. Coptis grows in tree-shaded locales in the mountains of Central China.

- *Energetics*. Very bitter, astringent, cold, dry, decongesting, calming, stimulating, and restoring.[9]
- *Strength*. Medium strength with moderate chronic toxicity.
- *Key constituents*. Goldenseal: Alkaloids, including berberine 3.5% to 6%, hydrastine essential oils, resins, lipids, chlorogenic acid, potassium, sugar, and starch. Coptis: Alkaloids, including berberine 5% to 8%, coptisine, obakulactone, and trace minerals including selenium. (High alkaloid content of these herbs requires a 1:3 55% to 65% ethanol percentage in tinctures.)
- *Actions*. Numerous. (1) Foremost, stimulates activated protein kinase (AMPK), an enzyme inside cells that plays a protective role in diabetes, insulin resistance, cancer, mitochondrial dysfunction, obesity, neurodegeneration, and chronic inflammation, all of which lay the groundwork for chronic diseases.[15] (2) Broad-spectrum antimicrobial: clears damp heat. Interferes with adherence of bacteria to mucous membranes, particularly GI and respiratory tree. (3) Astringent quality dries up mucus, discharges, diarrhea, excessive sweating, and lessens bleeding. (4) Cholagogue quality increases bile flow and stimulates liver. (5) Antipyretic for lowering fever. (6) Immune stimulant. (7) Oxytocic, because it promotes labor and delivery. (8) Vulnerary, because it is an excellent mucous membrane tonic, heals wounds, and acts as an antiinflammatory by inhibiting cyclooxygenase-2 (COX 2), an enzyme that increases inflammation. (9) Cardiotonic, hypolipidemic, antiarrhythmic, and vasoconstrictive. (10) Antitumoral, because it inhibits actions of carcinogens and increases action of carcinogenic drugs. (11) Hypoglycemic and helps insulin resistance, as shown in a number of studies.[1–5]
- *Indications, syndromes, and disorders*. (1) Broad-spectrum antimicrobial for bacteria, virus (induces interferon), yeast, fungus, and amoebas. All acute, damp heat conditions of any body system. (2) GI: normalizes intestinal flora. Helps burning, pus, heat, chronic loose stool enteritis, gastric ulcers, dysentery, hemorrhoids, and any inflammatory bowel disorder, especially with bleeding, Crohn's, parasites, *candida*, and *giardia*. In diabetes type 2, normalizes blood sugar. (3) Eyes, ears, nose, throat: resolves sinus infections, nosebleeds, sties, and conjunctivitis. (4) Female pelvis: clears vaginal yeast, fibroids, ovarian cysts, endometriosis, menorrhagia with short cycles. (5) Skin: relieves itching, burning, acute dermatitis, allergic eczema, burns, boils, abscesses, breast pain and swelling, measles, chicken pox, and varicose veins. (6) Liver: for damp heat of gallstones, gallbladder infections, jaundice, hepatitis, and cholera.
- *Dose*. For short-term use. Small doses stimulate and warm the liver. Medium doses are mucostatic, decongestant, antiseptic, and antiinflammatory. Large doses are stimulating and cooling.[9] Tincture: 1:3 proportion 2 to 5 mL per day; 1:5 proportion 3.5 to 8 mL per day.
  - For the alkaloids to be truly effective, they must come in direct contact with the mucous membranes. Very effective for internal GI use. Topical use is excellent, because the alkaloids touch the infected tissue.[13] May be used as a compress, eyewash, douche, or vaginal suppository. If using as an eyewash, make very sure *all* the marc is strained out, so it does not irritate and burn the eyeballs.
- *Side effects*. May deplete intestinal flora with long-term use. Always supplement with probiotics or miso soup or fermented veggies. Large amounts can cause diarrhea because of its cholagogue effect.
- *Contraindications*. (1) Pregnancy, a uterine stimulant. Not for breast feeding. Not for jaundiced infants. (2) Goldenseal may cause hypertension due to vasoconstriction. (3) Coptis Huang Lian and Goldenseal are for short-term acute use only for the earlier stated and other reasons. Overdose can cause kidney and liver damage. (4) Because the berberine herbs are drying, they are not for yin deficiency. We don't need to add more dryness to an already dry constitution. If person is yin deficient, balance out the formula with a demulcent, such as Marshmallow root or Comfrey root.
- *Commission E*. There is no monograph for Goldenseal. In the Commission's opinion, there is no evidence for the benefit of the herb, and there are risks involved. However, it was safely used by the Eclectics and has a long history of use in the United States by Native Americans. It is official in the National Formulary USP 26-NF 21 2003, as well as on the UK General Sale List.

Editorial. There are at least five major plants from the East and West containing the cold, yellow berberine alkaloid. All are anti-infective. Medium strength Goldenseal root and Coptis Huang Lian (Goldthread root) belong to the Buttercup family. Phellodendron Huang Bai (Siberian Cork Tree bark) hails from the Rutaceae/Rue family. Oregon Grape root and Barberry root of the Berberidaceae family are milder remedies.

All of the mentioned berberines are very good for infection and are used to clear damp heat. Goldenseal is popular but is an endangered, overharvested, and expensive American plant, whereas Chinese Coptis Huang Lian (Goldthread root) is plentiful, much less costly, and easily available from Chinese pharmacies and herb companies. The two are therapeutically interchangeable, although Coptis contains slightly more berberine and is a bit stronger. Western Oregon Grape and Barberry are very effective, easy to purchase or harvest, and are not endangered. Of course, if you care to obtain cultivated Goldenseal for a high price, feel free.

Hypericum perforatum L. (St. John's Wort)

Trigger words. * **Mild to moderate depression** * **Neuralgia** ***Antiviral** * **Nervine** *

Botanical name. Hypericum perforatum L. (Fig. 11.13)

Common name. St. John's Wort, St. Joan's Wort

Less common names. Witches' herb, Klamath weed

Pinyin name. None

Family. Hypericaceae

Part used. Herb, especially the aerial flowering parts

- *Growth and harvest.* Opposite, oblong, paired leaves, yellow flowers with five petals and many stamens. Whitish glandular oil dots visible on leaf undersides. It is considered an invasive species according to the U.S. Department of Agriculture, crowding out native plants. It grows in disturbed ground, roadsides, and meadows. That said, St. John's Wort is a valuable herb, well worth gathering fresh. Harvest when the flowers are in bud or full. Best used fresh.
- *Energetics.* Somewhat bitter, sweet, astringent, cool, dry, relaxing, restoring, stimulating.

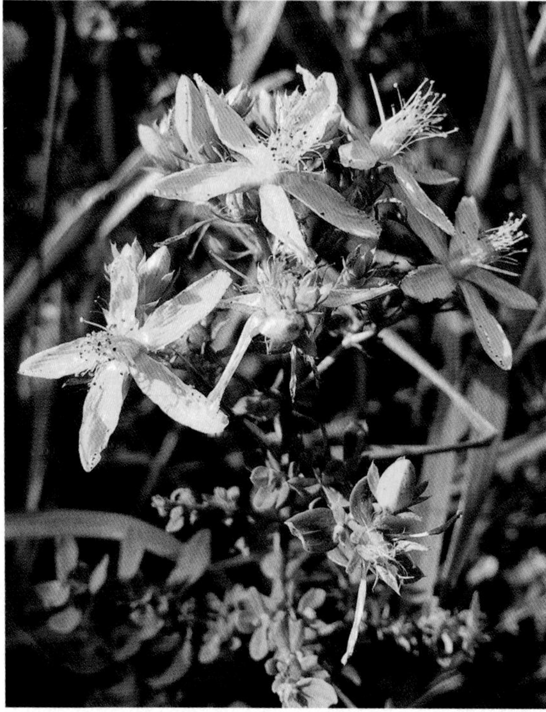

• **Fig. 11.13** A beautiful *Hypericum perforatum* (St. John's Wort) flowering top. This is the perfect stage for wildcrafting.

- *Strength.* Mild with minimal chronic toxicity.
- *Key constituents.* Many volatile essential oils, red dianthrones (plant was named for red colored hypericin and pseudohypericin), and flavonoids including rutin, resins, carotenoids, pectin, hyperforin. (Tincture with medium ethanol percentages of 50%–75%.)
- *Actions.* There are many qualities: (1) Antiinflammatory, analgesic (blocks qi stagnation), astringent, vulnerary, ***nervine*** (affects the nervous system). (2) Antimicrobial, due to presence of hyperforin. Antiviral, antifungal, antibacterial for damp heat. (3) Antidepressant exact mechanism of action is not definitively determined. Over the years, it was thought to be a MAO inhibitor, a tricyclic antidepressant, and then a serotonin-reuptake inhibitor (SSRI), as found in the popular drugs Prozac and Zoloft. These categories are all drug classifications for antidepressants.
- *Indications, syndromes, and disorders.* (1) Neuralgic for nerve pain, including from injury, sciatica, shingles, herpes, and fibromyalgia. (2) Mild to moderate depression. Safe alternative to pharmaceuticals.[1–5] (3) All damp heat-type viral infections, including *Herpes simplex 1* (cold sores), *Herpes simplex 2* (genital herpes), *Varicella zoster* (chickenpox) and *Herpes zoster* (shingles). Other damp heat afflictions include cystitis, dysentery, intestinal parasites, dermatitis. (4) Important topically in creams/lotions/poultices. Used for antiviral, vulnerary effects (blocks qi stagnation) because of its cooling and antiinflammatory traits. Brings down swelling and burning in bites and stings, burns, ulcers, sores, sunstroke, bruises, breast lumps, and engorgement. (5) Astringency makes it useful for bed wetting, hemorrhage, and discharges. (6) Its nervine, *anxiolytic* (antianxiety), sedative, and ***hypnotic*** (an herb that cause drowsiness) activity is due to the hypericin. Helps anxiety and irritability, especially in menopause.
- *Single dose.* Tincture: 2 to 4 mL 3 times per day in a 1:5 40% solution. Infusion: 1 to 2 teaspoons dried herb to 1 cup boiling water. Standardized: 3% to 5% hyperforin extract is 300 mg 3 times per day. Takes about 4 to 8 weeks to kick in if treating for depression. Gentle and good for children and the elderly.
- *Side effects.* Rare photosensitization in doses exceeding normal range. Avoid excessive sunlight or UVA light exposure in fair-skinned individuals taking high doses. Rare increased sensitivity to heat, cold, and pain in the hands and feet. Safe for pregnancy and lactation.
- *Contraindications.* (1) Not for psychosis or severe depression. (2) Not with use of other photosensitizing drugs. (3) Increases liver's cytochrome P450 detoxification system, resulting in increased breakdown and/or reduced intestinal uptake of some drugs.
- *Commission E.* For psychovegetative (psychoautonomic) disturbances, depressive moods, anxiety, and nervous unrest. Use oil preparations externally for contusions, myalgia, and first-degree burns; use internally for dyspepsia.[16]

Editorial. Named for the fresh herb's association with blood and the distinctive bright-red dye from the hypericum that appears on the knife and cutting board when chopping up or crushing the fresh plant. It's gorgeous. Never mind that said blood refers to John the Baptist's severed head (St. John). ***Wort*** is the Old English name for herb or plant. As far as I'm concerned, the fresh wort provides best results.

Shingles is a viral *Herpes zoster* infection that causes horrible numbness, tingling, and burning nerve pain affecting nerve roots. St. John's Wort is the perfect remedy for this common affliction (Chapter 25). It's a common, essential ingredient in first-aid creams and poultices for all damp heat conditions, especially viral.

St. John's Wort takes 4 to 8 weeks to work for depression, so combine with fast-acting Rhodiola root plus other nervines such as Passionflower, Melissa, Milky Oat, or Skullcap herb. St. John's Wort has been described as "nature's Prozac," and is given allopathically as an adjunct to antidepressant drugs in stubborn cases. The old paranoia about combining the herb with antidepressant drugs no longer applies. However, if a client wants to stop use of selective SSRIs, wean off slowly with permission of a physician while gradually increasing the St. John's Wort dosage.

Mentha x piperita L. (Peppermint leaf) and *M. arvensis* L. Bo He (Field Mint herb)

Trigger words. * **Wind Heat/Wind Cold** * **Carminative** * **Antimicrobial** * **Diaphoretic** * **Spasmolytic** *

Botanical name. Mentha x piperita L., *M. arvensis* L. (Figs 11.14 and 11.15)

Common name. Peppermint, Field Mint, Poléo Mint

Less common names. Menthe

Pinyin name. Bo He *Mentha arvensis* L. (Asian Field Mint herb)

Family. Lamiaceae/Labiatae (Mint)

Part used. The leaf

- *Growth and harvest.* Mint family plant with characteristic square stem and opposite leaves. Flower spike is pinkish mauve with numerous congested whorls. Leaves are rough textured, lighter on underside. Has pungent peppermint scent. Easily grown and spreads like crazy.
- *Energetics.* Pungent, somewhat sweet, aromatic, warm with potential secondary cooling effect, dry, stimulating, dispersing, restoring, and relaxing.[9]
- *Strength.* Medium strength with mild chronic toxicity.
- *Key constituents.* Essential oils including menthol, menthyl acetate, terpenes, azulene, limonene, tannin, flavonoids, carotenoids, rosmarinic acid, and resins. (Tincture at 1:4 in 60%–90% ethanol, because of its high volatile essential oil content that is not water soluble.)
- *Actions.* (1) Seemingly contradictory warming and cooling energetics. (2) Warming: its pungency creates warming by stimulating arterial circulation. (3) Cooling: when taken internally in a large dose of hot tea, it has a diaphoretic effect that causes sweating and cooling, making it antipyretic. (4) Carminative: stimulating to the GI, to help old-fashioned tummy aches or nausea/vomiting when we overeat. (5) Spasmolytic: thereby helping GI, Liver, and uterine cramping. (6) Drying: Peppermint essential oil can dry up breast milk. (7) Stimulating: to liver, bladder, stomach, pancreas, and nervous/cardiovascular system. (8) Antimicrobial: antibacterial, antifungal. (9) Local analgesic, antiseptic, ***antipruritic*** (inhibits itching).
- *Indications, syndromes, and disorders.* (1) GI and Liver: carminative and spasmolytic action for nausea/vomiting, dyspepsia, flatulence, colic, Stomach Qi Stagnation, irritable bowel syndrome, and gallstone spasms. (2) Respiratory: for bronchitis, cough, wind heat, wind cold onset colds and flu. (3) Neuro: for headaches and nervous disorders, migraines. (4) Menses: for spasmodic dysmenorrhea. (5) Topically: for arthritic pain, burns, acne, boils, bug bites, poison ivy, and eczema. (6) Insect repellent: for mosquitos, gnats, and ants.
- *Dose.* Infusion: 3 to 7 g per dose of dried leaf. Tincture: 1 to 3 mL per dose. Essential oil: 1 to 2 drops in gel cap with olive oil. Topical essential oil: massage Peppermint mixed in a carrier oil. Steams: 1 to 3 drops essential oil or 2 teaspoons dried herb to a pot of water. Topical compresses: Make up a strong tea for compresses or liniments for arthritis, neuralgia, skin inflammation, itching.

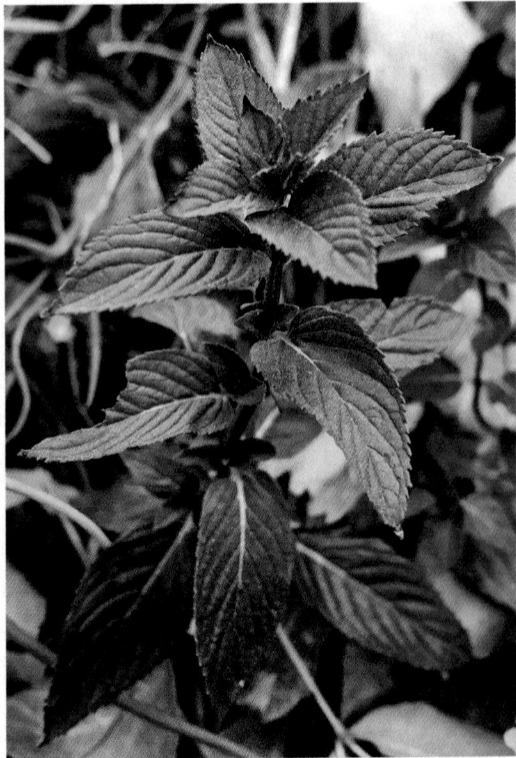

• **Fig. 11.14** Pungent and aromatic *Mentha x piperita* (Peppermint leaf) pictured in the fall. It opens the airway when used in a steam.

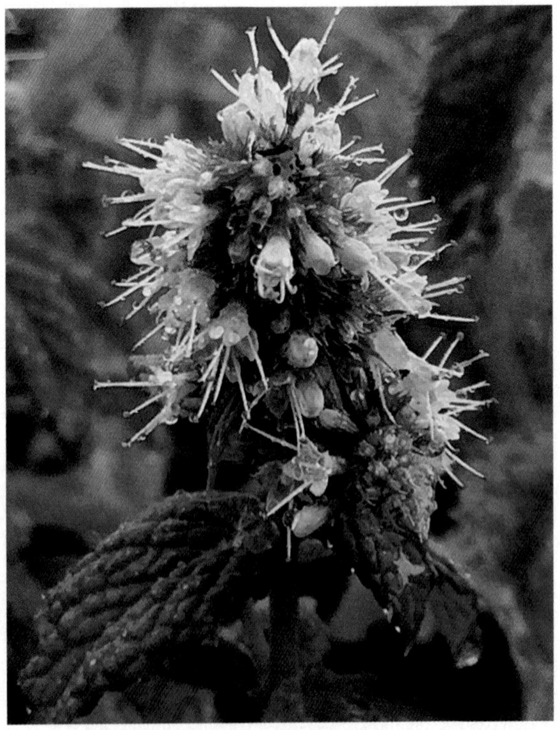

• **Fig. 11.15** *Mentha* spp. (Mint) has tiny lavender flowers arranged in compact whorls from middle to upper leaf axils.

- *Side effects.* Essential oil on children could cause burning, so test site first. Oral intake of the oil can cause heartburn. Dilute in capsules or use enteric coated.
- *Contraindications.* (1) Yin deficient dry conditions. (2) Gastric hyperacidity and esophageal reflex because it is a GI stimulant. (3) Essential oil in nursing because it could dry up milk production. (4) Large continued doses in those prone to epilepsy may bring on a seizure (even the tea). (5) In babies, do not use essential oil on face or around nose or chest, because it could cause laryngeal and bronchial spasms.[1–5]
- *Commission E.* Use Peppermint leaf for GI, gallbladder, and biliary tract cramping. Essential oil internally for spastic discomfort of GI tract, gallbladder, and biliary tract. Essential oil externally for myalgia and neuralgia.

Editorial. Peppermint is a perennial aromatic herb that is a natural hybrid of *Mentha aquatica* L. (Water Mint) and *M. spicata* L. (Spearmint).[17] Hence, the *x* in *Mentha x piperita*, means a cross between the two. Peppermint is a medium-strength herb, whereas its cousin, Spearmint, is a milder remedy that also causes sweating and lowers fever, settles the stomach, and is useful for respiratory infections. It works well in a steam.

Versatile Peppermint leaf is a convenient herb to keep in the kitchen cabinet for easy access, when you are feeling "iffy" and have no energy, or lack the mental capacity to even think about a complicated remedy. It's a useful herb in cough syrups. As a steam, it opens the airway (combine with Eucalyptus essential oil). Use as a tea if coming down with a cold. If the essential oil is placed on a cotton ball, it will repel ants and also smell divine. Just put it where you don't want them to be and watch those ants march away, vacating the premises.

Serenoa serrulata L. (Saw Palmetto berry)

Trigger words. * **Male tonic** * **Reproductive restorative** * **BPH** * **Anabolic** *

Botanical name. Serenoa serrulata L. (Fig. 11.16)

Common name. Saw Palmetto berry

Less common names. Dwarf palm, Sabal berry

Pinyin name. None.

Family. Palmaceae

Part used. Ripe, dried fruit

- *Growth and harvest.* A small, low-growing palm tree, native to southeastern North America, particularly Florida.
- *Energetics.* Somewhat sweet, oily, moist, warm, astringent, restorative, pungent, and stimulating.
- *Strength.* Mild with minimum chronic toxicity.
- *Key constituents.* Fatty oil with fatty acids (FAs), esters, phytosterols, and polysaccharides. (Tincture at 1:3 with 60%–80% high ethanol content because of the large amount of non-water-soluble FA constituents.)
- *Actions.* (1) Diuretic, antiinflammatory, antiandrogenic. (2) Urinary: antiseptic and shrinks prostate in benign prostatic hypertrophy (BPH) and for that reason is standardized into an extract of its liposterolic content. Mechanism of action for BPH is as follows: Testosterone is a major male hormonal androgen that enhances prostate cell growth. ***5-Alpha-reductase (5-AR)*** is the enzyme that converts testosterone to the more potent dihydrotestosterone (DHT). Saw Palmetto berry inhibits 5-AR in prostate tissue, slowing down growth, in the same way that the prostate drug Proscar does.[1–5] (3) Reproduction: helps conception, lactation, and libido. Nourishes male and female reproductive organs. (4) Anabolic, in that it builds muscle mass and helps nutrient absorption, the best herb for this in Western herbalism.

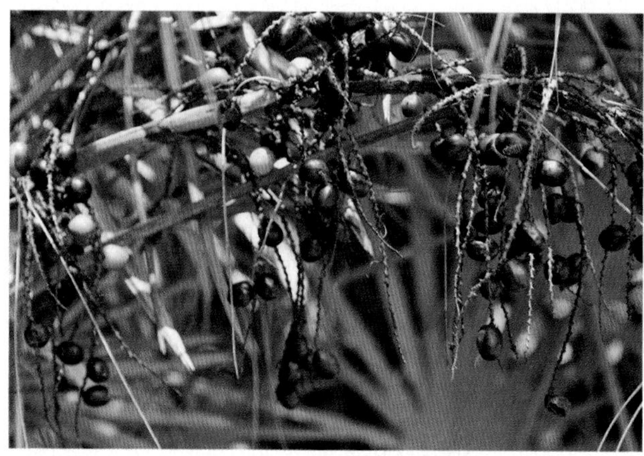

• **Fig. 11.16** *Serenoa serrulata* (Ripe Saw Palmetto berry) with large palmate, fan-shaped leaf in background. A reproductive restorative for men and women. (iStock.com/credit: NoDerog.)

- *Indications, syndromes, and disorders.* (1) Kidney Yang deficiency. Men: for BPH, urinary leakage/irritation, weight loss, decreased libido, and decreased muscle density. Women: for polycystic ovaries that exhibit with excess androgenic hormonal symptoms, such as facial hair (hirsutism), infertility, acne, and amenorrhea.
- *Dose.* Extract: (1:2 45%) 1 to 3 mL per dose. Decoction: 4 to 8 g per cup. Suppositories: for prostate conditions 2 times per day. Standardized: Fatty acids 160 mg 2 times per day.
- *Side effects.* In rare cases, stomach problems.
- *Contraindications.* None known.
- *Commission E.* Antiandrogenic and antiexudative activity. Relieves the symptoms associated with an enlarged prostate without reducing the enlargement. (This will most likely change, because new data indicates Saw Palmetto also shrinks prostate size.)

Editorial. Saw Palmetto berry has a long history of European and American use for BPH. It was an official drug, listed in two editions of the USP from 1906 to 1916, and in the *National Formulary* from 1926 to 1950. BPH use is supported by many studies. A good herb to combine with Saw Palmetto berry for this purpose is Nettle root. The Eclectics used Saw Palmetto for upper and lower respiratory tract problems, prostatic irritation, and enlarged gonads.

Silybum marianum Gaertner (Milk Thistle seed)

Trigger words. * **Hepatoprotective** * **Hepatic tropho-restorative** * **Antioxidant** *

Botanical name. Silybum marianum Gaertner or *Carduus marianus* L. (botanical synonyms) (Fig. 11.17)

Common name. Milk Thistle

Less common names. St. Mary's Thistle, Lady's Thistle, Lady's Milk

Pinyin name. None

Family. Asteraceae (Compositae, Daisy)

Part used. Fruit/seed

- *Growth and harvest.* Native to Mediterranean but naturalized throughout North America. Likes dry, rocky ground with full sun. A biennial thistle (same tribe as the Globe Artichoke)

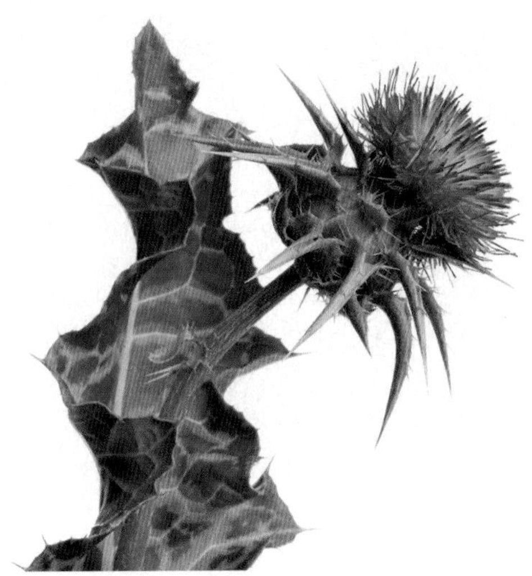

• **Fig. 11.17** Notice that *Silybum marianum* (Milk Thistle seed) has distinctive milky-veined leaves, unlike many other purple-flowered thistles. (iStock.com/credit: vencavolrab.)

with dark green, oblong leaves with spiny margins. White veins give leaves a mottled look. Flower heads are deep violet and spiny and sit above spiny bracts.

- *Energetics*. Pungent, bitter, warm, dry, situating, restoring, dissolving, and softening.[9]
- *Strength*. Mild with minimum toxicity.
- *Key constituents*. Many flavolignins including silibinin, silydianin, and silychristin, which are collectively known as *silymarin*, fixed oils consisting of flavonoids, taxifolin and sterols. The fixed oils can give a milky color in liquid extracts and could separate out or precipitate.[1–5] (Tincture at 1:3 65%–75% high ethanol, because of its many alcohol-soluble oils and sterols.)
- *Actions*. (1) Milk Thistle has been widely studied and established as a hepatoprotective and first-class liver restorative. (2) Constituent silymarin reduces cellular damage in the liver caused from oxidative stress because it activates glutathione and superoxide dismutase (SOD), both powerful cell antioxidants. (3) Detoxifies by reducing cytochrome P450 liver enzymes (Chapter 19). Showed good survival rate when given IV after Death Cap mushroom poisoning. (4) Protects liver by inhibition of inflammatory leukotrienes in Kupffer cells. Inhibits inflammatory cell proliferation in hepatitis C and lessens scarring in cirrhosis. (5) Protective effect in pancreatic cells for diabetes type 1 and type 2.[1–5]
- *Indications, syndromes, and disorders*. (1) For Liver Qi Stagnation with cold, jaundice, and many liver conditions, such as acute and chronic hepatitis. Protective against ethanol ingestion, fetal alcohol syndrome, alcoholic and nonalcoholic liver disease, cirrhosis, esophageal varices, and fatty liver. (2) Environmental exposure to chemicals and solvents, paints, glues, and anesthesia. (3) Adjunct therapy in cancer to protect liver cells from chemotherapy. (4) Put in any formula if person requires liver detoxification. (That could be almost everyone.)
- *Dose*. Decoction: 8 to 14 g per cup. Liquid extract: 2 to 4 mL per dose of 1:2 proportion. Tincture: 3 to 4 mL 3 times per day of a 1:3 to 1:5 proportion. Standardized extract dose is 3 to 4 tablets per day containing 140 mg silymarin.
- *Side effects*. Milk Thistle is a very safe herb with no side effects. Safe in pregnancy and lactation.
- *Contraindications*. None except for known allergies to any of its constituents or to any other plants of the Compositae/Asteraceae (Daisy) family.
- *Commission E*. For dyspeptic disorders (crude herb), supportive for toxic liver damage and cirrhosis in *formulation*, meaning the extract standardized to at least 70% to 80% silymarin.

Editorial. This plant has the best reputation in the West as an all-around liver remedy. It restores and protects liver cells, as well as stimulating the liver to do its work. It is a definite choice for any liver disease or liver damage or problem stemming from poor liver detoxification. Pair with Dandelion root for a more stimulating effect and for use in menstrual problems caused from poorly deconjugated hormones. It's a no-brainer for any herbalist's Materia Medica.

Taraxacum officinale Weber (Dandelion root and leaf) and *T. mongolicum* Handel-Mazzetti Pu Gong Ying (Mongolian Dandelion root and leaf)

Trigger words. * **Liver/gallbladder stimulant** * **Clears Damp Heat** * **Diuretic** * **Detoxifier** *

Botanical name. *Taraxacum officinale* Weber (Fig. 11.18)

Common name. Dandelion

Less common names. Puffball, Lion's tooth, Wet the Bed

Pinyin name. Pu Gong Ying (*Taraxacum mongolicum*)

Family. Asteraceae/Compositae/Daisy

Part used. Root and leaf

- *Growth and harvest*. Found around the world, up to 12 inches tall with oblong, green, sharply toothed leaves (Lion's tooth) in a rosette. Distinctive yellow flowers that bloom year-round. Flower turns into a fuzzy white, globe-shaped cluster that contains seeds for propagation.
- *Energetics*. Bitter, somewhat salty, and a little sweet, cold, dry, softening, dissolving, restoring, decongesting, calming, and sinking.[9]
- *Strength*. Mild with minimal chronic toxicity
- *Key constituents*. Bitter glycosides; bitter resins, including taraxacerin and taraxerol, FAs, essential oils, inulin, saponin, citric acid; high mineral content, including potassium, sodium, phosphorus, and iron; vitamins A, C, choline, niacin; and gum. (Tincture at 1:4 in 45% ethanol.)
- *Actions*. (1) Dandelion is a liver/gallbladder ally. It stimulates the liver to detoxify, and therefore clears damp and toxic heat. It dissolves bile and kidney stones, because of its salty nature. (2) Diuretic, it drains water, especially the leaf. (3) Bitter taste stimulates stomach acid and pancreatic enzymes, creating digestive stimulation. (4) ***Galactagogue*** (stimulates oxytocin, which causes milk ejection) and *cholagogue* (stimulates bile from the liver) action helps move damp heat and move bowels. (5) Restorative: its sweetness and high mineral content restores the liver and pancreas. (6) Alterative, due to its cleansing nature.
- *Indications, syndromes, and disorders*. (1) Detoxification for damp or toxic heat with indigestion and constipation; boils, sores, ulcers, and eczema; arthritis; or infections, including herpes simplex and pelvic inflammatory disease. (2) Liver: for congestion, jaundice, hepatitis, gallstones, toxicity. (3) To restore and protect the liver, gallbladder, and pancreas. (4) GI:

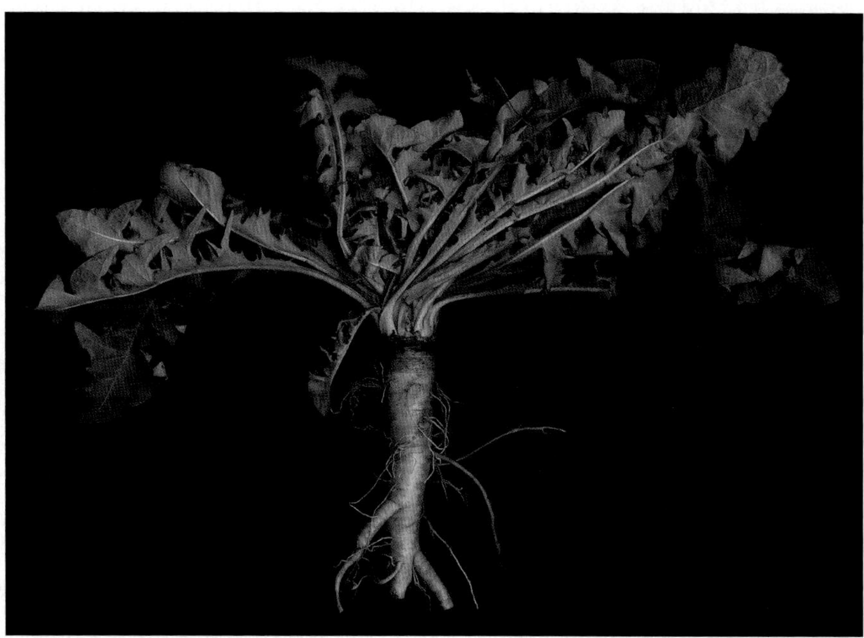

• **Fig. 11.18** *Taraxacum officinale* (Dandelion root and leaf) showing deep taproot. (Copyright Lang/Tucker Photography. Photographs loaned with permission from *The Botanical Series* are copyrighted by Jennifer Anne Tucker and Gerald Lang from the Studio at Hill Crystal Farm. www.jennifer-tucker.com.)

as a bitter digestive stimulant, to support diabetes; dyspepsia; mild laxative.

- *Dose*. Tincture: 2 to 5 mL 3 times per day. Decoction: 6 to 16 g. Leaves: may juice, tincture, or eat raw. Roasted root: used as coffee substitute, like Chicory. All doses are detoxicant. Small doses for restoring; larger doses for cooling and draining.
- *Side effects*. Large continuous doses may cause mild diarrhea, heartburn, or nausea.
- *Contraindications*. Bile duct obstruction.
- *Commission E*. For disturbances in bile flow, stimulation of diuresis, loss of appetite, and dyspepsia.[18]

Editorial. Dandelion root is used in Chinese Medicine, and Western and Ayurvedic herbalism. The Chinese species is *T. mongolicum*. It has a universal healing history. All varieties are interchangeable. Because it probably grows in your (one hopes) unsprayed backyard, use it. Westerners consider it a bitter digestive stimulant, liver tropho-restorative, diuretic, and detoxicant. The Chinese use it as an antiinflammatory that clears heat toxins for conditions such as boils, abscesses, and throat inflammation. Ayurvedic tradition values Dandelion as a digestive bitter and detoxicant.

Dandelion leaf has similar constituents to the root but with more potassium.[9] This makes it an excellent diuretic for edema or hypertension. Don't forget to include Dandelion greens in a spring salad as a bitter, nourishing, cleansing tonic food similar to Lamb's Quarters herb. New, young leaves picked before the plant goes into flower are best. Juicing is a good option. The leaves should be eaten or tinctured fresh because they quickly lose potency when dried.

Urtica dioica L. (Nettle herb)

Trigger words. * **Nutritive tonic** * **Antiallergenic** * **Styptic** * **BPH (roots)** *

Botanical name. *Urtica dioica* L. (Fig. 11.19)

Common name. Nettle, Nettles, Stinging Nettles

Less common names. Scaddie, Ortie, Slender Nettle

Pinyin name. None

Family. Urticaceae

Part used. Leaf, root, and seed

- *Growth and harvest*. Leafy, stemmed, erect perennial up to 2 feet tall. Four-sided hairy stem, opposite serrated leaves with stinging hairs. Flowers green or pinkish clusters hang from upper leaf axils. Grows in moist, rich disturbed sites.
- *Energetics*. Astringent, somewhat sweet and salty, bitter, cooling and dry, nourishing, restoring, astringing, and dissolving.[9]
- *Strength*. Mild with minimal toxicity but a medium-strength hemostatic.
- *Key constituents*. Flavanol glycosides, especially rutin, proteins, magnesium, sulfur, iron, linolenic acid, iron, beta carotene, and lots of silicon in the stinging hairs. (Tincture at 1:3 with medium ethanol percentage of 40%–55%.)
- *Actions*. (1) Nutritive tonic high in iron, minerals, and vitamins A and C, and chlorophyll. (2) Antiallergenic, a natural antihistamine, particularly in a freeze-dried preparation. (3) Astringent, reduces bleeding; the root helps shrink the prostate in BPH but also contains a phytoandrogen for prostate health. (4) Diuretic and helps detoxification. (5) Fresh leaves are a counter-irritant and a ***styptic*** (stops external bleeding).
- *Indications, syndromes, and disorders*. (1) Nutritive tonic and antioxidant for adrenals (including burnout), PMS, menopause, and any trace mineral deficiency. Builds blood and treats anemia, because of its content of chlorophyll, trace minerals, proteins, and enzymes. (2) Astringency helps dry up draining wounds, bedwetting, diarrhea, bleeding from heavy menses, shrinks hemorrhoidal tissue. (3) Immediate allergy symptoms of hay fever, food allergies, and asthma. (4) Detoxification support because it eliminates metabolic wastes through the kidneys. (5) Dissolves kidney stones, tumors, and hard deposits due to its salty taste. (6) Arthritis relief when fresh herb is rubbed on skin. This action is known as *urtication*.

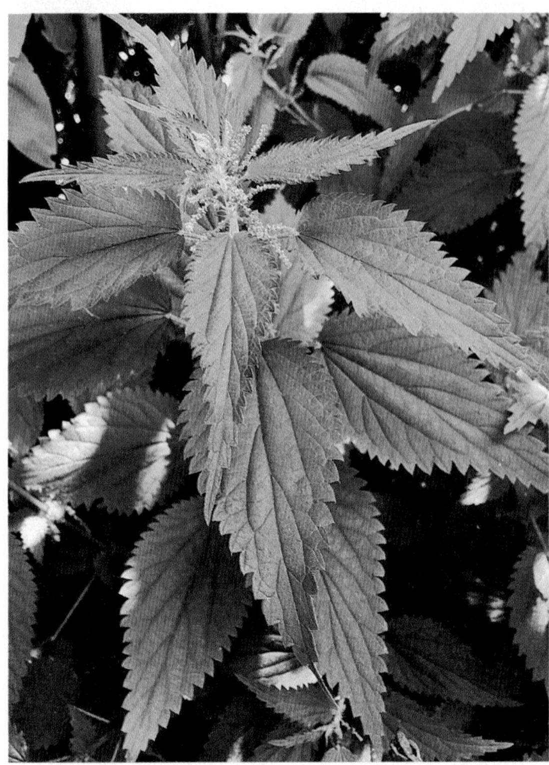

• **Fig. 11.19** *Urtica dioica* (Nettle herb) is a nutritive tonic that grows in wet, disturbed sites.

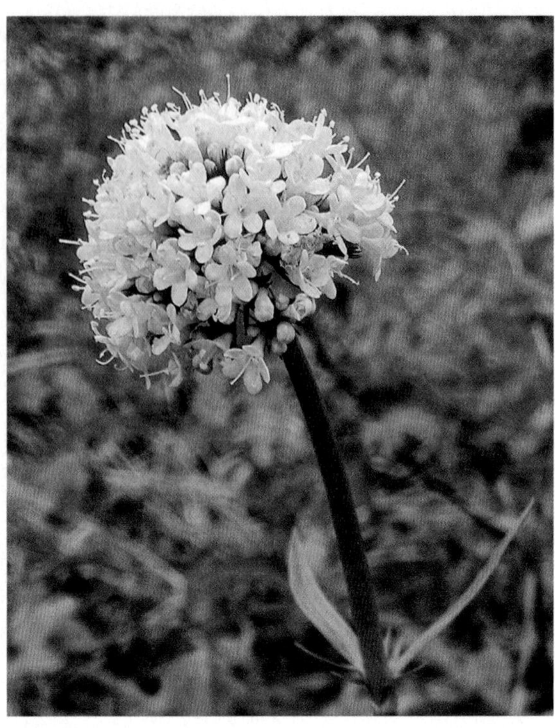

• **Fig. 11.20** Western Valerian flower ranges in color from light pinkish-lavender to white.

- *Dose.* Tincture 4 to 6 mL 1:3 30%. A shot of fresh Nettle juice is very nourishing. Freeze dried, especially for allergies. Brush fresh plant on skin topically for arthritis; expect it to sting.
- *Side effects.* Safe in pregnancy and lactation. Histamine effect (urticaria, or hives) is caused by many organic acids, including formic acid, silicon, and neurotransmitter/inflammatory modulators, including histamine, serotonin, and acetylcholine in the fresh Nettle hairs.[19] These effects clear up in a few minutes.
- *Contraindications.* When used topically, Nettle stings individuals who are allergic to it.
- *Commission E.* Use the root for mild BPH and the herb in supportive treatment for rheumatism and kidney gravel.

Editorial. Nettle is an incredibly useful, indispensable, and versatile plant. Herbalist Brigitte Mars serves this superfood all spring and summer from her garden in smoothies and baked in quiches and casseroles. (Use small young leaves, because older ones may cause digestive disturbances.) Handle and harvest the fresh plant with gloves; touching it causes an instantaneous burning rash from its formic acid content. But this rash also serves as a topical counterirritant. If the fresh leaves are intentionally brushed on the skin, it brings blood to the skin and helps arthritis and muscle pain. The sting doesn't last long and really helps. As a styptic in a compress, it stops bleeding. Nettle root inhibits cellular growth of the prostate in BPH and is diuretic.

The fresh leaves were used as a spring vegetable, much like spinach, throughout history and helped prevent scurvy. Two cups of strong nettle infusion substitutes as a multivitamin and is a nutritious woman's ally. The stinging hairs from the formic acid are inactivated when cooked or thoroughly dried. The seed oil was used for burning in ancient Egypt, and the herb is currently used as a commercial source of chlorophyll.

Valerian officinalis L. (Valerian root)

Trigger words. * **Calming, anxiolytic** * **Sleep** * **Empty Heat** * **Spasmolytic** *

Botanical name. Valerian officinalis L. and spp. (Fig. 11.20)

Common name. Valerian

Less common names. All-heal, Capon's tail, Setwell

Pinyin name. None.

Family. Valerianaceae

Part used. Rhizome/Root

- *Growth and harvest.* Perennial with knobby roots that creep along under the ground and that could smell rank. Leaves opposite, slender, and lance-shaped, and some basal. Small pinkish to white flowers in dense cymes. Up to 2 feet tall. Likes moist soil (Fig. 11.21).
- *Energetics.* Sweet, bitter, pungent, warm with cooling potential, dry, relaxing, restoring, stimulating, and decongesting.[9]
- *Strength.* Medium strength with moderate chronic toxicity
- *Key constituents.* Many essential oils including valerianol acid (iridoids), monoterpenes, sesquiterpenes, flavonoids, amino acids, and lignins. (Tincture at 1:4 with 50%–60% ethanol, due to alcohol-soluble essential oil content.)
- *Actions.* (1) Sedative and anxiolytic effect because of various flavonoids. (2) Spasmolytic as a smooth-muscle relaxant. (3) Anticonvulsant for seizures. It clears internal wind.
- *Indications, syndromes, and disorders.* (1) Anxiety, as in neurosis; stress-related conditions, depression, heart yin deficient phobias. (3) Insomnia caused by exhaustion when recuperation is needed; but, not exhaustion from overstimulation. (4) Menopause and PMS manifesting as yin deficient symptoms (not from hyperfunctioning), such as in hot flashes (known as empty heat), insomnia, fatigue, depression, anxiety, and cold

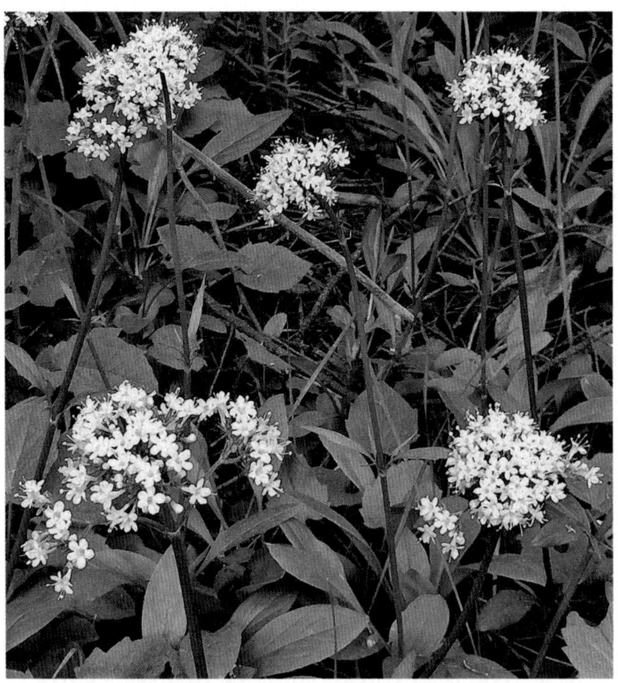

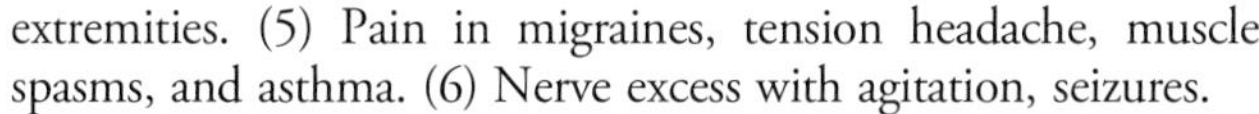

• **Fig. 11.21** *Valerian occidentalis* (Western Valerian) habit, spring flowering in Colorado mountains.

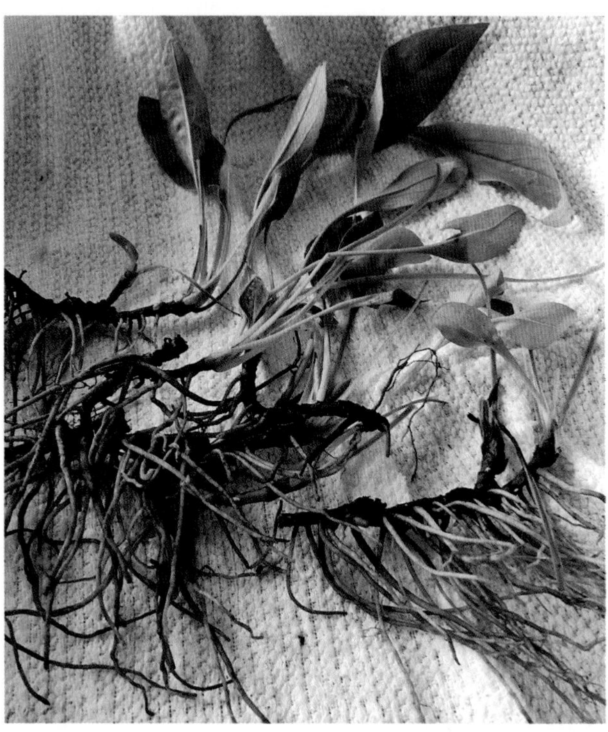

• **Fig. 11.22** *Valerian occidentalis* (Valerian root), freshly dug, with plantlets attached.

extremities. (5) Pain in migraines, tension headache, muscle spasms, and asthma. (6) Nerve excess with agitation, seizures.

- *Dose.* Tincture: low, single-dose tincture is restorative for depression 0.5 to 1 mL; medium single-dose tincture is stimulating and relaxing for anxiety and empty heat 1 to 2 mL; large single dose is more sedating 2 to 5 mL.
- *Side effects.* Large doses can have a ***paradoxical effect***. It may cause the opposite of the intended calming action if used for full heat conditions such as fever, inflammation, and overstimulation. (This could be embarrassing for the herbalist who does not correctly assess the condition.) In very high doses, could cause unwanted drowsiness and dependence (if taken over long periods). Safe in pregnancy and lactation. In Sweden, it is the most commonly used herb during pregnancy.
- *Contraindications.* May *potentiate* antianxiety and sleeping medications (making the pharmacological response greater than the herb or drug used separately) but not conclusively proven. Best not to combine. Valerian is for empty heat and yin deficiency. It is not for full heat conditions, except in migraines or seizures.[9] Not for children under 3 years old.
- *Commission E.* For restlessness and sleeping disorders based on nervous conditions. The World Health Organization approves Valerian as a milder alternative, or a possible substitute, for stronger synthetic sedatives, e.g., benzodiazepines, in the treatment of states of nervous excitation and anxiety-induced sleep disturbances.[20]

Editorial. Valerian root has the reputation of being a stinky-smelling herb because the dried root has a dirty-sock odor, reminiscent of football locker rooms or teenage boys' bedrooms, because of its pungent, warming, and stimulating qualities (Fig. 11.22). This reputation is not as true of the fresh root, newly dug from the forest, which is cooler, more restorative, and less odiferous. Therefore the fresh root is more predictable and forgiving for hot conditions, with less chance of a paradoxical effect.

Valerian combines well with *Melissa officinalis* (Lemon Balm herb), *Passiflora incarnata* (Passionflower herb) and *Humulus lupulus* (Hops flower) for sleep disorders. For kids over 3 years of age, combine with Lemon Balm. This medium-strength herb is not appropriate for younger children or babies. Substitute Lemon Balm or California Poppy for the little ones.

Vitex agnus-castus L., *V. negundo* L. Mu Jing Zi (Chastetree berry)

Trigger words. * **Progesteronic** * **Pituitary regulation** * **PMS** * **Menopause** * **Infertility** *

Botanical name. Vitex agnus-castus L. (Fig. 11.23)

Common name. Chastetree berry, Chaste Lamb, Five-Leaf Chaste tree Berry

Less common names. Monk's Pepper, Cloister Pepper

Pinyin name. Mu Jing Zi (*Vitex negundo* L.)

Family. Verbenaceae (Verbena)

Part used. The fruit/berry

- *Growth and harvest.* Indigenous to southern Europe and Mediterranean areas, now widely cultivated. Shrub grows up to 9 feet tall with five large, dark-green leaves radiating from hairy stalk. Whorls of violet flowers result in blue-gray berries.
- *Energetics.* Bitter, pungent, somewhat astringent, aromatic, neutral to warm, and dry.
- *Strength.* Mild with minimal chronic toxicity.
- *Key constituents.* Essential oils, flavonoids, iridoid glycosides (Tincture at 1:3 with 60%–75% ethanol, due to large essential oil content.)
- *Actions.* (1) Indirectly increases progesterone. Mechanism of action: Vitex reduces prolactin secretion from the anterior pituitary. Too much prolactin shortens the luteal phase, causing PMS, breast

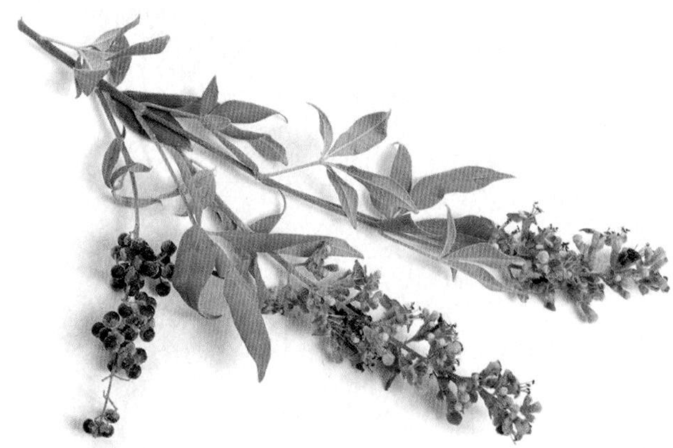

• **Fig. 11.23** *Vitex agnus-castus* (Chastetree berry) is used as a reproductive herb in the West and V. *negundo*, Mu Jing Zi, as a respiratory herb in the East. (iStock.com/Credit: spline_x.)

pain, benign breast tumors, and infertility[21] (Chapter 28). A longer luteal phase means more progesterone is released from the corpus luteum, and fewer PMS symptoms occur. (2) Relaxing and astringent; relieves muscle pain and dries up phlegm and vaginal secretions. (3) Galactagogue.

- *Indications, syndromes, and disorders*. (1) Progesterone deficiency with probable estrogen dominance in many women's issues, including PMS with sore breasts, dysmenorrhea, and estrogen dominance manifesting as uterine fibroids, endometriosis, or ovarian cysts. (2) Menstrual problems, like amenorrhea, metrorrhagia, and irregular menstrual cycles from a shortened luteal phase. (3) Infertility in women with low progesterone levels. (4) Perimenopause and menopause with low progesterone levels presenting as painful, lumpy breasts; fatigue; introverted personality; and sleep problems. (5) Hormone replacement therapy withdrawal. (6) Helps lactation; a galactagogue. (7) Men: for hypogonadism, breast cysts, and BPH. (8) Acne in women and men.
- *Dosage*. Tincture: 1 to 5 mL of a 1:5 tincture daily. Extract: 1 to 3 mL of 1:2 45% extract daily. May use Vitex in biphasic dosing: meaning, for use in the last half, or luteal phase, of menstrual cycle to enhance phyto-progesteronic effects. Takes about 6 months to create hormonal changes.
- *Side effects*. Rarely: nausea and rashes. Safe in pregnancy and lactation.
- *Contraindications*. Best not to take with hormone replacement therapy (HRT) or progesterone drugs to be on safe side, but safely given with over the counter (OTC) low dose 0.1% progesterone cream. May counteract effects of birth control pills.[22]
- *Commission E*. For menstrual cycle irregularities, PMS, and mastodynia (breast pain).[23]

Editorial. Vitex is a go-to long-term herb for women with PMS, menopausal, and menstrual disorders caused by progesterone deficiency. This problem presents as withdrawn personality with loss of self-esteem, fatigue, and fibrocystic, painful, and lumpy breasts. Combine it with Yarrow flower to enhance progesterone effect. Think of it as acting on the pituitary and as a first-rate hormone balancer.

Spicy, peppery-tasting Vitex was used in place of Black Peppercorns to dampen a monk's libido in monasteries of the Middle Ages, hence the common name "Chaste tree." In China, other *Vitex* species (*V. negundo*, *V. rotundifolia*, and *V. trifolia*) are used very differently from the way they are used in the West. They are used as a respiratory bronchodilator, expectorant, and antitussive.[4] Western Vitex can be used similarly.

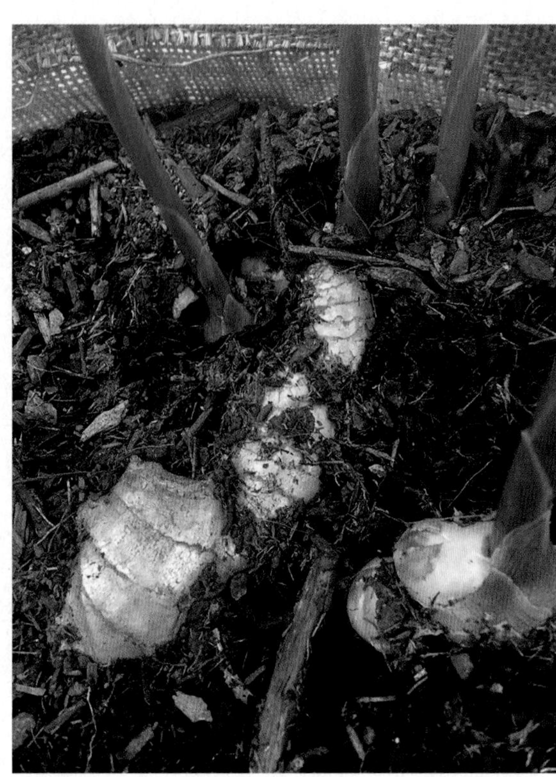

• **Fig. 11.24** *Zingiber officinalis* (Ginger root) growing in burlap.

Zingiber officinalis Roscoe Gan Jiang (Ginger root)

Trigger words. * **Warm and Pungent** * **Antiemetic** * **Diaphoretic** * **Blood Mover** *

Botanical name. Zingiber officinalis Roscoe (Figs. 11.24 and 11.25)
Common name. Ginger
Less common names. Common Ginger, East Indian Ginger
Pinyin name. Gan Jiang (dried), Sheng Jiang (fresh), Pao Jiang (quick-fried), Jiang Pi (peel)
Family. Zingiberaceae (Ginger)
Part used. Rhizome/root

- *Growth and harvest*. Ginger grows with erect, leafy stems and narrow leaves. Terminal spike has irregular yellow-green, purple-streaked flowers. Rhizome is grayish white with light-brown rings.
- *Energetics*. Very pungent, aromatic, sweet, hot, dry, stimulating, relaxing, restoring, and dispersing.[9]
- *Strength*. Mild with minimum chronic toxicity.
- *Key constituents*. Oleoresins, essential oils including zingiberene, pungent hot principles, gingerol, gingerdiols, sulphur, and lignin. (Tincture root with 1:3 60%−80% higher ethanol percent, because of its high essential oils and resins.)
- *Actions*. (1) Diaphoretic for wind cold, especially the fresh rhizome in a tea. (2) Antimicrobial: antiviral, antibacterial,

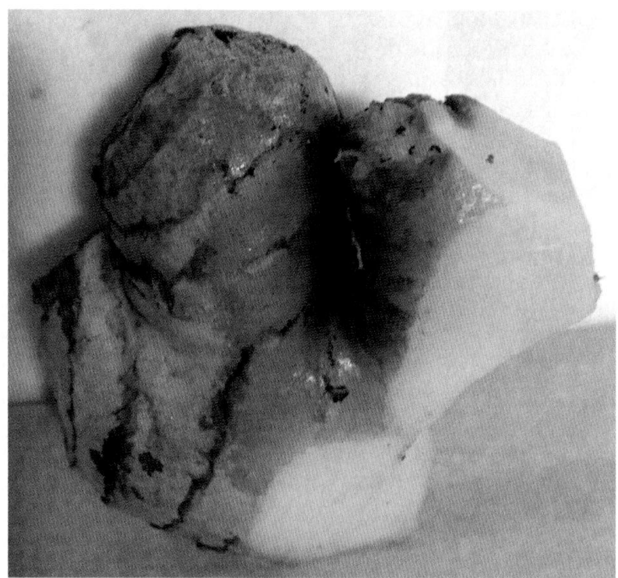

• **Fig. 11.25** Fresh decocted Ginger root is hot, dispersing, and diaphoretic, just right for early onset colds and flu.

and immunostimulant. (3) GI: digestive stimulant/relaxant, ***antiemetic*** (stops nausea and vomiting), and carminative (helps digestion). (4) Arterial stimulant for arteries (moves blood). (5) Lung stimulant for expectoration. (6) Analgesic, because it is spasmolytic and antiinflammatory (inhibits inflammatory prostaglandins and leukotriene formation).

- *Indications, syndromes, and disorders.* (1) Early-onset colds and flu, external wind cold. (2) Stomach qi stagnation: helping flatus, nausea, vomiting, enteritis, morning sickness, and motion sickness. (3) Menses: for cramps and delayed or absent periods (not due to pregnancy), because it moves blood. (4) Increases circulation, helping to warm up cold hands and feet.
- *Dose.* Tincture: 0.5 to 2 mL 1:4 70%. Decoction: 1 to 3 g fresh or 3 to 10 g dried per cup. Essential oil: 1 to 2 drops in gel cap with olive oil. Topically: a compress over sore joints and muscles; foot soak for athlete's foot; additive in baths for chills, muscles soreness, sciatica, and poor circulation.
- *Side effects.* None known.
- *Cautions.* Only use for passive bleeding in cold conditions. Avoid in yin deficiency (dryness), stomach or lung heat, or during early pregnancy, except as an antiemetic for morning sickness.
- *Contraindications.* (1) Gallstones and pregnancy and lactation.
- *Commission E.* For dyspepsia and prevention of motion sickness. For morning sickness, not to exceed 2 g daily.[24]

Editorial. Ginger is widely used in the major herbal traditions around the world: Chinese, Western, Ayurveda. It is a necessary herb in any apothecary. In Chinese Medicine, it is a minor but important part of many formulas, but not the major component. It is used to add warmth, movement, and increased tropism, and to help minimize toxicity of other herbs. It is used in four forms: the fresh rhizome is the most dispersing and diaphoretic—perfect in hot teas to bring on sweating in early-onset wind cold conditions, with watery, foamy white sputum and cold hands and feet. The dried rhizome is hotter and longer lasting for cold conditions. The fried rhizome is the strongest of the three and used locally to stop bleeding.[1–5] The peel is considered more cooling.

For damp heat in the GI and skin, use Ginger and pair with Coptis Huang Lian (Goldthread root), Goldenseal, or Oregon Grape root and Scutellaria Huang Qin (Baikal Skullcap root). The Huang Qin species has a very different use from that of Western Skullcap, which is a nervine. For liver damp heat, combine Ginger with Coptis Huang Lian, Chinese Gardenia Shan Zhi Zi, or Western Blue Flag root.

Summary

In this chapter, a basic Materia Medica was presented. These herbs are very important for any herbalist's apothecary. It is not a conclusive list but provides a starting point. I use these herbs repeatedly and retincture them often.

Monographs

Actaea racemosa L. Sheng Ma (Black Cohosh root)
Achillea millefolium L. (Yarrow herb)
Bupleurum chinensis de Candolle Chai Hu (Bupleurum root)
Crataegus oxyacantha L. Shan Zha (Hawthorn berry)
Curcuma longa L. Jiang Huang (Turmeric root)
Echinacea spp. L. (Echinacea root)
Ginkgo biloba L. Yin Xing Ye (Ginkgo leaf)
Glycyrrhiza glabra and *G. uralensis* L. Gan Cao (Licorice root)
Hydrastis canadensis L. (Goldenseal root) and Coptis chinensis Franchet Huang Lian (Goldthread root)
Hypericum perforatum L. (St. John's Wort herb)
Mentha x *piperita* L. (Peppermint leaf) and *M. arvensis* L. Bo He (Field Mint herb)
Serenoa serrulata L. (Saw Palmetto berry)
Silybum marianum Gaertner (Milk Thistle seed)
Taraxacum officinale Weber (Dandelion root and leaf) and *T. mongolicum* Pu Gong Ying (Mongolian Dandelion root and leaf)
Urtica dioica L. (Nettle herb and root)
Valerian officinalis L. (Valerian root)
Vitex agnus-castus L. (Chastetree berry)
Zingiber officinalis Roscoe, Gan Jiang (Ginger root)

Review

Fill in the Blanks

(Answers in Appendix B.)

1. What is Black Cohosh root's action on skeletal muscles? ___.
2. Name three therapeutic effects of Yarrow herb and a condition or symptom for each. ___ for ___, ___ for ___, ___ for ___.

3. Name four actions of Hawthorn berry: ___, ___, ___, ___.
4. The action of Chinese Scutellaria Huang Qin (Baikal Skullcap root) is very different from that of Western Skullcap, which is a ___. It has actions similar to ___ root and ___ root.
5. St. John's Wort is known to treat mild to moderate depression. What is less known is its ability to treat ___ infections in diseases such as ___, ___, and ___. These infections are known in Chinese Medicine as the syndrome ___, ___.
6. *Taraxacum officinalis* stimulates and protects the liver and also treats damp or toxic heat for skin ailments such as ___ and ___.
7. *Taraxacum officinalis*'s temperature is ___; taste is ___; and moisture is ___.
8. Give herbal choices. ___ would be a choice for estrogen deficiency, whereas ___ would be a choice for progesterone deficiency. To balance them both, ___ would be a good choice.
9. Some of the side effects/cautions from continuous intake of Gan Cao could be ___ and ___.
10. The Latin name for this important Western heart tonic is ___, ___. Two actions for this herb are ___ and ___.
11. Choosing from our basic Materia Medica, one could use ___ to help memory loss and ___ in an arthritis formula to bring down inflammation.

Critical Concept Questions

(Answers for you to decide.)

1. Why is Valerian root an unusual nervine? Why can its therapeutic effect backfire?
2. Why is information about Commission E included in the monographs for each herb?
3. Name 10 good starter herbs for your apothecary and the rationale for each choice.
4. Compare nature and uses of Western Skullcap herb versus Chinese Scutellaria Huang Qin (Baikal Skullcap).
5. Discuss berberine content and relative potencies of Coptis Huang Lian, Barberry root, Goldenseal root, and Oregon Grape root.
6. Discuss the merits of Nettle herb as a superfood.
7. What is the mechanism of action in *Serenoa serrulata* L. to shrink the prostate?
8. A client asks the difference between using Dandelion leaf and root. You answer?
9. Is Licorice candy the same or as good as *Glycyrrhiza glabra* for a sore throat?
10. What does the *x* mean in *Mentha x piperita*?

References

1. Holmes, Peter. *Energetics of Western Herbs* (Boulder, CO: Snow Lotus Press, 2006).
2. Holmes, Peter. *Jade Remedies: A Chinese Herbal Reference for the West* (Boulder, CO: Snow Lotus, 1996).
3. "The ABC Guide to Clinical Herbs Online." American Botanical Council. http://abc.herbalgram.org/site/PageServer?pagename = The_Guide (accessed October 13, 2019).
4. Bone, Kerry and Simon Mills. *Principles and Practice of Phytotherapy* (London, U.K: Elsevier, 2013).
5. Alfs, Matthew. *300 Herbs: Their Indications and Contraindications* (New Brighton, MN: Old Theology, 2003).
6. "Expanded Commission E, Black Cohosh root." American Botanical Council. http://cms.herbalgram.org/expandedE/BlackCohoshroot.html (accessed October 11, 2019).
7. "Expanded Commission E, Yarrow." American Botanical Council. http://cms.herbalgram.org/expandedE/Yarrow.html (accessed October 11, 2019).
8. Vail, Karen and Mary O'Brien. *Edible and Medicinal Plants of the Southern Rockies* (Leaning Tree Tales, 2015).
9. Blumenthal, Michael, et al. *The American Botanical Council's Complete German Commission E Monographs: Therapeutic Guide to Herbal Medicines* (Austin, TX: American Botanical Council, 1998). and published in cooperation with Integrative Medicine Communications, Boston, Mass.
10. Shoba, G, et al. https://www.ncbi.nlm.nih.gov/pubmed/9619120 (accessed October 11 *Influence of piperine on the pharmacokinetics of curcumin in animals and volunteers* (PubMed.gov U.S. National Library of Medicine, National Institutes of Health, 2019).
11. Ringman, John, et al. http://www.ingentaconnect.com/content/ben/car/2005/00000002/00000002/art00006 (accessed October 11 A Potential Role of the Curry Spice Curcumin in Alzheimer's Disease (Ingenta Connect, 2019).
12. "Expanded Commission E: Echinacea angustifolia herb and root/Pallida herb." American Botanical Council. http://cms.herbalgram.org/expandedE/EchinaceaAngustifoliaherbandrootPallidaherb.html (accessed October 11, 2019).
13. Buhner, Stephen Harrod. *Herbal Antivirals* (North Adams, MA: Storey, 2013).
14. "Expanded Commission E: Licorice root." American Botanical Council. http://cms.herbalgram.org/expandedE/Licoriceroot.html (accessed October 11, 2019).
15. Lee, Yun S, et al. https://diabetes.diabetesjournals.org/content/55/8/2256 (accessed October 12 *Berberine, a Natural Plant Product, Activates AMP-activated Kinase with Beneficial Metabolic Effects in Diabetic and Insulin-Resistant States* (American Diabetes Association, 2019).
16. "Expanded Commission E: St. John's Wort." American Botanical Council. http://cms.herbalgram.org/expandedE/StJohn27swort.html (accessed October 12, 2019).
17. "Expanded Commission E: Peppermint Leaf." American Botanical Council. http://cms.herbalgram.org/expandedE/Peppermintleaf.html (accessed October 12, 2019).
18. "Commission E Monographs: Dandelion Root with Herb." American Botanical Council. http://cms.herbalgram.org/commissione/Monographs/Monograph0081.html (accessed October 12, 2019).
19. Ganora, Lisa. *Herbal Constituents: Foundations of Phytochemistry* (Louisville, CO: Herbalchem, 2009).
20. "Expanded Commission E: Valerian root." American Botanical Council. http://cms.herbalgram.org/expandedE/Valerianroot.html (accessed October 13, 2019).
21. Ruth, Trickey. *Women, Hormones & the Menstrual Cycle* (St. Leonard's, Australia: Allen and Unwin, 1998).
22. Simon, Mills and Kerry Bone. *The Essential Guide to Herbal Safety* (UK: Elsevier, 2005).
23. "Expanded Commission E: Chaste Tree Fruit." American Botanical Council. http://cms.herbalgram.org/expandedE/ChasteTreefruit.html (accessed October 12, 2019).
24. "Expanded Commission E: Ginger Root." American Botanical Council. http://cms.herbalgram.org/expandedE/Gingerroot.html (accessed October 12, 2019).

12

Materia Medica Groupings

"...Now we turn to all the Medicine herbs of the world. From the beginning they were instructed to take away sickness. They are always waiting and ready to heal us. We are happy there are still among us those special few who remember how to use these plants for healing. With one mind, we send greetings and thanks to the Medicines and to the keepers of the Medicines."

—from the Thanksgiving address by John E. Echohawk

CHAPTER REVIEW

- Sorting out the laundry list: Choosing the best herb in a particular category.
- Calming herbs for the nervous system.
- Demulcents or yin tonics.
- Common adaptogens.
- Alterative herbs that help detoxification.
- Expectorants, bronchodilators, and antitussives.
- Women's allies.
- Infections and toxicosis.

KEY TERMS

Adaptogens
Alteratives
Anhidrotic
Anticoagulant
Antineoplastic
Antitussive
Anxiolytics
Demulcents
Diaphoretic
Diuretic
Dysuria
Enuresis
Hematuria
Hypnotics
Hypoglycemic
Oxytocic
Purulence
Yin tonics

In this chapter, we consider a few key herbal groupings, a sampler, using three approaches. One is the Western herbalism, action-oriented methodology that would describe Burdock root as an *alterative*. Another is the allopathic model of assigning names to diseases, like *pneumonia* or *eczema*. Finally, the Chinese Medicine approach, which uses energetics—*warmth, taste, moisture*—and syndromes, such as *Damp Heat* or *Wind Cold*. Western herbology, allopathic medicine, and Chinese Medicine descriptions are used back and forth—the intention being to single out the best herbal choice for a specific situation, and to distinguish one tradition from another.

As always, herbal indications, dosage, and safety reflect traditional and historical consensus and modern information based on research. No matter what, and if in doubt, consult the latest sources for up-to-date safety information.

Sorting Out the Laundry List

Given five common nervous relaxants, which is the best choice for your client? They are not all the same, and although any one plant might do an ok job, why not choose wisely to complement the person's condition? Instead of using herbs in an automatic "this-for-that" mentality, such as Goldenseal for infections or Lemon Balm for anxiety, how about being more specific and effective? The idea is to avoid picking at random from a list.

Furthermore, what if that nervine/calmer-downer could accomplish more than one function? If a person is anxious and stressed from an asthma attack, we might choose Lobelia herb because it opens the airway to help stop bronchial wheezing in the respiratory tree in addition to being a calming nervine. If there is stress because the head feels like it's stuck in a vise, Skullcap would be better than

Lobelia, because it relieves muscle spasms in that specific area, and calms emotional stress. Two birds; one stone.

Let's take a look at some groups or categories, so we can consistently obtain good results, taking the guesswork out of herbalism.

Calming Herbs for the Nervous System

Scutellaria lateriflora L. (Skullcap herb)

Matricaria recutita L. (Chamomile flower)

Melissa officinalis L. (Lemon Balm leaf)

Lobelia inflata L. (Lobelia herb)

Humulus lupulus L. (Hops flower)

Ziziphus spinosa Hu, Suan Zao Ren (Sour Jujube seed)

General trigger words.

* **Nervous sedative** * **Spasmolytic** * **Insomnia** *

Specific trigger words

- *Skullcap herb.* Restores nerves.
- *Chamomile flower.* Pain, spasms, sleep aid, good for kids.
- *Lemon Balm* or *Melissa Balm leaf.* General relaxant.
- *Lobelia herb.* Medium strength. Spasmolytic, used to quit smoking, high doses called Puke Weed (Fig. 12.1).
- *Hops flower.* Medium strength, estrogenic, cooling.
- *Ziziphus Suan Zao Ren seed.* Means *sour dates;* insomnia caused by worry.

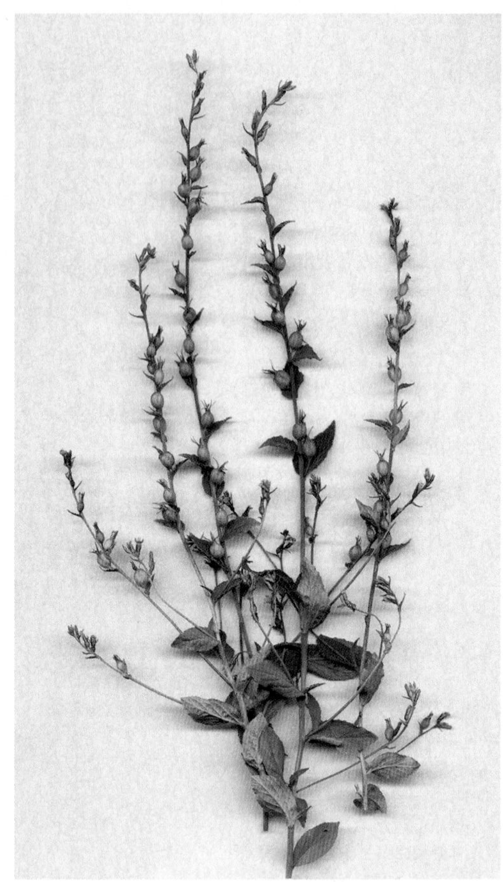

• **Fig. 12.1** *Lobelia inflata* (Lobelia herb) is a medium strength herb that should be administered with care, and is best in formula. It is extremely useful in relaxing the lungs with spasmodic coughing, and in laryngitis and asthma with panic and difficulty breathing. It can also cause violent emesis in high doses. (Copyright Lang/Tucker Photography. Photographs loaned with permission from *The Botanical Series* are copywritten by Jennifer Anne Tucker and Gerald Lang from the Studio at Hill Crystal Farm. www.jennifer-tucker.com.)

Families

- *Skullcap herb.* Lamiaceae/Labiatae/Mint.
- *Chamomile flower.* Asteraceae/Compositae/Daisy.
- *Melissa Balm leaf.* Labiatae/Lamiaceae/Mint.
- *Lobelia herb.* Lobeliaceae.
- *Hops flower.* Cannabaceae.
- *Ziziphus Suan Zao Ren seed.* Rhamnaceae.

Growth and Harvest

- *Skullcap.* Small herbaceous perennial mint with ridged leaves and tiny two-lobed flowers ranging in color from purple and blue to pink and white.
- *Chamomile.* Annual, with delicate, lobed, alternate leaves. Flowers are tiny white rays surrounding a yellow mounded disc center.
- *Melissa Balm.* Wrinkled, ovate, medium-green, lemon-scented leaves appear in typical Mint family fashion with paired leaves on a square stem (Fig. 12.2). White flowers with two lobes.
- *Lobelia.* Grows in dry open fields with small blue or violet flowers, inflated capsule tinted yellow on the inside. Stems are covered in tiny hairs. Leaves ovate and toothed.
- *Hops.* This vine is dioecious, so male and female flowers develop on separate plants; the female flower matures into the cones called *strobiles*, which consist of membranous stipules and bracts attached to a zigzag, hairy axis. The stipules and bracts resemble one another closely but are actually numerous shining lupulin glands.
- *Ziziphus* Suan Zao Ren. Low shrub or tree, yellow to green flower, alternate leaves with basal prominent veins. Fruit is a sweet date-like drupe. Grows in temperate and subtropical regions. Originated in northern China.

Strength

- *Mild.* Skullcap, Chamomile, Melissa Balm, and Ziziphus Suan Zao Ren have minimal chronic toxicity.
- *Medium.* Lobelia and Hops have moderate chronic toxicity.

Key constituents

- *Skullcap herb.* Essential oils, fixed oils, and flavonoids, including scutellarin, albumin, tannin, lignin, and many minerals. (Tincture 1:3 45%–50% ethanol.)

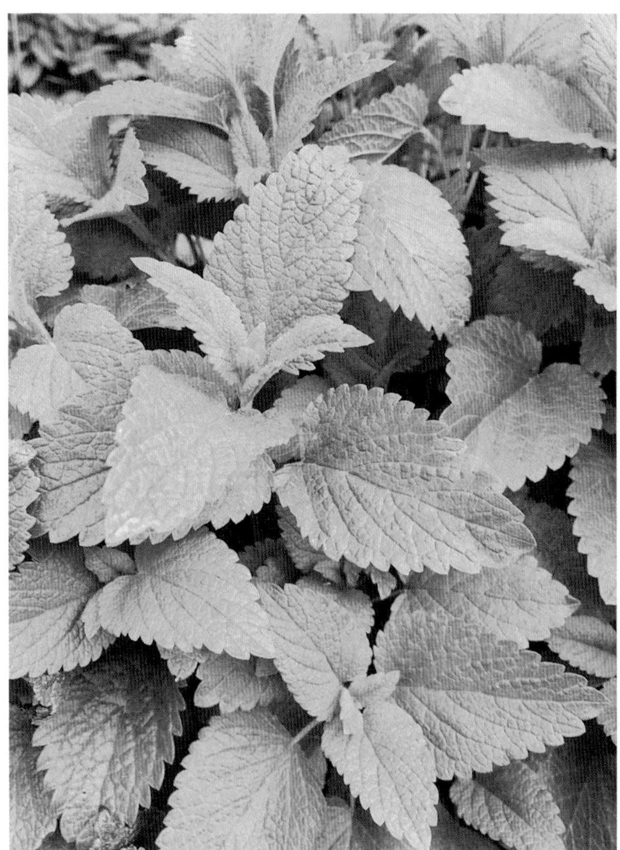

• **Fig. 12.2** *Melissa officinalis* (Lemon Balm, Melissa Balm herb) is lemony smelling, uplifting, antidepressant, and antiviral.

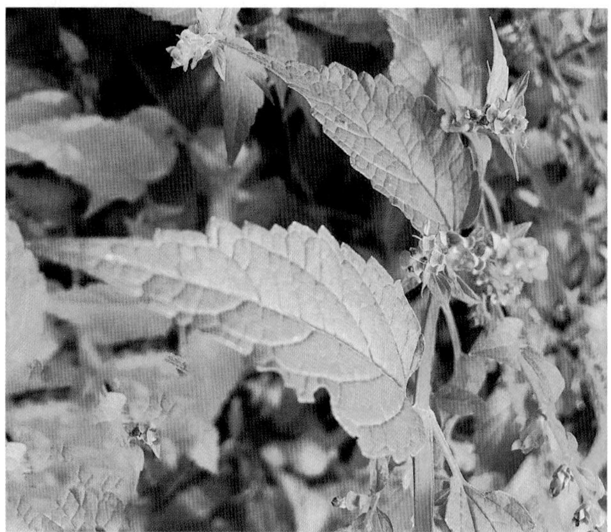

• **Fig. 12.3** *Scutellaria lateriflora* (Skullcap herb) has tiny flowers and grows by streams and swamps. It treats headaches that feel like a tight band around the skull.

- *Chamomile flower.* Essential oils, hydrocarbons (including blue chamazulene), alcohols, sesquiterpenes, flavonoids, coumarin, tannins, and malic acid. (Tincture 1:3 60% ethanol.)
- *Melissa balm.* Essential oils (including citronella, limonene, and pinene), bitter compounds, tannins, organic acids, and minerals. (Tincture 1:3 45% ethanol.)
- *Lobelia herb.* 14 pyridine alkaloids, essential oils, resin, lignin, potassium, lime, and ferric acid. Puke weed is a well-earned common name. The Eclectics used Lobelia for purging therapies. (Tincture 1:4 40%–45% ethanol.)
- *Hops flower.* Bitter resin compounds, including lupulic acids and humulone, essential oils, monoterpenes and sesquiterpenes, alkaloids, flavonoids, phytoestrogens, gamma linolenic acid (GLA), and vitamin C. (Tincture 1:3 65% ethanol.)
- *Ziziphus Suan Zao Ren seed.* Saponins, flavonoids, triterpenes, acids, fatty oil, sterols, vitamin C, and manganese. (Tincture 1:3 65% ethanol.)[1–5]

Energetics, actions, indications, dosages, safety

Skullcap herb (Figs. 12.4 and 12.5)

- *Energetics.* Bitter, astringent, cool, dry, relaxing, restoring, stabilizing, stimulating.
- *Actions.* (1) Major restorative to nerve cells. (2) Nervous system: hypotensive, analgesic, sedating and relaxing, and hypnotic (helps sleep). (3) Estrogenic. (4) Clears empty heat of heart and kidney yin deficiency.

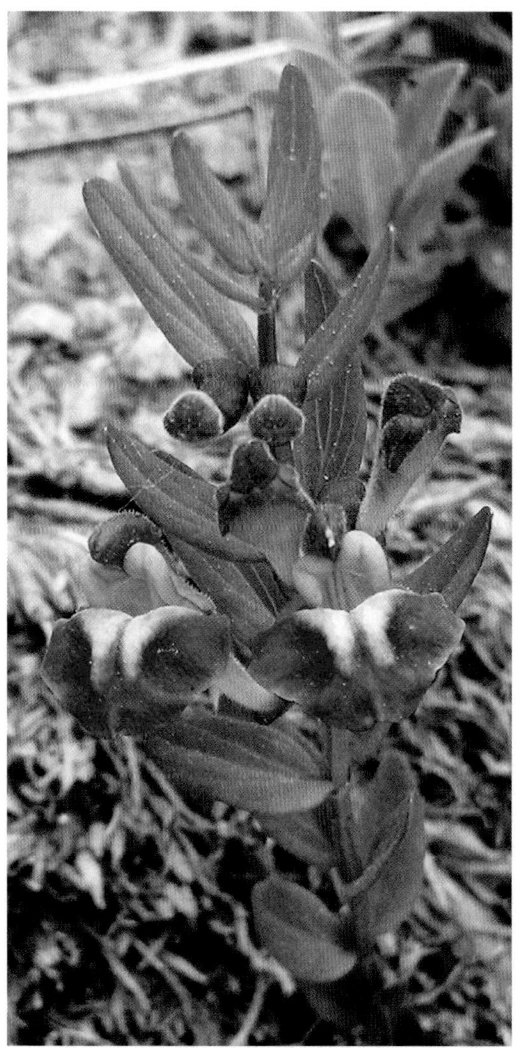

• **Fig. 12.4** *Scutellaria brittonii* (Skullcap herb), flowering. This species grows in drier areas than *S. lateriflora*. Both are cooling and drying. They are calming and restorative to the nervous system.

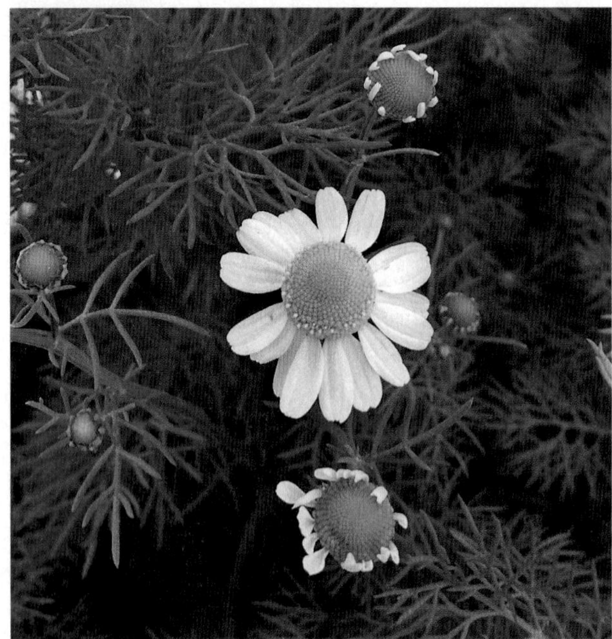

• **Fig. 12.5** Gentle *Matricaria recuitita* (Chamomile flower), shown with buds and finely cut leaf, is good for anxiety, insomnia, stomach aches, and colic. Safe for infants, children, and adults.

- *Indications.* (1) Neuro: restores and calms for depression and all chronic stress-related conditions, mental and physical: insomnia, panic attacks, palpitations, hypertension, restlessness, intense dreams, wet dreams, and exhaustion. (2) Menopause: for hot flashes and empty heat; it is cooling and estrogenic. (3) Internal wind: in tremors, seizures, and twitches. (4) Muscular spasms and pain.
- *Dosages.* Tincture: 2 to 4 mL at 1:3 45% ethanol. Long infusion: 8 to 14 g.[1–5]
- *Side effects.* Hormone precursor. Don't use in pregnancy.
- *Contraindications.* Pregnancy, as it has steroid precursors.
- *Commission E.* No listing.

Chamomile flower (Fig. 12.5)

- *Energetics.* Bitter/sweet, cool, neutral, relaxing, stimulating, restoring, decongesting, and dissolving.
- *Actions.* (1) Antiinflammatory: It inhibits leukotriene production. (2) Spasmolytic for peripheral nerves and muscles. (3) Analgesic and mild sedative. (4) Gastrointestinal (GI): antiulcer, carminative. (5) Vulnerary and helps itching (antipruritic), and mild antimicrobial. (6) ***Diaphoretic*** (causes sweating) for hot conditions.
- *Indications.* (1) GI: for Liver Spleen Disharmony as in diarrhea, infantile colic, dyspepsia, indigestion, irritable bowel syndrome (IBS). (2) Neuro: for stress, anxiety, insomnia, neuralgia in shingles, fibromyalgia, tension headaches and migraines, infantile seizures. Calming down kids with stomach aches, fever. (3) Skin: for damp and toxic heat—vulnerary for dermatitis, eczema, wound healing, shingles, boils, and in a teabag for eye irritations, if not allergic. (4) Women: for spasmodic dysmenorrhea, PMS. (5) Respiratory: for wind heat with mucus, allergy, flu with fever, acute asthma.
- *Dosages.* Tincture: 2 to 4 mL of 1:3 60% ethanol. Infusion: 3 to 4 g per cup. Essential oil: 1 to 2 drops in capsule mixed with olive oil. Use in gargles, steams, baths, salves, compresses, eyewashes.[1–5]
- *Side effects.* Pregnancy, a uterine stimulant, so not to be used as a simple.
- *Contraindications.* Topical application with sensitivity to plants in the Compositae family. Infusion should not be used near the eyes, if allergic.
- *Commission E.* For external use of mouth sores, gums, infections, respiratory steams, baths and washes to anal and genital areas, GI spasms, inflammatory bowel disease.[4]

Melissa Balm or Lemon Balm herb (Fig. 12.2)

- *Energetics.* Bitter, sour, astringent, cool, dry, relaxing, stimulating, restoring.
- *Actions.* Many. Carminative, nervous system relaxant, antispasmodic, antidepressant, diaphoretic, antimicrobial, antiviral, and vulnerary.
- *Indications.* (1) GI: flatulence, dyspepsia. (2) Neuro: depression, anxiety, stress, restorative. (3) Heart: mildly hypotensive because of vasodilation. (4) Respiratory: with immediate allergy, or onset of flu with fever, because it dispels wind heat. (5) Skin: wound healing, for nosebleed (it is astringent), eye inflammations, stings, mumps, tumors.
- *Dosages.* Tincture: 2 to 6 mL per dose: 1:5 40% ethanol. Infusion: 2 to 4 g/cup.[1–5]
- *Side effects.* May decrease action of thyroid hormones. Caution in pregnancy, a mild uterine stimulant, immediate allergies have been reported.
- *Contraindications.* None.
- *Commission E.* For nervous sleeping disorders and functional gastrointestinal complaints.[6]

Lobelia herb (Fig. 12.1)

- *Energetics.* Pungent, somewhat bitter, warm with cooling potential, relaxing, stimulating, restoring.
- *Actions.* Lobelia can relax or stimulate depending on body's condition and dosage. This seeming contradiction is not unusual in the herb world—explained in later section under *dosages.* (1) Balances autonomic nervous system: it helps excess yang and deficient yang, a qi regulator. (2) Neuro: spasmolytic and relaxing, calms the nervous system and relieves pain. (3) Respiratory and reproductive: it dispels Wind Heat in colds, flu, laryngitis, and relaxes bronchioles. It is stimulating and clears stagnation in delayed menses or stalled labor. (4) Heart: a vasodilator for hypertension. (5) Vulnerary: it antidotes poison and has a vulnerary action with bites, stings, eczema, herpes.
- *Indications.* (1) Lungs: spasmolytic and relaxant quality helps Lung qi constraint as in dyspnea caused by asthmatic and panic attacks, with labored breathing. Clears heat for colds and flu. For wheezing, dry, hard coughing (expectorant), croup, pneumonia. For tobacco withdrawal, helps to quit smoking. (2) GI: colic, dyspepsia, IBS. (3) Neuro: seizures and calming. Helps in fainting, coma, and shock, heatstroke, chronic exhaustion caused by yang deficiency, and so regulates the autonomic nervous system (ANS). (4) Gynecology: for eclampsia in high-risk pregnancy and other heart conditions with hypertension, and to bring on menses or labor. (5) Stimulating: Lobelia's stimulating effect can create emesis in very large doses, move stool along in constipation.
- *Dosages.* Smaller doses are more stimulant and larger doses are more relaxant. Best to use in a combination formula. Regular

tincture: 0.5 to 2 mL of 1:5 60% ethanol. Tincture to induce therapeutic emesis: 4 to 5 mL. Tincture for inability to progress in labor when there are strong but ineffective contractions: 1 to 2 mL every half hour.[1–5]
- *Side effects.* Overdosing causes nausea, emesis, diarrhea, salivation, vision or hearing disturbances, mental confusion, weakness. Warning signs of Lobelia overdose is vomiting, a signal to back off. Take short-term only. Not for pregnancy, except to help stalled labor.
- *Contraindications.* (1) Heart issues, as in dyspnea from enlarged or fatty heart, arrhythmias, hypertension. (2) Lung problems like hydrothorax. (3) Not in pregnancy or lactation. (It is used to bring on labor that has failed to progress by dilating the cervix and relaxing the uterus, so contractions will be effective.) (4) Use in individuals with tobacco sensitivity.
- *Commission E.* No listing.

Hops flower (Fig. 12.6)

- *Energetics.* Bitter, pungent, astringent, cold, dry, calming, relaxing, restoring, dissolving.
- *Actions.* (1) Neuro: Hops is pungent, anxiolytic, calming, and relaxing. (2) GI: bitter resins make it a digestive aid like its cousin, Gentian. (2) Its cold quality allows it to clear empty heat in yin deficiency, but it also clears full and damp heat because it is antiinflammatory, antiseptic, and detoxicant. (3) Women: it is estrogenic and helps in estrogen deficient PMS and dysmenorrhea, and clears empty heat in yin deficient hot flashes. It is also a *galactagogue* that stimulates the secretion of milk in nursing mothers.
- *Indications.* (1) Neuro: use Hops as a calmer-downer in relieving anxiety, nervous strain, sleep loss, spasms, pain, stress, and upset stomach. (2) GI: as a digestive bitter and appetite stimulant. (3) In damp heat for eczema, oozing skin eruptions, *Herpes simplex* (cold sores), acne, blemishes. (4) Women: for estrogen-deficient PMS and hot flashes in menopause, and to stimulate milk flow.
- *Dosages.* Tincture: 1 to 3 mL per dose of 1:3 60% ethanol. Infusion: 6 to 9 g freshly dried flowers (strobiles).[1–5]
- *Side effects.* Caution in pregnancy; don't use unless in formula, because its bitterness has a downward energy. But yes, use for lactation if milk is scarce. Being medium strength, use for short term only.
- *Contraindications.* (1) Do not combine with sedative medications, such as phenobarbital, as it is medium strength to begin with. Do not use as a simple for longer than 6 weeks.
- *Commission E.* For mood disturbances, such as restlessness and anxiety, sleep disturbances.[7]

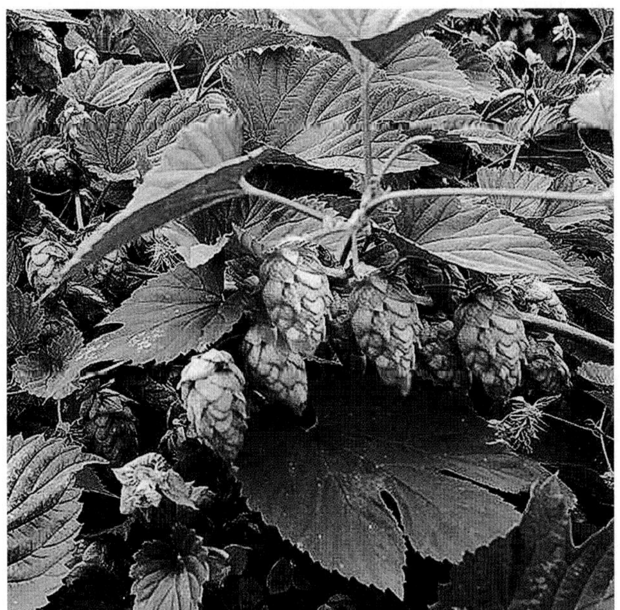

• **Fig. 12.6** Medium strength *Humulus lupulus* (female Hops flower or strobile) is collected for medicine or beer. It is best tinctured fresh or newly dried, no older than 6 months, to retain its active lupulin content.

Ziziphus Suan Zao Ren seed (Sour Jujube seed)

- *Energetics.* Sour, sweet, cool, moist, calming, relaxing, stabilizing, sinking.
- *Actions.* (1) Neurocardiac sedative, hypnotic, analgesic, anticonvulsant. (2) Cardiac relaxant: brings down blood pressure. (3) ***Anhidrotic*** (dries up sweat), demulcent laxative, and an oxygenator.
- *Indications.* (1) Neuro and emotional: Liver Yang Rising and heart blood toxification—with unrest and irritability, anxiety, apprehension, palpitations, sleep loss, insomnia, hot spells, night sweats (it's anhidrotic). For the person who can't sleep because of anxiety. (2) GI: Demulcent laxative for dry stool and constipation. (3) Oxygenator for high-altitude sickness with fatigue and vomiting.
- *Dosages.* Tincture: 2 to 4 mL per dose. Decoction: 10 to 18 g.[1–5]
- *Side effects of Ziziphus.* Full heat and severe diarrhea, as it is used for constipation and dry stool.
- *Contraindications.* None.
- *Commission E.* No listing.

Editorial

- *Skullcap herb.* Skullcap addresses a certain type of headache, a feeling of a tight cap or band around the skull, or muscle pain up the back of the neck and into the head. *Scutellaria lateriflora* (Western Skullcap herb) is a systemic relaxant or calming nervine. Do not confuse this remedy with a different species, the Chinese *Scutellaria baicalensis* Huang Qin (Baikal Skullcap root), which has a very different action, and is used as a antimicrobial to clear heat in acute infections.
- *Chamomile flower.* This sweet little flower might be the most widely used nervine in the Western world, being safe for all kinds of anxiety- and stress-related conditions. A gentle children's herb for colic, tummy ache, excitability, or the *Birthday Party Syndrome.* Chamomile tea is a natural for digestive upsets (a bitter), anxiety, late-night insomnia, colds, teething, pain. Keep in the kitchen cabinet next to your Peppermint.
- *Melissa Balm herb.* Gentle, feminine, and uplifting, lemony-smelling Lemon Balm is perfect in an antidepressant formula. It is a lovely nervous system restorative, like Skullcap herb and St. John's Wort. Beware that cheap Melissa essential oil is sometimes a fake—cut with less expensive lemon grass, citronella, and lemon oils as main ingredients.[8]
- *Lobelia herb.* This herb is foremost a respiratory and cardiac relaxant that is spasmolytic and vasodilating. It is a first

choice for panic and difficulty breathing caused by an asthma or anxiety attack. But treat Lobelia with respect. Puke weed is its well-earned common name. The Thomsonians used it for dramatic purging/emetic therapies, giving it and themselves a bad reputation thanks to bad press from establishment physicians of the time. But it is a valuable and safe herb when attention is paid to proper dosing and individual constitutions. Therapeutic effects differ, depending on both.

- *Hops flower*. Holmes points out that Hops, being very cold, is best used for anxiety with signs of heat (red tongue, fast pulse), whereas Valerian root is better for those with signs of cold (pale tongue, slow pulse). Furthermore, dried Hops flowers more than 6 months old can oxidize and break down their lupulin content, resulting in paradoxical stimulating rather than calming effects.[1] The takeaway is to tincture Hops with fresh or newly dried flowers, called strobiles.
- *Ziziphus Suan Zao Ren seed*. This useful hypnotic complements Passionflower and Hops. I have found that the addition of Ziziphus Suan Zao Ren in sleeping formulas makes all the difference. For high altitude sickness, it can be used with Schisandra Wu Wei Zi (Five Taste berry).
- *Symptomatic relief for anxiety and insomnia*. Some tried and true herbs that relieve insomnia and cause drowsiness (***hypnotics***) and anxiety (***anxiolytics***) pure and simple, are medium-strength Passionflower herb, discussed earlier, and the mild, child-friendly, nonaddictive *Eschscholzia californica* (California Poppy herb).
    - Mention must be made of medium-strength *Piscidia erythrina* (Jamaican Dogwood root bark), which is the best in the West for pain, muscle tension, anxiety, and uncontrollable coughing. Its Chinese Medicine analgesic counterpart for any type of pain is Corydalis Yan Hu Suo (Asian Corydalis corm). The two make great pain relief partners. This is *not* the Corydalis species that grows in the West.

Demulcents or Yin Tonics

Asparagus officinalis L. (Asparagus root), *A. cochinensis* (Lour.) Merr. Tian Men Dong, *A. racemosus* (Bresler) Baker, (Shatavari)

Symphytum officinale L. (Comfrey leaf and root)

Ulmus fulva Michaux (Slippery Elm bark)

Althea officinalis L. (Marshmallow root)

Verbascum thapsus L. (Mullein leaf, flower, and root)

General trigger words

* **Demulcents** * **Tonify yin** * **Moisten dryness** *

Specific trigger words

- *Asparagus root:* Renowned yin tonic. (All species interchangeable.) Nourishing.
- *Comfrey leaf and root*. Wound and bone healer. Called Knitbone, Boneset. Nourishing.
- *Slippery Elm bark*. Stomach restorative. Nourishing.
- *Marshmallow root*. General, all-purpose demulcent.
- *Mullein leaf, root, flower*. Leaf is lung specific, root is urinary specific, and flower is ear specific.

Families

- *Asparagus root*. Liliaceae
- *Comfrey leaf and root*. Boraginaceae
- *Slippery Elm bark*. Ulmaceae
- *Marshmallow root*. Malvaceae
- *Mullein flower, leaf, and root*. Scrophulariaceae

Growth and harvest

- *Asparagus root*. Perennial garden vegetable bulbs (or other forms of enlarged underground stem) from which grow erect clusters of narrow, grasslike leaves or leafy stem. The leaves reduce to small scales.
- *Comfrey leaf and root*. Perennial grows 1 to 4 feet tall. Oval leaves with protruding midvein. Bristly leaves and stem. Flowers are bell-shaped white, pink, or purple, in curled clusters.
- *Slippery Elm bark*. Deciduous tree native to central North America. Bark deeply furrowed, brownish gray; leaves alternate, unequally toothed, covered with hairs. Becoming endangered.
- *Marshmallow root*. Perennial herb grows in damp lowlands. Downey, lobed leaves, pink to purple flowers.
- *Mullein flower, leaf, and root*. Biennial. First year a rosette. Second year a tall spike, some over 6 feet tall. Flowers densely packed, looks like a corn cob. Leaves velvety, fuzzy.

Strength

- All five are mild with minimal chronic toxicity.

Key constituents

- *Asparagus root*. Saponins, flavonoids, glycosides, asparagose, purines, amino acids, calcium, iron, potassium, trace minerals, Vitamin A, B, C. (Tincture 1:3 35%–40% ethanol.)
- *Comfrey leaf and root*. Mucilage, including mucopolysaccharides, allantoin (provides cell proliferation), saponins, tannins, inulin, alkaloids (especially potentially toxic pyrrolizidines), choline, protein, nicotinic acids, gums, resins, triterpenes, minerals, trace minerals, and vitamins A, B, C, E. (Tincture 1:3 with about 60% ethanol for gum, resin, alkaloid extraction.)
- *Slippery Elm bark*. Mucilage up to 50%, starch, tannins, calcium oxalates, calcium, and vitamin C.
- *Marshmallow root*. Mucilage up to 35%, pectin, starch, sugar, tannins, saponin, malic acid, calcium, trace minerals. (Tincture 1:4 with low ethanol, maybe 30%, in this chiefly water-soluble herb.)

- *Mullein leaf, flower, and root.* Mucilage, gum, resin, essential oils, saponins, flavonoids, carotene, tannins, trace minerals. (Tincture 1:5 40%–50% ethanol because of its essential oil content.)[1–5]

Energetics, actions, indications, dosages, safety

Note: In Chinese Medicine, ***yin tonics*** strengthen yin and are cool, moist, and nourishing. ***Demulcents*** are cooling and moist but not always nourishing. These two terms are often used interchangeably, although not with strict accuracy.

Asparagus root

- *Energetics.* Sweet, salty, cool, moist, restoring, nourishing, dissolving, stimulating, relaxing.
- *Actions.* This root is much more than a simple demulcent and mucogenic. (1) For yin-deficient men and women. In Ayurvedic medicine, Shatavari is "The Queen of Herbs," a primary remedy in women's health, used as a pregnancy and fertility tonic and galactagogue.[9] (2) Excellent restorative, moist yin tonic for reproductive system, lungs, and GI mucosa. (3) Mucolytic expectorant and ***antitussive*** (suppresses cough reflex), because it is cool and moist. (4) Antilithic and antitumoral quality, because of its salty and dissolving qualities. (5) ***Diuretic*** (increases urination). (6) Adaptogenic.
- *Indications.* (1) Respiratory: demulcent for dry coughs, thirst, dry throat, croup, Lung Yin Deficiency. (2) Reproductive tonic for vaginal dryness, infertility, and pregnancy. Good as a nourishing, reproductive restorative or yin tonic for low backache and impotence (low sperm count). (3) GI: demulcent laxative for dry stool and chronic constipation, particularly in kids and elders. (4) Moisturizing for fluid deficiency of dehydration, heat exhaustion. (4) Urinary: diuretic quality helps ***dysuria*** (pain on urination), scanty urination, stones (dissolvent). (5) Adaptogenic to enhance immune system.
- *Dosages.* Tincture: 2 to 5 mL per dose. Decoction: 6 to 14 g per dose.[1–5]
- *Side effects.* Very safe. In India, Shatavari is used as a tonic for pregnant women.
- *Contraindications—Asparagus.* (1) Not for diarrhea and cold conditions; not in acute urinary tract infections (UTIs). (2) Avoid in gout and rheumatoid arthritis, because of high purine content.[10]
- *Commission E.* For irrigation therapy for inflammatory diseases of the urinary tract and for prevention of kidney stones.[10]

Comfrey leaf and root (Fig. 12.7)

- *Energetics.* Sweet, bitter, astringent, cool, moist with drying effect, softening, astringing, solidifying, restoring, nourishing.
- *Actions.* Tonifies yin and moistens mucosa as other demulcents do. (1) Claim to fame: vulnerary and connective tissue restorative. (2) GI: moistens and restores mucosa. (3) Astringent: stops discharges and bleeding.
- *Indications.* (1) Connective tissue healer: for weak muscles, ligaments, fractures, ligaments in arthritis, thickens bones in osteoporosis, strengthens muscles in muscular dystrophy. (2) GI: As a yin tonic, it cools and restores mucosa in acute and chronic ulcers and intestinal permeability, hiatal hernia, ulcerative colitis, chronic constipation with dry hard stool, leaky gut. (3) Astringency stops bleeding, hemorrhage, ***hematuria*** (blood in urine). (4) Wound repair for cuts, bruises, abrasions, cracked nipples, anal fissures, hemorrhoids, boils, burns, acne. Topically in ointments and creams. Prevents scarring.

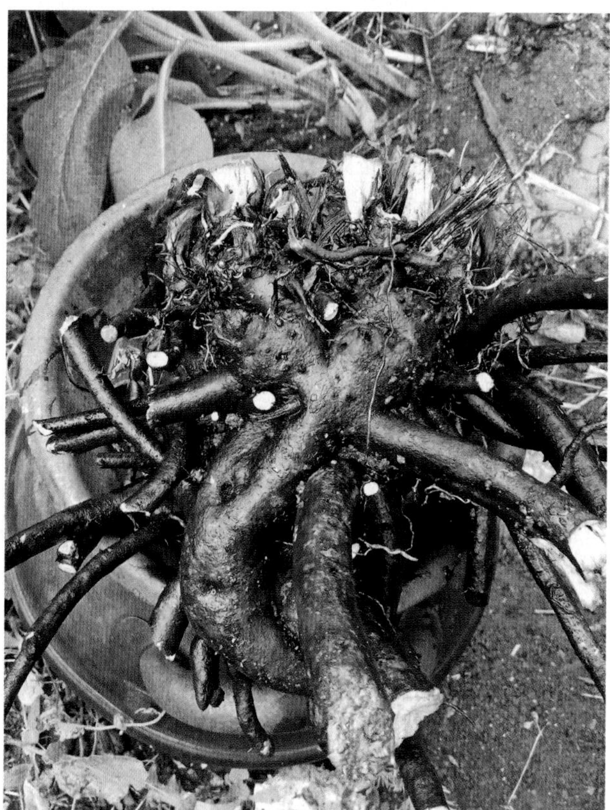

• **Fig. 12.7** Freshly dug and rinsed Comfrey root and leaf. *Symphytum officinale* is an exemplary vulnerary and connective tissue restorative.

- *Dosage.* Tincture: 2 to 5 mL 3 times per day. Decoction: 1 to 3 teaspoons per cup water. Famous externally as fresh leaf poultice, plaster, warm compress, or ointment. Combine with internal tincture for best results.[1–5]
- *Side effects.* Lengthy internal use as a simple (more than 6 weeks) is discouraged because of the risk of liver toxicity from pyrrolizidine alkaloids (PAs) (Chapter 8). External application results in only slight PA absorption.[8] The root contains the most pyrrolizidine, and young leaves contain more than older ones.[11] There are more hepatotoxic PAs in Comfreys that are grown without a real winter, e.g., in California.[12]
- *Contraindications.* (1) Do not use as a compress with deep wounds, because its amazing tissue repair action could cause tissue to form over the wound before it is healed underneath, leading to abscess.[12] (2) Do not use in pregnancy or nursing, or as a simple for over 6 weeks.
- *Commission E.* External use only, on bruises, sprains.[13]

Slippery Elm bark

- *Energetics.* Sweet, bland, cool to cold, moist, nourishing, thickening, astringing, stabilizing.

- *Actions.* (1) Coats mucosa of stomach, lungs, and urinary tract. (2) Nutritive restorative; tonifies digestive qi by enhancing absorption. (2) Antiinflammatory. Clears damp heat and toxic damp heat.
- *Indications.* (1) Lungs: yin tonic and demulcent for sore throat, coughing, laryngitis, chronic bronchitis. (2) GI: for gastric acidity, ulcer, gastroenteritis, chronic diarrhea; tonifies digestion to help weight gain when malnourished. (3) Urinary: helps cool mucosa and decrease pain from cystitis.
- *Dosage.* Paste or gruel for infants and children with diarrhea (mix finely powdered in a little milk). Long infusion: 6 to 14 g. Mix into cough syrups for thickening and demulcent action.[1–5]
- *Side effects.* Use in weak stomachs could cause damp. Mucilaginous quality could interfere with absorption; allergies have been reported.
- *Contraindications.* None, except in case of allergic response.
- *Commission E.* Not listed.

Marshmallow root

- *Energetics.* Sweet, cool to cold, moist, softening, thickening, relaxing.
- *Actions.* General, multipurpose demulcent. (1) Clears damp heat in GI, urinary and respiratory systems. (2) Mucogenic. Stimulates mucus. (3) Emollient. Draws pus and stops skin irritation.
- *Indications.* (1) GI: for peptic ulcers and gastritis. (2) Respiratory: for coughs, pleurisy, whooping cough. (3) Urinary: clears and soothes damp heat in cystitis, stones, chronic infections. (4) Topically: for boils, stings, abscesses, breast lumps, sprains.
- *Dosages.* Overnight cold infusion: 2 to 4 g per 1 cup water (ideal preparation). Tincture: 2 to 4 mL per dose 1:5 30% (best for urinary irritation/stones).[1–5]
- *Side effects.* None.
- *Contraindications.* None
- *Commission E.* For irritation of the oral and pharyngeal mucosa and associated dry cough, and for mild inflammation of the gastric mucosa.[14]

Mullein leaf, root, and flower (Fig. 12.8)

- *Energetics.* Sweet, astringent, cool, moist with secondary drying effect, restoring, thickening, astringing, softening, relaxing.
- *Actions.* All-round moist, a yin go-to respiratory herb, more for symptoms than an outright cure. (1) Mucolytic expectorant, reduces allergy, moisturizes, antiinflammatory. (2) Clears damp heat by cooling and moisturizing in GI, lungs, and urinary systems. (3) Externally: a skin emollient/demulcent. Draws pus, stops irritation, softens boils. (4) The root strengthens the trigone muscles at the base of the bladder, like Kegel exercises, to help alleviate incontinence.
- *Indications.* (1) Lungs: broad-acting respiratory remedy for dry, sticky, hacking coughs with or without mucus, and for expectoration of white or yellow sputum. Pleurisy, whooping cough, spasmodic asthma, immediate allergies. (2) GI: for peptic ulcers, painful diarrhea, enteritis, gastritis. (3) Urinary: clears damp heat in cystitis, stones, chronic infection, pain, and inflammation. The root for urinary incontinence. (4) Topically: for fire toxins in boils, open sores, stings, rashes, abscesses, breast lumps, sprains. Draws out pus from thorns and splinters.

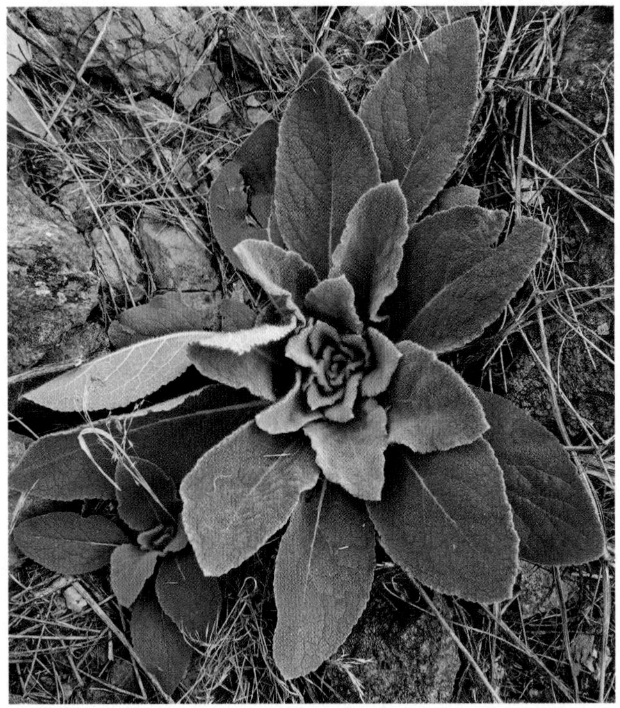

• **Fig. 12.8** *Verbascum thapsus* (Mullein leaf), first-year rosettes in the fall. The leaf has a tropism to the lungs, the root to the urinary tract, and the flower to the ears.

- *Dosages:* Tincture: 2 to 4 mL per dose of 1:3 30% ethanol. Decoction: 6 to 14 g per dose. (Strain decoction to remove hairs.) Topically in oils, ointments, and creams.[1–5]
- *Side effects.* None.
- *Contraindications.* None.
- *Commission E.* For catarrhs of the respiratory tract.[15]

Editorial

This is an ambitious grouping and contains herbs that all herbalists should know. They have a lot in common. All five demulcents are sweet, cool, and moist, but they are not interchangeable. Asparagus, Comfrey, and Slippery Elm are nourishing. If you get a handle on their differences, the best demulcent to pick will become obvious. Furthermore, most are usually combined in formula as helper herbs to provide cool, yin moisture.

- *Asparagus root.* This is a complicated demulcent that is also adaptogenic. In China, *Asparagus chinensis* Tian Men Dong is mainly a respiratory restorative. In the West, *Asparagus officinalis* is used as a detoxicant diuretic for kidneys and as a mucosal moistener and nutritive for dry GI and respiratory conditions.[1] In Ayurvedic, *Asparagus racemosus* (Shatavari root), meaning *she who has one hundred husbands*, is used as a major fertility and pregnancy tonic in women's health and as a galactagogue to bring on breast milk. In reality, these three species are interchangeable.
- *Comfrey leaf and root.* Comfrey was famously used by barbers, country bonesetters, Native Americans, and surgeons in the American Civil War for bone and wound healing. Combine in plasters with the resins of Camphor, Turpentine, or Frankincense. In liniments and lotions, combine with other vulneraries like Arnica flower, Plantain leaf, St. John's Wort, or Calendula flower. Its tannins stop bleeding. Its mucilage

reduces pain, bruising, and inflammation. The allantoin content heals tissue and can prevent need for sutures. Holmes says Comfrey leaf is better as a respiratory demulcent, and the root is a better nutritive and restorative.[1]

- *Marshmallow root.* The most useful overall mucogenic for relieving dryness. It is a pure, thick, moistening, soothing, and calming remedy. For damp heat, combine Marshmallow root with cold, heat clearing herbs that are antiinfective and antiinflammatory, such as the berberines, Horsetail, or Uva ursi herb.
- *Slippery Elm bark.* This nutritive demulcent is perfect for someone who is dry and malnourished. It has been used as a survival food. (Mix with a carminative like Fennel seed so that it doesn't get stuck and cause damp in the stomach.) It also is useful for soothing in skin damp heat with fire toxins appearing as rashes, boils, burns, and oozing sores. Here use both internally and externally in a compress/poultice. It does the job as a general yin tonic for the lungs and GI and much more.
- *Mullein leaf, root, and flower* (Fig. 12.9). Good old reliable Mullein is a European transplant that grows prolifically all over. Because of its availability, it is included it in our Materia Medica. The leaves are a broad-acting respiratory remedy, acting as a respiratory bronchodilator and relaxant for asthma (when smoked). The tannins in the root are notoriously helpful for ***enuresis*** (bedwetting) in children and elders, and the flowers make a famously wonderful ear oil for middle ear infections, with or without the addition of freshly chopped Garlic clove (Box 21.3).

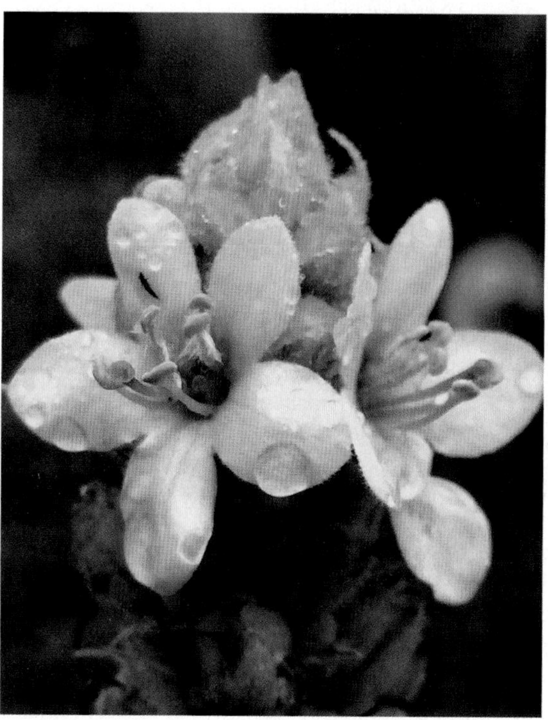

• **Fig. 12.9** *Verbascum thapsus* (Mullein flower) can be infused in oil to make an external remedy for ear infections.

Common Adaptogens

Eleutherococcus senticosus Ruprv. et Maxim, Ci Wu Jia (Eleuthero root)

Ganoderma lucidum Leyss. ex Fr., Ling Zhi (Reishi mushroom)

Astragalus membranaceus Fischer, Huang Qi (Astragalus root)

Withania somnifera L. (Ashwagandha root)

Schisandra chinensis Turcz, Wu Wei Zi (Five Taste berry)

Rhodiola rosea L. (Rhodiola root)

General trigger words

* **Adaptogens** * **Tonics/Restoratives** * **Neuroendocrine/immune balance** *

Specific trigger words

- *Eleutherococcus Ci Wu Jia root.* The King
- *Ganoderma Ling Zhi mushroom.* Spirit Plant (Fig. 12.10)

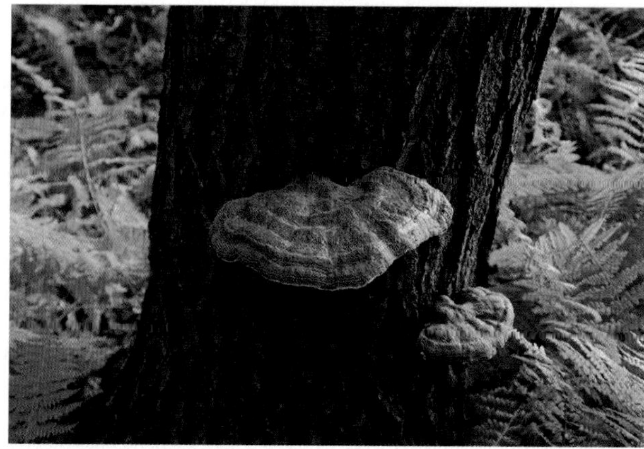

• **Fig. 12.10** Ganoderma Ling Zhi (Wild Reishi mushroom) growing on a hemlock tree in the forest. (iStock.com/Credit: James Mahan.)

- *Astragalus Huang Qi root.* Yellow Leader
- *Ashwagandha root.* Strong as a Horse
- *Schisandra Wu Wei Zi berry.* Five Taste berry
- *Rhodiola root.* The Queen

Families

- *Eleutherococcus Ci Wu Jia root.* Araliaceae
- *Ganoderma Ling Zhi mushroom.* Polyporaceae
- *Astragalus Huang Qi root.* Fabaceae/Leguminosae/Pea
- *Ashwagandha root.* Solanaceae/Nightshade
- *Schisandra Wu Wei Zi berry.* Magnoliaceae
- *Rhodiola root.* Crassulaceae/Stonecrop

Growth and harvest

- *Eleutherococcus Ci Wu Jia root.* Eleuthero, commonly called Siberian ginseng (even though it's not a ginseng) is a creeping, thorny plant that grows in far eastern Siberia and Russia.
- *Ganoderma Ling Zhi mushroom.* Reishi mushroom grows on decaying logs and tree stumps, purplish-brown with a long stalk, brown spores, and a fan-shaped cap with a shiny, varnish-coated appearance.
- *Astragalus Huang Qi root.* Astragalus is a long taproot usually cut into tongue depressor shaped slices, hairy stems, pinnate ferny looking leaves with 12 to 18 leaflets, pea family flowers with banner, wings, and keel.
- *Ashwagandha root.* A small shrub with yellow flowers and red fruit, smooth, bottle-green leaves, narrow, with pointed tip.
- *Schisandra Wu Wei Zi berry.* Five Taste berry is a deciduous woody vine with oval pink leaves and bright red berries.
- *Rhodiola root.* A perennial high alpine plant low to the ground, with gorgeous red, pink, or yellowish flowers, succulent leaves and shoots, rose-smelling rhizome, as in its species, *rosea*.

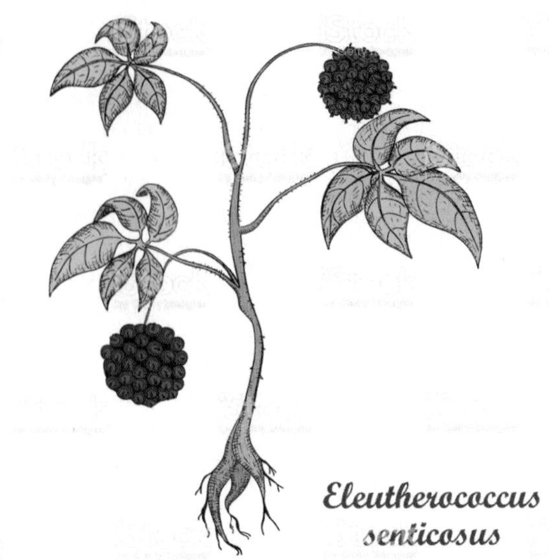

• **Fig. 12.11** Eleuthero Cu Wu Jia leaf, berry, and root is sometime called Siberian ginseng, although the plant is not a member of the panax genus. (iStock.com/Credit: Marakit_Atinat.)

Strength

- All mild. Adaptogens have minimal chronic toxicity and can be taken long term.

Key constituents

Note: Prepare all adaptogens as *dual extractions* to get the most out of these chemically complex important herbs. Prepare a 1:3 95% dual extraction straight ethanol maceration with no water, then double the calculated water, and simmer pressed marc down to half (Chapter 7).

- *Eleutherococcus Ci Wu Jia root.* Steroidal glycosides (eleutherosides, the major adaptogenic constituent) resin, triterpene saponins, lignins, polysaccharides, essential oils, many minerals.
- *Ganoderma Ling Zhi mushroom.* Triterpenes, polysaccharides, soluble proteins (32 amino acids), polypeptides, fungal lysozyme, acid protease, sterols, lactones, alkaloids, coumarin.
- *Astragalus Huang Qi root.* Flavonoids, choline, betaine, saponins, triterpenoids, polysaccharides, sitosterol, asparagine, androgens, fatty acids, trace minerals, and 19 amino acids.
- *Ashwagandha root.* Alkaloids, steroidal lactones, including with anolides, saponins, and iron.
- *Schisandra Wu Wei Zi berry.* Essential oils, lignins known as schisandrins, triterpenoids, stigmasterol, citric/malic/tartaric acids, saccharides, tannins, resin, vitamins C and E, and minerals.
- *Rhodiola root.* Phenylpropanoids, rosavins, tyrosol, flavonoids, tricin, rutin, quercetin, monoterpenes, triterpenes/sterols, phenolic acids.[1–5]

Energetics, actions, indications, dosages, safety

Note: ***Adaptogens*** are herbs that restore, build, nourish, and help the body balance stress.

Eleuthero Cu Wu Jia root (Fig. 12.11)

- *Energetics.* Somewhat pungent, bitter, neutral. Restoring, relaxing, calming, dissolving.
- *Actions.* (1) Immune enhancer. Tonifies the righteous qi and normalizes all human functions, more so than any other adaptogen, regardless of body type or constitution with no side effects.[9] A no-brainer. (2) Numerous actions: adaptogenic, anabolic, antitoxic, radio-/chemo-protective, neuroprotective, antiviral, gonadotrophic, antidiabetic. (3) Hormones and blood pressure: will normalize blood pressure, blood sugar, thyroid hormones, when either too high or too low. (4) Provides energy.
- *Indications.* (1) Any neuroendocrine deficiency: of essence, blood and qi, with exhaustion, anxiety, frequent or chronic infection, depression, dizziness, palpitations, poor sleep. (2) Imbalances: adrenals (with or without burnout), hyper or hypo thyroid, glucose imbalances of the pancreas (Chapter 27). (3) Yin deficiency of the liver, adrenals. (4) Any type of stress for any reason.
- *Dosages.* Solid root extract: Ideally, standardized to 1% eleutheroside B. Siberian Eleuthero root is far superior and more potent than same herb from China. Siberian root contains the active eleutheroside B, and the Chinese root has none.[9] Dual extraction: 1 to 5 mL per dose. Decoction: 4 to 16 g.[1–5]
- *Side effects.* Caution in yin deficiency conditions with signs of empty heat and with severe hypertension, fast pulse, or arrhythmias.
- *Contraindications.* In Chinese Medicine, most adaptogens are not taken during acute infections because they are thought to drive the infection in deeper.
- *Commission E.* Not listed.

Ganoderma Ling Zhi mushroom

- *Energetics.* Bland, bit sweet and bitter, neutral. Restoring, calming, relaxing, dissolving.

- *Actions.* (1) Adrenocortical restorative/regulator. (2) Antioxidant that inhibits free radicals. (3) Broad-spectrum antiallergenic. (3) Antilipemic: Lowers cholesterol. (3) Hypotensive: Angiotensin-converting enzyme inhibitor (ACE) that lowers blood pressure through the kidneys (Chapter 26). (4) Protects the liver and kidney in chemotherapy and radiation therapy. (5) Oxygenates in high altitude sickness.
- *Indications.* (1) Deficiency of yin, qi, blood. The perfect adaptogen for the modern world stereotype of a metabolically toxic person under constant stress. (2) Cancer treatment: minimizes symptoms of chemo and radiation therapy; antitumoral in early stages. (3) Immune enhancer: for frequent or chronic infections, autoimmune issues, immediate allergies, and immunodeficiency problems, like chronic fatigue syndrome and AIDS. May also be taken during acute infections, an exception to the usual adaptogen rule that forbids this. (4) Neuro-/cardiac restorative: for loss of memory and mental capacity, high blood pressure, high cholesterol. (5) Liver restorative in Chinese Medicine. Used for chronic hepatitis B.
- *Dosages.* Tincture: 0.5 to 2.5 mL per dose. Decoction: 2 to 6 g daily.[1–5]
- *Side effects.* Major detoxifier, so may produce minor side effects, such as loose stool, skin rash, dry mouth, because of its cleansing action. This is annoying but not necessarily bad.
- *Contraindications.* None.
- *Commission E.* Not listed.

Astragalus Huang Qi root

- *Energetics.* Sweet, bit warm, dry, restoring, astringing. Solidifying, stabilizing.
- *Actions.* (1) Immune: Superbly strengthens wei qi (defensive energy) because of its polysaccharide content. (2) GI: tonifies spleen qi (digestion) with diarrhea, poor appetite, anorexia, fatigue. (3) Strong tonic to build energy and stamina. (4) Inhibits cancer cells and is chemo/radiation protective. (5) Hepatoprotective. (6) Astringent.
- *Indications.* (1) Immune: for immune (qi) deficiencies, including chronic fatigue and AIDS. (2) GI: spleen qi deficiency with fatigue, appetite and weight loss, diarrhea, malabsorption. (3) Liver restorative for evening exhaustion, chronic hepatitis. (4) Astringency helps prolapses, hemorrhage, chronic diarrhea, excessive sweating. (5) Adrenals: restorative for fatigue, lack of stamina. (6) Heart strengthener.
- *Dosages.* Tincture: 2 to 5 mL per dose. Decoction: 10 to 30 g daily.[1–5]
- *Side effects.* Careful in yin deficiency with empty heat, full heat, spleen damp, initial stages of boils, and nursing mothers.[1]
- *Contraindications:* Acute infection.
- *Commission E.* Not listed.

Ashwagandha root

- *Energetics.* Warming, sweet, bitter, pungent, sharp. Restoring, calming.
- *Actions.* (1) Immune: restorative. (2) Neuroprotective by scavenging free radicals, antiinflammatory. (3) Increases libido. (4) Liver protective and cardioprotective. (5) Warming quality: raises metabolism, stimulates digestion, clears mucus, improves circulation. (6) Antiparasitic. (7) Cancer protective: restorative after chemotherapy and radiation, restores white blood cells. Inhibits cancer angiogenesis (blood supply to tumors) and cancer cell migration in breast tissue.
- *Indications.* (1) Immune stimulant for the sickly. (2) Neuro/endocrine restorative: especially in adrenal burnout with poor quality sleep. (3) Nervous exhaustion: calming for anxiety, bad dreams, mild obsessive-compulsive disorder, insomnia, as long as person does not show signs of heat. (4) Adjunct to cancer therapy: with chemo and/or radiation. (5) Infertility: enhances libido and semen potency.
- *Dosages.* Decoction: 20 to 30 g added to heated cow's milk. Tincture: 2 to 4 mL per dose.[1–5]
- *Side effects.* Very large amounts have caused nausea, vomiting, GI upset, and abortifacient properties. Caution in pregnancy. If person is very warm, combine with cooling herbs.
- *Contraindications.* Acute infection.
- *Commission E.* Not listed.

Schisandra Wu Wei Zi berry (Fig. 12.12)

- *Energetics.* Sour, bitter, sweet, pungent, salty (five tastes), warm, dry. Restoring, stimulating, stabilizing.
- *Actions.* (1) Restorative/tonic: liver, kidney and lungs. (2) Endocrine/immunomodulator stimulates/restores nervous system, antiallergenic, enhances athletic stamina and performance in high stress occupations. (3) Liver tropho-restorative by protecting and enhancing cytochrome P-450 detoxification system. (4) GI: detoxifier, regulates gastric hydrochloric acid (HCl), be it hyper or hypo. (5) Respiratory: restorative, expectorant, and antitussive. (6) Oxygenator. (7) Anhidrotic: decreases excess sweating because of its astringency.
- *Indications.* (1) Neuroendocrine deficiency: for insomnia, depression, forgetfulness, vision/hearing problems, fatigue, chronic infection. (2) Liver: for yin deficiency in liver diseases, hepatitis, toxicosis. (3) Adrenals: for deficiency with fatigue/burnout. (4) Lungs: for shallow breathing, wheezing, allergies. (5) Urogenital: restorative with incontinence, enuresis. (6) Astringency helps discharges and sweating.
- *Dosages.* Tincture: 2 to 5 mL at 1:2 45% ethanol per dose. Decoction: 4 to 10 g.[1–5]

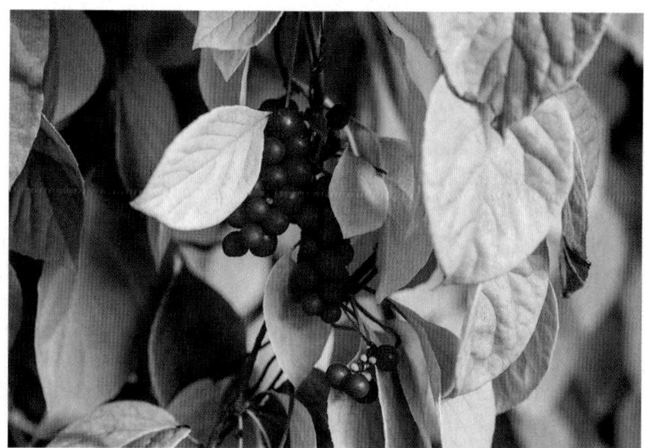

• **Fig. 12.12** Schisandra Wu Wei Zi (Five Taste berry). The five tastes traditionally refer to the five Chinese yin organs: Lungs (pungent), Spleen (sweet), Heart (bitter), Kidney (salty), and Liver (sour). (iStock.com/Credit: Geshas.)

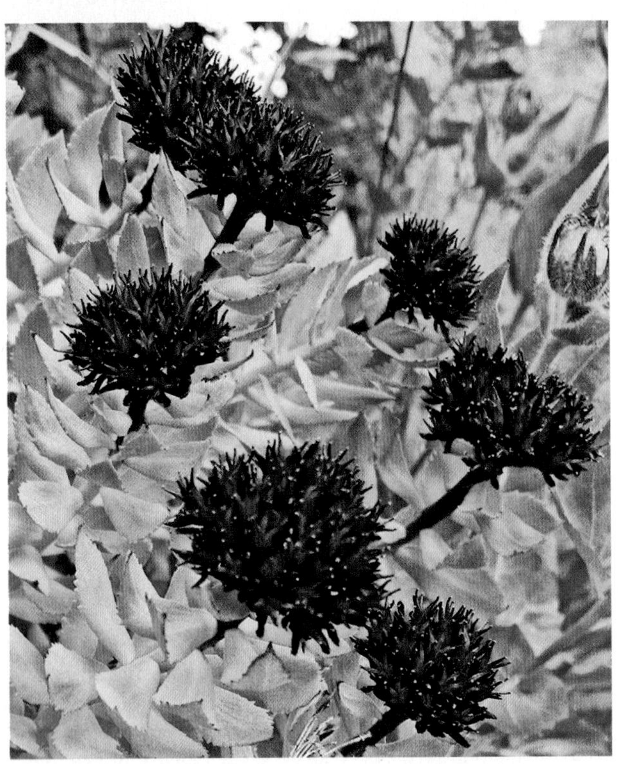

• **Fig. 12.13** Flowering *Rhodiola rosea* (Rhodiola root) is a high alpine, water-loving adaptogen. The succulent is quick acting for depression.

- *Side effects.* Cleansing action may produce temporary mild symptoms of loose stool, skin rash, dry mouth.
- *Contraindications.* Acute infection.
- *Commission E.* Not listed.

Rhodiola root (Fig. 12.13)

- *Energetics.* Very astringent and drying. Pungent, sour, a bit bitter, cool, restoring, stimulating, calming.
- *Actions.* (1) Immunostimulant. (2) Antidepressive: the best adaptogen around when there is depression. (3) Antioxidant, antimutagenic, cardioprotective, aids learning and memory. (3) Enhances physical performance. Olympians and serious athletes should take this one instead of steroids. (4) Antiinflammatory: lowers the inflammatory marker, C-reactive protein.
- *Indications.* (1) Endocrine/immune deficiency: with chronic hormonal insufficiencies of thyroid, thymus, adrenal, pancreas, and ovaries, testes. Increases estrogen and testosterone. (2) Neuro: for depression, mental fog, memory and learning challenges, poor physical endurance, anxiety, insomnia. (3) Cancer: chemo/radiation protection. (4) Discharges: as an astringent, it dries up discharges, sputum, shrinks hemorrhoids. (5) Cardiac: restorative.
- *Dosages.* Tincture: 0.25 to 2 mL of a 1:3 45% ethanol per dose. Decoction: 1.5 g per cup. Fast-acting herb that does not require high doses.[1–5]
- *Side effects.* It is very drying, so use with other adaptogens to balance.
- *Contraindications:* Acute infection.
- *Commission E.* Not listed.

Editorial

Adaptogens are precious, restorative plants, and very safe if you stay within dosage range. They are cross-cultural, the supreme, elite, revered tonics that maintain health and help the body adjust to stress and modern chronic diseases, including autoimmune. The common names of many countries' adaptogens often have the word *ginseng* in them (even though they're not true ginsengs) to honor and imply their therapeutic similarity to the genuine "ultimates": Asian *Panax ginseng* Ren Shen, and American *Panax quinquefolius* Xi Yang Shen. Cases in point are *Eleutherococcus senticosus* (Siberian ginseng root), *Rhodiola rosea* (Tibetan ginseng root), *Pfaffia paniculata* (Suma or Brazilian ginseng root). Asian and American ginsengs do not appear in this Materia Medica because of their exorbitant price. However, Chinese Medicine frequently uses a mild, weaker non-ginseng substitute in triple doses for the same purpose.[16] The herb is *Codonopsis pilosula* Dang Shen (Downy Bellflower root), sometimes called *Poor Man's Ginseng.*

Adaptogens are mild tonics that can, and probably should, be taken indefinitely for maximum prevention and health. They work well in combination with one another. All are warm or neutral, except the more cooling Rhodiola. True adaptogens support the hypothalamus-pituitary-adrenal (HPA) axis (Chapter 27).

- *Eleutherococcus Ci Wu Jia root.* This invaluable Siberian adaptogen is the most studied herb in the world. Use it for any type of constitution or body type. It normalizes all systems.
- *Ganoderma Ling Zhi mushroom.* Reishi mushroom is the longevity elixir mushroom. It has been revered and used by Chinese emperors since the time of the Ming dynasty (CE 1590) because it is reputed to prolong life. It is a go-to adaptogen for people under constant stress. And for those with cancer, Reishi counteracts the toxic effects of chemotherapy and is protective to healthy cells during radiation therapy.
- *Astragalus Huang Qi root.* This woody root is routinely used in soups and stews in China for its sweet-tasting, energy-building, rich amino acid and trace mineral content. It is very popular in the United States and was one of the first Chinese herbs to become available in the West. It is foremost an immune modulator that enhances energy and stamina, safe for babies, children, the sick, and elders. Astragalus excels in combination with other adaptogens.
- *Ashwagandha root.* This is a well-balanced herbal adaptogen and brain food for most people. It is sharp, pungent and warming, and—helps digestion, circulation, and clearing of mucus. Think Ashwagandha when energy is needed: combine with Milky Oat berry or Nettle herb for adrenal burnout. Conversely, it can also help to relax and aid sleep. For heat signs, combine with cooling herbs because this is a warm, stimulating plant. In female sexuality issues, combine with Asparagus root (Shatavari) from India. Ashwagandha is libido-enhancing for women and men, aptly named "like a horse," whether a mare or a stallion.
- *Schisandra Wu Wei Zi berry.* In Chinese Medicine, the five tastes of this herb traditionally reflected the five visceral yin organs, Lung (pungent), Spleen (sweet), Heart (bitter), Kidney (salty), and Liver (sour). Schisandra is best for nervous exhaustion, fatigue, liver detoxification, insomnia, depression, forgetfulness, and vision problems. Its tonic action goes to the Chinese Liver, Kidneys, and Lungs. It is also antiallergenic.
- *Rhodiola root.* The classic candidate for Rhodiola is a person who is depleted, depressed, and has no energy. It is the best adaptogen for depression, and as a bonus, is fast acting. When

combined with St. John's Wort, it works quickly, whereas the other takes its time and kicks in over 6 to 8 weeks. Good quality Rhodiola root should smell like roses. Use with Hawthorn berry as a cardiac restorative.

Alterative Herbs that Help Detoxification

Rumex crispus L. (Yellow Dock root)

Arctium lappa L. (Burdock root), Niu Bang Zi (Burdock seed)

Galium aparine L. (Cleavers herb)

Trifolium pratense L. (Red Clover flower)

Apium graveolens L. (Celery seed)

General trigger words

* **Alteratives** * **Detoxifiers** * **Skin** * **Autoimmune** *

Specific trigger words

- *Yellow Dock root.* GI, bitter, liver.
- *Burdock root.* Detoxicant diuretic, urinary restorative. Seed: wind heat, demulcent.
- *Cleavers herb.* Lymphatic drainer.
- *Red Clover flower.* Estrogenic.
- *Celery seed.* Kidneys. Diuretic, detoxification.

Families

- *Yellow Dock root.* Polygonaceae
- *Burdock root and seed.* Asteraceae/Compositae
- *Cleavers herb.* Rubiaceae
- *Red Clover flower.* Leguminosae
- *Celery seed.* Umbelliferae

Growth and harvest

- *Yellow Dock root.* Perennial 1 to 3 feet high, mature flower/seed stalk is reddish-brown, green leaves are crispy and curly (common name Curly Dock), large yellow taproot. Habit, open fields.
- *Burdock root and seed.* Dull green, 3 to 4 feet; lower leaves can be huge—up to 1 foot across, with furry underside, and smaller upper leaves; flowers thistle-like, purple blossoms on top of the tall stalks. Bristly, sticky burrs (the inspiration for velcro) follow the flowers as a method of seed dispersal. Biennial: the first year is a rosette and the second year, a flowering stalk (like Mullein).
- *Cleavers herb.* Straggling climber covered in hooked hairs that stick to animal fur and clothing. Leaves whorled. Flowers tiny white with four petals.
- *Red Clover flower.* Leaves alternate, trifoliate (three leaflets), pale chevron in the outer half, dark pink flowers in dense cluster, beloved by bees.
- *Celery seed.* Pungent, slender, erect biennial, leaves shiny, pinnate with toothed leaflets, white flowers in compound umbels.

Strength

- These are all mild herbs with minimal chronic toxicity.

Key constituents

- *Yellow Dock root.* Anthraquinones, quercetin, tannins, essential oils, calcium, oxalate, resin, high in minerals including calcium, phosphorus, iron, and vitamins A, B, and C. (Tincture 1:4 45%–55% ethanol in order to extract its tannins, essential oils, and resins.)
- *Burdock root.* Bitter glycosides, flavonoids, polysaccharides, lignans, alkaloids, inulin, resin, mucilage, vitamins A and C, mineral and trace mineral rich. (Tincture 1:4 40%–60% ethanol.)
- *Cleavers herb.* Citric and other acids, red dye with anthraquinones, saponins, coumarins, chlorophyll, tannins, trace minerals. (Tincture 1:4 in only 35% ethanol, because of its many water-soluble constituents.)
- *Red Clover flower.* Caffeic, silicic, oxalic, salicylic acids, essential oils, glycosides, including genistein and daidzein (estrogenic), coumarin, resins, tannins, chlorophyll, minerals, vitamin C, tocopherol. (Tincture in 40%–50% ethanol.)
- *Celery seed.* Essential oils, flavonoids, choline, alkaloids, many minerals and trace minerals, and vitamins A, B, C, and E. (Tincture in 1:3 40% ethanol.)[1–5]

Energetics, actions, indications, dosages, safety

Note: All ***alteratives*** (also called *depuratives*) enhance overall absorption and assimilation of nutrients and elimination of waste products of cellular metabolism through the liver, lungs, kidney, bowel, or skin. They are cooling, restorative, and dissolving. Some alteratives have affinities for certain body systems.

Yellow Dock root

- *Energetics.* Bitter, astringent, cold, dry. Dissolving, decongesting, restoring.
- *Actions.* (1) Broad-spectrum, dry, and cooling detoxifier/alterative that works to eliminate wastes through the liver, kidneys, colon, and lymph. (2) Its bitter taste stimulates the GI to release digestive enzymes, and the liver to release bile (a cholagogue). (3) Laxative because of bile stimulation in the liver. (4) High in minerals, notably iron. (5) Dissolvent for stones, swollen glands.
- *Indications.* (1) Skin damp heat: especially for chronic eczema, psoriasis itching, redness, vesicles, boils, and abscesses of skin; inflammations of the eyes and mouth. (2) For swollen glands and ovarian cysts because of its lymph draining property. (3) For anemia; it has lots of iron. (4) Aids elimination of metabolic waste products through the kidneys, bladder, and colon. Use for chronic arthritis and gout, and in any general detox formula. (5) Liver detox for those with chronic constipation and food allergies or jaundice. (6) Kidney, diuretic, and dissolves stones.
- *Dosages.* Tincture: 2 to 4 mL per dose of 1:5 45%. Decoction: 1 to 2 teaspoons per cup.[1–5]
- *Side effects.* Not in pregnancy or lactation, caution with kidney stones.
- *Contraindications.* Not for renal failure, diabetes, inherited elevated blood iron (hemochromatosis) or electrolyte abnormalities.
- *Commission E.* Not listed.

Burdock root (Figs. 12.14 and 12.15)

- *Energetics.* Root: Somewhat bitter, pungent cool, dry. Dissolving, stimulating, restoring. Seed is pungent, bitter, moist, and cooling.
- *Actions.* (1) Kidney affinity: the skin is considered the third kidney (Chapter 25). When the kidneys are overloaded, toxins leech out through skin eruptions and can proceed into joints, causing many types of arthritis. All of this is considered damp in Chinese medicine. Therefore Burdock is a general detoxifier of damp and toxic heat. For skin, kidneys, and arthritis. (2) It dissolves deposits, decongests lymph flow. (3) Its polysaccharides help immune regulation and immediate allergies. (4) Galactagogue, diaphoretic, immune stimulant. (5) Liver: promotes bile flow to stimulate digestion.
- *Indications.* (1) Think Burdock root for skin, bladder, and arthritis, because of those organs' physiological relationship to detoxification. (2) Kidneys for frequent UTIs, stones, bladder irritations, dysuria. In arthritis for gout, rheumatoid (RA), and osteoarthritis (OA). (3) Skin damp heat: for eczema, psoriasis, infectious wounds, skin ulcers, bites, stings, boils, eye inflammations. (4) Allergies: its immuno regulation helps food allergies and allergic dermatitis. (5) Chinese Medicine use of seeds: Wind Heat for common cold/flu onset, because of its diaphoretic, antiinflammatory, and demulcent action. (6) Galactagogue, stimulates bile flow, and helps constipation, stomach aches, and intestinal dysbiosis.
- *Dosages.* Tincture: 1 to 4 mL per dose; Decoction: 6 to 12 g.[1–5]
- *Side effects.* Possible cleansing reactions such as skin eruptions. If this occurs, add stronger diuretics such as Cleavers herb, Dandelion root, or Poria Fu Ling to enhance toxin elimination through the kidneys.
- *Contraindications.* Pregnancy, a gentle uterine stimulant.
- *Commission E.* Not listed.

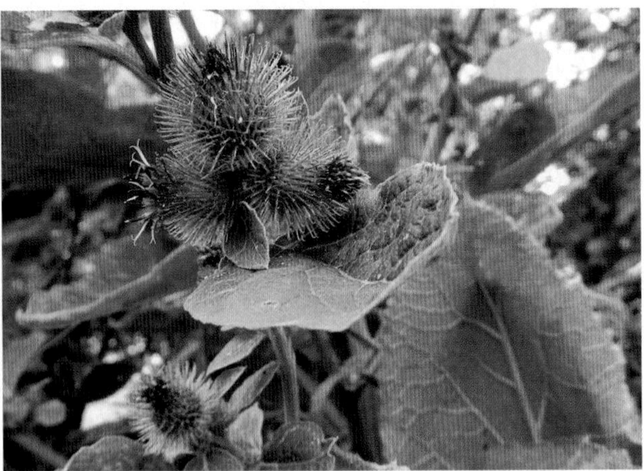

• **Fig. 12.14** *Arctium lappa* (Burdock root and seed). The plant has large, soft leaves and a hooked spiny flower calyx holding many tiny seeds.

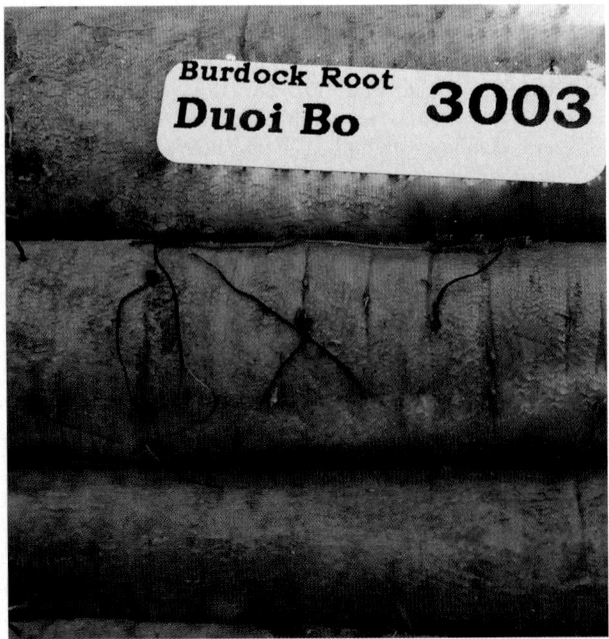

• **Fig. 12.15** Burdock root wrapped for sale in a Chinese market. The roots often end up in a stir fry or soup pot in Asia, and in the West, as a diuretic detoxicant and urinary restorative in a tincture.

Cleavers herb

- *Energetics.* Somewhat bitter, sweet, salty, cold, dry. Softening, dissolving, diluting, decongesting, restoring.
- *Actions.* (1) Lymphatic drainer. Dissolves clots, deposits. (2) Clears toxic heat, relieves pain and inflammation in skin eruptions. (3) Refrigerant for heat. (4) Urinary sedative/diuretic.
- *Indications.* (1) Detoxicant/lymphatic drainer/skin repairer for burns, wounds, eczema, tumors, tonsillitis, measles. (2) Urinary damp heat for stones, diuresis, cystitis, UTIs, prostatitis. Use as a urinary demulcent with Cornsilk or Marshmallow root. (3) Liver damp heat for jaundice, hepatitis. (4) Refrigerant for fevers.
- *Dosages.* Tincture: 2 to 5 mL per dose. Decoction: 8 to 16 g. Requires long-term use for chronic conditions.[1–5]
- *Side effects.* None.
- *Contraindications.* None.
- *Commission E.* Not listed.

Red Clover flower (Fig. 12.16)

- *Energetics.* Somewhat sweet and bland, neutral with cooling potential, moist. Softening, dissolving, diluting, nourishing, astringing, relaxing.
- *Actions.* (1) Detoxicant, dissolvent, nutritive. (2) Repairs tissue and reduces pain and inflammation. (3) Relaxant to respiratory and urinary system. (4) Estrogenic because of its flavonoids, genistein and daidzein.
- *Indications.* (1) Tissue repair: detoxicant for skin damp/toxic heat for chronic eczema, many types of arthritis. (2) Superb respiratory relaxant for acute/chronic bronchitis, wheezing, asthma, laryngitis, spasmodic uncontrollable coughing. (3) Relaxes bladder spasms. (4) Estrogenic and moistens dryness in yin deficient/estrogen deficient PMS, dysmenorrhea, menopause. (5) Dissolvent for tumors of skin, breast, ovaries.

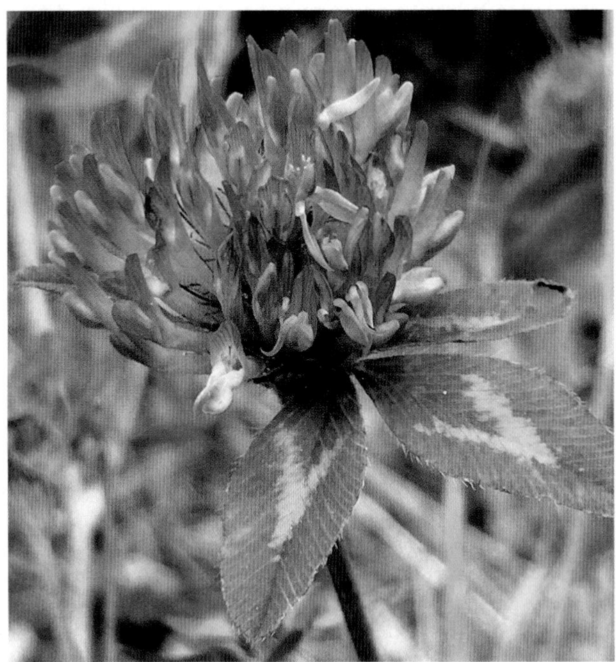

• **Fig. 12.16** Red Clover flower and leaf. Collect flowers and first three leaves for the most complete medicine. *Trifolium pratense* is an alterative that also excels as a respiratory relaxant in acute and chronic bronchitis and spasmodic coughing.

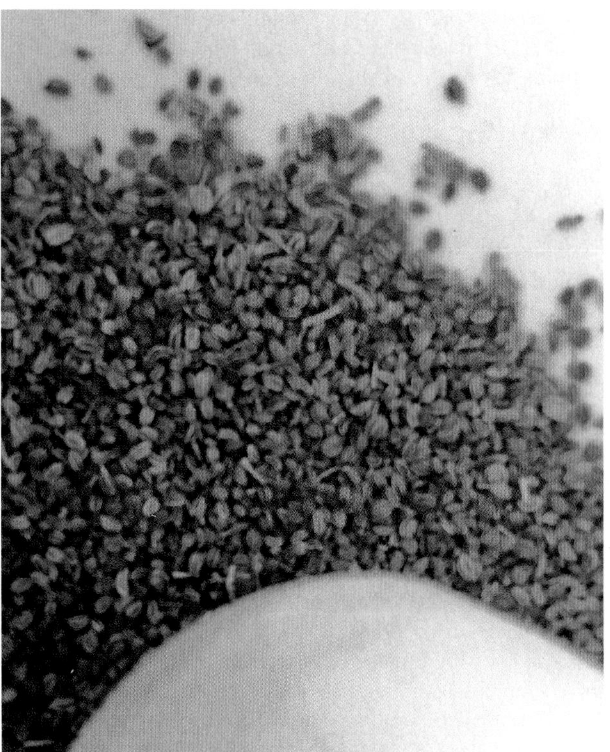

• **Fig. 12.17** *Apium graveolens* (Celery seed) is a diuretic detoxifier, shown with mortar and pestle ready for grinding.

- *Dosages.* Tincture: 2 to 5 mL per dose at 1:3 50% (could triple this as needed). Infusion: 10 to 16 g. May use as fresh juice; topically in first aid creams, enema, sponges, or pessaries for vaginal itching; and in syrups for coughs. Must take faithfully, long term, for detox/tumor resolving effects to occur.[1–5]
- *Side effects.* None.
- *Contraindications.* Not during pregnancy—estrogenic.
- *Commission E.* Not listed.

Celery seed (Fig. 12.17)

- *Energetics.* Somewhat bitter, sweet and pungent, neutral to cool, moist. Dissolving, stimulating, restoring, nourishing.
- *Actions.* (1) Detoxicant/alterative, diuretic, and dissolving, works on a kidney level. (2) Regenerating restorative for the kidneys, nerves, adrenals, and reproductive organs. (3) Galactagogue, like Fennel seed. (4) Clears damp heat.
- *Indications.* (1) Kidneys: dissolves stones, diuretic that helps dry damp in edema, especially of lower limbs and face and in UTIs. (2) Detoxification: through kidneys for arthritis, gout, bone spurs, and excellent for acute flare-ups of fibromyalgia and chronic fatigue. (3) Female health for low libido, low breast milk, delayed or irregular periods, and restorative postpartum. (4) Clears damp heat in acute UTIs and fever. (5) Adrenal/nervous restorative for burnout from stress along with adaptogens. (6) Celery stalk eaten regularly has a cooling, detoxicant, restoring action.
- *Dosages.* Tincture: 2 to 5 mL per dose. Decoction: 8 to 14 g. Essential oils: 1 to 2 drops in gel cap with olive oil.[1–5]
- *Side effects.* None.
- *Contraindications.* Caution during pregnancy, a uterine stimulant. Not with organic kidney disease present.
- *Commission E.* Potential allergy reactions.

Editorial

The designation—*alteratives*—is a rather antiquated and vague herbal category, said to *alter* the body. They are used for treating toxicity, most famously from skin eruptions but also for arthritis and infections. Alteratives were widely used by the Eclectics and Thomsonians who called them *blood purifiers*, although not quite accurately. Alteratives help eliminate waste products of metabolism by stimulating the body's natural avenues of detoxification. The body detoxifies all the time through the lymphatics, liver, kidneys, skin, and bowels. The result is so-called *cleaner* blood, because the blood is the transport system that carries waste products of cellular metabolism to those organs for removal. Hence, blood purifiers are actually detoxifiers. True alterative/depurative herbs not only aid detoxification, but also facilitate proper nutrient assimilation, which has a normalizing action on overall physiology.

- *Yellow Dock root.* This one is a multipurpose detoxicant, except for those who have abnormally high iron levels in the blood (hemochromatosis). Good in combination with others of this class, it is the damp heat clearer-upper, along with Dandelion root. Damp heat shows up as skin rashes, joint pain, acute (hot) arthritis, indigestion, constipation, thirst, dark urine, red tongue with possible oily yellow or gray fur, and rapid pulse.
- *Burdock root.* Think kidney detox for Burdock. In the West, Burdock root is a cooling hepatic and kidney remedy, used for detoxicant, diuretic, and urinary restorative properties.

The need for kidney detoxification implies that the liver and kidneys are overloaded and could be doing a better job of filtering toxins out of the blood or the kidneys are in need of a boost. Signs of this are skin eruptions and eczema that won't go away.

- In Chinese Medicine, *Arctium lappa* Niu Bang Zi (Burdock *seed*) is used, mainly as a respiratory demulcent, expectorant, and for infections in external wind heat. This is the same plant that is used in the West, but here the seed is used as opposed to the root.[5]

- *Cleavers herb.* Cleavers and *lymph mover* go hand in hand. In doing this one thing, it detoxifies and helps skin damp heat and related ills. Its dissolving, softening attributes make it an excellent member of a kidney stone or benign breast lump formula.
- *Red Clover flower.* The two standout functions for Red Clover are as a chronic bronchitis relaxant and as a mild estrogenic. For maximum phytoestrogenic benefit, include the first three leaves under the flower head in a tincture, because the leaves have been chemically analyzed to have the estrogenic component, whereas the flowers are more detoxifying. This is where wildcrafting excels, so we can pick and choose which parts to use. Herb companies typically harvest blossoms only. It is standard operating procedure to use Red Clover in first aid creams and healing lotions for skin damp heat and wounds.
- *Celery seed.* Chronic stress with adrenal burnout is a key description of a Celery seed-type person. They're exhausted, overworked, stressed, and anxious, with bad digestion, low sex drive, perhaps damp, and most likely in need of detoxification. Although not technically an adaptogen, Celery seed would pair nicely with Eleutherococcus Ci Wu Jia (Siberian ginseng root), Rhodiola root, Milky Oat berry, or Rosemary leaf. For kidney problems, combine with Burdock root as a dissolvent for deposits and any water retention. Excels in the female department.

There are so many alterative/depurative/detoxifying herbs not detailed here that address various body systems and problems or complement those covered. For skin detox, use Burdock root, Yellow Dock root, Jamaican Sarsaparilla root, Cleavers herb, Red Clover flower, or Figwort herb. For lymphatic drainage/detox, try Burdock root, Marigold flower, Walnut leaf, Echinacea root, Blue Flag root, Poke root, or Chinese Lonicera Jin Yin Hua (Honeysuckle flower) or Forsythia Lian Qiao (Forsythia valve/capsule). For antiarthritic action, try Celery seed, Parsley seed, Red Clover flower, Horsetail herb, or Pipsissewa (Wintergreen herb.)

Expectorants, Bronchodilators, Antitussives

Thymus vulgaris L. (Thyme herb)

Tussilago farfara L. (Coltsfoot herb), Kuan Dong Hua (Coltsfoot flower)

Prunus serotina Ehrhart (Wild Cherry bark)

Xanthium sibiricum Patrin, Cang Er Zi (Siberian Cocklebur fruit)

Chrysanthemum x *morifolium* Ramatuelle, Ju Hua (Chrysanthemum flower)

Platycodon grandiflorum de Candolle, Jie Geng (Balloonflower root)

General trigger words

* **Antitussive** * **Bronchodilator** * **Expectorant** *

Specific trigger words.

- *Thyme herb.* Broad-spectrum antimicrobial. Drier-upper.
- *Coltsfoot herb.* Multipurpose coughs. Hot or cold, expectorant, antitussive, demulcent.
- *Wild Cherry bark.* Antitussive. Nutritive.
- *Xanthium Cang Er Zi fruit.* Upper respiratory. Sinuses. Allergies.
- *Chrysanthemum Ju Hua flower.* External Wind Heat.
- *Platycodon Jie Geng root.* General coughs, Expectorant.

Families

- *Thyme herb.* Lamiaceae/Mint
- *Coltsfoot herb.* Asteraceae/Compositae
- *Wild Cherry bark.* Rosaceae
- *Xanthium Cang Er Zi fruit.* Asteraceae/Compositae
- *Chrysanthemum Ju Hua flower.* Asteraceae/Compositae
- *Platycodon Jie Geng root.* Campanulaceae

Growth and harvest

- *Thyme herb.* Small, highly aromatic, shrub-like with square woody stems finely covered with hair. Tiny ovate opposite leaves with bluish-purple or pink two-lipped flowers.
- *Coltsfoot herb* (Fig. 12.18). Grows in dry and wet areas along streams. Yellow flowers blossom before rounded, heart-shaped, serrated leaves develop and are said to resemble a colt's foot.
- *Wild Cherry bark.* Large tree or bush, smooth reddish bark with lenticels when young, and darker, rough bark when mature, oval serrate leaves, white flowers in long, erect, terminal racemes.
- *Xanthium Cang Er Zi.* Annual, from 1 to 3 feet high, grows worldwide, lanceolate leaves, undersides covered with thick white down, small flowers, rough burrlike fruit.
- *Chrysanthemum Ju Hua flower.* Widely cultivated, flower head in densely packed cluster of numerous, small, flowers. Yellow and white flowers used in Chinese Medicine, leaves alternate, lobed.
- *Platycodon Jie Geng root.* A 1- to 2-foot ornamental perennial, beautiful purple-blue flowers. Buds puff up like balloons (Balloonflower) before bursting open into upward-facing, bell-shaped flowers with five pointed lobes. Ovate, toothed, blue-green leaves.

Strength

- Thyme herb, Coltsfoot herb, Wild Cherry bark, Chrysanthemum Ju Hua flower are mild with minimal chronic toxicity.

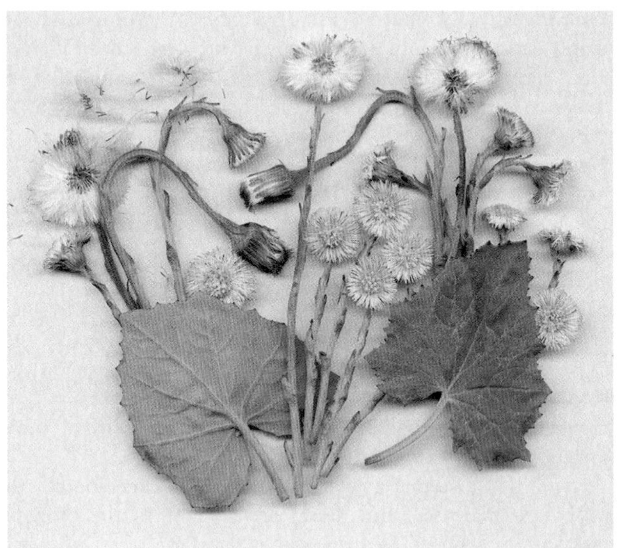

• **Fig. 12.18** *Tussilago farfara* (Coltsfoot herb) is a species that grows in the Eastern US. Western Coltsfoot is a different variety, used similarly. Coltsfoot flower is a relaxant/stimulant expectorant. The leaf is demulcent for dry lung conditions. Both are antitussive, antispasmodic, and antiinflammatory cough remedies. (Copyright Lang/Tucker Photography.) (Photographs loaned with permission from *The Botanical Series* are copywritten by Jennifer Anne Tucker and Gerald Lang from the Studio at Hill Crystal Farm. www.jennifer-tucker.com.)

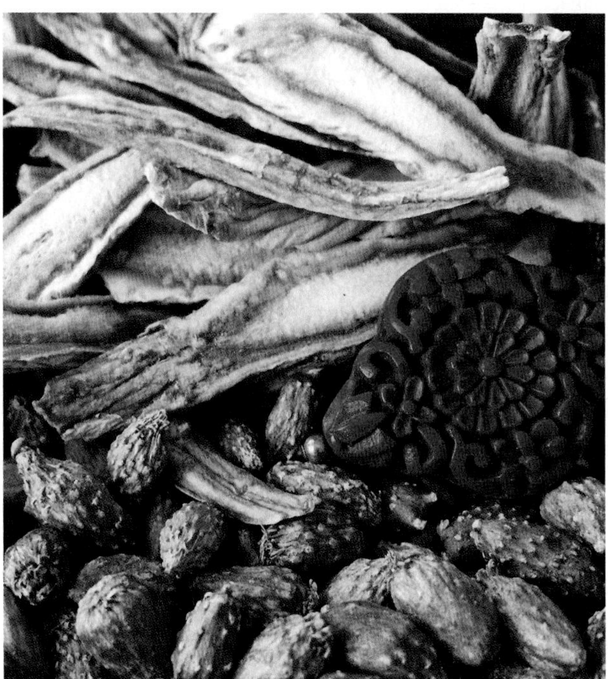

• **Fig. 12.19** Platycodon Jie Geng (Balloonflower root) is a moist expectorant that is a natural in a cough syrup (top), and Xanthium Cang Er Zi (Siberian Cocklebur fruit) (lower) is a go-to for upper airway respiratory allergies.

- Xanthium Cang Er Zi fruit is medium strength with some chronic toxicity.

Key Constituents

- *Thyme herb*. High content of many essential oils, notably thymol and carvacrol, which are both antimicrobial. Carnosol and rosmanol are antioxidant. Bitter tannins, flavonoids, saponins. (Tincture 1:3 in 70%–75% ethanol due to extremely high essential oil content.)
- *Coltsfoot herb*. Essential oils, mucilage, inulin, up to 17% tannins, bitter glycosides, flavonoids, hormonal substances, gallic acid, alkaloids, sitosterol, minerals, and trace minerals. (Tincture 1:4 in 45% ethanol.)
- *Wild Cherry bark*. Cyanogenic glycosides, coumarins, tannin, gallic/azulic/benzoic acids, essential oils, starch, lignin, gallitannins, resin, minerals. (Tincture 1:3 in 60% ethanol.)
- *Xanthium Cang Er Zi fruit* (Fig. 12.19). Glycosides (xanthostrumarin), fatty oils (linoleic and oleic), xanthenol, resin, alkaloids, organic acids, vitamin C. (Tincture in 1:3 50% ethanol.)
- *Chrysanthemum Ju Hua flower*. Many essential oils, alkaloids, flavonoids, adenine, choline, amino acids, vitamins B1 and E, trace minerals. (Tincture 1:3 in 50% ethanol.)
- *Platycodon Jie Geng root*. Eighteen kinds of triterpenoid saponins including platycodon, sterols, botulin, inulin, platycodonin, platycogenic acids. (Tincture 1:3 in 50% ethanol.)[1–5]

Energetics, actions, indications, dosages, safety

Thyme herb

- *Energetics*. Pungent, bitter, astringent, very aromatic, warm, dry. Stimulating, dispersing, restoring, relaxing, astringing.
- *Actions*. (1) Expectorant function is because of its thymol essential oil content. (2) Antimicrobial function is because of thymol. (4) Anti-everything: antibacterial, antifungal, antiviral, antiparasitic, antioxidant, and antiinflammatory. (3) Spasmolytic for coughs. (4) Rubefacient. (5) Uterine stimulant. (6) Adrenal tonic.
- *Indications*. (1) Lungs: Thyme is foremost for coughs and wheezing, sore throats, infections of the cold variety. (2) Mucolytic. It dries up mucus supremely. (3) Its many actions are tailored to Wind Damp Cold and tense conditions; everything that's needed for early upper or lower respiratory infections with sneezing, chills, fatigue, spasmodic cough with white sputum, sore throat, clear rhinitis, muscle aches, laryngitis, or sinusitis. (4) GI: Warms and relaxes, relieves gas and diarrhea, intestinal dysbiosis, colitis with mucus. For intestinal parasites like tapeworm, hookworm. (5) Externally for lice and scabies. (6) Adrenals: tonic/restorative effect for adrenal deficiency, fatigue. (7) Women: for amenorrhea and discharges.
- *Dosages*. Tincture: 3 to 4 mL dose 1:5 45%. Infusion: 3 to 12 g a day. Essential oil: 1 to 2 drops in a capsule with olive oil carrier. Use in gargles, steams, douches, compresses, for antimicrobial properties. As a mouthwash, decreases pain in mouth, gums, and teeth problems.[1–5]
- *Side effects*. Careful in dry conditions or yin deficiency. (Thyme is very drying.)
- *Contraindications*. Pregnancy, because of its uterine stimulant properties. In children, keep the essential oil away from mouth and nose, as could cause reflex spasm.[4]
- *Commission E*. For symptoms of bronchitis and whooping cough and phlegm of the upper respiratory tracts.

Coltsfoot herb

- *Energetics*. Somewhat astringent, bitter, pungent, and sweet; cool, dry/moist. Restoring, stimulating, decongesting, relaxing.

- *Actions.* Symptomatic relief. (1) Lungs and cough: expectorant, antitussive, antispasmodic, demulcent, anticatarrhal. (2) Diuretic. (3) Vulnerary.
- *Indications.* (1) Lungs: for lung phlegm heat with white/yellowish sputum, bronchitis, asthma, wheezing of any type. For coughing, sore throats of the warm, dry variety, because it is cool and moist. (3) Moistens the lungs in all dry, scratchy sore throats. (4) Tissue repair in chronic wounds or ulcers.
- *Dosages.* Tincture: 2 to 4 mL 3 times per day 1:5 45%. Infusion: 2 teaspoons dried herb/1 cup water. May smoke dried for asthma, along with Thyme herb.[1–5]
- *Side effects.* Avoid in pregnancy and lactation because it contains small amounts of PAs, the same constituent as in Comfrey, but in smaller amounts.
- *Contraindications.* Pregnancy and breast feeding due to PAs.
- *Commission E.* Not listed.

Wild Cherry bark

- *Energetics.* Bitter, astringent, somewhat pungent, cool, dry. Relaxing, restoring.
- *Actions.* (1) Antitussive, antispasmodic (powerful cough reflex sedative), expectorant. (2) Astringent. (3) Nervine. (4) Restoring to the nervous system.
- *Indications.* (1) Lungs: for irritating coughs of any type. Dry harsh coughing, in bronchitis, wheezing, whooping cough. It sedates the reflex, but it is a bit dry, so a moist herb needs to accompany. (2) Astringent: to help diarrhea, clear up weepy eye infections with Goldenrod or Eyebright. (3) Restorative for chronic stress.
- *Dosages.* Tincture: 2 to 4 mL 1:5 40% ethanol. Decoction: 1 teaspoon to 1 cup water. Use in cough syrups and lozenges.[1–5]
- *Side effects.* None.
- *Contraindications.* Pregnancy because of its teratogenic cyanogenic glycoside.[1]
- *Commission E.* Not listed.

Xanthium Cang Er Zi fruit

- *Energetics.* Sweet, bit bitter and pungent, warm. Restoring, stimulating.
- *Actions.* (1) Ear, nose, and throat remedy. Antiallergenic, mucostatic, decongestant (from a diuretic action), antiinflammatory, antiinfective. (2) Restores nasal mucosa. (3) Stops itching (antipruritic). (4) Analgesic for joints and muscle aches.
- *Indications.* (1) Upper respiratory: head Damp Cold conditions with rhinitis, sinus congestion, chronic and allergic sinusitis, itching. (2) Analgesic for arthritic and joint conditions, muscle aches called Wind Damp Obstruction.
- *Dosages.* Tincture: 2 to 4 mL per dose. Decoction: 3 to 9 g per day.[1–5]
- *Side effects.* Very rarely causes vomiting, diarrhea, abdominal pain, hypotension with continuous long-term use.
- *Contraindications.* None.
- *Commission E.* Not listed.

Chrysanthemum Ju Hua flower

- *Energetics.* Sweet, a bit bitter, cool. Calming, relaxing.
- *Actions.* (1) Expels External Wind Heat with fever, headache, and red, painful, dry eyes. (2) Vasodilation.
- *Indications.* (1) Upper respiratory: cooling, antiinfective, and diaphoretic for External Wind Heat with fever, headache, dry red eyes, conjunctivitis, bronchitis. (2) Vasodilating for hypertension. (3) Eyes: calms the Liver, which opens to the eyes. For blurry vision, dizziness, tinnitus, and floaters. (4) Nervous relaxant for headache, vision problems, dizziness, tinnitus.
- *Dosages.* Tincture: 2 to 5 mL per dose. Infusion: 5 g per cup.[1–5]
- *Side effects.* None.
- *Contraindications.* None.
- *Commission E.* Not listed.

Platycodon Jie Geng root

- *Energetics.* Sweet, a bit bitter and pungent, neutral, moist. Stimulating, restoring.
- *Actions.* (1) Respiratory stimulant and expectorant that reflexively increases and dilutes secretion from the bronchial mucosa, making it easy to discharge. (2) It is antitussive, demulcent, even an antiinflammatory detoxicant with some antihistamine action. (3) Dispels throat and lung pus, a strong herb for abscesses in the lung and throat. (4) Mild nervous sedative. (5) Helps lower blood sugar (***hypoglycemic***), cholesterol, and lipids.
- *Indications.* (1) Lungs: for External Wind Cold or External Wind Heat and coughing, with or without sputum. For acute or chronic bronchitis. (2) Throat infections: dry, itchy, perhaps with laryngitis, wheezing, repeated coughing that makes the chest hurt, pneumonia, or tonsillitis. (3) Lung abscesses, especially with pus. (4) GI: for ulcers as an antacid, and hypoglycemic. (5) Cardiac: systemic hypertension with anxiety and palpitations.
- *Dosages.* Tincture: 2 to 4 mL per dose. Decoction: 3 to 20 g.[1–5]
- *Side effects.* None.
- *Contraindications.* Diseases such as tuberculosis and with blood-streaked sputum or coughing up blood.[2]
- *Commission E.* Not listed

Editorial

- *Thyme herb* (Fig. 12.20). This one does it all for beginning upper and lower respiratory infections, as long as the condition is on the cooler, moist side, with no fever or heat. It dries up watery drippy noses, thin white or sticky sputum, and helps sweat out the infection. Not only that, Thyme herb calms stubborn coughs, and breaks up and pushes out mucus. It relieves muscle aches and fights any type of infection. Not bad for one herb.
- *Coltsfoot herb.* Better for warmer, wetter coughs than Thyme but can be used for cold conditions also. Coltsfoot herb is a versatile respiratory herb used as cough suppressant, antitussive, expectorant, and demulcent. (The word *tussive* means all-purpose cough dispeller.) It is a natural player with White Horehound herb and Wild Cherry bark in a cough syrup. Mildly diuretic, Coltsfoot could go in a cystitis blend. A go-along herb to complement others in formula. Excellent choice if you're not sure if the condition is hot or cold. The Chinese use Coltsfoot flower (Kuan Dong Hua) for similar purposes.
- *Wild Cherry bark.* A multipurpose symptomatic cough choice in the West. It relaxes and has an additional *restorative*

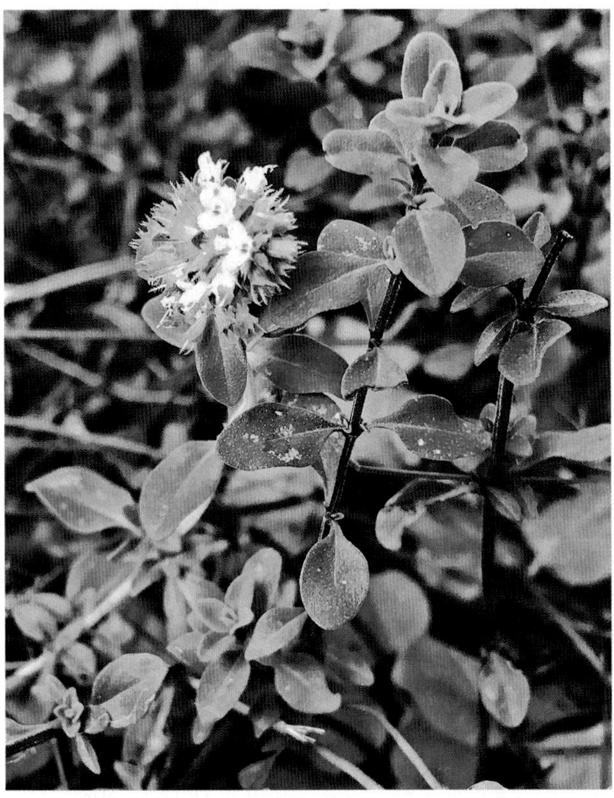

• **Fig. 12.20** Warming and drying *Thymus vulgaris* (Thyme herb) excels in cold, wet productive coughs with thin, white mucous.

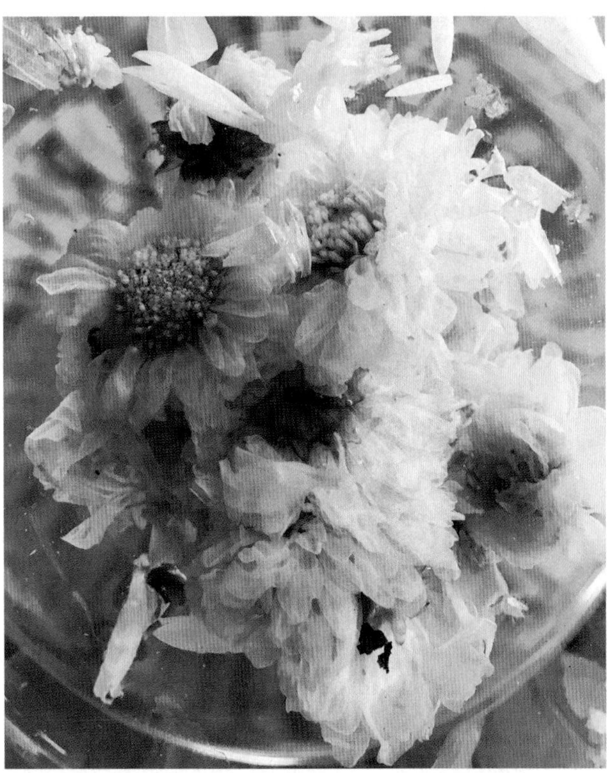

• **Fig. 12.21** Chrysanthemum Ju Hua flowers rehydrating in tea. These yellow blossoms are a popular Chinese antiinfective and diaphoretic for External Wind Heat.

benefit, like Mullein leaf. *Prunus serotina* (commonly called Wild Cherry, Black Cherry, Chokecherry, and Virginia prune bark), is the perfect antiinflammatory, antitussive, and bronchodilator. It's a must for cough syrups. A bit drying, so to counteract, could add moisturizing Licorice root or Slippery Elm bark, White Horehound or *Grindelia robusta* (Gumweed flower) into the formula.

- *Xanthium Cang Er Zi fruit*. This is the main Chinese herb for respiratory allergies and chronic sinusitis with nasal obstructions and discharge.[17] It dries up runny eyes and noses and is one of my go-to herbs for upper respiratory conditions, especially paired with Western Goldenrod herb and Chinese Medicine's pungent Magnolia bud Xin Yi Hua. Specifically, Xanthium Cang Er Zi fruit is more for chronic conditions, Goldenrod is more for acute, whereas Magnolia bud opens the airway just as aromatic Eucalyptus leaf does.
- *Chrysanthemum Ju Hua flower* (Fig. 12.21). A very important Chinese herb for upper respiratory infections, as an ear, nose, and throat relaxant, sedative, and diaphoretic. The two most popular flowers used as single herbs are Chamomile in the West and Chrysanthemum in the East; both in the Daisy family and have similar properties. Dried, flattened Chrysanthemum flowers transform when dropped into boiling water, unfolding into glorious yellow flowers. It is a daily tonic tea popular in China to nourish Liver and Kidney yin, benefit the essence, and brighten the eyes when used in combination with *Lycium* Gou Qi Zi (Goji berry or Wolfberry). It is also an important cardiac relaxant and vasodilator used for hypertension with dizziness and anxiety.
- *Platycodon Jie Geng root*. This sweet, moist, respiratory demulcent/expectorant, widely used in China, pops up in numerous patent formulas. The forgiving thing about Balloonflower is its use in varied conditions, be they hot or cold, with or without sputum, acute or chronic. It's an obvious choice for cough syrups, blending well with Licorice. Platycodon Jie Geng root is also used in Chinese formulas to treat early morning (cock's crow) diarrhea.

Women's Allies

Rubus idaeus L. (Raspberry leaf)

Angelica sinensis Oliv., Dang Gui (Angelica root)

Paeonia lactiflora Pallas, Bai Shao Yao (White Peony root)

Viburnum opulus L. (Cramp bark)

Rehmannia glutinosa Gaertner, Shu Di Huang (Prepared Rehmannia root)

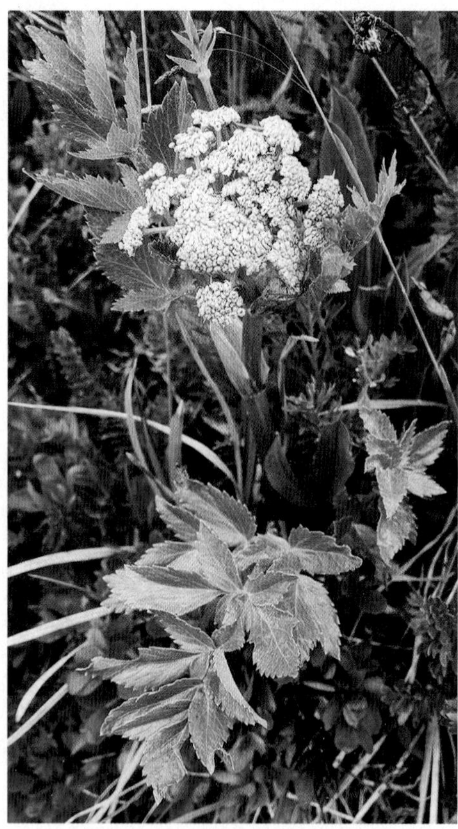

• **Fig. 12.22** *Angelica grayi*, shown growing in high Colorado mountains, looks similar to the Chinese Angelica Dang Gui/Dong Quai. The former is used as a respiratory and GI herb; the latter a blood tonic and uterine stimulant.

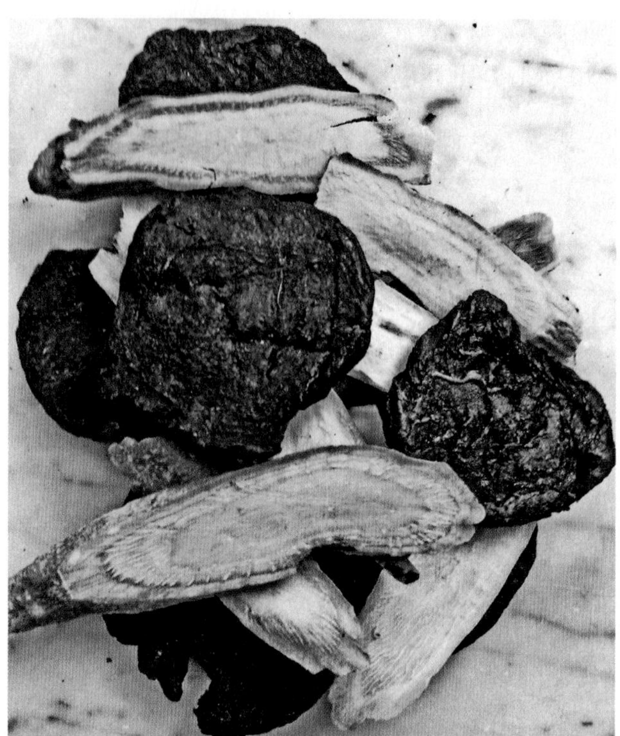

• **Fig. 12.23** Paeonia Bai Shao Yao (White Peony root) and dark, leathery Rehmannia Shu Di Huang (Prepared Rehmannia root) are women's allies. Bai Shao Yao is often used for menstrual cramps and Shu Di Huang for adrenal, Kidney and blood deficiencies during menopause.

General trigger words

* **PMS** * **Menopause** * **Yin Deficiency** *

Specific trigger words

- *Raspberry leaf.* Uterine restorative.
- *Angelica Dang Gui root.* Nourish Blood.
- *Paeonia Bai Shao Yao root.* Dysmenorrhea.
- *Cramp bark.* Dysmenorrhea. Nourish blood. Restore liver.
- *Rehmannia Shu Di Huang root.* Pituitary, adrenals, liver.

Families

- *Raspberry leaf.* Rosaceae
- *Angelica Dang Gui root.* Umbelliferae
- *Paeonia Bai Shao Yao root.* Ranunculaceae
- *Cramp bark.* Caprifoliaceae
- *Rehmannia Shu Di Huang root.* Scrophulariaceae

Growth and harvest

- *Raspberry leaf.* Brambly shrub with long, overhanging branches covered in thorns, pinnate leaves, white flowers in clusters. The fruit is actually an aggregate of many tiny berries in a cluster.
- *Angelica Dang Gui root.* Grows in cool high mountains in China. Can get 10 feet high, white umbels, hollow stems, thin conical roots. Likes to grow near running water.
- *Paeonia Bai Shao Yao root.* Beautiful, large delicate white flowers, large compound leaves, thick storage roots.
- *Cramp bark.* Deciduous shrub that grows in wet lowland northern forests. Large white flower clusters maturing into red berries. Bark harvested in fall, before leaves change colors, or in spring before leaves open.
- *Rehmannia Shu Di Huang root.* Perennial grows in moist, well-drained soil. Basal leaves, erect stem, tubular five-lobed flowers mixed with yellow and purple stripes. Root surface is brownish-black or pitch black, lustrous and sticky.

Strength

- All mild with minimal chronic toxicity.

Key constituents

- *Raspberry herb.* Tannin with gallic and ellager acids, lactic acid, ferric citrate, alkaloid, flavone farfarin, vitamins A and C, calcium, phosphorus, iron, trace minerals. (Tincture 1:4 65% ethanol.)
- *Angelica Dang Gui root.* Essential oils (45%), falcarinol, sitosterol, phytosterol six polysaccharides, nicotinic acid, folic acid, ferulic acid, coumarins, 24 minerals and trace elements, vitamins A, B_{12}, and E. (Tincture 1:3 65%–70% ethanol to extract the fat-soluble steroidal sitosterols.)

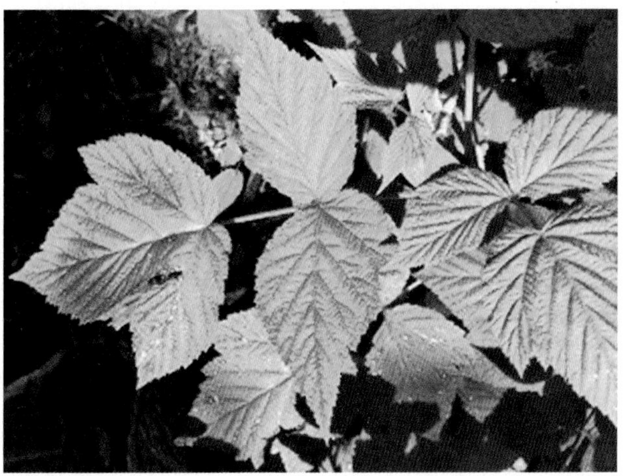

• **Fig. 12.24** *Rubus idaeus* (Raspberry leaf) is a gentle, forgiving woman's uterine restorative that is safe in any stage of reproduction, including pregnancy, labor and delivery.

- *Paeonia Bai Shao Yao root.* Essential oils including paeonol, alliflorine, steroids, dicosterol, and sitosterol, benzoic acid, tannin, asparagin, glucosides, minerals including zinc, magnesium, iron, and selenium. (Tincture 1:3 60% ethanol.)
- *Cramp bark.* Valerianic acid, salicosides, arbutin, bitter (viburnin), resins, and tannins. (Tincture 1:3 60% ethanol.)
- *Rehmannia Shu Di Huang root.* Simple sugars (including glucose, galactose, fructose, sucrose), alcohols (including mannitol and sitosterol), over 20 amino acids, aminobutyric acid, iridoid catalpol, 23 glycosides, rehmannin, tannin, resins, iron, trace minerals, vitamin A. (Tincture 1:3 75% ethanol. It contains lots of fat-soluble oils, alcohols, and resins.)[1–5]

Energetics, actions, indications, dosages and safety

Raspberry leaf (Fig. 12.24)

- *Energetics.* Astringent, cool, dry; restoring, astringing, stimulating.
- *Actions.* (1) Women: nutritious, uterine tropho-restorative, harmonizes menses, pregnancy, delivery. (2) Astringes and dries damp.
- *Indications.* (1) Women: dysmenorrhea, all stages of pregnancy and birth, habitual miscarriage and morning sickness, eases delivery, eases postpartum bleeding, increases milk. (2) GI: for diarrhea and colic in infants. (3) Dries discharges, diarrhea.
- *Dosages.* Tincture: 2 to 4 mL per dose of 1:3 35% ethanol. Diffusion: 8 to 14 g.[1–5]
- *Side effects.* None. Safe for all stages of pregnancy.
- *Contraindications.* None.
- *Commission E.* Not listed.

Angelica Dang Qui root (Fig. 12.22)

- *Energetics.* A bit sweet, pungent, bitter, warm, moist; stimulating, restoring, relaxing, calming, diluting, softening.
- *Actions.* (1) Women: uterine stimulant and emmenagogue. Balances hormone levels and relaxes uterine muscles. Mixed evidence of it being estrogenic and progesteronic. (2) Cardio-relaxant, restorative, vasodilator, antilipemic, and ***anticoagulant*** (increases clotting time and decreases blood clots). (3) Immune regulating and antitumoral, because of its polysaccharide content. (4) GI demulcent, mild laxative. (5) Liver restorative/protective.
- *Indications.* (1) Women's tonic. Relieves menstrual cramps, brings on delayed periods, increases scanty menses (emmenagogue) in Uterus Qi Stagnation, Blood deficiency. Helps PMS, as long as flooding is not the problem, and enhances fertility. (2) Pregnancy: fetal relaxant in threatened miscarriage. (3) Cardiac: heart restorative and relaxant for high blood pressure and high cholesterol; anticoagulant. (4) Immune: immediate allergies, hives, allergic rhinitis. (5) GI: mild laxative for constipation/hard dry stool. (6) Liver: protects and restores.
- *Dosages.* Tincture: 10 to 20 mL daily in divided doses of a 1:5 50%. Decoction: 3 to 25 g per day.[1–5]
- *Side effects.* Bleeding. Caution with warfarin (Coumadin), a blood thinner.
- *Contraindications.* Flooding, heavy menses, very damp conditions. Not for menopause with Yin-deficient heat (hot flashes), as this is a warming herb.
- *Commission E.* Not listed.

Paeonia Bai Shao Yao root (Fig. 12.23)

- *Energetics.* Bitter, sour, astringent, cool, dry. Relaxing, restoring, astringing, decongesting, calming.
- *Actions.* (1) Uterine relaxant. (2) Spasmolytic for smooth and striated muscles. (3) Nervous sedative because of its relaxing action. (4) Anhidrotic because of its astringency. (5) Antipyretic because it is cooling. (6) Immunostimulant.
- *Indications.* (1) Women: uterine blood congestion and qi constraint, thereby helping any type of menstrual cramps. (2) Cooling and anhidrotic for yin-deficient hot flashes, night sweats. (3) Nervous sedative for PMS, menopause, and general anxiety. (4) Spasmolytic action branches out in GI for colic, diarrhea, and in muscular-skeletal system for leg cramps. (5) Cooling for low-grade fevers.
- *Dosages.* Tincture: 2 to 4 mL per dose. Decoction: 8 to 18 g daily.[1–5]
- *Side effects.* Caution in diarrhea from deficient conditions with cold.
- *Contraindications.* None.
- *Commission E.* Not listed.

Cramp bark (Fig. 12.25)

- *Energetics.* Bitter, somewhat astringent, cool, dry; relaxing, calming, astringing, stabilizing.
- *Actions.* (1) Spasmolytic for smooth and skeletal muscles. (2) Women: regulates uterus qi, relieves pain during menses or ovulation. (3) Men: for all kinds of muscle pain.
- *Indications.* (1) Women: Analgesic for spasmodic and congestive dysmenorrhea and during ovulation. For threatened miscarriage and possible eclampsia-type seizures. (2) Lungs: clears wind and stops spasms in irritating dry cough and asthma. (3) Bladder: for dysuria.
- *Dosages.* Tincture: 3 mL up to 4 times per day of 1:5 50%. Decoction: 8 to 14 g. To prevent miscarriage: medium doses 2 to 3 weeks before anticipated and well into second

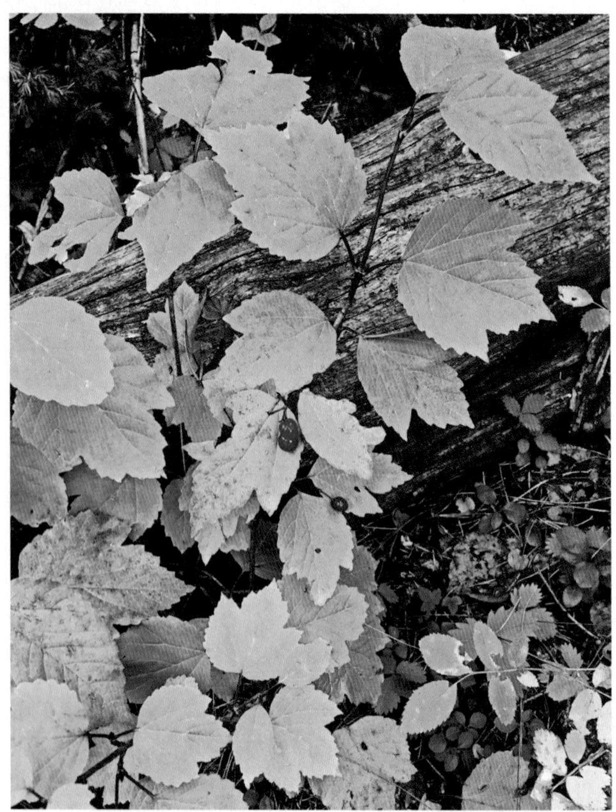

• **Fig. 12.25** *Viburnum opulus, V. edule* (Cramp bark/Highbush Cranberry bark) growing in the Colorado mountains. Its spasmolytic and relaxing properties help it excel for pain and spasms in the uterus, skeletal muscles, intestines, and lungs.

trimester. Threated immediate miscarriage: one teaspoon tincture every hour. Threatened third trimester eclampsia-related seizures: medium doses during last 2 months of pregnancy.[1–5]

- *Side effects.* None.
- *Contraindications.* None.
- *Commission E.* Not listed.

Rehmannia Shu Di Huang root (Fig. 12.23)

- *Energetics.* Sweet, oily, warm and moist. Restoring, nourishing, thickening, dissolving.
- *Actions.* (1) Pituitary/adrenal, HPA axis restorative. (2) Liver protective and restorative. (3) Menstrual regulator. (4) Detoxicant, diuretic. (5) Heart tonic, hemostatic, hypotensive. (6) Hypoglycemic and antilipemic. (7) Radiation protective.
- *Indications.* (1) Adrenals: restores HPA, making it important in menopause, fatigue, hormone production, Kidney Yin and Liver Yin/Blood deficiencies (Chapter 28). (2) Liver: restores and protects in Liver Yin/Blood deficiency, antiinflammatory, helping hepatitis. (3) Women: menstrual regulator, being hemostatic for bleeding. (4) Heart tonic: hypotensive, antilipemic. (5) Pancreas: hypoglycemic.
- *Dosages.* Tincture: 2 to 4 mL per dose. 1:3 75%. Decoction: 10 to 30 g daily.[1–5]
- *Side effects.* Too much of this herb alone could be cloying, too rich and sweet, and hard to digest,[18] causing loose stool and bloating. When used in formula, this problem is resolved. Could increase mucus because of its oily, moist nature.
- *Contraindications.* None.
- *Commission E.* Not listed.

Editorial

Even though the enriching herbs in this category are placed under the heading *Women's Allies*, they are also appropriate for men who are blood deficient. This applies to the entire list, with the exception of the muscle relaxant *Viburnum opulus* (Cramp bark), appropriate for both sexes for smooth muscle relief but not for blood deficiency.

- *Raspberry leaf.* Gentle all-purpose uterine tonic for women in any stage of reproduction, whether for menses, pregnancy, delivery, or postpartum. It is chock full of vitamins and trace minerals.
- *Angelica Dang Gui root.* This major women's herb in Chinese Medicine is sometimes called *women's ginseng* but is not a true ginseng. It's a sweet, pungent blood-building tonic, especially when combined with Astragalus Huang Qi. Dang Gui is a member of the famous *Four Substances/Things Decoction* for PMS and anemia (Chapter 28). An added benefit for women is its Liver restorative aspect. Caution: it's an emmenagogue and should not be used in situations with heavy bleeding or flooding, which can happen in early menopause or in abnormal menses. Dang Gui/Dong Quai also does well for cardiovascular problems, as a coronary restorative, anticoagulant, antilipemic, and vasodilator for hypertension.
- *Paeonia Bai Shao Yao root.* Peonies are such beautiful flowers, a prized ornamental in China and elsewhere. White Peony root is a highly esteemed women's remedy for menstrual pain, both spasmodic or congestive (Chapter 28). It relaxes smooth uterine muscles if the problem is spasmodic, and its astringency helps the congestive type, where blood tends to pool in the uterus, giving a feeling of heaviness or downward pressure before onset of period. Also, a great herb to use for uterine fibroids with heavy congestive bleeding.
- *Cramp bark.* This herb stops menstrual cramps and other muscle pain in both women and men. It works well with Pasque flower or Paeonia Bai Shao Yao (White Peony root) or Motherwort herb. It is simple, straightforward, and uncomplicated, and it relaxes smooth and striated muscles. It is perfectly safe in small doses throughout pregnancy for threatened miscarriage or seizures, along with Raspberry leaf.
- *Rehmannia Shu Di Huang root.* Prepared Rehmannia root is dried, steamed, and redried repeatedly or cooked in wine until it becomes black as ink and shiny as lacquer; it looks and feels like soft, sticky, oily leather, as opposed to Rehmannia Sheng Di Huang (raw), which is sun-dried, colder, and heat clearing. Prepared Rehmannia makes a superb Kidney/adrenal/Liver yin tonic. It's a very important Chinese herb in menopause formulas, where the adrenals are called on to produce reproductive hormones that are barely being made in the shrinking ovaries and where the liver must be healthy enough to carry out high order detoxification. A woman's ally, for sure.
- The Wise Woman's tradition has experimented with and identified countless herbs to help women. In Chapter 11, we detailed Vitex berry, Ginger root, Yarrow herb, Dandelion root, Red Clover flower, Black Cohosh root, Saw Palmetto berry, and Licorice root, all very useful in women's formulas (but absolutely not limited to that use). Not formally

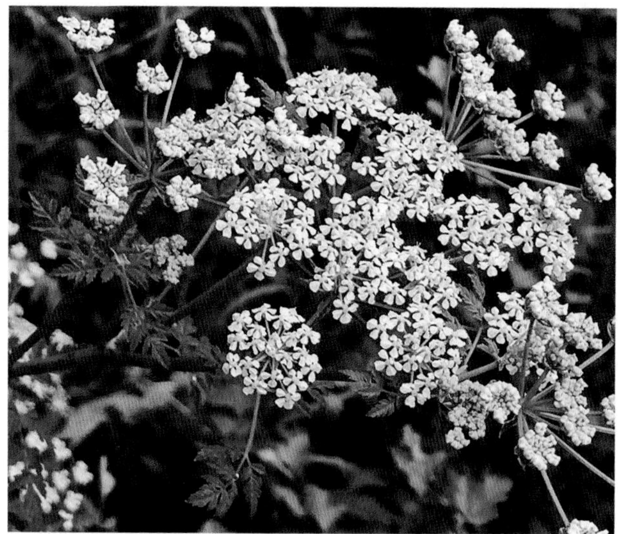

• **Fig. 12.26** *Ligusticum porteri* (Osha root) flowers are compound umbels, typical of the Parsley family. The root is warming, antiviral, and diaphoretic.

introduced, but also relevant here, are Blue Cohosh root, Wild Yam root, Kava root, Pasque flower, and Anemarrhena Zhi Mu (Know Mother root).

Infections and Toxicosis

Lonicera japonica Thunberg, Jin Yin Hua (Honeysuckle small flower or bud)

Allium sativa L. (Garlic bulb), Allium Da Suan

Andrographis paniculata Burman f., Chuan Xin Lian (Heart-Thread Lotus leaf)

Arctostaphylos uva ursi L. (Bearberry or Kinnikinnick leaf)

Ligusticum porteri Coulter and Rose (Osha or Colorado Cough root)

Artemisia absinthium L. (Wormwood herb)

General trigger words

* **Antimicrobials** * **Wind Heat** * **Wind Cold** * **Damp Heat** *

Specific trigger words

- *Lonicera Jin Yin Hua bud.* Broad-spectrum antimicrobial, External Wind Heat and fire toxins.
- *Garlic bulb.* Hot, antimicrobial, hypoglycemic.

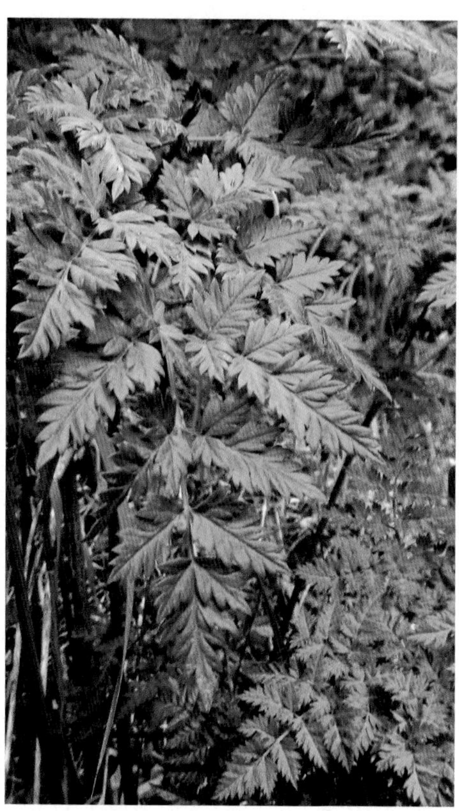

• **Fig. 12.27** Osha leaf veins extend out to the points of the compound, lacy leaves. Sometimes leaves are used in smoke mixtures or soups.

- *Andrographis Chaun Xin Lian leaf.* Sinus infection, Damp Heat.
- *Uva ursi leaf.* Urinary infections, Damp Heat.
- *Osha root.* Early-onset upper respiratory, Wind Cold.
- *Wormwood herb.* Parasites, food poisoning, cholagogue, Toxic Heat.

Families

- *Lonicera Jin Yin Hua bud.* Caprifoliaceae
- *Garlic bulb.* Liliaceae
- *Andrographis Chuan Xin Lian leaf.* Acanthaceae
- *Uva ursi leaf.* Ericaceae
- *Osha root.* Apiaceae/Umbelliferae
- *Wormwood herb.* Asteraceae/Compositae

Growth and harvest

- *Lonicera Jin Yin Hua flower bud.* Asian Jin Yin Hua is a semievergreen vine with oval-shaped, opposite leaves on the branches. Flowers are tubular, yellow-white; black berries.
- *Garlic bulb.* Aromatic compound bulb consisting of numerous cloves grouped together between papery scales and enclosed within a whitish skin, holding them in a sac. Leaves are long and grasslike, flowers dense with spherical, greenish-white clusters.
- *Andrographis Chuan Xin Lian leaf.* Annual bushy shrub; grows prolifically in tropical and subtropical China in all types of

soil. Leaves opposite, oval or lanceolate; small, hairy flowers, white to rosy.
- *Uva ursi leaf.* High mountainous small ground shrub with leathery evergreen leaves, darling white to pinkish urn-shaped flowers with red edges in small drooping clusters. Its red berries are beloved by bears.
- *Osha root.* Grows in the Rockies from Canada to Mexico above 7000 feet. Resembles Parsley family's Wild Carrot and Poison Hemlock, but it has a distinctively lovely pungent celery-like *Osha smell.* Hemlock smells mouselike. Osha has a tell-tale collar of dead leafy material surrounding the root crowns. Leaf veins extend out to the points of the compound, lacy leaves; Hemlock veins go to the leaf cuts or notches. Osha grows in Aspen groves.
- *Wormwood herb.* Erect annual with brownish stem and leaves divided by deep cuts into two to three small leaflets; flowers are small, yellowish-green. Highly aromatic; grows in sunny, warm places.

Strength

- *Mild.* Lonicera Jin Yin Hua bud, Garlic bulb, Andrographis Chuan Xin Lian leaf, Uva ursi leaf, and Osha root have minimal chronic toxicity.
- *Medium. Artemisia absinthium* has some chronic toxicity.

Key constituents

- *Lonicera Jin Yin Hua bud.* Chlorogenic and isochlorogenic acids, saponins, flavonoid luteolin, inositol, tannins, essential oils. (Tincture 1:3 in 50% ethanol.)
- *Garlic bulb.* Sulfurous compounds including allicin, garlicin, allistatine, many essential oils, phytohormones, allinase, cholin, silicic aid, mucilage, fructose, many trace elements, vitamins A, B, C. (Tincture freshly chopped at 1:2 95%–100% ethanol.)
- *Andrographis Chuan Xin Lian leaf.* Diterpenoid lactones (andrographolides), flavonoids, polysaccharides PB and PA, diterpene dimers. (Tincture in 1:3 50% ethanol.)
- *Uva ursi leaf.* Flavonoids (including 5%–18% arbutin), quercetin, gallic and ellagic tannins, gallic, malic, ursolic and other acids, triterpenoids, resin, allantoin, minerals, trace minerals. (Tincture harvested leaves no older than 9 months old to assure adequate arbutin content in 1:3 50% ethanol.)
- *Osha root.* Essential oils including cineole and monoterpenes, resin, glycoside, silica, bitters. (Tincture 1:3 in 60%–75% ethanol to extract essential oils and resin.)
- *Wormwood herb.* Many essential oils including 45% thujones, terpenoids, sesquiterpenes, absinthin, tannins, and flavonoids. (Tincture 1:3 in 50%–75% ethanol because of its high essential oil content.)[1–5]

Energetics, actions, indications, dosage, safety

Lonicera Jin Yin Hua bud (Fig. 12.30)

- *Energetics.* Sweet, astringent, cold, dry. Stimulating, astringing, dissolving.
- *Actions.* (1) Cooling broad-spectrum antimicrobial. Dispels External Wind Heat and fire toxins, reduces fever, inflammation, and swollen glands. (2) Immunostimulant. (3) Lymphatic decongestant because of its dissolving action.
- *Indications.* (1) Broad-spectrum antiinfective for acute External Wind Heat as in colds, flu, herpes, HIV, pneumonia, fungal/yeast infections. (2) Dissolving and lymphatic decongestion action for acute swelling infections/fire toxins with fever, inflammation, and possibly ***purulence*** (containing pus) from glands, boils, abscesses, laryngitis, mastitis, fibrocystic breasts, tonsillitis, tumors.
- *Dosages.* Tincture: 2 to 5 mL per dose. Decoction: 10 to 60 g.[1–5]
- *Side effects.* None.
- *Contraindications.* Pregnancy, sores with clear exudate caused by low immunity, chronic cold ulcers. Not for use in diarrhea because loose stools are a cold condition.
- *Commission E.* Not listed.

Garlic bulb

- *Energetics.* Pungent, sweet, aromatic, hot, dry; stimulating, decongesting dispersing.
- *Actions.* (1) Broad-spectrum antimicrobial (parasites, bacteria, viruses, fungus infections, amoebas), antiinflammatory with a hot, pungent nature. (2) Immunostimulant, antitumoral. (3) Diaphoretic (causes sweating). (4) Anticoagulant, lowers blood pressure and cholesterol. (5) Hypoglycemic.
- *Indications.* (1) All kinds of acute and chronic infections. (2) Respiratory: bronchitis, bronchial asthma, emphysema. (3) GI: for dysbiosis and *Candida albicans*, bloating, food poisoning, toxicosis, signs of Spleen Damp Cold. Intestinal parasites of all types. (3) Diabetes: hyper-/hypoglycemia. (4) Cardiac: congestive heart failure, hypo-/hypertension, angina, hyperlipidemia, atherosclerosis.
- *Dosage.* Eaten raw: for acute infections, 3 fresh raw cloves per dose up to eight cloves a day. Large doses are needed. Crush first, then swallow quickly. Crushing converts alliin into the beneficial allicin which decomposes rapidly. Tincture: 0.5 to 2 mL per dose. Prevention: cooked or fresh raw small doses.[1–5]
  - Fresh Garlic: causes sweating, which is needed in Wind Cold early-onset respiratory infections. Chew raw or drink in decoction. Dried Garlic: promotes warmth and dries up internal cold and damp.[1]
- *Side effects.* Flatulence, if dysbiosis present with sensitive stomachs. Combine with a carminative, like Peppermint herb or Ginger root.
- *Contraindications.* Pregnancy or lactation, and hot, dry conditions, deficient yin and fluids, spontaneous bleeding, premature ejaculation.
- *Commission E.* For elevated levels of lipids in the blood and as a preventive measure for age-dependent vascular changes.

Andrographis Chuan Xin Lian leaf

- *Energetics.* Very bitter, astringent, cold, dry; astringing, stimulating, sinking.
- *Actions.* (1) Broad-spectrum cooling antiinfective for acute Damp Heat infections. (2) Immunomodulating, ***antineoplastic*** (inhibits tumors by increasing T-lymphocyte activity). (3) Liver protective and stimulant. (4) Antipyretic, detoxicant, expectorant, and antiinflammatory.
- *Indications.* (1) Respiratory: viral and bacterial infections of acute sinusitis, damp heat of acute colds and sore throats with

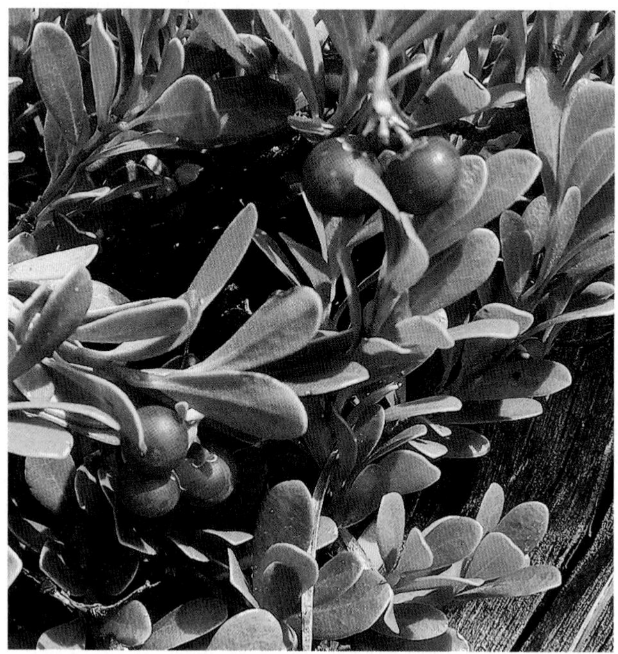

• **Fig. 12.28** *Arctostaphylos uva ursi* (Bearberry/Kinnikinnick leaf) has red fall berries that bears enjoy eating. Known for use in acute urinary tract infections.

thick, green-yellow mucus, viral pneumonia, tonsillitis, laryngitis. (2) Fever. (3) Prevention of colds and UTIs in low continuous doses. (4) GI: ulcerative colitis, enteric infections, and in small doses as a bitter digestive aid. (5) Gallbladder/Liver Damp Heat for dysentery, hepatitis, cholecystitis.

- *Dosages.* Tincture: 12 mL per day of a 1:2 extract. Decoction: hard to take because of extreme cold and bitterness. Chinese Medicine practitioners use 7 to 9 g. Dried leaves have been standardized to andrographolides.[1–5]
- *Side effects.* Energetically cold. Combine with warming herbs like Ginger root, Astragalus Huang Qi root or Holy Basil (Tulsi herb) in cold constitutions. Otherwise, safe.
- *Contraindications.* Early pregnancy; not in hyperacid states, such as duodenal ulcers because of its bitterness; not in esophageal reflux.
- *Commission E.* Not listed.

Uva ursi leaf (Fig. 12.28)

- *Energetics.* Astringent, cold, dry, astringing, solidifying, stabilizing, restoring, calming.
- *Actions.* (1) Antiinfective. Clears urogenital damp heat and infection, particularly in acute UTIs. (2) High astringency/tannin effect stops discharges, incontinence, and bleeding. (3) Vulnerary. (4) Promotes contractions, labor, and delivery.
- *Indications.* (1) Urinary: acute UTIs with damp heat; pain, blood/pus in urine, stones, bleeding, prostatitis, glomerulonephritis, nephritis, dysuria. (2) GI: dysentery, enteritis, colitis. (3) Astringency for uterine bleeding, blood in urine (hematuria), bedwetting (enuresis), hemorrhoids, genital and urinary discharges.
- *Dosages.* Tincture: 1 to 3 mL per dose. Infusion: 4 to 8 g. Also use in suppositories, sitz baths, sponges, and douches for postpartum perineum trauma and to prevent infection.[1–5]

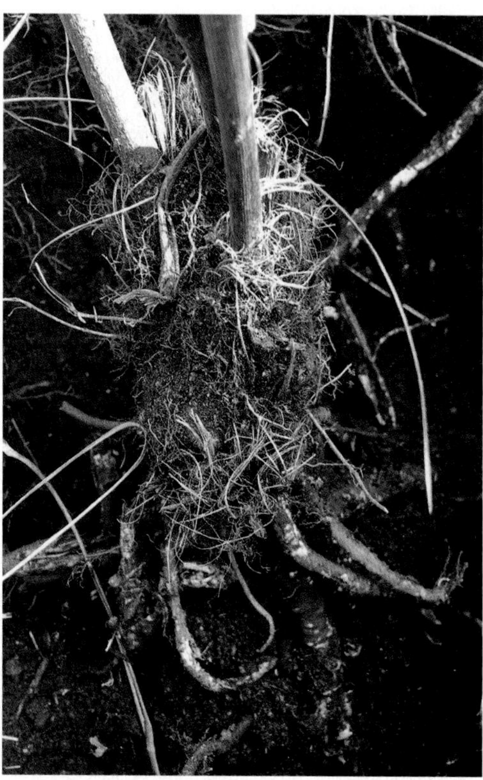

• **Fig. 12.29** *Ligusticum porteri* (Osha root) in the ground, showing dried dead material surrounding the root crowns. This feature helps give it a positive ID, distinguishing it from Poison Hemlock.

- *Side effects.* Use over a few days can upset stomach because of its tannin content, so combine with a demulcent, like Licorice root or Marshmallow root.
- *Contraindications.* Not in pregnancy, as it is ***oxytocic***, a uterine stimulant.
- *Commission E.* For inflammatory disorders of the efferent urinary tract.

Osha root (Figs. 12.26, 12.27, and 12.29)

- *Energetics.* Pungent, somewhat bitter, aromatic, warm, dry; stimulating, relaxing, restorative.
- *Actions.* (1) Antiviral, antiseptic, spasmolytic, diaphoretic. (2) Lung warmer, stimulant expectorant, diaphoretic, nasal decongestant, restorative, and prevents lung scar tissue because of its silica content. (3) Digestive stimulant. (4) Uterine stimulant and spasmolytic.
- *Indications.* (1) Primarily for respiratory: pungent, warm expectorant and diaphoretic for upper respiratory with External Wind Cold, as in cold/flu onset that is not yet hot and with sneezing and coughing up of white or clear sputum, sinus congestion. Relaxant for wheezing, bronchitis, lung TB, emphysema. (2) GI: relaxing for colic, colitis, gastroenteritis with pain, bloating, loose stool (drying). (3) Uterus: can use as a stimulant and spasmolytic for dysmenorrhea/amenorrhea, failure to progress during labor, and for retained placenta.
- *Dosages.* Tincture: 0.5 to 3 mL. Cold infusion or short decoction: 3 to 8 g.[1–5]

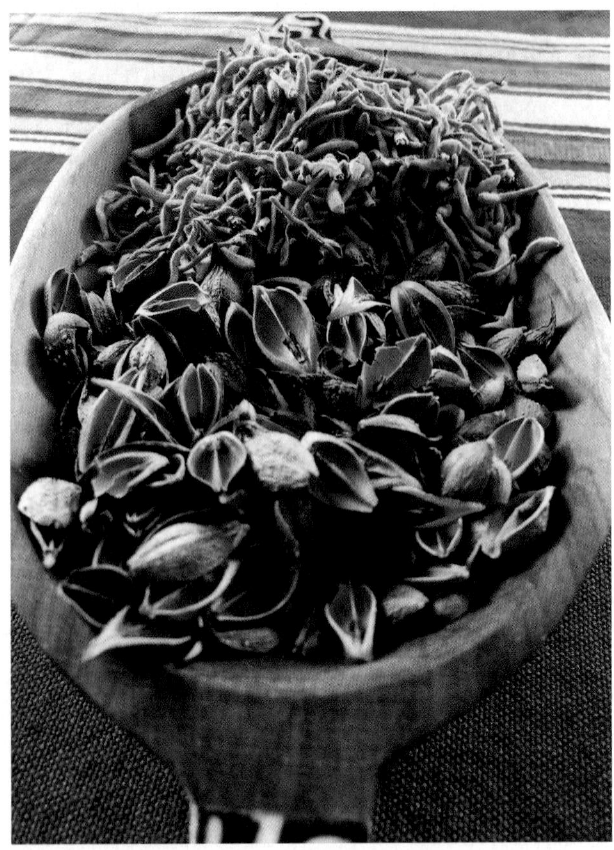

• **Fig. 12.30** Forsythia Lian Qiao (Forsythia valve) (lower) and Lonicera Jin Yin Hua (Japanese Honeysuckle flower) (upper) are frequently combined in Chinese formulas to eliminate heat in early respiratory infections.

- *Side effects.* None.
- *Contraindications.* Pregnancy, as it stimulates the uterus. In those with hot constitutions, as it can overheat the body. In that case, combine with cooler herbs.
- *Commission E.* Not listed.

Wormwood herb

- *Energetics.* Bitter, pungent, cool, dry, and astringent. Stimulating, restoring, decongesting.
- *Actions.* (1) Cold, antiinfective, antiparasitical, antihelminthic, antipyretic, antiinflammatory. (2) GI: stimulates gastric secretions, bitter quality improves appetite and digestion. (2) Liver: cholagogue, increases bile flow.
- *Indications.* (1) For damp heat infections of stomach and liver. (2) GI: for intestinal parasites (helminths), especially roundworms and pinworms, food poisoning, gastritis, indigestion, constipation, Spleen Damp Heat. (3) Liver: for infections such as hepatitis with jaundice, Liver and Stomach Qi Stagnation.
- *Dosages.* Infusion: 4 oz per day. Tincture: 1 to 2 mL. Larger doses clear heat, but do not use for over 4 weeks, because of its medium strength.[1–5]
- *Side effects.* None.
- *Contraindications.* Uterine stimulant. Not in pregnancy or breast feeding. Do not exceed traditional doses.
- *Commission E.* For loss of appetite, dyspepsia, biliary dyskinesia. Thujone, the active component of the oil, acts as a convulsant poison. Therefore the Wormwood essential oil must not be used except in combinations.

Editorial

There are numerous antimicrobial bug killers in the herbal realm. The sampler presented is enough to get an herb lover started. Lonicera Jin Yin Hua (Japanese Honeysuckle flower), often paired with Forsythia Lian Qiao (Forsythia valve) are a dynamic duo in Chinese Medicine and star players in the famous formula Yin Chiao (Chapter 17) for early-onset colds and flu. Uva ursi is a primary evergreen leaf in the West for acute UTIs. Andrographis Chuan Xin Lian (Heart-Thread Lotus leaf) goes straight to the sinuses. Osha root grows high in the Rockies and is one of my go-to plants for early onset upper respiratory gunk before heat sets in. Wormwood herb is a valuable intestinal parasite eliminator. Lonicera Jin Yin Hua (Japanese Honeysuckle flower) is a broad-spectrum anti-infective and detoxicant; it is one of the most important Chinese herbs used for eliminating heat and accumulated toxins. It is a different species from the many other Honeysuckles occurring worldwide. Pair with Western *Calendula officinalis* (Marigold flower) or Eastern Forsythia Lian Qiao (Forsythia valve).

- *Garlic bulb.* This is an ancient and legendary superfood and remedy. Warm, dry, pungent Garlic has many constituents and uses, particularly in people who are damp and cold. It is placed in the antimicrobial section because of its sulfurous and essential oil content, but it could easily have been listed in a cardiac section because of its anticoagulant, antihypertensive, and antilipemic actions.
  - Controversy exists as to the benefits of raw Garlic versus dried Garlic supplements. Scientific consensus holds that odorous *allicin,* the active ingredient that forms in about 10 seconds when Garlic is pressed, chopped, or chewed, decomposes rapidly and is best consumed raw on the spot. Fresh Garlic can be refrigerated or placed in water for about a day before the allicin destabilizes. A freeze-dried or enteric coated pill has a decent chance of remaining effective.[19] Garlic used in cooking is best crushed or minced and added close to serving time.
  - *Garlic breath* is caused by gaseous sulfur (allyl methyl sulfide). It is absorbed into the blood when metabolized and exhaled from the lungs, creating stinky breath. Some of the sulfur is also excreted from skin pores, resulting in Garlic skin.
- *Andrographis Chuan Xin Lian leaf.* This plant appears in the Materia Medica of India, China, and Southeast Asia. In Ayurvedic medicine, Andrographis is known as "the King of Bitters;" in the West, Gentian root is considered "the Queen of Bitters." Chuan Xin Lian is a go-to herb for all types of acute hot infections and is a classic for acute sinusitis. Of similar ilk is Chinese Scutellaria Huang Qin (Baikal Skullcap herb), Coptis Huang Lian (Goldthread root), and Goldenseal root from the West.
- *Uva ursi leaf.* Bearberry is a terrific botanical for acute UTIs when combined with a nice demulcent, like Marshmallow root, and something for pain, such as White Willow bark. When using Uva ursi for UTIs, an alkaline diet rich in vegetables is recommended, because the active antiseptic and antiinflammatory ingredient, albutin, must be transformed into hydroquinone in an alkaline pH environment.[4]
- *Osha root* (Fig. 12.31). Colorado cough root is bear medicine. Bears love Osha, just as cats love Catnip. They are known to

roll around in it. If you ever become acquainted, you will fall in love with Osha. Anything that smells so good and pungent must be good medicine. Osha is a Native American plant, often smoked in ceremonial pipe blends. It is a powerful, straightforward remedy for cold, early onset of upper respiratory infections and a natural in cough syrups.

- *Artemisia absinthium (Wormwood herb). A. absinthium* is mainly used in the West as a cholagogue, bitter gastric stimulator, and worm remedy. There are many species, and they are easily confused. A couple are *A. annua* Huang Hua Hao (Sweet Annie herb), which is probably the most famous antimalarial herb in the world (Chapter 10) and Chinese *A. argyi* Ai Ye (Asian Mugwort leaf) that is hemostatic, used for uterine bleeding and burned as moxa.

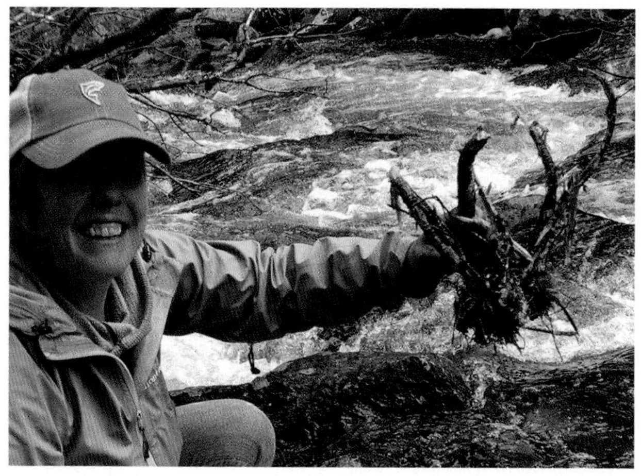

• **Fig. 12.31** Sarah with freshly dug and river-washed Osha root.

Summary

A few key herbal groupings that an herbalist returns to again and again were considered. Important Western and Chinese herbs were included. The intention was to provide some common herbs with similar but nonidentical actions to provide a format for intelligent selection, based on energetics and matched to the patient's condition: warming plants for cool conditions; drying herbs for dampness; pungent remedies to disperse congestion; sour taste for astringing, and so on.

Monographs

Calming Herbs for the Nervous System

Scutellaria lateriflora L. (Skullcap herb)
Matricaria recutita L. (Chamomile flower)
Melissa officinalis L. (Melissa herb)
Lobelia inflata L. (Lobelia herb)
Humulus lupulus L. (Hops flower)
Ziziphus spinosa Hu, Suan Zao Ren (Sour Jujube seed)

Demulcents or Yin Tonics

Asparagus officinalis L. (Asparagus root)
Symphytum officinale L. (Comfrey leaf and root)
Ulmus fulva Michaux (Slippery Elm bark)
Althea officinalis L. (Marshmallow root)
Verbascum thapsus L. (Mullein leaf, root, and flower)

Common Adaptogens

Eleutherococcus senticosus Rupr. Et Maxim, Ci Wu Jia (Eleuthero root)
Ganoderma lucidum Leyss. ex Fr., Ling Zhi (Reishi mushroom)
Astragalus membranaceus Fischer, Huang Qi (Astragalus root)
Withania somnifera L. (Ashwagandha root)
Schisandra chinensis Turcz., Wu Wei Zi (Five Taste berry)
Rhodiola rosea L. (Rhodiola root)

Alterative Herbs That Help Detoxification

Rumex crispus L. (Yellow Dock root)
Arctium lappa L. (Burdock root and seed)
Galium aparine L. (Cleavers herb)
Trifolium pratense L. (Red Clover flower)
Apium graveolens L. (Celery seed)

Expectorants, Bronchodilators, and Antitussives

Thymus vulgaris L. (Thyme herb)
Tussilago farfara L. (Coltsfoot herb)
Prunus serotina Ehrhart (Wild Cherry bark)
Xanthium sibiricum Patrin, Cang Er Zi (Siberian Cocklebur fruit)
Chrysanthemum x morifolium Ramatuelle, Ju Hua (Wild Chrysanthemum flower)
Platycodon grandiflorum de Candolle, Jie Geng (Balloonflower root)

Women's Allies

Rubus idaeus L. (Raspberry leaf)
Angelica sinensis Oliv., Dang Gui (Angelica root, Dong Quai)
Paeonia lactiflora Pallas, Bai Shao Yao (White Peony bark)
Viburnum opulus L. (Cramp bark)
Rehmannia glutinosa Gaertner, Shu Di Huang (Prepared Rehmannia root)

Infections and Toxicosis

Lonicera japonica Thunberg, Jin Yin Hua (Honeysuckle small flower and bud)
Allium sativa L. (Garlic bulb)
Andrographis paniculata Burman f., Chuan Xin Lian (Heart-thread Lotus leaf)
Arctostaphylos uva ursi L. (Uva ursi leaf)
Ligusticum porteri Coulter & Rose (Osha root)
Artemisia absinthium L. (Wormwood herb)

Review

Fill in the Blanks

(Answers in Appendix B.)

1. ___ herb is a good choice for an asthma attack. ___ is a gentle children's relaxant.
2. As far as demulcents go, ___ is a good yin tonic for women, whereas ___ is a prime choice for wound healing, its active ingredient being ___. Another word for wound healing is ___.
3. An Ayurvedic adaptogen is ___. A Chinese adaptogen is ___. Name two mushroom adaptogens: ___ and ___. An adaptogen especially good for depression is ___.
4. Name three adaptogenic super foods. ___, ___, and ___. Name three companion adaptogenic herbs: ___, ___, ___.
5. Name two alteratives that work on a kidney level. ___ and ___. Name one that moves lymph. ___.
6. ___ is very warming and drying, so could be used for a ___ and ___ cough with ___ colored sputum. Someone coughing up dark yellow-green sputum would do better with more cooling expectorants, such as ___ or ___.
7. Two multipurpose cough expectorants are ___ and ___.
8. Give a good herbal choice for pregnancy ___, menopause ___ and dysmenorrhea ___.
9. A person has an allergic sinus infection with profuse green rhinitis. Chinese Medicine herbal choices could be ___ for infection and ___ to dry up secretions.
10. In terms of heat and taste, Lonicera Jin Yin Hua is ___ and ___. Garlic bulb is ___ and ___. Andrographis Chuan Xin Lian is ___ and ___. Osha root is ___ and ___. Wormwood herb is ___ and ___. Uva ursi leaf is ___ and ___.

Critical Concept Questions

(Answers for you to decide.)

1. Why do you get better herbal results by matching the energetics of the herb to the patient's condition?
2. How and why can Lobelia herb be both a relaxant and a stimulant?
3. Why should adaptogens be prepared as dual extractions?
4. Why might you choose Codonopsis Dang Shen (Downy Bellflower root) over Panax Xi Yang Shen (American ginseng root)?
5. Discuss relationship between alteratives and skin eruptions.
6. What are the *Four Substances* in the Chinese patent formula, and what do they do?
7. What causes garlic breath? Discuss the pros and cons of Garlic bulb cooked, raw and in supplements.
8. When and why would you choose Osha root over Lonicera Jin Yin Hua (Honeysuckle flower) for a respiratory antimicrobial herb, and vice versa?

References

Dosages, energetics, and/or key constituents for monographs compiled from references 1–5

1. Holmes, Peter. *Energetics of Western Herbs* (Boulder, CO: Snow Lotus, 2006).
2. Holmes, Peter. *Jade Remedies: A Chinese Herbal Reference for the West* (Boulder, CO: Snow Lotus Press, 1996).
3. "The ABC Guide to Clinical Herbs Online." American Botanical Council. http://abc.herbalgram.org/site/PageServer?pagename = The_Guide (accessed October 13, 2019).
4. Bone, Kerry and Simon Mills. *Principles and Practice of Phytotherapy* (London, UK: Elsevier, 2013).
5. Alfs, Matthew. *300 Herbs: Their Indications and Contraindications* (New Brighton, MN: Old Theology, 2003).
6. "Expanded Commission E: Lemon Balm." American Botanical Council. http://cms.herbalgram.org/expandedE/LemonBalm.html (accessed October 3, 2019).
7. "Expanded Commission E: Hops." American Botanical Council. http://cms.herbalgram.org/expandedE/Hops.html (accessed October 13, 2019).
8. Hoffman, David. *Medical Herbalism: The Science and Practice of Herbal Medicine* (Rochester, VT: Healing Arts, 2003).
9. Yance, Donald. *Adaptogens in Medical Herbalism* (Rochester, VT: Healing Arts, 2013).
10. "Expanded Commission E; Asparagus root." American Botanical Council. http://cms.herbalgram.org/expandedE/Asparagusroot.html (accessed October 15, 2019).
11. Mars, Brigitte. *The Desktop Guide to Herbal Medicine* (Columbus, OH: Basic Health, 2016).
12. "Comfrey hepatotoxicity." Henriette's Herbal. http://www.henriettes-herb.com/faqs/medi-2-15-comfrey.html (accessed October 15, 2019).
13. "Commission E Monographs: Comfrey herb and leaf." American Botanical Council. http://cms.herbalgram.org/commissione/Monographs/Monograph0072.html (accessed October 13, 2019).
14. "Expanded Commission E: Marshmallow root." American Botanical Council. http://cms.herbalgram.org/expandedE/Marshmallowroot.html (accessed October 13, 2019).
15. "Expanded Commission E: Mullein flower." American Botanical Council. http://cms.herbalgram.org/expandedE/Mulleinflower.html (accessed October 13, 2019).
16. Dharmananda, Subhuti. "Codonopsis: Medicine and Food." Institute for Traditional Medicine. http://www.itmonline.org/arts/codonopsis.htm (accessed October 13, 2019).
17. "Xanthium Fruit: Cang Er Zi." Acupuncture Today. http://www.acupuncturetoday.com/herbcentral/xanthium.php (accessed October 13, 2019).
18. Dharmananda, Subhuti. "Rehmannia." Institute for Traditional Medicine. http://www.itmonline.org/arts/rehmann.htm (accessed October 17, 2019).
19. Ganora, Lisa. *Herbal Constituents: Foundations of Phytochemistry* (Louisville, CO: Herbalchem Press, 2009).

13 Herbal Safety

"First, do no harm."

—Hippocrates, Father of Western Medicine

CHAPTER REVIEW

- General considerations about herbal safety. When it comes to herbs, be safe, not paranoid.
- Allergic reactions.
- Herbal constituents that can help or harm.
- Herbal actions that can help or harm.
- Adverse herb and drug interactions.
- Cytochrome P450 liver interactions with drugs and herbs.
- Pregnancy and lactation guidelines.

KEY TERMS

Abortifacients
Anaphylactic shock
Antitussive
Cardiac glycosides
CNS depressants
Cyanogenic glycosides
CYP450 system
Cytochrome P450 (CYP450)
Good Manufacturing Practice (GMP)
Hypoglycemics
Lectins
Monoamine oxidase inhibitors (MAOIs)
Oxalates
Pyrrolizidine alkaloids (PAs)
Photosensitizing
Potentiation
Pseudoaldosteronism
Salicylates
Serotonin syndrome
Selective serotonin reuptake inhibitors (SSRIs)
Synergy
Teratogenesis

This chapter is designed to provide a general awareness of what can go wrong when using botanicals for healing. It is not meant to scare anyone off or give false alarms—but to help us all be informed clinical herbalists. Herbal medicine has an excellent track record over time for being surprisingly safe.

In the United States, herbs are regulated as dietary supplements (Chapter 29). This regulation could lull one into the false assumption that they are perfectly safe, with no side effects in any amount or dose. Not so. Even beans and other commonly consumed foods can cause allergic reactions and toxicity. In Europe, Canada, and Australia, herbs are registered as medicinal products or classified as herbal medicine, even drugs. Because herbs contain a complex array of chemicals, they have physiological and pharmacological properties and are not inert. No matter their legal classification, have respect.

Presenting every side effect for any herb you might encounter is an unrealistic goal. Many reliable references are dedicated to this topic and represent contemporary knowledge. It is recommended that you include one or two in your library. Those listed in the bibliography and endnotes are good places to start. It is always the practitioner's responsibility to determine the best treatment and dosage for each client and to appreciate that idiosyncratic and allergic reactions can be unpredictable. Herbal safety and drug interaction data are constantly changing. What is presented is a broad overview with guidelines and consensus (if one can be found) based on tradition, experience, and new information.

We are interested in general topics, such as herbs that might cause bleeding, raise blood pressure, or are contraindicated in pregnancy. The Materia Medicas (Chapters 11 and 12) also give specific safety considerations. We must all use herbs rationally and wisely, and above all, be safe.

General Considerations Regarding the Safety of Herbs

- *Herbs are not inert substances.* If they were inert, they would have no therapeutic effect. For that reason, use mild to moderate strength only, nothing that is extremely dangerous or highly toxic. Most herbs are generally safe—if used with knowledge. But don't get too cavalier. There are legitimate reasons to be respectful of our allies. Follow dosage ranges and a client's reaction and condition.
- *Opinions vary on safety.* Not enough pure research has been done on humans. Sources range from being overly reactionary to excessively casual. Some claim that any remotely possible adverse effect is cause for alarm, whereas others insist that because herbs are natural substances, they are harmless. Don't be fooled. Both extremes are unacceptable.
- *Don't believe everything you hear.* Check out and analyze the research, if any. At times, warnings are based on theoretical conjectures that have never been studied. Sometimes toxicity studies are designed by feeding abnormally high quantities of an herb or an isolated constituent to a lab animal. Whole herbs have a large array of chemicals, many canceling out the potential toxicity of others. The many constituents in a whole herb work together in a manner known as ***synergy***, and their combined effect can be different, and often safer, from that of a single one by itself. The takeaway is to be discerning and critical of studies and media reports, particularly those on TV and websites. Realize that information is constantly changing.
- *Quality.* Knowing a good herb when you see and smell one is important. Use organic, wildcraft in safe places at least 50 to 100 yards away from roads. Use reliable Chinese herbal sources that import organic, contaminant-free herbs that do not contain heavy metals or pathogenic organisms. Order from reputable companies that make no substitutions to cut corners, misidentify, or use the wrong plant part. Make sure herbs are fresh. Sometimes herbs are adulterated with drugs or other, cheaper substances. There could be a bad batch. It's best to use companies that are ***Good Manufacturing Practice (GMP)*** certified, which are those that have their products periodically, independently analyzed (Chapter 30).
- *Pregnancy.* This is a loaded topic, with many books leaning toward paranoia. Numerous references go far overboard. There is no general consensus or much research. Many of the few studies have been done on animals, not humans. There are inconsistences and misinformation. Countless herbs have been historically and safely administered and used in pregnancy, e.g., in the Wise-Woman tradition.
- *Safety classification systems.* Books and references use diverse lettered classifications or categories to designate risk from safest to absolutely forbidden. This text doesn't use these designations; it just writes out the information in words. Three reputable references follow.
  - *Essential Guide to Herbal Safety* by Simon Mills and Kerry Bone[1] uses pregnancy categories adapted from the *Australian Therapeutic Goods Administration Classification for Drugs in Pregnancy* (which includes herbs). Their system ranges from *A*, meaning safe, to *X* for high risk.
  - *The Botanical Safety Handbook* by Michael McGuffin et al.[2] has its own categories from "Class 1" (those safely consumed when used appropriately) to "Class 2d" (other specific use restrictions as noted).
  - *Herb Contraindications and Drug Interactions* by Francis Brinker[5] is an excellent resource on the herbal-drug interaction aspect. This text does not use a numbering system.
- *Learn to evaluate studies.* Safety information typically applies to one herb used in isolation, not in combination. If an herb is in formula, the cautions are probably overstated because one chemical tends to cancel out the toxicity of another. Research rarely applies to herbs used as foods or spices, which are generally added to recipes in less-than-therapeutic amounts. Further, be aware of which plant part and dosage is employed in a study. Results could be based on testing a root, when it's the leaf that that is actually used. Some studies do not even specify which plant part is being tested. Dosages used in studies are frequently much higher than in normal usage, skewing results. Furthermore, make sure the study states the botanical name, not the common name of the herb in question.
- *Herb-drug interactions.* They sound negative but are not always a bad thing. Herb-drug interactions can be used beneficially.
  - *Potentiation.* Sometimes when an herb is combined with a drug, the overall effect of the two together is revved up exponentially, becoming far greater than the sum of its parts. This situation is known as ***potentiation***. In such case, either the herbal dose or the drug dose would need to be adjusted, decreased, or discontinued to maintain a safe therapeutic effect. Since many drugs are extremely toxic, increasing the herbal dose and lowering the drug dose might be desirable. This is where working with an open-minded prescribing health care provider would be necessary.
  - *Sometimes an herb decreases a drug's effect.* Bulk laxatives actually decrease the effect of a drug by hindering absorption, the opposite of potentiation.
- *Dosage.* Never change a drug dose on your own. Always work with the prescribing health care provider. End of story.
- *Monitoring.* Occasionally, an herb-drug combination requires monitoring, such as for blood pressure, blood sugar levels, coagulation studies, or potassium levels.
- *Overdose versus therapeutic dose.* Adverse effects apply to herbs given in the therapeutic range, not in outrageously large quantities.

Allergic Reactions

Allergic reactions are the most common adverse effects related to herbs and drugs. It is theoretically possible for any herb to cause an immune response, ranging from contact dermatitis all the way to anaphylactic shock. These responses are mostly unpredictable. However, if your client has any previous history of allergies in the plant department, take precautions.

Out of all allergic responses, contact dermatitis is most common. Plant families commonly causing skin reactions are Ranunculaceae (Buttercup), Euphorbiaceae (Spurge), and Asteraceae (Daisy). Causes are from chemical irritants in the plants, including alkaloids, saponins, and anthraquinones.[1] Some of these plants are frequently used as vulneraries in first-aid creams. Arnica flower (Fig. 13.1), German and Roman Chamomile flower, Garlic bulb, Peppermint herb, and Lavender flower are examples. None is completely harmless in

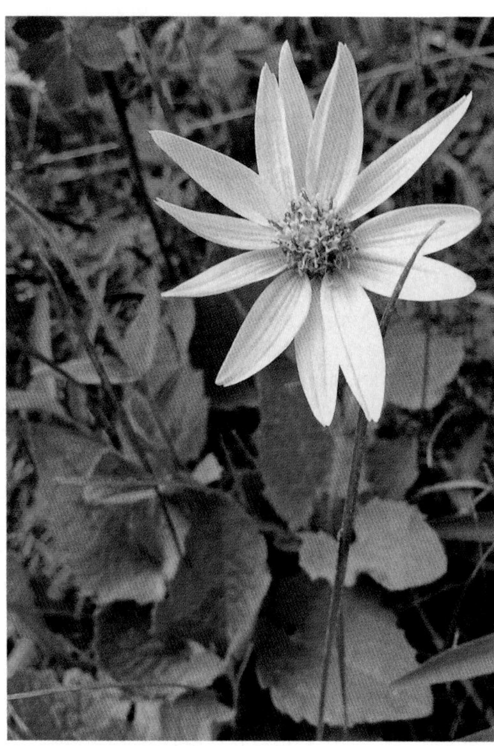

• **Fig. 13.1** *Arnica* spp. (Heart-leaf Arnica leaf and flower) is a valued Daisy family vulnerary that could cause contact dermatitis with external use in susceptible individuals.

susceptible individuals. Other reported offenders are Licorice root, Tea Tree essential oil, Cayenne pepper, and Echinacea root.

Allergic reactions can also cause asthma, eye reactions, or oral lip blisters. Always ask clients about plant allergies and for those with positive histories, look into cross-reactivity between species belonging to the same family. Most allergic reactions resolve when the herb is discontinued. Rarely, but possibly, there could be a history of a serious type 1 immediate sensitivity allergic reaction (***anaphylactic shock***) with hives, face swelling, swollen tongue, difficulty breathing, or respiratory arrest. This reaction is life threatening and requires an immediate emergency room visit.

Herbal Constituents That Can Help or Harm

The chemicals listed in this section occur in many herbs. They can be a problem, or they can be used to therapeutic advantage.[2] If you come across an herb with these chemicals, know that in the wrong situation, with the wrong dose, you might get into trouble. A few myths are cleared up, particularly the confusion over coumarins and salicylates.

- *Berberines* are amazing bright yellow alkaloids found in many herbs, such as Coptis Huang Lian, Phellodendron Huang Bei, Goldenseal root, Barberry root, and Oregon Grape root. They are used as antimicrobials, bitters, and antipyretics. They are not recommended in pregnancy or neonatal jaundice, because they're purported to be a uterine stimulant and also hypertensive.
- *Cardiac glycosides.* ***Cardiac glycosides*** are steroidal glycosides containing digitoxin and digoxin, both of which strengthen the function of the heart muscle and decrease heart rate (Chapter 8). Cardiac glycosides are a class of drugs used in Western medicine to treat certain arrhythmias and congestive heart failure (CHF), a very common problem.
  - *Digitalis toxicity* can cause excess calcium to be released into the heart muscle, resulting in life-threatening arrhythmias and cardiac arrest. For this reason, there is some concern with calcium supplementation in conjunction with cardiac glycosides. Any drug (or herb) that acts as a cardiac glycoside sends a streak of caution and sometimes fear through the hearts of doctors and nurses. The synthetic drugs digoxin and lanoxin were derived from *Digitalis* spp. (Foxglove herb and root). These medications are strong and toxic, and a therapeutic dose is just a tiny bit lower than a toxic dose. Anytime amounts are that critical, you better know exactly how much you're giving. Blood monitoring and drug titration is essential.
  - *Herbs containing cardiac glycosides.* Foxglove should never be used by modern herbalists, although it was used until 1868, when digitalin was isolated from it. The entire plant of medium-strength *Convallaria majalis* (Lily of the Valley herb) can be used by experienced herbalists for CHF, although 4 days should elapse between taking the synthetic drugs and the herb. If given as a simple, allow a 10-day break after 10 days of continuous use.[3] Other herbals containing cardiac glycosides are Squill bulb leaf scale, Dogbane seed, root, and bark, Pleurisy root, Oleander root and herb, and Night Blooming Cactus stem.
- *Coumarin and anticoagulants.* This story is convoluted. Coumarin occurs in many plants that are antioxidant and antiinflammatory and tonic to venous and lymphatic vessels, but coumarin is *not* anticoagulant (Chapter 8). The trouble and/or confusion about coumarin started with *Melilot officinalis* (Sweet Clover herb) in the 1920s. When the coumarin in Sweet Clover molds in hay or is dried improperly, it turns into dicoumarol, which happens to be a powerful hemorrhagic, 1000 times stronger than coumarin. It is used in rat poison to make rats bleed to death. The dicoumarol discovery led to the use of the potent synthetic blood-thinning drug, Coumadin (warfarin), which contains coumadin, not coumarin, which are close but not the same. Coumadin inhibits vitamin K, a necessary cofactor in blood clotting, so much so that coagulation levels are required when taking.
  - *The takeaway.* Coumarin-containing herbs not spoiled from mold or bacteria have little effect on clotting one way or the other.[4] Such herbs are Meadowsweet herb, Sweet Clover herb, Saw Palmetto berry, and Willow bark. Even so, be cautious.
- *Cyanogenic glycosides (cyanide).* ***Cyanogenic glycosides*** are sugar compounds that yield cyanide on hydrolysis in the digestive tract and, speculatively, might cause teratogenic effects (birth defects). They are common in the Rosaceae (Rose), Fabaceae (Pea), and Asteraceae (Daisy) families, among others. The culprit here is *amygdalin*, which is found in the seeds of stone fruits (not the fleshy fruit part) of many *Prunus* species, notably peach, apricot, and bitter almond pits, as well as in cherry pits and apple, pear, and loquat seeds. They can be fatal with moderate consumption.[4] The body can metabolize and detoxify low levels but ultimately succumbs to cyanide poisoning with continued use. *Prunus serotina* (Wild Cherry bark) is an example of a very useful cough suppressant (***antitussive***) that contains low levels of cyanogenic glycosides. The amount varies with the type of bark, thickness, and time of collection. For that reason, dose

should not exceed 1.5–6 grams per day of dried bark per infusion, or 2–4.5 mL a day as a 1:2 liquid extract, nor should it be taken over long-term use, or in pregnancy.[1]

- *Iodine.* Iodine is essential for good thyroid functioning and hormone production. Lack of iodine in mined salt in the Great Lakes, Appalachian, and northwestern regions of the United States used to cause enlarged thyroid glands or goiter before salt was enriched with iodine. Sea veggies (seaweeds) are rich sources of iodine, living as they do in salty trace mineral-rich water. *Laminaria* spp. (Dried Kelp thallus) has the highest natural iodine content of them all. Dulse and Irish Moss also provide this important trace mineral. The worry is that these herbs can potentiate thyroid medications and make thyroid hormones too high. Concurrent use requires monitoring. Wouldn't it be lovely if your client could get off Synthroid, the most prescribed drug in the United States? But use caution with the iodine. Please note that excess iodine can cause goiter and other symptoms in adults (Chapter 27). Excessive salt consumption in pregnant women has caused infantile goiter.
- *Lectins and clotting.* **Lectins** are potentially toxic glycoproteins that cause blood cells to clot. They are found mainly in seeds of Fabaceae (Bean) and Euphorbiaceae (Spurge) families. These plants possess the deadly property of causing red blood cells to agglutinate (bind together) causing clotting. Therapeutically, they are immune-stimulating and have anticancer properties. Even two to four ingested *Ricinus communis* (Castor bean) (Fig. 13.2) seeds are highly poisonous and can be lethal because of the very toxic lectin called *ricin*, although Castor bean oil contains no ricin and is safe.[2] Other lectin-containing herbs include *Viscum album* (Mistletoe leaf), used in hypertension and CHF, and *Phytolacca americanum* (Poke root), a medium-strength herb contraindicated in pregnancy and with immunosuppressant drugs. Obviously, remaining in proper dose range is paramount. Even foods such as red kidney beans, soybeans, green beans, and lentils have slightly toxic lectins that are destroyed in cooking. Peanuts have lectins, too. Lectins also contribute to intestinal permeability.
- *Oxalates.* **Oxalates** are a salt or ester of oxalic acid that can be toxic to the kidneys for those at risk for calcium oxalate kidney stones and fat malabsorption problems (Chapter 26). They combine with calcium to form crystals that mechanically injure the kidneys. Oxalates run high in Skunk Cabbage root and Jack in the Pulpit root and less so in Shepherd's Purse herb, Chickweed herb, Lamb's Quarter herb, Yellow Dock root, and even spinach and rhubarb. These plants contain more oxalates when fresh than when dried.
- *Pyrrolizidine alkaloids (PAs).* Large amounts of ***pyrrolizidine alkaloids (PAs)*** can cause liver toxicity (Chapter 8). Herbs such as Comfrey root and leaf, and less so Coltsfoot herb, contain varying amounts of this alkaloid. In Comfrey, the largest concentration is in the roots and to a lesser extent in the young leaves. Most sources say to use Comfrey externally only. It certainly can be and has been used internally, but monitoring and care are needed. It is not recommended for long-term use.
- *Safroles.* These appear as an essential oil in Sassafras root bark, Nutmeg seed, Cinnamon bark, Camphor tree, and Basil herb. Isolated doses were found to be carcinogenic in rats.[2] But in teas or eggnog, ground nutmeg and cinnamon are not a problem.
- *Salicylate glycosides and the clotting myth.* ***Salicylates*** are a group of chemicals derived from salicylic acid (Chapter 8). The saga of salicylates concerns herbs containing naturally occurring salicylates including: Sweet Birch bark, Willow bark, Wintergreen herb and root, Meadowsweet herb, various Poplars, including Aspen bark (Fig. 13.3). These botanicals are antiinflammatory and used in arthritis, fevers, and headaches. They also have a *faulty* reputation for inhibiting platelet aggregation, slowing down clotting, just as aspirin does. Aspirin (now a generic name) is used prophylactically in various drugs as an anticoagulant therapy to prevent heart attacks. Aspirin contains the acetyl group, acetylsalicylic acid, which is the anticlotting property. The herbs just mentioned do *not* contain this acetyl group. They are *not* aspirin alternatives. They are *salicylates.* Therefore, despite standard warnings in herb books and elsewhere, cautions about these herbs in combination with anticoagulant drugs are unwarranted.[1]

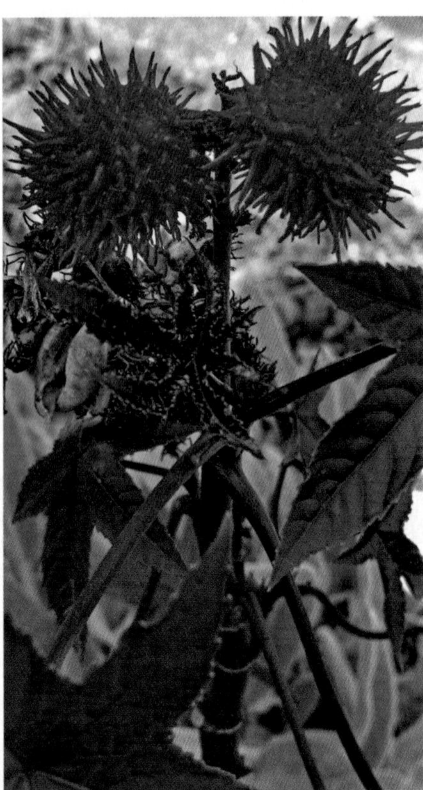

• **Fig. 13.2** *Ricinus communis* (Castor bean) seed pods and leaf. The seeds are highly poisonous because of a toxic lectin called ricin.

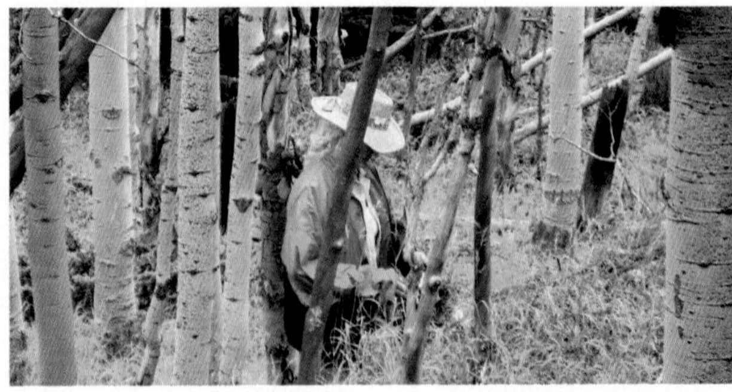

• **Fig. 13.3** Meditation in the Aspens. *Populus tremuloides* (Aspen bark) is antiinflammatory and contains naturally occuring salicylates.

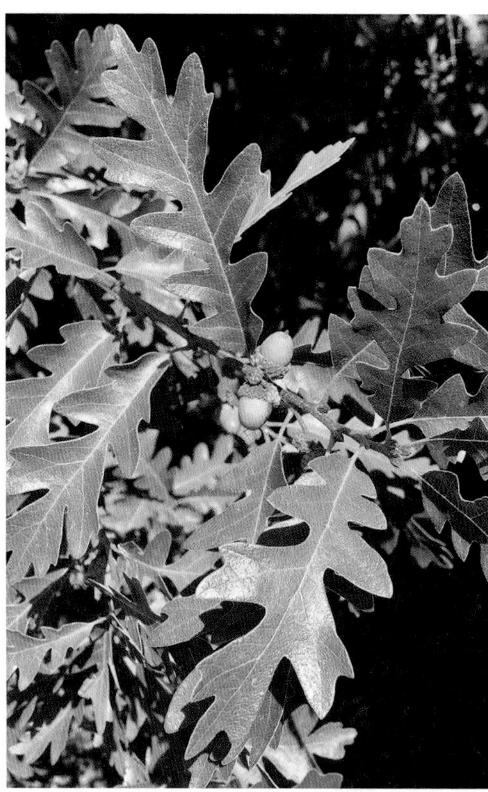

• **Fig. 13.4** *Quercus gambelii* (Gambel, Scrub Oak bark, leaf, and acorn) is very high in tannins and could cause GI nausea, vomiting, and stomach irritations in those with pre-existing intestinal damage. *Quercus alba* (Eastern White Oak) has the same precautions.

- *Tannins.* Tannins have astringent properties. The main side effects of herbs that contain high levels of tannin are nausea, vomiting, and stomach irritation. These effects occur when used in those with already irritated GI problems or kidney damage. Internally, tannins bind with and precipitate proteins to force dehydration and tightening of mucosal tissues. Externally, the same action allows for formation of a hard, protective cellular layer, as well. The Fagaceae (Oak family) (Fig. 13.4) has the highest tannin content of all. A plant needs to contain at least 10% tannins to be relevant to adverse side effect discussions.[2] Notable high-tannic herbs (greater than 10%) are White Oak bark, White Willow bark, Witch Hazel bark and leaf, Bearberry leaf, Eucalyptus leaf, Yellow dock root, Rhubarb root, St. John's Wort, and *Camilla sinensis* (Tea leaf).
- *Thujone.* This is a monoterpene component of volatile oils present in extracts and essential oils of Wormwood herb, Garden Sage leaf, Feverfew herb, and Thuja (various Cedars). Long-term or high-dose thujone can cause nervous system effects, such as dizziness, tremors, and seizures. Thujone oil is not easily extracted in water, so teas of these herbs are not a problem.

Herbal Actions Can Be Therapeutic or Harmful

Herbs have therapeutic actions; otherwise they would not be useful. However, with each positive action may come a negative action. For this reason, it is important to understand the *mechanisms of herbal actions* (how they work in the body). The following list shows general herbal classifications and commonly stated interactions you will frequently see in the literature.

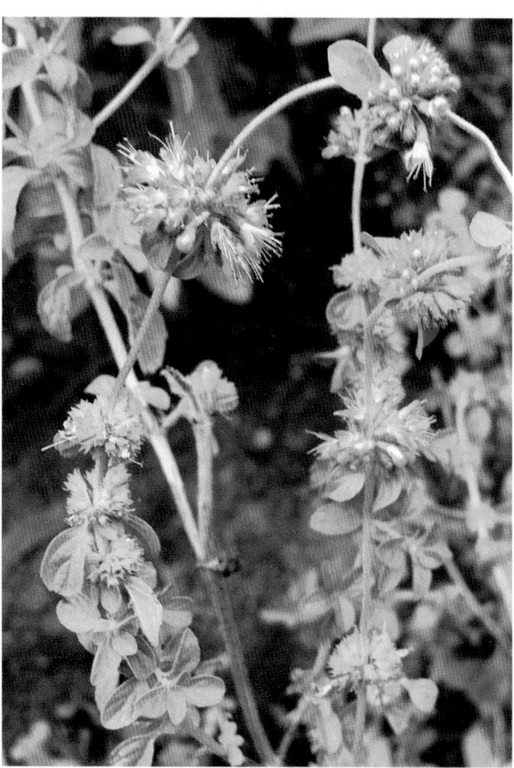

• **Fig. 13.5** Pennyroyal herb flowering. The essential oil of the Mint family's *Mentha pulegium* is an abortifacient, contraindicated in pregnancy.

- *Abortifacients.* Obviously, use of herbs that can cause abortion (***abortifacients***) are 100% contraindicated in pregnancy when the fetus is forming. They act in different ways and come in different strengths, but they can ultimately stimulate the uterus strongly enough to cause abortion. Some herbs become abortifacients only if used above therapeutic dose range. Examples are Andrographis Chuan Xin Lian and the adaptogen, Ashwagandha root, if normal dosages are exceeded. Blue Cohosh is used in labor and delivery to bring on contractions but may also be used outside pregnancy as a uterine relaxant for dysmenorrhea, along with Motherwort herb or Cramp bark. Many volatile essential oils, such as Tansy, Pennyroyal (Fig. 13.5), and Rue are very strong and toxic and should be absolutely avoided by pregnant women, but this contraindication does not apply to their weaker extracts.[1]
- *Anticoagulants.* Anticoagulants have various mechanisms of action. Some inhibit platelet aggregation, preventing red blood cells (RBCs) from clumping together and forming a clot. A few herbs implicated here are also used as foods that require large amounts and continuous use to prolong clotting time, such as, garlic, ginger, onion, cayenne pepper, and turmeric rhizome. Coumarin-containing herbs (discussed and listed in earlier section) do not contain coumadin and are actually very low risks in causing bleeding. They have been confusingly and erroneously linked to the acetylsalicylic acid anticlotting property in aspirin but do not contain that substance, either.

- *Bulk-forming laxatives*. These are the safest type of herbal laxatives: Psyllium husk or Flax seed, Guar gum or Agar (found in Red Seaweeds and used as a thickener). Think of Metamucil, which is mainly *Plantago* spp. (Psyllium husk). Psyllium expands on contact with liquid and increases bulk and water content of the stool, thus helping evacuation.
  - *Minus side of bulk laxatives*. They must be taken with plenty of water (at least 8 oz or a full glass), so they don't cause paradoxical constipation, bowel or esophageal obstruction, and gagging. If this happens, drink more water or stop taking. They can also decrease absorption of nutrients and drugs, such as aspirin, digitalis, anticoagulants, antibiotics, and cardiac glycosides.[2] So don't combine with those drugs —and monitor drug levels if combined for long periods. Long-term laxative use is not recommended anyway.
  - *Advantages of bulk laxatives*. They are not absorbed in the GI tract and pass right on through, pulling toxins along with them. This action can decrease hunger by giving a feeling of fullness, and it can bring down cholesterol and blood sugar levels.
- *Stimulating laxatives*. They relieve constipation by local stimulation and contraction of the smooth muscle of the colon, resulting in increased peristalsis that causes the bowel to empty quickly. Side effects are intestinal cramping, uterine contractions, and watery diarrhea. Long-term use leads to dependency, dehydration, and electrolyte imbalance.[2] Herbs include: Cascara sagrada bark, Aloe resin (Fig. 13.6), Senna leaf, and Rhubarb root.
- *GI irritants*. Their therapeutic action is to irritate and inflame the gut, causing bowel movements, so they are thus used short-term for severe and chronic constipation. They are strong herbs, like Coffee, Cola, and Rue. In sensitive folks, they can cause cramping, colic, or bloody diarrhea. Some stimulate the uterus and should not be used if pregnant. Coffee grounds are sometimes used for a few days only, as a bowel irritant in detoxifying enemas.
- *Coagulants*. There's a group of herbs (and some foods) which actually are mild coagulants. They aid clotting because of their high vitamin K content. Fat-soluble vitamin K is necessary for clotting to occur. (If blood didn't clot where and when it's supposed to, we would bleed to death from slight injuries.) Mild coagulant-type foods include beet roots and greens, cabbage, Brussels sprouts, and kale. Plantain leaves have vitamin K and are also filled with tannins, both instrumental in first aid to stop bleeding from wounds and trauma. Vitamin K-rich Shepherd's Purse herb is used for heavy menstrual bleeding in menorrhagia.
- *Emmenagogues* (*uterine stimulants*). They work in various ways, bringing on delayed menses (Chapter 28). Many work directly on the uterus by stimulating the surrounding vasculature of the myometrium to promote menses. However, it does not follow that all emmenagogues are necessarily abortifacients.[1] Emmenagogues encourage menses but do not cause abortion. *Vitex agnus-castus* (Chastetree berry) works indirectly on the pituitary level. Chinese Medicine *blood movers* are described as herbs that invigorate the blood, causing uterine blood vessels to vasodilate and stimulate circulation and menstrual flow. Some of these are Carthamus Hong Hua (Safflower), Yarrow herb, and Prickly Ash bark. Modern herbalists make good use of emmenagogues in nonpregnant women to boost reproductive health, improve fertility, stabilize pregnancy, and provide optimal recovery from pelvic infections and procedures.[2] Uterine stimulants are contraindicated in menorrhagia or pregnancy, unless one is well versed in their use.

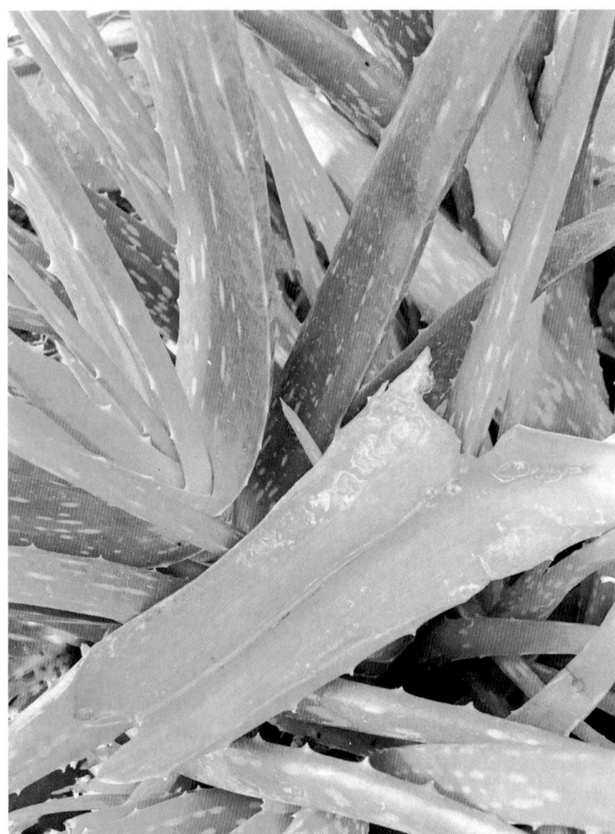

• **Fig. 13.6** *Aloe vera* with leaf split open to reveal its gentle wound healing gel. The resin in the leaf itself is a stimulating laxative that causes severe smooth muscle colon contraction, making that part of the plant a last-resort purgative.

- *Urinary irritants*. If the urinary mucosa is already inflamed from a urinary tract infection (UTI) or other condition, these herbs could make it worse. Some are Coffee seed, Asparagus rhizome, Celery seed, Cinnamon bark, Eucalyptus leaf, Juniper berry, and Thyme leaf.[5]
- *Photosensitization*. This side effect (***photosensitizing***) is caused by ingestion of certain substances combined with excessive periods of sunlight or cosmetic or therapeutic UV light exposure. Skin irritations could appear as allergic dermatitis with rashes, blisters, swelling or hyperpigmentation. The culprits are *furanocoumarins* and *psoralens* found in species of the Apiaceae (Parsley), Rutaceae (Rue), and Fabaceae (Pea) families. Common herbs that can cause photosensitivity, and then only at doses much higher than recommended, are St. John's Wort, Celery seed, *Angelica* spp., Bitter Orange peel, and Rue herb. St. John's Wort gets a lot of bad press, warranted or not.

Adverse Herb and Drug Interactions

Allopathic drugs are very strong medicine. Increasingly, people use herbs without knowledgeable guidance or combine them with prescription drugs. Naturally, this circumstance is worrisome for herbalists, nurses, and doctors. It is a hot topic, because we want our patients to be safe. How does this fare when combined with herbs that may potentiate or interfere with those actions? Drugs, such as Coumadin that prolong clotting time or digoxin used in heart failure, must be monitored closely. There is a lot of misinformation out there, and most texts and resources written for herbalists and doctors err on the side of extreme caution. The *Physician's Desk Reference for Herbal Medicine* is in its fourth edition at this printing and takes an extremely conservative viewpoint.

Herbalists are not expected to know every drug in existence, nor their side effects. Even doctors, nurses, and pharmacists constantly look up information. So, two points: (1) Always get a drug history from your clients, both for prescription and over-the-counter products. (2) Purchase a good drug handbook that is not too complicated. Recommended are Mosby's *Nursing Drug Reference* or Saunders *Nursing Drug Handbook.* Both are updated every year. And there is always the internet. The top 10 medications by number of monthly prescriptions in 2016 are listed here.[6] The drug categories don't change much from year to year.

- *Synthroid (levothyroxine).* Synthetic thyroxine (T4) thyroid hormone for hypothyroidism.
- *Crestor (rosuvastatin).* A statin that lowers cholesterol.
- *VHFA (albuterol).* Bronchodilator for bronchospasms, as in asthma.
- *Nexium (esomeprazole).* Proton pump inhibitor for acid reflux (GERD).
- *Advair Diskus (fluticasone).* Bronchodilator for wheezing and asthma.
- *Lantus Solostar (insulin glargine).* Long-acting insulin for type 1 diabetes.
- *Vyvanse (lisdexamfetamine).* CNS stimulant for ADHD and binge eating.
- *Lyrica (pregabalin).* Anticonvulsant for seizures and fibromyalgia.
- *Spiriva HandiHaler (tiotropium).* Bronchodilator for spasms and COPD.
- *Januvia (sitagliptin).* Oral antidiabetic for type 2 diabetes.

As you see from this preceding list, low thyroid, high cholesterol, asthma, diabetes, and indigestion are rampant health issues. These can often be helped by herbal remedies accompanied by lifestyle modifications such as diet and exercise. Frequently prescribed anticoagulants, antihypertensives, cardiac glycosides, analgesics, and antibiotics round out the top-10 list and have appeared there in other years.

Some Common Categories of Herb-Drug Interactions

Listed here are some categories of herb-drug interactions and what they mean. They are often cited in herbal safety books, and some knowledge of physiology, pharmacology, and chemistry is needed to understand these herb-drug combinations and why they might be a problem. A few of the specific herbs that could be implicated in these reactions are shown in Table 13.1. Some are substantiated by studies, and others are theoretical.

- *Blood pressure interactions.* If a person is concurrently on pharmaceutical antihypertensives and herbs that accomplish the same thing, blood pressure (BP) can get too low. The best bet is to slowly wean down the drugs and gradually increase the herbs, all with the cooperation of the health care provider. Frequent BP monitoring is a must.
- *Blood sugar interactions.* ***Hypoglycemics*** (herbs that lower glucose) are generally given for type 2 diabetes when the pancreas is still producing a little insulin (Chapter 27). Use of blood glucose lowering herbs may lower the necessary doses of oral hypoglycemic prescription medication such as Metformin, or eliminate the need for such drugs altogether. Always work with a health care provider when incorporating this treatment. If patient has metabolic syndrome with high insulin levels and is not on prescription medication, the herbs could fix it. Always include a hypoglycemic diet and exercise in the equation. Hypoglycemic herbs combined with insulin in those with type 1 diabetes could drive sugar levels dangerously low. In this case be careful and always monitor glucose levels. Hyperglycemic herbs that raise blood sugar usually contain caffeine: Cocoa, Coffee, Cola seeds, and black tea leaf.[5]
- *Monoamine oxidase inhibitor (MAOI).* Monoamine oxidase enzymes are chemicals that break down mood-enhancing neurotransmitters, such as, dopamine, serotonin, and norepinephrine. ***Monoamine oxidase inhibitors (MAOIs)*** are a drug classification used for depression that blocks breakdown of this enzyme, thus elevating mood. Drugs, such as Nardil and Parnate are examples of MAOIs that are used for depression and anxiety. Herbs that the medical establishment has speculated might interfere with these drugs include St. John's Wort, Ephedra Ma Huang (Ephedra stem), and Nutmeg seed. Convincing evidence for this interference is slim,[2] but nurses and doctors can become very nervous about this issue.
- *Potentiation with central nervous system (CNS) depressants.* The drug classification that depresses the nervous system and slows down brain activity are ***CNS depressants*** that may be enhanced by nervous sedatives and anxiolytic herbals, including Kava root and Valerian root. CNS depressant drugs cover a very large category used for pain, anxiety, insomnia, and seizures. Many are physically and psychologically addictive. Whenever possible, wean down on the drugs and increase use of the herbs
  - *Examples of CNS depressant drugs.* These drugs include sedatives, tranquilizers, analgesics, sleep medications, antihistamines, and antiseizure medications. Examples are benzodiazepines, like Ativan or Xanax, used for anxiety, acute stress, and panic attacks; narcotic/opioid analgesics, like morphine and codeine and the many brands made from them; barbiturates, such as Seconal or Nembutal; anticonvulsants, such as Lyrica or Dilantin; antihistamines (antiallergy drugs), like Benadryl that make you sleepy; and, of course, alcohol, which slows down brain functioning. Caution must be taken if the drugs and herbs are combined because they can potentiate each other.
- *Pseudoaldosteronism and the Licorice root connection.* The somewhat complicated physiology behind Licorice root's reputation for increasing blood pressure and potassium in the blood follows. Too much aldosterone, called *hyperaldosteronism,* is caused by a benign adrenal tumor. The condition increases renin from juxtaglomerular kidney cells, causing vasoconstriction, and pulls excess water and sodium into blood, increasing blood volume and blood pressure. This scenario results in edema, hypertension, low potassium, high sodium, and cardiac involvement.
  - *Large and prolonged Licorice root dosing* (with no adrenal tumor) can mimic these symptoms in susceptible individuals, including those with edema and water imbalances. The

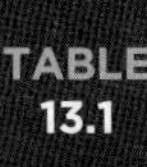

TABLE 13.1 **Possible Adverse Herb-Drug Interactions with Some Common Herbs**[1]
(List includes drug concerns/contraindications with a few frequently used botanicals to provide an idea of the issues. Always refer to more complete sources when needed.)

Herb	Drug or Generic	Possible Interaction	Herbalist Action
Andrographis paniculata Chaun Lian herb	Coumadin (anticoagulant)	Potentiate bleeding	Low risk, monitor coagulation
Astragalus membranaceus Huang Qi root	Cyclophosphamide (chemo and immuno-suppressants)	Might reduce effectiveness	Low risk, monitor
Vaccinium myrtillus Bilberry berry and leaf	Coumadin (anticoagulant)	Potentiate bleeding	Low risk at high doses >100 mg per day anthocyanins
	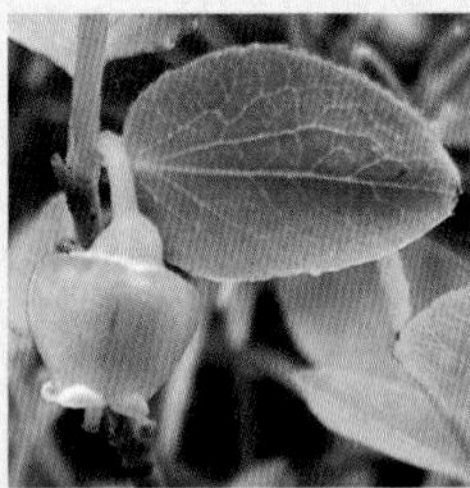 *Vaccinium scoparium* (Broom huckleberry, Bilberry leaf and flower).		
Fucus vesiculosus Bladderwrack and other sea veggies	Carbimazole for hyperthyroidism	Theoretically, might decrease effectiveness because of its iodine content	*Contraindicated*
Lycopus virginicus Bugleweed herb (Raises thyroid level)	Radioactive iodine used in tests, thyroid hormones	Could potentiate drugs that treat hyperthyroidism	*Contraindicated* with thyroid drugs to lower thyroid
Cardioactive glycosides: Lily of the Valley Squill bulb Foxglove herb Pleurisy root	Digoxin to treat heart failure and others that increase cardiac output; calcium supplements	Theoretically, may potentiate cardiac glycosides per Commission E	Monitor, low risk
Apium graveolens Celery seed	Thyroxine—hormone used for hypothyroidism	Potentiates	Very low risk
Salvia miltiorrhiza Dan Shen (Cinnabar Sage root)	Warfarin (anticoagulant)	May potentiate	*Contraindicated* per case report
Diuretics: Horsetail herb Juniper berry Corn Silk Uva ursi leaf	Lithium salts used for bipolar disorder	May potentiate based on case study	Monitor, low risk
		Juniper berry.	

(*Continued*)

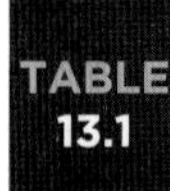

TABLE 13.1 Possible Adverse Herb-Drug Interactions with Some Common Herbs[1]
(List includes drug concerns/contraindications with a few frequently used botanicals to provide an idea of the issues. Always refer to more complete sources when needed.)—cont'd

Herb	Drug or Generic	Possible Interaction	Herbalist Action
Angelica sinensis Dang Gui root	Warfarin	May potentiate based on case report	Monitor coagulation, low risk
Echinacea spp. root	Immunosuppressant medications	Theoretically may decrease effectiveness	*Contraindicated*
Trigonella foenum-graecum Fenugreek seed	Iron supplements	Inhibits iron absorption	Take 2 hours before or after iron supplementation
High-fiber herbs: Psyllium seed Marshmallow root Slippery Elm bark	Iron, lithium, vitamin B_{12} Carbamazepine for seizures	May decrease absorption	Take at least 2 hours before or after meds
Allium sativum Garlic bulb	Aspirin, warfarin, HIV protease inhibitors	Could increase bleeding time, per case reports and clinical study	Fresh Garlic *contraindicated* in warfarin doses >5 grams per day; monitor the other drugs
Ginkgo biloba Ginkgo leaf	Anticonvulsants	May decrease drug effect	Medium risk, monitor
	Antiplatelet, anticoagulants: aspirin, warfarin	Increased bleeding tendency	Monitor, aspirin low risk; warfarin medium risk
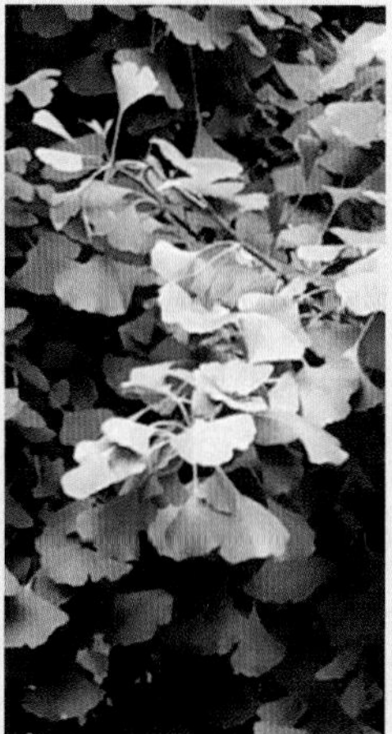 Ginkgo tree.	SSRIs	Could cause sedation	Monitor SSRIs, very low risk
	Haldol	Potentiate	Caution: confer with health care provider for schizophrenia patients taking Haldol
Camellia sinensis Green Tea leaf	Warfarin	Low risk to decrease effectiveness	Monitor coagulation
Crataegus oxyacantha Hawthorn berry	Beta blockers like Atenolol and other hypotensives, digitalis	May increase effectiveness of drug	Monitor, low risk
Hypoglycemic herbs: Gymnema leaf Fenugreek seed Goat's Rue herb	Hypoglycemic drugs and insulin	Theoretical concern	Monitor blood sugar, might need health care provider to reduce drug dose

(Continued)

TABLE 13.1 Possible Adverse Herb-Drug Interactions with Some Common Herbs[1]
***(List includes drug concerns/contraindications with a few frequently used botanicals to provide an idea of the issues. Always refer to more complete sources when needed.)*—cont'd**

Herb	Drug or Generic	Possible Interaction	Herbalist Action
Piper methysticum Kava root	CNS depressants	Potentiation—theoretical concern	Monitor, low risk
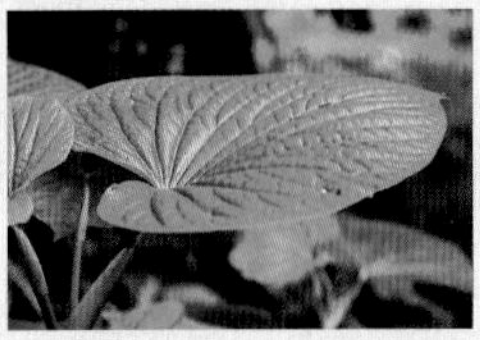	L-dopa and other Parkinson's drugs	Possible dopamine antagonist	*Contraindicated* or watch closely
Kava leaf. (iStock.com/Credit: Female photographer from Thailand.)			
Laxatives with anthraquinones: Aloe resin Cascara sagrada bark Senna leaf Yellow Dock root	Antiarrhythmics, cardiac glycosides, potassium-depleting diuretics, and Licorice root	May affect if low K+ (potassium) from long-term use per Commission E	Monitor K+, low risk. Maintain high K+ diet
	With other Rx meds	May decrease absorption time	Monitor, low risk
Glycyrrhiza glabra *G. uralensis* Gan Cao Licorice root	Antihypertensives	Pseudoaldosteronism (edema and high BP)	Theoretical case with Licorice candy
	Prednisolone and cortisol	Potentiation from decreased drug metabolism	Theoretical, low risk, monitor
	Digoxin	With Licorice intake could cause low K+ making drug toxic	Avoid long-term Licorice use dose >100 mg/d. High K+ diet
	Thiazide diuretics and other potassium-depleting drugs	With Licorice possible K+ loss in urine	Same as with digoxin
Filipendula ulmaria Meadowsweet herb	Warfarin	May potentiate	Monitor, low risk
Piperine-containing herbs like Black and Long Peppercorn	Prescribed medication	Enhances bioavailability	Monitor, low risk
Polyphenolic and Flavonoid herbs: Peppermint herb Verbena herb Pennyroyal herb Green Tea leaf Chamomile flower Rosemary leaf	Iron supplements	Can inhibit absorption 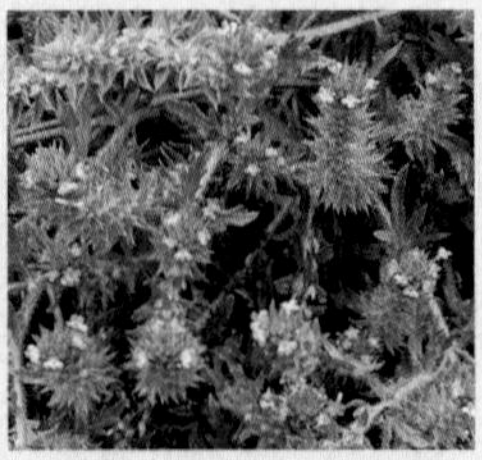 Verbena herb flowering.	Don't take these herbs simultaneously with meals or iron supplements

(*Continued*)

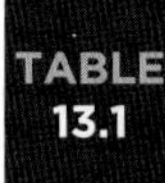

TABLE 13.1 Possible Adverse Herb-Drug Interactions with Some Common Herbs[1]
***(List includes drug concerns/contraindications with a few frequently used botanicals to provide an idea of the issues. Always refer to more complete sources when needed.)*—cont'd**

Herb	Drug or Generic	Possible Interaction	Herbalist Action
Serenoa serrulata Saw Palmetto berry	Warfarin	May potentiate	Monitor, low risk
Schisandra chinensis Wu Wei Zi (Five Taste berry)	Any med Rx	Theoretically may increase Phase I/II hepatic metabolism	Monitor, medium risk
Eleutherococcus senticosus Ci Wu Jia (Eleuthero, Siberian ginseng root)	Digoxin	Interfered with digitalis assay	Monitor, very low risk
Hypericum perforatum St John's Wort	Amitriptyline, Simvastatin, Digoxin	Decreased drug levels	Monitor, medium risk
	Antihistamines, benzodiazepines	Decrease drug levels dependent on dose	St. John's Wort contraindicated with Digoxin at >1 grams per day dried
St. John's Wort flower and buds.	Warfarin, immunosuppressives like Cyclosporine, HIV protease inhibitors, Phenprocoumon	Decreases drug levels	All Contraindicated
Tannins, as in: Cranesbill root Grape seed extract Green/black tea St. John's Wort Mint herb Meadowsweet herb Hawthorn berry Raspberry leaf Willow bark Uva ursi leaf	Alkaloids and alkaline drugs, minerals, especially iron and thiamine	May reduce absorption, especially iron in heavy black tea drinkers	Take at least 2 hours away from medication Uva ursi leaf and berry.
Curcuma longa Turmeric rhizome	Aspirin, warfarin	Potentiates antiplatelet activity	Monitor, low risk at normal doses. Contraindicated >15 grams per day dried tuber
Valerian officinalis root	CNS depressants and alcohol	May potentiate	Monitor, very low risk level
Willow bark	Warfarin	May potentiate	Monitor, low risk

glycyrrhizin in Licorice root contains steroids similar to the adrenocortical ones, which can cause what's known as ***pseudoaldosteronism***. The resulting high blood pressure reverses itself when the herb is discontinued.

- *Selective serotonin reuptake inhibitors (SSRIs) and serotonin syndrome.* Serotonin syndrome is an adverse side effect caused from ***selective serotonin reuptake inhibitors (SSRIs)***, a drug classification used to fight depression. They work by increasing

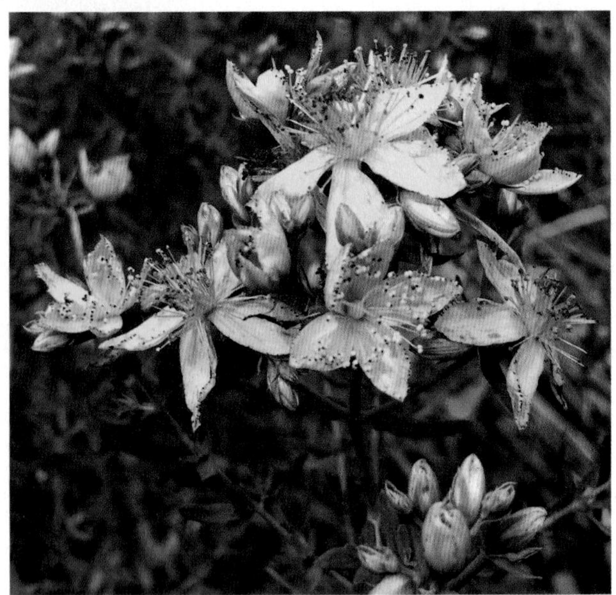

• **Fig. 13.7** Saint John's Wort blooming. *Hypericum perforatum* can decrease blood levels of the drugs theophylline and digoxin because of its effect on the liver's CYP450 detoxification system.

serotonin, a feel-good neurotransmitter, in the blood, which elevates mood and calmness. Adverse effects cause diarrhea, sweating, shaking, and seizures, known as ***serotonin syndrome***. Examples of SSRIs are Celexa, Prozac, and Zoloft. Saint John's Wort (Fig. 13.7), combined with SSRIs, has been implicated in causing serotonin syndrome, despite little convincing evidence.[2] However, you may still find dire warnings about St. John's Wort and serotonin syndrome in some herbals.

- *Vitamin K and Coumadin.* Vitamin K is necessary for clotting. The drug Coumadin (generic name is warfarin) competes with vitamin K and inhibits liver production of prothrombin, an essential clotting factor. That's why warfarin is used to prevent blood clots in heart disease. So if one eats enormous, and I mean huge, amounts of plants high in vitamin K, then the drug might be less effective. So don't worry about collard greens, Chinese cabbage, broccoli, Brussels sprouts, and beet roots and greens; they're very nutritious (Table 13.1).

Cytochrome P450 Enzyme System and Herb–Drug Interactions

Fat-soluble drugs, herbs, foods, hormones, chemical pollutants and other substances are broken down, metabolized, and detoxified through the ***cytochrome P450 (CYP450)*** family of enzymes, mainly in the liver (Chapter 19). This action is significant because this breakdown can affect how well a drug or herb does (or doesn't) work when used in combination with others. Some enzymes inhibit, and some potentiate, a drug's effect. It could make the difference between an overdose or an ineffective dose.

Various herbs, drugs, and foods, alone or in combination, react differently in this system and have an affinity to certain enzymes. There are 14 families of enzymes in the system, and it is hard to predict which enzyme does what—which drug-drug, herb-drug, food-drug, or food-herb combination will cause reactions and which ones won't. Some enzymes cause no reaction at all. Many substances have not yet been studied, so the jury is out. There are also pronounced individual and racial differences in drug-metabolizing activity. A drug-drug or drug-herb combination can interact with CYP450 enzymes and be either an inhibitor or an inducer of the substance with which it is combined.[7] Here are the terms and process involved.

- *Substrate.* This is the therapeutic drug, herb, or food that is acted on by the CYP450 enzyme.
- *Inducing agent.* Enzyme in the CYP450 system that *increases* the rate of the substrate's metabolism and thereby shortens its half-life, causing drug blood levels to drop. The drug leaves the body too quickly and isn't therapeutic.
- *Inhibiting agent.* Enzyme in the CYP450 system that *decreases* the rate of the substrate's metabolism and thereby prolongs half-life, causing blood drug levels to rise. The drug stays in the body too long, leading to a potential overdose.
- *Dose adjustments.* In either case, dosage needs monitoring to maintain therapeutic levels.

Examples of the CYP450 System Working Positively and Negatively

The CYP450 system can work in positive or negative ways on the body, depending on which substrate combines with which agent, and on which enzyme. For instance, the flavonoid *naringenin* in grapefruit or grapefruit juice activates enzymes in the liver's detoxification system that decreases certain drugs' rates of elimination from the body, altering their clinical activity and toxicity. An 8-oz glass of grapefruit juice contains enough *naringenin* to decrease CYP450 detoxification activity by a large amount. This boils down to an increase in the drug's bioavailability, and can lead to overdose when the juice is taken with statins, antiarrhythmics, calcium channel blockers, and immunosuppressive agents. That's why those drug labels say *not* to take with grapefruit juice. However, grapefruit juice on its own can be quite a healthy drink because of its vitamin C, minerals, and antibacterial activity.

Another example is Dandelion root, which inhibits the substrate/drug theophylline (bad effect) but also inhibits alcoholic intoxification (good effect). Umbelliferous herbs of the Apiaceae family, like Celery seed or Osha root, can inhibit the therapeutic effect of calcium channel blockers and antihistamines. Many drugs but very few herbs have been studied regarding their CYP450 interactions. The most-studied herbs and therefore most implicated in affecting CYP450 enzymes, up or down and for better or for worse, are Ginkgo leaf, Kava root, and St. John's Wort. For instance, St. John's Wort decreases blood levels of theophylline and digoxin, but Ginkgo, Kava, and St. John's Wort increase blood levels of Dilantin and progesterone.[1] An increased level of Dilantin can lead to an overdose (bad effect) but an increase in progesterone in a menopausal woman may be considered a favorable outcome.

Indole 3-carbinol is a sulfurous compound found in cruciferous herbs and brassica vegetables, such as broccoli, cauliflower, Brussels sprouts, and bok choy (Chapter 28). Indole 3-carbinol is a key nutrient for CYP450 liver detoxification in both Phase I and Phase II, speeding up excretion of toxins. Thus cruciferous veggies are important foods to include in any well-thought-out detoxification program. They are extremely useful in treating cancer and for reproductive health in men and women. Indole 3-carbinol selectively binds to estrogen receptors blocking the *bad* estrogen (estrone) from building up in the body, which can cause breast, uterine, cervical, and prostate cancers.[8]

Our understanding of the CYP450s has been increasing since the first enzyme in the system was identified by Julius Axelrod and Bernard Brodie in 1955. As time goes on, herbalists can take advantage of new findings and incorporate them into their therapies. Diet seems to play an important role, as do herb-drug interactions.

Pregnancy and Lactation Guidelines

Nothing strong or toxic should be ingested during pregnancy, and special care should always be taken in the first trimester, when risk of miscarriage is highest. Other concerns in pregnancy are risk of toxicity of the mother that can influence the child, fetal toxicity, developmental malformations (***teratogenesis***), and health effects on the child later in life. The fewer herbs and drugs ingested in pregnancy, the better. Many herb books give huge lists of herbs contraindicated in pregnancy. That said, sometimes they are safe and indicated (Table 13.2).

Consensus as to which herbs are safe in pregnancy varies greatly. Some of the most common herbs given by midwives in a survey of North Carolina–certified nurse midwives were Ginger root for nausea (although you'll see this one contraindicated in some books and also by Commission E), Raspberry leaf, Peppermint herb, Chamomile flower (Fig. 13.8), Evening Primrose oil, and Black and Blue Cohosh roots near labor and delivery time. Among naturopaths, popular herbs to administer were Echinacea root, Raspberry leaf, and Nettle herb.[1] Many pregnant women take herbs on their own with no ill effects. This practice is common throughout the world. In general, follow these suggestions and refer to trusted herb books.

- *Avoid herbs with known toxicity or abortifacients.* This category includes herbs such as Aconitum Fu Zi (prepared Sichuan

TABLE 13.2 Some Herbs to Avoid in Pregnancy[a]

Herb	Reason to Avoid
Actaea racemosa (Black Cohosh root)	Emmenagogue, used during labor and delivery
Aloe vera leaf (resin from the leaf)	Uterine vasodilating, very strong purgative
Angelica archangelica (Angelica root)	Emmenagogue, moves blood
Angelica sinensis (Dang Gui root)	Moves blood, can cause miscarriage
Apium graveolens (Celery seed)	Uterine stimulant
Berberis spp. (Barberry root)	Stimulating laxative, uterine stimulant, hypertensive
Cascara sagrada root	Strong, stimulating laxative
Caulophyllum thalictroides (Blue Cohosh root)	Stimulates soughing of uterine lining, used during labor and delivery
Foeniculum vulgare (Fennel seed)	In excess, a uterine stimulant
Gossypium hirsutum (Cotton Root bark)	Abortive, emmenagogue, stimulates tissue that responds to oxytocin
Iris versicolor (Blue Flag root)	Cathartic
Sanguinaria canadensis (Bloodroot)	Uterine vasodilator
Symphytum officinale (Comfrey root)	External use OK; questionable PA safety
Thymus vulgaris (Thyme herb essential oil)	Large dose may be uterine stimulant
Turnera diffusa (Damiana herb)	Uterine vasodilator
Tussilago farfara (Coltsfoot herb)	Possible carcinogen, questionable PA safety
Verbena officinalis (Vervain herb)	Uterine stimulant
Xanthoxylum americanum (Prickly Ash bark)	Uterine vasodilator

[a]List provided by author and herbalist, Brigitte Mars, AHG certified.

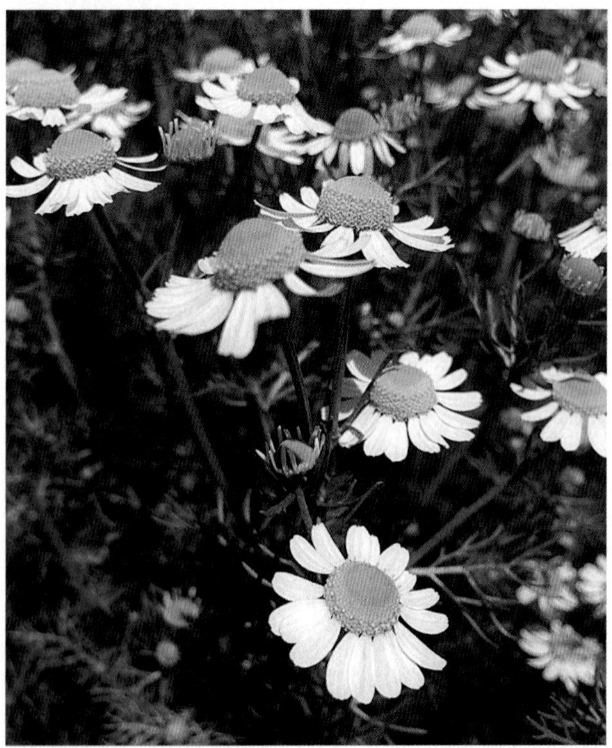

• **Fig. 13.8** Chamomile flowering. *Matricaria recutita* is one of the most common and safest herbs used by midwives when caring for pregnant women, although in essential oil form it can be abortifacient.

Aconite root), Bloodroot, Ephedra Ma Huang (Ephedra stem), Poke root, Lobelia herb, Rhubarb root, Yarrow herb, and essential oils of Tansy, Pennyroyal, Rue, and Chamomile.

- *Essential oils and pregnancy*. Essential oils, in general, are very strong and should not be taken internally in pregnancy. They are commonly at least 50 times more concentrated than the raw herb, and most need to be diluted that much. Chamomile essential oil is said to be 200 times stronger than the dried plant. (All of this information does not apply when used in cooking or flavoring of food.) Some are very toxic and known abortifacients and should never be taken in pregnancy: Rue, Pennyroyal, and Tansy.
- *Lactation*. There is little understanding as to how secondary plant metabolites pass into breast milk or affect the infant. For this reason, it is probably best to give the herb directly to the infant, rather than hoping it will pass through the mother's milk. It is unlikely that normally recommended doses taken by the mother will have much therapeutic effect on the infant.[9] The takeaway is for breast feeding moms to use the following method when giving herbs to their infants.
  - *Administering herbs to babies while breastfeeding*. The best way is to mix the appropriate herbal extract with about 5 mL of expressed milk, draw into a syringe, and apply with steady pressure to the back of the baby's mouth. It can also be mixed into formula or a bottle (Chapter 21). Anything toxic or poisonous must be avoided. The American Academy of Pediatrics classifies drugs used in lactation as "ND," meaning no data available. Most drugs, by far, come under this heading. "C" designates compatible with breastfeeding; "CC" means Compatible with breastfeeding but use caution; "SD" Strongly discouraged; and "X" means Contraindicated. You may see these symbols used in herb books.
- *History of miscarriage*. More caution must be taken for high-risk pregnancies than for a normal one. Go easy here. Raspberry leaf or Wild Yam root are always safe bets to restore the uterus and strengthen the tissue.
- *Strong laxative herbs* containing anthraquinones such as Aloe resin, Cascara bark, Senna leaf or pod, and Rhubarb root must be avoided in high doses. Commission E contraindicates these at any dose.

Summary

As a rule, available information about herbal safety errs on the side of caution. We must be discerning, keep up with research, and evaluate the validity of studies. Respect for our herbal allies is in order, but do not be overly paranoid. Confidence is tempered with knowledge and common sense. Trust your intuition. If you have reservations, don't use that herb.

Allergic reactions are the most common side effect any herbalist will encounter, and of those, contact dermatitis heads the list. Dosage, herb quality, and the occasional need for monitoring blood pressure, coagulation, or glucose levels were examined. Certain herbal constituents such as tannins, lectins, and herbs that act as cardiac glycosides can present potential problems.

Herbs may potentiate or inhibit drug actions and vice versa. Strong allopathic drugs can be problematic when combined with herbs. The liver's cytochrome P450 system of enzymes can also inhibit or potentiate drug and herb dosages. In pregnancy and lactation, nontoxic herbs are recommended. Children and infants can be given a wide variety as long as dosage parameters are followed (Chapter 21).

Review

Fill in the Blanks

(Answers in Appendix B.)

1. The most common herbal side effect is ___.
2. Name three herbs that contain coumarin. ___, ___, ___.
3. Name three herbs that contain natural salicylates ___, ___, ___.
4. Cardiac glycosides act by increasing ___ and lowering ___. They are used in treating ___. The drugs are ___ and ___ derived from the chemical ___. Two herbal examples are ___ and ___.
5. Name three herbal actions or categories that could cause miscarriage. ___, ___, ___.
6. Four side effects of stimulating laxatives ___, ___, ___, ___. Three herbal examples are ___, ___, ___.
7. Aldosterone is a hormone made in the ___. Tumors in this area may cause a syndrome called ___. Four symptoms of

this are ___, ___, ___, ___. The herb ___ can mimic this in susceptible people. The syndrome is then referred to as ___.

8. Name five potential abortifacients to absolutely avoid in pregnancy. ___, ___, ___, ___, ___.
9. Two herbs that contain PAs are ___ and ___. The worry is that this alkaloid can cause ___.

Critical Concept Questions

(Answers for you to decide.)

1. Your client asks, "Will taking this Meadowsweet cause me to bleed or bruise?" Discuss.
2. Why is St. John's Wort so often implicated in herb-drug interactions? Issues?
3. Is Comfrey root a safe herb? Discuss.
4. Give an example of when the so-called adverse effect of an herb might actually be used to therapeutic advantage?
5. What are the benefits and pitfalls of psyllium fiber in Metamucil? What is its mechanism of action? What are the cautions?
6. Why is grapefruit juice contraindicated with antiarrhythmic drugs? Relate this to liver detoxification.
7. What are some guidelines for using herbs with pregnant women?
8. What adverse effect could be caused from excessive intake of pure Licorice candy? What chemical is involved?
9. If a client is on warfarin, which factors would you consider as to herb choices?

References

1. Mills, Simon and Kerry Bone. *The Essential Guide to Herbal Safety* (Philadelphia, PA: Elsevier, 2005).
2. McGuffin, Michael, Christopher Hobbs, et al., eds. *American Herbal Products Association's Botanical Safety Handbook* (New York: CRC Press, 1997).
3. Holmes, Peter. *Energetics of Western Herbs* (Boulder, CO: Snow Lotus Press, 2006).
4. Ganora, Lisa. *Herbal Constituents: Foundations of Phytochemistry* (Louisville, CO: Herbalchem, 2009).
5. Brinker, Francis. *Herb Contraindications and Drug Interactions* (Sandy, OR: Eclectic Medical Publications, 1998).
6. "The 10 Most Prescribed and Top-Selling Medications." WebMD. http://www.webmd.com/news/20150508/most-prescribed-top-selling-drugs (accessed October 18, 2019).
7. "The Cytochrome P450 System: What Is It and Why Should I care?" Davis's Drug Guide. http://www.drugguide.com/ddo/view/Davis-Drug-Guide/109519/all/The_Cytochrome_P450_System:_What_Is_It_and_Why_Should_I_Care (accessed October 19, 2019).
8. Meschino, James. "Indole 3 carbinol: Key cancer preventative natural agent in food and supplements." http://meschinohealth.com/article/indole-3-carbinol-key-cancer-preventive-natural-agent-in-food-and-supplements/ (accessed October 19, 2019).
9. Santich, Rob and Kerry Bone. *Phytotherapy Essentials: Healthy Children, Optimizing Children's Health with Herbs* (Warwick, Queensland, Australia: Phytotherapy Press, 2008).

14 Formulating, Dispensing, and Dosing

"Always dispense the correct formula, to the correct person, at the correct time, in the correct dose."

—Rachel Lord, your author, herbalist, and nurse

CHAPTER REVIEW

- Herbal formulations. General considerations for making up an herbal blend and principles of formulation. Creating a formula with proportions for each herb.
- Dispensing. Bottle sizes, calculations, and labeling.
- Dosage: General principles. Approximate adult dosages for mild to moderate strength preparations. Dosages for infusions, decoctions, tinctures, essential oils, syrups, and capsules.
- Conversions. Metric and U.S. customary units.
- Common abbreviations pertaining to dosing.

KEY TERMS

Apothecary
Conversions
Dispensary/dispensing
Formulation/formulating
Part
Proportion
Signs
Symptoms
Therapeutic principles

Formulating is the art of making up a personalized herbal blend. For individualized *formulations*, an herbalist must know the criteria for composing a generic herbal formula—*any* formula. This chapter is not about which specific herbs to use but rather the philosophy of choosing herbs, concocting a well-balanced herbal combination, and prioritizing and deciding herbal proportions in a remedy. How many parts of Dandelion root versus how many parts of Marshmallow root should go into the bottle, and why?

A ***dispensary*** is a dedicated space, such as an herbal apothecary, where herbs are prepared, combined (formulated) and provided. The process of formulating consists of deciding on which herbs to use, calculating correct herbal proportions, and accurately measuring and labeling. Proper calculation involves figuring out the amount of each herb needed for any bottle size based on decided ***proportions*** (how much of one herb is needed in relation to another). The exact same formula must be dispensed, regardless of container size.

Dispensing is ideally done in a dedicated room containing all herbs and supplies, called the ***apothecary***—or in modern allopathic terms, a *pharmacy*. The space contains the tools of the trade: dry herbs, tinctures, measuring tools, bottles, droppers, and labels, all in one convenient location. Actual preparations are made up in the apothecary and presented correctly to the client. Accurate measurement and labeling are key.

Proper dispensing—handing out the remedy—involves deciding on appropriate dosage along with providing clear instructions on how to take the herbs. How much should a client take, how is that done, and when? Another detail is knowing which size bottle to dispense and the length of time it will last. If the client needs to take the formula for 2 weeks, it is best to dispense the appropriate amount so that they don't run out or have too much left over.

Conversions, (changing medical measurements back and forth from English to metric), and medical abbreviations are part of formulating. A knowledge of metric measurements and English equivalents are vital when negotiating the world of herbal delivery. Standard Latin medical abbreviations simplify life and communication. Speak the language. Walk the talk.

Herbal Formulation

General Formulating Considerations

There are various considerations when making any herbal formula, regardless of client or condition.

- *Therapeutic principle(s)*. What is the main intention? What is the herbalist trying to accomplish? These are the ***therapeutic principles***. Are you trying to banish infection, dry damp, nourish the lungs, help sleep, or accomplish a combination thereof? Prioritize and list these principles in order of importance. Link the herb with the pathology, syndrome, or condition(s).

- *Signs and symptoms. **Signs*** pertain to objective information about a client's condition that can be observed or measured, such as external bleeding, blood pressure (BP), swollen ankles or lab results. ***Symptoms*** are the subjective evidence of disease, perceived by the client that the observer cannot see, such as pain, anxiety, or depression. Consider both types of information and choose appropriate herbs.
- *Constitution.* Is the person weak, strong, dry, or damp? Do they need restoratives? Is it acute or chronic, hot or cold?
- *Age.* Pediatric patients, elders, or very sick people require mild herbs. Choices should be age appropriate.
- *Amounts or proportions.* The most important therapeutic principle (or intention) in a formula requires the largest proportion of herb. Intentions of secondary importance will require a smaller herbal proportion, and so on down the line.
- *Duration.* Acute conditions change rapidly. Begin with a week's worth and revise the formula as needed. If using medium-strength herbs as a simple, take for 2 to 3 weeks at a time only. Tonics can be used indefinitely except during acute flare-ups. Even for chronic conditions, a few days break every few weeks is appropriate.

Principles of Herbal Formulation

The general principles in organizing a formula are the same in Western herbalism, Eastern, or otherwise. Once an assessment has been made of the client, the principles of formulating are as follows.

- *Principle/sovereign herb(s).* This herb represents the *primary therapeutic action* or therapeutic principle. It is your best choice. What is or are the most important thing(s) to accomplish? The principle herb addresses the main condition or symptom being treated. It is the herb used in the largest quantity.
- *Secondary/minister herb(s).* This herb comes next. In Chinese Medicine parlance, the minister reinforces the king or sovereign's desire. The secondary herb enhances or compliments the effect of the principle action and perhaps has another important function as well. The secondary herb is used in a smaller quantity but still addresses the chief therapeutic principle.
- *Assistant herb(s).* These herbs help and address any signs or symptoms not yet covered. Amounts here are even smaller. Assistants help the minister.
- *Helpers/envoy herb(s).* This is the fine-tuning part: the work of the messenger or envoy. You might want to increase the tropism to a certain organ or meridian, blend the formula together, and detoxify or balance out the herbs to adjust an energetic problem. Examples might be to protect and restore the stomach mucosa with Slippery Elm bark or prevent nausea with Citrus Chen pi. If the formula is too cold energetically, perhaps adding warming Ginger root would balance it out. If the formula is extremely bitter and unpalatable, a sweetener like Cinnamon bark (drying) or Licorice root (moisturizing) could be used. Helper herbs are dispensed in the smallest amounts.

Creating a Formula with Proportions for Each Herb

Proportion refers to how much of one herb is used in relation to another. Each proportion is referred to as a ***part***. Parts in a formula remain constant regardless of amount of formula required. What changes is the number of milliliters used, depending on the container size. A gallon jar of a given formula always contains the same proportions or parts as a 1-oz bottle of the same formula. (If it didn't, the formula would have changed.)

Examples show the principles of formulation, using formulas, with the principle, secondary, assistants, helper herbs, and the number of parts for each herb (Tables 14.1 and 14.2).

Dispensing

Bottle Sizes and Steps in Dispensary Calculations

When we have decided on the herbs in our formula and proportions or parts of one herb to another, we need to dispense them to our clients. Become familiar with standard bottle sizes. Boston rounds (BRs) in different sizes are typically used (Box 14.1).

The following are the various steps in dispensing a formula to a client. The steps assume that the formula has been decided upon, and the dose, and proportion/parts of each herb has been determined.

TABLE 14.1 Principle, Secondary, Assistants, and Helper Herbs with Parts *(Example is formula for an acute common cold, copious clear rhinitis, and dry cough, known as External Wind Cold)*

Role	Parts	Herb	Therapeutic Principle
Principle herb	3 parts	Osha root	To fight virus and decongest airway.
Secondary herb	2 parts	Echinacea root	To fight infection and detoxify.
Assistant herb	2 parts	Thyme herb	To dry up secretions.
Assistant herb	2 parts	Coltsfoot herb	To decongest, loosen cough, aid expectoration.
Helper herb	1 part	Licorice root	To moisten airway, decongest lungs, sweeten.
	10 parts total		

TABLE 14.2 Formula Showing Principle, Secondary, Assistants, and Helper Herbs with Parts
(Example is a formula for indigestion and heartburn, known as Spleen Qi Deficiency)

Role	Parts	Herb	Therapeutic Principle
Principle herb	4 parts	Meadowsweet herb	To decrease acidity, heal stomach.
Secondary herb	3 parts	Codonopsis Dang Shen	To balance and restore flora.
Assistant herb	2 parts	Irish moss thallus	To soothe and heal/restore gut.
Assistant herb	1 part	Slippery Elm bark	To soothe pain, heal mucosa, cool stomach.
Helper herb	1 part	Licorice root	To moisten, heal gut mucosa, sweeten.
	11 parts total		

• BOX 14.1 Boston Rounds

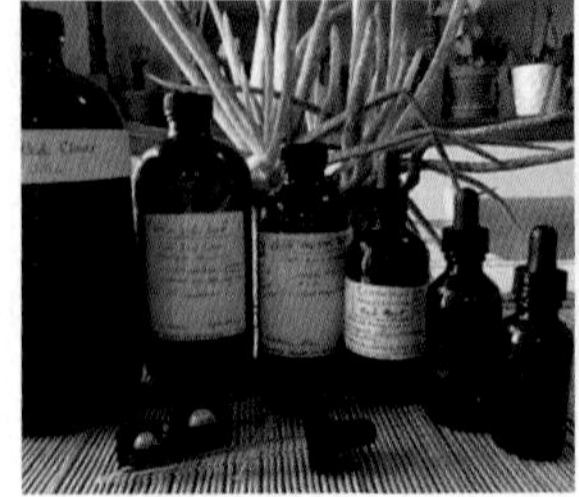

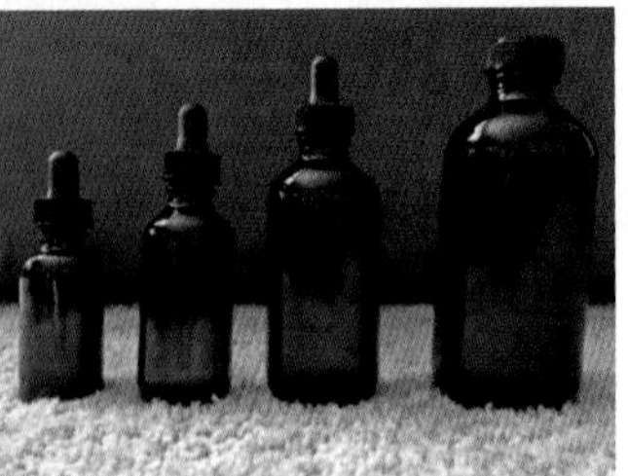

Boston round bottles in assorted sizes with lids and droppers.

- 30 mL = 1 oz (1-oz Boston round bottle)
- 60 mL = 2 oz (2-oz Boston round bottle)
- 120 mL = 4 oz (4-oz Boston round bottle)
- 240 mL = 8 oz (8-oz Boston round bottle)
- 480 mL = 16 ounces (16-oz Boston round bottle; this and a larger 32-oz size is usually reserved for storage.)

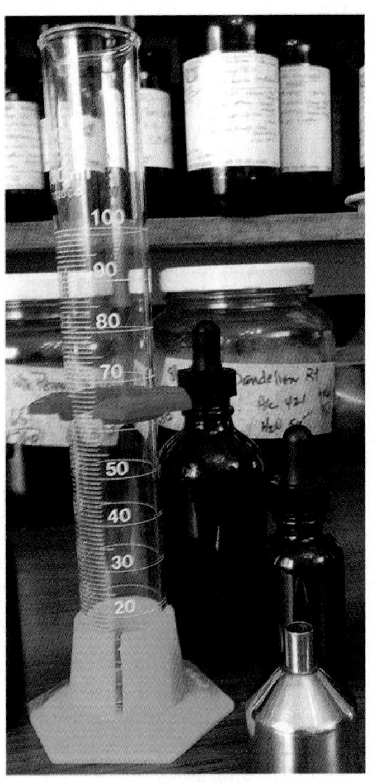

• **Fig. 14.1** Dispensary tools showing 100 mL graduated cylinder, Boston rounds, funnel, and herbs in background.

- *Determine bottle size.* The dose and duration of administration determines the size of the bottle needed. How often is the dose taken and over how many days? For example, if the dose is 4 mL 3 times a day for 30 days, we would need 12 mL per day given 30 times, or *360 mL of total tincture*. BRs come in many sizes. The ones used in dispensary are traditionally 1-oz, 2-oz, 4-oz, or 8-oz bottles. Checking out equivalencies in BRs (Box 14.1), we see that an 8-oz BR holds 240 mL and a 4-oz BR holds 120 mL. Added together, they hold the required 360 mL. So, we choose a 4-oz and an 8-oz BR to dispense.
- *Determine number of milliliters for each herb* needed to total the 360 mL of tincture in example just discussed. To accomplish this, we need to know the total parts in the formula. Then that number is divided into the total milliliters. For instance, if there are 10 parts, then 360 mL of total tincture is divided by 10. This equals 36 mL for each part. If you needed 1 part of Osha root, that's 36 mL. If you needed 2 parts of Red Clover flower, that's 2 times 36, or 72 mL of Red Clover, and so forth.
- *Uneven parts.* In real life, one part does not always come out to an even number. As a rule, round up if it is 0.5 mL or greater; round down if under 0.5 mL. Sometimes we might do the opposite if the numbers just won't work out. We are trying to get as close as possible to the proportions and still fill our bottle. It's not rocket science, and a milliliter more or less of a mild to medium-strength herb is not critical.
- *Measure each herb into a graduated cylinder and transfer it into a measuring cup.* Graduated cylinders are metered out in milliliters, and the largest one pictured in Fig. 14.3 is 250 mL, which is not quite big enough to hold the required 360 mL in our example. One solution is to measure out each herb in a graduated cylinder and then transfer, one by one,

into a larger temporary container such as a 500-mL (2-cup) measuring cup.

- *Stir and pour into Boston rounds.* Stir up the herbs in a temporary container and pour from spout or with funnel into an 8-oz and a 4-oz BR, which together hold the required 360 mL (Figs. 14.1 and 14.2).
- *Label.* (Labeling is discussed in the next section.)
- *Dispense to client with instructions.* The dose should be clearly written on label. Show them how to take the tincture. Have them ingest the first dose before they leave so that you can watch. Typically, dose is measured with the dropper into a small cup with a little water added to improve taste and absorption. Then the client should drink it down. Use a plain water chaser, as needed. Practice dispensary calculations are shown in Tables 14.3 through 14.7.

Labeling

Labels must be precise. Labels should include the name of the client, date, concentration of the tincture (as in 1:4 50%).

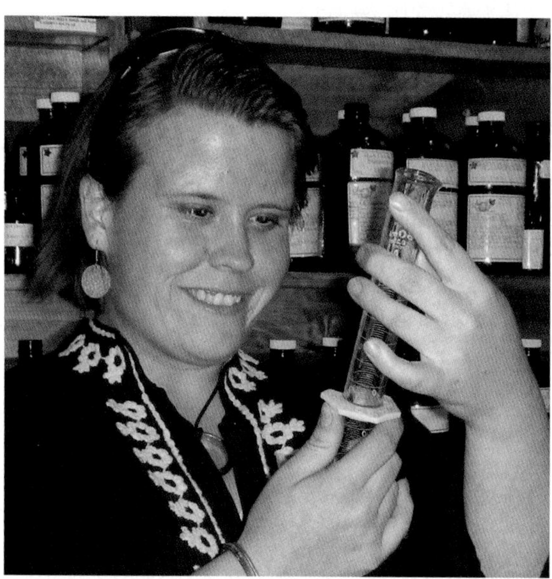

• **Fig. 14.2** Amanda dispensing in apothecary.

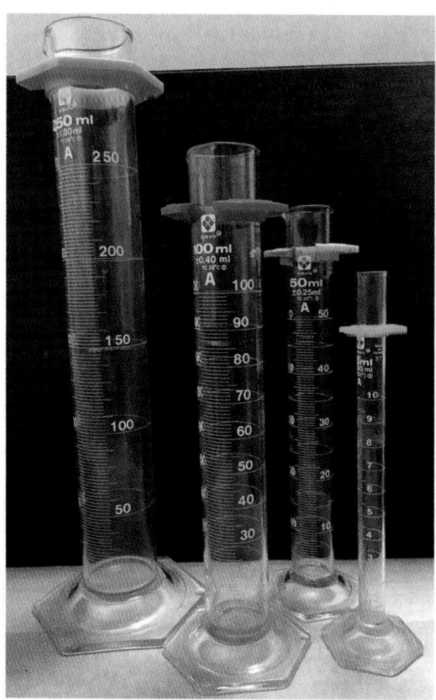

• **Fig. 14.3** Graduated cylinders in various milliliter sizes.

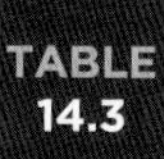

TABLE 14.3 Problem #1 Dispensary Calculation to Determine Milliliters of Each Herb Needed for a Given Bottle Size

Calculate: Number of milliliters needed per herb? The number of parts is given. Formula needs to fit into a 4-oz bottle (120 mL)

Solution: Total parts = 12. 120 mL ÷ 12 parts = 10 mL per part. Multiply number of parts × 10 mL to get number of milliliters per herb. Formula is going into a 4-oz bottle that holds 120 mL.

4 parts	Milk Thistle herb	4 parts × 10 mL	= 40 mL
3 parts	Dandelion root	3 parts × 10 mL	= 30 mL
3 parts	Astragalus root	3 parts × 10 mL	= 30 mL
2 parts	Licorice root	2 parts × 10 mL	= 20 mL
12 parts total	Fits perfectly. It all comes out even.		120 mL total = 4 oz

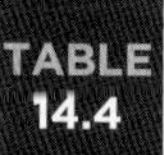

TABLE 14.4 Problem #2 Dispensary Calculation to Determine Bottle Size and Total Amount of Each Herb Needed Per Day/Per Dose

Calculate: How many milliliters needed per herb for formula below. What size bottles should be used? The parts are given.
Dose: 4 mL every 2 hours when awake, for 7 days.

Solution: Assuming the person is awake for 16 hours, that's 8 doses needed per day or 4 × 8 = 32 mL a day. 7 days × 32 mL = 224 mL total needed. An 8-oz Boston round holds 240 mL. This works, even though the bottle will not be filled exactly to the top. No big deal. 224 mL ÷ 10 parts total = 22.4 mL per part.

3 parts	Osha root	3 × 22.4 mL	= 67.2 mL
2 parts	Echinacea root	2 × 22.4 mL	= 44.8 mL
2 parts	Thyme herb	2 × 22.4 mL	= 44.8 mL
2 parts	Coltsfoot herb	2 × 22.4 mL	= 44.8 mL
1 part	Licorice root	1 × 22.4 mL	= 22.4 mL
10 parts total	Pour into 8-oz bottle, not quite full.		224.0 mL tincture

TABLE 14.5 **Problem #3 Dispensary Calculation to Determine Bottle Size and Total Amount of Each Herb Needed Per Day/Per Dose**

Calculate: How many mL needed per herb? What size bottles?
Dose: 5 mL 3 × day for 30 days, between meals.

Solution: 3 doses a day = 15 mL a day × 30 days = 450 mL total needed. There are 12 parts total. One 8-oz Boston round holds 240 mL, so need two 8-oz bottles. 450 mL ÷ 12 parts = 37.5 mL per part. Multiply each part times the number of parts for each herb to get amount of each herb needed.

4 parts	Meadowsweet herb	4 × 37.5	= 150 mL
3 parts	Codonopsis Dang Shen	3 × 37.5	= 112.5 mL
2 parts	Irish Moss thallus	2 × 37.5	= 75 mL
1 part	Slippery Elm bark	1 × 37.5	= 37.5 mL
2 parts	Licorice root	2 × 37.5	= 75 mL
12 parts total	One 8-oz bottle fills to top; other 8-oz bottle slightly lower.		450 mL total

TABLE 14.6 **Problem #4 Dispensary Calculation to Fit a Formula Into a Given Size Bottle**

Calculate: Need the following formula to fit into a 4-oz bottle which holds 120 mL. Parts are given. How many mL are needed per herb?

Solution: 120 ÷ 13 parts = 9.2 mL per part. Round part down to 9.0 mL. Multiply part amount in milliliters times number of parts to get total number of milliliters needed for each herb.

4 parts	Red Clover flower	4 × 9	= 36 mL
3 parts	Nettle herb	3 × 9	= 27 mL
3 parts	Dandelion root	3 × 9	= 27 mL
2 parts	Peppermint leaf	2 × 9	= 18 mL
1 part	Licorice root	1 × 9	= 9 mL
13 parts total	Total tincture is pretty close to a full 4-oz bottle.		117 mL total

Additional Question: If dose is 3 mL 3 × day, how long will the bottle last?

Solution: 3 mL × 3 = 9 mL needed per day. 120 mL ÷ 9 mL = 13 days plus one dose left over

Ingredients must be listed (Box 14.2). Herbalist's contact information should appear. Dosage should be clear. Any additional instructions must be listed. There are laws regarding labeling that specify what you can and cannot claim. Most claims must be exceedingly vague. Here's what to have on your label.

• BOX 14.2 Sample Label

For: Mary Smith Date 00-00-00

FEMALE BALANCE

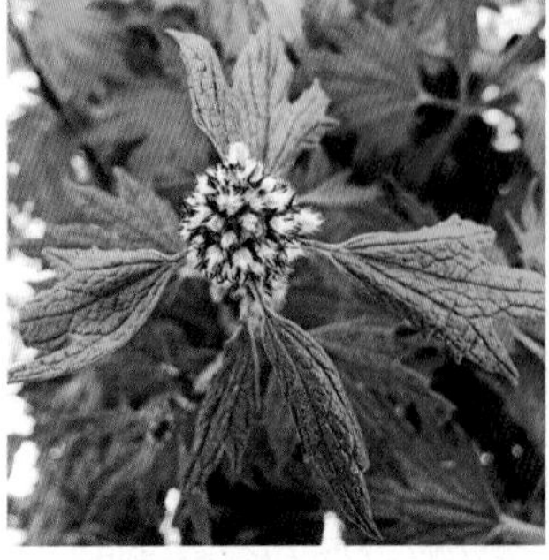

Woman's ally, *Leonurus cardiaca* (Motherwort herb) is an ingredient in our formula for this sample label.

Contents: *Actaea racemosa* (Black Cohosh root), *Vitex agnus-castus* (Chasteberry), *Angelica* Dang Qui (Dong Quai root), Rehmannia Shu Di Huang (Prepared Rehmannia root), *Leonurus cardiaca* (Motherwort herb), *Passiflora incarnata* (Passionflower), *Stellaria media* (Chickweed herb), *Glycyrrhiza glabra* (Licorice root) in ethyl alcohol and water.
Dose. 3 squeezes 3 times per day in a little water between meals. Shake before using.
Contact. Mother Earth Herbals, Lily Green, MH 000-000-0000
Motherearthherbals@xxxxx.com 8 oz

- *Herbalist or company name and contact information.* This information can take the form of a logo with your name, plus a phone number, email address, website, or all of them. The client/customer should have access to quick contact info in case they need to call or have a question. Responsible herbalists make themselves available.
- *Client name and date dispensed.* This information is basic. Who is it for? Provide date compounded or dispensed.
- *Formula name.* As an herbalist, we cannot diagnose, treat, or prescribe, so labels must not say that the formula is for an ulcer or for diabetes (Chapter 29). That is why herb labels in health food stores are so ambiguous. The company WishGarden Herbs in Louisville, Colorado, has cutesy formula names like "Kick-Ass Immune" and "Kung Fu Fighter." Companies like Mountain Rose Herbs offer "Aphrodite Aroma Oil," and HerbPharm formulas plainly state its use, like "Herbal Detox" and "Menopause Health." The names give a clue as to what the formula accomplishes, but they do not mention a diagnosis. You can't either. So dream up a name for your formula that is descriptive but inexact, like, for example, "Sweet Dreams" for an insomnia formula or "Female Balance" for your menopausal lady's blend.
- *Ingredient list.* List herbs in descending order of amount used, just as food labels are done. The primary herbal ingredient—the herb used in the largest amount—comes first. The botanical with the smallest amount comes last. A commercial label lists the common name and usually the botanical name. If it's a formula for a personal client, you can use common name. If it's a Chinese herb, list the pinyin as well. Include the nonmedicinal contents, such as "Mixed in ethyl alcohol and spring water or with bee's wax and olive oil."
- *Proportions.* If the tincture is a simple, the label should list the proportion, such as 1:4 40% ethanol. You'd be surprised by how many commercial herbal tincture labels don't include

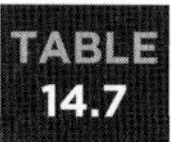

Problem #5 Dispensary Calculation to Convert Formula Given in Grams Into Milliliters

Calculate: You are making up your own 4-oz tincture of the following Chinese patent formula that is typically presented in a range of grams for each herb. Need to know how many milliliters of tincture are needed for each herb to approximate the given grams.

Jade Windscreen Decoction
(Prevents respiratory infections, stabilizes the interior)

Herb	Part	Use this column as your worksheet
Ledebouriella Fang Feng	6–9 g	
White Atractylodes Bai Zhu	9–15 g	
Astragalus Huang Qi	6–20 g	

Solution: This problem is a little more complex, so need to complete three steps. Remember that according to the weight to volume equivalent, 1 gram (weight) equals 1 mL (liquid). One gram is equal to one part.

1. Average out the number of grams (parts) for each herb. Add grams together and divide by 2 to get average. Round up or down.
2. Calculate how many milliliters there are per part. Add grams together for a total number of parts and divide into 120 mL (the size of the 4-oz bottle).
3. Calculate how many milliliters are needed of each herb. Multiply number of grams times each part in milliliters. Round number up or down.

Ledebouriella Fang Feng	7 g	(6 + 9 g = 15 ÷ 2 = 7.5 average g rounded down)
White Atractylodes Bai Zhu	12 g	(9 + 15 g = 24 ÷ 2 = 12 g)
Astragalus Huang Qi	13 g	(6 + 20 g = 26 ÷ 2 = 13 g)
	32 g or total parts	120 mL ÷ 32 parts 3.75 mL per part
	The 4-oz bottle gets the following amount in milliliters	
Ledebouriella Fang Feng	7 g × 3.75 mL	= 26 mL
White Atractylodes Bai Zhu	12 g × 3.75 mL	= 45 mL
Astragalus Huang Qi	13 g × 3.75 mL	= 49 mL
		120 mL total tincture in 4-oz bottle

this important information. If a formula containing many herbs is dispensed, listing a different proportion for each plant is a bit impractical.

- *Dose.* Naturally, the dose must be on the label. Example: 3 to 4 dropperfuls or squeezes of dropper 3 times daily between meals, or 2 squeezes every 2 hours when awake, or 1 teaspoon before bedtime as needed. Include any other dispensing instructions, such as "Take in a little water."
- *Amount.* Include the amount of product dispensed, such as 4 oz.

Dosage

General Principles

Herbal dosing is one of the most variable aspects of modern herbalism. Doses have differed among herbal traditions throughout the course of history, in pharmacopoeias of various countries, and in established pharmacological and clinical research. Herbal texts usually show a wide range. If an herb is used in a formula with 10 others, the dose of each individual herb will be smaller.

In the United States, doses tend to be conservative and small; in the United Kingdom, they are larger. In Chinese Medicine, doses tend to be extremely high, yet still safe. Herbalist Michael Moore, who ran the Southwest School of Botanical Medicine for many years, typically recommended tinctures at a 1:5 proportion with ethanol percentages dependent on constituent solubility. His tincture dosage varied from Asparagus root at 30 to 60 drops 3 times per day to Sarsaparilla and Burdock root at 30 to 90 drops 3 times per day.[1]

The point is that as long as you stick with nontoxic mild- to medium-strength herbs, dosing can be on the high end rather than low. I have personally found that higher dosing (within limits) obtains better results.

- *Strength of herb.* Dosage depends on the strength of an herb.
  - *Mild herbs* such as Nettle leaf or Marshmallow root are foods and have minimum toxicity, so you can go high. Mild herb doses range from 2 to 4 g of herb or 2 to 4 mL of tincture 3 times a day. Exact dosing is not critical.[2]
  - *Medium-strength herbs* like Coptis Huang Lian or Valerian root have some potential toxicity, and care should be taken, but no need to get paranoid. There is no dangerous toxicity, but perhaps a side effect could occur that is easily reversed with a

lower dose. Medium-strength doses of the simple range from 1 to 2 g of herb or 1 to 2 mL of tincture 3 times a day.[2]

- *Strong herbs* are just that: strong. They are more like toxic allopathic drugs, such as Digitalis, and great care must be taken in dosage because they could cause severe side effects or even death. The toxic generic nitroglycerin that lowers blood pressure is dispensed in hospitals at 5 mcg per minute in continuous IV infusion.[3] That's a minuscule amount. One thousand micrograms equal 1 mg. Aconite or Foxglove can be very toxic if care isn't taken, so take them seriously, and don't play around.
- *Toxic plants.* This text does not include highly toxic plants in its Materia Medica. A legitimate problem of using strong, toxic herbs is that it is hard to know how much is actually being dispensed because of the variability of plant constituents. Unless each batch is chemically tested, there is no assurance of dose when exact amounts count. Mild- to moderate-strength herbs are much more forgiving.

- *Age and constitution.* A very frail, sick person obviously needs a smaller dose than a strong healthy adult. Children's doses must be smaller than those for adults (Chapter 21).
- *Weight* is a factor because a thinner, smaller person cannot tolerate as much as a heavier person. Men generally need higher doses than women. As a person ages, there is higher percentage of body fat and less body water content. Therefore the rate of absorption is reduced but not the amount of absorption. It just takes longer to get there and delays onset of action. Furthermore, elders have decreased liver function, so herbs are metabolized and excreted more slowly. The same is true for renal function and excretion. In general, elders and children require smaller doses, as do the very sick and frail. They also do better with mild herbs and tonics.
- *Type and form of remedy.* Whether an herb is given as a simple or in a formula makes a difference. Translation of one remedy form to another is not equal. Doses given for decoctions and infusions are not the same as for stronger tinctures and extracts. A tea is rarely as strong as a tincture; a tincture is weaker than an equivalent amount of extract. The dosage suggested in most Materia Medicas imply that the herb is used alone and dispensed as a simple, and should indicate which form is used for that dose, whether it is a decoction, tincture, or whatever. When using a formula or an infusion with many combined herbs, the dosage for a simple no longer applies. Furthermore, the dosage delivered depends on the concentration of the tincture. Many variables need be considered.
- *Traditional Chinese Medicine.* High dosing is usual. Decoctions and infusions consisting of many raw herbs are generally around 3 to 10 g taken 3 times per day.
- *Other traditions and countries.* Ayurveda uses complex formulas and range from 1 to 6 g a day of powders or tinctures. The Eclectics used higher doses than those used by others at the time.[2] Germany's Commission E monographs give daily doses of teas from 2 to 10 g. The United Kingdom currently uses average doses of 1:5 tincture at 2.5 to 5 mL 3 times per day.

Approximate Adult Dosages for Mild- to Moderate-Strength Preparations

The takeaway from the preceding dosage discussion is that there is a lot of leeway as long as you are using mild- to medium-strength herbs. The dosage ranges listed next are the ones that I have personally found to work safely and effectively and were used by students in the school I ran (Table 14.8 and Appendix A). I tend to go on the higher side because the results are better in individuals who can tolerate such. This approach is especially true with the strong superbugs and stubborn infections that are starting to inundate our world. But always know or get to know your client by starting conservatively. The dose can always be increased later. Honor your judgment.

- *Doses.* Refer to mild- to medium-strength herbs, unless otherwise stated in a reliable reference.
- *With or without food.* If on a 3-times-a-day schedule, tinctures and capsules are best taken on empty stomach or 20 minutes before meals. They absorb better. But if there is a lot of nausea when taking, try them *with* food to temper the nausea. If on an acute schedule, like every half hour, the food factor becomes irrelevant.

Infusions and Decoctions Dosage

The weight of dried herb used in a tea is the important measurement, not the amount of water used. Debate arises whether to go by weight or by volume when measuring out dried or raw herbs for a tea. Weight is more accurate. It's been done this way in Chinese Medicine for thousands of years. However, a few grams of a dry, fluffy herb like Calendula or Chrysanthemum flower is an incredible amount of volume to fit in 1 little cup of tea. In such cases, many herbalists go with 1 tablespoon per cup and call it a day. If going by grams when dispensing a bag of tea to your client to make up at home, you can translate the gram amount for them to use into tablespoons (3 level teaspoons equal 1 tablespoon).

- *Dosage for long-term chronic problems.* Three to 4 cups daily for several weeks.
- *Dosage for acute problems.* One-quarter to one-half cup throughout the day up to 3 to 4 cups.
- *To prepare a hot or cold infusion by weight.* (Add extra water for evaporation.)
  - *Dried herb.* One ounce to 1 pint of boiling water equals 2 cups of infusion or decoction.
  - *Fresh herb.* Two ounces to 1 pint boiling water equals 2 cups of infusion or decoction.
- *To prepare one cup of infusion or decoction by weight.* (Add extra water for evaporation) 0.5 to 5 g dried herb per cup of water (250 mL).
- *To prepare 1 cup of infusion or decoction by volume.* One teaspoon to 2 tablespoons per cup, depending on fluff factor.

Tinctures Dosage

When a problem is acute, the dose must be given frequently, such as every half hour to every 2 hours. Examples of acute problems include onset of infectious diseases, such as colds or flu, migraines, toothaches, bleeding, or burns. If the problem is chronic, the dose is reduced to steady amounts at 2 to 3 times daily. Chronic situations exist in ailments such as diabetes, deficiency syndromes, long-standing allergy or bronchitis, back pain, arthritis, or autoimmunity. Some conditions may start chronic and then flare-up to acute, or vice versa, all of which necessitates changing around the regimen frequency and also the formula.

Furthermore, the stronger the concentration of the tincture or extract, the less you need. The doses stated earlier by Michael Moore were usually based on a 1:5 proportion. I rarely make a 1:5 these days because better results seem to be obtained with stronger preparations, such as 1:3. Then, smaller doses may be given if need be.

If a tincture consists of mild-strength herbs, dose on the high end. If a tincture consists of mostly moderate-strength herbs, dose

TABLE 14.8 Average Adult Doses for Teas and Tinctures
(Medical abbreviations explained in Table 14.11. Doses and abbreviations also appear in Appendix A)

Average Adult Dose Ranges for Acute Situations	Average Adult Dose Ranges for Chronic Situations
Tea	**Tea**
Infusions. 1/4–1/2 cup throughout the day q 2 h up to 3–4 cups.	*Infusions.* 1 cup t.i.d. for several weeks.
Decoctions. 1/4–1/2 cup throughout the day q 2 h up to 3–4 cups.	*Decoctions.* 1 cup t.i.d. for several weeks.
Tinctures in formula.	**Tinctures in formula.**
For tinctures in acute-onset infections. 24 mL q 2 h when awake. or 1–2.5 mL q 30–60 min (1/4–1/2 tsp q 30–60 min).	Tinctures in formula. 1–5 mL t.i.d. Fluid extracts in formula. 1–4 mL t.i.d (1:1 or 1:2).
To stop or decrease diarrhea and hemorrhage. 1/2–2 tsp q 15 min PRN.	
Pain. 1 tsp or 5 mL q 15–30 min PRN.	
For insomnia. 4 mL HS; then 2 mL q 15 min PRN up to 2 h, then STOP.	
For stalled labor. 1/4–1/2 tsp q 30 min up to 3 × max.	
Fluid extracts in formula. (1:1 or 1:2) Varies. Look up individual herbs.	

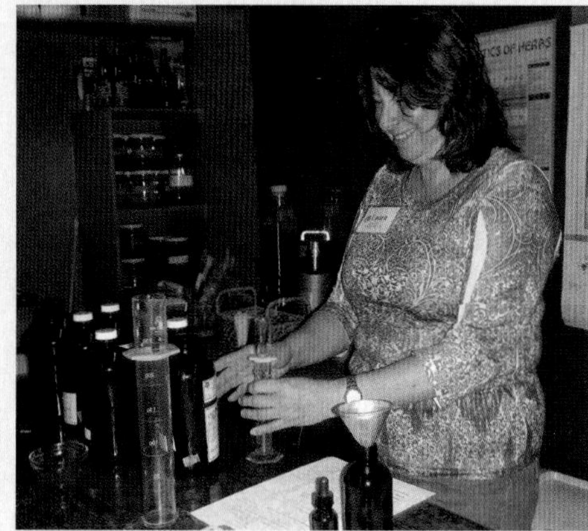

Laura dispensing a formula.

on the low end. Include a dose range on the label and have client start low and slowly build up to test the waters. More isn't always better. Good judgment consists of gearing dosage to client's constitution and sensitivity.

- *Tinctures with acute problems.* Dosage should be 3 to 5 mL every 2 hours *or* 1 to 2.5 mL every 30 to 60 minutes (1/4–1/2 teaspoon every 30 to 60 minutes, usually up to a certain amount).
- *Tinctures with chronic problems.* Dosage should be 3 to 5 mL 3 times a day or 1/2 to 1 teaspoon 3 times a day (1:3–1:5 proportions).

Essential Oil Dosage

Make sure all essential oils taken internally are safe to do so. Consult a reliable text, such as *The Complete Guide to Aromatherapy* by Salvatore Battaglia (Bibliography). Also, be sure to use high-quality pure oils with no adulterants (Chapter 6). For average adult essential oil dosages, see Box 14.3.

- *Internal dose of essential oils in tinctures.* Essential oils of the ingestible category may be added to tinctures for therapeutic effect and to improve taste and smell, approximately 1 drop per ounce of tincture.
- *Internal dose of essential oils in teas.* Use 2 to 4 drops in warm water or mild herbal tea, 2 to 3 times daily.
- *Internal dose of essential oils in capsules.* Some essential oils are irritating to the mucosa and must be encapsulated with a neutral carrier oil. They are too harsh to swallow and could burn on the way down. Use 1 to 2 drops topped off with a carrier such as olive or flaxseed oil. Examples for internal use are Oregano, Cinnamon, and Thyme essential oils. (Check respected essential oil texts for dosages.)
- *Essential oils for external massage.* Add 10 to 25 drops per 1 oz of carrier vegetable oil, such as olive, almond, avocado, or grape seed oil.

• BOX 14.3 Average Adult Essential Oil Dosages

Make sure all essential oils taken internally are safe for that use. Consult a reliable text. Make sure to use high-quality pure oils with no adulterants.

- ***Internal dose in tinctures.*** Approximately 1 drop per ounce of tincture.
- ***Internal dose in teas.*** 2–4 drops in warm water or mild herbal tea 2–3 × daily.
- ***Internal dose in capsules.*** Some essential oils are irritating to the mucosa and must be encapsulated with a carrier oil. They are too harsh to swallow and could burn on the way down. Use 1–2 drops topped off with a carrier such as olive or flaxseed. Examples of potential skin irritants are Oregano, Cinnamon, and Thyme.
- ***Topical or external dose on skin.*** 1 drop neat (if tolerated) or 1–3 drops diluted into 1/2 teaspoon vegetable carrier (fixed) oil. Douches, 20 drops to 1 pint warm water daily × 1 wk.
- ***For massage.*** Add 10–25 drops per ounce of carrier vegetable oil such as olive, almond, avocado, or grapeseed fixed oil.

Syrup and Capsule Dosages

- *Typical syrup dose.* One teaspoon as needed.
- *Capsule doses.*
  - *Acute problems.* One 00 (large) capsule every hour until symptoms subside and then wean down. Children: not feasible.
  - *Chronic problems.* Average adult dose is two 00 caps 2 to 3 times daily. For children, use one 00 cap or two of the smaller 0 size caps (easier to swallow), 2 to 3 times daily. Take with juice or water as you would any pill.

Conversions

Because most nonmedical folks in the United States use English measurements of cups, teaspoons, and ounces and the rest of the medical world uses metric, it is helpful to have some equivalents at your fingertips. When a dropper or pipette is inserted into a tincture bottle and squeezed once, the dropper fills nearly to one-half. This is considered to be 1 mL (30 drops). So if the dose is 60 drops, the dropper is squeezed twice to deliver that dose. The equivalency of 30 drops to 1 mL refers to *drops of water*. Tinctures are a bit more viscous and will take up varying amounts of room in the dropper. That is why this is all approximate, not rocket science. For mild- to moderate-strength herbs, it's fine.

The equivalents provided in Box 14.4 are the most-used conversions for herbalists when making and dispensing preparations. They allow herbalists to figure out dosages for clients and to painlessly travel back and forth from metric units to English units and to weight-to-volume units. Tables 14.9 and 14.10 give other useful conversions, going from teaspoons to droppers to milliliters, and from grams to tincture equivalents.

• BOX 14.4 Post These Conversions in Apothecary

Important Equivalents Used in Dispensary

- 1 mL = 1 dropperful (1 squeeze) = about 25 to 30 drops = 1 g.
- 1 tsp = 5 mL = 5 squeezes = 180 drops of 60% alcohol tincture.
- 1 tbsp = 15 mL = 15 squeezes
- 29.573 mL to 30 mL = 1 oz. (30 mL to 1 oz is the rounded-up version. It is easier to calculate and more commonly used.)
- 1 g = 1 mL = 1 part (weight to volume)
- 1 oz = 30 g approximately. (Rounded up unless you need to be totally exact because 1 oz = 28.3495231 g precisely.)

Milliliters to Ounces

- 30 mL = 1 oz (1-oz Boston round bottle)
- 60 mL = 2 oz (2-oz Boston round bottle)
- 120 mL = 4 oz (4-oz Boston round bottle)
- 240 mL = 8 oz (8-oz Boston round bottle)

U.S. Customary Units to Metric

- 1 tsp = 5 mL = 5 squeezes
- 3 tsp = 15 mL = 1 tbsp = 15 squeezes
- 8 oz = 1 cup = 250 mL
- 2 cups = 1 pint = 500 mL
- 2 pints = 1 quart = 1000 mL or approximately 1 L (1 L = 0.946353 of a quart.)
- 4 quarts = 1 gallon = 4000 mL

TABLE 14.9 Teaspoons to Droppers to Milliliters *(In case client is using a regular measuring spoon instead of dropper)*

Teaspoon	Squeeze of dropper and total drops	Milliliters
1/4	1 squeeze = 30 drops	1.0 mL approximately
1/2	2.5 squeezes = 75–88 drops	2.5 mL approximately
1	5.0 squeezes = 150–175 drops	5.0 mL approximately

Abbreviations

The medical establishment uses many convenient Latin abbreviations that make life easier when writing your own notes. However, when writing instructions on labels for clients, it is best to use, for example, "3 times daily," rather than "t.i.d.," written out in plain English (Table 14.11).

TABLE 14.10 Tincture Equivalents to Grams of Dried Herb

Tincture proportion	Tincture dose	Equivalent of dried herb in grams
1:3 (33% w/v tincture)	100 mL	33 g
1:4 (25% w/v tincture)	100 mL	25 g
1:5 (20% w/v tincture)	100 mL	20 g
1:10 (10% w/v tincture)	100 mL	10 g
1:2 Fresh plant tincture	100 mL	50 g[4]

TABLE 14.11 Common Abbreviations Pertaining to Dosing

As needed = **PRN**	Ointment = **ung.**
Bedtime = **H.S.**	Suppository = **supp.**
Before meals = **a.c.**	Tablespoon = **tbsp.**
By mouth = **p.o.**	Teaspoon = **tsp.**
Capsule = **cap.**	3 times a day = **t.i.d.**
Drop = **gtt.**	Tincture. = **tinc.**
Every = **q**	2 times a day = **b.i.d.**
Every day or 1 × daily = **q day**	With = **c**
4 times day = **q.i.d.**	Without = **s**
Hour = **h**	

Examples Applying the Abbreviations

3 squeezes of dropper 3 × day = 3 mL t.i.d
4 squeezes 2 × day and before bed = 4 mL b.i.d & HS
1 suppository each evening before bed = 1 supp. q HS
2 drops every 1/2 h = 2 gtts. q 1/2 h
1 cup every morning = 1 cup q AM
1 tablespoon 3 × day with juice = 1 tbsp t.i.d. c juice
2 squeezes 4 × daily before meals = 2 mL q.i.d. a.c.
1-inch ointment to affected area 2 × daily = 1-inch ung. to affected area b.i.d.

Summary

Considerations when making up a formula include intention (therapeutic principles), symptoms, age, constitution, proportions of one herb to another, and duration of treatment.

The traditional philosophy for making formulas divides the thought process into four areas. The *principle/sovereign* herb or first best choice addresses the chief complaint. The *secondary/deputy* herbs reinforce the effects of the principle. *Assistant* herbs attend to symptoms or problems not yet covered. The *helpers/envoys* round it all out, correcting energetic imbalances. Once these herbs are chosen, proportions are assigned to each.

A dispensary is a dedicated space where herbs are prepared, formulated and provided. Formulation consists of deciding on your herbs, their proportions, and determining amounts needed to fit in the correct sized bottle. Deciding on safe, yet effective dosages is an extremely variable aspect of modern herbalism. As long as mild- or medium-strength herbs are used, there is a lot of leeway. Ranges were provided for various preparations.

Herbalists should have the ability to use basic metric measurements and medical abbreviations, along with making wise dosage determinations. This important information is further summarized in Appendix A.

Review

Fill in the Blanks

(Answers in Appendix B.)

1. An intention in formulation (what you are trying to accomplish) is known as a ___ ___. (two words)
2. The principle herb is the one used for ___. (phrase)
3. The secondary herb's job is to ___. (phrase)
4. The assistant herb(s) purpose is to ___. (phrase)
5. The helper herbs(s) role is to ___. (phrase)
6. A formula is 50/50 Passionflower to Hops. How many mL of each herb for a 4-oz bottle? ___ mL of Passionflower. ___ mL of Hops flower.
7. A formula is 3 parts Dandelion root, 2 parts Bupleurum Chai Hu, 1 part Milk Thistle seed, to be dispensed in an 8-oz bottle. One part = ___ mL. We will need ___ mL Dandelion root, ___ mL Bupleurum root and ___ mL Milk Thistle seed.
8. Average adult decoction dose for a chronic problem is ___.
9. Average adult infusion dose for an acute problem is ___.
10. Average adult tincture dose for a chronic problem is ___.

Critical Concept Questions

(Answers for you to decide.)

1. Discuss leeway in herbal dosing.
2. Give some factors to consider in determining dosage.
3. What is the problem with dispensing a very strong (potentially toxic) herb?
4. How does one choose the principle herb(s) in a formula?
5. What do secondary herbs accomplish?
6. What does fine-tuning a formula mean? Examples?
7. You are dispensing 00 capsules to an adult. How many are needed to give her a 7-day dose t.i.d.?
8. Ms. G. wants to use her kitchen measuring spoons to administer her tincture. If her dose is 5 mL, what do you tell her? If dose is 4 mL? If dose is 2 mL? (These will be approximate amounts.)
9. How would you administer Thyme essential oil p.o.?
10. Why does an herbalist need to know the metric system?

References

1. "Clinical Herb Manuals by Michael Moore." Southwest School of Botanical Medicine. Web site generously shares Moore's former school manuals and publications with the public free of charge. http://www.swsbm.com/ManualsMM/MansMM.html (accessed October 24, 2019).
2. Bone, Kerry and Simon Mills. *Principles and Practice of Phytotherapy* (London, UK: Elsevier, 2013).
3. "Nitroglycerin Dosage." Drugs.com https://www.drugs.com/dosage/nitroglycerin.html (accessed October 24, 2019).
4. Green, James. *The Herbal Medicine Maker's Handbook* (Berkeley, CA: Crossing, 2000).

15 History, Assessment, and Documentation

"It is more important to know what sort of person has a disease than to know what sort of disease a person has."

—Hippocrates (460–377 BCE)

CHAPTER REVIEW

- Intake: Principles, preparation, the correspondences, and the 24-hour clock.
- Herbal Health History form: Taking a health history and rationale for questions.
- Physical assessment: Review of tongue and pulse and cheat sheets.
- Blood pressure: How to take and pertinent facts.
- Herbalist's Assessment form: SOAP charting and explanation.
- Herbal Consult Suggestions form: Explanation of instructions given to client.
- Record keeping: Health Insurance Portability and Accountability Act (HIPAA).

KEY TERMS

Blood pressure (BP)
Chief complaint
Correspondences
Diastolic
Herbal Health History and form
Herbalist's Assessment and form
Health Insurance Portability and Accountability Act (HIPAA)
Herbal Consult Suggestions and form
Nutrigenomics
SOAP
Systolic
Therapeutic principles
24-hour clock

The time has come for action, to be a practicing herbalist. We covered a lot of basics, and the tools are in place. The next step is to meet and greet a real, live client, figure out what to do for her, and what to recommend. We will give wise and effective advice and do no harm. The nitty gritty can be scary but exciting.

A tried and true method is to follow what all medical professionals do. If you have ever visited a doctor, you know the routine. Practitioners gather information in the form of a written and verbal health history. We conduct a physical assessment, arrive at a conclusion as to the problem or syndrome at hand, and compose a health plan. We dispense herbs, if any, and finally document what was done so that we have a record. This process allows for a thoughtful, consistent follow up for the next visit.

Intake: Principles to Use for a Health History

Preparation

Get ready. Wash your hands. Set your priorities. *Center* and get *grounded*. Say a prayer or put out an intention for the greatest and highest good of all concerned. It is imperative to clear your mind of your own worries, anxieties, concerns, and to-do lists before you can be fully present for your client. Now breathe in deeply, blow out slowly. Allow the breath to wash over you and go down through your soles to Mother Earth. Cleanse and connect. Be receptive. Put out love. You are now ready to meet your client.

First Impressions

When meeting a client for the first time, the person is a blank slate. Who is this person who walks into your office or clinic? You begin an unbiased, sizing-up process on a physical and vibrational level the moment the person appears. Does the client appear healthy and strong, weak or sick? Observe the walk, posture, and gait. Is it loose, relaxed, and easy going? Does the person appear in pain; use a cane, crutches, or favor one side? Is the client of average weight, overweight, or thin as a rail? What feeling is emitted? Is there sadness, depression, exaggerated cheerfulness, stress, confidence, or insecurity? How is the qi? Is there exhaustion or energy and liveliness? Is the voice strong, small, or normal? Is the person glad to be here or were they talked into it?

Use your senses. Observe, feel, smell, and listen. Observe skin and complexion. Does it shine or have an inner glow, or is it dull and pasty? Are there blemishes, eczema, or acne? Is the color very red, overly pale, or bluish? Are the eyes clear, or are deep circles underneath? What do you pick up? If it is part of your repertoire, how is their aura? Are there unusual body odors? Is the voice true and clear, overly soft or loud, or are words swallowed and inhaled? This nonjudgmental assessment speaks volumes in a short time.

Greet them and shake their hand, feeling their body heat or lack of it. Is the hand hot, warm, dry, or rough like sandpaper? Or is it cool, cold, or wet and sweaty? Is hand clasp strong or weak and flabby? Does person feel predominantly excess or deficient, warm or cold, dry or moist? Even now, in the first couple of minutes, clues are picked up. By the time the health history is completed, a blood pressure, pulse and tongue assessment done, an energetic pattern begins to emerge, and things start to add up.

Revisit the Table of Correspondences

In the *Table of Correspondences* from the Chinese Medicine Five Element System, each of the five yin organs, plus their yang partners, has a color, taste, emotion, smell, and sound that are open to a sense organ and rule a tissue (Chapter 9). For example, the Liver's emotion is anger/flow, taste is sour, sense organ is the eyes, and the tissues it influences are the joints, tendons, ligaments, and nails. So this gives clues. If the person is loud, angry, and extroverted and has sore joints and unhealthy nails, their Liver is calling. All things being equal, a Liver-related herb would be considered in the formula, particularly when other aspects of the health history and physical assessment point in the same direction (Table 15.1).

The 24-Hour Organ Clock

The yin/yang organ pairs have a time of day when they are dominant, called the 24-hour clock (Box 15.1). The ***24-hour clock***

• BOX 15.1

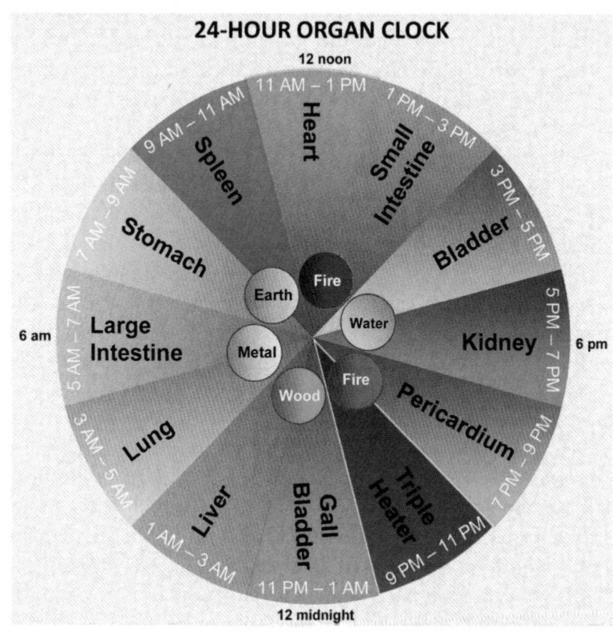

The 24-hour organ clock illustrates one complete cycle of qi flowing through the body's meridians.

TABLE 15.1 Five Elements and the Correspondences

Yin Organ	Yang Organ	Environment	Season	Element	Taste	Color	Sense Organ	Tissue	Emotion and Sound
Liver	Gall Bladder	Wind	Spring	Wood	Sour	Green	Eyes	Joints Tendons Ligaments Nails	Anger/Frustration-Flow Shouting
Heart	Small Intestine	Heat	Summer	Fire	Bitter	Red	Tongue	Heart Blood Vessels	Joy-Sorrow Laughter
Spleen	Stomach	Damp	Late Summer	Earth	Sweet	Yellow	Mouth or Lips	Muscles	Worry-Spaced Out Singing
Lungs	Large Intestine	Dryness	Fall	Metal	Pungent	White	Nose	Skin Body Hair	Grief-Mourning/Recovery Crying
Kidney	Bladder	Cold	Winter	Water	Salty	Dark Blue or Black	Ears	Bones Head Hair	Fear/Vulnerability-Courage Groaning

represents the time of day when each organ is functioning optimally and has the most energy. The qi in that meridian is peaking. If the organ is healthy, all is well, and the organ is busy doing its job. But if that organ is challenged, a person could have adverse symptoms in the exact time slot related to that particular organ. There are six organ pairs. Each organ has a 2-hour period when it dominates. Four hours for each pair adds up to 24 hours. This is useful information in your assessment.

The organ at the opposite side of the clock from the dominant one, 12 hours away, has waning energy and is at its lowest. When the Liver peaks at 1 to 3 in the morning, the Small Intestine's energy is at its lowest because its peak time is 1 to 3 in the afternoon. At 3 a.m. the Liver is busy detoxifying, so give it a chance and don't eat. However, at 1 to 3 in the afternoon, the Small Intestine is queen, a great time for eating and digestion. That's why the wisdom is to have the heaviest meal of the day at lunch. The 24-hour clock helps us to know the best times to exercise, eat, have sex, rest, and sleep.

Every organ has a physical and emotional component, a lovely holistic mind-body view. If an individual repeatedly wakes up coughing at 4 a.m., it's Lung time. There could be a physical Lung problem. If a person wakes up at 4 a.m. grieving for their dog who just died, it's a Lung emotion. The Kidney filters blood and balances electrolytes but emotionally represents fear and insecurity. Use the 24-hour clock to assist healing on all levels. Often, if the emotional issue is not addressed, it will manifest later in the physical body in increasingly serious ways. The 24-hour organ clock is a powerful tool.

The 24-hour clock relates to the Western concept of biorhythms or the circadian rhythms of day and night. If we honor that flow and live our lives accordingly, stress will decrease, and well-being will increase. When I was a night shift intensive care nurse, my flow of qi was completely backward. I was completely off kilter for years and never knew the day or the time. No wonder. I slept all day and was up all night. Following the clock as much as possible gives us proper times for life's activities.

- ***Lung/Large Intestine time 3 a.m. to 7 a.m.***
  - *The Lungs (3 a.m. to 5 a.m.).* The Lungs move air and qi around the body through the meridians and protect the immune system. On an emotional level, the Lungs deal with grief and loss. If a person gets sick frequently or wakes up wheezing, coughing, or wracked with sorrow and loss, it's time for Lung attention.
  - *Large Intestine (5 a.m. to 7 a.m.).* This is an ideal time to move the bowels, first thing in the morning. Or is there constipation or dry stools? If so, this is a *letting-go* problem. From an emotional standpoint ask, "What are you holding on to?" Is it a relationship, a possession, a resentment, or an emotion?
- ***Stomach/Spleen Time 7 a.m. to 11 a.m.***
  - *Because the Stomach (7 a.m. to 9 a.m.)* breaks down and digests food, have a decent and healthy breakfast. Digestion problems such as indigestion, bad breath, and belching begin here. Fermented foods are a must. An emotional pain in the gut can be a physical pain, too.
  - *The Spleen (9 a.m. to 11 a.m.)* transforms food into energy and transports it to other organs. Bloating, sweet cravings (because the Spleen taste is sweet, and cravings occur if unbalanced), loose stools, and low energy are clues to poor function. With regard to emotions, there can be worry or low self-esteem. This is the ideal time to exercise and do any heavy, exerting work. Use energetic morning time to go to yoga class or exercise.
- ***Heart/Small Intestine Time 11 a.m. to 3 p.m.***
  - *The Heart (11 a.m. to 1 p.m.).* This is lunch time. The Heart pumps nutrients around through the blood to provide nutrition to the cells. Extreme joy or sadness manifest here. Research shows that 70% of heart attacks occur during this time frame.[1] A strong heart responds to joy and enthusiasm, whereas sadness and walling in emotions weaken the heart.
  - *The Small Intestine (1 p.m. to 3 p.m.)* This is the time to digest lunch. Do light tasks or exercise after lunch. It is a vulnerable time for feelings of abandonment or insecurity.
- ***Kidney/Bladder Time 3 p.m. to 7 p.m.***
  - *The Bladder (3 p.m. to 5 p.m.)* is when metabolic waste moves toward the Kidneys for filtration and elimination. Drink a lot of water. An afternoon energy slump is possible at this time.
  - *The Kidneys (5 p.m. to 7 p.m.)* deal with electrolyte balance. Detoxification is occurring. Take a walk. Slow down. Know that fear can come with the sunset and darkness.
- ***Pericardium/Triple Heater Time 7 p.m. to 11 p.m.***
  - *The Pericardium (7 p.m. to 9 p.m.)* is related to circulation when nutrients go to the capillaries, which is a quiet time to read and relax and a good time for sex and conception.
  - *Triple Heater (9 p.m. to 11 p.m.)* is considered the endocrine system peak. Enzymes replenish and adjust. Prepare for sleep and rejuvenation.
- ***Liver/Gallbladder Time 11 p.m. to 3 a.m.***
  - *The Gallbladder (11 p.m. to 1 a.m.)* helps self-esteem and decision making, and on the physical level, stores bile. If you are churning over decisions, lie awake, or have indigestion after a fatty meal during these times, address the Gallbladder.
  - *The Liver (1 a.m. to 3 a.m.)* is connected to anger, resentment, and frustration. Physically, it balances menses and anemia and is associated with frontal headaches, joint aches and pains. If one frequently wakes up between 1 a.m. to 3 a.m. with hot flashes or bad, angry, or frustrating dreams, the Liver needs help. And so it goes around and around, back to Lungs—the 24-hour cycle.

Taking a Health History

There are many ways to obtain a health history. Over the years, I've tried many combinations and various intake forms. One option is to have a client fill out a written form. Another is to ask questions face to face and jot down notes as you go along. Sometimes a combination works best. Either way, it is important to have an organized method, so nothing is left out. I ask the client to fill out a written questionnaire and bring it with them to their first visit. This initial health history form includes general demographics, covers the body systems, and asks for their pressing problems, the reason for the visit, or the chief complaint. I then review the history with them and take my own additional notes on a separate sheet. Both the client's written (and signed) history, plus my handwritten notes, go into their folder or chart. This information provides a baseline for future visits.

Herbal Health History: The Intake Form

There is no perfect health history form out there. Whatever you ask, something is always forgotten. A sample ***Herbal Health History form*** is provided, but you are all encouraged to develop your own, as experience is gained. Furthermore, it is human nature for a client to leave out sensitive written and verbal information until trust has been achieved. Sometimes people just plain forget certain facts. Others are reluctant to share intimate details, such as sexual concerns or bathroom habits, until they feel comfortable. As time goes on, you will develop a chemistry with your client and find out whatever is needed. The more you know, the better you can devise a good treatment plan. A warm, safe environment that is neat but homey helps. Privacy and a peaceful setting are important.

The Herbal Health History form (Table 15.2 and Appendix A) covers the bases. Going through this with a client will take about an hour and a half. It could easily take longer, depending on the complexity of the case and if the client is talkative. It is easy to get sidetracked and drift off topic. Stay focused and gently steer the conversation back on target. Venting is often therapeutic but set limits because the conversation could stretch out all day. Obtaining a good history is an art and skill that improves with practice.

Rationale for Herbal Health History Questions

- *Demographics*. Obviously, accurate contact information is needed. Add new clients to a mailing or email list right after each one leaves.
- *Birthday and place raised*. I always (privately) consider their astrological sign. You might send out birthday cards. Age tells what stage of life they're most likely going through. "Place raised" may have health ramifications. If they grew up in the humid East Coast and now live in dry Arizona, they may develop dry skin or nose bleeds. Folks with heart problems who move from sea level to the mountains could get into trouble because of high altitude and low oxygen.
- *Occupation*. This section is significant if the client reports a job that involves exposure to environmental toxins. Likely suspects are house painters, road workers, auto body workers, dry cleaners, etc. Does the job have physical hazards such as those for construction workers, massage therapists, and police officers? Is the job spiritually/emotionally toxic? It is not healthy to hate going to work.
- *Referred by*. Always thank that person if you know them. Cards are thoughtful. If a client sends you many people, perhaps a gift certificate is in order. Build a network with other kinds of practitioners and refer back and forth. Keep the names of any allopathic healthcare providers you like and respect who are open to herbal/holistic remedies. This record is valuable to have when your client asks (and they frequently do), "Do you know a good doctor?"
- *Living situation*. Worth exploring and opens up the conversation to relationship and stress issues. There are so many options. Traditional nuclear families are a declining breed. Some folks live alone and love it. Others are lonely and yearn for a partner. Marriages could be fulfilling or filled with stress. A single mom with five young kids might be taxed emotionally and financially. Be open-minded and nonjudgmental. Furthermore, support at home could mean the difference between success and failure with all the new things they will soon be asked to do.
- *Height/weight*. This is an interesting question, fraught with self-image issues. How many people are actually happy with who they are or with their appearance? This may or may not be a medical concern.
- *Practitioners*. Never change a prescription medication on your own, but conferring with a client's primary healthcare provider is certainly an option. If a person sees five other holistic practitioners, they could just be shopping around. Are they serious about an herbal alternative?
- *Treatment goal(s)*. This is a very important section of the health history. Know the main reason for the visit and what they want to accomplish, the ***chief complaint***. Determining treatment goals works best if the client describes their experience, rather than presenting a diagnosis they may have gotten from Dr. Google. If they have a long laundry list, set priorities together. Perhaps, the goal is to help digestion before beginning anything else. Can't do it all or at not least all at once. However, if the person is in pain, I know from experience that if it isn't dealt with first and foremost, they won't come back.
- *Stressors and exercise*. Countless illnesses are related to chronic stress. A major job of any herbalist is to pinpoint these stressors and help in that area. Hence the stress-level question on the health history and the "How do you relax?" question are important ones. Some folks are out of touch with their bodies and don't know what true relaxation feels like. Exploring this is worthwhile. Exercising is one method to relieve stress and important for other health reasons. Weight-bearing exercise is key for osteoporosis prevention. Relaxation techniques or referrals to yoga, meditation classes, and others should be in an herbalist's bag of tricks.
- *Energy level*. This question goes back to the 24-hour clock. A midafternoon slump after Small Intestine time (1 to 3 p.m.) could indicate bad digestion or poor lunchtime food choices. Proteins sustain energy; simple carbs are metabolized quickly, followed by a rapid decline in blood sugar, resulting in fatigue. Trouble waking up in the morning could mean habitual late-night snacking or excessive alcohol intake that has overtaxed the liver and compromised nighttime detoxification and rejuvenation.
- *Past illnesses, accidents, and hospitalizations*. This section is standard and important information for any health history. Even if these issues are now resolved, they could point to body weakness for which restorative herbs would be helpful. Tonsillectomies, appendectomies, or splenectomies caused by trauma mean less lymphatic tissue remaining to help the immune system's first line of defense. Dental surgery, wisdom teeth, and abscess removal can open the body up to bacteria.
- *Prescription medications, herbs, and supplements*. Going over this information could take a while. It is important to know what they're taking and why. Often the answer to *why* is "I heard it is good for you." Some people don't have a clue about their prescription medications, or why they're on them. If they're on prescription medications, be alert for herb-drug interactions (Chapter 13). If you don't know a drug, look it up or ask. Sometimes symptoms are from drug side effects Always inquire if their goal is to get off any of these meds. If *yes*, work with the healthcare provider, and if *no*, use supportive herbs and supplements.
  - *Supplement assessment*. I always request that clients put all their over-the-counter (OTC) supplements and prescription medications, etc., into a bag and bring them to the first visit. Then I line them up, and we take a look. Don't forget your drug book, such as *Saunders Nursing Drug Handbook* or *Mosby's Nursing Drug Reference*, for quick reference (Bibliography).
  - *Too many supplements*. Often people take handfuls of supplements for no valid reason. Try to get them down to a reasonable number and eliminate redundancies. There could be duplications, such as calcium in three or four

TABLE 15.2 Herbal Health History
(See Appendix A, Fig. A.1, for reproducible form)

Today's Date_______________
Last Name:___________________________ First Name: ____________________ Middle_______
Address:_____________________________________ City: __________ State:_______ Zip________
Phone: Cell: ______________ Home:___________________ Work: ________________________
Email: ______________________________
Date of Birth: ________________ Age: ______ Place raised:_____________________________
Occupation:_______________________________ Employer _________________________________
Referred By: _______________________

Who do you live with? Myself ☐ Other(s) ☐ (Adults and relationship to you)
____
____
____
____

Children: Name(s), Age(s), Living with You?
____
____
____

Height: _______Weight:_______ Happy With Weight?_________ Desired weight: ________
Allergies:_____________________________ Food Sensitivities _____________________________
____

Do you have a Primary Care Practitioner? ☐ No ☐ Yes Name and Title ____________________
____ Phone __________________ For what?
____

Other Current Practitioners
Name/Title:_________________________Address:________________________Phone:_____________
Name/Title:_________________________Address:________________________Phone:_____________

Herbal Treatment Goals: Why did you come in today?

1. ____
2. ____
3. ____

Stressors in your life: (Rate stress level 1–10; Ten is the worst.) Family: ______ Social: ______Work related: ______ Stress in your body? _____Other? ________________________
Where do you hold your tension? _____________________________________
How do you relax? ____
Do you exercise? ☐ Yes ☐ No What type? _______________ How often?______________
____________How long is each session? _______________ Weight bearing? ______

Energy level and pattern? (least and most productive time of day)
____
____
____

Are you pregnant? ____________Due date: ___________
Serious Past Illnesses?
____
____
____

Accidents, Injuries and Dates
____
____
____

Hospitalizations and Dates
____
____
____

Current prescription medications and what condition is being treated?
____
____

(Continued)

TABLE 15.2 Herbal Health History
(See Appendix A, Fig. A.1, for reproducible form)—cont'd

____
____

Current herbs and supplements and why are you taking them?
____
____
____
____

Current Medical Concerns

☐ Asthma	☐ Headaches	☐ Multiple Sclerosis
☐ Blood Clots	☐ Heart Problems	☐ Osteoarthritis
☐ Breast Lumps	☐ Hemophilia	☐ Osteoporosis
☐ Cancer	☐ HIV	☐ Rheumatoid Arthritis
☐ Chronic Fatigue	☐ Infections	☐ Stomach Ulcers
☐ Diabetes	☐ Liver Problems	☐ Other: ____________
☐ Epilepsy	☐ Lupus	____________

Family History

☐ Arthritis	☐ Obesity	☐ Ovarian Cancer
☐ Heart Disease	☐ Thyroid	☐ Depression/Anxiety
☐ Diabetes	☐ Epilepsy	☐ Mental Health Disorders
☐ Alcoholism	☐ Breast Cancer	☐ Other ______
☐ Asthma	☐ Prostate Cancer	

Wellness Continuum (Please mark where you think you fall on this wellness continuum)

Sick ------------------------------------**Your Optimum health**

| Getting sick | | OK | | Good | Healthy |

Addictions or Frequent Habits			
☐ Sugar	☐ Smoking tobacco/marijuana	☐ Alcohol	☐ Drugs
☐ Caffeine	How many a day? ________	How much? ________	What? ________
☐ Salt	How long? ________	How long? ________	How Long? ________

Insomnia: ☐ Yes ☐ No ☐ Can't fall asleep ☐ Can't stay asleep What time do you wake up? _____ How often does this happen? ____________ Average hours sleep per night. _______ Do you feel rested in the morning? _______

Frequent headaches or migraines? ☐ No ☐ Yes Describe type of pain like stabbing, aching.

____

Relationship to Food

Cravings: ☐ Salt ☐ Sweets ☐ Carbs ☐ Fats ☐ Chocolate

How much water do you drink a day? ____________

How much soda do you drink a day? ____________

How many cups of coffee do you drink a day? ________

How many cups of tea do you drink a day and what kind? ____________________

What are your favorite snacks? ______________ How often do you partake? _________

What kind of cooking oil do you use? ____________________

Are you on any specific kind of diet? (gluten-free, vegetarian, vegan) ________________

Do you buy organic? _____

How many times a day/week/month do you eat the items in the following list? Indicate how often.

Red Meat ____	Syrup ____	All vegetables ____	Miso _____
Poultry ____	Honey ____	Organic? _____	Sauerkraut _____
Fish ____	Refined Sugar ____	Yellow/orange veggies ___	Umeboshi _____
Pork _____	Brown Sugar ____	Green veggies ____	Kimchi _____
Wild Meats ____	Agave ____	White/purple veggies ____	Pickles _____
Quinoa ____	Candy ____	Coconut/rice milk_____	Sprouts _____
Soy Foods ____	Ice Cream ____	Rice white or brown _____	Salads _____
Beans ____	Baked goods ____	Millet ______	Vinegar _____

(Continued)

TABLE 15.2 Herbal Health History
***(See Appendix A, Fig. A.1, for reproducible form)*—cont'd**

Eggs ____ Mushrooms ____ Nuts ____ Dairy – organic? ____ Yogurt _____ Kefir ____ Cheese ____Nuts _____		Package cereal _____ Oats _____ Barley _____ Bulgur ______ Pasta _____ Bread ________ Type? ________ White Flour _____	Crackers _____ Chips _____ Pretzels _____ Green smoothies ___ Seaweeds ____

Symptom Survey

General:
☐ General fatigue
☐ Loss of or excessive gain in weight
☐ Motion Sickness
Other: ___________

Respiratory
☐ Allergies
☐ Sinus Problems
☐ Difficulty breathing deeply
☐ Nosebleeds
☐ Frequent coughing
☐ Frequent colds/sore throats
☐ Asthma

Cardiovascular
☐ Rapid or skipped beats
☐ Varicose veins
☐ Bruise easily
☐ Chest pain
☐ Cold hands/feet
☐ Shortness of breath with activity
☐ High blood pressure

Neuromuscular
☐ Headaches
☐ Muscle pain – Where? _____________
☐ Muscle cramping
☐ Weakness in arms or legs
☐ Swollen joints
☐ Painful joints
☐ Frequent dislocations
☐ Jaw/pain tension (TMJ)
☐ Frequent bone fractures
☐ Memory loss
☐ Absent minded
☐ Numbness/tingling Where?_______________
Other:__________________________________

Skin
☐ Skin eruptions
☐ Excessive sweating – Where?___________
☐ Dry or oily skin
☐ Hair loss
Other: __________________________________

____

Urinary
☐ Frequent urination
☐ Involuntary escape of urine
☐ Burning/discharge on urination
☐ Weak urine stream
☐ Difficulty starting urine
☐ Constant urge to urinate
☐ Bedwetting
☐ Flank pain

Senses
☐ Hearing Loss
☐ Earaches
☐ Ringing in ears
☐ Glasses/Contact Lenses
☐ Eye Problems _____

Digestive
☐ Frequent indigestion
☐ Heartburn
☐ Gas/bloating
☐ Nausea/vomiting
☐ Abdominal cramps
☐ Frequency of bowel movements____________
☐ Alternating constipation/diarrhea
☐ Consistency of stools: hard, firm, soft, loose
☐ Pain/itching in rectum
☐ Hemorrhoids
☐ Excessive or loss of appetite
Other:___________________________

Endocrine
☐ Swollen glands
☐ Excessive thirst, hunger, sweating, urination
☐ Slow/fast metabolism
☐ Blood sugar imbalances
☐ Thyroid problem such as low energy
Other: ______________________________

For Women:

Menses
Do you have periods? ☐ Yes ☐ No
☐ Frequency and duration
☐ Amount of bleeding: scant, average, heavy, spotting
☐ Color: bright red, dark red, pink
☐ Clots? Color: _______________
☐ Bleeding between periods
Other: _____________________________

PMS
☐ Breast Lumps
☐ Sore breasts
☐ Irritable
☐ Depressed
☐ Emotional swings
☐ Bloating
☐ Other ___________________________

Menopause
☐ Do you think you have started? ☐ Yes ☐ No
☐ Irregular cycle time frame: _____________
☐ Anxiety or Depression? _______________
☐ Spotting
☐ Hot flashes

(*Continued*)

TABLE 15.2 Herbal Health History
***(See Appendix A, Fig. A.1, for reproducible form)*—cont'd**

☐ Number of times awaken in night to urinate_____
☐ Frequent urinary tract infections
Other:________________________________

For Men:
☐ Burning/discharge on urination
☐ Lumps/swelling of testicles
☐ Pain in prostate or testicles
☐ Sores on penis or scrotum
☐ Hernia
☐ Impotence
☐ Erectile Dysfunction
Other:________________________
____
____
____
____

☐ Vaginal dryness/itching

Childbirth
☐ Number of pregnancies: ____________
☐ Number of births: ____________
☐ Miscarriages: ☐ Yes ☐ No
☐ Premature births
☐ Cesareans
☐ Abortions

Other
☐ Vaginal pain/rash/irritation
☐ Vaginal discharge __Color:
____

Muscular-Skeletal
☐ Arthritis
☐ Pain _______
☐ Stiff neck
☐ Mobility limitations
☐ Spinal curvature
☐ Other _______

Cancellation Policy

So that I may better serve my clients, 24-hour notice is required for cancellation. You will be charged the full session with less than a 24-hour notification.

Disclaimer

1. I understand that this work does not constitute, and it is not a substitute for, medical treatment but rather is a form of health maintenance. I realize that this herbalist is not a doctor and does not diagnose, prescribe, or treat any specific conditions.
2. I understand and agree that I am responsible for keeping my herbalist informed of any changes in my physical condition because this could affect the treatment I receive.

Signature ________________________________ Date ______

products, totaling far too many milligrams. Have a good supplement reference book on hand with recommended dosages. One such is the *Encyclopedia of Nutritional Supplements* by Michael T. Murray, N.D. (Bibliography).

- *Current medical concerns and family history.* Medical concerns single out red-flag areas that may have been missed. Family history items such as heart disease, diabetes, and arthritis are potentially hereditary. It is not a given that if mom had breast cancer the client will also. Gene expression is frequently determined by lifestyle. Help clients to make wise nutritional choices to protect themselves from having that myocardial infarction that runs in the family. The role of nutrition and its effect on gene expression and DNA is a field called ***nutrigenomics***. It turns out that many foods, such as greens or blueberries, can be thought of as medical foods. What we eat has a large bearing on health.
- *Wellness continuum.* It is very interesting to see how clients perceive their health, and if this jives with your assessment. Sometimes people are hypochondriacs, whereas others are in denial.
- *Addictions and habits.* There is nothing good about smoking cigarettes. It affects the lungs and the heart and it can cause breast, lung, jaw, and esophageal cancer; osteoporosis; and wrinkles. It raises cortisol (stress) levels and lowers estrogen and progesterone in menopausal women.[2] Coffee is not harmful in moderation (2 cups per day) and does contain antioxidants. But beyond that, coffee can deplete the adrenals and B vitamins, and it can decrease estrogen and progesterone.[3] Opiate addiction is on the rise, especially with teenagers and in atypical populations. A promising herb called *Mitragyna speciosa* (Kratom leaf) is known to safely help withdrawal and recovery from opioid and

alcohol addiction and has been in and out of favor with the U.S. Food and Drug Administration. There is no official consensus yet on its safety,[4] but opinions are heated. Stay up to date on its safety.

- *Insomnia.* This problem is practically epidemic. There are no guaranteed herbal knockout drops, but various nervines can work. In Chinese Medicine, the problem is often blamed on restless shen (Heart). If it's hard to fall asleep, it's considered an imbalanced Liver; but if you sleep too lightly, it could be a Heart or Spleen deficiency. A good bet is Zizyphus Suan Zao Ren (Sour Jujube seed) that helps to enrich the blood that flows to the heart and liver and regulates and calms the liver meridian.[5] Other causes for insomnia are bad nighttime habits or problems that keep the mind churning. This issue requires experimentation.
- *Headaches.* A lot of detective work is necessary. A headache (HA) is a symptom of something else (Chapter 23).
  - *Headaches, Western style.* In Western medicine, there are cluster headaches, tension headaches, migraines, and others. Causes include stress, dehydration, indigestion, head injuries, sinus pressure, infection, tight neck muscles, temporomandibular joint (TMJ) syndrome, or anything ranging from a brain tumor to a hangover. Ask how long it has been going on, where it hurts, when it hurts, and the type of pain, such as dull, sharp, heavy, and better or worse with pressure. Sometimes an MRI from a healthcare provider is necessary to rule out a dangerous cause, such as a brain tumor or cancer.
  - *Headaches, Chinese Medicine style.* In Chinese Medicine, there are perhaps 10 types of HAs. Type of pain indicates a possible syndrome and the meridian the pain travels through gives more information. Consider the time of day the headache occurs and use the 24-hour clock described earlier. When does the HA occur? What organ is peaking? Is there a pattern? Recurring headaches are a puzzle, a symptom of something else requiring a full assessment.
- *Relationship with food.* There are many food-related queries in our healthy history. Whatever is checked can trigger a conversation or an opportunity to teach. The questions request the frequency of healthy and unhealthy choices. In general, determine whether the client eats out or cooks their own meals. Finding healthy restaurant choices can be challenging. After the initial food history, what's next depends on other information, particularly the state of digestion. Food choices are intricately intertwined with health. General advice includes frequent and many-colored vegetables, very few simple carbs and sugary foods, organics when possible, and healthy fats. Gear specifics to the problems at hand, where food is treated as medicine. This process takes additional thought and research.
  - *Examples.* If clients eat compulsively or consume a lot of bagels and muffins, there could be insulin resistance. Drinking with meals dilutes digestive enzymes. (Best to drink 15 to 20 minutes before or after meals, not during.)
- *Food cravings.* In a perfect world, a body craves what it needs. If a real protein deficit exists, protein is needed and desired. But what if one yearns for sugar, salt, fat, or chocolate? The body has become out of balance. Foods such as gluten, sugar, and caseins in dairy have narcotic properties that bind to opioid receptors, so we want to eat them. This can lead to an *addiction.* The feel-good hormone, dopamine, decreases and the munchies increase. Resistance to insulin and leptin (the hormone that curbs appetite) builds up.[6] Signals to turn off hunger and sugar cravings go away. Weight loss becomes difficult, and the body wants more and more sugar and fat in a vicious cycle. The best fix is to eat unprocessed foods and introduce cruciferous vegetables and bitter herbs. The body weans off sugar, and the need disappears.
- *Food cravings, Chinese Medicine style.* From the Chinese perspective, cravings are attributed to imbalances related to the organs and their related tastes, leading us back to the Table of Correspondences. If the client has sugar (*sweet*) cravings, the Spleen and digestion need work, so they should eat naturally sweet foods like sweet potatoes, brown rice, or dates in moderation and lay off simple carbs. *Salt* cravings are the Kidney's domain, so turn to naturally salty fish and seaweeds. The Liver is wood energy, the *sour* taste. This organ often correlates to fat cravings; sour and bitter foods are good to eat in Liver imbalances. The *bitter* taste corresponds to Heart fire energy and is associated with anxiety, depression, and nightmares. Even though this taste is rarely craved, bitter foods and herbs will help these problems. Chinese Medicine fixes are not that different from the Western methods.
- *Symptoms survey.* This section of the health history goes through body systems and covers key questions in each area. Symptoms are alerts for medical problems that need investigating, or that may not have been previously mentioned. Although *Health Goals* and *Current Medical Concerns* sections were already addressed, other areas may need attention in order to achieve good outcomes. For instance, hypothyroidism is often linked to menstrual or menopausal health; heart health is linked to insulin resistance; and autoimmune illnesses cannot be addressed without a good look at diet.

The Physical Assessment

Once the interview is complete, it is time to do a physical assessment. This process consists of Western and Eastern techniques and any other known system. In a good assessment, a BP will be obtained, and a pulse and tongue analysis will be done. Information gained in the written and verbal Herbal Health History is compared with physical findings. The more signs and symptoms that line up, the greater the assessment accuracy. If tongue is purplish in the liver area and there is history of hepatitis or menstrual problems, you are getting liver clues. If the stomach area on the tongue map is yellow and greasy, there is damp and probably heat. These symptoms indicate digestive issues that most likely have already surfaced on the intake form. Having a red tongue and a fast pulse means heat. Having a pale tongue or a slow pulse means cool or cold (Chapter 9).

Tongue Cheat Sheet

The tongue reflects the body's condition and is observed for color, texture, size, and shape (Fig. 15.1). We look at its body under the coating (also called the fur or moss) and its shape. Finally, we see if there's any correlation with the tongue map in relation to the organs. Table 15.3 is a handy reference to keep in the clinic.

Pulse Cheat Sheet

The primary location is the radial pulse on each wrist on the thumb side (Fig. 15.2). The wrists should always be below heart level when you are taking pulses. Both parties should be relaxed. Three pulses are palpated on each wrist. Hook your middle (longest) finger over styloid process until your fingertip

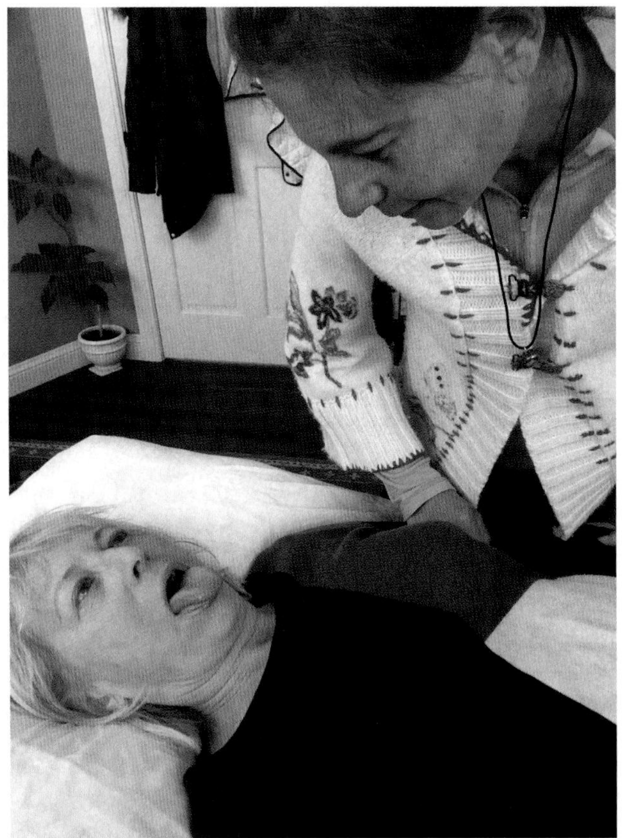

• **Fig. 15.1** Tongue diagnosis by Cheryl Harris, M.S., L.Ac., owner of Therapeutic Acupuncture.

finds client's radial pulse. Place your index finger over the radial pulse between longest finger and client's wrist. Third finger should naturally slip over the radial pulse next to longest finger toward the person's elbow. Table 15.4 provides a quick review.

Blood Pressure Assessment

Blood pressure (BP) is the pressure of the blood within the arteries as the heart pumps blood. When the right ventricular valve in the heart contracts, it produces the high number, called ***systolic*** pressure, as blood is pushed out into circulation. When the ventricular valve muscles relax, the pressure is at its lowest, which is measured as ***diastolic*** pressure. The pressure is measured in millimeters of mercury (mm Hg). A typical BP is written as systolic over diastolic, e.g., 120/80 and stated as "one-twenty over eighty."

BP is measured with a sphygmomanometer, an inflatable cuff with a gauge attached that is wrapped around a limb right above a radial pulse. The most common site is the brachial artery at the inner elbow. Another site is on the leg just above the popliteal artery behind the knee. The cuff is inflated so that blood flow is cut off. Then it is slowly released while you listen to the pulse with a stethoscope and watch the gauge. The top heart sound or beat is the systolic pressure; the bottom or last sound heard is the diastolic pressure. Although there are many electronic cuffs out there, the most accurate readings are taken by hand with a cuff and your ears to a stethoscope.

When arterial pressure is too high, the client has hypertension, which increases the risk of dementia, Alzheimer's, stroke, and coronary heart disease that leads to heart attack. This is particularly true when present with other risk factors. High blood pressure can occur in children or adults, but it's more common among people over age 35. Risk factors include being of African-American descent; being middle-aged and elderly; being obese; being a heavy drinker; having a history of insulin and leptin resistance, gout, or kidney disease; and taking birth control pills. It may run in families but not always. Cardiovascular risk begins to increase steadily as BP rises from 115/75 mm Hg to higher values. The American Heart Association guidelines designate normal BP to be below 120/80 (Table 15.5).

Directions for Taking a Blood Pressure

- *Client sits* with feet flat and uncrossed, back and arm supported, and arm slightly flexed at elbow at heart level. (Brachial artery too high above heart level gives false low reading; artery too low below the heart gives a false high reading.) Place the bag over brachial artery on inside of arm on skin, not clothes. Lower border should be about 2.5 cm above antecubital crease.
- *Inflate cuff* to about 30 mm Hg above level at which radial pulse disappears. This is the palpatory systolic pressure and helps you avoid being misled by the *auscultatory gap*, which is a silent interval between systolic and diastolic pressures in some patients, usually those with hypertension.
- *Deflate cuff.*
- *Place stethoscope over brachial artery* in antecubital space. (Just medial to biceps tendon.) It should not touch clothing or cuff.
- *Inflate cuff again* to about 30 mm Hg above the palpatory systolic pressure. Then deflate the cuff slowly, allowing pressure to drop at a rate of about 3 mm Hg per second. Level at which you hear sounds of at least two consecutive beats is systolic pressure. Continue lowering pressure slowly until sound becomes muffled. This point is the diastolic pressure.
- *Take in both arms*, at least initially. Normally, there may be a difference in pressure of 5 mm Hg. Subsequent readings should be made on the arm with the higher pressure.[7]

Blood Pressure Facts

- *White-coat effect.* Many people with Stage I hypertension have elevated blood pressure only in the presence of a physician. This *white-coat effect* is more common in older men and women (who are probably the most stressed and worried about it). Stress and fear associated with hospital and doctor's visits do not reflect accurate results.
- *Gold standard BP cuff.* The original mercury sphygmomanometers are considered the most accurate, but they are being phased out by aneroid and electronic devices. These days most clinics and hospitals use electronic cuffs. But many cardiologists (and nurses) don't trust this method and take a manual BP. If the electronic reading seems really off, take BP the old-fashioned way by listening for the pulse sounds with a stethoscope.
- *Proper cuff size.* This factor is critical for accurate measurement. The bladder length and width of the cuff should be 80% and 40% respectively of the arm circumference. BP measurement errors are generally higher when using cuffs that are too small than when using those that are too big. Overweight people need large cuffs to prevent false high readings. Cuffs come in infant, children, average adult, and large sizes.
- *Positioning.* Blood pressure measurement in sitting and recumbent positions is acceptable. The diastolic blood

TABLE 15.3 Tongue Cheat Sheet

TONGUE MAP

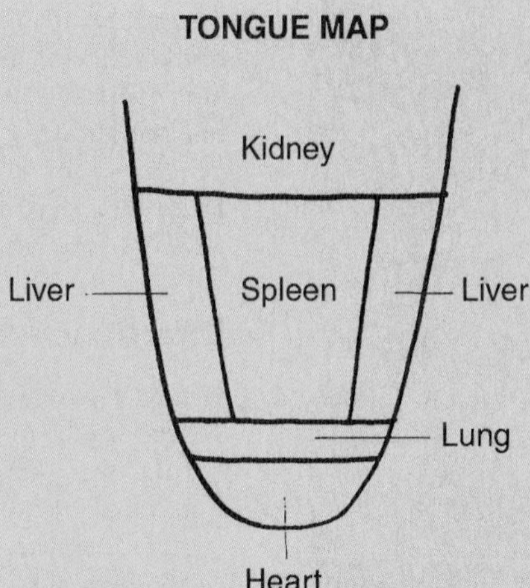

The five-organ tongue correspondence map can be useful in identifying the affected organ. (Illustration by Matthew Berk, L.Ac., MSTOM, and Reviewer for Chinese herbal portion of book.)

Body Color	Body Shape	Coat Quality	Coat Color
Light red Normal	**Moderate size, no cracks or teeth marks** Normal	**Thin, slightly moist** Normal	**White** Normal
Pale Deficient blood, qi or yang	**Thin and narrow or small** Deficient blood and/or yin	**Thick** Dampness or phlegm	**Yellow** Heat
Very pale, blue hue Interior cold	**Stiff or deviating** Heart fire or internal wind	**Absent coating** Yin or fluid deficiency	**Brown or black** Extreme heat
Bright red, entire tongue Excess heat	**Quivering** Spleen qi deficiency	**Geographical or peeled** Stomach yin deficiency	
Bright red, tip only Excess heat	**Lengthwise cracks** Yin or essence deficiency	**Greasy, curdlike** Dampness	
Dark red Heat in deeper levels, blood or yin	**Crosswise or random cracks** Longstanding heat and deficiency (could be hereditary, normal)	**Very wet** Spleen or yang deficiency	
Dark red with sores Heart fire	**Large or long** Excess heat		
Lavender or dusky Qi stagnation	**Scalloped edges** Damp or spleen qi deficiency		
Purple or dark blue Qi and blood or blood stagnation			

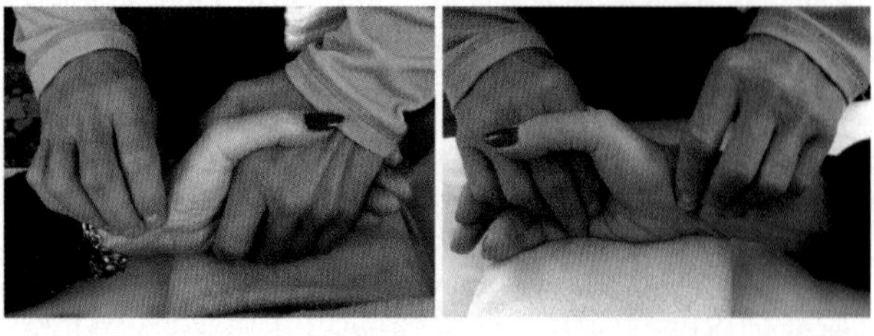

• **Fig. 15.2** Pulse taking. The practitioner lines up her three middle fingers along the radial pulse on each wrist.

pressure can be expected to be about 5 mm Hg higher when sitting.

- *Arm difference.* Difference in blood pressure between the two arms can be expected in about 20% of patients. The higher value should be the one used in treatment decisions. Those with a difference of 10 to 15 points systolic have a greater risk of developing heart disease and related complications during the next 13 years.[8]
- *BP readings in the emergency room.* These do not accurately predict hypertension on subsequent healthcare provider visits. Talk about the stress factor in play here.

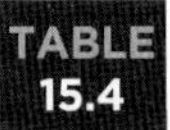

TABLE 15.4 Pulse Cheat Sheet. Basics Of Pulse Palpation

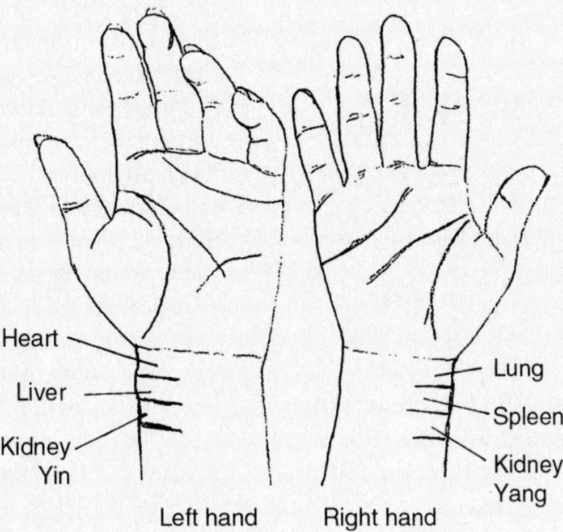

Pulse positions showing the yin organs on each wrist. (Illustration by Matthew Berk, L.Ac., MSTOM, and Reviewer for Chinese portion of book.)

Fast (>5 beats per breath) = Heat	———	Slow (>4 beats per breath) = Cold
Superficial = External, acute	———	Deep = Internal, chronic
Empty/thin = Deficient	———	Full = Excess

Depth	Strength	Quality
Floating Distinct when barely touches skin and fades with pressure. Exterior conditions, elderly.	**Weak** Hardly presses back. Qi and blood deficiency.	**Slippery** Feels rubbery, soft, and rolling as if pencil is spinning inside vessel. Borders indistinct or poorly defined. Dampness or phlegm or pregnant.
Deep Only distinct with considerable pressure. Interior disease.	**Strong** Forceful and pounding. Excess, a pathogen is present.	**Choppy** Irregular form like grains of sand moving through a straw or teeth on a fine saw blade. Congealed blood, stagnant qi, or deficient blood.
		Wiry Guitar string that pushes back. Hits fingers at same time. Liver conditions and pain.
		Fine Small, thin like thread, thinner than wiry. Blood and yin deficiency.
		Irregular. Hasty, knotted, intermittent Disorders of Heart qi, dangerous in sick, can occur in health with mental or emotional strain.

- *Public BP machines*. Frequently inaccurate.
- *Nighttime*. Evening home readings are usually lower than daytime pressure.
- *Stress and diet*. Diets high in sugar, fructose, and fatty foods can increase BP. Laughter, breathing, yoga, exercise, and meditation can reduce stress and BP.
- *When is BP too low?* When it becomes symptomatic as evidenced by dizziness, lightheadedness, or nausea. Athletes often have lower BPs, which is normal. Approximately, low BP is anything less than 90/60. Check for symptoms. Other factors such as illness, prolonged bed rest, and drugs can make it low.

Herbalist's Assessment Form

The ***Herbalist's Assessment form*** (Table 15.6 and Appendix A) is designed for the herbalist to use for initial visits and follow-up appointments and is separate from the Herbal Health History

TABLE 15.5 Blood Pressure Parameters

Systolic	Diastolic	Category
Below 120	Below 80	Normal
120–139	80–89	Prehypertension
140–159	90–99	Stage I Hypertension
160 or higher	100 or higher	Stage II Hypertension[9]

form. It is where herbal formulas are designed and where records are kept of what was asked, observed and recommended at each visit. A new form is used for every session; use a form for the initial client assessment and for all others.

In subsequent follow-up visits, applicable areas are filled out and the rest left blank. First time visits will take about an hour and a half, whereas follow-up appointments should be perhaps a half hour unless there are major new developments. Follow-ups are concerned with the goal for today, the chief complaint, primary problem(s) being addressed, or anything new and different. Because a detailed health history has been already obtained, there is no need to do it again.

Any health professional, herbalists included, must always keep good records and make sure any dispensed herbal formula is on file. It is not unusual to hear from a client 1 or 2 years down the road with a request for a refill of that wonderful cold formula you gave them eons ago. Of course, their bottle with label of ingredients is long gone.

SOAP

The Herbalist's Assessment form follows a very particular format and uses an acronym called ***SOAP***, which stands for *subjective, objective, assessment, and plan*. SOAP notes are a style of charting that is frequently used in medical professions. It is found in clinics and hospitals and used by doctors, nurses, physical therapists, and others; and it is a method of organizing information and going through a logical thought process to arrive at a treatment strategy.

- *S stands for subjective*. Subjective is information the client *says*. It's their report, their version, their account. They might say, "I have terrible pains in my stomach when I eat." Or "I have bad menstrual cramps with clotting." Or "My father died of a heart attack." Or "I eat at Burger King five times a week." *S* consists of all the verbal information you obtain from a client in that visit. There is no right or wrong or judgment here because it's their story. The most important thing for the herbalist is to build trust, be present, listen closely, and ask the right questions in the right way. If it's the first visit, the subjective part will take longer than the follow-ups, because you are getting it all (within reason) and sorting out the information.
- *O stands for objective*. Objective is the part *observed*. Objective information consists of tongue and pulse assessment and BP. It involves observations made as to skin, complexion, posture, affect, body temperature, hair, nails, facial analysis, or any other observations and techniques you might know and choose to use. If you have the skill, listen to the client's heart, lungs, and bowel sounds with a stethoscope. Part of *O* includes any lab reports the client has brought in from a healthcare provider, x-rays, MRI or ultrasound results, or any other objective findings from other practitioners. It includes the herbs, supplements, and drugs they are taking and that they have been asked to bring into their appointment.
- *A stands for assessment*. After considering what the client said and what was objectively observed, a *conclusion* is reached. This might be a list of symptoms they have, a disease name that has been diagnosed from an M.D., D.O., or D.C., or a Chinese syndrome based on pulse and tongue assessment, such as damp or heat or lung dryness or liver congestion. Assessments are also arrived at by consideration of any predisposing causes or triggers that might be setting off the problem. The more accurate the assessment, the better the herbalist's chance for success. This process is what student clinics are all about: practice, practice, practice to arrive at a plausible conclusion.
- *P stands for plan*. The ultimate goal is deciding the *now what* part. Good plans are holistic in that they consider not only herbs, but diet, exercise, supplements, lifestyle changes, and spiritual and emotional issues. A plan might use essential oils and make referrals for massage, acupuncture, chiropractic, or psychotherapy. A plan is useless unless it's realistic. Suggest only what can be handled. If a client is overwhelmed or too stressed, they'll give up fast. Negotiate. What is reasonable given lifestyle, emotional state, and budget? Set priorities. Recommend a little at a time. Formulate short, medium, and long-term goals, even though they could be subject to change.

What Subjective Entails

- *Chief complaint*. This is the "Why are you here?" part. What is the goal, the *chief complaint*, or the main problem? Ask about signs and symptoms. How often does each occur? Is there a pattern? What makes it better or worse? What has been tried? Was a healthcare provider consulted, and if so, what was the diagnosis? What drugs were prescribed? Are there any labs or medical tests to share? Obtain a timeline. When did it begin? Were there particular triggers such as extreme stress, a personal trauma, an accident, or a major life event when it all began? Mind-body connection plays a part, and if issues are not dealt with when they happen, they can get worse and manifest in the physical body. Attitudes, beliefs, daily thought patterns, and emotions have a profound effect on our health.[10]
- *Secondary problems*. What else is going on? Is this other problem related to the chief complaint? A chief complaint of menopausal symptoms could be directly related to the secondary problem of sore joints or hypothyroidism. Sometimes there are too many issues to deal with at once. An herbalist needs to prioritize and have a therapy plan of what to address and in what order. First things first.
- *Body systems history*. This section is included to jog a client's memory and is most useful at the initial consult. It covers all body systems, so nothing is omitted. If positive findings pop up, ask the same type of questions laid out under the chief complaint bullet of the SOAP heading.
- *Emotional/mental health*. This is an important and sensitive area. Anxiety and depression are epidemic. Emotional health includes sexual history and whether the client is sexually active. Ask about dreams, nightmares, abuse, and mental illness. Inquire about spiritual paths or importance of religion.

TABLE 15.6 Herbalist's Assessment Form
(See Appendix A, Fig. A.2, for reproducible form)

S. Client Name ____________________________ Date ________ Sex _____ Age____

Chief Complaint or status since last visit ____________________

Secondary Problem(s) or status since last visit ____________________

Body Systems: Initial history or status since last visit.

Respiratory____________________

Cardiovascular____________________

Nervous____________________

Urinary____________________

Endocrine____________________

Gastrointestinal____________________

Urinary____________________

Skin____________________

Musculoskeletal____________________

Reproductive ____________________

Emotional/Mental Health

____

____

____

General Questions:

Body pain____________________

Headache ____________________

Digestion ____________________

Stools ____________________

Thirst ____________________

Sleep ____________________

Energy Level ____________________

Menses/Menopause

____

EENT/Phlegm ____________________

Emotions ____________________

Lifestyle ____________________

Exercise ____________________

Are they taking the herbs/supplements?

____

Typical diet or dietary progress since last visit

____

____

____

H2O intake________ Favorite foods ____________________ hot or cold ______ raw_______

cooked______ caffeine_______ dairy______ gluten_______

Breakfast	Lunch	Dinner	Snacks

(*Continued*)

TABLE 15.6 Herbalist's Assessment Form
***(See Appendix A, Fig. A.2, for reproducible form)*—cont'd**

Overall reported progress since last visit
□ Much Improved □ Slightly Improved □ No change □ Slightly worse □ Much worse

O. Pulse rate________ Blood Pressure ___________
Tongue body/color/shape ____
Tongue coat/color____

Right Pulses	Left Pulses
Overall Depth Overall Strength Overall Quality	Overall Depth Overall Strength Overall Quality
Lung	Heart
Spleen	Liver
Kidney Yin	Kidney Yang

Other Physical Findings (complexion, heart/lung/gut auscultation, lab results, etc.).
____
____
____
____

A. Conditions: (Circle what applies)
Hot or Cold Dry or Damp Tense or Weak Hard or Soft Interior or Exterior Excess or Deficient
Chinese Syndromes ____
Western Syndromes (Signs/symptoms, healthcare provider diagnosis)
____
Predisposing Causes/Triggers
____

P. Therapeutic Principles (Herbal, dietary, supplements, lifestyle)
Herbal Formula Name ______________________________
Dose ____
Instructions ____

Part	Herb	Rationale

Supplements, Dietary Changes, Lifestyle Suggestions
____
Treatment Priorities and Sequence ______________________________
____
____
Return visit/referrals ____
Herbalist Signature and Date __________________________________

Connection to some type of higher power, whether God, Nature, or inner self has been shown to add years to our lives. The holistic way is to mesh mind, body, and spirit.

- *General questions.* This section applies to topics that should be addressed in every visit. How are they doing with digestion, diet, sleep, exercise, energy, and herbal compliance? Any new stressors or lifestyle changes?
- *Dietary progress.* This topic requires constant discussion, encouragement, and fine tuning.
- *Self-assessment.* Meant for follow-up visits, to track subjective progress. It's good to get the client's take. Has there been any improvement, how much, or is there a need to start over in a different direction?

What Objective and Assessment Entail

- *Pulse, tongue evaluation and BP measurement.* In each visit, pulse and tongue should be evaluated. BP needs rechecking in follow-ups if that is an issue. Any other physical evaluations are done here.
- *Assessment and reassessment.* Based on history and physical findings (Subjective and Objective), what do you come up with? Western symptoms, Chinese syndromes, new healthcare provider's diagnosis? Assessments change as conditions change.

What the Plan Entails

- ***Therapeutic principles.*** This section is a list of what you are trying to accomplish with a client or in a formula. To stay organized, always list these before dispensing any herbs. Once intentions are clear, a coherent plan can be devised. No floundering around. Examples: clear heat, decrease infection, or begin a gluten-free diet.
  - *Listing therapeutic principles is the best way to compose an herbal formula.* For instance, pretend the client came in with a clear runny nose, sinus headache, and sore throat with a dry cough, and you came up with the Chinese syndrome External Wind Cold with dryness. Then the therapeutic principles might be to: (1) decrease infection/inflammation; (2) Dry secretions; (3) Moisten cough and increase expectoration; (4) Decrease pain; and (5) Help sinuses to drain. Then herbs would be chosen to cover these bases. To round out the holistic plan, the herbalist might suggest a throat gargle and perhaps some vitamin C (to help immune coverage).
- *Herbs.* The initial formulas with proportions and rationales are worked out. Dispense enough herbs to last until the next appointment. For follow-ups, you might need to change the herbs. I have found that subsequent formulas invariably need adjustments, revisions, or tweaks. Entirely new ones might be added, or old ones discontinued. If something tastes too awful, rethinking is in order. If you need time to research and think about a formula, ask your client to return later or the next day to pick up their herbs. No harm in that.
- *Supplements.* Too many bottles of things to consume are overwhelming, not to mention expensive. Narrow choices down to top picks.
- *Diet.* Negotiate. Ask what a client is willing to do. Introduce only one or two new foods at a time. What is most important? It may be to drink more water or cut out gluten; if so, that's plenty for a while. New elaborate diets and foods can be too much. Be creative. If a person eats out or doesn't have time to cook, they may need guidelines on what to order and where to go. Suggest easy, healthy snacks. If possible, get the whole family involved. It is hard to make changes if everyone else is indulging in chips and cookies.
- *Lifestyle.* Suggestions must be realistic. Exercise, therapy referrals, and classes go in this section. Lifestyle changes must be affordable and something that the client will actually do.
- *Treatment priorities and sequence.* This is the long-term therapy plan. List sequence of goals in order while they are fresh in your mind. Often getting the gut healthy is the first priority before any herbs or supplements.
- *Follow-up appointments and referrals.* Always reschedule before a client leaves. An electronic reminder the day before the next appointment is often appreciated. Refer to other practitioners, if pertinent. Network with others and keep their contact information accessible.

Herbal Consult Suggestion Form

The ***Herbal Consult Suggestions form*** (Table 15.7 and Appendix A) is a form for you to write out the client's instructions for them to take home. I fill this out as I go along and make a copy for my records. They'll never remember it all, and calmly indicating that you're writing it all down takes away the stress. Be sure your contact information appears on the form so that they can call with any questions. Of course, being available and promptly returning calls is a given. At the follow-up appointment, review this form with them to determine what was actually done and accomplished.

Explanation of Consult Suggestion Form

- *Herbs (instructions).* No need to relist formula contents. This list is on the dispensed bottle. Write down formula name, dose, and any special instructions, such as to take between meals with juice or water. If you are asking them to buy loose herbs for a tea from the health food store, here's where to list them with common name, botanical name, and brewing instructions. Are they supposed to purchase a ready-made tincture? Give particulars.
- *Dietary.* List suggested foods but be realistic and practical. If a food is brand new, explain where to buy and how to prepare. Be explicit. Cooking instructions, such as "Quinoa can be found in bulk at blank store. Prepare like rice, 1 cup grain to 2 cups water." Or say, "Gluten-free grains are quinoa, millet, corn, rice, amaranth, and buckwheat." Remember to emphasize a varied diet with a rainbow-colored plate, remind the client to chew well, and discourage microwaving. Encourage eating at home and cooking organic, using foods that are free of genetically modified organisms (non-GMOs), and choosing healthy snacks. If client is not the type to frequent a health food store, list healthy choices available in a conventional supermarket.
- *Supplements.* Don't pile on too many. Make them relevant to the condition. If there are heart problems, Fish oil caps or CoQ10 could be indicated. Suggest medicinal foods such as broccoli, flax seeds, or GMO-free soy products.
- *Lifestyle.* This lumps together exercise suggestions, classes such as yoga or meditation, massage therapy, taking a hot bath in the evening with essential oils, sitting down to eat at a table without the news on, taking a walk, going out with friends, or taking time for self.
- *Aromatherapy.* An interesting area, depending on your expertise. Many people respond beautifully to scents, because essential oils work on both an emotional level and a physical level. Carrying around a pretty bottle of Lavender and inhaling it now and then

TABLE 15.7 Herbal Consult Suggestions
(See Appendix A, Fig. A.3, for reproducible form)

Name ______________________________	**Date** ______________
Herbs (instructions) ______________________________	
______________________________	
Dietary ______________________________	
______________________________	
Supplements ______________________________	
______________________________	
Lifestyle ______________________________	
Aromatherapy ______________________________	
Referrals ______________________________	
Next Appointment Date/Time ______________________________	

for stress or rubbing a drop on the temples for a headache is very therapeutic.

- *Referrals*. Respect your intuition and know your limits. Your mantra should be "When in doubt, refer it out." Any client whose condition is beyond your expertise or who makes you uncomfortable presents a signal to refer. If you're not making progress after several visits, it's time to move them on. Certainly, any red flags, such as suspected cancer, undiagnosed lumps, chest pain, or difficulty breathing must be referred to a qualified healthcare provider. Uneven pupils, slurred speech, droopy mouth, or loss of movement could mean a stroke. Gastrointestinal bleeds with black, tarry stools might suggest a bleeding ulcer. Back pain? Refer to a chiropractor or osteopath. Mental illness? Have a therapist's number in your phone.
- *Next appointment*. Always reschedule before the client leaves and send a reminder. With a new client, call to check in a couple of days after the initial visit.

Keeping Records

The client has been seen. You now have three paper (or electronic) forms. The client filled out their (1) Herbal Health History form. A verbal interview and a physical assessment were completed. You, the herbalist, filled out your own sheet, the (2) Herbalist's Assessment form, where you followed a SOAP format. You arrived at a plan and dispensed the herbal formula. You presented said client with her herbs and an (3) Herbal Consult Suggestions form to take home. You made a copy for your own records.

All that paperwork is confidential. It now becomes a medical record that must be kept in a locked file cabinet and locked office. What was said in the consult room stays there. No blabbing on the elevator, bus, or internet to a friend or family member about your client. Electronic records must be protected. Confidentiality and right to privacy are not only a moral obligation but a law. ***HIPAA, the Health Insurance Portability and Accountability Act*** of 1996 and the HIPAA Privacy Rule that followed the Act, protect a patient's written and electronic medical records and health information.

The only time HIPAA does not apply is when the client or a legal guardian has given written permission/authorization to share it with another health professional, facility, insurance company, attorney, or billing agency. Patients have a right to examine and obtain a copy of their health records and to request corrections.[11] This all amounts to a client's right to privacy and the need for discretion. Sounds obvious; worth saying.

What if you want to get some help and confer with another herbalist or health professional about a case? Of course, you may. Just do not use the client's name. Consults are done all the time. The only times you are required to disclose medical information without a client's permission are situations involving court orders, fraud, or mental health problems where the client presents some danger to self or others. Never give out information to anyone without making sure.

Summary

The entire process of how an herbalist operates in real time was covered. First was the initial intake, where the client filled out the Herbal Health History form. A rationale was provided for each question. Physical assessment includes (at the least) taking pulse, examining the tongue, and obtaining a BP. The cheat sheets provided for pulse and tongue may be copied for clinic use.

The Herbalist's Assessment form is where the practitioner's notes and findings are recorded and where a holistic course of action involving diet, exercise, herbs, and such is decided on. The assessment form is divided into a classic SOAP format (subjective, objective, assessment, and plan). Formulating the plan begins with listing the therapeutic principles. Then the herbal formula is designed, complete with parts, herb, rationale, and dose. Dietary changes, supplements, lifestyle changes, and any other recommendations are listed. The Herbal Consult Suggestions form is given to the client, and a follow-up appointment is made.

Every practicing herbalist should appreciate the importance of keeping medical records safe and the need for maintaining trust and privacy. HIPAA regulations and where herbalism fits into this scheme were covered.

Review

Fill in the Blanks

(Answers in Appendix B.)

1. Name the three herbalist forms described in this chapter. ___, ___, ___.
2. Name four items on the table of correspondences. ___, ___, ___, ___.
3. On the 24-hour clock, give the times for Liver ___, Heart ___, Spleen ___, Kidney ___, Lungs ___, and Pericardium ___.
4. SOAP stands for ___, ___, ___, and ___.
5. What are five risk factors for high blood pressure? ___, ___, ___, ___, ___.
6. HIPAA stands for ___.
7. Name five red flags for a need to refer out. ___, ___, ___, ___, ___.
8. Pulses from right wrist toward elbow are ___, ___, ___. Pulses from left wrist toward elbow are ___, ___, ___.
9. When assessing a pulse, the three aspects are ___, ___, ___.
10. When assessing a tongue, the four aspects are ___, ___, ___, ___.

Critical Concept Questions

(Answers for you to decide.)

1. A client frequently wakes up with hot flashes around 2 am. What organ is involved? What might you deduce?
2. What is the reason for listing therapeutic principles? How do they help with devising an herbal formula?
3. Pulse is fast, tongue is very red, person is anxious. What does this tell you?
4. Discuss the statement *"Herbalists must respect their intuition and know their limits."*
5. What dietary advice would you give to a 45-year-old, overweight, single man, who frequents fast food joints?
6. Discuss what *setting someone up for failure* means related to suggestions for a client.
7. What is the mind-body connection?
8. Describe an office or setting that would help make a client feel safe and likely to share sensitive information.
9. How does a follow-up appointment differ from the initial intake?
10. Discuss a patient's right to privacy and HIPAA.

References

1. "Chinese Body Clock". Spiritual Coach. http://www.spiritualcoach.com/chinese-body-clock/ (accessed January 10, 2021).
2. "Cigarettes Can Sabotage Hormone Balance." Women in Balance Institute. https://womeninbalance.org/2012/10/26/cigarettes-can-sabotage-hormone-balance/ (accessed October 26, 2019).
3. Flint, Margi. *The Practicing Herbalist: Meeting with Clients, Reading the Body* (Marblehead, ME: EarthSong Press, 2013).
4. Yearsley, Connor. "Kratom: Medicine or Menace?" HerbalGram: Journal of the American Botanical Council. 2016, Nov 2016–Dec 2017.
5. "Traditional Chinese Medicine Encourages Restful Sleep: Alternative Treatment for Insomnia, Nightmares, or Fitful Sleeping." Pacific College of Oriental Medicine. https://www.pacificcollege.edu/news/blog/2015/02/03/traditional-chinese-medicine-encourages-restful-sleep-alternative-treatment-insomnia-nightmares-or-fitful-sleeping (accessed October 26, 2019).
6. Kittrell, Hannah. "How to Control Your Hunger Hormones, To Lose Weight Fast, According to Experts." Eat This, Not That! https://www.eatthis.com/hunger-hormones-weight-loss/ (accessed January10, 2021).
7. Bates, Barbara. *A Guide to Physical Examination* (Philadelphia, PA: Lippincott, 1979).
8. "Blood Pressure: Can it be higher in one arm?" Mayo Clinic. https://www.mayoclinic.org/diseases-conditions/high-blood-pressure/expert-answers/blood-pressure/faq-20058230 (accessed January 10, 2021).
9. "Blood Pressure Chart: What Your Reading Means." Mayo Clinic. http://www.mayoclinic.org/diseases-conditions/high-blood-pressure/in-depth/blood-pressure/art-20050982 (accessed October 26, 2019).
10. Northrup, Christiane. *The Wisdom of Menopause* (New York: Bantam, 2001).
11. "HIPAA Rules Explained." WebMD. https://www.webmd.com/healthy-aging/news/20030422/hipaa-rules-explained#1 (accessed October 27, 2019).

16 Maintaining the Body in Health

"Nurture life, wherever you find it."

—Hildegard von Bingen

CHAPTER REVIEW

- Optimum health, an herbalist's responsibility.
- The microbiome: functions, dysbiosis, diet, and herbal categories to build the flora.
- Inflammation: acute and pathological.
- Oxidative stress.
- Food guidelines to maintain health: Rainbow, Mediterranean, Paleo diets, and GAPS protocol.
- A healthy immune system.
- Materia Medica to maintain health: restoratives, adaptogens, and Chinese tonics.
- Common conditions with case histories to maintain health: dysbiosis and indigestion, weak immune system, and assorted problems.

KEY TERMS

Acute inflammation
Adaptogens
Antioxidants
Bitters
Cholagogues
Demulcents
Dysbiosis
Free radicals
Functional foods
Functional medicine
GAPS protocol
Gluten
Intestinal permeability (IP)
Intermittent fasting
Lactose
Leaky gut
Mediterranean diet
Microbiome
Oxidative stress
Paleolithic diet
Pathological inflammation
Prebiotics
Probiotics
Rainbow diet
Restoratives
Tonics
Tropho-restoratives
Vegetarian diet

An herbalist's highest mission is to maintain health by the practice of preventative measures or to recognize what optimal health could look like for any given individual and help them attain that goal. This chapter is a crash course in ***functional medicine***, which addresses the underlying causes of disease using a systems-oriented approach that engages client and practitioner in a therapeutic partnership. Everyone is unique. Some days are better than other days. Herbalists use functional medicine concepts, restoratives, tonics, adaptogens, bitters, appropriate dietary principles, supplements, and lifestyle suggestions to facilitate maintaining the body in health.

A fundamental aspect of prevention is supporting the gut microbiome. Use of functional foods and herbs geared toward healthy gut function heads the list and is given prime time. The role of inflammation and oxidative stress is explained in relation to the gut. Healthy food guidelines and proven diets play a role.

Case histories following the SOAP format (Chapter 15) will be used to arrive at individualized herbal formulas for typical situations and include diet and lifestyle recommendations to maintain a healthy state. Practice case histories culminate in real-life herbal consults. That's where we're headed.

Optimum Health

Every person is biochemically unique. Optimum health is a continuum and different for everybody depending on life choices and what was dealt at birth. Individual metabolism depends on genetic expression, age, environment, activity levels, and the physical and spiritual nutrition we give our bodies. An herbalist's greatest calling is to help her or his clients live up to their unique health potential through *preventative medicine*, the ultimate kind of healing. Maintaining this coveted state involves mindfulness: consciousness in respect to food, herbs, exercise, sleep, spirituality, service, action, and stillness. It is a process and a life's work. To facilitate this state, an herbalist uses restoratives, tonics, adaptogens, appropriate diet, lifestyle suggestions, and intuition.

The Microbiome

Good health begins in the gut. The gastrointestinal (GI) tract is considered one of the most complex microbial ecosystems on Earth. The bacteria, viruses, fungi, and other critters that reside there outnumber the cells in our body by 10 to 1. There are more bacteria in our intestines, particularly the colon, than cells in the entire body. In fact, that collection of little bugs weighs over 2 pounds. This community of organisms that resides in the intestines of humans and animals is known as the ***microbiome*** or *gut flora*. Unbelievably, more than 10,000 species of bacteria are found in the gut. They perform a wide variety of functions and need to be fed, balanced, and nourished if we expect to maintain physical and mental well-being. They make or break our health. There is no one ideal gut microbiome or flora. We are all different, just as we all have different gene combinations or genomes.[1]

Certain autoimmune diseases, like multiple sclerosis (MS) or type 2 diabetes and arthritis, are showing up with specific patterns or signatures of gut bacteria. The *Human Microbiome Initiative* sponsored by the National Institutes of Health is a research initiative to improve the understating of microorganisms found in healthy and diseased humans. Distinct, signature bacterial colonies have been found in people with some types of cancer, mental illness, obesity, or *Clostridium difficile* infections. That is enormously empowering news. The clinical pearl for herbalists is to make a priority of balancing out the gut in themselves and in each and every client. Some of the gut's many functions are summarized below.

A Few Impressive Gut Flora Functions

- *Counteracts inflammation.* Healthy gut flora increases immune function by decreasing inflammatory *cytokines* (messaging immune cells that can cause disease). When cytokines get out of control, they become inflammatory markers that can travel along the vagus nerve to the brain. Once at the brain, they signal the rest of the body to begin a nonproductive inflammatory cascade.
- *Healthy flora keeps harmful organisms, including yeast, under control.* This process occurs on the gut mucosal barrier, which would be the size of a tennis court if spread out flat.
- *Ferments dietary fiber into short-chain fatty acids (SCFAs).* SCFAs, such as *butyrate*, are produced by healthy gut microbes as they ferment fiber in the colon. They provide energy for the cells lining the colon and fight inflammation and cancer. Eating fiber-rich foods, such as fruit, vegetables, and legumes typical of a Mediterranean diet, increases inflammation-fighting SCFAs. Pectin in apples, oranges, and legumes is especially effective.
- *Synthesizes vitamins.* Vitamins, notably the B-complex and K, are synthesized by gut flora and helps mineral absorption.
- *Reduces risk of allergies and autoimmune diseases.* The flora trains the immune system to distinguish between pathogens and nonharmful antigens and to respond appropriately.
- *Antibody production.* Flora increases the good guys, the antibodies that fight infection such as IgA, IgE, and T and B immune cells.

Unbalanced Gut Flora or Dysbiosis

If the intestinal flora gets out of whack with too much yeast or the wrong combinations or types of bacteria (***dysbiosis***), many acute and chronic diseases occur. Gut cell wall junctions become widened, leading to ***intestinal permeability (IP)*** or ***leaky gut***, which are different names for the same thing. Undigested large protein food particles (macromolecules) leak out between the cell walls into the blood circulation, acting as environmental antigens. They travel to weak places in the body, setting up shop and causing inflammation and autoimmune responses. Resulting problems are asthma, arthritis, mental health disease, lupus, and so many more.

Signs and symptoms of leaky gut are all over the map, depending on which organ or body system is weakened or susceptible. As time goes on, major diseases can manifest: irritable bowel syndrome (IBS), Crohn's disease, attention deficit hyperactivity disorder (ADHD), multiple sclerosis (MS), and other autoimmune problems. If you come across a client with bizarre signs and symptoms in many body systems with no apparent reason, the best approach is to start at gut level. When it is healthy, many of their symptoms and problems described in the following list will miraculously disappear.

- *Constant fatigue.* This is perhaps an underlying complaint.
- *Seasonal allergies.* Included are hay fever and pollen allergies.
- *Brain fog.* The person can't think straight.
- *Skin problems.* Included are eczema, acne, and rashes.
- *Autoimmune diseases.* This category consists of a huge array of chronic illnesses that have become societal epidemics, such as multiple sclerosis, osteoarthritis, type 2 diabetes, lupus, and Hashimoto's hypothyroidism.
- *Digestion problems.* Diarrhea, constipation, bloating, and belching; irritable bowel syndrome; inflammatory bowel disease (IBD); and colic in babies are a few.
- *Food intolerances.* These include gluten sensitivity, lactose intolerances, and many others.
- *Depressed immunity.* The gut is a huge immune organ; when in balance, it keeps us healthy.
- *Mental illnesses.* Depression, anxiety, and other psychiatric problems are caused by dysbiosis. *Probiotics* (live, friendly gut organisms that make up healthy digestive systems) help in treating them.
- *Muscle aches and pains.* Body hurts all over.
- *Obesity.* There are differences in bacterial strains between normal and overweight bodies. *Lactobacillus rhamnosus* seems helpful for weight loss in women. What a find.

Dysbiosis and its resultant health problems are rampant in our society. The causes are everywhere and can be hard to avoid. Unless we and our clients are educated and conscious about these triggers in our food and drug supply and elsewhere, it is easy to develop an unbalanced microbiome (Table 16.1).

TABLE 16.1 Causes of Dysbiosis

Genetically modified organisms (GMOs)	**Refined sugars**	**Agricultural chemicals**
Foods with altered DNA occurring in processed foods and drinks. Frequently in corn, beet sugar, and soy crops. Foreign to the human genome.	Processed high-fructose corn syrup (HFCS) starring in salad dressings, soda, candy, junk foods, bread, canned fruit, and sweetened yogurt.	Herbicides, pesticides. Grow organic; frequent farmer's markets.
Conventionally raised meats and chickens	**Gluten and processed foods**	**Antibiotic use**
Those fed antibiotics and genetically engineered feed.	Sugar and dead nutrients feed bad gut microbes and yeast.	Only if really necessary. Afterwards, reforest gut with probiotics.
Nonsteroidal antiinflammatory drugs (NSAIDs)	**Proton pump inhibitors**	**Chronic stress**
Habitual use of drugs like Ibuprofen, Celebrex, or Motrin disrupts energy production in the mitochondria and causes intestinal permeability.	These are the popular antacid drugs that block stomach acids in gastroesophageal reflux disease (GERD), such as Prilosec, Prevacid, or Nexium.	Increases cortisol (stress hormone) and decreases insulin sensitivity.
Food allergens	**Chronic constipation**	**Elevated hormone levels**
Food sensitivities, such as to gluten or lactose, are setups for leaky gut.	Leads to and/or causes disrupted flora.	Birth control pills and steroid hormones cause leaky gut.

A Good Diet Builds the Microbiome

Gut flora is as individual as a fingerprint or a snowflake, but certain foods have a huge impact on its health. Fibers in foods that feed the gut flora are known as ***prebiotics***, whereas ***probiotics*** are actual live, friendly gut organisms, like *acidophilus* or *bifidobacteria*, that live long and prosper when fed a good diet of prebiotics. Prebiotics *heal and seal* the gastrointestinal tract, provide fiber for bowel health, and provide probiotics for healthy gut bacteria. Care and feeding of the microbiome with specific prebiotic and probiotic foods follow.

- *Brightly colored fruits and veggies feed the gut.* Prebiotics include carrots, tomatoes, eggplants, and fruits such as raspberries (surprisingly high in fiber) and blueberries (high in anthocyanins and other antioxidants).
- *High-fiber foods.* Fruits, veggies, and legumes build SCFAs to fight inflammation.
- *Fermented foods.* These cost-effective foods are an absolute *must* to build healthy flora. The microorganisms they contain are highly prolific and viable and are not killed off by the stomach's own hydrochloric acid (HCl). Foods such as kefir (fermented grass-fed, organic milk), plain Greek yogurt, miso, tempeh, pickles, sauerkraut, and natto (fermented soy) all have natural microflora. They add vitamin K_2, a vital co-nutrient to vitamin D, and calcium. Fermented foods provide a wide variety of microflora. The microbial strains will always be different, depending on which veggies are used and whether the growing conditions are anaerobic or aerobic, or which wild organisms are in the air. But that's fine. A variety of these foods provide a well-rounded array of beasties. Box 16.1 provides a protocol for introducing fermented food into the diet.
- *What not to eat.* Avoid antibiotics, whenever possible, because they indiscriminately kill off both good and bad bacteria and lead to yeast overgrowth. Say *no* to processed foods, chlorinated water, antibacterial soap, and foods sprayed with carcinogenic Roundup (a glyphosate weed killer). These culprits kill off the good with the bad.

• BOX 16.1 Tips of the Trade: The Gut and Fermented Kefir

A clinical herbalist frequently begins by helping clients fix the gut even before a single herb is administered. When digestion functions properly, herbs can be absorbed and utilized efficiently.

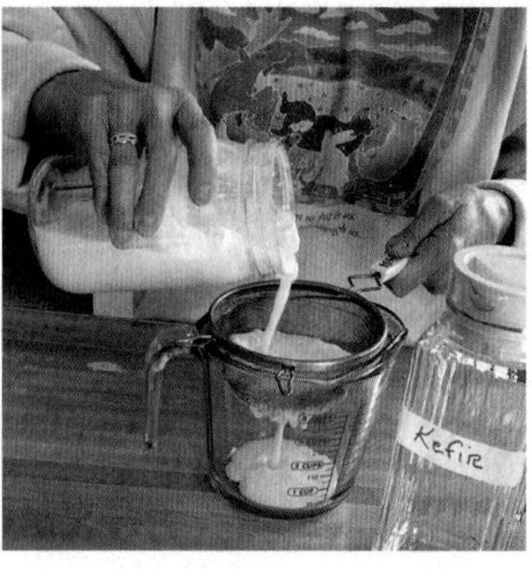

Rachel straining fermented kefir.

A nifty way to fix the gut is with all kinds of fermented foods, starting with lactose-free kefir. Kefir is fermented milk made with a culture that can be easily and economically made at home with a little instruction. It is rich in viable probiotics that aid digestion and snuff out gut inflammation. Kefir kills unfriendly bacteria, yeasts, and fungi while adding the good stuff, an amazing way to improve digestion. A plain, unsweetened kefir smoothie, sometimes with fruits and veggies added, provides a nourishing morning digestive aid, so any morning supplements can be better absorbed.

Fermented foods protocol.[2]

- Fermented foods must be taken *every day* to make a difference. Begin user-friendly kefir slowly, with ¼ cup for 4 days, then ½ cup for 4 days, up to 1½ to 2 cups per day.
- Encourage adding fermented veggies—like sauerkraut or kimchi on a sandwich or rice cracker—to the diet. Include pickles. Clients can ferment their own cauliflower, carrots, onions, and cabbage. Once done, they should store these fermented vegetables in the fridge. Add to salads and other foods at lunch and dinner.
- The goal is to work up to daily kefir and one large forkful of fermented veggies 2 times daily.

Herbal Categories That Build Up the Microbiome and Help Leaky Gut

The following is a list of herbal categories that might be chosen in a leaky-gut formula (Table 16.2). Generally, pick one or two from each category as needed, depending on the person's condition. Nothing is written in stone, and a good assessment is needed for each person so that formulas can be individualized. More on this in Chapter 18.

- *Bitters.* Herbs with a bitter taste are called ***bitters***, such as Dandelion leaf, Turmeric root, or Hops strobile. They stimulate digestion and have long been used in various cultures in cocktails and tonic waters, and taken before meals to get digestive enzymes, saliva, and bile flowing. Bitter taste receptors have actually been found in the gut, indicating that the intestines are hungry for that taste. Bitters stimulate hepatic and biliary function, help fat digestion and bowel movement, and bring down elevated blood hemoglobin A1C that occurs in metabolic syndrome/insulin resistance. Common food sources are dark greens like kale or arugula, coffee, hops, olives, and dark chocolate. Some bitters have specific prebiotic properties and feed the flora with needed fructo-oligosaccharides. Bitters are forbidden in hyperacidity, especially with duodenal ulcers.[3]
- *Cholagogues.* Herbs that promotes discharge of bile from the gallbladder are ***cholagogues***. Examples are Barberry root, Wild Indigo root, or Blue Flag rhizome (Fig. 16.1). Bile salts stimulate growth of gut bacteria[3] and help bowels move. Cholagogues also increase liver function and fat metabolism.
- *Antimicrobials and antiinflammatories.* All kinds of microorganisms can overload the gut, including yeast overgrowth (*Candida albicans*), bacteria, fungus, and viruses. Pick the appropriate herb if you know the offending organism or choose broad-spectrum antibiotic herbs to cover the bases, such as Scutellaria Huang Qin (Baikal Skullcap root), Echinacea root, or *Usnea* spp. (Old Man's Beard thallus). Cooling antimicrobials tend to be anti- inflammatory.

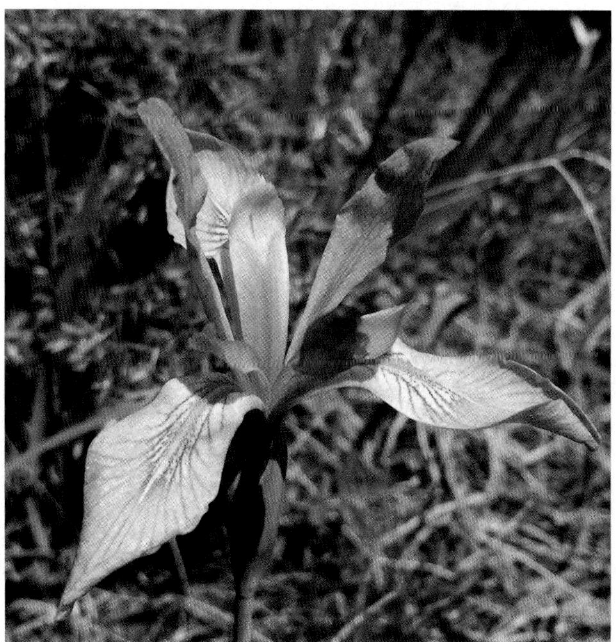

• **Fig. 16.1** Blue *Iris versicolor* (Blue Flag/Wild Iris) blooms in wet areas. The rhizome is a strong cholagogue that stimulates bile flow and growth of friendly gut bacteria.

- *A protocol for broad-spectrum antimicrobials* is called the "weed and feed" approach—out with the bad and in with the good, but just not at the same time. The idea is to alternate and separate the times that bad gut bacteria, fungi, and protozoa are being killed off from the times the gut is being fed. The method makes flora imbalances less likely and has a dampening effect on the regrowth of pathogenic bacteria.
  - *Two formulas are used.* A broad spectrum *weeding* antimicrobial formula is given in high doses for 3 days—for example, Saturday, Sunday, and Monday—to destroy bad bacteria (try Garlic bulb, a berberine such as Coptis Huang Lian, and Oregano herb). Then the *feeding* formula is given the rest of the week to nourish the gut (Slippery Elm bark, Green Tea leaf, and Grape seed extract).[3] Continue for a minimum of 6 weeks. Give the herbs along with prebiotic and probiotic foods already suggested.
- *Restoratives.* Any weak and damaged tissue needs to be healed and then nourished and reconditioned to its original good condition. A good formula includes a restorative, such as Milk Thistle seed (liver) or Mullein leaf (lungs).
- *Demulcents.* Herbs that help to cool and moisten (***demulcents***) are used to decrease inflammation in a damaged intestinal tract. They also feed the gut, although it takes a high dose to be effective for this; use Slippery Elm bark or Irish Moss thallus.
- *Drying herbs for Spleen Damp.* In Chinese Medicine, *dysbiosis* with overproduction of mucus is a classic Spleen Damp situation. The fix is to reduce damp by using dry, warm, and pungent antimicrobials. Examples are Cinnamomum Rou Gui (Cinnamon bark), Thyme herb, and fresh Horseradish (both tinctured and in edible form). Magnolia Hou Po (Magnolia bark), Eugenia Ding Xiang (Clove bud), Thyme herb, and Garden Sage leaf are especially drying. Atractylodes Cang Zhu (Black Atractylodes root) kills damp like nobody's business and tackles all types of gut microbes, especially yeast overgrowth which is common when antibiotics are overused (Chapter 18).

Inflammation: The Good and the Bad

When working properly, ***acute inflammation*** is the body's normal attempt at self-protection and promotes the removal of harmful stimuli, including damaged cells, irritants, or pathogens. When we have an infected cut finger, the inflammatory cascade gets busy. The finger becomes red, hot, swollen, and painful. The immune system reacts normally. White blood cells remove pathogens; blood and lymph remove excess edema and fluid. Alarm substances are released: prostaglandins, interleukins, leukotrienes, and eicosanoids. These trigger the *inflammatory cascade* or pathway. Our finger heals, pain is resolved, and the inflammatory response ends. All's well that ends well.

Chronic, ***pathological inflammation*** is another story and can last month or years. In this case, the inflammatory response is triggered when there are no foreign invaders to fight off. The body responds as if normal tissues are infected or somehow abnormal. But they're not. The immune system won't shut off. This response is misdirected inflammation, and it sets the person up for chronic disease and pain, cognitive decline, heart disease, and autoimmune reactions where inflammation attacks healthy tissue, such as the joints, the heart, brain, uterus, pancreas, or any individual weak area.

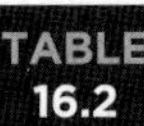

TABLE 16.2 Herbal Categories that Heal the Gut Mucosa and Balance the Microbiome

The two traditional Western bitters that help digestion *Gentiana lutea* (Gentian root) *Artemisia absinthium* (Wormwood herb) **Other bitters** *Hydrastis canadensis* (Goldenseal root) *Coptis chinensis* Huang Lian (Goldthread root) *Berberis vulgaris* (Barberry root) *Menyanthes trifoliate* (Bogbean herb) *Citrus aurantium* Zhi Shi (Bitter Orange fruit) *Cinchona* spp. (Cinchona bark) Source of the antimalarial quinine, bitter digestive aid *Matricaria recutita* (Chamomile flower) *Taraxacum officinale* (Dandelion root and leaf) Small doses work well for digestive aids 5–10 drops of a 1:5 tincture	**Antimicrobials to weed out bad bacteria and clear heat and inflammation** **The berberines** *Coptis chinensis* Huang Lian (Goldthread root) *Hydrastis canadensis* (Goldenseal root) *Mahonia aquifolium* (Oregon Grape root) *Phellodendron amurense* Huang Bai (Siberian Cork Tree bark) **Other antimicrobials** *Allium sativum* (Garlic bulb) *Larrea divaricata* (Creosote bush) *Syzygium aromatica* (Clove bud) *Thymus vulgarus* (Thyme essential oil) *Cinnamomum cassia* Rou Gui (Cinnamon bark) – especially anti-fungal *Magnolia officinalis* Hou Po (Magnolia bark) – classic gut antimicrobial *Armoracia rusticana* (Horseradish root) *Atractylodes lancea* Cang Zhu (Black Atractylodes) – especially kills *Candida albicans*
Bitter prebiotics that feed the gut *Artemisia absinthium* (Wormwood herb) *Taraxacum officinalis* (Dandelion root/leaf) *Cichorium intybus* (Chicory root) **Other gut feeders** *Origanum vulgare* (Oregano essential oil) *Camellia sinensis* (Green tea leaf) Grape seed extract—purchase this one	**Traditional Western stomach/leaky gut healers** *Matricaria recutita* (Chamomile flower) *Filipendula ulmaria* (Meadowsweet herb) *Ulmus fulva* (Slippery Elm bark) *Glycyrrhiza glabra* (Licorice root) *Calendula officinalis* (Calendula flower) *Symphytum officinale* (Comfrey root)
Cholagogues help produce BMs and gut flora *Citrus reticulata* Chen Pi (Ripe Tangerine peel) *Citrus reticulata* Qing Pi (Green Tangerine peel) *Artemisia vulgaris* (Mugwort herb) *Curcuma longa* (Turmeric root) *Iris versicolor* (Blue Flag rhizome) *Gentiana lutea* (Gentian root) Decongests liver	**Nutritive gut restoratives** *Arctium lappa* (Burdock root) *Chondrus crispus* (Irish Moss thallus) *Stellaria media* (Chickweed herb) *Urtica dioica* (Nettle herb) *Taraxacum officinale* (Dandelion root) *Avena sativa* (Milky Oat berry) *Trifolium pratense* (Red Clover flower)
Mucilages feed healthy bacteria and cool inflammation: They must be taken in large doses to be effective *Ulmus fulva* (Slippery Elm bark) *Althea officinalis* (Marshmallow root) *Aloe vera* (Aloe gel) *Trigonella foenum-graecum* (Fenugreek seed)	**Resolve mucous damp with drying herbs** *Allium sativum* (Garlic bulb) *Salvia officinale* (Garden Sage leaf) –antimicrobial *Eugenia caryophyllata* Ding Xiang (Clove bud) – antimicrobial *Thymus vulgarus* (Thyme essential oil) –antimicrobial

Chronic inflammation is caused primarily by dysbiosis. Contributing factors are poor diet, toxins, stress, heavy exercise, trauma, and even fasting and cleanses. Chronic inflammation can also be caused from chronic infection, adrenal exhaustion, poor immune functioning, and toxic environmental exposures. The fix is to normalize gut flora and indulge in an antiinflammatory diet with lots of veggies. Add whole grains, grass-fed meat, and healthy fats, including cold water marine fish and oil, and back way off processed foods, sugar, high-fructose corn syrup, and junk foods. It's the same old mantra.

Huge lists of herbs in the literature cite antiinflammatory botanicals. Most are useless because they're too general. A few herbs have tropisms to particular body systems and help reduce pain and inflammation. Think energetics. Inflammation is a hot condition, so most cooling herbs automatically tend to help inflammation. For instance, Scutellaria Huang Qin (Baikal Skullcap root) is a cold, bitter herb and a broad-spectrum antimicrobial and antiallergic. It is used in heat stages of infection and acute allergy (which is also hot), so by its very nature it is antiinflammatory by default. When choosing Huang Qin, we are adding the antimicrobial piece and inadvertently addressing inflammation. This is an elegant use of a single herb to accomplish a lot. Some of the best dietary choices to help inflammation are the use of omega-3 FAs and antiinflammatory foods (Table 16.3).

Oxidative Stress

When chronic inflammation takes hold, free radical damage or ***oxidative stress*** occurs at the cellular level. This process damages

TABLE 16.3 Superfoods and Herbs to Help Snuff Out Pathological Inflammation

Herbs	Supplements/Foods
Boswellia serrata (Frankincense tears) Muscular skeletal tropism	Omega 3 Fatty Acids (EPA/DHA)
Zingiber officinale (Ginger root) Gut-related	Cold water marine fish and their oils—salmon, tuna, cod, herring, kippers, anchovies
Curcuma longa (Turmeric root) Brain food for Alzheimer's and pain	Golden Flax seeds (ground)
Scutellaria baicalensis Huang Qin Baikal Skullcap root Allergies/skin/gut, infection/toxicosis	Probiotics *Lactobacillus acidophilus* and *Bifidobacterium* spp. and others, to be well-balanced
Solidago canadensis (Goldenrod herb) This herb goes to kidneys	Brightly colored veggies: carrots, tomatoes, squash, blueberries, all cruciferous
Matricaria recutita (Chamomile flower) Topical use	Walnuts (omega-3)
Melaleuca alternifolia Tea Tree essential oil (topical use)	Pumpkin seeds (omega-3)

DNA and cell membranes and is implicated as a cause of premature aging and degenerative diseases, including cancer.

Oxidative stress begins in the liver (Chapter 19) with the formation of rogue, unstable molecules called *reactive oxygen species* (ROS). As the liver detoxifies, it breaks down metabolites into ***free radicals***, which are unstable oxygen molecules that have lost an electron, but need that extra electron to remain stable. A well-functioning liver (with the help of antioxidant-containing foods) eventually breaks down free radicals into water-soluble molecules that can be harmlessly excreted through the bowel and bladder.

If the liver becomes overwhelmed with its normal load and by too many added exogenous toxins, it becomes overworked (and underpaid in nutrients). It can't keep up with the large influx of free radicals, which cause a destructive molecular chain reaction as they attempt to pick up their missing electrons. They steal electrons from one another, and more and more free radicals develop, playing havoc in the body. Damaging oxidation or oxidative stress is similar to how oxygen causes iron to rust. This alarming scenario is the result of chronic inflammation.

A healthy liver that detoxifies free radicals efficiently is helped along by antioxidants. ***Antioxidants*** are substances that inhibit oxidation by donating electrons to neutralize free radicals. They include vitamins C and E, selenium, and flavonoids. They are available in supplement form, but the best sources are from herbs and whole foods: fruits and vegetables. The purer the diet (minimizing food additives, preservatives, and drugs), the fewer free radicals are produced and the less oxidative stress occurs. Foods and herbs that potentially have an effect on health beyond basic nutrition are called ***functional foods*** or superfoods. They reduce oxidative stress, may be prebiotics or probiotics, are filled with antioxidants, vitamins and minerals, and promote optimal health (Box 16.2).

BOX 16.2 Some Functional Foods (Superfoods) That Reduce Oxidative Stress

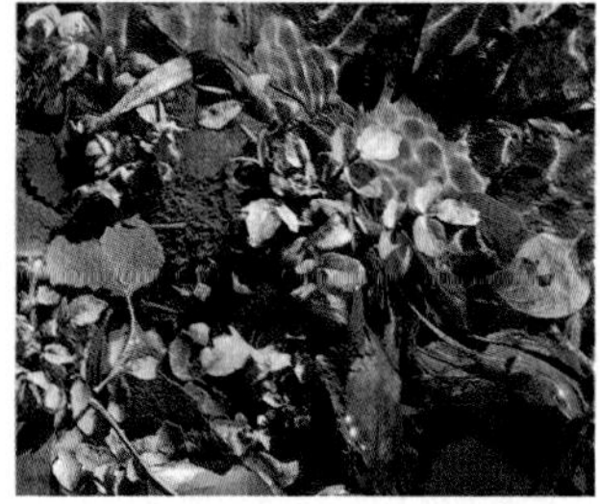

Watercress in early winter growing in shallow, slow-moving, cold mountain stream. It is a pungent Mustard family superfood filled with chlorophyll, vitamins, and minerals.

Urtica dioica (Nettle herb) Liver/blood/kidneys.
Nasturtium officinale (Watercress herb) Neuroendocrine and immune system.
Lentinula edodes (Shitake mushroom) Stimulates immune T cells.
Grifola frondosa (Maitake mushroom) Another superior immune food.
Sesamum indicum (Sesame seed) Nervous system, cholesterol reduction, skin health.
Allium sativa (Garlic bulb) Immune, infection, dysbiosis.
Spirulina spp. and *Chlorella* spp. (Microalgae) Contain vitamins, minerals, essential FAs.
Granum floris pollinis (Flower pollen) Allergies, immune, broad-spectrum antibiotic.
Camellia sinensis (Green Tea leaf) Antioxidant, repairs DNA.
Sambucus nigra (Elderberry) Immune function and inhibits colds and flu.
Vitis spp. (Grape seed and skin) Contains resveratrol, anticancer effects.
Lycium Gou Qi Zi (Goji or Wolfberry) Tonic, antioxidant, longevity.
Red, *Blue*, and *Black berries*, the queens of flavonoid antioxidants.

General Food Guidelines to Maintain Health

Our epidemic of obesity in children is accompanied by early-onset type 2 diabetes, allergies, and food sensitivities, autoimmune diseases, and eventual chronic dementias. All are testaments to the typical Standard American Diet (SAD) that is filled with sugar, saturated fats, and fast foods. It's no wonder that the first three letters in the word *diet* are *d-i-e*.

Healthy food choices are not really complicated. The following are generalities for healthy food choices and habits:

- *Dietary habits.* Which diet does one choose and why? There are some benefits to most, but no one kind fits all. Here are some food idiosyncrasies and general dietary guidelines.
  - *Vegetarians.* The ***vegetarian diet*** is a broad category that excludes meat protein from the diet. *Vegans* consume no animal protein whatsoever. *Lactovegetarians* eat plant foods and dairy but no eggs. *Ovo-lactovegetarians* eat plant foods, dairy, and eggs.
  - *Gluten-free* folks steer clear of ***gluten***, the sticky, allergy-producing protein found in wheat products, barley, rye, triticale, and oats. Instead, they choose gluten-free grains such as rice, amaranth, quinoa, millet, or buckwheat. Going gluten-free often helps with bloating, indigestion, and weight loss in susceptible individuals.
  - *Lactose-free.* ***Lactose*** is the sugar present in milk and dairy to which many are sensitive. Dairy products fermented with lactic acid bacteria like *Lactobacillus* are more digestible. Kefir, yogurt, cheese, and buttermilk are examples of fermented dairy foods.
- *How often and what?* It's surprisingly easy to have a boring diet when eating the same few foods most every day. Keeping a food diary helps to get a handle on what one really consumes. No cheating or omissions are allowed for this enlightening project. If diet is an issue, have clients keep a food diary as a homework assignment after the first consult. Record *all* foods ingested over a period of weeks, including snacks and mindless munching. A *rotating diet* fills in nutrient gaps and ensures a well-rounded array. Clients should not get into a food rut.
- *Rainbow diet.* Have a multicolored plateful, and you can't go wrong. The ***rainbow diet*** with varied colored foods translates into a full selection of vitamins and antioxidants.
  - *Carotenoids* contain a group of *orange* and *yellow* antioxidants: carrots, butternut squash, yellow and orange bell peppers, pumpkin, corn, and sweet potatoes. Carotenoids help vision, skin, bones, heart, and the immune system.
  - *Lycopenes* are *red* nutrients found in raspberries, apples, beets, red peppers, radishes, red onions, rhubarb, and tomatoes that boost immunity, memory, and urinary health.
  - *Anthocyanins* are the *blues* and *purples* found in blueberries, eggplant, plums, purple cabbage, purple peppers, purple potatoes, and purple onions; anthocyanins are antiinflammatory and reduce risk of cardiovascular disease, benefit cognitive function, and prevent some types of cancer.
  - *Chlorophylls* are the *greens* that help prevent cancer and are found in collards, asparagus, broccoli, celery, peas, spinach, and zucchini.
- *How much water?* This one varies, but two-thirds of the body is made up of water and for babies, even more. We require water for metabolism, digestion, and elimination. A urine check is a good way to tell. It should be light yellow and mild smelling. If it's dark and stinky, dehydration is present. If we are thirsty, we are already dehydrated. Symptoms of dehydration include chapped lips, dry skin, dry sticky mouth, headache, weakness, dizziness, palpitations, fainting, decreased urine output, and no sweating.[4] Aside from poor intake, dehydration can be caused by diarrhea, vomiting, sweating, and diabetes. Clients with such symptoms should be advised to carry a bottle of water around and drink, especially when exercising.
  - *What should we drink?* Coffee is a dehydrating diuretic. Sports drinks contain high-fructose corn syrup. Sugary juices and colas are very sweet and unhealthy. The best choice is plain water or with a lemon slice thrown in to stimulate the liver. Herbal teas are a close second. Next best comes coconut water or some unflavored sparkling water. It is best to drink water between, rather than with meals.
- *Eating out.* If this is a frequent habit, beware. It is hard to come by healthy choices in most restaurants. Learning to cook is a better option, because you have knowledge and control of ingredients. But stay clear of the microwave.
- *Beans.* Generally, these are a healthy form of carbohydrates. It is best to soak in water overnight to remove the phytic acid in their skins which blocks mineral absorption. Rinse before and after cooking to decrease and dispose of the phytic acid and to reduce the gas factor caused by their oligosaccharide content that the body cannot metabolize. Kidney, black, adzuki, and pinto beans are good options. Previously cooked organic canned beans that are packed in water (no sugar added) are quick options. Rinse before using.
- *Red meat.* Grass-fed, organic, and free-range meat is an eater's choice. Vegetarians often lack vitamin B_{12}, which comes only from animal protein such as meat, chicken, fish, and shellfish. Sometimes soy, a good source of protein, is fortified with vitamin B_{12}.
- *Intermittent fasting.* The ***intermittent fasting*** approach involves restricting daily eating to 14 to 16 hours a day, allowing the gut time to chill out, empty, and shift from burning sugar to burning fat as its primary fuel.
  - *Fat is slow burning* and will prevent the typical glucose highs and lows that accompany insulin resistance. By burning fat, nutritional ketosis is achieved.[5] Burning fat helps with obesity, hypertension, sugar cravings, high cholesterol, dementia, oxidative stress, and cancer.
  - *Nighttime is the worst possible time to eat* because that is the GI system's 24-hour Chinese clock moment to detox and rejuvenate. The gut needs about 12 hours of rest with no food intake at all to burn up the sugar stored as glycogen in the liver.
  - *Intermittent fasting protocol.* The idea is to maintain a healthy diet but to eat only two meals a day, making sure the last meal is 3 whole hours before bedtime. No late-night snacking and no grazing throughout the day. Otherwise the gut has no time to rest. It's not that hard. This schedule can be individually tailored. If breakfast is skipped, make lunch the first meal of the day. Eat lunch at 11:00 a.m. and finish dinner before 7:00 p.m. If you eat breakfast, the window might be between 8:00 a.m. and 4:00 p.m. Even intermittent fasting 1, 2, or 3 days a week is beneficial and better than nothing.

Types of Diets

The least food faddy, gimmicky diets follow. They are based on sound principles and research, and have been around for a good long run.

- *Mediterranean diet.* The much-studied, antiinflammatory ***Mediterranean diet*** began in the 1960s, making it less a fad and more of a go-to lifestyle, which can be modified as needed. It was based on the dietary traditions of Crete, Greece, and southern Italy at a time when the rates of chronic disease in that region were among the lowest in the world, and adult life expectancy was the highest. The Mediterranean diet has been shown to reduce the risk of heart disease, certain cancers, diabetes, Parkinson's, and Alzheimer's. It is the typical antiinflammatory diet that can be tailored to many individual requirements, such as vegetarian, vegan, lactose, or gluten-free diets.

- *Protocol.* It consists of primarily fresh plant-based foods, such as fruits and vegetables, whole grains, legumes, and nuts. It emphasizes healthy fats such as olives, olive oil, avocados, coconut oil, moderate consumption of fish, shellfish, poultry, and whole grains. Red meat is kept at a minimum. It even includes a glass of antioxidant red wine daily, if so inclined.

- *Paleolithic diet.* This is also called the paleo, cave dweller, or Stone Age diet and is based on the premise that our digestion hasn't changed that much since prehistoric times, so why push it? The ***Paleolithic diet*** hunter-gatherer approach forces one to cut back on processed foods, simple carbs, additives and chemicals and to eat a clean, healthy diet.
  - *Protocol.* A paleo diet uses whole foods: a lot of meat, organ meats, veggies, fruits, nuts, seeds, roots, and healthy fats. It excludes agricultural grains, sugar, legumes, processed foods, salt, alcohol, and coffee. Many find this approach provides more energy, helps with insulin and leptin resistance, and achieves weight loss when it seems those last 10 pounds won't ever melt away. It can be quite beneficial.
- *Gut and Psychology Syndrome (GAPS) protocol.* The ***GAPS protocol*** and lifestyle change program was developed by Dr. Natasha Campbell-McBride and is a good bet for the toughies like severe digestive and neurological issues, autoimmune diseases, IBD, hyperactivity, chronic depression, and anxiety. It establishes a connection between the digestive system and the brain, the gut-brain connection (Chapter 23), and was originally and successfully used for children and adults with several neurological and psychiatric conditions, including autism, attention deficit, bipolar disorders, and depression.[6] Its use now extends to autoimmune problems in just about any body system and even to problems such as chronic eczema and tooth cavities.
  - *Protocol.* GAPS is an elimination diet that proceeds in various stages, slowly reintroducing more and more foods. The intention is to heal and seal a leaky gut and eventually build the flora (Chapter 18). It begins with meat stock, simmered meats or poultry and their bones and joints, good-quality fat, and easily digested nonfibrous vegetables. Further stages proceed to raw, cultured dairy products and ghee, and then to lacto (lactic acid)-fermented vegetables. Finally, soaked nuts, certain beans and seeds, and to a lesser extent, grains, are added. *Bone broth* simmered for many hours is introduced during the transition diet at the very end of the protocol.[7] The process can take up to 2 years or more, but the results can be outstanding. GAPS is strict but can work miraculously when all else fails. It is a great tool to have in your pocket.

A Healthy Immune System

Maintaining a healthy, vigorous immune system includes keeping the microbiome balanced, keeping inflammation and oxidative stress to a minimum, and maintaining a good antiinflammatory diet. Those measures help keep us relatively flu- and cold-free most of the time. They are important physical-level factors.

Particular foods that boost immunity are vitamin C-rich: red bell peppers, kiwi, papaya, strawberries, and citrus and dark greens, such as spinach. Garlic, onions, and ginger are classics. The antiinflammatory magical mushrooms, such as turkey tail, shitake, maitake (Hen of the Woods), Ganoderma Ling Zhi (Reishi mushroom) are rich in antioxidants, B vitamins, and polysaccharides. They modulate inflammatory cytokines, boost immunity, balance blood sugar, and fight cancer and aging. Not only that, they are delicious and flavorful (Box 16.3). Many are available in farmers' markets, health food stores, and Asian food markets.

There are also emotional, spiritual, and environmental stressors to consider. Situations come along that are one-time events and cause us to become run down and then sick. But if someone develops infections on a regular basis, such as three or more colds a year regardless of external factors, then the immune system is shouting for attention. Tips for good immune function include:

- *Keep stress/emotional/mental health in check.* First, listen well. Suggest stress-management techniques tailored to the client.

• BOX 16.3 Delicious Immune Soup (Adapted from Andrew Weil's Eight Weeks to Optimum Health)[8]

Some of the best foods for the immune system include Lily family Onions and Garlic, antiinflammatory Ginger root, adaptogenic Astragalus Huang qi root, and nutrient-filled mushrooms (not the white button variety).

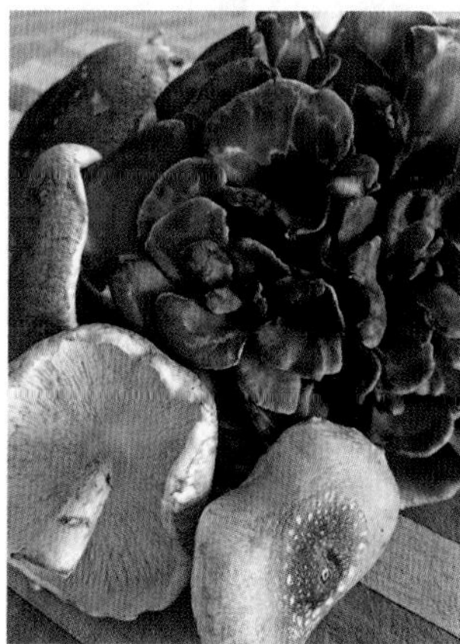

Lentinula edodes (Shitake mushroom) and *Grifola frondosa* (Maitake/Hen of the Woods mushroom) are key players in our immune soup.

2 cups fresh Shiitake mushrooms (or 1 cup dried, woody stems removed)
1 large Reishi and/or Maitake mushroom
5 pieces sliced Astragalus Huang Qi root
1½ piece of freshly grated Ginger root
1 onion, diced
1 garlic bulb, diced
8 cups water
1 tablespoon olive oil
1½ cups salted vegetable broth, bone broth, or soup stock
Cayenne powder if desired

Instructions.

Bring water to boil in large pot. Heat olive oil. Sauté garlic, onions, and ginger until soft and aromatic. Add the maitakes and shitakes to the sauté. Add veggie broth, sautéed items, and Reishi mushroom to the water. Simmer covered for 2 hours. Remove Astragalus pieces and Reishi. Add salt and pepper to taste, then just enough cayenne powder to bring about a light sweat.

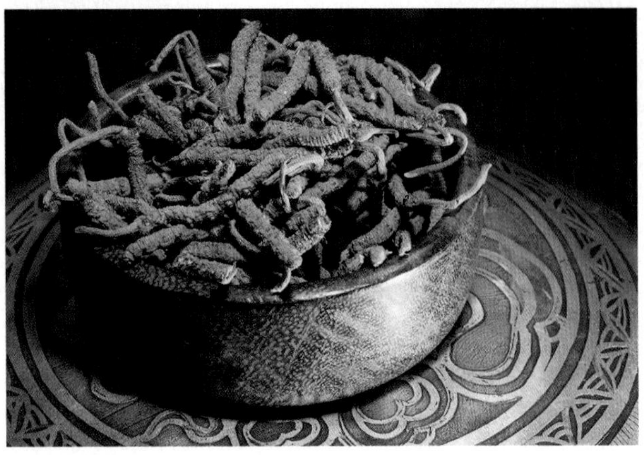

• **Fig. 16.2** Cordyceps Dong Chong Xia Cao (Chinese Caterpillar mushroom fruiting body) is an adaptogen with an affinity to the lungs. (iStock.com/IgotChus).

Exercise, meditation, essential oils, breathing, massage, and taking walks. Refer clients to a psychotherapist as needed. Often, symptoms like depression and anxiety lessen when the body is in balance.

- *Spiritual connection.* This factor is important. Longevity and good health are frequently linked to a connection with a spiritual other. It doesn't matter who or what, just that it's there.
- *All my friends and relations.* Having good friends and family ties makes us healthier and is linked to longevity. People in committed, meaningful partnerships seem to have stronger immunity than those living alone.
- *Good-quality sleep.* This has been associated with increased immune killer cells, more resistance to infection, and whole-body health. A good 8 hours is needed to rejuvenate, regenerate, and sort out yesterday's stress and problems. Lack of sleep is linked to obesity, chronic illnesses, cancer, heart disease, and decreased learning and memory. It is critical for

TABLE 16.4 Some Exceptional Trophorestoratives per Body System *(Superfoods and herbs with specific tropisms)*

Gastrointestinal	Endocrine	Reproduction and Nervous	Liver
Glycyrrhiza spp. Gan Cao Licorice root For ulcers *Atractylodes macrocephala* Bai Zhu White Atractylodes root *Codonopsis pilosula* Dang Shen Downy Bellflower root *Medicago sativa* Alfalfa herb High in minerals.	*Ginseng* spp. All ginsengs support the glands. *Withania somnifera* Ashwagandha herb General to all glands. *Glycyrrhiza* spp. Licorice root Glycyrrhiza Gan Cao For Adrenal support. *Urtica dioica* Nettle herb Adrenal support. **Sea veggies** Kelp Irish Moss Iceland Moss All for thyroid support.	*Serenoa serrulata* Saw Palmetto berry *Avena sativa* Milky Oat berry and straw Bee Pollen *Glycyrrhiza* spp. Gan Cao Licorice root *Panax* spp. Ginsengs are noted to support the adrenals. *Urtica dioica* Nettle herb Mineral-rich.	*Taraxacum officinale* Dandelion root *Silybum marianum* Milk Thistle seed *Cynara scolymus* Artichoke leaf *Urtica dioica* Nettle herb *Schisandra chinensis* Wu Wei Zi Five Taste berry *Lycium chinense* Gou Qi Zi Wolfberry *Astragalus membranaceus* Huang Qi Beets – liver food.
Kidney/Lungs/Skin	**Immune**	**Muscular-Skeletal/Connective Tissue**	**Heart**
Solidago spp. Goldenrod herb Kidney and skin. *Galium aparine* Cleavers herb Kidney and skin *Cuscuta chinensis* Ti Si Zi Asian Dodder seed Kidney. *Astragalus membranaceus* Huang Qi Lungs. *Cordyceps sinensis* Dong Chong Xia Cao Chinese Caterpillar mushroom Lungs and general adaptogen.	*Echinacea* spp. All species are adaptogens. *Atractylodes macrocephala* Bai Zhu White Atractylodes root *Astragalus membranaceus* Huang Qi *Salvia officinalis* Garden Sage herb Adrenal/immune support.	*Equisetum arvense* Horsetail herb Trace minerals/lungs. *Eucommia ulmoides* Du Zhong Builds bones and sinews. *Eleuthero senticosus* Ci Wu Jia Siberian/Eleuthero ginseng root Misnomer, not really a ginseng. *Symphytum officinale* Comfrey root	*Crataegus* spp. Hawthorn berry *Ligusticum wallichii* Chuan Xiong Sichuan Lovage root *Ginkgo biloba* Ginkgo leaf *Salvia miltiorrhiza* Dan Shen Cinnabar Sage root *Allium sativa* Garlic clove

brain development in children and teenagers. Sleep flushes out neurodegenerative toxins in the spaces between brain cells that develop when we're awake.[9] One of these toxins is beta-amyloid, prevalent in Alzheimer's. A good sleeping environment is cool, dark, and free of electromagnetic disturbances from a TV, cell phones, and such.

- *Low environmental toxins.* Exposure to outside pollutants such as smoke, dust, industrial toxins, or exhaust from cars does not do our immune system any favors. These factors are the hardest to control, unless we have the unusual luxury of being able to relocate to a clean, pristine area. Detrimental factors include living near high-power electric and magnetic fields (EMFs); exposure to emissions from radio towers, power plants, and low-frequency electronic devices; and use of cell phones, computers, TVs, and electric blankets. Turn off what you're not using.
- *Wash your hands.* Sounds obvious. Good handwashing habits certainly help prevent spread of microorganisms. The Centers for Disease Control say keeping hands clean is one of the most important steps we can take to avoid getting sick and spreading germs to others.[10] This includes cleanliness for doorknobs, keyboards, and phones, all objects that are frequently touched. As a former nurse, I can testify that the simple act of handwashing is not religiously carried out in hospital settings, causing many infections to be contracted when patients are hospitalized.
- *A little dirt doesn't hurt.* On the other hand, go easy on hand sanitizers because they can cause children to lose the ability to build up resistance to bacteria. Being too clean makes the immune system lazy.[11] Dirt is a healthy part of childhood, and overzealous hygiene is detrimental.
- *Limit antibiotic use.* The microbiome can easily develop toxic yeast overgrowth caused by antibiotics that kill bacterial friends and foes alike. Over the last 70 years or so, excessive antibiotic use has led to the development of *superbugs* that are resistant to many antibiotics, such as methicillin-resistant *Staphylococcus aureus* (often referred to as MRSA). Bacterial resistance is a serious world health problem that has resulted

TABLE 16.5 Adaptogens Are the Ultimate Balancers

Primary Adaptogens	Secondary Adaptogens	Companion Adaptogens
Studied and proven to definitely tonify and vitalize the HPA axis and the neuroendocrine system.	***Meet most criteria of primary adaptogens, but not as extensively studied, so we don't know definitively. Have been used for centuries. Indispensable and by all means, combine with the primaries.***	***These go along with, enhance, and synergize effects of adaptogens. Many superfoods and other nutritious herbs are in this category.***
Panax quinquefolium Xi Yang Shen American ginseng root Adrenals and gut, yin deficiency	*Astragalus membranaceus* Huang Qi Restores liver	*Glycyrrhiza* spp. Gan Cao and Western Licorice root Immune, hyperglycemia, adrenals, and gut
Withanea somnifera Ashwagandha root	*Bacopa monnieri* Bacopa stem/leaf	*Lycium chinensis* Gou Qi Zi Goji berry Antioxidant
Panax ginseng Ren Shen Asian ginseng	*Centella asiatica* Ji Xue Cao Gotu Kola leaf Central nervous system	*Codonopsis pilosula* Dang Shen GI/Spleen restorative Need large doses
Rhodiola rosea Rhodiola root Antidepressant	*Polygonum multiflorum* He Shou Wu Neuro/slows aging process	*Echinacea* spp. Increases WBCs/immunity
Schisandra chinensis Wu Wei Zi Liver	*Ocimum tenuiflorum* Holy Basil or Tulsi herb Ayurvedic/woman's repro	*Cinnamomum cassia* Rou Gui Cinnamon bark Balances glucose, yang tonic
Eleutherococcus senticosus Ci Wu Jia Siberian ginseng root Nervous system	*Panax notoginseng* San Qi Wound healing and bruising	*Crataegus* spp. Hawthorn berry Primary Western heart tonic
Ganoderma lucidum Ling Zhi Reishi mushroom	*Asparagus racemosus* Shatavari root Yin tonic	*Salvia officinalis* Garden Sage leaf Western longevity, elixir, qi tonic
Aralia spp. Manchurian Spikenard root	*Rehmannia glutinosa* Shu Di Huang For Liver, builds blood	*Zizyphus jujube* Da Zao Red Date Liver/GI restorative[11]

in many truly needed wonder drugs becoming no longer effective for treatment of life-threatening infections.

- *Regular exercise.* Moving around improves health, increases circulation of immune cells throughout the body, and aids in elimination of toxins. Exercise may or may not actually increase the actual number of immune cells, but it definitely benefits heart, mental status, and other chronic diseases.
- *The sun and full-spectrum lighting.* We all need sunlight, including the full electromagnetic spectrum, from infrared to near-ultraviolet light. These types of light encompass all the visible colors of the rainbow. Sunlight exposure activates immune T cells and helps decrease depression and stress. Sunlight also optimizes vitamin D production, which is crucial for immune function.
- *Immune fighting supplements.* Vitamin D_3 is essential, especially to fight the flu. Many doctors will order blood levels drawn when requested. If results come out very low, below 45 to 60 ng/mL, 8,000 to 10,000 international units (IUs) a day for at least 3 months should bring levels up. Then recheck blood and adjust dose as needed. Vitamin D is a fat-soluble vitamin, and excessive accumulated amounts can cause indigestion and elevate blood calcium, leading to bone loss and osteoporosis.
- *Other supplements.* Use zinc picolinate, but no more than 20 mg a day, because higher amounts can lower levels of copper, an important trace mineral. Use vitamin C in the form of *acerola*, because this natural form does not cause diarrhea, which others do in large doses. Because vitamin C is water soluble, doses can be high: up to 7 to 10 g per day if sick or on the verge. You cannot overdose on vitamin C. Being a water-soluble vitamin, a person just pees out any excess.

Materia Medica to Maintain Health

We're aiming to get the body healthy and practice preventative herbalism. An important way to do this is to incorporate *restoratives*, *adaptogens*, and *tonics*, the foundational herbs that maintain health. Herbs in these three categories have a lot of overlap. Many restoratives are thought of as adaptogens, and in some circles Chinese tonics are also considered to be like Western restoratives. Superfoods such as red, blue, and black berries, algae, bee pollen, and Milky Oat berry fit into the tonic/restorative classifications.

TABLE 16.6 Chinese Tonic Herbs and Western Equivalents

Qi	Blood	Yin	Yang
Panax ginseng Ren Shen Asian ginseng root Premier Chinese herb for qi deficiency	*Angelica sinensis* Dang Gui Angelica/Dong Quai Premier Chinese herb for blood deficiency	*Rehmannia glutinosa* Shu Di Huang (prepared) Sheng Di Huang (unprepared)	*Epimedium saggitatum* Yin Yang Hu Horny Goat Weed For Kidney yang deficiency, low libido
Codonopsis pilosula Dang Shen Spleen and lung qi deficiency	*Medicago sativa* Alfalfa herb Liver and blood deficiency, post-partum, pregnancy	*Ophiopogon japonicas* Mai Men Dong Lung yin deficiency	*Eucommia ulmoides* Du Zhong Builds bones and sinews
Salvia officinalis Garden Sage leaf Tonifies qi, blood, neuroendocrine	*Urtica dioica* Nettle herb Liver and blood deficiencies	*Panax quinquefolius* Xi Yang Shen American ginseng root For lung yin deficiency	*Cordyceps sinensis* Dong Chong Xia Cao Kidney yang and lung tonic
Astragalus membranaceus Huang Qi For lung qi deficiency	*Trifolium pratense* Red Clover flower Blood and yin tonic. For skin and lungs	*Polygonum vulgaris* Solomon's Seal root Yin and Spleen qi deficiency	*Cuscuta chinensis* Ti Si Zi Asian Dodder seed Low libido, urogenital discharges
Atractylodes macrocephala Bai Zhu White Atractylodes root Spleen qi deficiency	*Rehmannia glutinosa* Shu Di Huang Prepared, wine cured Tonifies Liver and blood	*Stellaria media* Chickweed herb Tonifies yin and blood	*Cervus nippon* Lu Rong Deer Antler Kidney yang tonic
Glycyrrhiza uralensis Gan Cao Licorice root	*Paeonia lactiflora* Bai Shao Yao White Peony root	Black Sesame seed For Kidney and Liver yin and blood	*Rosmarinus officinalis* Rosemary leaf Helps memory
Zizyphus jujuba Da Zao Jujube berry Liver qi and blood deficiency	*Cynara scolymus* Artichoke leaf Builds blood and liver	*Asparagus officinalis* Root interchangeable with Chinese Tian Men Dong and Ayurvedic Shatavari	*Atractylodes macrocephala* Bai Zu White Atractylodes root GI tropism
Dioscorea opposita Shan Yao Mountain Yam root Spleen and lung qi deficiency	*Taraxacum officinalis* Dandelion root Builds blood and liver yin	*Symphytum officinale* Comfrey leaf/root For connective tissue, throat, and gut	Chai tea Warming and builds yang

CASE HISTORY 16.1

Case History for Dysbiosis and Indigestion

S. Rosa is a 35-year-old single mom. She has two school-aged kids and holds down two jobs to make ends meet. She complains of chronic bloating, flatus, diarrhea, and stomach cramps. Sometimes she "can't think straight." She describes her life as very stressful. Most days, she resorts to fast-food take-out to get dinner on the table.
O. **P** Slippery and slow. **T** Sticky white coat.
A. Dysbiosis/Spleen Qi Deficiency/Damp and cold.
P. *Specific therapeutic principles.* (1) Warm and restore gut (Spleen). (2) Dry damp and resolve diarrhea. (3) Help indigestion, gas, and bloating with carminatives. (4) Decrease stress with essential oils.

Sample Formula and Dose: 4 mL 3 times per day between meals

Parts	Herb	Rationale
3	Atractylodes Bai Zhu White Atractylodes	Restore Spleen, warming tonic.
2	Magnolia Bark Hou Po	Dry Spleen damp/restore. Kill gut microbes.
2	Poria Fu Ling	Dry damp, help diarrhea.
2	Citrus Chen Pi Ripe Tangerine rind	Bitter, warming, carminative.
2	Meadowsweet herb	Heal gut, restore flora.
1	Thyme herb	Warming, drying.
1	Slippery Elm bark	Soothe inflammation/prebiotic, heal mucosa.

Other Suggestions

- Diet: Antiinflammatory Mediterranean with walnuts, green tea, and less fast food. Include lots of fermented foods. Fermented veggie: one forkful a day. Chai tea to warm and dry gut.
- Supplements: EPA/DHA (fish oil) to help inflammation. Also, begin probiotics in 1 month after gut is more healed.
- Lavender essential oil for stress.

CASE HISTORY 16.2

Case History for Weak Immune System

S. Janine is a 40-year-old attorney who is always traveling. Another business trip is pending. She has had five "colds" since January (it's May). She takes Tylenol when needed, frequent Emergen-C packets that contain 1000 mg of vitamin C, antioxidants, zinc, manganese, and B vitamins. She averages 6 hours sleep a night, and her energy is down. She rarely cooks; tries to eat "healthy" restaurant food when away.
O. **T** Pink. **P** Weak. She has dark circles under her eyes; skin is pale.
A. Weak Immune System, run down. Wei qi or protective qi deficiency.
P. *Specific therapeutic principles.* (1) Boost immunity with adaptogens, nutritive herbs, qi tonic herbs. (2) Gut restorative and blood building herbs. Inflammation.

Herbal Formula and Dose: 5 mL every a.m. and p.m. and before meals for 3 months, minimum

Parts	Herbs	Rationale
3	Astragalus Huang Qi	Boost wei qi and lungs/ adrenals.
2	Reishi Ling Zhi	Boost Immune and qi/ adrenals.
2	Nettle herb	Nutritive restorative/blood builder.
2	Lycium Gou Qi Zi	Companion adaptogen/ antioxidant.
2	Licorice root	Gut/adrenals/immune support/ qi tonic.

Other Suggestions

- Diet: Antiinflammatory. Try grocery store plain yogurt with added fresh fruit and nuts. Include salads, hard-boiled egg, or a whole piece of fruit at lunch. Discuss what healthy restaurant choices mean. Limit eating out to minimum. Raw nuts for snacking (walnuts, cashews). Medicinal mushrooms, such as shitake and maitake.
- Supplements: Liquid vitamin D_3 daily for immune health, EPA/DHA 1000 mg daily to help inflammation, Spirulina 2 times per day. Multivitamin with minerals daily.
- Sleep: Work towards 8 hours a night.
- Lunchtime: Walk in the sunshine.
- If sick, Emergen-C daily.

Restoratives

Restoratives are used in Western herbalism to target specific tissues or body parts to heal and build, improve function, and support vital energy. Some restoratives fall into the adaptogenic category, and others simply enhance the effects of adaptogens. Restoratives rebuild and strengthen tissue and are full of nutrients. Energetically, restoratives tend to be sweet, harmonizing, and balancing and are mild, nontoxic herbs safely used for long periods (Fig. 16.2). A particularly interesting immune-stimulating mushroom is Cordyceps Dong Chong Xia Cao (Chinese Caterpillar Mushroom fruiting body), which is parasitic on dead insect larva rather than on live or nonliving plant matter, like most other fungi. It is notably restorative to the lungs and bronchi but acts on the entire hypothalamic-pituitary-adrenal axis (HPA) as well (Chapter 27).

Some restoratives are general, in that they provide global nutrition for the entire body, much like a multivitamin. Others are sometimes called ***tropho-restoratives***, because they have an affinity for a specific organ and improve structure and function (Table 16.4). In a broad sense, restoratives can be considered tonics in the Chinese sense, because they address deficiency conditions. They are extremely useful for postpartum issues, mental stress, grief and worry, and weak constitutions.[12] In many formulas, restoratives are used solely for protection.

Adaptogens

This word is relatively new. It was coined in Russia in 1962 with the study of *Panax ginseng*, and then with *Eleutherococcus senticosus*, which was nicknamed Siberian or Eleuthero ginseng root. This common name led to confusion, because Eleuthero is not even in the ginseng family. ***Adaptogens*** reduce signs of the fight or flight phase of the immediate stress response and also help with long-term stress. Because stress causes so much disease and illness, we are blessed to have these botanicals. Their three major functions are that they normalize the HPA axis that deals with stress, decrease cortisol (an adrenal cortex stress hormone), and enhance the immune response.[13]

Additionally, they balance out all hormones and the nervous system and so are vitally important herbs to maintain health. Adaptogens are mild herbs that can be taken over a long term. The most studied adaptogens are from China, but that does not detract from those traditionally used for centuries in other major herbal traditions (Table 16.5).

Chinese Tonics

In China, ***tonics*** are targeted to build and maintain the broad categories of qi, blood, yin, and yang (Table 16.6). They are used when the body is deficient and weak and needs vital energy; they are important herbs that increase longevity. Some schools of thought say that tonics are not appropriate during acute illnesses because they could drive infection deeper into body. But I have personally found this not to be true, and that tonics can be taken safely over long periods of time, sick or not. This is especially the case with Astragalus Huang Qi and Ganoderma Ling Zhi (Reishi mushroom) which boost immune function during illness.

- *Qi tonics are nutrient-dense* and are used to enhance energy in chronic injury and illness, in cases of improper diet, and after childbirth. They help absorption and increase mitochondrial production of adenosine triphosphate (ATP), the energy molecule. Most adaptogens are considered qi tonics, and combine well with other tonic categories. Someone who requires a qi tonic would have **Pulse (P)** Weak and **Tongue (T)** Pale.
- *Blood tonics contain vitamins, minerals, amino acids, and enzymes.* They address nutritional deficiency and promote tissue growth. By doing this, they are said to *build blood,* enhance the *quality* of blood, but not necessarily increase the *quantity* of blood cells. They often target the Heart, Liver, and Spleen, when a person has palpitations, dizziness, pale complexion, and anemia or is underweight. **P** Fine. **T** Pale.
- *Yin tonics are cool, moist, sweet, and mucogenic.* They address hormones connected with the parasympathetic nervous system that increase secretions. They are needed when the mouth, skin, and orifices are dry. **P** Fine and rapid. **T** Red with little fur.
- *Yang tonics are warm, pungent, and stimulating.* They increase metabolism and enhance hormones associated with the sympathetic nervous system. They are indicated in a slow metabolism, low energy, coldness, or low libido. **P** Deep and weak. **T** Pale.[14] Many yang tonics double as qi tonics. In both situations the body needs energy and warmth.

CASE HISTORY 16.3

Case History for Assorted Problems

S. Joe drives a truck cross-country and lives on truck-stop and restaurant food. He belches, burps, and has a lot of gas and bloating. Furthermore, he has had many colds the last 2 years, more than usual. Takes no supplements or herbs but is willing to "give it a try." He has at least 3 energy drinks a day and drinks copious amounts of coffee. Sometimes his heart races, and he can feel it beat. He weighs 285 pounds and would like to lose 50 pounds.

O. **P** Slippery, strong. **T** Scalloped, yellow center/red body.

A. Dysbiosis, Spleen damp heat, lowered immunity, inflammation.

P. *Specific therapeutic principles.* (1) Normalize gut flora with bitters, cholagogues, restoratives, fermented foods. (2) Dry damp, cool gut. (3) Restore/detox liver caused by fast food and excessive caffeine intake. (4) Boost immunity with adaptogens, superfoods. (5) Lower inflammation and cool down heat with clean diet/herbs.

Herbal Formula and Dose: 5 mL 3 times a day between meals (Large dose; he's heavy.)

Parts	Herb	Rationale
4	Ashwagandha root	Immunity/energy in place of caffeine.
3	Schisandra Wu Wei Zi	Detox liver/immune restore/hypotensive.
2	Scutellaria Huang Qin	Bitter/gut restore/cooling/bitter.
2	Goldenrod herb	Dry damp/diuretic/toxicosis – cooling.
1	Citrus Chen Pi (ripe Tangerine rind, or Ching Pi (unripe, green Tangerine rind)	Ripe and unripe tangerine rinds/peels are both cholagogue/bitter/digestive aids, but unripe is considered more relaxant and anti-spasmodic.

Other Suggestions

- Diet: Mediterranean. Shop in grocery stores for fresh veggies, fruit, carrots, celery, yogurt, and hummus to take in truck. Keep kefir in truck cooler.
- Fast, easy food: Look for healthier fast food options such as Subway, Tokyo Joe's. When eating out, choose grilled fish and meats rather than fried foods, and choose veggies and baked potatoes rather than french fries. Use olive oil and vinegar, rather than creamy salad dressings. If diet is followed, client will probably lose weight.
- Healthy snack foods: Look for those available at truck stops, such as trail mixes with raw walnuts, other nuts/pumpkin/sunflower seeds, and dried fruit to increase EFAs/decrease inflammation; canned tuna, salmon, herring; hard-boiled eggs; boxed salads; plain yogurt; apples or oranges; and dark chocolate.
- Drinks: Replace caffeinated drinks with Chai/Green tea/Black tea, lemon water, or sparkling water.
- Breathing exercises: Practice when driving for stress.
- Supplements: Zinc 20 mg a day for immunity; EPA/DHA 1000 mg for inflammation/gut.

Common Conditions to Maintain the Body in Health

Each case history in this chapter, and thoughout Part Four (Therapeutics and Formulations) is presented in SOAP format. This organizational principle gets us from A to B in a logical sequence, covering all bases. There is no one right answer or definitive herbal formula for any given scenario. Case histories presented are representative to maintain the body in health. Many different herbs and strategies could arguably be used and would not be wrong. The general situations have been discussed in this chapter. (Case Histories 16.1, 16.2, and 16.3).

Summary

Optimum health can look very different for each person. Maintaining a healthy microbiome is an important mission for every herbalist. Processed foods, GMOs, and stress contribute to dysbiosis and intestinal permeability, bitters, GI restoratives, cholagogues, antimicrobials, and herbs to dry damp are often used to keep the flora in check. Important additions are prebiotics and probiotics (especially fermented foods).

Acute inflammation is a normal process the body uses to deal with injury that sends out alarm substances via the inflammatory cascade. However, chronic inflammation is pathological and causes heart, brain, and autoimmune diseases. Poor diet, dysbiosis, toxic overload, stress, and trauma are contributing factors. Oxidative stress is a result of too many free radicals, causing DNA and cellular damage. Intake of antioxidants, eliminating processed foods, and enjoying a clean environment are helpful.

Dietary guidelines to maintain health include a rainbow diet and plenty of fresh water. Herbalists should be familiar with the Mediterranean and paleolithic diets, and the Gut and Psychology Syndrome (GAPS) protocol for hard-to-treat mental and autoimmune problems. There are many tools to boost immunity to keep clients relatively free of infection. The techniques include physical, emotional, and spiritual measures. Herbally, adaptogens balance stress, restoratives build and strengthen tissue, and tonics tonify qi, blood, yin and yang.

Review

Fill in the Blanks

(Answers in Appendix B.)

1. Name three inflammatory cascade chemical triggers: ___, ___, ___.
2. Leaky gut is also called ___ and ___. Three causes are ___, ___, ___.
3. Four herbal categories used to treat IP are ___, ___, ___, ___.
4. Oxidative stress and cellular damage cause ___ and ___.
5. Name an herbal tropho-restorative for the liver ___, GI ___, adrenals ___, lungs ___, heart ___, kidneys ___.
6. Name four bitter foods: ___, ___, ___, ___.
7. Name five ways to improve immunity other than herbs: ___, ___, ___, ___, ___.
8. What two functions must a major adaptogen have? ___, ___.
9. Name three important categories of herbs that maintain health: ___, ___, ___.
10. The four types of Chinese tonics are ___, ___, ___, ___.

Critical Concept Questions

(Answers for you to decide.)

1. Explain the concept that optimum health is a continuum.
2. Is inflammation always bad? Explain.
3. What is the connection between fermented foods and gut health? How do they work?
4. Describe the kefir protocol for IP. What are its advantages in treating leaky gut?
5. Describe a generally healthy diet to your client. Include recommendations for water, healthy fats, meats, veggies, and snacks.
6. In China, Ganoderma Ling Zhi (Reishi mushroom) has been called an "imperial herb." Why do you think this is so? What does it do for the body?
7. Answer these client questions. "What is leaky gut? Why is it so bad? Do I have it?
8. Discuss use of bitters in herbal medicine.
9. What are functional foods? Name some and explain their purpose.
10. Explain the concept of intermittent fasting. What are the benefits?

References

1. Bland, Jeffery. "The Gut Mucosal Firewall and Functional Medicine." U.S. National Library of Medicine, National Institutes of Health. https://www.ncbi.nlm.nih.gov/pmc/articles/PMC4991645/ (accessed October 27, 2019).
2. As told to author by Valerie Blankenship, herbalist and owner, Sage Consulting & Apothecary, Colorado Springs, CO.
3. Bone, Kerry and Simon Mills. *Principles and Practice of Phytotherapy* (London, UK: Elsevier, 2013).
4. "What is Dehydration? What Causes It?" WebMD. http://www.webmd.com/a-to-z-guides/dehydration-adults#1 (accessed October 29. 2019).
5. "What the Science Says About Intermittent Fasting." FitnessPeak, Presented by Mercola. http://fitness.mercola.com/sites/fitness/archive/2013/06/28/intermittent-fasting-health-benefits.aspx (accessed October 29, 2019).
6. "GAPS™-What Is It?" Gut and Psychology Syndrome. http://www.gaps.me/gaps-what-is-it.php (accessed October 29, 2019).
7. Corrado, Monica. *The Complete Cooking Techniques for the GAPS™ Diet* (Fort Collins, CO: Selene River Press, 2019).
8. Weil, Andrew. *8 Weeks to Optimum Health* (New York: Random House, 2013).
9. "Brain May Flush Out Toxins During Sleep." National Institutes of Health. https://www.nih.gov/news-events/news-releases/brain-may-flush-out-toxins-during sleep (accessed October 29, 2019).
10. "Show Me the Science. Why Wash Your Hands?" Centers for Disease Control and Prevention. https://www.cdc.gov/handwashing/why-handwashing.html (accessed October 29, 2029).
11. Lieberman, Daniel E. *The Story of the Human Body* (New York: Vintage Books, 2014).
12. Holmes, Peter. *Energetics of Western Herbs* (Boulder, CO: Snow Lotus Press, 2006).
13. Yance, Donald. *Adaptogens in Medical Herbalism* (Rochester, VT: Healing Arts, 2013).
14. "What is Tonification (bu fa) and Why Is It Used?" Shen Nong. http://www.shen-nong.com/eng/lifestyles/tcmrole_bufa.html (accessed October 29, 2019).

17

Infection and Toxicosis

"Doctors put drugs of which they know little into bodies of which they know less for diseases of which they know nothing at all."

—Voltaire

CHAPTER REVIEW

- Infection and toxicosis: About antiinfective herbs, herbs for infection and toxicosis worth honorable mention.
- Bacteria and Materia Medica.
- Biofilms and Materia Medica.
- Viruses and Materia Medica.
- Therapeutic principles for treating bacteria, virus, and biofilm infections. Case Histories for upper respiratory viral infection and early-onset respiratory infection, organism type unknown.
- Parasites and Materia Medica. Therapeutic principles for treating parasites. Case History for fungal infection.
- Chinese Medicine perspective on infections with major syndromes.

KEY TERMS

Acute
Antimicrobials
Antipyretics
Antiseptics
Bacteria
Biofilms
Broad-spectrum
Chronic
Die-off
Fire toxins
Fungi
Germ theory
Gram stain
Helminths/anthelminthics
Infection
Local
Parasites
Parasiticides
Systemic
Toxicosis
Vaccine
Vermicides
Vermifuges
Virus

We are transitioning into a discussion of a *dis-ease* state, such as when optimum health is off balance. An herbalist's first intention is prevention, and for that endeavor we use adaptogens, tonics, and restoratives. But if a harmful, infectious microorganism has arrived for any reason, we use the *anti*'s: antibacterials, antivirals, antifungals, antiparasitics, antiprotozoals, antiinflammatories, antihelminths, or antibiofilms. When wellness is restored, we rebuild the body using preventative strategies so that *dis-ease* doesn't come back to haunt us.

Specifics to address particular organisms include broad-spectrum and systemic herbs covering lots of territory. The berberines lean toward bacterial and fungal infections. *Usnea* spp. (Old Man's Beard lichen) is notorious for going after streptococcal bacteria, although it is still used for others. Many, including Scutellaria Huang Qin (Baikal Skullcap root) cross over, treating both viruses and bacteria. *Artemisia annua* (Sweet Annie herb) is antifungal and antiparasitic, especially for malaria (Box 10.3).

Why are some infectious diseases and organisms so hard to treat despite our best efforts? Superbugs and biofilms are explored as possible explanations.

Infection and Toxicosis

An ***infection*** is an invasion and multiplication of microorganisms such as bacteria, viruses, and parasites that are not normally present in or on the body. It can cause many symptoms or none at all. We are interested in both: those that cause symptoms and make us miserable and others that are temporarily dormant, particularly viruses. The presence of fever and inflammation implies the existence of infection, although these symptoms are not always present in the early stages. Infectious diseases range from *external* and superficial (on the skin) to *internal* or all the way down deep in the body. An ***acute*** infection is newly arrived, whereas a ***chronic*** one has been there a long time. In general, acutes are easier to treat. The longer they last, the deeper they go and the more stubborn they are.

Antimicrobials are generally taken internally, swallowed into the gastrointestinal (GI) tract, absorbed into the blood, and circulated to various organs, tissues, and cells where they fight the offending microorganism. ***Antiseptics*** destroy or inhibit the growth of microorganisms locally, in or on living skin or mucous membranes. A Garden Sage leaf gargle swishes directly on the throat tissue, killing off organisms residing there; an Eyebright herb or Goldenseal root eyewash does the same for eyes. When using an external, antiseptic remedy, also treat internally to approach in in both directions.

Infections don't magically appear out of nowhere. The body in health does a pretty good job of maintaining homeostasis, providing strength and vitality, known as *wei qi* or life-force. By remaining free of chronic unproductive stress and anxiety and maintaining an ecosystem of beneficial microbes, we increase chances of health. When dysbiosis occurs, we retain toxins and are more susceptible to infection. The first approach in treating infection is always prevention. The second or last resort is curative and remedial.

Toxicosis is the build-up of poisons from environmental (exogenous) factors and from factors that originate from within (endogenous). The body's many metabolic processes produce their own end-product toxins, which are normally eliminated through the bowel, bladder, or skin. When foreign microbes invade the body, they release their own toxins as they are killed off by the immune system. If the load becomes too great, host tissue is damaged, and immunity is disabled. Therefore, when treating infection, toxins need to be cleared out as part of the therapeutic strategy. Environmental toxins are an entirely different story and are responsible for many health problems but not usually part of the infectious disease process (Chapter 19).

About Antiinfective Herbs

- *Energetics*. Infections usually are accompanied by fever, inflammation, and in the case of the respiratory tract, mucus or phlegm. Therefore antiinfective herbs tend to be cold, bitter, astringent, drying, and sinking, such as Goldenseal root or Coptis Huang Lian (Goldthread root). The bitterness and coolness are due to the alkaloid content which fights infection. The astringency dries up the mucus and gunk. Coolness is needed to counter hot inflammation and possible fever.
- *Biochemistry*. Many antiinfective herbs contain strong bitter alkaloids that kill germs. They also contain essential oils and glycosides that act on the immune system.
- *Mechanisms of action*. Antiinfective herbs treat infection in various ways. Some kill off the bacteria, virus, or fungus directly at the site of a tissue or organ (***local***) with antiseptic action. A Goldenseal root mouthwash must actually touch the mucous membranes of the throat for a few seconds to kill any germs. Some are ***systemic***: they circulate through the bloodstream and affect the whole body. Most are *immunostimulant*, coaxing the immune system to respond to pathogens. Antiinfectives tend to be ***antipyretic*** (they bring down fever). They are antiinflammatory, inflammation being part of the infectious process.
- *Doses*. To be effective, antiinfective herbs need to be taken in frequent doses, every 1 to 2 hours. Dosage amounts range between 2 and 4 mL each time, depending on individual and age. Sometimes doses as high as 1 teaspoon (5 mL or 5 pipette/dropper squeezes) every 2 hours might be necessary. My experience is that larger doses are more effective.
- *Synergy*. A few antiinfectives used together enhance one another. Rather than using one herb only, it is useful to use two or three different antiinfectives together in one formula to potentiate their individual actions and obtain more powerful results, which is called synergy. This combination will increase the odds of a having broader spectrum medicine that covers the bases, especially if you do not know the specific offending organism.
- *Gut flora and antiinfective herbs*. I am happy to report that plant-based antibiotics work with the organism's own defense functions, not against them. They do not get the flora out of balance or weaken the immune system as prescription antibiotic drugs do. In fact, they actually enhance the flora, especially when they are bitter. Bitters are indicated in building up helpful gut microorganisms.
- *Prevention and cure*. The sooner you treat, the better. If taken immediately, at the first indication of an infection, antibiotic herbs can stop bugs in their tracks, being preventative. If the infection is a couple of days old, they still work, but more slowly.
- *Broad- versus narrow-spectrum herbs*. Many herbs that treat viruses also treat bacteria. Some have affinities for one but also treat the other. Herbs are often ***broad-spectrum***, meaning they are general for a large variety of organisms, rather than specific for one in particular (narrow-spectrum). The drug penicillin is broad-spectrum; Vancomycin is narrow, for gram-positive bacteria only. Which medication treats which infection is always interesting information, but without lab cultures, urine, or sputum tests, etc., herbalists usually don't know which organism is being dealt with. Research can tell us definitively which herb snuffs out which infection. For example, clinical trials in China found that Isatis Ban Lan Gen (Isatis root) is extremely broad-spectrum and is actually active against many A and B influenza strains, SARS, chickenpox, shingles, herpes simplex (cold sores), and more. Nice to know. However, many Western infectious disease names actually fall under External Wind Heat/Cold or Damp Heat in Chinese Medicine designations, and we could've/would've used Isatis root anyhow.
- *Systemic versus localized nonsystemic herbs*. Oral antibiotic herbs cross the GI tract and circulate throughout the bloodstream, reaching every cell in the body. Most antibiotic herbs are systemic; they go everywhere.
  - *Nonsystemics* are localized and do not easily cross the GI tract. They are limited to the GI tract itself and the organs through which they are eliminated. Garlic is eliminated through the lungs, hence the creation of Garlic breath and the herb's ability to heal throat infections. Juniper berry metabolizes through the kidneys, so it is great for urinary tract infections. The berberines localize on gut mucous membranes and others that they touch. The primary localized nonsystemic herbal antibiotics are the berberines, and also Juniper berry, Usnea thallus, and honey.[1]

Herbs for Infections and Toxicosis Worth Honorable Mention

An *Herbs Worth Honorable Mention* section will appear throughout Part IV, Therapeutics and Formulations (Chapters 16–28). These herbs are not listed in Part II Materia Medica (Chapters 11–12), but are still very important and specific to the particular body system addressed.

- *Sambucus nigra*. (Elderberry and Elder flower). This lovely bush or small tree is spectacular in flower and when the dark purplish berries are out. Use this species, not the red *Sambucus racemosa* that is slightly toxic. Elderberry is a narrow-spectrum antiviral, specifically superior for *enveloped viruses*. Elder helps in flu (if begun at early onset), *Herpes* spp. (shingles and chickenpox), and viral hepatitis. Use in syrups and elixirs. It is kid-friendly for fevers, being diaphoretic and causing a sweat.
- *Larrea divaricata* (Creosote leaf, Chaparral leaf) (Fig. 17.1). Robust-smelling Creosote or Chaparral bush grows in the American Southwest. It is a cold, dry, industrial medium-strength detoxicant: antibacterial, antifungal, antiviral, and immunostimulant. It clears damp heat, tastes strong, smells strong (nicknamed little stinker), and acts fearlessly. It is a major remedy for infectious heat and fever. As an added bonus, it dissolves stones and relieves constipation. Although it has many merits, it is best used in formula and not taken for more than 3 weeks without a break because of possible hepatotoxicity in those with a history of liver damage.
- *Scutellaria baicalensis* Huang Qin (Baikal Skullcap root). Scute for short, is a go-to remedy for acute damp heat and fire toxins. It is a different species with a different use than the relaxing Western nervine known as *Scutellaria lateriflora* or *S. brittonii* (Skullcap herb). Huang Qin is an indispensable cold and bitter plant used for broad-spectrum damp heat, being antiviral, antibacterial, antifungal, immunostimulant, and resistant to biofilms. It works for bacterial infections in liver, lungs, kidneys, and bladder. It is antiallergenic and a good digestive bitter, and it limits the ability of microbes to develop resistance to antibiotic drugs.[2]
- *Forsythia suspensa* Lian Qiao (Forsythia valve). Lian Qiao is a broad-spectrum antibacterial, antiviral, antifungal, and immunostimulant for damp heat and fire toxins. It is often used with *Lonicera japonica* Jin Yin Hua (Honeysuckle flower). Honeysuckle and Forsythia appear in the famous formula for early-onset colds and flu, Yin Chiao (Box 17.1).
- *Isatis tinctoria* Ban Lan Gen (Isatis or Woad root). Cold and bitter, Isatis root is broad-spectrum antibacterial and antiviral for damp heat and fire toxins. Isatis root is specific for all strains of flu, viral pneumonia, meningitis, encephalitis, hepatitis B, and bacterial conjunctivitis (in eye drops).

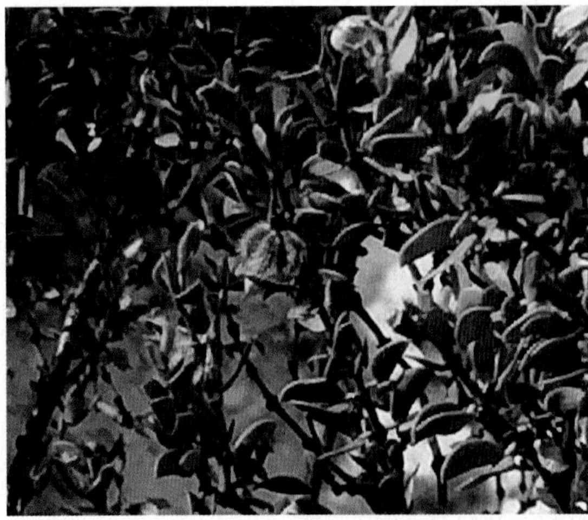

• **Fig. 17.1** *Larrea divaricata* showing leaf and seedpod. Chaparral or Creosote leaf treats a wide range of infections. It is dry and cold, making it appropriate for damp heat conditions.

• BOX 17.1 Yin Chiao Pien, Honeysuckle, and Forsythia Tablets for Early-Onset Colds and Flu

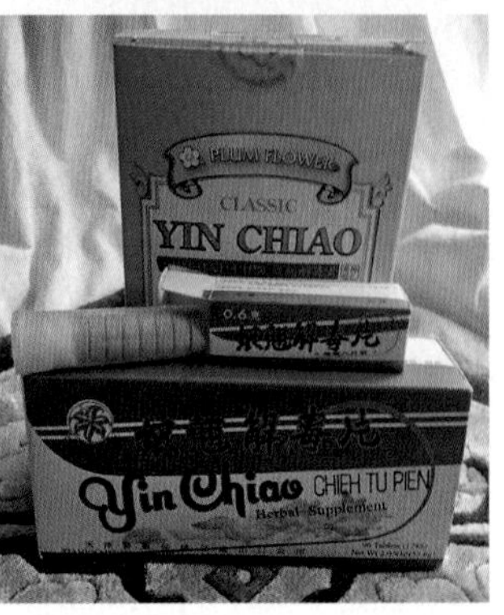

Yin Chiao Pien patent formula is often packaged, Chinese style, in individual vials of tablets.

This is a 200-year-old classic that is considered tried and true to ward off the external pernicious influences, such as wind and cold invading the lungs, External Wind Cold, and External Wind Heat. Use when exposed or likely to be exposed to external pathogens, sore throat, common cold, and other respiratory pathogens.[4] Honeysuckle and Forsythia flowers are known for their synergistic antimicrobial effects.

There are many versions of Yin Chiao with differing proportions. The first seven herbs are found in most of them. Be sure to include those. Some formulas include other herbs, such as Bamboo grass leaf and prepared Soybean.

Dose. Tincture 1:4 60%, 5 mL every 2 hours. **Patent**. Directions on label.

15 g	Lonicera Jin Yin Hua (Honeysuckle flower)	Antimicrobial, clears heat
15 g	Forsythia Lian Qiao (Forsythia flower)	Antimicrobial, clears heat
10 g	Arctium Niu Bange Zi (Burdock seed)	Clears fire toxins, expectorant, diaphoretic
10 g	Platycodon Jie Jeng (Balloonflower root)	Expectorant, antitussive
8 g	Schizonepeta Jing Jie (Chinese Catnip herb)	Pungent diaphoretic, cooling
8 g	Mentha Bo He (Field Mint herb)	Diaphoretic, aromatic, cool
8 g	Glycyrrhiza Gan Cao (Licorice root)	Expectorant, antitussive, sweet, moist
8 g	Lophatherum Dan Zhu Ye (Bamboo grass leaf)	Clear heat, nervous sedative
8 g	Glycine Dan Dou Chi (Prepared soybean) (Dan Dou Chi may be hard to find; if so, omit.)	Diaphoretic

Bacteria and Materia Medica

Bacteria are one-celled organisms that have a cell wall but lack organelles and an organized nucleus. They live everywhere, in and on plants, animals, and humans and in all environments, hot to cold, dry to wet, and desert to ocean. These are one of the oldest forms of life on planet Earth and are neither plants nor animals. Many are harmless; most are useful, covering the soil, causing fermentation, or inhabiting our gut. A few cause disease.

Bacteria have survived harsh environments, each other, and chemical assaults. Ever since Alexander Fleming developed penicillin in 1928, the "one drug for one bug" mentality was born. Antibiotics (meaning antilife) became the miracle drugs that could cure many dangerous bacterial infections like *Pneumococcal pneumoniae* (most common type of bacterial pneumonia), *Streptococcus pneumoniae* (causes bacterial strep throat), and *Clostridium difficile* (bacteria that affects the colon).

Unfortunately, antibiotic drugs have been overprescribed and overused, so much so that the bacteria have reacted as any self-respecting microbe would. They evolved, mutated, adapted, and changed form, generation by generation. For some bacteria, a new generation occurs every 20 minutes. Hence, many bacteria became resistant to antibiotics. In response, we keep changing the drugs to keep up with the mutations. Methicillin is no longer working against aptly named methicillin-resistant *Staphylococcus aureus* (MRSA). Bacteria have evolved into *superbugs* that are harder and harder to treat. Gonorrhea, tuberculosis, and other diseases, once presumed dead and eradicated, have returned, creating worldwide infectious disease crises.

Gram stains are a way to identify bacteria in the lab. In 1884, Danish scientist Hans Gram began applying a crystal violet stain to bacterial slides. If the cells showed up purple under the microscope due to a thick cell wall, they were dubbed *gram-positive*. If they didn't and showed up red, they were *gram-negative*. Gram-negative bacteria lose the crystal violet stain and take on the color of a red counterstain.[3]

When applied to antibiotics, certain drugs and antimicrobial herbs are active against major gram-positive microbes like *Clostridium difficile*, *Staphylococcus aureus*, *Streptococcus* spp., and *Mycobacterium tuberculosis*. Others treat major gram-negative bacterial microbes such as *Klebsiella pneumonia*, *Pseudomonas aeruginosa*, *Escherichia coli*, and *Salmonella* spp. Unless a drug or herb is broad-spectrum (most are), they are specific for certain microorganisms within one gram type or the other. Of course, this is known only if the studies have been done.

The Antibacterial Materia Medica table (Table 17.1) provides an overview of a few extremely useful herbs, information about broad- versus narrow-spectrum, systemic versus nonsystemic, and a little on gram-positive or gram-negative designations.

Biofilms and Materia Medica

Biofilms are communities of bacteria species that live together within a protective slimy coating. They stick to each other, and often adhere to tissue surfaces. The normal state for bacteria is to coexist with many other species. Biofilms secrete a slimy matrix, chiefly a polysaccharide, that protects them from bacteria in other biofilm communities and from antibiotic penetration. The bacteria in a biofilm colony work together collectively to protect themselves. Biofilms have been compared to multicellular organisms, because there is so much interaction between the individual cells. In the 1980s, biofilms were discovered growing on medical implants, heart valves, stents, catheters, and pacemakers, causing infection. They can cause infective endocarditis and pneumonia in cystic fibrosis patients.

Biofilm theory explains why so many bacteria are resistant to antibiotic drugs and why certain diseases return repeatedly despite many rounds of antibiotic drug treatment.[5] Consider chronic ulcers, stubborn urinary tract infections, and sinus infections that won't clear up. Many bacterial species (but not all) live together in this fortified, protective slime, their biofilm community. This film protects them from antibiotics as they build up resistance, alter genetic expression, mutate, and change.[6] To be fair, some biofilms are actually beneficial. For instance, *Lactobacillus* in the gut forms a biofilm that is protective for humans against malicious bacterial overgrowth.

Pertinent Biofilm Facts

- *Biofilms reside throughout the body.* They live on the mucous membranes of the respiratory and urinary systems, vagina, placenta, the mouth (oral plaque), and on the skin.
- *The germ theory versus biofilms* (Fig. 17.2). Developed by Louis Pasteur and Robert Koch in the 1800s and still believed today, the ***germ theory*** assumes that one specific microorganism causes a specific disease, a revolutionary concept at the time. Kill that bug and the disease is cured. This does not always work. In some cases, the germ theory may be phasing out.
- *Why the biofilm approach makes sense.* Sometimes an antibiotic kills off the upper layers of microbes within the film but doesn't penetrate down deep where other species reside and hide. These inner layers can't even be found on a culture swab. (Cultures only scrape the surface.) The infection clears up temporarily but then returns, causing a chronic condition. This situation is creating an infectious disease health crisis where antibiotics are less and less effective. Is the biofilm approach the answer to infectious disease eradication?

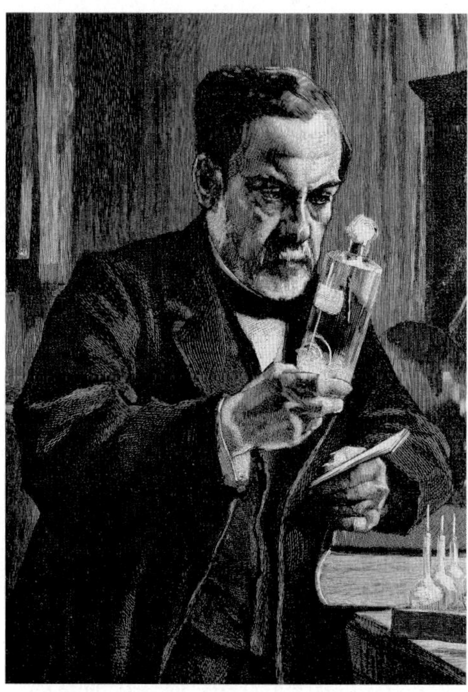

• **Fig. 17.2** Louis Pasteur (1822–1895) in his laboratory. He is famous for the germ theory, that microscopic bacteria cause disease. (iStock.com/Credit: Suteishi.)

TABLE 17.1 Antibacterial Materia Medica: A Few Superb Examples
(Most double as general crossover antimicrobials)

Herb	Notes
The berberines (all yellow roots) *Coptis chinensis* Huang Lian *Phellodendron amurense* Huang Bai (Siberian Cork Tree bark) *Hydrastis canadensis* (Goldenseal root, cultivated) *Berberis vulgaris* (Barberry root) *Mahonia aquifolium* (Oregon Grape root) Tincture 1:5 70% alcohol and water with a pH of 1–6.[2] If water pH is 7–14 (alkaline hard), add 1 tablespoon apple cider vinegar to menstruum.	**Strongest to weakest:** Coptis Huang Lian, Goldenseal root, Phellodendron Huang Bai, Barberry root, Oregon Grape root. All berberines are nonsystemic herbs. Great for GI and sore throat because they directly contact the tissue. Antifungal and effective for resistant bacteria of many types, including *Staphylococcus* spp. and *Streptococcus* spp. (Stops microbe adherence to mucous membranes.) For hepatitis B, *Trichomonas vaginalis*, yellow fever, *H. pylori* in ulcers. Use topically in douches, sprays, eye washes, gargles.
Artemisia annua Ging Hao Sweet Annie herb	Fresh plant is strongest. Globally antimicrobial: antibacterial, antifungal, antiviral, antiparasitic, antitumoral, antiprotozoal (malaria). Excels at GI problems. Nonsystemic: the alkaloids stay in the GI tract and on the skin.
Juniperus spp. Juniper berry and essential oil.	Nonsystemic. Active against at least 57 bacterial species. Also, antiviral, antifungal, anthelmintic, antiseptic, carminative, diuretic. Classic for urinary tract infections because it comes in direct contact with the mucosa.
Usnea spp. Song Luo Old Man's Beard lichen	Used systemically and locally. Inhibits biofilm formation. Antibacterial against resistant and nonresistant gram-positive strains, especially upper respiratory infections such as strep throat, and urinary tract infections. Antiviral, antiparasitic, immunostimulant. Wind Heat, Fire toxins. Good for washes, gargles, nasal sprays, and douches. Dual extraction best.
Glycyrrhiza glabra or *G. sinensis* Gan Cao Licorice root	Antibiotic for gram-negatives. Licorice is a moisturizing synergist, enhances effect of the primary antibiotic. For use in formula, rarely as a simple.
Zingiber officinale Gan Jiang Ginger rhizome	Antimicrobial. A warming circulatory stimulant, potentiates other herbs, creates sweating. Use fresh tea for best results for wind cold, early-onset antibacterial action. A synergist.
Ligusticum porteri Osha root	Antimicrobial, pungent, warm diaphoretic and expectorant for colds and flu, wind cold.
Origanum vulgare Oregano herb and essential oil	Antibacterial, antiviral, antifungal, warming for wind cold. In essential oil, use 2–4 drops in a gel cap plus a carrier oil.
Essential oils Ravensara, Myrrh, Pine, Spruce, Oregano, Tea Tree, Thyme, Winter savory, Eucalyptus, Myrrh, Lavender, Lemon	All antibacterials. 2–4 drops in gel caps with carrier oils. Add to tinctures; 1 drop per oz.
Andrographis paniculata Chuan Xin Lian Heart-Thread Lotus leaf	Broad-spectrum antibacterial, antiviral, immunostimulant for Wind Heat and Damp Heat, fire toxins. Classic for sinuses and chronic respiratory infections.
Scutellaria baicalensis Huang Qin Baikal Skullcap root	Broad-spectrum antibacterial, antiviral, immunostimulant, antifungal, Damp Heat, fire toxins.
Isatis tinctoria Ban Lan Gen Isatis root	Broad-spectrum antibacterial, antiviral. For Damp Heat and fire toxins.
Lonicera japonica Jin Yin Ha Honeysuckle flower	Broad-spectrum antibacterial, antiviral, antifungal, immunostimulant. Damp Heat, fire toxins.
Forsythia suspensa Lian Qiao Forsythia valve	Broad-spectrum antibacterial, antiviral, antifungal, immunostimulant. Damp Heat, fire toxins.[1,2]

- *Quorum sensing within biofilms protects bacteria.* Bacteria do many things to protect themselves. One is called *quorum sensing*. Quorum sensing chemicals are signaling molecules that tell bacterial DNA to change gene expression and switch function. Once enough bacteria are living together—called a *quorum*—a cell population density is reached. Then a chemical message is sent out via cell-to-cell communication to secrete a protective biofilm.[7]
- *The multiple-drug-resistant efflux pump (MDR) protects bacteria.* This is a protective survival mechanism used by bacteria to actually spit out harmful substances[8] and to expel the very antibiotic drugs that were intended to do them in. Smart bacteria.

- *Aerobic versus anaerobic bacteria.* Aerobic bacteria require oxygen, and anaerobic types do not. The outer layers of biofilms are aerobic bacteria, whereas the inner core consists of anaerobic bacteria. This creates a problem because antibiotics generally attack either one or the other, not both kinds and thus doesn't get them all.
- *Antibiofilm drugs.* Drug companies are working on antibiofilm agents to treat biofilm-associated infections. These might be the next category of *miracle drugs*. Antibiotics that work on a single bug are becoming ineffective and perhaps obsolete.
- *An effective biofilm herb or drug needs to accomplish many tasks.* Ideally, any effective drug, herb, or herbal combination must do all of the above jobs just mentioned, plus inhibit the nitric oxide pathway.[10]

In summary, an effective biofilm herb or drug needs to accomplish many tasks:

- Must be a multiple drug/herb-resistant pump inhibitor (MDRi).
- Must be able to target quorum sensing.
- Must be able to fight both aerobic and anaerobic bacteria.[9]
- Must be able to inhibit the nitric oxide pathway.[10]

This list is a tall order, but you'll find that many of the antimicrobial herbs already discussed actually fit this criterion. One example is Andrographis Chuan Xin Lian (Fig. 17.3).

- *Consider the biofilm theory when infections reoccur.* The clinical takeaway is that whenever there are chronic or persistent infections in your client (with impaired immune function ruled out), consider the existence of a biofilm, a multiple drug resistant (MDR) situation. Make use of broad-spectrum, antibiofilm herbs shown in the Antibiofilm Materia Medica (Table 17.2).

TABLE 17.2 Antibiofilm Materia Medica

Herb	Action
Angelica sinensis Dang Gui Angelica root, Dong Quai	For qi stagnation, builds blood, antimicrobial. Interrupts nitric oxide cycle that bacteria use to make biofilms.
Paeonia lactiflora Bai Shao White Peony root	For qi stagnation, builds blood. Interrupts nitric oxide cycle in biofilm formation.
Paeonia suffruticosa Mu Dan Pi Tree Peony root	Cools heat, clears blood. Interrupts nitric oxide cycle that bacteria use to make biofilms. Inhibits many microbes.
Seaweeds: *Sargassum* spp. Hai Zao (Sargassum seaweed) *Laminaria* spp. Kun Bu (Kelp thallus) *Fucus vesiculosus* (Bladderwrack thallus)	Resists biofilm formation. Slimy and help prevent bacteria sticking to mucous membranes.
Andrographis paniculata Chuan Xin Lian Heart-Thread Lotus leaf	Clears damp heat and fire toxins. Resists biofilm formation. Broad-spectrum antibacterial, antiviral. Shines for head/sinus congestion.
Scutellaria baicalensis Huang Qin Chinese Baikal Skullcap root	Clears damp heat, fire toxins. Resists biofilm formation. Limits ability of microbes to develop resistance to medication.
Silver	Used as a coating to reduce bacterial adhesion on living material.
Sodium bicarbonate Baking soda	Antibiofilm. Also alkalizing to raise pH of urine, defending against UTIs.
The Berberines: Goldenseal root Oregon Grape root Barberry root Coptis Huang Lian (Goldthread root) Phellodendron Huang Bai (Siberian Cork Tree bark)	Broad-spectrum for biofilms. An MDR pump inhibitor, not systemic, nor absorbed. Internal use for GI works best. Use externally when in direct contact with infected tissue. The herbs probably contain constituents other than the berberines that are effective. Historically, used internally and externally. Combine two together.
Echinacea angustifolia root	MDRi, detoxifier, immunostimulant.
Allium sativum (Garlic bulb)	MDRi. Anthelmintic, antiprotozoal.
Plantago lanceolata (Plantain leaf)	MDRi.
Arctostaphylos uva ursi (Bearberry leaf)	MDRi.
Usnea spp. (Old Man's Beard thallus)	Biofilm inhibitor. Note: Usnic acid has been found to be liver-toxic when used in isolation. But the whole herb is extremely safe for herbal use.[1]

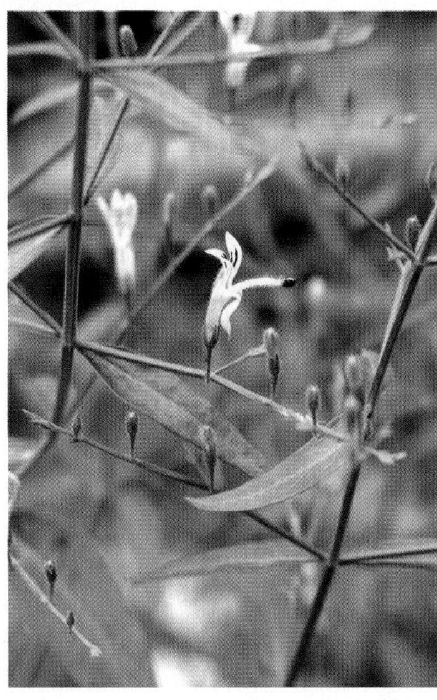

• **Fig. 17.3** *Andrographis paniculata* Chuan Xin Lian (Heart-Thread Lotus leaf) is a broad-spectrum antimicrobial that is splendid for sinus infections, and effective against biofilms. (iStock.com/Credit: mansum008)

Viruses and Materia Medica

Viruses are unique life forms—the ultimate survivalists. Unlike bacteria, viruses have no nucleus or cell wall. They are a simple strand of DNA or RNA surrounded by a protein coat or capsid, so small they cannot be seen with an electron microscope and can reproduce only within a host cell. Each type of virus has a specific shape.[2] Viruses can enter cells, snip off sections of its DNA or RNA, and weave the sections into their own genetic structure. This allows them to alter themselves and be extremely adaptable. Like seeds or spores, they can hang out for years on their own or exist in host cells in a state of hibernation and dormancy. When conditions are right, they come to life and multiply. They don't break apart and divide like *normal* cells. Instead, they insert their genetic material into their host's nucleus, literally taking over its functions.

Viruses are travelers. Some are spread by respiratory droplets, as with colds and flu. Some travel on ticks, such as Rocky Mountain spotted fever, or on mosquitoes, causing dengue fever, yellow fever, West Nile virus, and Zika virus illnesses. In humans, they often travel via immune system cells in search of preferred locations. The Epstein-Barr virus looks for B cells, and the human immunodeficiency virus (HIV) searches out T4 lymphocytes. Others prefer certain organs. The *hepatovirus* species that causes hepatitis goes to the liver, and the *Herpes* spp. virus

TABLE 17.3 Antiviral Materia Medica: A Few Wise Choices

Herb	Action
Scutellaria baicalensis Huang Qin Baikal Skullcap root	This is *not* Western Skullcap, the nervine. Huang Qin is for damp heat, a broad-spectrum antiviral and adjunct for bacterial infections in liver, lungs (flu), UTIs. Antiallergenic. This is a must-have bitter herb.
Sambucus nigra Elderberry and Elder flower	Narrow-spectrum antiviral, specifically superior for enveloped viruses, especially flu (when begun early), *Herpes* spp. (shingles and chickenpox), and hepatitis. Make the Elderberry elixir (Box 20.2).
Zingiber officinale Gan Jiang (Fresh Ginger rhizome) (Only fresh root works well as an antiviral. If using dried, constituents are mostly lost for this purpose.) Chinese Medicine considers fresh and dried as different medicines with different actions.	Respiratory antiviral circulatory sweater-outer, reduces fever, stops cough. Specific for flu and colds as fresh Ginger juice/tea (Box 17.2). Dried root tincture is for digestion, stomach cramps, nausea, diarrhea.
Isatis tinctoria Ban Lan Gen Woad root and leaf For best antiviral results, use 2:1 dried leaf to root. Dual extraction. 1:5 25%.[2]	Specific for all strains of flu (use leaf), viral pneumonia, meningitis, encephalitis, hepatitis B, bacterial conjunctivitis (in eye drops). Also, antibacterial.
Glycyrrhiza glabra or G. sinensis Gan Cao Licorice root	Broad-spectrum antiviral. For flu, colds, and great when combined with Chinese Skullcap. Best as a synergist, not alone.
Larrea divaricata Creosote leaf, Chaparral leaf	Antiviral, antibacterial, clears Damp Heat, and detoxicant. Industrial-strength liver cleanser.
Lonicera japonica Jin Yin Hua Honeysuckle flower	Broad-spectrum antiinfective. Dispels wind heat, Damp Heat, and fire toxins.
Forsythia suspensa Lian Qiao Forsythia valve	Forsythia and Honeysuckle are go-together herbs.
Hypericum perforatum (St. John's Wort)	Important for herpes (cold sores, shingles).
Andrographis paniculata Chaun Xin Lian Chronic respiratory problems.	Broad-spectrum antimicrobial, antiviral, antibacterial, immunostimulant.

travels to the brain and spinal cord, causing encephalomyelitis. Once viruses find a compatible host cell, they break off pieces of themselves and send them to the host's nucleus where they quickly replicate.

But don't consider all viruses on Mother Earth to be a horror show. Most live in the soil, the water, and in and on us quite symbiotically and happily. The healthy microbiome in the gut and on our skin are examples of places where bacteria and viruses live with us harmlessly and beneficially. Viruses, like other microorganisms, represent our origins and beginnings of life. They were here first and still remain. We evolved from them and are dependent on them, so we best get along. That means not madly and obsessively washing them from our skin and countertops. Hygiene is important, but no there is need for fanaticism.

No really effective antiviral drugs exist, and those that do tend to be very strong with nasty side effects. Thankfully, this is not so with antivirals in the plant kingdom. An Antiviral Materia Medica appears in Table 17.3. The main Western medicine weapons for viral infections are vaccines. ***Vaccines*** stimulate the production of our own antibodies against the disease in question, providing immunity most of the time. Early vaccines eradicated deadly smallpox and polio. Tetanus and measles vaccines have practically eliminated those threats. Today there is a movement against vaccinations. Doubt, controversy, and strong opinions exist about contaminants, heavy metals (especially mercury), and claims that vaccines actually cause, rather than prevent, the disease or make us sicker. It is a loaded topic and one where it's best to steer clear and let parents and individuals decide for themselves.

Therapeutic Principles for Treating Bacteria, Viruses, and Biofilm Infections with Case Histories

Fortunately for us, many herbs are quite effective against general infection and biofilm communities because the plants have learned to fight off their own microbe invasions and contain chemicals that can do this. Strategies for biofilms are similar as for general infection. Basically, the therapeutic principles for an infectious disease formula should include the following components.

- *Antiinfectives* are the chief herbs in the formula. Since you may not know which species are involved in any given infection and because biofilms comprise a variety of microbe species, it makes sense to use a few broad-spectrum antibiotic herbs to cover the bases. Use about two herbs, whether antibacterial or antiviral. If the organism is unknown, or you are not targeting a specific elimination pathway, use broad-spectrums.
- *Immunostimulants*. These should be part of the formula. Most antiinfective herbs are immunostimulant, as well. Some good ones used during acute infections are Echinacea root, Ganoderma Ling Zhi (Reishi mushroom), Garlic bulb, Elderberry flower and berry, Boneset herb, and Usnea thallus. They work safely on immune function during *active* infections, covering two therapeutic principles with one herb.
- *Detoxicant (alteratives)*. The intention is to help the body eliminate endogenous toxins or poisons. Toxicosis occurs from metabolic wastes generated by the body, and also from bacteria that have either caused or contributed to the infection. Detoxicant choice depends on site of infection. For instance, lymph movers like Cleavers herb, Red Root, Burdock root, or Calendula flower drain swollen glands. Dandelion root, Jamaican Sarsaparilla root, or Cleavers herb, and the docks are for skin. Milk Thistle seed, Dandelion root, or Artichoke leaf cleanse the liver. Goldenrod herb or Cleavers herb have a tropism to the kidneys. Broad-spectrum, antiinfective detoxifiers include Garlic bulb, Horseradish root, Oregon Grape root, Chaparral leaf, Wormwood herb, and Pau d'arco bark.[11]
- *Restoratives*. If there is tissue damage, use one of the many restoratives, depending on tropism. Examples could be Mullein leaf for the lungs, Hawthorn berry for the heart, Licorice or Parsley root for the gut, Raspberry leaf or Saw Palmetto berry for reproductive. Tissue damage is frequently involved with long, chronic infectious processes.
- *Synergists*. These are the finishing touch (Fig. 17.4). Use small amounts to enhance the work of the other herbs and to pull the formula together, such as Licorice root or Ginger root, *Piper nigrum* (Black Peppercorn) or *P. longum* (Long Peppercorn). Licorice root helps absorption and moves herbs into the bloodstream.[11] Its sweet taste improves compliance and balances the formula because most antimicrobials are bitter. An added reason for its inclusion in many formulations is its ability to lessen toxicity of other potent herbs that may be present. Ginger root is a good blender to add warmth and protect against stomach upset. Peppercorn is warm, pungent, and antibacterial. Refer to

• BOX 17.2 Sweating It Out *With Fresh Ginger Juice/Tea*

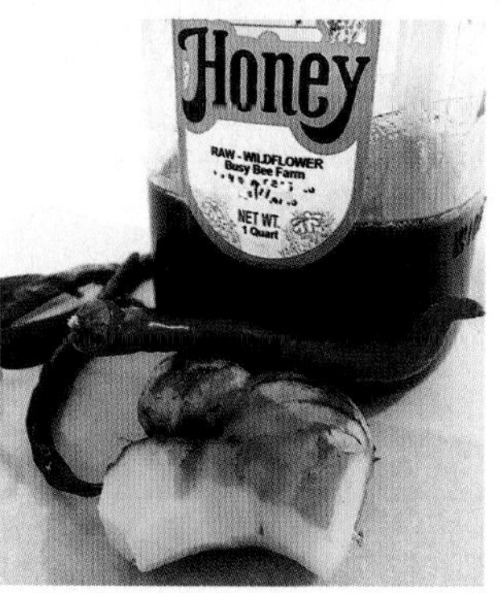

Fresh Ginger root (*Zingiber officinale*), Cayenne pepper, and honey are the main ingredients in this diaphoretic remedy for early-onset colds and flu.

The most effective way to use Ginger root for early-onset antiviral purposes is to make a fresh tea. That way, the active compounds enter the blood stream in about 30 minutes, peaking in 60, and get the sweat going.

Directions with juicer. Juice a large piece of fresh rhizome, the size of a medium carrot or 4 thumb-sized pieces. Combine ¼ cup fresh juice with 12 oz hot water. Add 1 tablespoon wild honey, ¼ of a squeezed lime as juice, and ⅛ teaspoon ground Cayenne pepper.

Directions for tea. Grate or finely chop a thumb-sized piece of Ginger. Steep covered in 8–12 oz hot water for at least 20 minutes, and then strain. Add honey and ground Cayenne pepper. Spicy, hot-tasting, and yummy for a Wind Cold condition.

Yield. One cup or a little more. It's easier to double or triple this to last for a day's worth, especially if sick and feeling very sleepy. Just reheat/simmer tea, as needed, throughout the day. Add the honey and Cayenne separately each time.

Dose. One cup every 2 to 3 hours in acute conditions to keep blood levels high.

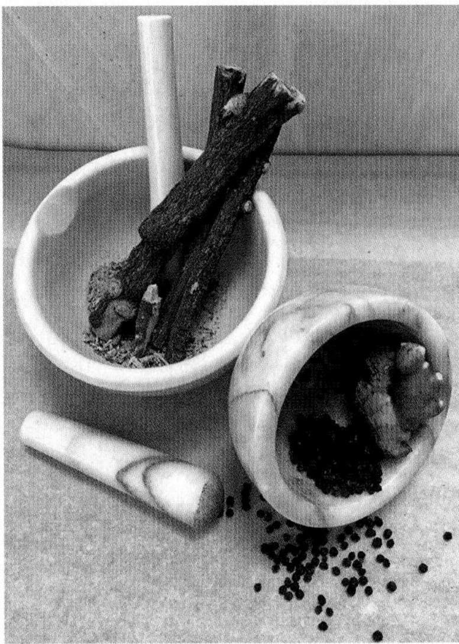

• **Fig. 17.4** Synergists to pull a formula together—*Glycyrrhiza glabra* (Licorice root), *Piper nigrum* (Black Peppercorn), and *Zingiber officinalis* (Ginger root).

CASE HISTORY 17.1

Case History for Upper Respiratory Viral Infection

S. Roy seems to have had "the same cold" many times this season. It comes and goes. Low grade fever averages 101°F when it occurs. Rhinitis with clear mucus. Complains of headache and pressure around the eyes. He has been using Echinacea tincture from the health food store and vitamin C. Throat culture and sensitivity was negative for bacteria.
O. **P** Rapid. **T** Red. Temperature 100°F. Lungs clear to auscultation.
A. Depressed immune system (Wei qi). Wind Heat. Resistant upper respiratory/sinus/viral infection.
P. *Specific therapeutic principles.* (1) Eliminate infection and fever with strong, cooling antibiofilm, antiviral herbs. (2) Increase immunity with immunostimulants. (3) Nervine for headache and relaxation. (4) Restorative for respiratory.

Herbal Formula and Dose. 4 mL every 2 hours when awake.

Parts	Herbs	Rationale
3	Andrographis Chuan Xin Lian	Sinus antiviral, immunostimulant, cool.
1	Elderberry berry and flower	Antiviral, decrease fever.
2	Isatis Ban Lan	Antiviral for sinus, cooling.
2	Passionflower	Headache and relaxation.
1	Marigold flower	Detoxification.
2	Mullein leaf	Respiratory restorative, soothing.
1	Licorice root	Antiviral, soothing, blending, immune support.

Other Suggestions

- Steam. 2 drops Eucalyptus essential oil and 2 drops Peppermint essential oil added to pot of just boiled water. Steam in a.m. and p.m.
- Supplements:
  - Vitamin C 1000 mg 3 times per day
  - Zinc 10 mg 2 times per day for immunity.
- Good hydration to help sinus drainage.
- When infection resolved, begin adaptogen formula for at least 3 months and continue vitamin C and zinc.

CASE HISTORY 17.2

Case History for Early-Onset Respiratory Infection, Microorganism Type Unknown

S. Stefanie came down with chills the previous night. Her throat is scratchy and tickly. She wants to "get right on it" before she is "really sick." There is no fever or thirst. Stomach feels "queasy," and she is a little nauseated.
O. **P** Tight. **T** Normal; thin, white coat. Forehead cool and sweaty. No fever.
A. Wind Cold. Early-onset infection, microorganism unknown.
P. *Specific therapeutic principles:* (1) Dispel wind cold/infection with warm, stimulant diaphoretics. (2) Ginger juice/tea to "sweat it out." (3) Soothe throat. (4) Settle stomach. (5) Stimulate immunity.

Herbal Formula and Dose. 2 mL every 2 hours when awake.

Part	Herbs	Rationale
3	Osha root	Expectorant, pungent, warm diaphoretic, antiseptic. Expels wind damp cold.
2	*Echinacea angustifolia*	Antiviral, antibacterial, immunostimulants, detoxifier.
2	Peppermint leaf	Warming, diaphoretic, antiviral, relax GI.
2	Magnolia Xin Yi Hua bud	Opens airway, antiviral.
2	Mullein leaf	Soothe throat, cooling.
1	Ginger root	Warming diaphoretic; protects stomach.

Other Suggestions

- Ginger juice/tea: Fresh Ginger root, honey, and cayenne (Box 17.2). Sweating.
- Supplements:
  - Vitamin C 1000 mg 3 times per day.
  - Zinc 20 mg 2 times per day to stimulate immune system.

Case History 17.1 for Upper Respiratory Viral Infection and to Case History 17.2 for Early-Onset Respiratory Infection, Microrganism Type Unknown.

Parasites and Materia Medica

Parasites are organisms that live on others and obtain nutrients from their host. The three types of parasites that cause human disease are helminths, protozoa, and ectoparasites. ***Helminths*** are worms—like roundworms, tapeworms, and pinworms—and can live in the GI tract or blood. *Protozoa* are one-celled organisms that can multiply in humans and elsewhere. *Trichomonas vaginalis* is a protozoan that infects the vagina. Malaria is caused by the protozoan parasite, *Plasmodium* spp. *Giardia* spp. is a microscopic protozoan parasite found in unsafe, unsanitary water. *Ectoparasites* are the bloodsuckers, including ticks, fleas, lice, and mites.[12]

Anthelminthics are herbs that kill and flush worms. They work as ***vermicides*** that kill parasites and as ***vermifuges*** that flush them out. Remedies called ***parasiticides*** treat parasites externally. These include Aloe Vera gel and Alum root and essential oils of Camphor, Thyme, Lemon, Lavender, and Eucalyptus. Inorganic substances are also used: calomel, realgar, litharge, and sulphur.

Fungi are neither plants nor animals. Some are parasites; some are not. They consist of mushrooms, yeasts, molds, mildews, smuts, and rusts; they live by breaking down and absorbing dead or live organic matter. They have no chlorophyll and reproduce by spores. Fungal infections can affect any part of the body. *Candida albicans* is one of the most common yeast infections that can infect the gut, the vagina, and the mouth (thrush). Other frequently seen fungal infections are athlete's foot and ringworm. Onychomycosis, also called *tinea unguium*, is a fungal infection that gets under the fingernails and toenails and is very hard to eradicate.

Therapeutic Principles for Treating Parasites

Parasites can be difficult to treat with herbs because they often accompany or hide behind other syndromes. Sometimes a specific diagnosis can be helpful, such as a positive ova and parasite (O and P) stool culture for worm eggs taken by a healthcare provider. Parasites might be a one-time problem, caused from drinking *Giardia*-infested water or from traveling to a foreign country and contracting a strange eye fungus. If that is the case, antifungal herbs should do the trick. See the Antiparasitic Materia Medica in Table 17.4. Case History 17.3 illustrates a typical fungal infection.

TABLE 17.4 Antiparasitic Materia Medica

Herb	Actions
Tabebuia avellanedae Pau d'arco bark	Antifungal, antiparasitic, antibacterial, yeast. Removes damp heat from urogenital and GI tracts.
Larrea divaricata Creosote, Chaparral leaf	Antifungal, antibacterial, antiviral. Clears damp heat in urogenital, GI, and dermal areas.
Mahonia repens Oregon Grape root	Mild antifungal, antiviral, antibacterial. Clears damp heat, especially from skin.
Olea europaea Olive leaf	Antifungal, antiparasitic, antibacterial; also stabilizes blood sugar.
***Artemisia* spp.** *A. annua* (Sweet Annie herb) *A. vulgarus* (Mugwort herb) *A. dracunculus* (Tarragon herb) *A. absinthium* (Wormwood herb)	All are antifungal, antibiotic, anthelmintic, antiamoebic, antiinflammatory, antiinfective, and insect repellant.
Allium sativum Garlic bulb	Anthelmintic, antiprotozoal, antifungal. Use externally in poultices/ear oil. Immunostimulant.
Gentiana lutea Gentian root	Anthelmintic, antiprotozoal, and for parasites in general.
Quercus alba Oak bark	Antiprotozoal.
Commiphora myrrh Mo Yao Myrrh resin	Antifungal of mouth, gums, throat, vagina. Antibacterial and antiviral. Gargles, douches.
Ruta graveolens Rue herb	Anthelmintic and for parasites in general.
Essential oils Thyme, Cinnamon, Oregano, Clove, Boldo, Black Spruce, Eucalyptus, Cajeput, Tea Tree	Anthelmintic and parasites in general. For topical use or in capsules with carrier oil or add to tincture, 1–2 drops per ounce.
Usnea spp. Old Man's beard thallus	Antifungal; clears toxic heat.
Calendula officinalis Marigold flower	Antifungal, antiamoebic. Clears toxic heat (mild).
Juglans regia Walnut hull and leaf	Anthelmintic for tapeworms and roundworms.
Cucurbita maxima Pumpkin seed (raw)	Anthelmintic. Blend raw seeds into a paste with almond or coconut milk and water.
Areca catechu Bing Lang Betel nut	Broad-spectrum anthelmintic, especially tapeworm.
Brucea javancia Ya Dan Zi Java berry	Anthelmintic, antiprotozoal, antiamoebic.
Melaleuca spp. Tea Tree essential oil	Antifungal. Very good topically for athlete's foot and others.

CASE HISTORY 17.3

Case History for Fungal Infection

S. Louise has red cracks between her toes. They itch, sting, and burn. She's had this since the summer when she went swimming. Over-the-counter athlete's foot powder didn't help. Reports gas, bloating, and indigestion on regular basis.

O. **P** Normal. **T** Thick, yellow coat. Feet have red cracks between the toes with flaking and sweaty skin that looks like it's breaking down.

A. Spleen Damp Heat. Fungal infection of the foot; probably athlete's foot (*Tinea pedis*). Compromised immunity due to dysbiosis.

P. *Specific therapeutic principles.* (1) Kill foot fungus. (2) Dry spleen damp. (3) Treat dysbiosis. (4) Strengthen immune system. (5) Treat herbally, externally and internally.

Internal Herbal Formula and Dose. 5 mL 3 times a day.

Part	Herbs	Rationale
3	Coptis Huan Lian	Antifungal, antibacterial, bitter for gut flora, dry.
2	Pau d'arco or Usnea	Antifungal.
2	Meadowsweet	Balance gut flora and restore gut.
2	Magnolia bark Hou Po	Balance gut flora, dry spleen damp.
2	*Echinacea angustifolia*	Immunostimulant, detoxifier.

External Foot Soak and Dose. 1 week to 1 month 2 times per day until rash is cleared.

Part	Herbs	Rationale
3/4	Warm water	Solvent.
1/4	Apple cider vinegar	Antifungal, acidic.
40 gtts	Tea Tree essential oil	Antifungal.

Other Suggestions

- Keep feet very dry. After soaks, sprinkle Garlic powder in dry white socks. Change after each soak.
- Diet: Prebiotics, fermented foods and/or yogurt. No sugar.
- Supplements: Probiotics.

More often parasites are sneaky, because they hide behind and accompany other problems like chronic skin outbreaks, dysbiosis, allergies, chronic infections, chronic fatigue, or cancer. Consequently, in addition to eliminating the actual parasites, it is necessary to treat the underlying deficiency.[11] This treatment includes using restoratives for the offending area, tonifying yin or yang as the case may be, nourishing the yin or blood. The microbiome has to be addressed. It takes good detective work and a wise assessment to puzzle it out. The basic therapeutic principles follow.

- *Antiparasitics are the primary herbs.* Use two to cover the bases. Unless you know the exact species of fungus, helminth, or amoeba, use broad-spectrum antiparasitics that are aimed toward that type of parasite. If it's worms, choose Wormwood herb or Rue herb; if it's athlete's foot fungus, use Tea Tree essential oil externally, and perhaps Usnea thallus internally. If it's vaginal amoebic *Trichomonas vaginalis*, perhaps use a Mugwort herb and Oregon Grape root douche, combined internally with Oak bark and a berberine.
- *For external parasites, also treat internally.* As well as using an external remedy on, say, ringworm or a tick bite, make up an internal formula to approach it from the interior with vulneraries and immunostimulants.
- *Treat underlying problem.* Unless there is a known history of direct exposure, parasites are usually caused by a root problem. Address possible causes by choosing bitters for dysbiosis, adaptogens for decreased immunity, adrenal restoratives such as Licorice root or Nettle herb for fatigue, and alteratives (skin detoxicants) like Yellow Dock root or Red Clover flower for skin outbreaks.
- *Flush out helminths.* Use lymphatics, diuretics, or blood movers to provide an escape route for the worms. A lymphatic mover might be Cleavers herb, Red Root, or Dandelion leaf for a diuretic and Salvia Dan Shen (Cinnabar Sage root) as a blood mover.
- *Immunostimulants.* Assume the immune system is weakened, or the parasite wouldn't be there in the first place. Try Echinacea root, Ganoderma Ling Zhi (Reishi mushroom), Lonicera Jin Yin Hua (Honeysuckle flower), Forsythia Lian Qiao (Forsythia valve), and others.

Intestinal parasitic die-off. This is a possible, but not an absolute, positive side effect of anthelmintic treatment. ***Die-off*** refers to toxins from dying pathogens (parasites, worms, candida, etc.), overwhelming the body's abilities to clear them out. It can cause nasty side effects: fever, muscle aches, headaches, skin rash, excess mucus, brain fog, and irregular bowels. Hence, an important therapeutic principle is to make sure the body can eliminate all the dead worms and their toxins. This is accomplished by including one or two lymphatic decongestants, such as Cleavers herb or Red Root, a qi and blood mover, a mild laxative, and/or a diuretic.

Chinese Medicine Perspective on Infections with Major Syndromes

In Chinese Medicine, many infectious syndromes have *wind* in their names, meaning microbes enter the body from the outside environment, *external wind*, or from the inside, *internal wind*. Herbs that treat these infections are broad-spectrum antiinfectives that also stimulate the immune system. Most are antipyretic, anti-inflammatory, and act as local antiseptics or systemic antimicrobials (Table 17.5).

- *Wind Cold.* In early-onset infectious processes that come on gradually, many infections are still cold and have not yet progressed to heat. There is no fever, phlegm is still clear or white, and inflammation is just beginning. This is known as Wind Cold. The infection is there, or we would not feel *inklings* and *warnings* like a scratchy throat or a headache. Herbs should be antiinfective, neutral, or warming to dispel Wind Cold, like Garlic bulb, Ginger root, Osha root, and/or Peppermint leaf. It's time to sweat it out by taking a hot bath or sauna to nip it in the bud. **Tongue (T)** Normal, thin, white coat. **Pulse (P)** Tight, superficial, especially in the Lung position.
- *Wind Heat.* At this stage, there is heat, manifesting as chills, fever, or feeling hot; mild thirst; yellowish phlegm. These require herbs to promote sweating, reduce any fever, and dispel Wind Heat. The energetics to accomplish these goals are cool and pungent herbs. Relaxant diaphoretics, sometimes called peripheral vasodilators, are also used: Catnip herb, Spearmint leaf, and Elderberry. **T** Red body; thin, white, or yellow coat. **P** Rapid, superficial.

TABLE 17.5 Herbs for Chinese Medicine Infectious Syndromes
(Notice that many of these herbs have more than one action, and appear in multiple lists)

Wind Cold	Wind Heat	Damp Heat	Fire Toxins
To treat: dispel wind cold and promote sweating. Use warm, stimulant diaphoretics and antimicrobials.	*To treat: dispel wind heat, cool the exterior, and promote sweating. Use pungent, cool, relaxant diaphoretics and antimicrobials.*	*To treat: dry damp and clear heat. Use bitter, cold, dry astringents, and antimicrobials.*	*To treat: clear damp heat and detoxify fire toxins. Use broad-spectrum antiinfectives, antiseptics, detoxicants, antipyretics, and immunostimulants.*
Zingiber officinale Ginger root and/or essential oil. Also for digestion, nausea.	*Lonicera japonica* Jin Yin Hua Honeysuckle flower	The berberine roots. Goldenseal, Oregon Grape root, Barberry, Coptis Huang Lian, Phellodendron Huang Bai.	The berberine roots. Goldenseal, Oregon Grape root, Barberry, Coptis Huang Lian, Phellodendron Huang Bai
Ligusticum porteri Osha root Diaphoretic, expectorant.	*Forsythia suspensa* Lian Qiao Clears toxins, moves lymph.	*Vaccinium* spp. Bilberry leaf and fruit.	*Andrographis* Chuan Xin Lian Heart-Thread Lotus leaf.
Mentha x piperita Peppermint leaf Cooling and warming.	*Nepeta cataria* Catnip leaf Very good for fever in infants.	*Gentiana lutea* Gentian root For liver/gallbladder.	*Forsythia suspensa* Lian Qiao often paired with *Lonicera japonica* Jin Yin Hua Honeysuckle flower
Magnolia liliiflora Xin Yi Hua. Magnolia bud Ear, nose, throat (ENT) tropism.	*Sambucus nigra* Elderberry and flower Excels in syrup for kids and adult kids.	*Arctostaphylos uva ursi* Bearberry leaf For bladder damp heat, UTI.	*Isatis tinctoria* Ban Lan Gen Isatis root
Xanthium sibiricum Cang Er Zi Siberian Cocklebur Nasal decongestant.	*Tilia cordata* Linden flower	*Larrea divaricata* Creosote/Chaparral leaf.	*Phellodendron* Huang Bai Phellodendron leaf
Perilla frutescens Zi Su Ye Perilla leaf. Nasal stimulant.	*Mentha spicata* Spearmint leaf and essential oil.	*Tabebuia avellanedae* Pau d'arco bark Also, for toxic heat, fungus, and parasites.	*Echinacea angustifolia* root Antibacterial and antiviral, but foremost clears toxins. Immunostimulant.
Angelica dahurica Bai Zhi Like Western *A. archangelica*	*Eupatorium perfoliatum* Boneset herb Very, very bitter.	*Scutellaria baicalensis* Huang Qin Baikal Skullcap root Broad-spectrum, biofilms.	*Calendula officinalis* Marigold flower Excels with tissue trauma, first aid.
Asarum canadense Wild Ginger root. Also, spasmolytic and relaxing	*Mentha* x *piperita* Peppermint leaf	*Gardenia jasminoides* Zhi Zi. Gardenia pod For liver damp heat.	*Plantago* spp. Plantain leaf Antifungal and antibacterial.
	Verbena officinalis Vervain herb	*Salix alba* White Willow bark. For pain.	*Usnea* spp. Old Man's Beard thallus *Streptococcus* specific.

- *Damp Heat.* Dampness has now come on board, along with heat and infection. This is a little more challenging. Intention is to dry damp and reduce fever and infection with bitter, cold, dry astringents such as berberines or Pau d'arco bark. **T** Red body; sticky, yellow coat. **P** Slippery and rapid.
- *Fire toxins.* In the Western sense, toxins are damaging proteins produced by bacteria, which target other bacteria or host cells. They are also formed as waste products of metabolism. In Chinese Medicine, ***fire toxins*** are infectious materials occurring in tissues in the form of pus and oozing, as seen in tumors, cysts, ulcers, boils, skin rashes, or eczema. Remedies are herbs that clear damp heat, drain pus and fluid, and kill infectious organisms from internal and external sores and abscesses. The Chinese have herbs that clear fire toxins.[13] Examples are Creosote/Chaparral leaf, Yellow Dock root, or Scutellaria Huang Qin (Baikal Skullcap root). **T** Deep red body; thick, yellow coat. **P** Rapid.

Summary

This chapter explored concepts regarding infection and toxicosis, which included bacteria, viruses, the many types of parasites, and their Materia Medicas. Antimicrobial herbs are usually cold, bitter, astringent, drying, sinking, and chemically rich in alkaloids. Chinese Medicine syndromes related to infection and toxicosis include: Wind Cold, Wind Heat, Damp Heat, and Fire Toxins.

Bacteria are one-celled organisms that can cause lethal diseases. They can be broad- or narrow-spectrum, systemic or nonsystemic, and gram-positive or gram-negative. They are becoming increasingly resistant to many antibiotic drugs, causing an infectious disease health crisis.

Viruses are incomplete cells made up of strands of DNA or RNA surrounded by a protein coat. They can lie dormant for years and come to life inside a healthy host cell's nucleus, replicating when the time is right. The chief allopathic treatment for viruses is vaccines; however, there are many antiviral herbal remedies.

Parasites live on other organisms and get their nutrients from their host. Helminths are parasitic worms that can live in the gut. When treating worms and other parasites, an important concept to address is die-off, in which toxins from dying pathogens can cause unpleasant symptoms in their host.

The *germ theory* was contrasted to the biofilm theory. Biofilms may be one explanation for why infections are resistant to antibiotics. It now seems that these entire microbe groups are often the culprit and explains why some diseases remain entrenched and chronic, despite repeated antibiotic treatment. Many broad-spectrum antimicrobial herbals are effective for biofilms, such as *Echinacea angustifolia*, the berberines, and Scutellaria Huang Qin.

Review

Fill in the Blanks

(Answers in Appendix B.)

1. Energetically, antimicrobial herbs are (four) ___, ___, ___, ___.
2. Name three systemic antibiotic herbs: ___, ___, ___.
3. Name three nonsystemic antibiotic herbs: ___, ___, ___.
4. Name four therapeutic herbal categories for infectious disease formulation: ___, ___, ___, ___.
5. Give five therapeutic principles when treating parasites. ___, ___, ___, ___, ___.
6. Name five immunostimulant herbs: ___, ___, ___, ___, ___.
7. Name four Chinese Medicine infectious disease syndromes: ___, ___, ___, ___.
8. Give five Western examples of a hot, wet, toxic condition: ___, ___, ___, ___, ___.
9. Name three ways biofilms protect themselves: ___, ___, ___.
10. Name five broad-spectrum, systemic herbals (give botanical names): ___, ___, ___, ___, ___.

Critical Concept Questions

(Answers for you to decide.)

1. What is the difference between a virus and a bacterium?
2. Discuss why bacteria are becoming resistant to antibiotics.
3. Why is drug resistance a health crisis?
4. What is the biofilm theory and why are scientists developing antibiofilm drugs?
5. Because herbal antimicrobials don't disrupt the microbiome, why should clients still take probiotics?
6. Discuss herbal rationale and dosing for infections.
7. What is the difference between an epidemic and a pandemic?
8. Explain what helminth die-off means.
9. Why is *Sambucus nigra* perfect for wind heat infections? Explain in terms of energetics.
10. How do vaccines work? Do you think they are a good idea? What would you recommend to your client?

References

1. Buhner, Stephen Harrod. *Herbal Antibiotics* (North Adams, MA: Storey, 2012).
2. Buhner, Stephen Harrod. *Herbal Antivirals* (North Adams, MA: Storey, 2013).
3. Shiel, William C. "Medical Definition of Gram Stain." MedicineNet. http://www.medicinenet.com/script/main/art.asp?articlekey = 9583 (accessed July 31, 2019).
4. Naeser, Margaret. *Outline Guide to Herbal Patent Medicines in Pill Form* (Ann Arbor: Edwards Brothers, 1990).
5. Donlan, Rodney M. and J. William Costerton. "Biofilms: Survival Mechanisms of Clinically Relevant Microorganisms." American Society for Microbiology. https://cmr.asm.org/content/15/2/167 (accessed July 31, 2019).
6. D'Adamo Peter. "Biofilms and Herbal Medicine." Official Website of Dr Peter D'Adamo. http://www.dadamo.com/txt/index.pl?1025 (accessed July 31, 2019).
7. Miller, MB and B.L. Bassler. "Quorum Sensing in Bacteria." PubMed. https://www.ncbi.nlm.nih.gov/pubmed/11544353 (accessed July 31, 2019).
8. Bergner, Paul, American Herbalist Guild seminar notes. Poole, K. "Efflux Pumps as Antimicrobial Resistance Mechanisms." Ann Med 39 (2007).
9. Bergner, Paul. "Botanicals, Biofilms, and Chronic Infections." Southwest Conference on Botanical Medicine. Tempe, AZ, April 2016.
10. Aroram DP, et al. "Nitric Oxide Regulation of Bacterial Biofilms." PubMed https://www.ncbi.nlm.nih.gov/pubmed/25996573 (accessed July 31, 2019).
11. Holmes, Peter. *Energetics of Western Herbs* (Boulder, CO: Snow Lotus, 2006).
12. "About Parasites." Centers for Disease Control and Prevention. https://www.cdc.gov/parasites/about.html(accessed July 31, 2019).
13. Holmes, Peter. *Jade Remedies: A Chinese Herbal Reference for the West* (Boulder, CO: Snow Lotus, 1996).

18
The Gastrointestinal System

"Hidden civilizations reside in the gut."

—Dr. Felice Gersch

CHAPTER REVIEW

- Gut functions: Digestion, microbiome, immune system, autoimmunity, gut-brain connection and mental health, endocrine organ, and detoxification.
- Chakras. The third chakra, the power center.
- Chinese Medicine perspective on the gut with major syndromes.
- Maintaining gut health: The Four-R program/protocol.
- Digestive system Materia Medica: Honorable-mention gastrointestinal (GI) herbs. Tropho-restoratives and Spleen tonics, bitters, antimicrobials, prebiotics, leaky gut healers, digestive aids (stimulants, relaxants, antacids, carminatives, demulcents). Antidiarrheals, hemostatics, and laxatives.
- Common GI conditions with case histories: Diarrhea, chronic constipation, simple dyspepsia/indigestion, inflammatory bowel diseases (Crohn's and ulcerative colitis), irritable bowel syndrome (IBS), ulcers, gluten sensitivity and celiac disease, intestinal yeast infection, and gastroesophageal reflux disease (GERD).

KEY TERMS

Autoimmune response
Bitters
Celiac disease
Chakra
Constipation
Crohn's disease
Diarrhea
Elimination diet
Enteric nervous system (ENS)
Four-R program
Gastroesophageal reflux disease (GERD)
GI stimulants
GI ulcers
Gluten sensitivity
Gripe
Gut and Psychology Syndrome (GAPS) diet
Gut associated lymphoid tissue (GALT)
Hemostatics
Inflammatory bowel disease (IBD)
Intestinal permeability (IP), leaky gut
Irritable bowel syndrome (IBS)
Laxatives
Microbiome
Prebiotics
Probiotics
Purgatives
Small intestinal bowel overgrowth (SIBO)
Spleen tonics
Transit time
Ulcerative colitis

The gastrointestinal or digestive system is so named because of its obvious function as a channel for food *digestion*, *assimilation*, *absorption*, and *elimination*, and the many ills associated with these roles. We need food to live, providing both nutrients and energy. The gastrointestinal (GI) system was first discovered and researched by U.S. Army surgeon, William Beaumont (1785–1853), known as the father of gastric physiology. We now know the GI system goes far beyond Beaumont's original understanding.

The gut affects whole body health because of the 2 ½ to 3 pounds of intestinal microbiome associated with health and/or disease. The gut profoundly influences the immune and nervous systems and can even affect our moods, because it is part of the gut-brain connection. The Four-R approach to gut health involves using herbs and foods to fix and maintain the microbiome and mucosa. Appreciation for a healthy intestinal flora and for keeping it healthy is a priority for herbalists.

From a mind-body perspective, the gut is the location of the third chakra, our personal energetic power center in relation to the external world and the seat of our emotions. When we know and feel a truth at gut level, it is unshakable and hard to deny. It must be confronted, no matter how painful or fearful. The third chakra relates to self-esteem and our perceived place in the world. Working with it is part of the healing journey.

In Chinese Medicine, the GI system involves the yin Spleen and its organ pair, the yang Stomach. The Spleen has many functions, some not really part of digestion. Consequently, you will also meet the Chinese Spleen in other chapters.

The Many Aspects of Gut Functions

The Gut Is a Digestive Organ System

We can live about 3 days without water and around 3 weeks without food. The digestive system extracts and synthesizes the nutrients from our food with the help of enzymes and hormones. It takes care of breaking down our food into the macronutrients —carbohydrates, proteins, and fats—so that they can be absorbed and transported throughout the bloodstream to every cell in the body. Carbohydrates supply energy; proteins are used for growth and repair; fats store energy. These are obviously crucial functions, and things can go quite wrong with this process, causing most commonly indigestion, constipation, diarrhea, infection, weight gain or loss, reflux, gallstones, celiac and Crohn's disease, ulcerative colitis, irritable bowel disease (IBD), hemorrhoids, diverticulitis, and other problems.

The Gut Houses the Microbiome

The ***microbiome***, addressed throughout this textbook, concerns the all-important 2 ½ or so pounds of roughly 1000 different species of microorganisms residing mainly in the large intestine (Fig. 18.1). These can get out of balance and make us very uncomfortable. The microbiome affects nutrient absorption, detoxification, moods, appetite, food cravings, chronic pain, and mental function. When it gets out of balance, we get inflammation, leaky gut or intestinal permeability, and the resultant ills of inflamed neurons, autoimmune and chronic diseases, obesity, insulin resistance and diabetes, hormonal problems, anxiety, depression, and brain fog.[1] Add to this list arthritis, allergies, and food intolerances. Any and all body systems may be affected. Maintaining and/or healing intestinal permeability is paramount in dealing with these problems. Further on we'll look at the specifics of doing this on a nutritional and herbal level.

The Gut Is an Immune Organ

At least 70% of the immune system is in the gut. The gut is constantly threatened with antigens, which are foreign invaders from the diet and any other infectious bacteria that get in the mouth by whatever means. Even in our cleanliness-obsessed society, no food is sterile. Utensils and countertops are quite germy. Who knows what comes in contact with our hands before they reach our mouths? Don't even think about what babies touch and eat and somehow live through it. How come we don't (usually) get sick?

The colon has developed an amazing barrier to deal with these threats, the ***gut-associated lymphoid tissue (GALT)***, which is an important part of the immune system. The GALT is only one single cell wall thick yet guards against the penetration of microbes from outside sources. It traps bacteria in its rich protective mucus, kills and expels foreign invaders, and activates many types of immune cells.

A well-balanced colon microbiome provides essential immune protection and is necessary for mucosal health. Commensal, friendly microbes compete with potential pathogens for space and food. Furthermore, good gut flora regulates maturation of the mucosa and activates immune functions in the GALT, whereas pathogenic gut flora causes immune dysfunction, increasing inflammation that leads to leaky gut, and resulting in disease formation.

When exposed to pathogenic microbes in spoiled or bad food, we can get food poisoning. Should this occur, the gut wall secretes the inflammatory response chemical, *histamine*, which is detected by the ***enteric nervous system (ENS)***, a meshlike system of neurons that governs the function of the gastrointestinal tract. Nausea, vomiting, or diarrhea ensues in attempts to expel the bad bugs.

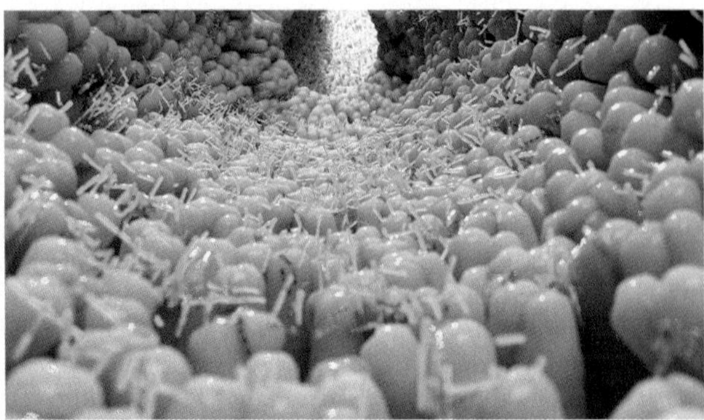

• **Fig. 18.1** Highly magnified view of various microorganisms residing in a healthy gut. (iStock.com/Credit: Marcin Klapczynski.)

The Gut Is an Autoimmune Organ

The autoimmune disease list keeps growing. Here's the physiology. When spaces form between the cell walls of the intestinal lining because of microbiome imbalance or dysbiosis, ***leaky gut*** or ***intestinal permeability (IP)*** is created (Fig. 18.2). IP allows large undigested protein molecules to leak out between the cells and be absorbed across the intestinal lining into the bloodstream (just like digested food). These molecules are then transported all over the body. When they arrive at a weakened, susceptible organ, they initiate an inflammatory response. This sets up an antigen-antibody response. The body perceives the undigested food as an antigen—an enemy—and builds up antibodies to destroy the tissue. Essentially, this process is an ***autoimmune response***—the body is destroying itself. The gut wall is destroyed in Crohn's, ulcerative colitis, and celiac disease. The myelin sheath is destroyed in multiple sclerosis (MS). Joints deteriorate in arthritis. Pancreatic islet cells stop making insulin in diabetes. The thyroid gland enlarges in Hashimoto's hypothyroidism. All of these are autoimmune responses.

When the microbiome is balanced, and IP is healed and sealed, inflammation and the antigen-antibody response stops. The autoimmune condition is improved, if not cured.

The Gut Communicates with the Brain and Affects Mood

We used to think that all thoughts and emotions were in our head. Not so. The gut affects the brain, and the brain affects the gut. The gut is considered the *second brain*. Neurons composing the enteric nervous system (ENS) in the gut send out hormones and chemical neurotransmitters to the brain along the vagus nerve. These chemicals are responsible for originating the emotions and thoughts that

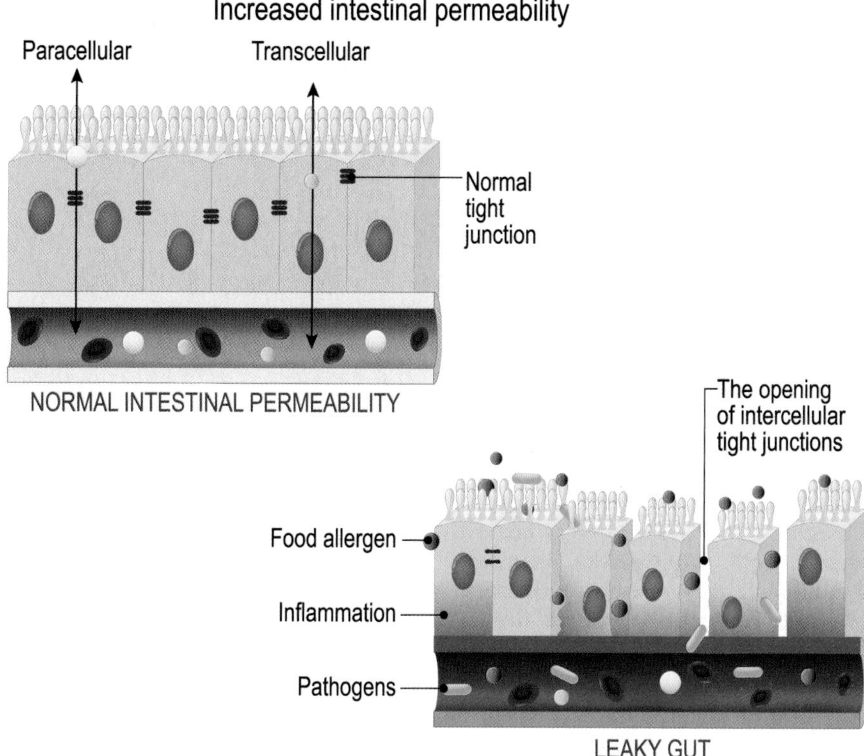

• **Fig. 18.2** Normal intestine showing tightly aligned cell walls, and an abnormal gut showing undigested particles leaking out between loose cell junctions into the bloodstream. (iStock.com/Credit: ttsz.)

the brain interprets. If we are joyous, nervous, or depressed, the actual chemicals released from the ENS send that message to the brain. In this way, mood and mental illness are influenced on a gut level. This connection is why the gut is considered the second brain.

The brain does the same thing in reverse. Sometimes the chemicals and neurotransmitters originate at the brain end, sending messages to the gut. However, more emotional messages originate in the gut than in the brain. This association is why so many GI illnesses are stress related (excessive cortisol production) and why stress gives us GI symptoms.

We literally "feel it in our gut," intuitively and physically, and this phenomenon affects our health for better or worse. Mental illness and exaggerated emotions are related to this phenomenon, egged on by intestinal permeability. Most mental illnesses, including attention deficit hyperactivity disorder (ADHD) and autism, are helped by healing dysbiosis and leaky gut.

The close connection between gut and brain explains why we can feel intestinal or GI pain or get a bout of diarrhea when stressed, because these issues all begin on a gut level. Nausea might result from appearing before an audience or presenting a paper. It's not all in our heads. Depression, anxiety, anger, happiness, and particularly stress have an influence on our health. Negative emotions can lead to GI inflammation, susceptibility to infection, and depressed immunity. Irritable bowel and other GI irregularities are more severe when there is stress. Stress makes pain worse.[2] Therefore, therapies for stress reduction such as meditation, yoga, psychotherapy, and other modalities can help reduce many inflammatory bowel diseases and improve immunity and overall well-being.

The Gut Is an Endocrine Organ

The gut and a healthy microbiome influence hormonal balances throughout the body, which then impacts women's health, thyroid problems, sleep patterns, diabetes, weight control, and appetite. For instance, gut flora plays a role in premenstrual syndrome (PMS) and menopause. When estrogen accumulates and is not properly eliminated by the liver each month, a situation called estrogen dominance occurs (Chapter 28). This is one cause of heavy periods, PMS, fibroids, and uterine cancer. Dysbiosis is a key player and makes the situation worse.

Hashimoto's thyroiditis is an autoimmune type of hypothyroidism, the most common kind. Autoimmune diseases are a well-established result of leaky gut. Healthy flora is essential for conversion in the thyroid gland (and liver) of thyroid hormone T-4 into the stronger and more bioavailable T-3 (Chapter 27).

The flora also affects mood and sleep. About 80% to 90% of the feel-good hormone, serotonin, is produced in the gut. Melatonin hormone production, which enhances sleep, is produced from serotonin. Therefore a good serotonin supply helps induce a good melatonin supply and ensures sound sleep.

Another example is appetite control. The wrong microbiome mix alters the way we store fat, balance blood glucose levels, and respond to hunger and satiety. *Leptin* hormone tells us we're full; *ghrelin* hormone increases hunger. With a wacky microbiome, we become leptin-resistant and don't get the signal to quit eating.[3] We plow on through that carton of ice cream.

The Gut Is a Detoxifier

The digestive system is a natural toxin eliminator that works 24/7 to sort through and eliminate waste. When it becomes overloaded, trouble begins. Normally, undigested, unabsorbed, and unusable food products are passed through the colon for elimination. If these pile up too fast, they overwhelm the gut. They break down, adhere to the colon wall, and, in time, seep back into the bloodstream, resulting in a toxic condition.

Bowels develop toxic overload from chemicals, fertilizers, antibiotics, pesticides, industrial waste, cleaning products, heavy metals, and drugs that permeate our food and water supply. The body tries hard to detoxify these contaminants through the bowel and liver but often can't keep up. Toxins can bind to cells in the immune, nervous, and endocrine systems. Inflammation and oxidative stress occur, even causing genetic alterations.[1] Symptoms can manifest in any body system. We might develop brain fog, impaired memory, autoimmune syndromes, metabolic prediabetic syndrome, and hormonal imbalances with PMS or hot flashes. Some of the more common symptoms are fatigue, cyclic breast tenderness, inability to lose weight even on a low-calorie diet, emotional swings, and digestive problems, all of which signal toxic overload.

All kinds of cleanses or detoxification programs exist: colonics, colema boards (a type of home enema), fasting, expensive supplements, and powdered foods, for example. Most cleanses work temporarily, and the person initially feels lighter, brighter, and more energetic and experiences weight loss. Too soon old symptoms return, and the need for detoxification creates a vicious cycle. Eventually, the thyroid resets the thermostat to slow down and store more fat. As the person reverts back to old eating habits, weight gain returns. Except in severe instances when all else has failed, we really don't need a heroic cleanse. Here are two conservative detoxification methods:

- *Permanent lifestyle changes*. Eat a wide variety of natural foods. Go organic as much as possible. Cut down use of chemically laden cosmetics and household cleaners and avoid unnecessary medications.[1] These measures are really lifestyle changes that give the digestive system a rest, allowing the gut wall to heal and remain healed. If healthy measures become a habit instead of a yearly 2-week marathon, an occasional cookie or piece of cake won't matter. Sometimes it is necessary to stay gluten or dairy free forever, but not always.
- *Occasional 1-day cleanse*. A fairly easy detoxification method is to take a day out of every 1 or 2 weeks, and drink only easy-to-digest alkaline vegetable juices. This modified fast gives the digestive system a vacation, providing it with a periodic rest-and-rejuvenation spa day. This ritual can become a *going within* opportunity, a spiritual cleanse as well. Add luxurious bathing, resting, meditation, a walk, and time out. Include herbs that help the gut and liver work better. Bitters for the gut are Burdock or Yellow Dock root, Turmeric root, and Bitter Melon. For the liver, there's Milk Thistle seed and Bupleurum Chai Hu, among others.

Chakras

Chakra is a Sanskrit word meaning *wheel*. Chakras refer to the spiritual energy center of the body (Fig. 18.3). There are seven major chakras in the form of spinning wheels or balls of light ascending from the base of the spine to the crown or top of the head and situated along major nerve bundles (a *plexus)* along the way, places where the physical body and consciousness meet. They are a linking of mind, body, and spirit and have everything to do with holistic healing. Each chakra is associated with the physical organs they are near and with various emotional and spiritual issues a person might be dealing with that is contributing to their illness.

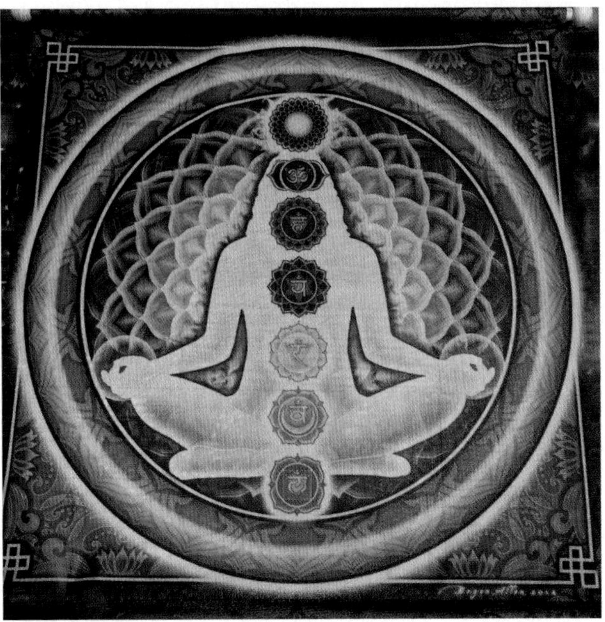

• **Fig. 18.3** The seven major chakras are the spiritual energy centers of the body. They are counted from the root (pelvis) to the crown (head).

These wheels of light are connected to one another, and energy can get blocked anywhere along the way. (A lot like Chinese meridians and qi.) So too, each spinning chakra can wobble on its axis, spin in the wrong direction (clockwise is normal) or stop moving altogether. If emotional issues are not dealt with, illness may eventually manifest on a physical level, because of the mind-body connection.

As we go through the Therapeutics and Formulations section, considering the body systems one by one, the chakra connected with that system will be included, along with its significance to total healing.

The Third Chakra, the Power Center

Gut-level feelings are nothing new. Metaphysically, they were always the case, and now science is chiming in with evidence that they are a physical fact (Fig. 18.4). The gut is related to the third chakra, our core and power center, called the *solar plexus*, located right below the diaphragm and connected energetically to the digestive organs.[4] It is the seat of our emotions, having to do with feelings, self-esteem, and how we view ourselves in the world. It is interesting that this intuitive metaphysical insight was around thousands of years before science became aware of the gut-brain relationship to emotions.

When we consider the mind-body connection, we realize that spiritual and emotional work must be done as effectively as the work we do to maintain physical structure. This requirement is especially true with autoimmune inflammatory bowel disease (IBD),

• **Fig. 18.4** The third chakra is our core and power center, called the solar plexus. It is associated with the organs of digestion.

irritable bowel syndrome (IBS), indigestion, ulcers, hepatitis, and eating disorders. It is important to take back our power and deal with issues, such as overcoming our fears, so that gut health can be realized.

Chinese Medicine Perspective: The Gut with Major Syndromes

The Chinese Spleen is different from the Western spleen. In Western physiology, the spleen is part of the immune system, a lymphatic tissue that stores blood and produces white blood cells, antibodies, and stem cells. In the Chinese Medicine realm, it is the main organ of digestion and much more besides.

- *The Chinese Medicine yin Spleen is the main organ of digestion.* It works with its yang partner, the Stomach. In this sense, it governs the transformation and transportation of food. It produces qi from the energy of the food it receives. Strong Spleen qi creates good digestion. Spleen Qi Deficiency or weakness results in indigestion, bloating, and burping, prevalent Western conditions. Digestion creates warmth. Spleen energy is warm and is in the Earth element.
- *According to correspondences,* the Spleen opens to the mouth and manifests on the lips. Healthy Spleen, bright lips; deficient Spleen, pale lips and dulled taste. Spleen controls the muscles and limbs. If Spleen is weak, muscles are weak and tired.
- *According to the correspondences, overthinking and excess worry* are Spleen problems, because the Spleen houses thought, intentions, and focus, called *yi.* When you can't think or remember anything or have brain fog, there is Spleen deficiency. If the mind won't be still and thoughts churn, the Spleen is to blame.
- *The Spleen holds things in place (raises qi).* It supports our organs. If the Spleen is weak or deficient, the organs can prolapse or sag—as in vaginal, uterine, or anal prolapse, weak vein walls, hemorrhoids, and varicose veins.
- *The Spleen produces and controls blood.* Not only does it actually make blood, it also keeps blood where it belongs. If Spleen qi is weak or deficient, we bruise easily from broken capillaries or have trouble with bleeding. Bleeding hemorrhoids is an example of the Spleen not controlling blood and of not holding the rectum firmly in place.
- *The Spleen likes to stay dry.* Spleen damp causes many problems. Heat combined with damp (Spleen Damp Heat) is even worse. It produces thirst without a desire to drink and loose smelly stools. On the other hand, if the Spleen is too dry, there could be constipation.[5] A balance must be reached. In general, the Spleen likes foods that are warm (in energy and temperature), e.g., meat, pepper, ginger, and orange peel. Too many cold foods cause Spleen dampness.

Chinese Medicine Major Spleen Syndromes

Please note that signs and symptoms listed for any given syndrome are all the ones that are possible, not all those required for that syndrome to exist. Furthermore, there are parallels in pulse and tongue that cross over to other syndromes. A person may also have one or more existing syndromes at the same time. (The same applies to Western signs, symptoms and diagnosis.)

- *Spleen Qi Deficiency.* This deficiency is a very common syndrome in the West. It translates as classic indigestion from stress, damp weather, excessive thinking or worry, having irregular eating habits, and eating too many cold or raw foods. The client with this deficiency also may crave sweets, the Spleen's taste. Symptoms include fatigue, bloating after eating, heavy limbs, sallow complexion, and loose stools (because if qi is deficient, the Spleen can't hold in gut contents). Ulcers and gastritis fit with this syndrome. **Pulse (P)** Weak, especially on the right side under the middle finger (the Spleen position). **Tongue (T)** Usually swollen and puffy. In severe cases, coat is thick, white, and greasy. The fix is to tonify and warm Spleen qi. Eat warm and cooked foods. Relax when eating. The *Four Gentlemen Decoction* is a classic formula to tonify Spleen qi (Box 18.1).
- *Spleen Yang Deficiency.* This syndrome is similar to Spleen Qi Deficiency but exhibits more severe symptoms: wet and cold, excess fluids, chilly with cold hands or feet, edema, loose undigested stool, heavy limbs, bloating, and fatigue. Might present with *Candida albicans,* food allergies, or chronic hepatitis. **P** Weak, slow, deep. **T** Pale, swollen, wet, and/or thicker white coat. Here, the fix is to tonify and warm Spleen yang, using Panax Ren Shen (Red ginseng root), Astragalus Huang Qi (Astragalus root), and Piper Hu Jiao (Black Peppercorn).
- *Liver Invading Spleen.* This problem could present as irritable bowel syndrome (IBS), with alternating constipation and diarrhea. Liver stagnation causes constipation. Stool is stuck. Weak Spleen qi can cause the opposite—diarrhea, where the client can't hold it in or keep it in the body. Both are often present and alternate back and forth. Abdominal pain that moves around is helped by bowel movements. There is lots of belching and gas. The condition is brought on by stress. This is a classic picture for IBS. **P** Wiry. **T** Thin, white coat; body color normal. To improve this condition, we must move Liver qi and tonify the Spleen. Specific herbs are chosen depending on symptoms.

• **BOX 18.1 Four Gentlemen Decoction**
Si Jun Zi Tang

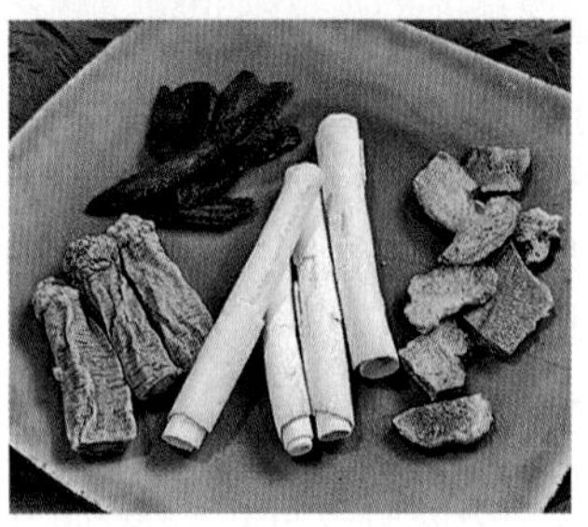

The Four Gentlemen are Poria Fu Ling (Hoelen fungus-center), Glycyrrhiza Zhi Gan Cao (Honey-fried Licorice-top left), Atractylodes Bai Zhu (White Atractylodes-right), and Codonopsis Dang Shen (Downy Bellflower root-bottom left).

The Four Gentlemen Decoction patent formula tonifies qi and strengthens Spleen (energy and digestion)

Si Jun Zi Tang is an elegant and essential energy-enhancing formula because of its yang and qi tonifying aspects. To have good energy, we must have good digestion. The formula addresses this, which is the root of many a problem. *Four Gentlemen* refers to the fact that each herb is equally important and together exhibit ideal behavior—a lovely *gentlemanly* Chinese concept, not that it is a men's-only formula. It is also useful for women.

Symptoms for the formula are fatigue, pale, quiet voice that results from lack of qi; possibly weak appetite and low body weight; and a tendency toward loose stools. All this involves a weakening of the central qi.[6] *Four Gentlemen* strengthens the immune system, digestion, and liver and gives more energy. Very useful for common ills of modern living.

Codonopsis Dang Shen (Downy Bellflower root)	9 g	Tonifies qi and Spleen.
Atractylodes Bai Zhu (White Atractylodes root)	6 g	Tonifies Spleen, dries damp.
Poria Fu Ling (Hoelen fungus)	6 g	Tonifies Spleen, dries damp.
Glycyrrhiza Zhi Gan Cao (Honey-fried Licorice root)	3 g	Does it all and blends.

Directions. 3 cups of decoction 3 × day or 5 mL of a 1:5 tincture 3 × day.

- *Damp Cold Invading Spleen.* This excess condition comes with the feeling of cold in epigastrium because qi is not moving. It improves with warmth. There is no thirst, no appetite, a sticky sweet taste in the mouth, heaviness in the head, loose thin stools, and sometimes white vaginal discharge. Excessive cold foods, hangover, and dampness overwhelm the Spleen, as do chronic illnesses, such as gastritis or colitis, ulcers, or hepatitis. **P** Slow and slippery. **T** Puffy or swollen, color pale, sticky and thick white coat. Dry up Spleen dampness by eating warming foods and eliminating dairy. Herbally, use a stimulating diuretic such as Poria Fu Ling (Hoelen fungus), bitter-pungent Magnolia Hou Pou (Magnolia bark), warming Zingiber Gan Jiang (Ginger root), Garlic bulb, aromatic Clove bud, and Atractylodes Cang Zhu (Black or Red Atractylodes root).[7]
- *Damp Heat Invading Spleen.* Excess condition with thirst, but no desire to drink, scant dark yellow urine, stuffiness in epigastrium, loose smelly stools with mucus, no appetite, burning dark-yellow urine, diarrhea, abdominal pain, occasional mouth sores, jaundice, bitter taste, low-grade fever, and headache. This condition could manifest as hepatitis, gallbladder disease, or acute gastroenteritis. **P** Slippery, rapid. **T** color normal or red, sticky, yellow coat. To reduce this condition, dry up dampness and clear heat with dry, cooling herbs like Coptis Huang Lian (Goldthread root) or Artemisia Yin Chen Hao (Wormwood herb). These also contain the needed antimicrobial properties.
- *Spleen Qi Collapse or Spleen Qi Sinking.* This is a prolapse syndrome where qi is deficient and can't hold up organs such as the uterus, colon, or anus. Even miscarriages with inability to hold up the fetus exhibit Spleen Qi Collapse. The abdomen feels heavy, with urgency of urination. **P** Empty or weak on right wrist, especially under Spleen point. **T** Normal or pale. Tonify Spleen qi to deal with this condition. Possibilities include Panax spp. (Ginseng root), Astragalus Huang Qi (Astragalus root), and Bupleurum Chai Hu (Asian Buplever root).
- *Spleen Not Controlling Blood.* Here the blood is in the wrong place, caused by weakness or deficiency. There could be bruising, small purple spots called *petechiae*, excessive menstrual bleeding, blood in urine, nosebleeds, and periodontal disease. **P** Weak, especially right wrist under Spleen point. **T** Pale. Tonify the Spleen qi and Liver blood to help resolve the condition. A classic formula is *Eight Treasure Decoction.* This consists of the previously mentioned Four Gentlemen Decoction (Box 18.1), plus Angelica Dang Gui (Dong Quai root), Ligusticum Chuan Xiong (Sichuan Lovage root), Paeonia Bai Shao (White Peony root), and Rehmannia Shu Di Huang (Prepared Rehmannia root) to build blood and stop bleeding.
- *Food Stagnation.* In this instance the client ate too much and is paying the price, with gas, abdominal pain, and bloating as symptoms. **P** Choppy or slippery. **T** Greasy coat. Carminatives are needed to move qi and remove indigestion: Fennel seed or Aniseed, and Peppermint leaf. Bitters help, too. The client should stop eating for a while and stay hydrated.

Good Gut Health

A happy digestive system requires a well-balanced gut microbiome. To prevent dysbiosis, diets rich in rainbow-colored foods provide a wide range of needed antioxidants, fiber, and nutrients. These ***prebiotics*** are essential to feed and grow the flora. Gut flora foods include fibrous veggies like onion, leeks, asparagus, garlic, chicory, and oats. The ***probiotics*** are the actual friendly bacterial strains a healthy gut requires. These can be supplied by fermented foods, such as unsweetened yogurt or kefir, miso, kimchee, and fermented veggies (Box 18.2). If a client refuses these foods, a last resort is a probiotic capsule filled with many live strains of bacteria. Foods first, pills later.

These basics are general dietary measures used to build and maintain the microbiome. When the microbiome is in disarray because of bad habits practiced over time, GI problems rage. Dysbiosis can be caused by many factors: excessive use of refined sugars, consumption of genetically modified organisms (GMOs), use of herbicides and pesticides, gluten, processed foods, consumption of conventionally raised animals and birds that were fed antibiotics and genetically engineered feed, chronic constipation, chronic stress, elevated hormones, and any or all food allergens or sensitivities. Often a Paleo diet that discourages grains and dairy does the trick (Chapter 16). Throw in small bowel bacterial overgrowth (SIBO) and bacterial, viral, yeast, and parasitical infections in the large intestine, and you'll see there are plenty of possibilities implicated in messing up the gut.

• BOX 18.2 Prebiotic and Probiotic Foods

Prebiotics are specific high fiber foods that are known to feed the friendly bacteria in the gut to help them divide and multiply. Examples are onions, asparagus, leeks, oats, garlic, Jerusalem artichokes, cabbage, jicama, legumes, apples, and apple cider vinegar.

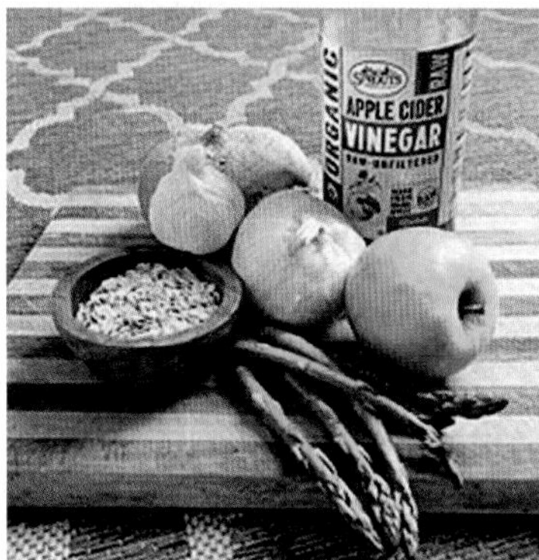

Prebiotic foods.

Probiotics are foods that actually reforest and replenish the microbiome, the good guys residing in the gut. Some of the best sources are fermented foods, such as sauerkraut, kimchi, natto, cabbage, carrots, and pickles (fermented veggies); miso and tempeh (fermented soybean products); kefir, buttermilk, and plain yogurt (fermented dairy); and apple cider vinegar (ACV) (fermented apples).

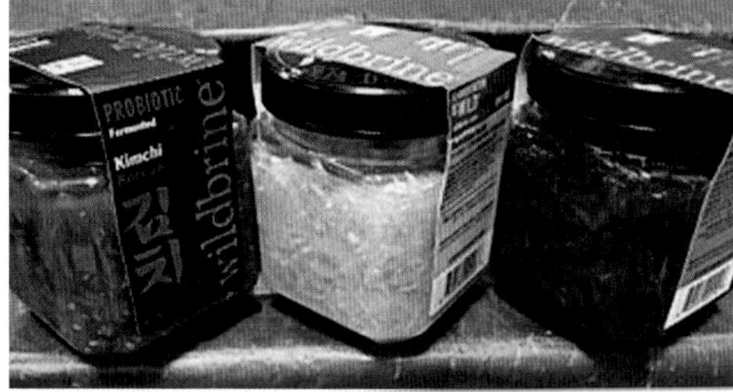

Probiotic fermented foods.

The Four-R Program: Remove, Replace, Reinoculate, Repair

How does herbal medicine deal with gut dilemmas? There is a systematic approach used in naturopathic and functional medicine circles developed by Jeffrey Bland, PhD., and his associates at the Functional Medicine Institute. Many variations of this program exist. The ***Four-R program*** has been successfully adapted by wise herbalists. The *remove* and *replace* categories have many choices to select from. Determining which categories to address takes a little detective work, however. The *repair* and *reinoculate* steps are pretty straightforward.

Remove and Replace

- *Remove offending foods (antigens) and triggers.* This approach means prevent intake of all foods that are known or likely to be harmful to the client's GI system, called an ***elimination diet***. (Later those categories will be reintroduced one by one to determine reactions.) Guidelines lay out an antiinflammatory regimen that determines food allergens—the most common being soy, gluten, dairy, corn, and egg white. This process could take a week or more.
  - *Protocol for elimination diet.* First, no white sugar, additives, fried foods, fruits, or alcohol. For the first week, eliminate gluten and cross-reactive grains such as barley, corn, oats, rye, and legumes that cause inflammation. Acceptable nongluten grains are brown rice, buckwheat, millet, and quinoa. You also may need to remove dairy. Healthy nuts and seeds are satisfactory, including cashews, almonds, pine nuts, pumpkin, sesame, and sunflower seeds. Include 2 servings a day of energy veggies: beets, parsnips, sweet potatoes, white potatoes, and winter squashes. Include plenty of rainbow-colored and green veggies. Meat-based, good-quality protein implies grass-fed beef, skinless organic chicken, lamb, turkey, low-mercury fish, or eggs (if not allergic).[1]
- *Remove and reintroduce a new food.* When the initial food removal time is finished, reintroduce a new food category every 3 days. Reintroduce foods in this order: first gluten, then corn, dairy, beans, nuts, nightshades (tomatoes, white potatoes, eggplant, peppers), yeasts and vinegars, and finally fruits.[1] Have client keep a food diary and notice and record symptoms, including any fatigue, brain fog, sleep disruption, mood changes, GI changes, joint pain, runny nose, watery or dark circles under eyes, rashes, cravings, and water retention. If any of these symptoms are present, then delete that food category for at least 3 months, possibly forever, depending on how the body reacts after the gut is healed. Wait until symptoms are completely gone, and then proceed to the next test-food group.
- *Remove environmental toxins.* Identify toxins such as mold, heavy metals, and mercury in the environment, and remove as much as possible. Indicators of toxic overload include frequent headaches, unexplained fatigue, food allergies, constipation, sensitivity to smells (e.g., perfumes and household cleaning products), intense PMS in women, and inability to sweat easily.[1] Good history-taking is necessary to pinpoint toxins. For example, ask when symptoms began. Could it have been when the client moved into a moldy, mildew-infested house, was exposed to water from lead pipes, or worked in an auto-body shop?
- *Remove* ***small intestinal bacterial overgrowth (SIBO)***. This problem is created by excessive bad bacteria in the small intestine. Occasionally, if a person is gluten intolerant, but a gluten-free diet doesn't seem to help, SIBO may be the reason. The majority of gut bacteria are supposed to reside in the colon, but low stomach acid or poor pancreatic enzyme production can lead to overgrowth in the small intestine. Signs and symptoms of SIBO include intense and painful gas, bloating, diarrhea, abdominal cramping, food intolerances, and sometimes the presence of IBS, or IBD, which have similar symptoms. SIBO leads to steatorrhea (fatty stools) with chronic diarrhea (less often constipation), nutritional deficiencies, and unintended weight loss.
  - *Treatment is complex.* In general, begin with Wormwood herb, the berberines (Coptis Huang Lian, Oregon Grape root), Black Walnut hull, and/or Garlic clove for 8 weeks. Use bitters and Spleen tonics to heal the gut. A specialized regime called the Low-FODMAP diet which eliminates

fermentable foods that are poorly absorbed in the small intestine can be helpful.

- *Remove yeast.* Common *Candida albicans* (yeast) symptoms can include brain fog, rosacea, bloating, extreme fatigue, and recurrent urinary tract and genital infections. If these are present, client must be on a yeast-free diet. This diet includes no sugar (breads, pastries, candies), because yeast cells feed on these substances, and no fermented foods, like wine, vinegar, yeast, soy sauce, and miso, because these fermented foods are created by yeast. Do not reintroduce fermented foods (which are normally desired and healthy) until yeast symptoms are under control.
- *Remove any intestinal worms.* These are more common than generally thought. Signs and symptoms are similar to yeast overgrowth: GI ills, muscle or joint aches, fatigue, skin rashes, hives, rosacea, or eczema. Additional clues are exposure to contaminated food or water, international travel, food poisoning, feeling hungry after meals, and grinding teeth during sleep. Remove worms with anthelminthics: Wormwood herb, Black Walnut hull, Turmeric rhizome, Garlic clove, Basil leaf, or essential oils of Melaleuca, Peppermint, and Thyme. (Dilute essential oils in a carrier oil and rub over stomach.)[1]
- *Remove the big four gut offending drug categories*: Antibiotics, nonsteroidal antiinflammatory drugs (NSAIDs), acetaminophen, and proton pump inhibitors (PPIs). One round of antibiotics can wipe out an entire species of gut flora permanently. NSAIDs, the ibuprofen sources, are drugs like Motrin and Aleve. They increase inflammation. Tylenol (acetaminophen) causes gut-bleeding and absorption troubles. PPIs used for GERD (reflux and heartburn), such as Prilosec and Nexium, cause detox problems and increase SIBO and inflammation.[1]
- *Replace digestive enzymes.* Signs of missing enzymes include bloating after eating and undigested food in stools (Fig. 18.5). Recommended selected enzymes at the start of each meal are bromelain, ginger, papaya, a bitters formula, or apple cider vinegar (ACV).
- *Replace stomach acid.* Many people are deficient in betaine hydrochloride (HCl) as they get older. This deficiency could cause bloating, belching, gas after meals, indigestion, diarrhea or constipation, acne, rectal itching, or chronic *Candida albicans*. How can you tell? Test for it as follows:
  - *Administer an acid test trial* to determine whether there is too much or too little acid being produced in the stomach. Supplement with 2 tablespoons ACV in water before meals, twice a day. If no stomach burning is experienced, then betaine HCl is deficient and supplement form is required. If a burning sensation occurs with the ACV, the betaine dose should be decreased until no burning is felt.
- *Replace prebiotics.* Have client ingest soluble fiber foods to feed the flora. This fiber bypasses the small intestine and goes to the colon, where most friendly bacteria reside. Fiber should consist of 2 cups of vegetables or dark leafy greens eaten twice daily. A tablespoon of ground flax seeds could be substituted for one of these portions. Various prebiotic herbs have the same function: Slippery Elm bark, Marshmallow root, Aloe Vera gel, Dandelion greens and root, and sea vegetables.

Reinoculate and Repair

- *Reinoculate.* Encourage friendly gut bacteria by having your client eat fermented foods or take supplementation. Unsweetened kefir (which aids in lactose digestion) or fermented vegetables are healing: ¼ cup once daily for a lifetime or a pill containing at least 10 billion colony-forming units (CFUs) or viable organisms per serving is recommended. The pill is the most expensive option and probably the least effective. If any of these measures cause increased gas or bloating, the client should return to using the herbal bug removers.
- *Repair gut lining.* Leaky gut and dysbiosis cause epithelial cell damage. Once all the damaging microorganisms are removed, clean up and repair lining damage, using fermented foods and herbs. An old standby is deglycyrrhizinated Licorice root (DGL), which has been successfully used to heal peptic and duodenal ulcer damage. The glycyrrhizin is removed, thus having fewer side effects for long-term use. DGL is an over-the-counter lozenge that is sucked before meals. Other gut healers are Slippery Elm bark, Marshmallow root, and fresh or dried Turmeric root. Fresh Turmeric added to smoothies is an option. Zinc maintains tight gut cell junctions at 30 mg daily, and the amino acid L-Glutamine heals the intestinal lining at 5 to 10 g of powder a day. Vitamin D3 is commonly deficient in inflammatory bowel diseases.

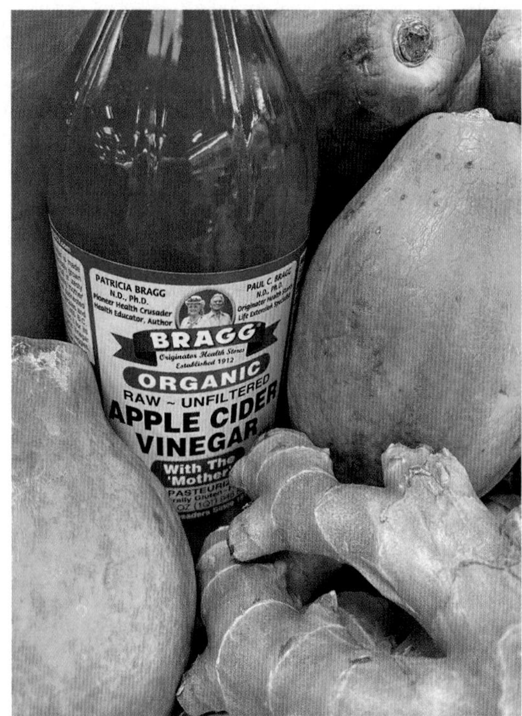

• **Fig. 18.5** Natural digestive enzymes: Papaya, Ginger, and apple cider vinegar.

Time Frames and Clinical Pearls for the Four-R Program

- *Total times vary.* On average, the entire Four-R program can take 6 weeks to 6 months, or even a year if symptoms are severe. Time frames are not written in stone, nor are they completely linear. Clients may need to repeat various segments of the protocol, depending on what occurs.
- *Microorganism removal time.* The average estimate is 4 to 8 weeks. Yeast infections may take longer because of die-off,

and removal is complete when no symptoms remain. Remove any yeast *before* beginning the reinoculation segment.

- *Replace*. Enzyme replacement herbs or supplements should be given before large meals. Hydrochloric acid (HCl) tablets need to be taken until the stomach makes its own acid, about 1 or 2 months. Then repeat the vinegar acid test and discontinue tablets when no longer needed.
- *Reinoculate*. Some form of probiotics must be eaten daily by everyone for life, leaky gut or not. If reinoculation causes gas or bloating, this step was begun too quickly. Back off, return to the protocols for removing foods and begin a broad-spectrum antibacterial removal herbal formula for another 4 to 6 weeks. Afterward, reintroduce the probiotics at a lower dose. If using supplements, switching brands might help.
- *Repair*. The intestinal lining renews itself every 5 days.[8] This is good news. Repair with Turmeric rhizome and Slippery Elm bark as chief herbs in a formula or use warm golden turmeric milk (Box 18.3).
- *How long for the antiinflammatory diet?* This diet may require a lifetime change to regain and remain healthy. As the gut heals, some of the original trigger foods might be reintroduced and tolerated. For some people, trigger foods such as gluten could be tolerated in small quantities or only a few times a week, within reason—or never, depending on the body's reaction. The body speaks loudly and clearly, so listen. If that beloved ice cream immediately creates gas, it may just have to be gone forever or the client will suffer the consequences. Consider substituting a coconut milk frozen dessert for dairy ice cream.

• BOX 18.3 Warm Golden Turmeric Milk

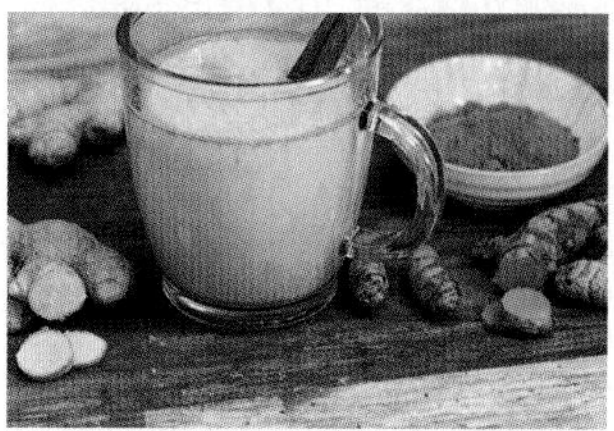

Golden Milk with fresh Ginger and Turmeric root. (iStock.com/Credit: Sarah Biesinger.)

Bright golden Turmeric milk is a traditional Ayurvedic staple. It heals the gut and has antiinflammatory and immune-building properties. There are many versions, but they should all be mixed in a fat-based liquid, because of Turmeric's fat solubility, and include Black Peppercorns, necessary for Turmeric absorption. Possible additives are Panax Xi Yang Shen (American ginseng root) or Ashwagandha root for stamina; Holy Basil leaf for stress; Lycium Gou Qi Zi (Goji or Wolfberry) or Zizyphus Da Zao (Jujube date) for antioxidants and sweetness; vanilla for flavor; and Cardamom pod to combat nausea, bloating, and gas. Be imaginative.

Ingredients

- 2 cups of regular milk (or nut milks of almond, pecan, or coconut) or bone broth.
- 1 tbsp. fresh or heaping teaspoon powdered Turmeric root.
- Pinch of Black Peppercorn to increase absorption and bioavailability of Turmeric.
- 1/2 tsp. cinnamon to normalize blood sugar and add sweetness.
- Tiny piece of fresh, peeled Ginger root or 1/4 tsp. Ginger root powder to support digestion.
- Pinch of Cayenne Pepper to taste (optional).
- 1 tsp. raw Honey (antibacterial and soothing) or maple syrup (optional) sweetening.

Blend all ingredients in high speed blender until smooth. Pour in saucepan and heat until hot but not boiling. Drink and enjoy daily.

Digestive System Materia Medica

GI Herbs Worth Honorable Mention

This list includes very valuable herbs for use in GI formulations that may not have been singled out in other parts of the text.

- *Gentiana lutea* (Great Yellow Gentian root). She is the Western "Queen of the Bitters," native to Europe's high mountain ranges (Fig. 18.6). The many Gentian species are one of the most bitter remedies known and are very strong, stimulating, and astringent. For this reason, only small doses are needed. The herb's bitter energy pulls downward and therefore is contraindicated in pregnancy. It is a cholagogue, promoting bile flow, and aids constipation in Stomach Qi Stagnation. Because Gentian is quite cold, it clears toxic and damp heat. It is healing to the gut microbiome. Use in a bitters formula for digestion and chronic ulcers.
- *Tabebuia avellanedae* (Pau d'arco inner bark). This antifungal and antiparasitic plant is from South America and is sometimes harvested indiscriminately and unethically, so please obtain it from responsible sources. Its inner bark is anthelminthic (kills worms), antiprotozoal, and antiparasitic. It is also antibacterial and antiviral, particularly for damp heat. All this makes it a go-to plant for intestinal yeast overgrowth with leaky gut. Its restorative and astringent properties help it seal and heal the gut, and its astringency makes it useful for damp heat with burning, urgent diarrhea, as in IBS or Crohn's.
- *Filipendula ulmaria* (Meadowsweet herb) (Fig. 18.7). This fragrant, sweet herb is well-named. Its silicon content heals and seals leaky gut and connective tissue. It builds intestinal flora. It is antacid and also good for gastroesophageal reflux disease (GERD). It is antiinflammatory, cooling, and good for stomach aches. Its salicylic acid content makes it analgesic in gut aches and in arthritic pain.
- *Codonopsis Dang Shen* (Downy Bellflower root). A classic sweet, moist, and nutritious digestive restorative tonic for Spleen Qi Deficiency. It aids absorption, is antacid, and is considered a "poor man's ginseng." Although not a *Panax*, a true ginseng, it has adaptogenic and immunostimulant properties with a bias for digestion. *Codonopsis* is far less expensive than *Panax* spp., but larger doses are needed for this purpose.
- *The Two Chinese Atractylodes*. This genus comes in a Black (or Red) and White species, both useful, but with quite different uses. *Atractylodes macrocephala* Bai Zhu (White Atractylodes root) is a sweet gut-restoring go-to Spleen qi tonic and carminative for Spleen Qi Deficiency with weakness, poor absorption, and indigestion. It is further notable as a Liver tonic. *Atractylodes lancea* Cang Zhu (Black or Red Atractylodes root) is a pungent, aromatic, drying and warming GI stimulant with broad-spectrum antimicrobial properties against viruses and fungi. Use the black one for SIBO, gut bacterial infections, and yeast overgrowth. It is a perfect candidate for the *remove* stage of the Four-R program.
- *Magnolia officinalis* Hou Po (Magnolia bark), a GI stimulant. This warm, pungent, spasmolytic, and astringent carminative is a natural for acute colic with abdominal pain, distention and nausea, diarrhea, indigestion, and food allergies.

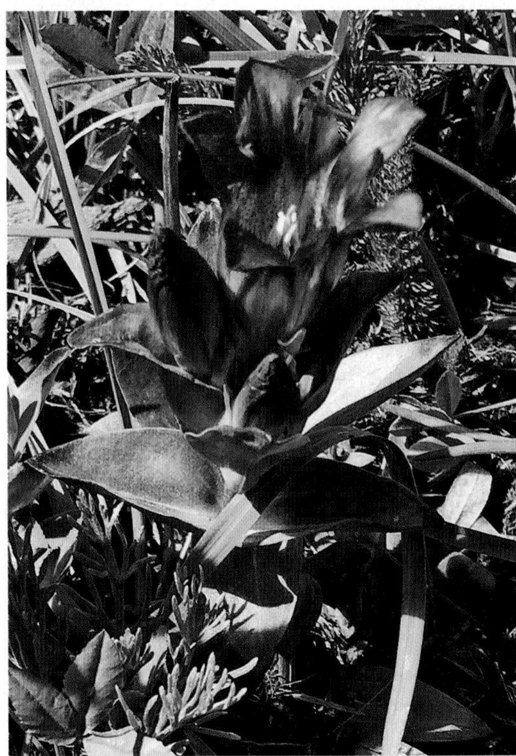

• **Fig. 18.6** *Gentiana parryi* (Bottle Gentian). Its purple flowers appear in late summer, a Colorado mountain native. *Gentiana* spp. root is bitter, cold, dry, and stimulating, making it effective in clearing damp and toxic heat, healing the microbiome and stimulating bile flow.

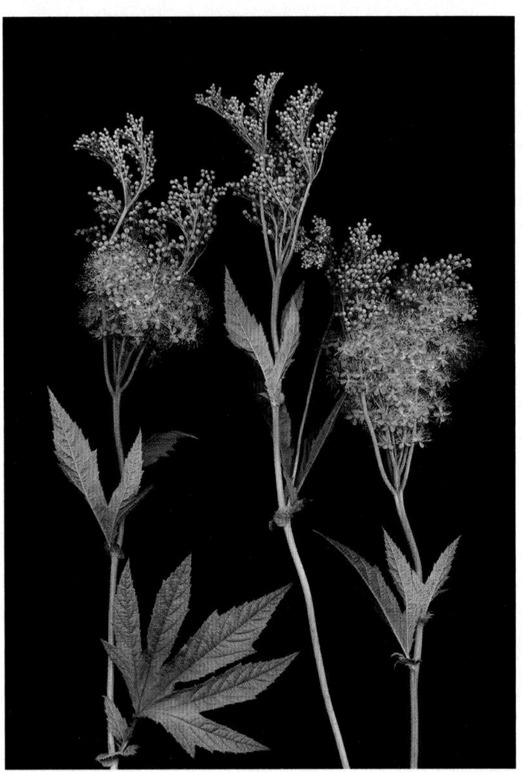

• **Fig. 18.7** *Filipendula ulmaria* (Meadowsweet herb) is superlative for GI problems. It heals and seals a leaky gut, restores the microbiome, and works as an antacid. (Copyright Lang/Tucker Photography. Photographs loaned with permission, from THE BOTANICAL SERIES are copywritten by Jennifer Anne Tucker and Gerald Lang from the Studio at Hill Crystal Farm. www.jennifer-tucker.com.)

Furthermore, it enjoys top billing as a broad-spectrum antimicrobial for dysbiosis or amebic dysentery.

- An entirely different species, *Magnolia liliiflora* Xin Yi Hua (Magnolia bud) is used in flower bud form as a respiratory aromatic and antiseptic, similar to Eucalyptus leaf.

Trophorestoratives, Spleen Tonics

GI trophorestoratives are nutritive, have an affinity for the gut, and heal and seal the intestinal lining over time. ***Spleen tonics*** include Chinese Medicine and Western herbs specific to digestive health. They treat deficient conditions and are predominantly sweet. The Spleen is associated with the sweet taste; thus general GI restoratives are sweet, as well. They can also be moist or drying. The moist, demulcent ones help with constipation or dry, hard stools. The dry ones address wet, loose, and frequent bowel movements. Spleen tonics work gradually over time, build the flora, contain nutrients, facilitate absorption, build tissue and physical strength, and help fatigue. Because they tonify Spleen qi, they are indicated in Spleen Qi Deficiency. They work for the Western disorders that we call enteritis, ulcerative colitis, and Crohn's (Fig. 18.8).[7] The big three Spleen tonics—Codonopsis Dang Shen (Downy Bellflower root), Atractylodes Bai Zhu (White Atractylodes root), and Panax Xi Yang Shen (American ginseng root)—appear at the head of the tropho-restorative list (Table 18.1).

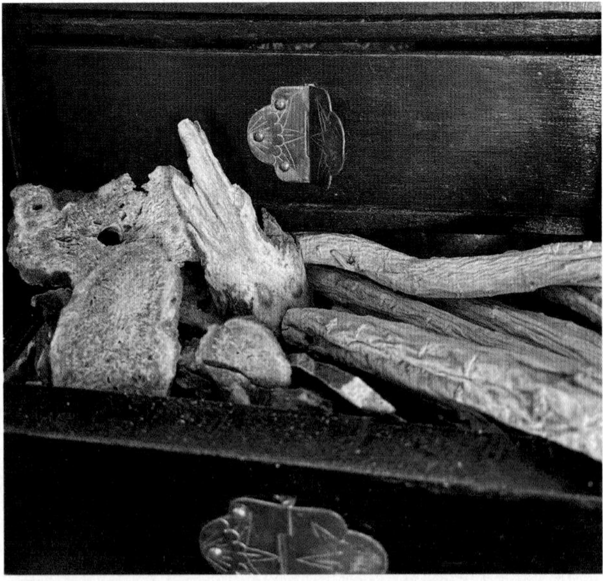

• **Fig. 18.8** Atractylodes Bai Zhu (White Atractylodes root) and long, twig-like Codonopsis Dang Shen (Downy Bellflower root) are indispensible sweet digestive tonics that restore the Chinese Spleen.

Bitters

A well-established fact of physiology, backed by centuries of tradition in the West, is that ***bitters*** (herbs with a predominantly bitter taste) trigger certain digestive juice production and processes. In fact, many of these processes need to be in full swing before foods such as heavy proteins and starches hit the stomach for healthy, robust digestion to occur. Bitter taste receptors are directly

TABLE 18.1 Tropho-Restoratives, Spleen Tonics (Used to "Restore" in the Four-R Program)

Herb	Notes
Codonopsis pilosula Dang Shen Downy Bellflower root	Sweet and moist, for Spleen Qi Deficiency. Ginseng substitute in larger doses. Builds blood, aids absorption.
Atractylodes macrocephala Bai Zhu White Atractylodes root	Sweet, bitter, and spicy, for Spleen Qi Deficiency. Versatile, for yin and yang deficiency, small intestine, and stomach.
Panax quinquefolius Xi Yang Shen American ginseng root	Sweet and moist, for Spleen Qi Deficiency, adrenal support, restores liver and nervous system.
Smilax officinalis Jamaican Sarsaparilla root	Sweet, warm, moist, for Spleen Qi Deficiency, malnutrition, weight loss, loose stool.
Dioscorea opposita Shan Yao Mountain Yam root This is not American Wild Yam.	Sweet, for Spleen Qi Deficiency, weight loss, loose stool.
Serenoa serrulata Saw Palmetto berry	Sweet, warm, moist, oily, and nutritive, for Spleen Qi Deficiency and those chronically underweight.
Glycyrrhiza glabra or *G. uralensis* Gan Cao Licorice root	Sweet, warm, and moist, for Spleen Qi Deficiency. Normalizes blood sugar, heals gut, restores adrenals. DGL form for ulcers. Used in formulas to protect the stomach.
Astragalus membranaceus Huang Qi Astragalus root	Sweet, warm, somewhat dry, for Spleen Qi Deficiency, malabsorption, and chronic underweight.
Arctium lappa (Burdock Root) *Chondrus crispus* (Irish Moss thallus) *Stellaria media* (Chickweed herb) *Urtica dioica* (Nettle herb) *Taraxacum officinale* (Dandelion root) *Avena sativa* (Milky Oat berry) *Trifolium pratense* (Red Clover flower)	Nutritive GI trophorestoratives with high vitamin and mineral content.
Medicago sativa Alfalfa herb	For Spleen Qi Deficiency. High in minerals. Increases absorption. Normalizes gastric pH.

connected to the digestive part of the stomach's functions. The centuries-old Swedish bitters tradition is based on this now well-proven information.

These days, herbalists use bitters for many purposes. Bitter is one of the five major tastes and has a downward, sinking energy. Bitter taste receptors are not only on the tongue but have been found in the smooth muscle cells of the stomach. Energetically, bitters are cooling and so relieve heat and toxins; drying, so they dry damp; and stimulating so they help liver detoxification. The alkaloids present in bitters provide an antimicrobial action. The concept and popularity of bitters is very Western; recall the Victorian penchant for bitter tonics as a digestive aid. Bitters also heal the gut, although the Chinese healer would include sweet restoratives as part of the rejuvenation process. In such cases, Codonopsis Dang Shen (Downy Bellflower root) or Atractylodes Bai Zhu (White Atractylodes root) would be used, neither of which are bitter.

Some bitters can be strong and overpowering, though bitters offer a continuum of strengths. Gentian is one of the strongest, famously present in Angostura bitters found in most bars worldwide. *Artemisia absinthium* (Wormwood herb) and *Ruta graveolens* (Rue herb) are also strongly bitter tasting. Strong, but easier-to-take notables are Goldenseal root and Oregon Grape root of berberine fame. Even milder ones include Dandelion root, Yarrow herb, or Chamomile flower (Table 18.2). The more bitter an herb, the less you need to use.

The bitter facts and actions:[9]

- *Digestive aid.* Bitters stimulate pancreatic digestive enzymes and increase bile flow from the liver and HCl from the stomach. This stimulation helps digestion by eliminating burping, bloating, and gas.
- *Support a healthy, normal appetite.* Bitters help us feel full without overeating. They help change our relationship to sweet carbs that are overemphasized in this society. Any time there is a problem with overweight and poor eating habits, bitters are important tools in an herbalist's pocket. If struggling with leptin resistance and weight gain, pull out the bitters. This approach includes consuming wild, weedy plants and bitter green foods, such as arugula, kale, and spinach in dark, leafy salads.
- *Carminative action.* Many bitters double as carminatives, increase peristalsis, and help with indigestion (e.g., Peppermint leaf, Fennel seed, Ginger root, Chamomile flower).
- *Dysbiosis and leaky gut repair.* Bitters are essential in gut repair work, necessitated from the results of leaky gut and dysbiosis. Intestinal permeability and unbalanced gut flora call for help here from antibacterial bitters. When removing foods from the Four-R program, try Usnea thallus or Oregon Grape root; when replacing foods, use Fennel seed, Dandelion leaf, Citrus Chen Pi (Ripe Tangerine rind); when restoring gut lining, turn to Chamomile flower, Nettle herb, or Iceland Moss thallus.
- *Antimicrobial and antiinflammatory.* Bitter alkaloids provide bug-killing action. This is particularly true of the berberines

TABLE 18.2 **Examples of Bitters and Their Relative Strengths**

Herb	Notes
Gentiana lutea (Gentian root) Very strong bitter. Use in small doses.	One of the most bitter remedies known. Stimulates bile flow, improves constipation, clears toxic heat, heals flora. Contraindicated in pregnancy.
Artemisia absinthium (Wormwood herb) Excruciatingly bitter. Medium strength.	Increases bile flow, clears toxic heat, a prebiotic. Use for chronic indigestion, food poisoning, worms, in Stomach or Liver Qi Stagnation.
The berberine roots, strong bitters. Goldenseal, Coptis Huang Lian (very strong). Phellodendron Huang Bai (very strong), Oregon Grape root, Barberry root (milder).	All very drying and antimicrobial. Clears heat and infection and helps digestion.
Carduus benedictus (Blessed Thistle herb) Middle of the road bitter.	Digestive stimulant. For jaundice, chronic gastroenteritis, and spiking fevers. Works like Boneset.
Chionanthus virginicus (Fringe Tree bark) Middle bitter.	Improves appetite. Stimulates bile flow. For dyspepsia.
Elettaria cardamomum (Cardamom pod) Middle bitter.	Settles stomach, helps dysbiosis. For acute gastritis, heartburn, and indigestion.
Curcuma longa (Turmeric root) Middle bitter.	Decongests liver, promotes digestion, helps constipation, heals flora. For inflammation of GI and liver.
Taraxacum officinalis (Dandelion root and Leaf) Mild bitter.	Digestive bitter, prevents reflux and heartburn, liver stimulant, clears toxins, and helps the skin. A prebiotic; feeds the gut.
Achillea millefolium (Yarrow herb) Mild bitter.	Mild, dry bitter, antimicrobial, diaphoretic. Good for kids.
Matricaria recutita (Chamomile flower) Mild bitter.	Helps digestion. Popular relaxing nervine, antispasmodic. Good for kids.
Citrus reticulata Qing Pi Unripe Tangerine peel Mild bitter.	Bitter, warm, and dry. For Liver Qi Stagnation, digestive stimulant for gas, indigestion, and constipation. Heals flora.

such as Oregon grape root, Coptis Huang Lian for broad-spectrum infections; *Artemisia* spp. such as Wormwood herb for helminths (worms) or *A. annua* (Sweet Annie), now famous for malaria.

- *Help maintain healthy blood-sugar levels.* Bitters lower Hemoglobin A1c (Chapter 27). For this reason, they become inevitable chief herbs in any diabetic formula: *Momordica charantia* Ku Gua Gan (Bitter Melon fruit) and Turmeric rhizome are specific no-brainers in this department (Fig. 18.9). They really work.
- *Stimulate liver to detoxify and release bile.* When the liver is stimulated, it works harder and increases detoxification pathway action. Increased bile flow helps in fat metabolism and healthy bowel clearing and provides hormones that stimulate gallbladder contraction so that bile can be released and fats can be digested. Dandelion root, Blessed Thistle, and the Docks have a liver affinity.

Contraindications for bitters include situations where there is increased stomach acid (HCl), accelerated peristalsis, or accelerated bile stimulation. Conditions include peptic or duodenal ulcer, kidney stones, gallbladder disease, gastroesophageal reflux, or hiatal hernia.[10] These are conservative contraindications that occur in the literature but are not always supported by actual research.

Dosages of bitters need not be large. All that is needed for digestive aid is a bitter taste. No need to be overwhelming: dispense 5 to 10 drops of a 1:5 tincture before meals. Generally, the health benefits of bitters require that taste to dominate in a formula. So don't drown out the bitter taste with other sweet herbs in hope of helping the medicine go down. The benefits do not occur unless the bitter herb is tasted.[9] For instance, prepare a separate bitters formula to take before eating and use sweet Spleen qi restoratives in a formula specific to that purpose, taken at a different time.

Gut Antimicrobials

The antimicrobials listed in Table 18.3 are the major bug-removers for the Four-R program. Most are broad-spectrum. They take care of unwanted SIBO, yeast, parasites, fungus, amoebas, viruses, and bacteria. Some are cooling and drying, the ticket to removing Spleen damp heat. Uses are for long-term dysbiosis, acute intestinal infections, bacterial and amoebic dysentery, food poisoning, flare-ups of Crohn's, and acute ulcerative colitis. Sometimes referred to as GI sedatives for infection, they are strongly antiinflammatory and antimicrobial. A few striking examples to eradicate unwanted microbes are the broad-spectrum berberines, Atractylodes Cang Zhu (Black Atractylodes root) for yeast and fungal infections, or Gentian root for worms and parasites.

Prebiotics and Leaky Gut Healers

The herbs listed in Table 18.4 repair the epithelial lining of the gut and tighten cell junctions. Herbs that heal and seal leaky gut are

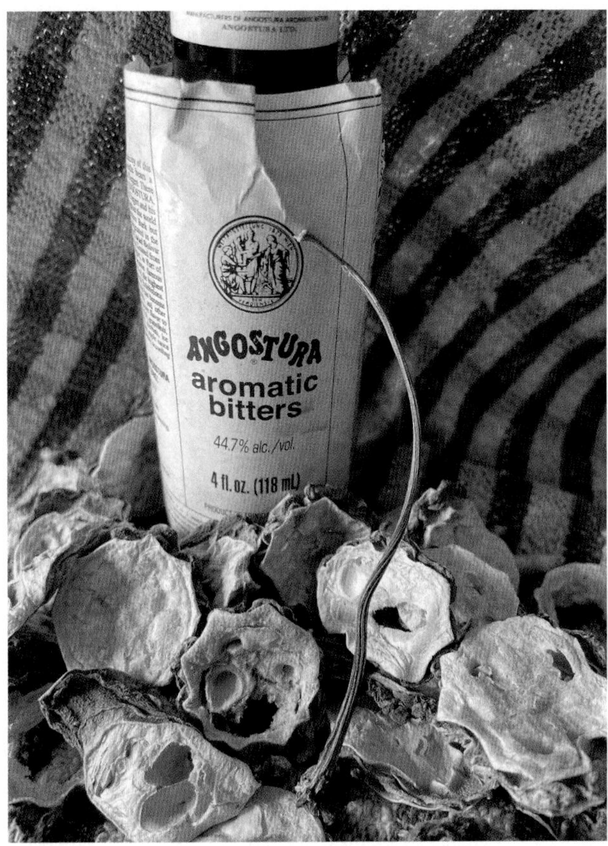

• **Fig. 18.9** Bitters help digestion. Examples are Angostura aromatic bitters containing Gentian root that are used in mixed drinks, and Chinese *Momordica charantia* Ku Gua Gan (Bitter Melon fruit).

our friends; sweet ones include Licorice root, Slippery Elm bark, Meadowsweet, and others. Many gut-healing herbs (but not all) happen to be bitter. Bitter-tasting gut healing herbs and roots include Gentian root, the *Artemisia* spp., the berberines, Blessed Thistle herb, and Turmeric and Dandelion root. These provide the many usual actions of all bitters. Refer to the earlier section on bitters to review.

When introducing a protocol for dysbiosis, do it in stages, using different formulas and herbal combinations at different times in the process. Once the gut lining is healed, it should usually stay that way, unless further abuses occur down the road.

Digestive Aids: GI Stimulants, Relaxants, Antacids, Carminatives, Demulcents

The plants listed in Table 18.5 are an array of herbals that help digestion, covering many categories. ***GI stimulants*** increase digestive processes, and by so doing, have a calming effect. They have an outward-moving, pungent taste. The warm-to-hot ones will either work or not, meaning reactions are quite individual. Some warm-to-hot ones are Black Peppercorn, Cayenne pepper, Clove bud, Ginger, and Horseradish root. Others are not as hot and more general: Magnolia Hou Po (Magnolia root), Kava root, and Atractylodes root Cang Zhu (Black or Red Atractylodes root). Some indications that pungent GI herbs are needed include dyspepsia (when the need is to help digestion and move food along) or when better peristalsis might help, as in nausea, projectile vomiting, and colic.[16]

The pungent taste could also help increase peripheral circulation, decongest the bronchia, or topically, reduce joint and muscle pain. Contraindications for hot GI stimulants occur with GERD or with very acid conditions, hepatitis, hot diarrhea with anal burning, and chronic nephritis.[16]

GI *relaxants* relax the gut. They relieve pain and take away the ***gripe***, an archaic word for sharp bowel pain and cramps. They ease painful smooth-muscle spasms by causing them to relax. They also relieve the pain of acute intestinal colic, gastritis, dyspepsia, IBS, enteritis, diarrhea, or constipation and stress. Alternately, they are called spasmolytics or intestinal analgesics. They circulate qi in the intestines (the middle burner) and induce gut relaxation. They help relieve symptomatic pain without necessarily getting to the root of the problem. Energetically, many GI relaxants tend to be warm, pungent, and stimulating. When they provide an outward moving energy, a tight gut relaxes; muscle spasms let go. Gone is the pain; in comes relief and relaxation.

Like any other remedies, GI relaxants have tropisms to particular organs and areas that are actually causing the cramping. Pain doesn't just happen for fun. Therefore Black Cohosh root, Cramp bark, St. John's Wort, or Tansy herb are useful spasmolytics with dysmenorrhea; gentle Chamomile helps children and elders with indigestion; Citrus Qing Pi (Green Tangerine peel) can be given when bile and liver need stimulation. Hops reduce stress or insomnia in hot conditions.

Herbal *antacids* relieve upset by alkalinizing gastric contents and can help with GERD. Some antacid herbs include Meadowsweet herb, Iceland Moss, and Chickweed herb. *Carminatives*, because of their volatile oils, aid indigestion by increasing peristalsis, moving gas, and relieving bloating. Consider using Cinnamon bark, Fennel seed or Cardamom pod. Bitters could easily have been included in this section but have been addressed separately because their uses go beyond digestion.

GI *demulcents* are moistening because of their saponins. They topically lubricate the gut wall, making them useful for constipation, dryness, and hard stools. They are also cooling and so can soothe inflammation, relieving stomach pain. Although Marshmallow root is a multipurpose demulcent, it is not restorative. Use others that have the added virtue of being nutritive and restorative, plus moistening to the gut mucosa: Slippery Elm bark, Licorice root, and Iceland Moss thallus do both. Pick your demulcent whenever cooling, moistening yin or pain relief is needed.

Antidiarrheals and Hemostatics

Most herbs that curb diarrhea are drying *astringents* that tighten connective tissue and mucous membranes (Table 18.6). They work because of their tannin content, which tightens cell junctions and pulls inward. If diarrhea is severe or chronic, dehydration becomes an issue. Astringents help prevent that danger by reducing water loss. Diarrhea is present in Spleen Qi Deficiency and Spleen Yang Deficiency, where there is not enough qi to hold the stool in place.

A good diarrhea formula should include astringents, plus a sweet Spleen restorative/tonic and anything else indicated to address the underlying cause. Use sweet Spleen restoratives, like Codonopsis Dang Shen (Downy Bellflower root) or Atractylodes Bai Zhu (White Atractylodes root). If there is exhaustion, include a neuroendocrine restorative, like Licorice root.[13]

TABLE 18.3 Gut Antimicrobials for Spleen Damp Heat *(Used to "Remove" in the Four-R Program)*

Herb	Notes
The berberines *Coptis chinensis* Huang Lian (Goldthread root) *Hydrastis canadensis* (Goldenseal root) *Mahonia aquifolium* (Oregon Grape root) *Phellodendron amurense* (Huang Bai root and inner yellow bark) *Berberis vulgaris* (Barberry root)	Broad-spectrum. Localized. They work by direct contact with any mucous membranes. Very specific to GI tract, SIBO, bacterial, fungal, and yeast infections. Also for skin, and vaginal douches.[14] Berberines are harsh and very drying; include a soothing demulcent in the formula.
The artemisias *Artemisia annua* (Sweet Annie herb) malaria specific *A. vulgaris* (Mugwort herb) *A. dracunculus* (Tarragon herb) *A. absinthium* (Wormwood herb)	Broad-spectrum. Localized. Very specific to all GI tract infections, and skin. Like the berberines, artemisias need direct contact with mucous membranes to work. All are antifungal, antibiotic, anthelmintic, antiamebic, antiinflammatory, insect repellant.[14]
Usnea spp. Usnea thallus	Broad-spectrum. More localized than not. Specific for *E. Coli* in food poisoning, *H. Pylori* in ulcers. Antifungal. Well known for urinary and throat infections.
Magnolia officinalis Hou Po Magnolia bark	Broad-spectrum. Very versatile. Classic Chinese Medicine gut antimicrobial. Also a spasmolytic gut relaxant and carminative. For dysbiosis.
Echinacea angustifolia Echinacea root	Broad-spectrum. GI infections, especially when detox is recommended as in typhoid, diphtheria. Antiviral, antibacterial, immune modulation.
Atractylodes lancea Cang Zhu Black or Red Atractylodes root	Broad-spectrum, aromatic, very drying. For yeast/fungus, *Candida albicans*, spleen damp.
Tabebuia avellanedae Pau d'arco bark	Broad-spectrum detoxifier, antifungal, antiparasitic, antibacterial. For yeast/fungus.
Eugenia caryophyllata Ding Xiang Clove bud	Antifungal. For *Candida albicans* and chronic dysbiosis.
Cinnamomum cassia Gui Pi Cinnamon bark Cassia and Ceylon species interchangeable.	For chronic dysbiosis, yeast, fungus, parasites, *Candida albicans*. Helps normalize blood sugar.
Larrea divaricata Chaparral leaf	Broad-spectrum antifungal, antibacterial, antiviral (*Herpes*). Detoxifying. Clears damp heat in GI, urogenital, and skin.
Cochlearia armora Horseradish root	Very hot and dry. Antifungal, antiparasitic. For dysbiosis, Spleen Yang Deficiency, and food stagnation.
Allium sativum (Garlic bulb)	Antiprotozoal, antifungal. For worms.
Gentiana lutea Gentian root	Antiprotozoal and antiparasitic. For worms and all parasites, in general.
Essential oils Thyme, Cinnamon, Oregano, Clove, Boldo, Black Spruce, Eucalyptus, Cajeput, Tea Tree	For worms, parasites, fungus. Use in capsules with carrier oil or add to tincture (1–2 drops per oz).
Juglans regia (Walnut hull and leaf)	For worms, tapeworms, and roundworms.
Cucurbita maxima Pumpkin seed raw	For worms. Blend raw seeds into a paste with almond or coconut milk and water.
Camellia sinensis Green Tea leaf	Tannin content binds proteins in the colon and inhibits pathological microbe growth.[16]
Vitis vinifera Grape Seed extract	Tannin content does same as Green tea. Rich in antioxidants.

TABLE 18.4 Gut Healers
(Used to "Repair" in the Four-R Program)

Herb	Notes
Prebiotics to feed the flora	
Ulmus fulva (Slippery Elm bark) *Althaea officinalis* (Marshmallow root) *Aloe vera* (Aloe gel)	
Taraxacum officinale (Dandelion greens/root) *Cichorium intybus* (Chicory root) *Arctium lappa* (Burdock root)	Dandelion, Chicory, Burdock, and other bitters double as prebiotics.
Chondrus crispus (Irish Moss thallus)	Irish moss is also a nourishing leaky gut restorative.
Camellia sinensis (Green tea leaf)	Green tea adds antioxidants.
Vitis vinifera (Grape seed extract)	Bitter, prebiotic, antibiotic.
Prebiotic food sources	
Asparagus, garlic, leeks, jicama, Jerusalem artichokes, all raw. Cooked onion, dandelion greens, chicory and burdock root, whole oats, barley, flax seeds, apples, green tea.	These specific foods contain important fibers that feed a healthy microbiome. They are sources of fructooligosaccharides (FOS) beta-glucans, and inulin.
Heal and seal the leaky gut	
Glycyrrhiza glabra (Licorice root)	Licorice: use deglycyrrhizinated licorice (DGL).
Ulmus fulva (Slippery Elm bark) *Cetraria islandica* (Iceland Moss)	Slippery Elm and Iceland Moss are praiseworthy nutritive demulcents.
Plantago major (Plantain leaf)	Plantain excels at tissue repair; heals ulcers.
Filipendula ulmaria (Meadowsweet herb)	Meadowsweet heals intestinal wounds, seals leaky gut, generates flora.
Symphytum officinale (Comfrey root)	Comfrey is a renowned wound/gut healer.
Urtica dioica (Nettle herb)	Nettle's silica content regenerates connective tissue.
Curcuma longa (Turmeric root)	Turmeric is classic for inflammation.
Calendula officinalis (Calendula flower) *Matricaria recutita* (Chamomile flower)	Calendula and Chamomile are classic tissue repairers.
Supplements	
L-Glutamine 20 g 2 × day with food × 2 months	Glutamine is a building block of protein.
Zinc picolinate 20–30 mg a day	Zinc, a trace mineral, heals gut, supports immunity.
Omega-3 Fatty Acids 1000 mg a day	Include combination of EPA and DHA.

Drying astringents can also be used to help curb internal GI rectal bleeding as might occur in a gastric ulcer. In such case the herbal choice would be a ***hemostatic***. Examples are Cotton root bark, Cranesbill root, Yarrow herb, or White Oak bark. Simple astringent hemostatics, like antidiarrheals, dry damp on a symptomatic level only and are not long-term solutions. They do not address the root cause, so herbs that do so should be included in the formula.

Laxatives

Laxatives are herbs that act mildly to gently relieve constipation. ***Purgatives*** are stronger and act more forcefully (Table 18.7). It is all a matter of degree. In addition to promoting bowel movements, laxatives have been used successfully for heat clearing, decongesting, detoxification, and draining of excess water. Even if these are not the main intent, they can be secondary effects. Laxatives

TABLE 18.5 Warm GI Stimulants, Relaxants, Analgesics, Carminatives, Demulcents *(Catch-alls for many GI woes)*

Herb	Notes
Eugenia caryophyllata Ding Xiang Clove bud	Hot, pungent, dry, stimulating, relaxing, carminative. For dyspepsia, colic, microbial dysbiosis.
Zanthoxylum bungeanum Chuan Jiao Sichuan Peppercorn	Hot, pungent, dry, stimulating, carminative. For colic, diarrhea.
Wasabia japonica (Wasabi stem)	Hot, pungent, dry. Used in Japanese sushi. Wonderful for digestion.
Armoracia rusticana (Horseradish root)	Hot, pungent, and dry. Used as a cheaper substitute for Wasabi. For chronic gastroenteritis and food stagnation.
Magnolia officinalis Hou Po Magnolia bark	Warm, pungent, and carminative. Gets top billing as a broad-spectrum antimicrobial for dysbiosis.
Amomum villosum Sha Ren Wild Cardamom pod	Warm, pungent, carminative, spasmolytic, antiemetic, and astringent. For indigestion.
Zingiber Gan Jiang (Dried Ginger root)	Warm, pungent, stimulating, carminative, antibacterial. For indigestion, nausea in morning sickness.
Common carminatives *Foeniculum officinalis* (Fennel seeds) *Pimpinella anisum* (Aniseed) *Zingiber officinalis* (Ginger root) *Rosmarinus officinalis* (Rosemary leaves) *Matricaria recutita* (Chamomile flower) *Menthe* x *piperita* (Peppermint leaf)	Carminatives relieve gas and bloating by increasing peristalsis. The common carminatives get food moving along, therefore for Stuck Stomach Qi.
Common antacids *Filipendula ulmaria* (Meadowsweet herb) *Cetraria islandica* (Iceland Moss) *Stellaria media* (Chickweed herb) *Glycyrrhiza glabra or G. uralensis* Gan Cao Licorice root *Codonopsis pilosula* Dang Shen Downy Bellflower root *Acorus calamus* (Calamus root) Apple Cider Vinegar (ACV)	Antacids neutralize stomach pH, make it less acid. This is helpful in acid reflux (GERD). Beware that indigestion is often caused by too little stomach HCl, not from too much. Need to establish which, by using the acid test. Notice that many of these herbs double as restoratives. Note: Native North American *Acorus calamus* (Calamus/Sweet Flag root) has long been used for all kinds of digestive problems. It is a warming and pungent antacid, antidiarrheal, carminative, and restorative. Contrary to bad press on and off throughout the years, it is a medium-strength herb that is safe and effective in formula. It is cumulatively toxic when used alone. Do not use as a simple or continuously.[13]
Common GI demulcents	Demulcents are not just for GI. See notes.
Althaea officinalis (Marshmallow root)	Marshmallow is a multipurpose demulcent.
Cetraria islandica (Iceland Moss thallus)	Iceland Moss is nutritive, for lungs, thyroid.
Symphytum officinalis (Comfrey root)	Comfrey is nutritive, for chronic diarrhea, lungs, connective tissue and wound healing.
Ulmus fulva (Slippery Elm bark)	Slippery Elm is nutritious, antacid, for lungs and damp heat.
Stellaria media (Chickweed herb)	Chickweed, for anemia, thyroid, tissue repair.
Glycyrrhiza glabra (Licorice root)	Licorice for ulcer healing, lungs, adrenals.

should not be used with clients in very weak conditions such as exhaustion, diarrhea, GI bleeding, or severe abdominal pain.[13] They also should not be used routinely. Find and fix the cause. We're supposed to go to the bathroom without help.

Bowel ***transit time*** refers to number of hours for food to move from the mouth to the end of the intestine or anus. To check, use the *dye test* or substance test. Have the client ingest beets, corn, or sesame seeds and have them observe the number of hours for these substances to be seen in the bowel movement. (Check the toilet. Beets turn the water fuchsia; undigested corn kernels come out whole.) Anything less than one bowel movement a day means toxins and waste are recirculating back into the bloodstream from the colon and may result in fatigue, headaches, gas, bloating, acne, allergies, and muscle and joint pain if constipation persists over time. A fast transit time (shorter than 10 hours) indicates food is passing through the system too quickly, suggesting nutrients are not absorbing properly.

Constipation is bowel frequency of less than 3 times a week, with the need to strain more than 25% of the time.[16] Some say two or more bowel movements a day are necessary. Regular,

TABLE 18.6 **Antidiarrheals**

Herb	Notes
Acorus calamus Calamus root	For chronic diarrhea and other discharges. More than a simple astringent, Calamus root is an important Spleen Qi restorative. Combines with many digestive herbs. (See cautions in Table 18.5.)
Geranium maculatum Cranesbill root	For chronic diarrhea, gastric acidity/heartburn.
Potentilla erecta (Tormentil Root)	Chronic diarrhea; restorative, aids absorption.
Quercus alba White Oak bark	Multiuse astringent for chronic diarrhea, menorrhagia, organ prolapse, excessive sweating, hot flashes, urinary/vaginal discharge.
Rubus idaeus Raspberry leaf	Mild astringent for children, elders. For diarrhea, leukorrhea; like others in the Rose family.
Achillea millefolium Yarrow herb	Astringent, cool and dry. For diarrhea, menorrhagia, dysmenorrhea. Hormonal aspect; estrogen and/or progesterone deficiency.
Four Gentlemen Decoction (Box 18.1)[6]	Classic Chinese formula for Spleen Qi Deficiency.

once-a-day movements seem to be a fine middle ground to keep us healthy. Before reaching for herbs, try the usual remedies first. Have the client consume adequate fluid and fiber, get plenty of exercise, reduce stress, listen to their body, and act on the urge.

Mild *bulk laxatives* work through enlarging, lubricating, and softening the stool. They are useful for hemorrhoids and constipation-dominant IBS and serve as a prebiotic to feed flora and slow absorption of sugars and cholesterol. Indications are for IBD, constipation, blood-sugar management, fluid retention, obesity,[16] and occasional use with atonic colon in sedentary or elderly folks. Psyllium husk is a good example of a bulk laxative. When mixed with water, it quickly thickens and slimes up into a bulky, mucilaginous gel before it is removed from the spoon. It is present in products like Metamucil.

Demulcent laxatives are mild, sweet, cooling, and moistening. Use for dry, hard stools when yin needs a boost. Demulcents are high in mucilage and, thus lubricating. Examples are the fruit kernels of peach, prune, and apricot. Cannabis goes in this category, as does flax seed. Demulcent laxatives are appropriate for pregnancy, children, and elders. *Sweet stimulating laxatives* are mild and gentle, good for children and elders as well. Licorice root, Tamarind pulp, and Ziziphus Da Zao (Black Jujube berry) gently stimulate peristalsis.

Saline laxatives are dissolvents that soften, moisten, and break up stool. Magnesium sulfate, better known as Epsom salts, the seaweeds, and liquid trace minerals work in this manner. They dissolve bowel accumulations and clear dry heat (Fig. 18.10). *Cholagogues* improve liver function and stimulate bile flow. They are bitter, cold, and useful in liver and gallbladder congestion. Dandelion root, Artichoke leaf, Milk Thistle seed, Yellow Dock root, and Burdock root reside in this category.

Stimulant anthraquinone-containing laxatives increase peristalsis by irritating the intestinal wall and causing large evacuations; they are the purgatives. Occasional *short-term* use is safe when nothing else works; long-term use can cause dependency. Find the cause, rather than allowing the client to become reliant on these laxatives. Purgatives are contraindicated in pregnancy and nursing because they stimulate the lower abdominal area. Examples in ascending order of strength include Senna and Cascara leaf, then comes Rhubarb root, and the strongest of all, Mayapple root.

Common GI Conditions

Diarrhea

Definition. Frequent liquid bowel movements that can be acute or chronic (***diarrhea***) are a symptom, not a disease. Look for causes like infection, food poisoning, drugs, and toxins. Chronic diarrhea is almost always from infection. Inflammatory bowel diseases like Crohn's or ulcerative colitis and IBS are likely suspects. Medications, food additives, and malabsorption are other possibilities.

- *Signs and symptoms.* Chinese Medicine differentiates types of diarrhea. A foul odor indicates heat or Liver involvement. No odor indicates cold. Pain implies Liver involvement or heat. Burning indicates heat. Chronic diarrhea is Spleen Yang or Kidney Yang Deficiency, not keeping it in. *Cock's crow diarrhea* (first thing in morning) is Kidney Yang Deficiency. If there is abdominal pain, it's cold. If mucus, it's damp. Loose with undigested food is Spleen Qi or Spleen Yang Deficiency.
- *Allopathic treatment.* Over-the-counter drugs such as Imodium and Pepto-Bismol. White rice, applesauce, toast. (The last three are helpful, especially in children.)
- *General therapeutic principles.* Treat symptoms. (1) Use berberines for microbes: Coptis Huang Lian or Phellodendron Huang Bai, or try Anise, Thyme, or Oregano essential oils in capsules. (2) Decrease inflammation, burning, or pain with demulcents: Slippery Elm bark and Marshmallow root. (3) Try tannic astringents: Yarrow herb, Cranesbill root, or White Oak bark (Case History 18.1).

Simple Constipation

Definition. Fewer than three bowel movements a week is considered to be ***constipation***. Can be caused by dehydration, lack of fiber, little exercise, being bedridden or post childbirth, having stress, or high alcohol consumption. Simple constipation can be occasional or chronic, but it is not inflammatory, and not in the IBS or IBD categories that are discussed further on.

TABLE 18.7 **Laxatives**

Herb	Notes
Ulmus fulva (Slippery Elm bark)	Bulk laxative.
Linum usitatissimum (Flax seed, ground)	Bulk laxative. Also a demulcent laxative.
Plantago psyllium (Psyllium husk)	Bulk laxative.
Sea vegetables *Laminaria* spp. (Kelp) *Pyropia* spp. (Nori) *Palmaria palmata* (Dulse)	Bulk laxatives and also salty, so they dissolve hard stools.
The kernels *Prunus armeniaca* (Apricot kernel) *Amygdalus persica* (Peach kernel) *Prunus domestica* (Prune kernel and juice)	Demulcent laxatives. For dry, hard stools.
Glycyrrhiza glabra (Licorice root)	Sweet, stimulating, but gentle laxative. Child and elder friendly.
Ziziphus jujuba Da Zao (Black Jujube berry)	Sweet, stimulating, but gentle laxative. Child and elder friendly.
Rumex crispus (Yellow Dock root)	Stimulating, gentle anthraquinone laxative. Helps atonic bowel function. Cholagogue.
Aloe vera (Aloe resin) Use the resin extracted from the leaf.	Stimulating anthraquinone laxative. For chronic constipation. Caution with hemorrhoids, pregnancy, heavy menses. Combine with carminatives.
Purges, the strong ones	These anthraquinone laxatives are stimulating.
Rhamnus purshiana (Cascara Sagrada bark)	Cascara, a cholagogue, clears heat.
Rheum officinale (Rhubarb root)	Rhubarb clears heat, and safest in this class for long-term constipation.
Cassia acutifolia (Senna leaf and pod)	Senna, for temporary constipation or amenorrhea.
Podophyllum peltatum (Mayapple root) Medium strength, very strong cholagogue.	Mayapple: is medium-strength, use very small doses only. A GI bitter. Large doses are emetic and purgative. Used in gallstone flushes.
All purges are contraindicated in pregnancy.	
Cholagogue laxatives *Berberis vulgaris* (Barberry root) *Carduus benedictus* (Blessed thistle) *Carduus marianus* (Milk Thistle seed) *Citrus reticulata* Chen Pi (Ripe Tangerine peel) *Curcuma longa* (Turmeric rhizome) *Cynara scolymus* (Artichoke leaf) *Gentiana lutea* (Gentian root) *Rumex crispus* (Yellow dock root) *Taraxacum officinale* (Dandelion root)	Stimulate insufficient bile flow, gastric and pancreatic secretions to break down and eliminate toxins and mucus, including stool. For Liver Qi Stagnation.

- *Signs and symptoms.* Dry, hard, or long narrow stools. Straining is involved, and there could be hemorrhoids and sometimes thirst.
- *From the Chinese Medicine perspective.* There are many types of constipation, some involving heat, some relating to cold, some involving deficiencies, and some indicating stagnation. Constipation with thirst implies heat. Dry stools with no thirst suggest Kidney or Stomach Yin Deficiency. Small clusters of fecal matter are indicators of Liver Qi Stagnation and Heat in Intestines. Abdominal pain indicates cold and is considered a yang deficiency. Little bowel movement without dryness is Liver Qi Stagnation. Constipation with alternating diarrhea is Liver Qi Stagnation Invading Spleen. Westerners might place IBS and IBD in this last category.
- *Allopathic treatment.* Fiber, Metamucil, fluids, exercise, and stool softeners are used.
- *General therapeutic principles.* (1) Gentle laxative; (2) Demulcent to lubricate bowel; (3) Find and treat root cause (Case History 18.2).

Indigestion, Food Stagnation

Definition. Dyspepsia. Pain or discomfort in the stomach from difficulty digesting food (Case History 18.3).

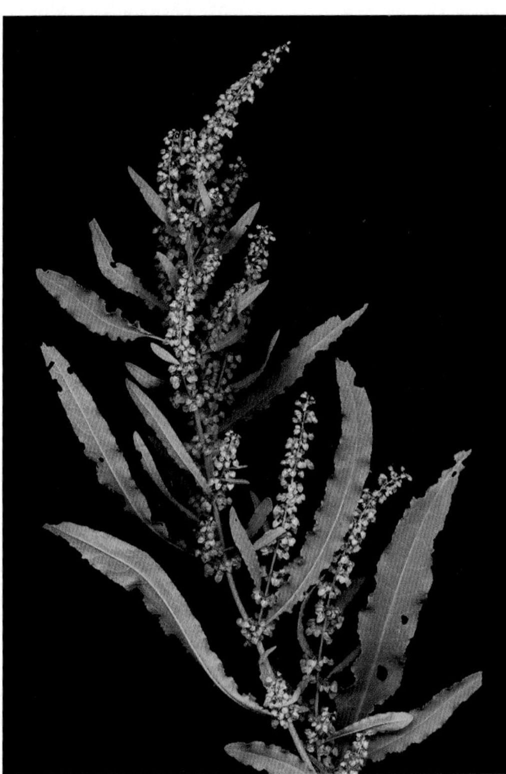

• **Fig. 18.10** *Rumex crispus* (Yellow Dock) root is a good cholagogue and a gentle anthraquinone laxative. (Copyright Lang/Tucker Photography. Photographs loaned with permission, from THE BOTANICAL SERIES are copywritten by Jennifer Anne Tucker and Gerald Lang from the Studio at Hill Crystal Farm. www.jennifer-tucker.com.)

CASE HISTORY 18.1

Case History for Diarrhea

S. Nancy ate some fresh oysters last night and now has foul smelling diarrhea, mucus, burning, and cramping. She feels weak.
O. P Weak. **T** Greasy, red coat.
A. Diarrhea with damp heat. Possible food poisoning.
P. *Specific therapeutic principles.* (1) Antimicrobials for food poisoning. (2) Astringents to curb diarrhea, dry damp. (3) Cooling demulcents to ease burning and pain. (4) Spasmolytics to ease cramping.

Sample Formula and Dose. 4 mL every ½ hour to 1 hour. Reduce as needed to 3 × day.

Parts	Herbs	Rationale
4	Magnolia Hou Po	Antimicrobial/food poisoning.
4	Calamus root	Astringent for diarrhea and gut restorative.
2	Irish Moss	Demulcent and cooling and restorative.
2	Cramp bark	Spasmolytic for pain.

Other Suggestion

Adequate fluids to prevent dehydration.

- *Signs and symptoms.* Epigastric pain, fullness, belching, bloating, excessive gas. From overeating, decreased GI enzymes, decreased peristalsis, smoking, swallowing air, or eating too fast.

CASE HISTORY 18.2

Case History for Chronic Constipation

S. Leslie is 70 years old and has had chronic constipation for years. Usually has one to two BMs a week with bloating, dry, hard stools that finally come after straining. She loves hot spicy foods. She has tried all kinds of laxatives, including Metamucil.
O. P Fine. **T** Red and dry.
A. Yin Deficiency. Chronic constipation.
P. *Specific therapeutic principles.* (1) Moisten and increase yin with a demulcent; (2) Gentle laxative. (3) Cholagogue to increase bile flow. (4) Carminative for bloating. (5) Gut restorative.

Sample Formula and Dose. 5 mL 3 × day.

Parts	Herbs	Rationale
3	Yellow Dock root	Cholagogue laxative.
2	Comfrey root	Cooling, moistening, restorative.
2	Slippery Elm bark	Moistening and restorative.
2	Peppermint leaf	Carminative for bloating.
2	Codonopsis Dang Shen	Gut restorative and moistening.
1	Licorice Gan Cao	Moistening, warming, restorative.

Other Suggestions

- *Diet.* Less hot, spicy foods. Oatmeal is moistening. Add seaweeds and ground flax seeds in foods. Figs are filled with fiber and are moistening. Avoid alcohol, refined foods, white flour, sugar, and iced drinks.
- *Supplements.* Fish oil capsules EPA/DHA 1000 mg daily.
- Better hydration.

- *From Chinese Medicine perspective.* Food stagnation, indigestion, dyspepsia.
- *Allopathic treatment.* Prilosec, Nexium, TUMS, and other antacids are used.
- *General therapeutic principles.* (1) Stimulate digestive enzymes with bitters; (2) Stimulate bile flow; (3) Use carminatives for gas; (4) Use Cascara if there is constipation; (5) With Liver congestion, use Celandine or Fringe Tree bark; (6) With dryness, use yin tonics, like Iceland Moss or Licorice root. (7) Use tummy-soothing digestive syrup (Box 18.4).

Inflammatory Bowel Disease (IBD)

Definition. ***Inflammatory Bowel Disease (IBD)*** is an umbrella term that involves two chronic autoimmune GI problems, both involving inflammation. Severity ebbs and wanes but continues for years, never disappearing. ***Ulcerative colitis*** involves long-lasting ulcerative sores and painful bleeding in the colon and rectum, whereas ***Crohn's disease*** involves inflammation, bleeding, and patchy damage through all layers of the gut wall anywhere in the GI tract (Case History 18.4).[15] These two must be treated with autoimmune protocols, adapted to the GI tract (Chapter 16).

- *Signs and symptoms.* Persistent diarrhea, abdominal pain, rectal bleeding, bloody stools, weight loss, and fatigue, not to mention the life-changing misery. It is painful and embarrassing, making a normal life impossible. Constant diarrhea makes it imperative to be near a bathroom.

CASE HISTORY 18.3

Case History for Simple Dyspepsia/Indigestion

S. Jack had lasagna, wine, and cheesecake for dinner and returned for seconds. Now he has epigastric pain, belching, bloating, and a heavy feeling.
O. **P** Slippery, wiry in mid position bilaterally. **T** Greasy, moist. Belching, gas.
A. Stuck Liver Qi, Food Stagnation. Indigestion.
P. *Specific therapeutic principles.* (1) Bitters. (2) Stimulate bile flow. (3) Carminatives for gas.

Herbal Formula and Dose. 2 mL every ½ hour as needed.

Parts	Herbs	Rationale
3	Blessed Thistle herb	Bitter, bile flow, and enzyme stimulation.
2	Calamus root	Restorative, relieves gas, bloating, epigastric pain.
2	Peppermint leaves	Carminative.
1	Citrus Chen Pi	Liver stimulant, cholagogue.
1	Ginger root	Warms stomach, relieves indigestion.

Red Flags

If indigestion is chronic, it could be from more serious GERD, ulcers, hiatal hernia, or gallstones.

Other Suggestions

- Avoid greasy fatty foods and cold drinks. Warming foods are best.
- Foods that help digestion: barley sprouts, papaya, pineapple.

• BOX 18.4 Tummy Soother Digestive Syrup

For upset stomach, acid reflux, and heart burn

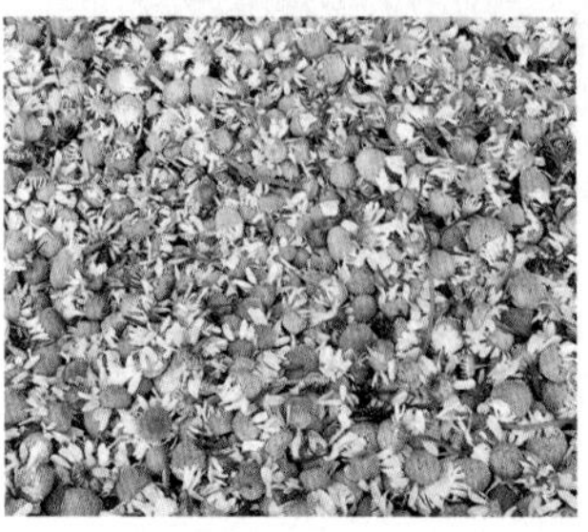

Drying Chamomile flowers. *Matricaria recutita* is a calming carminative that helps gas and bloating.

Ingredients:
1 oz Chamomile flower
1/4 oz Marshmallow root
1/4 oz Fennel seed
1/4 oz Ginger root
1/4 oz Meadowsweet herb
1 cup Honey
8 Tablespoons brandy
2–5 drops Peppermint essential oil
3 drops Tangerine essential oil

Directions:
Add herbs to 1 quart of water cold water and let sit 15–30 min (or even overnight); then cover and bring herbs to a simmer for 15–20 min. Strain and return liquid to pot. Over low heat, simmer to reduce liquid to 1 pint. It will be thick. Remove from heat. Add brandy for flavor and relaxant properties (1–4 tbsp. per cup). Add essential oils. Bottle and store in fridge. Keeps for 4–6 weeks (if it isn't gone by then).

- *Allopathic treatment.* Cortisone, surgery, and biologics (a class of protein-based drugs derived from living cells through recombinant DNA methods). The biologic for Crohn's blocks TNF alpha, a cytokine that causes inflammation.[12]
- *General therapeutic principles.* (1) Use autoimmune protocols. First and foremost, heal dysbiosis, using the Four-R program. Most often, the culprits are wheat and dairy. A GAPS diet might help. (2) Of specific proven value are antiinflammatory herbs: Wormwood herb, Frankincense resin, Cardamom seed, Calendula flower, and Turmeric root.[16] (3) Astringents to help stop blood loss and diarrhea. (4) Demulcents soothe irritation, especially Aloe gel. (5) Antispasmodics ease muscle cramping. (6) Antiinflammatories and immune support. (7) Nervous relaxants for stress. (8) Robert's Formula (Box 18.5).

Irritable Bowel Syndrome (IBS)

Definition. ***Irritable Bowel Syndrome (IBS)*** is the most common functional motility bowel disorder in the United States. It tends to flare up intermittently and then subside. Typically, it is triggered by stress and anxiety, food intolerances, leaky gut, too much fiber, parasites such as *Giardia* spp. or *Candida albicans*, enteric microbes, and inflammation (Case History 18.5). Unlike ulcerative colitis and Crohn's, no damage to the bowel tissues occurs, and it is not an autoimmune issue. *Note:* If there is bleeding, fever, weight loss, and persistent severe pain, it is not IBS but more likely one of the more serious autoimmune IBDs.

- *Signs and symptoms.* Cramping colon pain, gas, bloating, headaches, anxiety, alternating constipation and diarrhea (spastic colon), or constant diarrhea (mucous colitis), or constant constipation.
- *From Chinese Medicine perspective.* Various syndromes are involved, depending on how the symptoms manifest, whether related to the qi of the Liver or Spleen. Treatment depends on what's happening.
  - *Liver Qi Stagnation* presents with abdominal distention, constipation with small stools, and high stress levels. **P** Wiry (stress). **T** Dusky, distended sublingual veins—signs of stagnation in the Liver.
  - *Spleen Qi Deficiency* includes abdominal distention, diarrhea, or loose stools and is often related to worry, fatigue, and poor appetite. **P** Weak. **T** Dusky and scalloped because it's wet.
  - *Liver Invading Spleen* presents as alternating diarrhea and constipation because a little of both is going on. **P** Wiry and weak. **T** Pale dusky, thin white coat.
  - *Damp Heat.* If there's mucus, there's damp heat. **P** Slippery and rapid. **T** Greasy, yellow coat.
- *Allopathic treatment.* High fiber foods, fluids, exercise, sleep, antispasmodics, and even antidepressants are used.
- *General therapeutic principles.* (1) Intestinal sedatives, berberines Coptis Huang Lian or large doses of Barberry bark. (2) Astringents to reverse diarrhea or gentle laxatives for constipation. These could be separate formulas, depending on condition. (3) Bitters to help digestion and normalize bowel function. (4) Carminatives to help colic, cramping, and pain. (5) Antispasmodics for pain. (6) Nervines to help stress.

CASE HISTORY 18.4

Case History for Crohn's Disease

S. Louise has had Crohn's for 41 years, all her adult life. Her main symptom was almost continuous diarrhea with mucous and blood in the stool. She has lesions in her bowel per endoscopy, and no mainstream treatment has really helped. She has been on Prednisone for years.

O. P Wiry and rapid. **T** Dark red with a yellow, greasy coat.

A. Spleen Damp Heat, Spleen Qi Deficiency, Crohn's per healthcare provider, inflammation/diarrhea.

P. *Specific therapeutic principles*. (1) Eliminate microbes and heat. (2) Dry Damp. (3) Use astringents to stop bleeding. (4) GI Restoratives. (5) Antidiarrheals. (5) Cooling, soothing mucilage. (6) Nervous relaxant.

General Sample Formula and Dose. 5 mL 3 × day.

Parts	Herbs	Rationale
3	Wormwood herb	Antiinflammatory, antimicrobial, bitter, clear heat.
2	Cranesbill root	Astringent for bleeding and diarrhea.
2	Poria Fu Ling	Dry damp.
2	White Atractylodes Bai Zhu	Restore Spleen.
2	Aloe gel	Gut healing, cool demulcent, clear heat.
2	Passionflower	Nervous relaxant for stress.

• BOX 18.5 Robert's Formula for Ulcers and Inflammatory Bowel Diseases

Robert's Formula is a famous traditional Eclectic formula used for ulcers, IBS, Crohn's, ulcerative colitis, and any stomach inflammation. The story that has come down to us says that Robert was a sailor who learned about these herbs from healers in various ports. It helped him so much that he spread the word. This formula has stayed around, often with embellishments and changes, and is still recommended by naturopathic doctors today.

In ulcers, *Helicobacter pylori* is a biofilm that colonizes in the nonacidic mucous layer of the stomach. It becomes infectious when the mucous layer is damaged. This formula restores mucus and destroys the biofilm.[17] Originally, dried herbs were ground and placed in capsules, but this formula may also be dispensed as a tincture.

Parts	Herbs	Rationale
2	*Althea officinalis* (Marshmallow root)	Soothes, coats, and protects mucous membranes.
2	*Echinacea angustifolia*	Immunostimulant and antibacterial.
2	*Ulmus fulva* (Slippery Elm bark)	Soothing and coating.
2	*Geranium maculatum* (Cranesbill herb)	Astringency stops GI bleeding and diarrhea.
2	*Phytolacca americana* (Poke root)	Helps heal sores and ulcers.
2	*Hydrastis canadensis* (Goldenseal root)	Local antibacterial properties, bitter.
1	*Baptisia tinctoria* (Wild Indigo root)	Very bitter and antibacterial; its astringency stops diarrhea.

Dose: Flare-ups, 2 caps 3 × day as needed between meals. During remission: 1 cap 2 × day between meals.

Gastric or Duodenal Ulcers

Definition. ***Ulcers*** are open sores on the inside lining of the stomach (*peptic* or *gastric*) and the upper portion of the small intestine (*duodenal*) (Case History 18.6). Excess acid creates painful, open sores that may bleed or perforate, causing hemorrhage or leakage of gastric contents into the abdomen. Stomach wall perforation can lead to peritonitis, a medical emergency.

- *Causes*. Stress, hyperacidity, *Helicobactor pylori* (considered a biofilm), bacterial infections, trigger foods. Smoking is a strong risk factor as is habitual use of NSAIDs such as Ibuprofen, Aspirin, Motrin, and Advil. (Tylenol (acetaminophen) is *not* an NSAID.) These ulcers are usually diagnosed by endoscopy or upper GI barium x-ray.
- *Signs and symptoms*. Dull, sharp, or burning upper abdominal pain, and indigestion after eating, often relieved by antacids or further eating. Rectal bleeding is possible.
- *From Chinese Medicine perspective*. Caused by many syndromes and taken case by case.
- *Allopathic treatment*. Antibiotics, acid blockers, dietary changes, or surgery.
- *General therapeutic principles*. (1) GI demulcents to soothe gastric mucosa; (2) Antacids; (3) Antimicrobials for *H. pylori;* (4) GI restoratives, especially DGL; (5) GI relaxants for stress; (6) Stop any GI bleeding with hemostatics as needed; (7) Immune enhancer or Echinacea root; (8) GI antiinflammatories.

Gluten Sensitivity or Intolerance versus Celiac Disease

Definition (gluten sensitivity or *intolerance)*. ***Gluten sensitivity*** is a continuum that ranges from mild indigestion when gluten is consumed to flat-out celiac disease, in which gluten cannot be eaten under any circumstances. Both forms are on the rise, perhaps because of greater awareness or because of the prevalence of wheat-containing gluten not only in obvious foods like bread and other baked goods, but also in countless hidden sources, such as almost all processed foods, ice cream, gravies, soy sauce, and even beauty products. Gluten is hard to avoid. Just about everyone has some type of adverse reaction to gluten.

Definition (celiac disease). Sometimes called *sprue*, ***celiac disease*** is a long-term, genetic, autoimmune inflammatory disorder where the ingestion of the gluten protein triggers antibodies that release inflammatory cytokines, causing damage to villi in the small intestinal lining. Leads to severe malabsorption and long-term complications and is many steps up the ladder from simple gluten sensitivity. Although many people are not even aware of their sensitivities to gluten, 1 out of every 133 average, healthy Americans is diagnosed with celiac disease. In all cases of gluten sensitivity, ranging from discomfort to celiac disease, some amount of inflammation, intestinal permeability, and dysbiosis is involved.

- *Signs and symptoms (gluten sensitivity)*. Abdominal pain, nausea, diarrhea, constipation, intestinal distress, headaches, fatigue, skin problems, brain fog, mood changes, muscle pain, and neuropathy.
- *Signs and symptoms (celiac disease)*. Sometimes no initial symptoms show up, are slow to appear, and may or may not be numerous. They can lead to weight changes, abdominal pain, nausea, bloating, heartburn, headache, fatigue, foul-smelling fatty diarrhea (*steatorrhea*), or constipation, itchy rash, canker sores in the mouth, mood changes, and/or brain

CASE HISTORY 18.5

Case History for Irritable Bowel Syndrome (IBS)

S. Dave has a stressful computer programming job. For 10 years, he has had frequent alternating diarrhea and constipation, painful cramping, bloating, gas, and burping. He is anxious and gets headaches. He also eats fast foods and loves breads, pasta, and pizza. For the last 4 weeks, he's been constipated with a dry BM every 3 to 4 days.

O. P Wiry, especially in Spleen position. **T** Dry, thin white coat.

A. Liver invading Spleen, Liver Stagnation right now. Irritable Bowel Syndrome, dysbiosis.

P. *Specific therapeutic principles.* (1) Broad-spectrum antimicrobial: a berberine. (2) Spasmolytic for cramping. (3) Antianxiety herb. (4) Liver restorative and cholagogue. (5) Gut/Spleen restorative: White Atractylodes Bai Zhu or Calamus root. (6) Treat constipation with gentle cholagogues, like Dandelion root or Yellow dock, and a demulcent, like Comfrey root.

General Sample Formula and Dose. 5 mL 3 × day.

Parts	Herbs	Rationale
3	Coptis Huang Lian	Antimicrobial and bitter.
2	Hops flower	Antispasmodic and anxiolytic, bitter.
2	Artichoke leaf	Hepatic restorative/choleretic.
2	Valerian	Spasmolytic, and for pain and anxiety.
2	White Atractylodes Bai Zhu	Restore Spleen.
2	Comfrey root	Ease pain, restore and lubricate gut.
1	Licorice root	Soothe, restore and lubricate gut.

Constipation Formula and Dose. 4 mL every 2 hours; adjust as needed.

Parts	Herbs	Rationale
2	Dandelion root	Mild cholagogue. Liver repair.
2	Yellow dock	Cholagogue.
3	Slippery Elm	Soothing demulcent and gut healer.

Other Suggestions for Both IBS and All Inflammatory Bowel Diseases

- Begin Four-R program to treat dysbiosis and leaky gut.
- Diet: Antiinflammatory Mediterranean diet with elimination diet; first food to take out is gluten.
- Enteric-coated Peppermint essential oil capsules as a carminative for pain and cramping.
- Supplements: Sublingual vitamin D_3 1000 mcg a day is very important; often deficient in people with IBS. Fish Oil 1000 mg EPA/DHA every day for inflammation. This one also helps constipation if present. Zinc 30 mg every day. L-Glutamine at 5–10 g of powder a day.[1]
- If the IBS changes to diarrhea, stop the Constipation Formula and if needed, replace formula with Cranesbill root and Calamus root.

CASE HISTORY 18.6

Case History for Gastric or Duodenal Ulcers

S. Michael has a stressful job and home environment. He has gas, bloating after eating, general indigestion, and bright red rectal bleeding at night.

O. P Weak, wiry, deep. **T** Dusky, pale, teeth marks.

A. Possible GI ulcer. Healthcare provider consult for definitive diagnosis.

P. *Specific therapeutic principles.* (1) GI demulcents; (2) Antacids; (3) Stop infection with antimicrobials; (4) GI Spasmolytics for pain.

Herbal Formula and Dose. 6 mL 3 × day as needed.

Parts	Herbs	Rationale
3	Meadowsweet herb	Antacid, gut lining restorative, astringent for bleeding.
3	Coptis Huang Lian	Antiinflammatory and antimicrobial for *H Pylori.*
3	Chamomile flower	Decreases stress, antiinflammatory, spasmolytic.
2	Cotton root bark	Hemostatic.
1	Echinacea root	Immune stimulation.
1	Comfrey root or Licorice root Gan Cao	Heals and coats gut, antiinflammatory.
1	Irish Moss or Comfrey root	Demulcent, removes pain, heals gut.

Red Flag

Bleeding ulcers indicate bowel perforation, a medical emergency. It is evidenced by black tarry stools and/or red, black or coffee ground vomiting.

Other Suggestions

- *Elimination diet.* To detect any food triggers. Keep a food diary.
- *Stress management.* Yoga, meditation, exercise, breathing techniques.
- *Supplements.* Deglycyrrhizinated Licorice (DGL) over the counter to heal mucosa. Aloe Vera juice to soothe, cool, and heal gut.
- Marshmallow root overnight cold decoction taken before large meals.
- No smoking; quit.

fog. Eventually other complications can appear: malnutrition, weight loss, coldness, exhaustion, irritability, weakness, depression, infertility, depressed immunity and growth, osteoporosis, irregular menses, and miscarriages (Case History 18.7).

- *Diagnosis (gluten sensitivity).* History of elevated gluten antibodies.
- *Diagnosis (celiac disease).* Elevated antibody levels formed from contact with *gliadin*, one compound that makes up the protein gluten.
- *From Chinese Medicine perspective. Spleen damp*, deficiency of yin, yang, qi, or blood.
- *Allopathic treatment.* No cure other than a gluten-free diet for life.
- *General therapeutic principles.* (1) A strict gluten-free diet will allow the immune system to repair itself and keep symptoms from flaring up. The process can take anywhere from a few weeks to many months, depending on the severity. (2) Four-R program. (3) For stubborn cases, use the autoimmune protocol: The ***Gut and Psychology Syndrome (GAPS) diet.*** It begins with meat or fish stock and proceeds to other foods. (4) Use immune modulation (not stimulation) with Eleuthero Ci Wu Jia (Siberian ginseng) or Ganoderma Ling Zhi (Reishi mushroom).

Intestinal Yeast Infection

Definition. Candida albicans or yeast overgrowth in the gut occurs as a result of inflammation, intestinal permeability, dysbiosis,

CASE HISTORY 18.7

Case History for Possible Celiac Disease

S. Jack has had weight loss; foul-smelling, greasy stools; rectal itching; eczema-type skin breakouts; and abdominal cramping. He is forgetful and "can't think straight." This has been his norm for 5 years, He knows his trigger foods are pasta and bagels, but he loves them.
O. P Weak. **T** Pale and greasy.
A. Spleen damp and deficient. Malnutrition. Celiac disease or gluten intolerance with probable yeast infection.
P. *Specific therapeutic principles.* (1) Four-R program, gluten-free, antiinflammatory Paleo diet. (2) Antimicrobials. (3) Remove gut inflammation. (4) Restore gut lining. (5) Dry damp. (6) Immunomodulation. (7) Robert's Formula (Box 18.5).

Herbal Formula and Dose. 5 mL 3 × day

Parts	Herbs	Rationale
3	Pau d'arco or Magnolia Hou Po	Yeast removal.
2	Coix Yi Yi Ren (Job's Tears seed)	Diuretic, dry damp, immune-modulation.
2	Meadowsweet herb	Restores gut lining, strengthens Spleen.
2	Eleuthero Ci Wu Jia	Immune modulation.
2	Ginger root	Helps digestion, reduces inflammation, drying.
2	Poria Fu Ling	Dry damp.
2	Citrus Chen Pi (Tangerine peel)	Draining, aromatic.

Other Suggestions

- *Four R program.* Standard protocol. For replace portion, possible natural digestive enzymes to consider include papain, bromelain, papaya, and pickled Ginger root. If yeast is on board, make sure die-off is complete before adding probiotics.
- *GAPS diet.* Consider for difficult to treat autoimmunity situations like celiac, but not necessarily for plain gluten intolerance (Chapter 16).
- *Diet overhaul:* Antiinflammatory diet. Seasoning with Paprika decreases inflammation.
- *Beware of hidden gluten* sources in processed foods: gravy, soups, condiments.
- *Supplements.* Iron, calcium, and vitamin D3, zinc, B_6, B_{12}, and folate, which are common nutritional deficiencies caused by various degrees of malabsorption. Essential fatty acids EPA/DHA to decrease inflammation and coat gut lining. Aloe Vera gel daily to soothe and heal the gut.
- *Turmeric Golden Milk daily* (Box 18.3). Gut soother and healer.
- *Robert's Formula daily* (Box 18.5). Perfectly lovely Eclectic combo to heal gut and decrease inflammation.
- *Prognosis.* The protocol many require 6 months to a year to show improvement, or it may need to be followed for life. After 6 months, try reintroducing one food back every 3 days to identify triggers. The client will probably need some type of food modification for life. Maintain the client on bitters, gut healers, prebiotics, and probiotics. Give copious support.

weakened immune system, diabetes, antibiotic and cortisone use, and/or birth control pill use. Yeast infections can also appear on the skin, the vagina, rectum, penis, mouth (as thrush), and blood. In all cases, treat the root cause, the gut (Case History 18.8).

CASE HISTORY 18.8

Case History for Intestinal Yeast Infection

S. Jackie's stomach aches badly. She has had loose, smelly stools; rectal itching; gas; and bloating. She reports getting many colds over the last 2 years and losing weight. She feels hot. Though she has not changed her marginally standard American diet (SAD), she reports extreme fatigue and has had eczema on her elbows, knees, and hips for 6 months. Her stool tests positive for parasites.
O. P Rapid. **T** White coat and yellowish greasy center.
A. Spleen Damp Heat, Spleen Qi Deficiency. Probable stomach infection with intestinal parasites and diarrhea. Leaky gut and dysbiosis.
P. *Specific Therapeutic Principles.* (1) Antiparasitic herbs that should help underlying condition of eczema and fatigue. (2) Blood cleanser/alterative herbs for eczema. (3) Lymph movers and diuretics to flush out parasites. (4) Immunostimulant herbs. (5) Relieve cramping with carminative herbs. (6) Antidiarrheals, as needed (prn). (7) Restore and heal gut.

Herbal Formula and Dose. 4 droppers, 3 × day for 3 wk between meals

Formula #1 Remove Parasites, Stop Cramping and Diarrhea

Parts	Herbs	Rationale
3	Wormwood herb	Antiparasitic/antiviral/antibacterial, clears damp heat.
3	Oregon Grape root	Antiviral/antibacterial/antidiarrheal, clears damp heat, detoxification.
2	Calamus root	Antidiarrheal, Spleen restorative.
2	Chaparral leaf	Antiparasitic.
2	Fennel seed	Relieves cramping, carminative, relaxes GI.
2	Echinacea root	Detoxifier/immunostimulant.

Herbal Formula and Dose. 5 mL 3 × day for 2 wk between meals.

Formula #2 Drain Toxins, Treat Symptoms

Parts	Herbs	Rationale
3	Red Root bark	Alterative for skin, clears damp heat, moves lymph.
3	Cleavers herb	Lymph mover and cleanser, reduces fever, clears damp.
2	Burdock root	Alterative.
2	Dandelion root	Draining diuretic, clears liver.
2	Echinacea root	Immunostimulant.

Other Suggestions

- *Diet.* General Four-R protocol to remove parasites and yeast triggers. No sugar, alcohol, yeast, refined carbohydrates, gluten, or fermented foods. Begin by nourishing the Spleen with warming foods: sweet potatoes, yams, peas, mung beans, lentils, kidney beans, adzuki beans, carrots, beets, corn, butternut squash, spaghetti squash, acorn squash, zucchini, yellow squash, rutabaga, and pumpkin.[1]
- *Yeast die-off protocol.* Cycle through yeast-killing formula and detox formula 3 times.
- After parasite removal, continue on Four-R protocol for leaky gut/dysbiosis.
- Good hydration is important throughout.
- Lymphatic drainage, gentle manual therapy to clear lymph of the infection.

- *Signs and symptoms*. GI-related rectal itching and burning, gas, constipation, diarrhea, bloating, extreme exhaustion, cravings for sweets, gas and bloating, food sensitivities, headaches, brain fog, fever, and sinus infections.
- *Systemic symptoms*. Chronic sinus or allergy issues, food sensitivities, skin breakouts, weak immune system, bad breath, joint pain, hormone imbalance, vaginal itching, and recurrent urinary tract infections (UTIs) or vaginal infections that don't clear up with antibiotics.
- *From Chinese Medicine perspective*. Intestinal yeast infections are considered Spleen Damp Heat.
- *Allopathic treatment*. Antifungal drugs.
- *Die-off protocol*. Cycle through two herbal formulas to kill yeast and then to flush out toxins from the dying cells. Treat the yeast infection for 3 weeks and then detox with a draining, flushing formula for the next 2 weeks. Repeat pattern three times until all yeast egg cycles are exhausted. You will know this has happened when yeast die-off symptoms disappear. Each yeast cycle lasts about 18 days. If symptoms return, continue the regimen longer, because that indicates that the eggs are not all gone (Chapter 17).
- *General therapeutic principles*. Remove yeast and resume Four-R program. (1) Remove fermented foods and sugar from diet: sugar, alcohol, refined carbohydrates, and gluten. Nourish the Spleen with warming foods. (2) Use the two formulas for die-off: antiparasitics and then the detox flush. (3) For the flush, include alteratives, lymphatic drainers, and diuretics. (4) Relieve GI symptoms with carminatives. (5) Spasmolytics for cramping. (6) Antidiarrheals. (7) Immunostimulants. (8) When yeast growth has been resolved, continue Four-R program.

Gastroesophageal Reflux Disease (GERD)

Definition. In ***gastroesophageal reflux disease (GERD)***, hydrochloric acid comes up from the stomach into the esophagus through a weakened esophageal sphincter. This smooth muscle is supposed to close, but if it's weakened or relaxes inappropriately, the food goes back up. As a result, the stomach's HCl can damage the esophageal wall, thus leading to tissue breakdown and cancer. GERD is also called *acid reflux* or *acid indigestion* and is sometimes caused by a hiatal hernia, where the upper part of the stomach moves up into the chest (Case History 18.9). Common trigger foods are carbonated drinks, fatty or fried foods, tomato sauce, alcohol, chocolate, mint, garlic, onion, and caffeine.

- *Signs and symptoms*. Heartburn, burning in the throat and chest after eating or when lying down or bending over; bad breath; nausea or vomiting; and breathing problems. GERD is diagnosed through endoscopy, and is caused by stress, dysbiosis, obesity, smoking, medications like non-steroidal anti-inflammatory drugs (NSAIDs), including aspirin. GERD mimics a heart attack or *myocardial infarction* (MI) but is relieved with an antacid, whereas pain from an MI is not.
- *From the Chinese Medicine perspective*. Rebellious Stomach Qi (that is rising, rather than sinking).
- *Allopathic treatment*. Use of proton pump inhibitors (PPIs), like Nexium, Prilosec, and Prevacid decrease acid production. Acid (H2) blockers, such as Tagamet and Zantac inhibit the action of histamine on the cells and can reduce the production of acid by the stomach. Antacids like Mylanta, Maalox, and TUMS, which are alkaline and counteract stomach acidity, are also used. However, these common over the counter drugs do more harm than good. Surgery is a last resort. For author's comment on these GERD drugs, see *Author's Note* below.[a]
- *General therapeutic principles*. (1) Demulcents, such as Slippery Elm bark, relieve irritation. (2) Restoratives, such as Calendula flower and Comfrey root, help heal the esophagus. (3) Carminatives help digestion. (4) Use antacids, such as Chickweed herb and Calamus root. (5) Include antiinflammatories such as Calendula or Chamomile.

CASE HISTORY 18.9

Case History for GERD

S. Lucy has burning, acid regurgitation in her throat, and frequent burping after she eats a large meal. This makes her gaggy and nauseated. She fears she's having a heart attack, but antacids seem to help temporarily. She's been taking Maalox regularly for 5 years. She is overweight at 195 lb. but a nonsmoker. She is very stressed.

O. P Fast. **T** Red.

A. Heat and Rebellious Stomach Qi (that is rising instead of sinking).[1] GERD.

P. *Specific therapeutic principles*. Get her off OTC antacids. (1) Heat signs of red tongue, fast pulse, and burning require cooling down, e.g., with Coptis Huang Lian. (2) Demulcents to cool GI and decrease inflammation. (3) Decrease stomach inflammation. (4) Increase digestion with carminatives and decrease acidity. (5) Increase qi flow. (6) Decrease stress with nervous relaxants. (7) Use Spleen restoratives.

Herbal Formula and Dose. 6 mL 3 × day.

Parts	Herbs	Rationale
3	Chamomile flower	Carminative to relax stomach and for nervous/stress.
3	Slippery Elm bark	Moist, cool, anti-inflammatory, restorative.
2	Coptis Huan Lian	Cools gut, decreases inflammation.
2	Meadowsweet herb	Antacid.
2	Ripe Tangerine Peel/Qing Pi	Digestive stimulant for gas, indigestion; moves qi.
2	Licorice root/ Gan Cao	Heals and seals the gut; demulcent, restorative.

Other Suggestions

- *Four-R program*. After main symptoms are under control, begin treating dysbiosis.
- *Lose weight*. Suggest a Paleo diet. Take a walk after dinner.
- *Lifestyle Changes*. Sit up after eating until food is digested; no taking a nap or lying down for 2 hours after the meal. Avoid stooping over right away. Identify and avoid common trigger foods: chocolate, peppermint, fatty foods, coffee, alcohol. Decrease portion sizes.[1]
- *Manage stress*. Yoga, meditation, breathing, exercise, laughter.
- *Acupuncture*. Documented to be helpful.
- *Chamomile tea*. Take this during the day, as needed (prn), to help digestion.

[a]*Author's Note:* Acid reflux is epidemic. Countless ads appear about acid indigestion on TV during dinner hour. Antacid drugs are among the most commonly purchased OTC remedies, especially Nexium and Prilosec. They are not harmless. Acid blockers increase bacterial overgrowth, impair nutrient absorption, depress immunity, and increase cancer risk. Once the client stops taking these remedies, the situation rebounds and gets worse. Anything herbalists can do to get someone off this stuff is a blessing.

Summary

If all an herbalist ever did was to heal the gut, her or his service would be invaluable. Along with digestion, assimilation, absorption, and elimination, the GI houses the intestinal flora, a vital part of the immune system that plays a major role in the autoimmune epidemic. The gut influences mood and mental health via the gut-brain connection. It serves as an endocrine organ and detoxification center. The Four-R protocol is the core regimen for gut and body health that heals inflammation, dysbiosis, and intestinal permeability. Get this one down.

Esoterically, the gut is the home of the solar plexus chakra, our center of power and emotions. From the Chinese Medicine perspective, the Spleen and Stomach are the digestive organs. The Spleen also supports organs and holds blood in place. Prolapse indicates Spleen Qi Collapse, and abnormal bleeding and bruising indicate the Spleen is not controlling blood.

The GI Materia Medica is quite large and includes restoratives, which heal and seal the intestinal lining, and bitters with multiple actions. Antimicrobials clear up all kinds of infection, stimulants accelerate digestion and have a calming effect, relaxants decrease pain and smooth muscle spasm, and prebiotics feed the flora. Carminatives increase peristalsis and move stuck food, antacids alkalinize gastric contents, and demulcents cool, moisten, and soothe.

Review

Fill in the Blanks

(Answers in Appendix B.)

1. In Chinese Medicine the Spleen is the organ of ___. Its emotion is ___. Its taste is ___. It likes to be damp or dry? ___. Warm or cold? ___.
2. In Spleen Qi Deficiency describe the **P** ___ and **T** ___. Is there diarrhea or constipation? ___.
3. Name five things to remove in the Four-R program: ___, ___, ___, ___, ___.
4. Name three things to replace in the Four-R program: ___, ___, ___.
5. What are five actions of bitters? ___, ___, ___, ___, ___.
6. Name three Western gut tropho-restoratives ___, ___, ___. Name three Chinese Medicine gut restoratives ___, ___, ___.
7. Antidiarrheals work because of their ___ content and ___ action. Name three: ___, ___, ___.
8. Name four antacid type herbs: ___, ___, ___, ___.
9. Give four examples of food sources used for reinoculation: ___, ___, ___, ___.
10. Give six symptoms of a GI yeast infection: ___, ___, ___, ___, ___, ___.

Critical Concept Questions

(Answers for you to decide.)

1. A client wants to go on a bowel cleanse. What would you advise?
2. What is the Four-R program or protocol? Describe each step in detail.
3. What is DGL? How is it taken? What is it good for? Where do you get it? Can you make it?
4. Why are plants containing berberine so useful? Name five with common, botanical, and pinyin name, if applicable.
5. What does the endocrine system have to do with the gut?
6. Your client has been taking Prilosec before dinner for years for persistent indigestion symptoms. What's wrong with that? What would you suggest?
7. Explain the relationship between autoimmune illnesses anywhere in the body and the gut.
8. What is Food Stagnation and how is it handled?
9. Why is there so much IBS around these days?
10. What is the difference between celiac disease and gluten intolerance? How are they treated?

References

1. Romm, Aviva. *Adrenal Thyroid Revolution* (New York: HarperCollins, 2017).
2. "The Gut-Brain Connection." Harvard Health Publishing, Harvard Medical School. https://www.health.harvard.edu/diseases-and-conditions/the-gut-brain-connection (accessed August 11, 2019).
3. Wallis, Claudia. "How Gut Bacteria Make Us Fat and Thin." Scientific American. https://www.scientificamerican.com/article/how-gut-bacteria-help-make-us-fat-and-thin/ (accessed August 11, 2019).
4. Myss, Caroline. *Anatomy of the Spirit* (New York: Three Rivers Press, 1996).
5. "Spleen-Earth" Institute for Traditional Medicine. http://www.itmonline.org/5organs/spleen.htm (accessed August 11, 2019).
6. Dharmananda, Subhuti. "Understanding Qi: The Four Gentlemen Decoction." Institute for Traditional Medicine. http://www.itmonline.org/articles/si_junzi_tang/si_junzi_tang.htm (accessed October 17, 2019).
7. Holmes, Peter. *Jade Remedies: A Chinese Herbal Reference for the West* (Boulder, CO: Snow Lotus, 1996).
8. Park, Jung-Ha, et al. "Promotion of Intestinal Epithelial Cell Turnover by Commensal Bacteria: Role of Short-Chain Fatty Acids." U.S. National Library of Medicine, National Institutes of Health. https://www.ncbi.nlm.nih.gov/pmc/articles/PMC4883796/ (accessed August 11, 2019).
9. "About Bitters." Urban Moonshine, Organic Herbal Apothecary. https://www.urbanmoonshine.com/pages/about-bitters (accessed August 11, 2019).
10. Hoffman, David. *Medical Herbalism: The Science and Practice of Herbal Medicine* (Rochester, VT: Healing Arts, 2003).
11. Romm, Aviva. *Botanical Medicine for Women's Health* (St. Louis, MO: Elsevier, 2010).
12. Binion, David. "Biologic Therapies for Crohn's Disease." U.S. Library of Medicine, National Institutes of Health. https://www.ncbi.nlm.nih.gov/pmc/articles/PMC2886448/ (accessed August 12, 2019).
13. Holmes, Peter. *Energetics of Western Herbs* (Boulder, CO: Snow Lotus, 2006).
14. Buhner, Stephen Harrod. *Herbal Antibiotics* (North Adams, MA: Storey, 2012).
15. "What is Inflammatory Bowel Disease (IBD)?" Center for Disease and Control Prevention. https://www.cdc.gov/ibd/what-is-IBD.htm (accessed August 11, 2019).
16. Bone, Kerry and Simon Mills. *Principles and Practice of Phytotherapy* (London, UK: Elsevier, 2013).
17. Bergner, Paul. Class notes, Mountain West Herb Gathering. Breckenridge, CO. June 16-19, 2016.

19
The Hepato-Biliary System

"The Liver is the Commanding General."

—Chinese Medicine view

CHAPTER REVIEW

- Overview of liver functions: Portal circulation, chemical processing, bile and bilirubin, glucose regulation, clotting, immune function, and detoxification.
- Liver detoxification, gut and liver health.
- The Cytochrome P450 enzyme system. Herbs and foods for Phase I and II. How to tell if liver detoxification is needed. Signs and symptoms indicating metabolic overload.
- Heavy metal detoxification. General strategies to eradicate heavy metal poisoning.
- Chinese Medicine perspective: The Liver and Gallbladder with major syndromes.
- Hepato-biliary system Materia Medica: Liver herbs worth honorable mention. Hepatic categories: restoratives, stimulants (qi movers and cholagogues), stimulating detoxifiers, antiinfectives and antilithics.
- Common hepato-biliary conditions with case histories: Poor liver detoxifier, environmental toxicosis, acute and chronic viral hepatitis, cholecystitis, gallstones, and alcoholism-induced cirrhosis.

KEY TERMS

Antilithics
Bile
Bilirubin
Chelation
Cholecystitis
Cholagogues
Cholelithiasis
Cholesterol
Cirrhosis
Cytochrome P-450 enzyme detoxification system
Deconjugation
Endogenous
Exogenous
Free radicals
Gallstones
Gluconeogenesis
Glutathione
Gut-liver axis
Hepatocytes
Jaundice
Metabolism
Oxidative stress
Phase I liver detoxification
Phase II liver detoxification
Portal system
Wind

Hepato relates to liver, and *biliary* refers to bile. Nobody can live without a functioning liver, our main detoxification organ. Simply by being alive we create toxins from waste products given off through normal chemical reactions in the body (***metabolism***). Even if we had a pristine diet, breathed immaculately pure air, and lived on a remote mountaintop, the liver could never take a break.

We can live without a gallbladder but would not have optimal digestion. The gallbladder is tucked up under the two liver lobes, stores bile, and releases it in response to dietary fat intake. Bile emulsifies fats, preparing them for ultimate digestion and absorption into the blood. Hardened bile (gallstones) can form in the gallbladder or its ducts, causing excruciating pain and blockage.

Chinese Medicine is respectful and fond of the liver. Liver syndromes appear in many Western body systems, including the gastrointestinal, the hepato-biliary, neuro, kidney, and reproduction (notably women's health) systems.

A Liver's Work Is Never Done

As is famously touted in physiology books, the liver has over 500 functions, although rarely are they all listed; it is not called "the Commanding General" for nothing. The adult liver weighs close to 3 pounds, roughly the size and shape of a football. It is beloved in herbal and functional medicine circles and claims utmost importance in Chinese Medicine. We are always preaching to first fix the gut, but a well-functioning liver plays a close second. Almost any herbal formula could justifiably contain a good liver herb. A few liver highlights follow:

- *Private circulation, the liver's portal system.* A *portal system* is a system of venous channels that connect one capillary system with another. In the liver's private ***portal system***, digested food is first absorbed through the capillaries of the villi of the small intestine and then travels through the hepatic *portal* vein to the liver for initial cleaning, processing, and delivery of nutrients. Blood, containing the proper nutritional mix, is then released into the systemic circulation on its way to the heart and destinations beyond for cellular use.
  - The portal system is unique because all other veins bypass the liver and go directly to the heart. But in this case the liver processes absorbed nutrients first, either storing them for future use or passing them on, as needed. It makes sure the blood entering general circulation is free of toxicants and full of nutrients.
- *The liver is a chemical processing plant.* Thanks to the portal system, the liver (which holds about a pint of blood in its sinusoids at any given moment), performs a bit of alchemy. It metabolizes fats, carbohydrates, and proteins and then synthesizes, stores, and releases nutrients into the blood, based on the body's needs. It changes these macronutrients into one form for storage and another for immediate consumption, depending on demand.
- Every day the liver makes 1000 mg of ***cholesterol***, a valuable fat sterol used for production of bile, fat-soluble vitamins, and fatty hormones like estrogen, cortisol, and aldosterone.[1] The liver stores nutrients: fatty acids, vitamin B_{12}, iron, copper, and fat-soluble vitamins A, D, and K. It can convert carbohydrates and proteins into fatty acids and triglycerides. It makes plasma proteins, such as albumin. Busy.
- *The liver produces multifaceted bile.* ***Bile*** is a bitter, alkaline yellow-dark green substance made in the liver, stored in the gallbladder, and released by hormonal action into the duodenum, where it breaks down or *emulsifies* fats. Bile salts emptied into the duodenum neutralize acids and food material that has passed from the stomach. Bile also stimulates peristalsis that helps bowels to move. Herbs that increase bile flow are ***cholagogues***. Fringe Tree bark, Turmeric rhizome (Fig. 19.1), and Gentian root are examples.
- *The liver forms bilirubin.* An orange-yellow pigment (***bilirubin***) is formed in the liver by the breakdown (***deconjugation***) of iron-carrying and oxygen-carrying hemoglobin molecules in red blood cells (RBCs). Old, broken-down RBCs are excreted in the bile, and their pigment makes stools brown. In the process, the liver stores iron obtained from the hemoglobin. If the liver is metabolically overloaded or doesn't break down bilirubin efficiently, there is ***jaundice***, where the excess pigment leaks out into the skin, mucous membranes or sclera, coloring them bright yellow. This coloring is a sign of liver disease. In that case, liver restorative herbs and several others are in order: Milk Thistle seed, Dandelion root, and Schisandra Wu Wei Zi.
- *The liver regulates glucose.* The liver works with the pancreas in regulating blood glucose levels in two ways.
  - *It converts* excess glucose into *glycogen* for storage. When blood sugar falls or the body needs more glucose, the liver converts glycogen back into glucose for energy. This is known as ***gluconeogenesis***. Impaired liver function results in impaired gluconeogenesis and can cause fatigue, irritability, and depression. Once the proper amount of glucose is circulating, the pancreas takes over and fine-tunes glucose levels with the help of insulin (Chapter 27).
  - *The liver converts excess fat for storage.* It alters carbohydrates (glucose) and proteins into fatty acids and triglycerides, which are then exported and stored in fatty adipose tissue. In this way, it protects us from excess blood sugar levels when we overeat and gives the pancreas a little rest. Clinical pearl: Any self-respecting diabetes formula must include a liver stimulant, a bitter like Bitter Melon or Blessed Thistle herb.

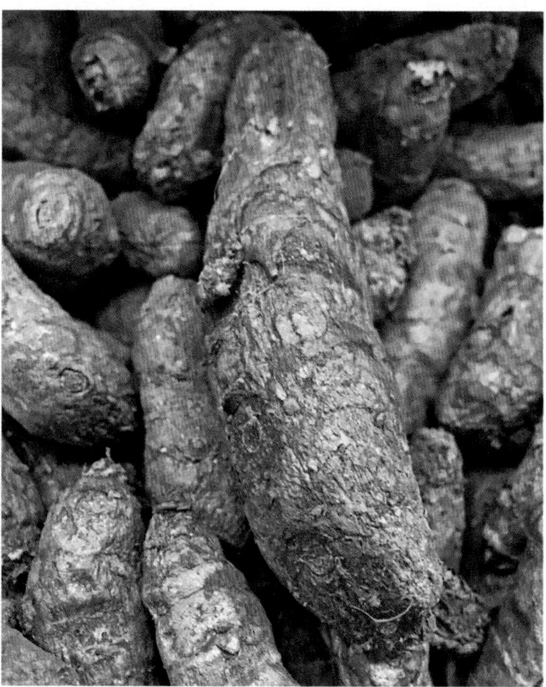

• **Fig. 19.1** *Curcuma longa* (Turmeric root) is a cholagogue that increases bile flow.

- *The liver converts ammonia into urea.* Unabsorbed protein in the small intestine is converted to ammonia and passed through the portal system to the liver. The liver changes ammonia into urea, which is excreted in the *urine* (from which urea gets its name and smell). Elevated blood ammonia levels reflect liver disease and affect the brain, producing foggy, muddled thinking (brain fog).
- *The liver regulates digestion.* In addition to regulating glucose, the liver is important in fat metabolism. It forms lipoproteins and cholesterol used in cell membranes and hormone production. It forms phospholipids, which are also needed in cell membranes. It converts a lot of carbohydrates into fat. Finally, the bile it produces breaks down fat, so it can be absorbed. Aromatic bitters are notorious in stimulating digestion and relieving qi congestion. (Stuck stomach qi results in indigestion.) Notable digestive aids are Turmeric root, Fennel seed, and various bitter citruses, such as Citrus Qing Pi (Green Tangerine peel) or Citrus Zhi Shi (unripe Bitter Orange fruit), and others.
- *The liver helps regulate blood clotting.* The liver stores and uses vitamin K to produce many clotting factors so we don't bleed to death. If there are coagulation or bleeding problems, the liver is often implicated as a root cause. In addition to tonifying the liver, we would also employ coagulants or anticoagulants as needed.

- *The liver is an immune organ.* Specialized Kupffer cells line the sinusoids in the liver. They capture and digest bacteria, fungi, parasites, worn-out blood cells, and cellular debris. Through the detoxification and elimination of metabolic poisons, immunity is helped.
- *The liver is crucial for detoxification.* The liver is a main avenue of detoxification, along with the gut, the kidneys, and the skin. It detoxes in three ways. The liver filters the blood to remove bacteria and toxins before it enters general circulation; it makes bile for excretion of fat-soluble toxins and cholesterol; and it uses the *Cytochrome P450 enzyme system* (see later section) to break down unwanted chemicals, drugs, alcohol, and waste products of metabolism. Measures to facilitate this process include intelligent use of herbs, foods, lifestyle choices, and maintaining a healthy gut microbiome.

Liver Detoxification, the Gut, and Liver Health

The liver is the largest metabolically active organ in the body. It is a garbage collector and recycler. In addition to processing nutrients and microorganisms from the gut and dealing with the normal end products of metabolic chemical breakdown reactions (***endogenous***), it handles toxins from the outside environment (***exogenous***) wastes: drugs, heavy metals, hormones, molds, and pollutants that are everywhere. The liver is assigned the huge job of deconjugating, transforming, and breaking down these toxins into harmless substances the body can excrete through the urine, bowels, and skin. If the liver isn't breaking down metabolites, and the kidneys aren't making good-quality urine, a person with such conditions will quickly die of sepsis in about a week. If the liver is off-kilter but not in failure, and the kidneys are doing all right, we live longer, but not in optimal health. End-stage liver failure from alcoholism, chronic hepatitis, or other factors is not a pretty sight.

The gut is related to the liver, and the liver is related to the gut. The two communicate in what is sometimes dubbed the ***gut-liver axis***.[2] It has been found that nonalcoholic fatty liver disease is positively correlated to intestinal permeability (IP). In other words, leaky gut can lead to liver disease and failure by overtaxing its detox pathways. A balanced microbiome, intestinal wall integrity and efficient liver detoxification are important aspects of whole-body health.

Unhealthy large intestine microbes and small intestine bacterial overgrowth (SIBO) excrete endotoxins that must be dealt with (Chapter 18). Foods, nutrients, and toxins are absorbed from the intestines, which happens either the right way across the villi into the capillaries or the wrong way through leaky gut junctions. Regardless of route, they go directly to the liver's portal system before entering general circulation. If all goes well, the liver handles the load as best it can and passes on cleaned-out blood and nutrients for delivery to all cells and tissues. If things go badly because of intestinal permeability and further toxic overload, many symptoms and chronic diseases can occur. We develop depressed immunity, brain fog, additional digestive problems, allergies, skin outbreaks, adrenal stress, hormone imbalances, and autoimmune syndromes.

Cytochrome P450 Enzyme Detoxification System

The liver's detoxification pathways occur through its ***Cytochrome P-450 enzyme detoxification system***. There are two phases or pathways, Phase I and II (Fig. 19.2). Both need to be properly balanced and in sync. The result is that toxic chemicals are converted

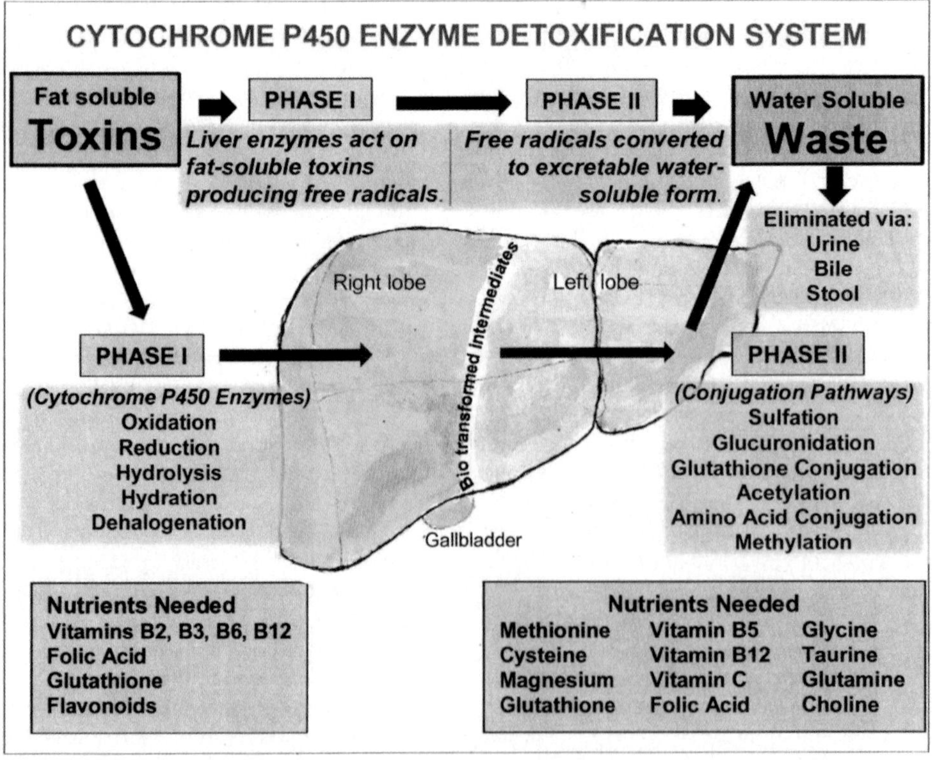

• **Fig. 19.2** Liver detoxification pathways, illustrating Phase I where fat-soluble toxins are broken down into biotransformed intermediates (free radicals), and Phase II where the free radicals are converted to easily excretable water-soluble form. (Credit Joan Zinn.)

into harmless substances the body can excrete. If not, there are increased incidences of allergies, asthma, environmental sensitivities, autoimmune diseases, skin outbreaks, food cravings, severe PMS, and hormone imbalances.

- *Phase I, where liver enzymes act on fat soluble toxins producing free radicals.* Phase I uses chemical reactions of oxidation, reduction, hydrolysis, and the Cytochrome P-450 family of enzymes (there are 50–100 enzymes) to break down fat-soluble toxins into biotransformed intermediates, better known as ***free radicals*** (unstable oxygen molecules with an unpaired electron). Excessive free radicals or reactive oxygen species (ROS) damage liver cells and DNA throughout the body. This process is known as ***oxidative stress***. (Chapter 16) Fat-soluble toxins come from environmental pollutants, exogenous estrogen, insecticides, drugs, alcohol, processed food, hormones, and normal metabolic body toxins, such as lactic acid from adenosine triphosphate (ATP) production. Oxidative stress damages the endocrine, nervous, and immune systems.
- *Phase II, where free radicals are converted to easily excretable water-soluble form.* Phase II uses the chemical reactions of methylation and sulfation, taking free radicals formed in Phase I and converting them into water-soluble form, easily excreted through the kidneys via urine and through the stool via bile. This is vitally important, because oxidative stress and chronic inflammation caused by free-radical DNA damage leads to premature aging, our epidemic of chronic diseases, and cancer.

Herbs and Foods for Phase I and II

- ***Phase I liver detoxification***: Excessive free radical production can be reduced by intake of a variety of colorful foods containing antioxidants, such as vitamins A, C, and E, and natural carotenoids like Pine and Grape seed extracts, all types of berries, and Artichoke leaf.
- ***Phase II liver detoxification***: This phase usually needs more of a boost (*up-regulation*) than Phase I, because it has to break down all the free radicals produced. There are functional medical lab tests to determine how well each phase is working, but in general Phase II usually takes the brunt and is the one needing up-regulation. Cholagogues and glutathione boosters are useful Phase II categories of herbs and foods that help detoxification.
    - *Cholagogues.* Herbs that stimulate bile flow to digest fats and increase bowel function are the *cholagogues*. Gentle, long-term cholagogues include Artichoke leaf, Dandelion root, Burdock root, and Yellow Dock root. Stronger cholagogues for short-term use include Boldo leaf, Celandine herb and root, and Black Radish root. Save the short-termers for a-once-or-twice-year liver cleansing. They empty the biochemical trash and help form glutathione.
    - *Glutathione boosters.* ***Glutathione*** is the primary antioxidant liver detoxifier, a protein containing three amino acids: glutamate, cysteine, and glycine. It takes the free radicals produced in Phase I and stops their chain reaction by quenching and scavenging. It changes free radicals into stable molecules that no longer destroy DNA and protects them from oxidative damage. Glutathione is not well-metabolized in supplement form because it is broken down by stomach HCl acid. It is more effective to use glutathione from herb and food sources. Notable glutathione-producing herbs are Milk Thistle seed, Turmeric root, and Platycodon Jie Geng (Balloonflower root). Superior foods include spinach, avocados, Brazil nuts, and cruciferous and/or sulfur-containing foods.

How to Tell if Liver Detoxification is Needed

People don't all detoxify at the same rate; some do it better than others. There are quite a few events that can cause the liver to be in *metabolic overload*, a sign that detoxification help is needed. One factor is a slow and steady dose of environmental toxins or a sudden influx of external pollutants and toxins that overwhelm the liver. Excessive drug and alcohol ingestion tax the liver. Another is a liver that does not have adequate nutrients to take on additional detoxification requirements.

Because of the liver's multiple responsibilities, one or more of these jobs done badly over time can create signs or symptoms that indicate attention is needed by herbalists. One sign may not be indicative, but three or four very well could be. Heeding subclinical early warning signs is far better than waiting for outright liver disease or failure. By the time liver function tests are elevated in a routine blood analysis, damage has already been done.

Signs and Symptoms Indicating Metabolic Overload

- *Chronic skin problems.* If the liver is in overload and can't handle toxic input, the garbage has to go somewhere. Often it comes out through the skin, causing outbreaks like dark skin spots, acne, rosacea, eczema, psoriasis, blotchy skin, and a lot of itching.
- *Signs of heat.* Redness and flushed facial appearance, rosacea, and excessive facial capillaries that are quite noticeable are signs of heat. **Pulse (P)** Full. **Tongue (T)** Red or purple. With excess heat comes sweating as the body tries to cool down. The person looks hot and feels hot.
- *Extreme fatigue.* Exhaustion, even with adequate sleep. This is quite typical of metabolic stress and poor detoxification.
- *Chemical sensitivity.* There is difficulty tolerating any alcohol and greater than usual intolerance of smells. Environmental toxins include pollution, pesticides, food additives, and fluoridated water. Specific offenders are fertilizers in nonorganic food; flame retardants; chemicals in new cars, drapes, and carpets; formaldehyde sources in insulation materials; tobacco smoke; and plastic bags. Lead comes from paint and gasoline. Mercury appears in seafood, dental and medical equipment, fertilizers, pesticides, and amalgam fillings.[3]
- *Brain fog and decreased nervous function.* Excessive chemical exposure inhibits brain function. There could be chronic headaches, mental confusion, muddled thoughts, or forgetfulness. These symptoms manifest in the nervous system, but root cause is the liver failing to detoxify properly.
- *Bitter taste* and *mouth odor.* Bile is bitter; sometimes a bitter taste in the mouth is bile-related, from chronically faulty fat metabolism. Bad breath is caused by excess ammonia produced by protein breakdown, which the liver neglected to convert into urea.
- *Digestive troubles.* Difficulty digesting fatty foods with a lot of belching and distress is related to faulty bile production and ejection. Abdominal bloating, water retention, weight gain, or problems losing weight, even with calorie restriction, and fat rolls around the abdomen are all signs of metabolic stress. Very foul, smelly, or clay-colored stools are a sign there could be a bile duct obstruction or gallstones.
- *History of gallbladder disease or removal.* Symptoms include right-sided pain or discomfort over, on, or under the liver; difficulty digesting fatty foods; and acid reflux. There could be *jaundice* (yellowish cast to the skin or sclera), dark urine filled with bilirubin, and diminished flow.

Heavy Metal Detoxification

Heavy metal exposure puts an enormous strain on the liver. The metals most concerning to human health include lead, mercury, cadmium, and inorganic arsenic. Heavy metals enter the body through eating nonorganic foods and fish, inhaled smoke and gasoline, lead paint exposure, mercury in tooth amalgams, exposure to air pollution, and more. Heavy metal overload is diagnosed from urine, blood, and hair analysis. Obtaining a thoughtful health history and asking the right questions can give the herbalist substantial clues to signal if this is a likely issue.

A *chelate* is any substance that attracts heavy metals. ***Chelation*** therapy is a form of heavy-metal detoxification, where heavy molecular-weight metallic ions chemically bind to ions of another substance, the *chelating agent*. They are both eliminated together through the kidneys. Plant allies acting as chelators include seaweeds (Fig. 19.3), algae, Garlic, Cilantro, and Milk Thistle seed.

General Strategies to Eradicate Heavy Metal Poisoning

- *Attend to gut health*. Use the Four-R program (Chapter 18). Enlarged epithelial cell junctions with leaky gut allow undigested food particles to enter the liver's portal system. These foreign substances create an antigen-antibody reaction, a setup for autoimmune diseases. The gut also loads the liver with all kinds of toxins: dirt, microorganisms from foods, endotoxins from the colon and small intestines (SIBO), drugs, alcohol, dirty water, and heavy metals. This large burden enters the liver's front door. It explains the *gut-liver axis* in a nutshell. Clean up the gut and attend to the liver.
- *Increase elimination through kidneys and skin*. Stay well-hydrated; drink lots of pure, clean water, so the kidneys make plenty of good-quality urine. After Phase II transforms intermediate free radicals into water-soluble substances, they have to get out somewhere. *Dry skin brushing* with a natural brush or luffa sponge loosens dry cells and toxins accumulated on skin surfaces. Follow this with dry heat, a sweat, or a sauna, which cleanses and pulls toxins out through the pores. Alternately, skin brush and take a hot bath with a large handful of Epsom salts added to the water.
- *Cleansing diet*. Fresh veggies in large supply increase glutathione, the primary antioxidant needed by the liver. Follow leaky gut dietary protocols with an emphasis on liver foods: dark, leafy greens, beets, shitake mushrooms, lemons, and artichokes.
- *Removal of mercury amalgams*. In some cases, mercury dental fillings (amalgams) may need removal by a qualified dentist. If done incorrectly, mercury can be released into the bloodstream, making the situation worse.

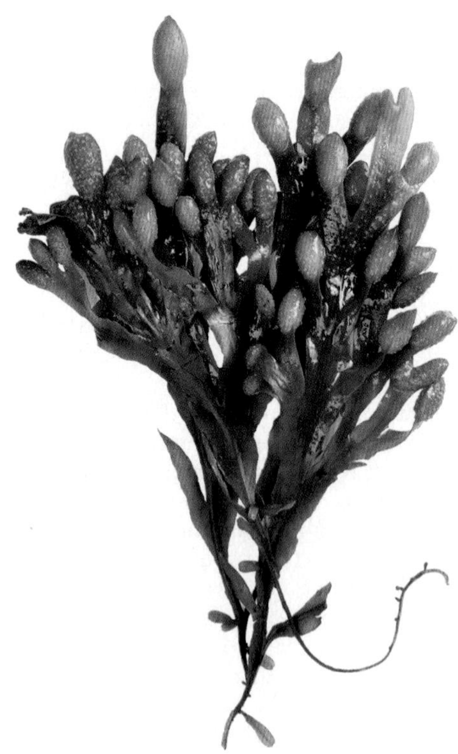

• **Fig. 19.3** *Fucus vesiculosus* (Bladderwrack thallus) is a familiar ocean seaweed that dissolves deposits and functions as a salty heavy metal chelating agent. (iStock.com/Credit: juniorbeep.)

Chinese Medicine Perspective: Liver and Gallbladder with Major Syndromes

The Liver is intricately related to a toxic world, anger, and stress. Because there is no shortage of these experiences, the Liver shows up in many conditions that are seemingly unrelated. The Liver is always lurking around women's menstrual problems and stress-related ailments that can affect any organ.

The Liver opens to the eyes, manifests in the nails, and is in charge of the tendons. Problems in any of these areas require Liver attention. Botanical medicine and the Liver go hand in hand. As part of their folk heritage, most people around the world recognize the importance of vegetables for a healthy liver. The bitter taste is prominent in liver botanicals because it specifically triggers secretion of bile, and bile is known to aid digestion and liver metabolism in general. A bitter taste in the mouth is also reported in various liver pathologies, because bile backs up into the mouth.

- *Liver and emotions*. The Liver is related to *anger* and its close relatives: resentment, frustration, unfulfilled desires, regrets, and repressed feelings. (Depression is considered anger turned inward.) If the Liver is emotionally balanced, we flow and easily glide through life without too much of a struggle.
- *Liver qi*. The Liver regulates the flow of energy, Liver qi. If we're uptight and angry for long periods, Liver qi slows down or even stops or stagnates, which is sometimes called stasis. Slowed down and stuck Liver qi can eventually become who we are, leading to anger, pain, and resentment as our *modus operandi*. If we flow through life, express our emotions, not allowing them to get in the way, we generally feel light and content. Slowed Liver qi manifests on a physical level around the chest, breasts, throat, head, hypochondrium, and epigastric regions. In women, stuck Liver qi leads to cysts, lumps, fibroids in reproductive organs, and tumors and lumps in the breast. From a physiological level, these are caused by toxin buildup that the liver cannot process and eliminate.
- *Rebellious Liver qi*. Liver qi can go in the wrong direction or *rebel* and flow upward instead of downward. If this happens, hot Liver yang rises over the top. Symptoms include irritability, headaches, and a quick temper. These are the folks who quickly

get irritable and impatient. (Recall that Stomach qi can also rebel in the wrong direction, producing nausea and vomiting.)

- *Liver stores the blood.* Because it stores blood, a deficiency of blood (either in quantity or nutritionally) can easily affect places under the Liver's influence.
- *Table of correspondences.* The Liver opens to the eyes, so if Liver blood is deficient, the eyes are not nourished, and vision problems can occur. Liver manifests in the nails; lack of nourishment and blood to the nails make them brittle. Liver body parts are the sinews (tendons). Muscle cramping, spasm, or weakness is a Liver area.
- *Liver's taste is sour.* Lemons have always been considered a prime liver and gallbladder food. Sour releases stagnation, stuck Liver qi. Sour foods include sauerkraut, Granny Smith apple, lemons, umeboshi (sour pickled plums), vinegar, and cherry. If the client doesn't like the sour taste, she or he probably needs it. Squeeze a little lemon on salad greens or cooked spinach and drink a glass of lemon water in the morning.
- *Liver's season is spring.* Its element is wood, the color is green, and spring is the time for new beginnings and growth. Spring would be ideal for a liver cleanse or tune-up.
- *Gallbladder time is 11 p.m. to 1 a.m. and Liver time is 1 a.m. to 3 a.m.* Going by the 24-hour organ qi cycle clock (Chapter 15), the Gallbladder and the Liver are most actively detoxing at those times. Detoxification has a better chance at being successful if we are asleep and fasting. If the liver is in mechanical overload and does not have enough time to detox during its active night hours, a person has a hard time getting up in the morning. (Assuming enough sleep and no stress.) This difficulty is a sign of Liver Qi Stagnation. If a woman in menopause repeatedly wakes up with night sweats during Gallbladder and Liver hours, she could use some liver stimulants to take in the daytime.
- *Headaches are related to the Liver.* Internally caused headaches (not from a neck spasm or injury) are related to the Liver and Gallbladder because of the position of their energy meridians. The paired Liver meridians go up through the middle of the eyes and over top of the head (vertex). Gallbladder meridians travel up through the sides of head, the temples (Box 23.3). Determining the location of the headache is a routine Chinese Medicine health history question.
- *Liver wind.* The Liver can cause internal or external movements and sudden shaking, called ***wind***, so-named because wind causes movement and change. Tremors, spasms, seizures, nystagmus, and bipolar episodes are examples. Uncaria Gou Teng (Gambir Vine twig) and Gastrodia Tian Ma (Celestial Hemp corm) are Chinese Medicine classics for Liver wind. You could also use Western Lobelia herb or Hops flower.
- *Gallbladder.* The Liver is yin; the Gallbladder is its yang partner. Liver's emotion is anger; Gallbladder's issue is *decision* or *indecision.* Having courage and taking initiative denotes a healthy Gallbladder on an emotional level.

Chinese Medicine Major Liver and Gallbladder Syndromes

- *Liver Qi Stagnation or Congestion.* This one is common. Liver qi is not circulating well because of toxic overload. Typical pattern relates to Liver emotions, a tendency to get depressed, frequent sighing, quick temper, anger, stress, and anxiety. Could be vertex headaches or headache over eyes, portal hypertension, jaundice, or varices. In women (Chapter 28), there is estrogen dominance with PMS, cramps, and irregular, heavy periods, fibroids, endometriosis, breast lumps or cysts, uterine cancer. **P** Wiry. **T** Normal body.
  - *Fix:* Move Liver qi, help detoxification, and increase bile flow. Noteworthy Chinese Medicine classics to move Liver qi are Bupleurum Chai Hu (Asian Buplever root), Paeonia Bai Shao Yao (White Peony root), Scutellaria Huang Qin (Baikal Skullcap root), and Dandelion root from East and West.
- *Liver Yin Deficiency.* Red cheeks, night sweats. **P** Thin, rapid. **T** Red, with no coat. Additional symptoms specific to the Liver are dizziness, irritability, and dry, irritated eyes. Toxic Liver overload is a Western scenario. Moisture and cooling are needed.
  - *Fix:* Tonify Liver yin with restoratives, such as Milk Thistle seed and Dandelion root, and clear heat, perhaps with a formula known as Qi Ju Di Huang Wan that contains Chrysanthemum Bai Ju Hua (Chrysanthemum flower), Lycium Gou Qi Z (Lycii/Goji/Wolfberry), and Rehmannia Shu Di Huang (Prepared Rehmannia root) as the main herbs.
- *Liver Blood Stagnation.* When blood slows down and stagnates, it gets thick and eventually clots. This one will show up frequently with women's health in uterine fibroids, cysts, and tumors. They go hand in hand with Liver Qi Stagnation. **P** Wiry. **T** Purple (more purple on the sides), possible purple spots.
  - *Fix*: Move blood with Angelica Dang Gui (Angelica/Dong Quai root), Paeonia Chi Shao Yao (Red Peony root), and Panax San Qi (Notoginseng root).
- *Liver Blood Deficiency.* Pale face and lips, tongue, anemia, dizzy, dry skin, hypotension from deficient blood volume. Eyes are itchy, with vision problems, blurriness, spots or floaters, or night blindness. Nails are pale or cracked. **P** Choppy, fine, thin. **T** Pale.
  - Women are particularly prone to Liver Blood Deficiency at puberty, after childbirth, and somewhat after each period, in scanty periods or amenorrhea.
  - Muscles: Numbness of the limbs, muscular weakness, spasms, cramps, brittle nails.
  - *Fix*: Tonify blood with the usual suspects: use blood tonics like Angelica Dang Gui (Dong Quai root), Rehmannia Shu Di Huang (Prepared/cooked Rehmannia root), Polygonum He Shou Wu (Flowery Knotweed root), and Ziziphus Suan Zao Ren (Sour Jujube seed), Nettle herb, Red Clover flower. Restore the Liver with Lycium Gou Qi Zi (Goji berry), and Milk Thistle seed.
- *Liver Yang Rising or Liver Fire.* Liver qi going in the wrong direction; anger. Yang is hot (yin is cold). Western syndromes include alcoholism, early-stage hypertension, hyperthyroidism, acute gallbladder, hepatitis, or ear infections. **P** Wiry and rapid. **T** Red cracked body.
  - *Fix*: Tonify yin and clear heat with Gentiana Long Gan Cao (Scabrous Gentian root), Scutellaria Huang Qin (Baikal Skullcap root), Bupleurum Chai Hu (Asian Buplever root), Gardenia Zhi Zi (Gardenia pod), Prunella Xia Ku Cao (Selfheal herb), and Chrysanthemum Ju Hua (Chrysanthemum flower). A classic Chinese Medicine formula for this is called Long Dan Xie Gan.
- *Gallbladder (GB) Damp Heat.* The gallbladder physically connects to the liver, and it doesn't like damp (neither does the Spleen). Gallbladder dampness interferes with the smooth

flow of Liver qi. Qi backs up and stagnates, causing hypochondrium (under the ribs) pain and distention, gallstones, cholecystitis. The heat causes nausea, vomiting, fever, bitter taste, and thirst without desire to drink, because there is dampness. Bile backs up, causing jaundice and dark-yellow urine. Expect long standing anger. **P** Slippery and wiry. **T** Red body with thick, sticky, yellow coating.

- *Fix:* Resolve damp, clear heat, and smooth out flow of qi.

Hepato-Biliary System Materia Medica

Liver Herbs Worth Honorable Mention

- *Carduus benedictus* (Blessed Thistle herb), a liver stimulant. This thistle is good for poor appetite and digestive problems. It is bitter, cool, and dry. For Liver and Gallbladder Qi Stagnation. It stimulates digestive enzymes and cholagogue action and promotes bile flow. A nice addition to a bitters formula. Blessed Thistle promotes sweating and clears heat.
- *Cynara scolymus* (Globe Artichoke leaf) (Fig. 19.4). Salty, cool, and moist, Artichoke leaf is filled with antioxidants—one of the very best liver restoratives, second only to Milk Thistle seed. Both are thistles, and both combine well. The thistles scream liver. They are nourishing and detoxifying to the liver and to build blood. Artichoke leaf is for liver toxicosis and any time liver is under stress or needs a boost. For Liver Qi Stagnation and Liver Yin Deficiency. Helps thyroid and pancreas and dissolves deposits.
- *Two Chinese citruses.* Dried tangerine peels must be included in this list because they are so often used in Chinese formulation as helper or secondary herbs in small amounts. They move stuck food and stool along whenever indigestion is occurring.
  - *Citrus reticulata* Chen Pi (Ripe Tangerine peel) (Fig. 19.5) and *C. reticulata* Qing Pi (Unripe or green Tangerine peel). Both are pungent liver and bile stimulants (cholagogues) and relieve liver and gallbladder congestion. Their essential oil spicy taste and citrus smell provide a carminative action for indigestion. What's the difference? Green Tangerine peel is considered stronger and harsher than the more relaxing Ripe Tangerine peel, so use with caution in those with weakness and fatigue.[4] Citrus peels, in general, are stronger dried than fresh, and the longer they're aged, the better. Syndromes are for Liver Qi Stagnation and Liver/Spleen disharmony.
- *Two Chinese berries.* Both of these sweet, moist, and delicious berries have liver affinities. *Lycium barbarum* Gou Qi Zi (Goji or Wolfberry), are a bit sour and sweet. *Zizyphus jujube* Da Zao (Jujube berry or date) come in dark-red and black varieties. Red ones are preferred to nourish the blood, whereas the dark ones are favored to tonify qi.[5] Eaten alone as a munchie, added to tonic teas, or in tincture, all these sweet berries are superb. They are restorative, nutritive, and protective tonics filled with antioxidants and high in vitamins and minerals and thus used in Liver and Kidney deficiencies.
- *Gardenia jasminoides* Zhi Zi (Gardenia pod). A bitter, cold, and astringent deep yellow-gold pod that excels in clearing damp heat of liver and gallbladder infections, such as acute hepatitis with jaundice, and liver abscesses. It is ***antilithic*** to dissolve gallstones, a cholagogue for liver congestion and constipation, antibacterial, and antiinflammatory.
- *Sea veggies and microalgae* are heavy-metal detoxifiers. *Laminaria* spp. (Kelp thallus) and *Fucus vesiculosus* (Bladderwrack thallus) are interchangeable ocean seaweeds. They are salty, cool, and moist. They are used for radiation exposure, and their saltiness dissolves deposits, chelates metals, and pulls out toxins.
- *Spirulina* spp. and *Chlorella* spp. are primitive superfoods, highly nutritious microalgae that serve as heavy-metal chelators and detoxifiers. *Spirulina* spp. is a blue-green alga

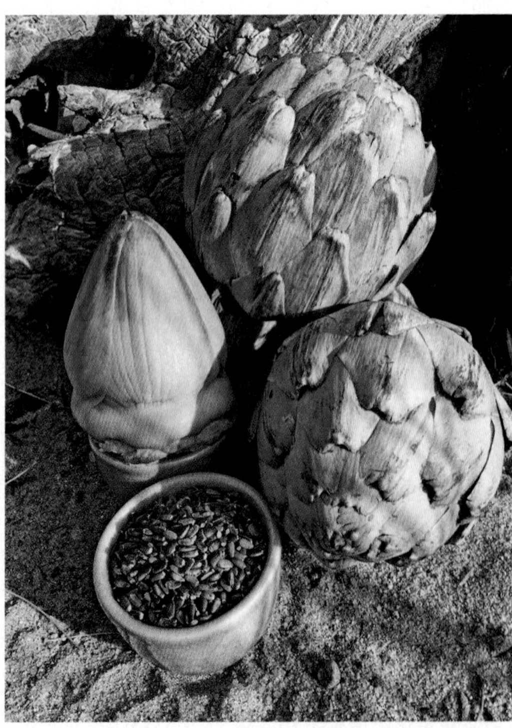

• **Fig. 19.4** *Cynara scolymus (Globe Artichoke leaf) stimulates digestive enzymes and bile flow, while Silybum marianum (Milk Thistle seed) is the best liver restorative the West has to offer.*

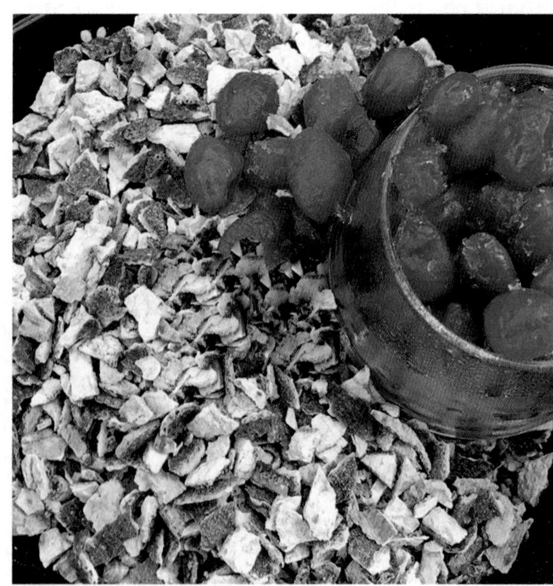

• **Fig. 19.5** Dried *Citrus reticulata* Chen Pi (Ripe Tangerine peel) is a stimulating liver carminative, and the delicious red berries of *Lycium barbarum* Gou Qi Zi (Goji or Wolfberry) restore and tonify Liver qi.

that lives in saltwater lakes, and *Chlorella* spp. is a freshwater green alga. Consider microalgae to be nutritious, antiinfective, and immune stimulating.

Hepatic Restoratives

Hepatic restoratives help liver cells (***hepatocytes***) regenerate and heal. The liver is the only internal organ that can regenerate. Only scarred, completely damaged liver cells (as in cirrhosis) will not heal. If too many cells are destroyed, a transplant is necessary. Restoratives are sweet and warm. They nourish and build moist Liver yin, the syndrome being Liver Yin Deficiency. A liver can't have too much yin. If the liver isn't detoxifying properly, restoratives are needed along with stimulants.

Specific indications for liver restoratives are a history of viral or bacterial hepatitis, adverse effects of alcohol consumption, exposure to toxic chemicals, long-standing drug use, cirrhosis and other chronic liver diseases, skin outbreaks, and chronic inflammatory diseases.[8] Symptoms could include constant all-day fatigue (adrenal burn-out), poor immune function, hypoglycemia, and headaches. Restoratives help with weight loss, malnutrition, anemia, frequent infections, and chronic hepatitis. Milk Thistle seed, Dandelion root, Bupleurum Chai Hu and Schisandra Wu Wei Zi are highly regarded restoratives (Table 19.1).

Hepatic Stimulants (Liver Qi Movers)

Liver stimulants encourage the liver to carry on its more than 500 functions (Table 19.2). They are the Liver qi movers that decongest sluggish or congested qi and are therefore called for in Liver Qi Stagnation, where Liver energy slows down or gets stuck. This condition can be caused by too much alcohol, poor diet high in fats and sugar, and inadequate exercise. Some stimulants are cooling; others are warmer and pungent. Many have a bitter taste (the bitters). In summary, hepatic stimulants increase liver activity. They are detoxifying because they stimulate Phase I and II detoxification pathways. Some cholagogues contain glutathione, an important liver antioxidant.

Choleretics are a subcategory of liver stimulants. The prefix *chol* and/or *chole* relates to bile and bile ducts. Technically, choleretics stimulate bile production and cholagogues stimulate bile ejection. In reality, herb categories with the prefix *chol* have both functions,

TABLE 19.1 Hepatic Restoratives
(To boost and restore Liver yin)

Herb	Notes (notables*)
Silybum marianum (Milk Thistle seed)	*Renowned in the West, boosts glutathione.
Taraxacum officinale (Dandelion root)	*Number one Western and Chinese Medicine (different species) that both restore, stimulate, and diurese.
Schisandra chinensis Wu Wei Zi Five Taste berry	*Top notch Chinese Medicine restorative, adaptogenic.
Bupleurum chinensis Chai Hu Asian Buplever root	*Excellent Chinese Medicine restorative, stimulant, detoxifier. Clears heat and relaxes muscles.
Cynara scolymus (Artichoke leaf)	*Top notch. Nourishes and detoxes. A must. Good for long-term use.
Rehmannia glutinosa Shu Di Huang Prepared Rehmannia root	Nourishes Liver blood, enriches Liver yin and clears heat. For adrenal burnout/stress and menopause.
Lycium barbarum Gou Qi Zi Goji or Wolfberry	Sweet, delicious, high in antioxidants, vitamins, and minerals. For eating or as tincture.
Astragalus membranaceus Huang Qi Astragalus root	Well-respected Liver restorative. Adaptogenic.
Cichorium intybus (Chicory root)	Liver blood nourisher. Coffee substitute.
Urtica dioica (Nettle herb)	*Nourishes everything. Loaded with vitamins, minerals, antioxidants. All-around detox support.
Medicago sativa (Alfalfa herb)	Important nutritive liver herb and food.
Zizyphus jujube Da Zao Jujube berry or date	Sweet, lovely antioxidant. Comes in dark-red and black varieties.
Atractylodes macrocephala Bai Zhu White Atractylodes root	Liver and Spleen tonic. Often needed in Liver Qi Stagnation with indigestion issues.

TABLE 19.2 **Liver Stimulants**
(Also known as decongestants or qi movers for Liver Qi Stagnation)

Herbs	Notes
Taraxacum officinale (Dandelion root) Mild stimulant, cholagogue, diuretic.	Dandelion does it all. Stimulant, restorative, cholagogue, bitter, glutathione enhancer. An essential cross-cultural liver herb. Safe for children and elders.
Curcuma longa (Turmeric root) Mild stimulant.	Bitter, cholagogue, stimulant. For viral and bacterial hepatitis. Glutathione booster.
Cynara scolymus (Artichoke leaf) Mild stimulant.	A little stronger than Dandelion. Cholagogue.
Scutellaria Huang Qin (Baikal skullcap) Mild stimulant.	Cold Liver stimulant that clears heat in infections. Antimicrobial. Antiallergenic.
Carduus benedictus Blessed Thistle herb Mild stimulant.	Good for poor appetite and digestive problems. Cholagogue.
Artemisia absinthium (Wormwood herb) Strong stimulant.	Strong bitter stimulant and cholagogue. Broad-spectrum antimicrobial, useful for acute hepatitis.
Citrus reticulata Chen Pi and Qing Pi Tangerine peel Chen Pi is ripe. Qing Pi is green. Mild stimulant.	Both green and ripe peels stimulate the Liver. Cholagogues. The ripe peels are a major part of many Chinese formulas.
Atractylodes macrocephala Bai Zhu White Atractylodes root. Mild stimulant.	Also, for Spleen Qi Deficiency.
Chionanthus virginicus Fringe Tree bark. Mild stimulant.	Getting stronger but for general use. General all-purpose use. Cholagogue.
Iris versicolor (Blue Flag rhizome) Stronger stimulant.	Not long-term; large doses toxic. Good for swollen glands, skin rashes. Cholagogue.
Podophyllum peltatum (May Apple root) Strongest liver stimulant.	Not for long-term use. Potential for chronic toxicity.
Bupleurum chinense Chi Hu Asian Buplever root Mild stimulant.	One of the most important Chinese Medicine Liver qi movers. Bupleurum has a cool energy, making it very useful for fevers and clearing heat.

and these days they are lumped together under the term *cholagogues*. Cholagogues stimulate peristalsis and thus reduce epigastric fullness, bloating, and constipation and are detoxifying because they carry out wastes through the bile.

Indications for cholagogues include nonimpacted gallstones, moderate gallbladder infection (cholecystitis), jaundice caused by decreased excretion of bile, chronic constipation, and indigestion caused by fatty foods.[8] Contraindications for cholagogues are for obstructed bile ducts from gallstones clogging up the works and for acute colic and spasms caused by the blocked duct. Cholagogues are not used for acute viral hepatitis with jaundice because they are too strong in such cases.[9] Most bitter herbs and liver stimulants are cholagogues by default. Strong cholagogues are Gentian root, Wormwood herb, Barberry root, Wild Indigo root, Blue Flag rhizome, and Goldenseal root. Milder ones include Dandelion root, Garden Sage herb, Fringe Tree bark, and Artichoke leaf.

Stimulating Hepatic Detoxifiers

Herbs that detoxify are stimulating. They help Phase I and Phase II along. Many are cholagogues and some provide the free radical-quenching antioxidant, glutathione. They are often found in foods. Herbalists should tuck these important allies into their detox repertoire and consciousness (Table 19.3). Indications for hepatic detoxifiers are when the liver is overwhelmed by external environmental toxins, heavy metals, and by internal microorganisms and metabolic overload.

TABLE 19.3 Hepatic Detoxification Herbs and Foods
(Cholagogues and glutathione enhancers[6])

Herbs	Liver Foods and Supplements
Silybum marianum (Milk Thistle seed) Big-time liver detoxifier and restorative. Boosts glutathione and quenches free radicals. Silymarin content helps to prevent glutathione depletion. This essential Liver herb stimulates and restores.	**All cruciferous and sulfur-containing vegetables in great quantity**. Liver Phase II detoxifiers. Supply indole-3-carbinol, which helps liver detoxify *bad* estrogen (Chapter 28). Cauliflower, broccoli, Brussels sprouts, bok choy, cabbage, collards, kale, onions, leeks, and raw garlic.
Curcuma longa (Turmeric root) Big-time glutathione producer and antioxidant.	**The primary three veggies containing glutathione:** Asparagus, spinach, and avocados.
Platycodon grandiflorum Jie Geng (Balloonflower root) Reduces oxidative stress; increases glutathione.	**Fresh and frozen fruits** Blackberries, blueberries, strawberries, watermelon. Rich in antioxidants.
Astragalus membranaceus Huang Qi (Astragalus root) Detox/tonic.	**Mushrooms** Shitake, Maitake. Reduces oxidative stress in the liver, restorative.
Vaccinium myrtillus (Bilberry berry)	Red beets and pomegranate seeds are are fabulous liver superfoods. (Fig. 19.6).
Pinus pinaster (Maritime Pine bark extract) Contains the free-radical quencher, pycnogenol.	**Supplements**
Vitis vinifera (Grape seed extract) Antioxidant pycnogenol is the free radical quencher.	Vitamins C and E and the B vitamins: B_6, B_{12}, folic acid, biotin, alpha lipoic acid (ALA).
Cordyceps sinensis Dong Chong Xia Cao (Caterpillar fungus) Lives inside a host insect, the caterpillar of the ghost moth, ultimately killing and consuming it. Expensive.	**Sour citrus** Lemons (sour is Chinese Medicine Liver taste). Drinking freshly squeezed lemon or lime juice in the morning is a stimulating liver wake-up call.
Ginkgo biloba (Ginkgo leaf) Brain antioxidant.	Brazil nuts (selenium source needed for glutathione production) and walnuts.
Bupleurum chinensis Chai Hu Liver protective and muscle relaxant.	Pomegranates, parsnips.
Cynara scolymus (Artichoke leaf) Detox and tonic.	Artichokes. Steamed as a veggie with fresh lemon juice.
Ganoderma lucidum Ling Zhi (Reishi mushroom) Liver detox.	Fresh fish and poultry.
Glycyrrhiza glabra, G. sinensis Gan Cao (Licorice root) Detox and tonic for Liver.	Watercress, which contains sulfur, increases bile flow and digestion.
Urtica dioica (Nettle Herb) Detox and tonic.	Daikon radish, notable liver food.
Lycium barbarum Gou Qi Zi (Wolfberry, Lycii berry, Goji berry)	Sweet, antioxidant-rich Lycii berry can be eaten in salads, oatmeal, or plain as a snack.
Schisandra chinensis Wu Wei Zi (Schisandra berry)	Pasture-raised eggs increase glutathione. Whey protein: Use unheated, undenatured form that is *not* a protein isolate.
Taraxacum officinale (Dandelion root)	Wasabi (Horseradish root or Wasabi root)
Bitters *Momordica charantia* (Bitter Melon) *Mahonia aquifolium* (Oregon Grape root) *Citrus aurantium* Zhi Shi (Bitter Orange peel)	**Clinical pearls** Cooking reduces glutathione. Raw veggies are best, whenever possible.

(*Continued*)

TABLE 19.3 Hepatic Detoxification Herbs and Foods *(Cholagogues and glutathione enhancers[6])*—cont'd

Herbs	Liver Foods and Supplements
Cholagogues	**Clinical pearls**
Mild cholagogues for long-term use. *Taraxacum officinale* (Dandelion root) *Arctium lappa* (Burdock root) *Rumex crispus* (Yellow Dock root) *Peumus boldus* (Boldo leaf)	Dairy, eggs, and meats should be as fresh as possible. Eat organic veggies. Longer shelf-life depletes glutathione. 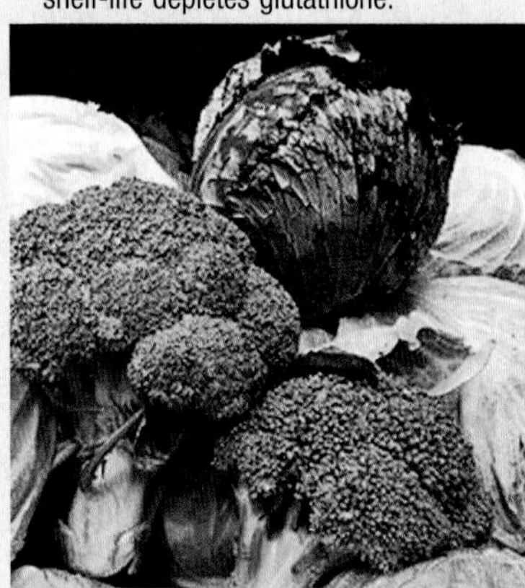 Cruciferous veggies supply glutathione and indole-3 carbinol.
Stronger for short-term use. *Chelidonium majus* (Celandine herb and root) *Raphanus sativus niger* (Black Radish root) *Iris versicolor* (Blue Flag rhizome) *Gentiana luteum* (Gentian root)	
Heavy metal chelators.	**Notes on chelators**
Laminaria spp. (Kelp thallus) *Fucus vesiculosus* (Bladderwrack thallus) *Spirulina* spp. or *Chlorella* spp. (Microalgae) *Allium sativum* (Garlic juice) *Silybum marianum* (Milk Thistle seed) *Coriandrum sativum* (Cilantro herb)	Sea veggies, Kelp, and Bladderwrack are interchangeable. Also use for radiation exposure. Microalgae are nutrient-dense foods that act as chelators. Garlic bulb, Milk Thistle seed, and Cilantro herb are proven heavy-metal detoxifiers.[7]

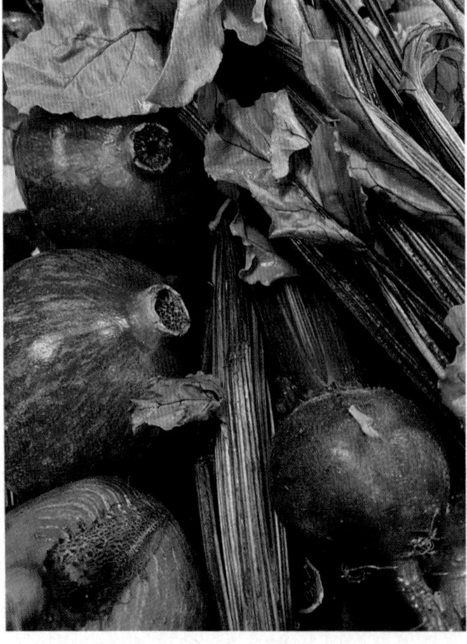

• **Fig. 19.6** Pomegranate seeds and beets contain antioxidants that help reduce oxidative stress. Consider them liver-restorative superfoods.

Hepatic and Gallbladder Antiinfectives and Antilithics

These are the ones for infection, inflammation, and possible fever (Table 19.4). They clear damp heat in the liver and gallbladder. They are sometimes called *sedatives*, because they cool heat and relax, in the sense that they cool a hot infection and stop gallbladder spasms. Some liver antiinfectives/sedatives work very well for generalized infections in other parts of the body, such as Scutellaria Huang Qin (Baikal Skullcap root). Western Liver Damp Heat diagnoses include acute hepatitis, cholecystitis (gallbladder inflammation with possible blockage), liver abscesses, and fatty liver.

Antilithics are used for gallbladder fire with gallstones. They have a moving and dissolving action and help prevent and/or break up stones. Signs of gallstones could be pain, pounding headache all over the head, dark urine, constipation or diarrhea, and possibly jaundice.

Common Hepato-Biliary Conditions

Poor Liver Detoxifier

- *Definition.* Liver overloaded from too many toxins, Cytochrome P-450 detox system upregulated or down-regulated in either phase (Case History 19.1). The liver doesn't build up or store nutrients.

Causes are numerous: malnutrition, anemia, chronic fatigue, chronic hepatitis, adrenal burn-out with constant fatigue, diabetes, hypoglycemia, and heavy metal toxicity. Often related to Liver Qi Stagnation, like endometriosis, fibroids, and heavy menses.

- *Signs and symptoms*. Many and various and could affect any or many body systems: rosacea and other skin outbreaks, feeling worn out, constant fatigue, bloating, brain fog, poor memory, muscle aches, allergies, asthma, gynecological problems, and hormonal imbalances.
- *Allopathic treatment*. Varied. Treats symptoms or diseases but does not address root.
- *General therapeutic principles*. (1) Liver stimulant/detoxifiers: Blue Flag rhizome, Scutellaria Huang Qin (Baikal Skullcap root), Citrus Chen Pi (Ripe Tangerine peel). (2) Glutathione antioxidant herbs: Milk Thistle seed, Turmeric root, and Platycodon Jie Geng (Balloonflower root). (3) Cholagogues to help detox and indigestion: Artichoke leaf, Fringe Tree bark, Blessed Thistle herb. (4) Liver restoratives: Schisandra Wu Wei Zi (Five Taste berry), Bupleurum Chai Hu (Asian Buplever root), Milk Thistle seed. (5) Diuretics to help kidneys unload water-soluble toxins: Dandelion root, Poria Fu Ling (Hoelen fungus), Goldenrod herb, Nettle herb. (6) Alteratives or blood

TABLE 19.4 Antiinfectives, Antilithics, Gallbladder Relaxants *(For infection, damp heat, and gallstones)*

Herbs	Notes
Scutellaria baicalensis Huang Qin Baikal Skullcap	Clears heat, dries damp, and *antimicrobial.* Good hepatitis herb.
Gardenia jasminoides Zhi Zi Gardenia pod	*Antilithic, antibacterial,* liver decongestant, antiinflammatory, dries damp, cholagogue. For nausea, jaundice, acute hepatitis.
Rheum palmatum Da Huang Rhubarb root	*Antilithic,* dries damp, biliary decongestant, cholagogue, cold and dry.
Gentiana lutea Gentian root	*Antimicrobial, antiviral,* cholagogue. Combines well with Boldo. For acute hepatitis.
Artemisia absinthium Wormwood herb, very bitter	Excellent for damp heat, acute hepatitis, parasites, and food poisoning. Diuretic.
Peumus boldus Boldo leaf	Specific antilithic, cholagogue. Combines with Gentian and Rhubarb for digestion.
Bupleurum chinense Chai Hu Asian Buplever root	Clears heat, antimicrobial and antilithic for gallstones.
Berberis vulgaris Barberry root	Specific antilithic, cholagogue, digestive bitter, and antimicrobial.
Coptis chinensis Huang Lian Goldthread root	Antibacterial. For damp heat, hepatitis, and gallstones.
Chionanthus virginicus Fringe Tree bark	*Antilithic,* mild cholagogue, antimicrobial. For acute hepatitis and cholecystitis.
Chelidonium majus Celandine herb	Cholagogue, antilithic. For chronic hepatitis.
Hypericum perforatum St. John's Wort	Antiviral, indicated in viral hepatitis.
Baptisia tinctoria Wild Indigo root	Cholagogue, antimicrobial. For fever, sepsis, and inflammation.
Essential oils of Thuja and Tea Tree	Antimicrobials.

cleansers: Burdock root, Red Clover flower, Chaparral leaf, Yellow dock root, Nettle herb. (7) Heavy-metal chelators, as needed. (8) Help any indigestion with bitters: Oregon Grape root, Gentian root, Yellow Dock root.

Environmental Toxicosis

- *Definition.* Exogenous toxicosis implies pollutants, chemicals, drugs, organisms, hormones, heavy metals, or toxic drinking water overwhelming liver detoxification pathways. Comes from bad air and water; heavy metals; molds; exogenous estrogens and other hormones; fertilizers; chemicals in clothing, dyes, carpets, drapes; plastics; gasoline fumes; paints; fragrances; cosmetics; cleaning supplies, etc. Anything out there that is toxic (Case History 19.2).
- *Signs and symptoms.* Many skin problems like eczema; extreme fatigue; depressed immunity; neurological symptoms, including brain fog and memory loss; gastrointestinal (GI) symptoms of belching and bloating; water retention; and bitter taste in mouth. Diagnosed by blood, urine, nail, or hair analysis. Usually occurs in people with multiple chemical sensitivities and/or compromised Livers.

CASE HISTORY 19.1

Case History for Poor Liver Detoxifier

S. John travels around farm country, selling fertilizer. He eats a lot of burgers, pizza, and fries on the road. He complains of extreme fatigue and fuzzy thoughts, sensitivity to smells, headaches over his eyes, and achy muscles. He has eczema on back of thighs and buttocks. There is bloating and indigestion when he eats fried chicken or donuts.

O. **P** Weak, thready. **T** Greasy, red coat.

A. Liver Yin Deficiency. Toxic Liver. Possible heavy metal overload.

P. *Specific therapeutic principles.* (1) Liver stimulants. (2) Liver restoratives. (3) Boost glutathione with Milk Thistle seed or Platycodon Jie Geng (Balloonflower root). (4) Cholagogues to move bile. (5) Help indigestion with Turmeric root, Meadowsweet herb, Citrus Chen Pi (Ripe Tangerine peel). (6) Heavy metal chelator.

Herbal Formula and Dose. 6 mL 3 × day.

Parts	Herbs	Rationale
4	Milk Thistle seed	Stimulant, restorative. Boosts glutathione, chelates heavy metals.
3	Turmeric root	Cholagogue, bitter for indigestion, enhance glutathione.
2	Dandelion root	Restore, stimulate liver, alterative, diuretic, cholagogue.
1	Nettle herb	Alterative and diuretic.
1	Artichoke leaf	Restore Liver, detox.

Other suggestions

- *Diet.* Liver restorative foods. Increase lemons, artichoke, beets, pomegranates, shitake mushrooms, Lycii berries, cruciferous veggies, and more veggies in general. Decrease/eliminate fatty foods, fast foods, coffee, alcohol. Cut out fatty foods.
- Lemon water on rising to stimulate liver and wake it up.
- Four-R program if indigestion doesn't improve with these measures.
- Skin brushing, sauna.
- Master Liver Cleanse (Box 19.1). Break morning fast with this drink for 1–2 weeks.

- *Chinese Medicine.* Liver Yin Deficiency.
- *Allopathic treatment.* Remove toxins, if possible.
- *General therapeutic principles.* (1) Liver restoratives: Milk Thistle seed, Schisandra Wu Wei Zi. (2) Liver stimulants: Dandelion root, Turmeric root. (3) Chelators: Kelp or Bladderwrack thallus. (4) Glutathione boosters: Milk Thistle seed, Turmeric root, and Platycodon Jie Geng (Balloonflower root). (5) Alteratives to move toxins: Nettle herb, Red Clover flower, Burdock root. (6) Diuretics to increase urine output: Goldenrod herb, Poria Fu Ling.

Acute and Chronic Viral Hepatitis

- *Definition.* Systemic inflammation of the liver where hepatocytes become damaged or die. Leads to anorexia, jaundice, and enlarged liver. Commonly caused by a virus but also by autoimmune conditions, drugs, alcohol, and bacteria. Can lead to liver disease, liver failure, and eventually, cancer. Livers will regenerate, but transplant might be the only option.
- *Kinds of hepatitis.* The three main viruses are hepatitis A, B, and C. A is acute. B and C can go chronic and destroy the liver.
  - *Hepatitis A Virus* (HAV): Acute and short-term, from fecal contamination, spread by consuming food or water contaminated by feces from a person infected with HAV or not washing hands. Very contagious. Curable.
  - *Hepatitis B Virus* (HBV): Contact with infectious body fluids such as blood, vaginal secretions, or semen. From injection drug use or sex with infected partner. Hep B can

• BOX 19.1 Master Liver Cleanse
Moves Liver qi and tastes good, too!

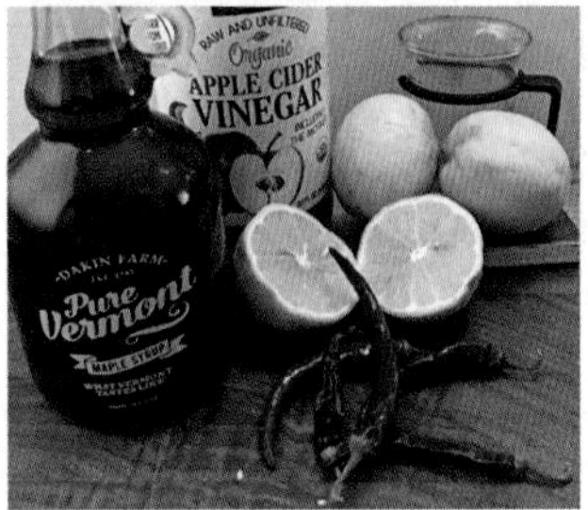

Stimulating liver cleanse ingredients include sour lemon juice, sweet maple syrup, acidic apple cider vinegar and a tiny bit of pungent cayenne pepper.

This cleanse is one of many versions of a traditional liver cleansing drink. It is stimulating and up-regulates the Phase II detoxification pathway. The Liver's season is springtime, and this would be an optimal time to partake, if intention is preventative. Any time will do if there are signs of metabolic overload.

Formula

- 2 tablespoons freshly squeezed lemon; the Liver's taste is sour, and this will stimulate the Liver.
- 1-2 tbsp. of Grade B maple syrup; filled with minerals and complements sourness.
- ⅛ tsp. Cayenne pepper; hot, pungent, stimulating, antiinflammatory.

1½ cups pure water or unsweetened organic apple cider vinegar; apple cider is healing to the gut.

Directions

Break morning fast with this for 1–2 weeks. Make up fresh each time. Keep well hydrated. Accompany with a cleansing veggie-packed diet. Include a restoring and stimulating liver formula taken 3 × day that includes Milk Thistle seed, Dandelion root, and Turmeric root.

CASE HISTORY 19.2

Case History for Environmental Toxicosis

S. Joseph is an auto mechanic. The job includes auto body repair work. His teeth are poor; he has many "silver" dental fillings and has smoked 1 pack per day (ppd) for 30 years. He complains of severe bloating, burping, chronic loose stools, memory loss, absentmindedness, water retention in his hands and feet, a bitter taste in mouth. He gets at least three colds a year. History of extensive Tylenol use, on and off for lower back pain. Now he is off Tylenol and gets massages instead, which help.

O. **P** Weak and deep. **T** Greasy, yellow in middle, red-tinged sides.

A. Dysbiosis, Spleen Qi Deficiency. Toxic Liver, environmental toxicosis.

P. *Specific therapeutic principles.* Auto shops have many toxins, including antifreeze, paints, oils, heavy metals, all types of chemicals. *Stage 1:* Do Four-R Program (Chapter 18) for a 4- to 6-month estimate. (1) Antidiarrheals. (2) Antimicrobials. (3) Gut restoratives. (4) Bitters for digestion/enzymes, bloating. *Stage 2:* Remove toxins with: (1) Hepatic stimulants. (2) Restoratives. (3) Hepatic chelators. (4) Glutathione boosters. (5) Diuretics. (6) Alteratives. (7) Address muscle pain to get him off Tylenol.

Stage One

Herbal Formula and Dose for Leaky Gut, Dysbiosis. 5 mL 3 × day between meals. Take either this bitters formula or apple cider vinegar with meals.

Part	Herbs	Rationale
3	Calamus root	Antidiarrheal, restorative.
2	Coptis Huang Lian	Broad-spectrum antimicrobial, bitter.
2	Atractylodes Bai Zhu	Bitter and restore Spleen/gastrointestinal (GI) tract.
2	Slippery Elm bark	Heal gut.
1	Licorice root	Heal and restore.

Stage Two

Herbal Formula and Dose for Heavy Metal Detox. 5 mL 3 × day.

Parts	Herbs	Rationale
4	Milk Thistle seed	Chelator, restorative, stimulant.
2	Kelp thallus	Hepatic heavy metal chelator.
2	Bupleurum Chai Hu	Liver restore and stimulate, helps muscles relax.
2	Dandelion root	Hepatic stimulate, restore, diuretic.
2	Platycodon Jie Geng	Reduces oxidative stress; adds glutathione.
1	Red Clover flower	Alterative, diuretic.

Other suggestions

Note: This will take a long time—a year or more. A challenge for client and herbalist. Needs planning in stages. Client has to be motivated, engaged, and ideally have a partner willing to encourage and help.

- *Plan.* Begin with Four-R program attending to leaky gut, dysbiosis, and diarrhea. If GI problems were less distressing, herbalist could omit Four-R Program and start with Liver detox. Not possible in this case. Make sure to remove Tylenol, which makes leaky gut worse. Second: When GI protocol complete and symptoms gone (6 months, perhaps), begin hepatic detoxification, using chelators, alteratives, diuretics, and Liver restoratives.
- *Diet.* Hopefully, some nontrigger foods have been reintroduced through the Four-R program. Continue on that diet with emphasis on foods high in glutathione and general Liver favorites: lemons, beets, artichokes, shitake mushrooms, dark greens. Very little or no alcohol.
- *Supplements.* Enteric-coated Garlic to detox. Alpha Lipoic Acid helps reduce lead, cadmium, and copper.
- *Environmental detoxification:* Remove the offending external toxins. Good history helps to deduce. In this case, a change of job would certainly help, if possible.
- *Smoking.* Support to quit. Stress-reduction plan.
- *Amalgams.* May have to get them replaced with composite resin.

go chronic and destroy the liver. Vaccines are available for HAV and HBV, but not C. It is usually mandatory for hospital workers to be immunized for Hep B (spread from contaminated blood). Hepatitis is diagnosed using ultrasound, biopsy, and liver function blood tests.

- *Hepatitis C virus* (HCV). HCV is very common and if untreated, can lead to liver failure and death. It was not identified until 1989. Before that, it was called non-A, non-B. There are now some fairly successful drug combinations used in treatment. Hepatitis C may not cause symptoms or be diagnosed for decades while it is quietly destroying the liver. Chronic hepatitis of any variety is *not* ok.
- Signs and symptoms.
  - *Beginning acute stage of any type.* Fatigue, flulike symptoms, pain between shoulder blades, headache (HA), weight loss, nausea and vomiting, malaise, fever (Case History 19.3).
  - *Clinical jaundice stage.* Later and more chronic. Extreme fatigue, dark urine, pale or clay-colored stool, jaundice, rashes, sharp abdominal pain, halitosis.
  - *Chronic stage:* May be few symptoms. Mainly run down, fatigue, undernourished, digestion issues. Jaundice, light stools and dark urine present in earlier stages tend to disappear. The liver is under chronic attack. (Case History 19.4).
- *Allopathic treatment.* Bed rest for 12 to 16 weeks, antivirals, hydration, high-protein meals, enteric precautions. HCV: antivirals and protease inhibitors that interrupt the viral replication cycle.[10]
- *Chinese Medicine.* Liver Damp Heat. Many syndromes can be involved.
- *St John's Wort.* This is an antiviral herb that is active against *enveloped viruses*, specifically HBV and HCV, but not against HAV, which is not enveloped.[8]
- *General therapeutic principles.* (1) Bitter antivirals for damp heat: Scutellaria Huang Qi (Baikal Skullcap root), Gardenia Zhi Zi (Gardenia pod), and Wormwood herb are all excellent. (2) Diaphoretics to clear heat: Yarrow herb, Elderberry berry. (3) Immune enhancers: Echinacea root or Andrographis Chuan Xin Lian (Heart-Thread Lotus leaf). (4) Liver restoratives: Bupleurum Chai Hu (Asian Buplever root), Milk Thistle seed, Dandelion root. (5) Antiemetics in separate formula, as needed.

Cholecystitis and Gallstones

- *Definition.* ***Cholecystitis*** is gallbladder inflammation with possible infection. There may or may not be gallstones. ***Cholelithiasis*** means formation of gallstones. ***Gallstones*** are hardened bile sediments or calculi in the gallbladder. They can be as small as a grain of sand or as large as a golf ball.[11] Stones are usually made of hardened calcium or hardened bilirubin. If small and sandlike, they are easily passed in the urine. If large, they can block narrow bile ducts that lead to the duodenum and be very

CASE HISTORY 19.3

Case History for Acute Viral Hepatitis

Part I

S. Lila is very ill. She has pain between her shoulder blades, vertex HA headache, temperature 102°F; feels too tired to get out of bed; has yellow-brown urine and yellowish cast to skin. She had recently visited a remote, natural hot springs. She was diagnosed with hepatitis from contaminated water.

O. P Rapid and wiry. **T** Body, red with dark-red dots. Coat, yellow, greasy.

A. Liver Damp Heat. Acute viral hepatitis.

P. *Specific therapeutic principles.* (1) Cold antivirals to clear heat, dry damp. (2) Diaphoretics to bring down fever. (3) Hepatic restoratives. (5) Decrease vertex headache pain.

Herbal Formula and Dose. 4 mL every 1–2 hours.

Parts	Herbs	Rationale
3	Scutellaria Huang Qin	Clear damp heat, antiviral, dry and cold.
3	Passionflower	Pain relief for headache.
2	Wormwood herb	Clear damp heat, antiviral, dry and cold.
2	Schisandra Wu Wei Zi	Liver restorative, immune modulation.
2	*Ligusticum sinense* Gao Ben Chinese Lovage root	Specific for vertex headaches.
1	Dandelion root	Dry damp/diuretic, hepatic restorative.

Other suggestions

- Bed rest, hydration, cool cloths.
- Diet: Light; bone broth, juices, toast, soups.

CASE HISTORY 19.4

Case History for Chronic Viral Hepatitis

Part II

S. Lila feels better. She has been on strong hepatitis herbs for 12 weeks. (Jaundice, fever, headache, and back pain are gone.) Urine is light yellow. She is now pale, run down, exhausted, in bed constantly. She has little appetite, and there is occasional nausea and vomiting. Blood test showed elevated Liver function enzymes.

O. P Weak. **T** Orangey **c**oat (blood deficiency), yellow sides.

A. Liver Qi Deficiency, Blood deficiency, Spleen Qi deficiency. Chronic viral hepatitis. Depressed immunity. Adrenal exhaustion. Liver function enzyme elevation means her Liver cells have become damaged.

P. *Specific therapeutic principles.* Intention is to prevent disease from becoming chronic and to lower Liver function enzymes. Will need long-term hepatic, adrenal, and energy restoratives and support. (1) Antivirals. (2) Heal Liver with restoratives. (3) Support immune system. (4) Increase energy with adrenal support/adaptogens. (5) Build blood. (6) Tonify Spleen as needed. (7) Carminatives for nausea as needed.

Herbal Formula and Dose. 6 mL 3 × day.
This will be long-term, maybe a year or more.

Parts	Herbs	Rationale
3	St. John's Wort	Antiviral.
3	Schisandra Wu Wei Zi	Restore Liver, stimulate, immune, adrenal support, energy.
2	Milk Thistle seed	Hepatic restorative.
2	Nettle herb	Build Blood, energy, nutrition.
2	Astragalus Huang Qi	Liver and immune support.
1	Licorice root	Coat stomach, immune/adrenal support, energy.

Separate Formula for Indigestion. 4 mL 3 × day (t.i.d.).

Part	Herbs	Rationale
3	Codonopsis Dang Shen	Restore Spleen/digestion, immune support.
2	Fennel seed or Peppermint leaf	Nausea and vomiting.
2	Citrus Chen Pi (Ripe Tangerine peel)	Carminative, help digestion.

Other suggestions

- *Diet.* Increase nutrition and energy with more proteins, grass-fed beef, green veggies. Foods to increase glutathione: mushrooms, Lycii berries added to foods. Lemons, beets, artichokes.
- *Green tea.* 1 cup 3 × day. Antioxidant to support/nourish liver.
- *Exercise.* Gentle yoga, walks.
- *Labs.* Repeat liver enzymes in 6 weeks and 6 months later, per healthcare provider.

painful. Often caused by an inflamed and infected gallbladder. Stones may result in duct blockage, pancreatitis, or cancer.

- *Signs and symptoms of cholecystitis.* Severe upper right quadrant (URQ) pain, radiating to between shoulder blades. Nausea and vomiting. Possible infection. This condition is often accompanied by gallstones, or a precursor to stones (Case History 19.5).
- *Signs and symptoms of gallstones.* None, if stones are tiny. If large, there is intense pain and gallbladder spasms. Severe pain in the URQ of the abdomen radiates between the shoulder blades. There is nausea, vomiting, indigestion, dizziness, jaundice, fever with chills, and itching. Attacks often follow fatty meals when bile is released and tries to get through a blocked bile duct but can't. Diagnosed by ultrasound or CAT scan. Cholecystitis may be present (Case History 19.6).
- *Allopathic treatment.* Surgery to remove gallbladder (*cholecystectomy*), and a low-fat diet for life. In 2011, cholecystectomy was the eighth most common surgery performed in the United States.[12] Surgery is usually done for cholecystitis and gallstones.
- *Digestion after gallbladder removal.* The liver constantly produces bile and releases it into the gallbladder holding tank. It then releases bile into the duodenum, as needed, after a fatty meal. If a gallbladder is removed, bile enters the duodenum continuously, needed or not, which may or may not create digestive problems. It's individual.
- *Chinese Medicine.* Gallbladder Damp Heat.
- *General therapeutic principles.* Cholecystitis and gallstones have similar treatment. (1) Use antilithics to dissolve and/or move stones, if present, and/or preventatively. (2) Antimicrobials with or without infection help immune support. (3) Antispasmodics to relieve spasms and pain. (4) Liver restoratives. (5) Relaxing nervines for stress and pain. (6) Cooling antiinflammatories to help pass stones, as needed. (7) Antipyretics and emetics, as needed. (Do not use strong cholagogues or bitters because they increase strength of peristaltic contractions and can make pain and spasms worse.)

CASE HISTORY 19.5

Case History for Cholecystitis

S. Jack is 43 and has severe upper right quadrant pain radiating to back between scapula, nausea, vomiting, stress, and no fever. Went to the hospital emergency room, and ultrasound showed no gallstones, but they wanted to remove his gallbladder. He eats a lot of fast food. He is anxious because he is missing work; does not want surgery.

O. **P** Tight, wiry. **T** Dusky.

A. Gallbladder inflammation and pain. Cholecystitis. Gallbladder Damp Heat.

P. *Specific therapeutic principles.* (1) Cold, drying antimicrobials. (2) Antilithics for stone prevention. (3) Hepatic restoratives. (4) Antispasmodics. (5) Antiemetics. (6) Relaxing nervines.

Herbal Formula and Dose. 5 mL 3 × day.

Part	Herbs	Rationale
3	Valerian root	Spasmolytic and relaxing nervine.
3	Scutellaria Huang Qin	Antimicrobial for damp heat.
2	Milk Thistle seed	Hepatic restorative.
2	Artichoke leaves	Antilithic, hepatic restorative.
1	Bupleurum Chai Hu	Hepatic restorative, detox, antispasmodic.
1	Ginger root	Gastrointestinal tonic, antiemetic.

CASE HISTORY 19.6

Case History for Gallstones

S. Betty had recurrent nausea, vomiting, and upper right quadrant abdominal pain, especially after a fatty meal; temp 99.5°F. An ultrasound showed small gallstones. She was given option to "wait and see" or have surgery. She opted for herbs. She was quite stressed.

O. **P** Wiry. **T** Dusky purple, thin white coat.

A. Gallbladder Damp Heat. Cholelithiasis or gallstones per ultrasound.

P. *Specific therapeutic principles.* (1) Antilithics to move and dissolve stones. (2) Cool, dry antimicrobial to clear heat, dry damp. (3) Antispasmodic for pain. (4) Antiemetic. (5) Calming nervine. (6) Soothing antiinflammatories to help stones pass.

Herbal Formula and Dose. 5 mL 3 × day.

Parts	Herbs	Rationale
2	Dandelion root	Antilithic, cooling, mild diuretic to dry damp.
2	Chamomile flower	Stop spasms, nausea, calming, antiinflammatory.
2	Fringe Tree bark	Antilithic, antimicrobial, for damp heat.
2	Artichoke leaf	Antilithic, liver restorative.
2	Bupleurum Chai Hu	Stop spasms and pain, protect liver.
2	Cornsilk or Couch grass root	Cooling, soothing antiinflammatory.
1	Ginger root	Stop nausea, vomiting.

Other suggestions (for both cholecystitis and gallstones)

- Lemon water before breakfast.
- Peppermint and Chamomile tea as needed for nausea, vomiting, and stress. Peppermint and Chamomile essential oils over abdomen if can't tolerate tea.
- Low-fat diet for now.

Cirrhosis and Alcoholic Liver Cirrhosis

- Definitions.
  - ***Cirrhosis*** is the widespread death of liver cells that perform no function. There is inflammation and fibrous thickening of tissue. It is most often a result of chronic alcohol abuse. Chronic HBV and HBC are other common causes.[9]

CASE HISTORY 19.7

Case History for Alcoholism-Induced Cirrhosis

S. Al has been a heavy drinker for 20 years. He has at least 8 to 16 oz of hard liquor a day. His face is red and puffy, nose is red; he is malnourished, is losing weight, has no interest in sex. He is impatient and irritable most of the time. He is trying to turn his life around. Has been through a detox program and joined AA.

O. **P** Full and rapid. **T** Red body, yellow coat. Red face, bloodshot nose.

A. Liver Yang Rising. Alcoholism with probable liver damage.

P. *Specific therapeutic principles.* (1) Liver restoratives. (2) Hepatic detoxifier. (3) Cool, draining diuretic. (4) Adrenal restorative. (5) Stress relief with relaxing nervine.

Herbal Formula and Dose

No alcoholic tinctures allowed.

Formula will have to be in a glycerite or capsules.

8 mL glycerite 3 × day between meals or 3 caps 3 × day.

Part	Herbs	Rationale
4	Milk Thistle seed	Restore liver cells, detoxifier.
3	Celery seed	Detoxicant, alterative, draining diuretic, adrenal restorative.
2	Schisandra Wu Wei Zi	Liver, adrenal, and nervous restorative, adaptogen.
2	Dandelion root	Hepatic stimulant, detox, restorative.
2	Passionflower herb	Nervous relaxant.

Other suggestions

- *Stop drinking alcohol.* The obvious first. Encourage AA attendance, counseling, support groups, detox centers, as needed. No herbs, mouthwashes, or cough syrups containing alcohol.
- *Nutrition.* Very important. Healthy diet with veggies, moderate organic protein and meat. Glutathione-rich foods. All simple sugars must go. Do this first and then begin the Four-R program. It would be hard to find an alcoholic who had a healthy gastrointestinal flora.
- *Supplements and rationales.* This list is long because malnourishment is a fact, and hepatic detoxification assistance is essential.
  - People with alcoholism are classically zinc deficient, and zinc is needed for detoxification. Vitamin A works with zinc.
  - B vitamins that help the nervous system are always low.
  - Carnitine, an amino acid compound, is recommended for fatty Liver because it is *lipotropic* (breaks down fat).
  - Vitamin C helps detox.
  - Alcoholism increases magnesium loss through the kidneys, so magnesium is needed.
  - Selenium and vitamin E regulate glutathione levels, which are low in people with alcoholism.
- *Supplement list.* Daytime with meals. Vitamin B complex 20 × the recommended daily allowance (RDA); vitamin A 25,000 IU a day; vitamin C 1 g 2 × day; Vitamin E 400 IU a day; L-carnitine 500 mg 2 × day; probiotics 1 tsp a day. Minerals do best when the body's at rest. At night: Magnesium 200 mg (to bowel tolerance because it can be a laxative) and zinc 30 mg. Slowly reduce supplements after client is off alcohol to 25% of these doses.[13]

Cirrhosis is the final outcome of a damaged liver from any cause, which can lead to liver failure and death.

- *Alcoholism* is the dependence on alcohol or repeated excessive use of alcoholic beverages resulting in withdrawal symptoms on reducing or ceasing intake. May have a genetic basis. The rate alcohol is metabolized by the liver varies. People with active alcoholism have fatty infiltration of the liver and eventually develop cirrhosis. Alcohol induces hypoglycemia, and the lowering of blood sugar triggers food cravings for sugar and alcohol, foods that quickly elevate blood sugar. People with alcoholism tend not to eat and substitute empty alcohol calories for real food. Malnourishment occurs.
- *Signs and symptoms of cirrhosis.* Usually none until it gets far along. First, there is weakness, anorexia, weight loss, malaise, and loss of libido. Later, multiple symptoms occur, including jaundice, fever, infection, bleeding from nose, gums, tarry stools, hair loss, and more (Case History 19.7). None of these are surprising, when you consider the many functions of the liver.
- *Allopathic treatment.* Liver transplant, medications.
- *Chinese Medicine.* Liver Yang Rising.
- *General therapeutic principles.* Herbalists will have better luck treating in very early stages. (1) Foremost, restoratives to improve liver function and heal cells. (2) Hepatic stimulants for detox. (2) Cooling alteratives to clear blood of toxins. (3) Increase elimination with lymphatics and diuretics. (4) Bitters for digestion and detox. (5) Relaxing nervines for stress and withdrawal. (8) Adrenal support.

Summary

A few of the liver's many functions include detoxification, the ability to transform one substance into another based on need, glucose regulation, bile and cholesterol production, regulation of digestion and blood clotting. The gut-liver axis refers to the relationship between the two organs. Many problems can occur if they are not working harmoniously. A leaky gut can lead to liver failure by overtaxing its detoxification pathways.

Detoxification involves the role of the cytochrome P450 enzyme pathways. This process can be helped through the use of cholagogues and hepatic stimulants, like Yellow Dock or Dandelion root, and the glutathione boosters Milk Thistle seed and Turmeric root. Metabolic overload is often related to environmental challenges, such as heavy metal toxicity. Remedies include herbal chelators, such as seaweeds, Milk Thistle seed, and Garlic.

In Chinese Medicine, the yin Liver deals with anger, opens to the eyes, and likes the sour taste, whereas the yang Gallbladder deals with decision or indecision. Liver Qi Stagnation has a role in toxic overload, Liver Yang Rising is connected to alcoholism, and Gallbladder Damp Heat is implicated in gallstones and cholecystitis.

Hepatic-biliary Materia Medica categories include restoratives that heal hepatocytes, stimulants that help detoxification, and sedative herbs that include antimicrobials and antilithics. When it comes to the liver, most herbalists will use detox measures the most. Gut dysbiosis and liver toxicity are the most pervasive causes of the chronic disease epidemic in our society. They are areas where allopathic medicine fails miserably.

Review

Fill in the Blanks

(Answers in Appendix B.)

1. Name five liver restoratives. Give botanical and common names. ___, ___, ___, ___, ___.
2. Six signs of toxic overload are ___, ___, ___, ___, ___, ___.
3. Name six substances or situations that can overload the liver: ___, ___, ___, ___, ___, ___.
4. Four heavy metals most detrimental to health are ___, ___, ___, ___.
5. Name four symptoms of environmental toxicity: ___, ___, ___, ___.
6. Name three mild cholagogues: ___, ___, ___ and three strong cholagogues: ___, ___, ___.
7. Name three Chinese Liver sedatives/antiinfectives: ___, ___, ___. Name three Western Liver sedatives/anti-infectives: __, ___, ___.
8. Gallstones are what syndrome? ___. Pulse is ___ and Tongue is ___.
9. Name four good antilithic herbs: ___, ___, ___, ___.
10. The main liver antioxidant is ___. Three foods that have it are ___, ___, ___. Three herbs that have it are ___, ___, ___.

Critical Concept Questions

(Answers for you to decide.)

1. How can you tell if someone has a liver in metabolic overload?
2. How does the liver regulate glucose metabolism?
3. Explain Phase I and Phase II liver detoxification pathways.
4. What is the relationship between gut and liver health? Discuss concept of root causes.
5. How do you decide whether to address the gut or liver first?
6. In Chinese Medicine, what does the Liver have to do with the eyes, headaches, seizures, and PMS?
7. Discuss the danger of chronic hepatitis, even if there are no symptoms.
8. Are gallstones always dangerous? Do they require surgery?
9. How would you decide whom to treat for heavy metal toxicity without any testing?
10. What is chelation? When would this be indicated? Are there any herbs that might work?

References

1. Andrews, Ryan. "All About Cholesterol: Understanding nutrition's most controversial molecule." Precision Nutrition. https://www.precisionnutrition.com/all-about-cholesterol (accessed January 30, 2021).
2 Kirpich, Irina, et al. "Gut-liver Axis, Nutrition, and Non-Alcoholic Fatty Liver Disease." PubMed. U.S. National Library of Medicine,

National Institutes of Health. https://www.ncbi.nlm.nih.gov/pubmed/26151226 (accessed November 8, 2019).
3. Sjoberg, Valerie. "Five Environmental Toxins and How to Reduce Your Exposure." Chopra Center. https://chopra.com/articles/5-environmental-toxins-and-how-to-reduce-your-exposure (accessed July 20, 2019).
4. Tierra, Lesley. "Citrus: Fruit or Peel?" Michael and Lesley Tierra's East West School of Planetary Herbology. https://planetherbs.com/blogs/lesleys-blog/citrus-fruit-or-peel/ (accessed July 20, 2019).
5. Holmes, Peter. *Jade Remedies: A Chinese Herbal Reference for the West* (Boulder, CO: Snow Lotus, 1996).
6. Berkheiser, Kaitlyn. "Ten Natural Ways to Increase Your Glutathione Levels." Healthline. https://www.healthline.com/nutrition/how-to-increase-glutathione (accessed July 20, 2019).
7. Bone, Kerry, and Michelle Morgan. "Herbs and Heavy Metal Detoxification." Medi-Herb. http://www.promedics.ca/site/downloads/Herbs%20and%20Heavy%20Metal%20Detox.pdf (accessed July 20, 2019).
8. Bone, Kerry and Simon Mills. *Principles and Practice of Phytotherapy* (London, UK: Elsevier, 2013).
9. Hoffman, David. *Medical Herbalism: The Science and Practice of Herbal Medicine* (Rochester, VT: Healing Arts, 2003).
10. Leuw, Philipp and Stephan Christoph. "Protease Inhibitors for the Treatment of Hepatitis C Virus Infection." U.S. National Library of Medicine, National Institutes of Health. https://www.ncbi.nlm.nih.gov/pmc/articles/PMC6301719/ (accessed July 20, 2019).
11. "Gallstones." Mayo Clinic. https://www.mayoclinic.org/diseases-conditions/gallstones/symptoms-causes/syc-20354214 (accessed July 20, 2019).
12. "Cholecystectomy." Wikipedia. https://en.wikipedia.org/wiki/Cholecystectomy (accessed July 20, 2019).
13. Murray, Michael and Pizzorno Joseph. *Encyclopedia of Natural Medicine* (Rocklin, CA: Prima, 1991).

20
The Respiratory System

"A cough is a symptom, not a disease. Take it to your doctor and he can give you something serious to worry about."

—Robert Morley, English actor

CHAPTER REVIEW

- Methods to keep breathing up to par.
- The fifth chakra, speaking your truth.
- Chinese Medicine perspective: The Lungs and major syndromes.
- Respiratory Materia Medica: Respiratory herbs worth honorable mention. Restoratives/tonics, expectorants (stimulating and relaxing), antimicrobials, diaphoretics, lymphatic drainers, antihistamines, and liver decongestants.
- About coughs.
- About permanent prevention of seasonal allergies.
- Common respiratory conditions with case histories: Laryngitis, sore throat, common cold, influenza, acute and chronic sinusitis, acute and chronic bronchitis, acute hay fever, bronchial asthma and acute asthma attack.

KEY TERMS

Anaphylactic shock
Antiasthmatics
Antihistamines
Antitussives
Arterial stimulants
Asthma
Bronchitis
Bronchodilators
Catarrh
Common cold
Cough
Demulcents
Diaphoretics
Expectorants
Hay fever
Histamine
Influenza
Larynx
Lymphatic drainers
Mucogenics
Pharynx
Sinusitis
Vasodilating
Wind, External wind, Internal Wind

Many thanks to the respiratory system for the breath of life. Unfortunately, common respiratory illnesses plague us like no other. Of all the remedies I personally formulate, these have top billing and are in highest demand. Herbs excel in treating numerous airway conditions, and effective combinations have been perfected over time in every culture. With judicious use, herbalists can have many successes and gain converts to botanical medicine in the process of eradicating a nasty cold.

Maintaining healthy lungs is paramount and reflects the health of our immunity. Respiratory Materia Medica categories are numerous, as are Chinese Medicine respiratory syndromes. Some of the more serious conditions are not covered here, such as chronic obstructive pulmonary disease (COPD) or tuberculosis (TB). In such cases, if they aren't hard-core herbal advocates, clients are probably at the hospital or seeking out a Western healthcare provider. The herbalist's role at that point, is to provide supportive treatment. If a respiratory problem doesn't resolve in a reasonable time, refer out for further assistance.

Methods to Keep Breathing Up to Par

We breathe in and out about 23,000 times a day and unless there is trouble rarely give it a thought. There are many obvious and not so evident measures to keep it that way. Genetics, smoking, and pollutants all play a part in hindering optimal breathing.

- *Hydration.* Drink plenty of water. This helps keep lung mucus and secretions liquefied and prevents sticky, gunky secretions clogging up the airway.

- *No smoking.* Once this addictive habit is established, it is hard to kick because of the nicotine. Nicotine is a brain-stimulating alkaloid found in Tobacco leaves of the nightshade family. Cigarettes are full of tar and chemicals that irritate, burn, and damage lung tissue, which can lead to COPD and cancer. Nicotine makes people feel good, stimulates the brain, and even relaxes the smoker in some cases. Nicotine, along with the effects of the smoke and burning, is bad news for the lungs.
  - *Vapes.* These are battery-operated electronic cigarettes or similar devices that heat up and vaporize a liquid or solid substance, which is then inhaled. Some vapes contain nicotine; others don't. Vape juices are available that contain only propylene glycol/vegetable glycerin and flavorings, so vaping without nicotine is definitely possible but not the norm. Candy-flavored vapes and others are extremely high in nicotine, their use is especially prevalent in the teenage culture. Vaping is not a harmless replacement for regular cigarettes, nor a substitute method to quit smoking. Their addictive nicotine content is extremely high.[1]
    - The danger of vaping is an evolving issue, with teenagers and young adults dying from respiratory failure caused by the presence of toxins and synthetic vitamin E (DL alpha tocopheryl acetate) used as an additive in the vape cartridges. This synthetic fat-soluble vitamin E has been found in patients' lung fluid, causing lung disease and death.[2] Natural vitamin E comes in eight chemical forms, but D-alpha tocopherol (present in nuts, whole grains, and green leafy veggies) is the only form that is recognized to meet human requirements.[3] It is a potent and healthy biological antioxidant when put on the skin and/or ingested into the gastrointestinal (GI) tract in therapeutic doses.)
    - *Herbal allies for quitting.* Nervous relaxants such as Lobelia herb, Passionflower herb, and Valerian root help reduce the stress associated with nicotine withdrawal. Add nervous system restoratives to the formula, such as Milky Oats and St. John's Wort; herbs to soothe and restore the respiratory tract, such as Licorice root and Mullein leaf; and Rhodiola root to help with anxiety, depression, and withdrawal symptoms.
    - *Non-nicotine smoke.* Sometimes an herbal substitute can help for a short time. A nice blend could include Mullein leaf, *Arctostaphylos uva-ursi* (Bearberry leaf, Kinnikinnick), Skullcap herb, and Coltsfoot leaf.[4]
- *Conscious breathing.* Polynesian *mana*, Hindu *prana*, and Chinese *qi* all refer to life energy. Yoga, pranayama (breath control), and meditation are all good techniques to fill the lungs to capacity, meaning all the way up to the top of the upper lobes at clavicle level. Normal breathing tends to be shallow. Teach clients diaphragmatic breathing, which involves inhaling from the belly up and exhaling from the top down. Benefits of breath work include stress reduction, less anxiety, better focus, better-quality sleep, lung health, and increased tolerance for exercise. Breathing with awareness is a cost-free consciousness-raising endeavor.
- *Green plants.* In addition to being beautiful and adding to the Feng Shui of any room, our green allies take in carbon dioxide and give off oxygen through photosynthesis. They absorb toxic air gases through their leaves and roots. (Rain forest destruction contributes to air pollution, smog, greenhouse gases, and less atmospheric oxygen.)
  - The best house plants for oxygenating and detoxifying the home environment include *Chrysanthemum morifolium* (Garden Mum), *Chlorophytum comosum* (Spider plants), *Dracaena* spp. (Dracaena), *Ficus benjamina* (Ficus), *Nephrolepis exaltata* (Boston Fern), *Sansevieria trifasciata* (Mother in Law's Tongue), *Aloe vera* (Aloe leaf), and *Crassula ovata* (Jade or Money plant).[5]
- *Aerobic exercise and fast walking.* Aerobic exercise that increases heart rate improves lung capacity and cardiac health. More oxygen increases capacity for more efficient muscle contraction. Benefits include healthier lungs, lower heart rate, and blood pressure.
- *Hot peppers.* Chili peppers, including Serrano, Jalapeño, and Poblano, all contain capsaicin. In addition to having a burning quality, they clear out clogged sinuses and airways. Hot chili makes your nose run and eyes water. This helps eliminate viruses, bacteria, cellular debris, and provides a hit of vitamin C.

The Fifth Chakra, Speaking Your Truth

The fifth chakra is located at the throat, and its energy connection to the physical body encompasses the throat, thyroid, parathyroid, trachea, esophagus, hypothalamus, neck vertebrae, mouth, jaw, and teeth—hence its inclusion in this respiration chapter that involves the throat (Fig. 20.1). Any physical illnesses and issues regarding these structures are under the auspices of the fifth chakra and most likely come from some form of speaking our truth and making decisions.

On an esoteric level, the fifth chakra involves the power (and illusion) of free will, finding your voice, having the courage to speak up and to act on it, regardless of consequences. It involves the power of choice, having authority with ourselves and not being out of control when it comes to another's power over us. It is the freedom to make our own life decisions about relationship, career choices, and money and includes realizing the consequences of these choices on our spiritual karma. This is a huge responsibility because if this is done with consciousness, by using our spiritual guidance we cannot blame anyone else for the results. It involves

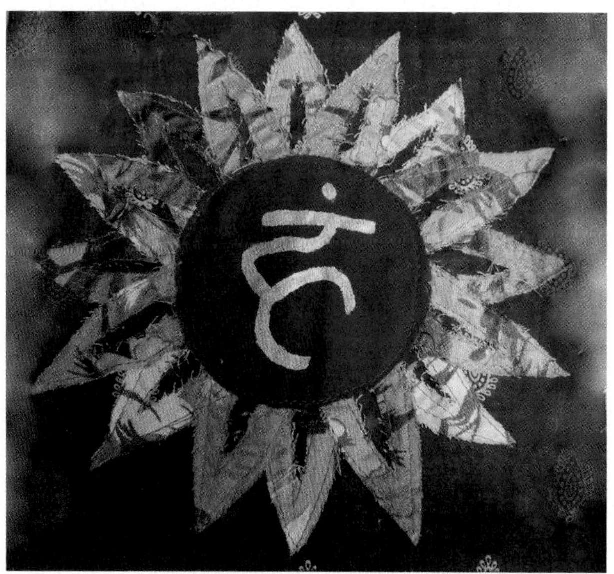

• **Fig. 20.1** The fifth chakra showing its Sanskrit symbol is also called the throat chakra. It corresponds to the physical structures in the neck, and is the seat of communication, growth, and speaking our truth.

faith and the courage to put our trust in Divine authority, and to commit to a decision.[6]

The pitfall of acting on our will is the danger of acting out of fear. If a decision is made only from fear, desire, or what we think we want, there may be unforeseen and unwanted consequences. The lesson is to give up needing to know why things happen as they do and trust that the unscheduled events of our lives are a form of spiritual direction.

Chinese Medicine Perspective: The Lungs and Major Syndromes

When assessing and formulating, it is useful to incorporate some common Chinese respiratory syndromes into the mix along with their accompanying pulse and tongue signs. If the Lungs are too dry, there's a deficiency of moist yin. If the Lungs are weak, there's not enough energy or qi. Lung phlegm, or catarrh, can be too hot and dry or too damp and moist.

A key respiratory concept involves the idea of ***wind*** (feng) and movement. ***External wind*** implies pathogens blowing in from the outside environment, *exterior* to the body. A superficial pulse accompanies this to show that the qi is on the surface, fighting the pathogen. If wind goes in deeply enough, it can affect and infect internal organs. It is best to stop external wind before that happens. (*Note*: ***Internal wind*** is different. It originates inside the body from the Liver and manifests as involuntary movements like tremors, dizziness, or spasms. It is associated with neurology in the West; in Chinese Medicine, there is no nervous system.)

Chinese Medicine Major Respiratory Syndromes[7]

- *External Wind Cold.* This is usually the early-onset stage of a respiratory infection. The symptoms can be subtle, such as a little extra clear or white phlegm in the morning and/or a slight stiffness in the neck. A person may have been chilled the previous day, sneezed several times in a row, or had very cold feet. **Pulse (P)** Superficial. **Tongue (T)** Normal body, thin white coat.
- *External Wind Heat.* If the wind cold isn't treated, it may develop into heat. This can occur as quickly as 2 hours after initial onset of wind cold or perhaps 2 days later. A person becomes warm, flushed or feverish, or has a sore throat. The sputum is yellow or greenish. **P** Superficial. **T** Body is red; coat is thin, white or yellow.
- *External Wind Damp Heat.* If there is copious mucus along with infection, it is now damp and hot. Sputum is sticky and hard to expectorate, and chest feels full. **P** Superficial. **T** Body is red; coat is sticky and yellow.
- *Lung Qi Deficiency.* Lung qi is too weak with no energy. There is shortness of breath (SOB); a weak, feeble cough; spontaneous sweating; hesitant, low voice; even depression. **P** Weak, especially in Lung position—client's right hand, under herbalist's right index finger. **T** Body is pale and scalloped; coat is thin.
- *Lung Yin Deficiency.* Lungs are too dry (not enough yin). There is an irritating cough, dry sticky sputum, dehydration, and dry stools. **P** Thin. **T** Body is red; coat is thin and dry.
- *Lung Phlegm Heat.* This applies to prodigious colored, sticky phlegm and goes along with Wind Heat. There is a cough with yellow/green sputum. **P** Rapid, slippery. **T** Body is red and swollen; coat is thick and sticky.
- *Lung Phlegm Damp.* This one applies to lots of white phlegm that goes along with Wind Cold. Therefore the sputum is copious and white and accompanies a chronic cough. **P** Slippery or weak. **T** Coat is thick and sticky or wet and white.

Respiratory Materia Medica

Many herbs, as usual, overlap and conveniently fit into more than one category. This is useful for efficient formulation. Licorice root is demulcent and cooling, and it is an immune modulator and anti-infective. Mullein leaf restores, moistens, and cools a sore throat. Thyme herb reduces infection, dries up mucus, and serves as an antispasmodic for asthma and coughs.

Respiratory Herbs Worth Honorable Mention

- *Ligusticum porteri* (Osha root). Colorado cough root, bear medicine. Osha merits top billing in the respiratory department. It is one of my all-time favorite Rocky Mountain plants; its noble masculine energy sends down deep stubborn roots among the aspens. It is a warm, pungent, and aromatic member of the Celery family and needs proper identification so as not to be confused with its poisonous cousins, the Hemlocks. Osha is a go-to expectorant for coughs and wheezing, and it is a good warming antimicrobial and diaphoretic pick for early-onset colds and flu, External Wind Cold that hasn't yet changed to heat. Not for pregnancy; a uterine stimulant.
- *Grindelia robusta* (Gumweed flower) (Fig. 20.2). The milky buds of this roadside attraction develop into a yellow,

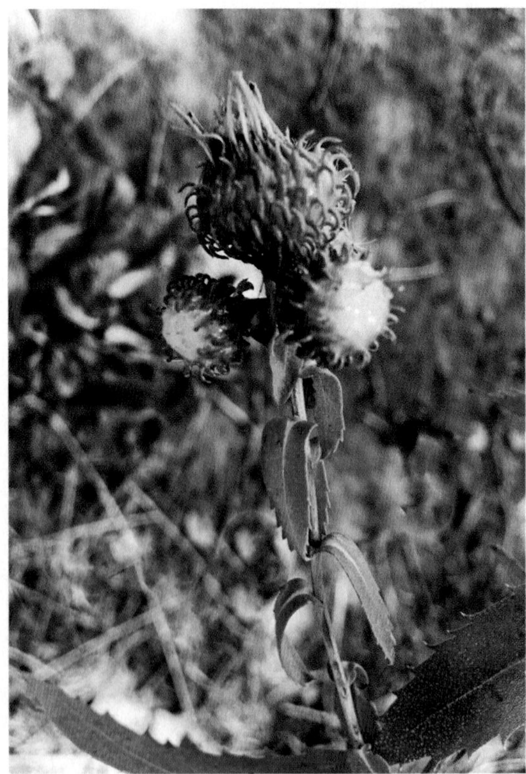

• **Fig. 20.2** *Grindelia robusta* (Gumweed flower) showing yellow petals folded up and drying inside its large, unique calyx. Below this are two milky buds in the perfect stage for collection. Tincture them fresh, for a pungent, cooling expectorant remedy.

TABLE 20.1 A Few Good Respiratory Restoratives (Tonics) and Demulcents ***(Tonifies yin and qi and moistens and cools the Lungs)***

Herb	Comment
Verbascum thapsus Mullein leaf	All-purpose restorative that tonifies yin. For phlegm damp, heat, full cough, allergies, bronchitis, wheezing.
Althaea officinalis Marshmallow root	Moistens lungs, tonifies yin, cools coughs. For bronchitis. Also, a gastric demulcent.
Ulmus fulva Slippery Elm bark	Nutritive and soothing. For cough, lung, and gastric dryness, and Lung Yin Deficiency.
Cetraria islandica Iceland Moss thallus (lichen)	Bitter, salty, cold, and moist. Tonifies yin. For thirst, dry mouth, tickle cough, chronic lung and gastric dryness and weakness.
Chondrus crispus Irish Moss thallus (seaweed)	Sweet and moist. For cough, Lung Yin Deficiency, but not for gastric deficiency, because it's sweet.
Asparagus officinalis Asparagus root	Mucolytic expectorant, tonifies yin, drains lymph, and detoxifies. For fluid deficiency.
Stellaria media Chickweed herb	Sweet, salty, cool, moist. Tonifies Lung yin and all fluid deficiencies. Also, for stomach dryness, and hot flashes.
Symphytum officinale Comfrey leaf and root	Sweet, astringent, cooling, moist. For dry coughs, scratchy throat, laryngitis. Also, for stomach and large intestine dryness.
Glycyrrhiza spp., *G. glabra* and *G. uralensis* Gan Cao Licorice root	Very sweet, neutral, moist, all yin tonics. For dry cough and nose, tickle throat, wheezing, and viscous sputum.
Ophiopogon japonicas Mai Men Dong Dwarf Lilyturf root Chinese Medicine classic	Cool, moist, restoring, mucolytic expectorant, bronchial demulcent, antitussive. For dry chronic cough, Lung phlegm dry and yin deficiency.
Polygonatum spp. Huang Jing Solomon's Seal root	Cool, moist, restores Lung Yin and Lung Qi Deficiency. Mucogenic. Lung restorative.
Codonopsis pilosula Dang Shen Downy Bellflower root	Sweet, moist, neutral, restoring qi tonic. For Lung Qi Deficiency and Spleen Qi Deficiency.
Astragalus membranaceus Huang Qi Astragalus root	Sweet, a bit warm and dry. The qi/energy tonic. For Lungs, Spleen, Liver, adrenals. Adaptogen.
Panax quinquefolius Xi Yang Shen American ginseng root	A bit sweet and bitter, cool and moist, adaptogen. For Lung and Spleen Qi Deficiency.

daisylike flower. The white, gummy mass, which is hard to wash off, is the therapeutic part. Gumweed usage is easy and straightforward. It's a loosening expectorant for sticky gunky phlegm that won't come up. (It kind of looks like it, an example of the Doctrine of Signatures philosophy.) It is pungent, cool, and moist, and it will liquefy secretions admirably to help a stubborn, dry cough.

- *Sambucus nigra* (Black Elderberry). These cool, drying, and sweet/sour, dark-blue berries are classic for colds and flu with fever, External Wind Heat. Give it to kids and adults in elixirs, syrups, and tincture. Works for sinusitis, rhinitis, and laryngitis. Also resolves toxic heat in local infections with pus. A go-to for fevers because of its vasodilatory and diaphoretic actions. It's mucostatic and diuretic. Red Elderberry, a different species, is considered somewhat toxic.
- *Ophiopogon japonicas* Mai Men Dong (Dwarf Lilyturf root). A cool, moist, and restoring Chinese classic for dry, chronic, and hacky unproductive coughs and spasms. Think of Mai Men Dong as a mucolytic expectorant that moisturizes and relieves dry coughs, much like Grindelia.
- *Pinellia ternata* Ban Xi (Prepared Pinellia corm). This Chinese herb is both restorative and antitussive and a no-brainer for

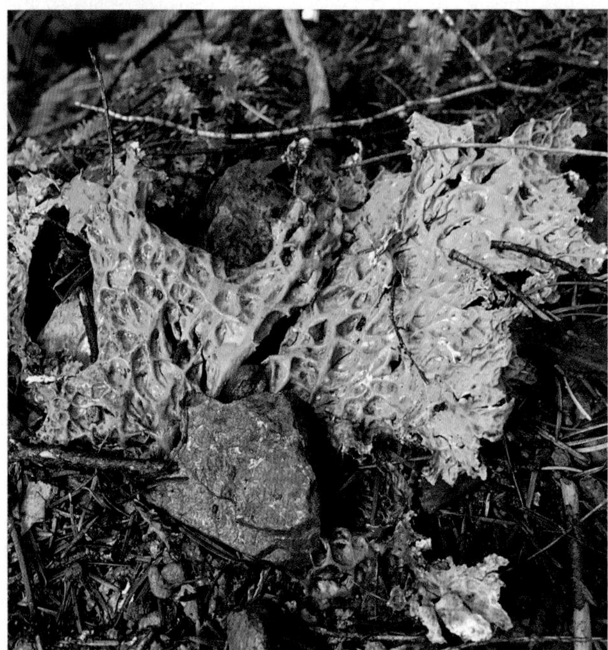

• **Fig. 20.3** *Sticta pulmonaria* (Lungwort thallus) is a moist, relaxing expectorant that soothes persistent, dry, wheezing coughs.

sputum and mucus, regardless of type. It appears in many a patent cough syrup. For warm, dry, or damp phlegm. A respiratory stimulant, expectorant, and antitussive for acute or chronic bronchitis, it is also an immune regulator, antiallergic, and antiemetic. It seems to do it all. Make sure to use the prepared (fermented) form, as its raw form is somewhat toxic.

Respiratory Restoratives/Tonics in Chinese Medicine and the West

There are two types of Lung tonics/restoratives in Chinese Medicine. One type is moist and cooling (demulcent) and tonifies the yin by addressing Lung Yin deficiency. The other type is more warming (adaptogen) and addresses Lung Qi deficiency, a lack of lung energy. Use either or both types, depending on condition (Table 20.1). Because lungs like to be cool and moist, respiratory restoratives do their jobs by tonifying yin (increasing moisture and coolness). If lungs become too hot and dry, there is inflammation and irritation with dehydration, thirst, dry tongue and throat, nonproductive irritating cough, and dry sticky sputum. There may be hard, waterless stools, fatigue, and possibly fever. These all point to the syndrome Lung Yin Deficiency, described earlier.[8]

- *Lung Yin Deficiency tonics.* Herbs that tonify Lung yin are sweet, cool, and moist. They do this locally on the respiratory tissue and systemically throughout the body. They tend to be ***demulcents*** (herbs that cool and moisten) and ***mucogenics*** (herbs that break up mucus). Chinese Medicine examples are Ophiopogon Mai Men Dong (Dwarf lilyturf root), and Fritillaria Chuan Bei Mu (Sichuan fritillary bulb). Then there's moist but confusing *Polygonatum* spp. (Solomon's Seal root). Two species are used in Chinese Medicine (Huang Jing and Yu Zhu) and one in the Western pharmacopeia, *Polygonatum vulgare* (not to be confused with Western *Maianthemum racemosum* (False Solomon's Seal), a different plant entirely). Other Western yin tonics are Irish Moss and Iceland moss, Mullein leaf, Asparagus root, Chickweed herb, and Comfrey leaf and root. These lung tonics double as demulcents. *Sticta pulmonaria* (Lungwort thallus) soothes persistent, dry, wheezing coughs (Fig. 20.3).
- *Lung Qi Deficiency tonics.* Lung Qi Deficiency comes from severe infections or long-term, chronic situations that weaken the lungs, such as in allergies, asthma, chronic bronchitis, tuberculosis, pneumonia, and emphysema.[7] In these cases, Lung qi needs to be increased/tonified. Herbs that do this are our adaptogenic friends, Astragalus Huang Qi (Astragalus root), Codonopsis Dang Shen (Downy Bellflower root), and Panax Xi Yang Shen (American ginseng root). These three also restore the gut, or in Chinese Medicine terms, tonify Spleen qi.
- *Western lung restoratives.* These are the cool, relaxing expectorants that are in the demulcent list: herbs like Licorice root, Grindelia milky flower bud, and Lungwort lichen.

Expectorants

Expectorants move mucus up and out of the lungs. In Western herbalism, they are a large and varied bunch. They can be stimulating or relaxing. They can be both stimulating and relaxing at the same time. They can be warming or cooling. The takeaway is that they either liquefy the mucus, help in its expulsion from the respiratory tree, or do both (Table 20.2).[9]

Abnormal mucus, known as sputum (***catarrh***), can narrow the airway and become thick, sticky, and difficult to clear out. Catarrh contains bacteria and viruses. Catarrh-filled, used nose wipes are very contagious items that should be stored in a closed paper bag. Basically, expectorants push up the gunk and stop mucus and infection from spreading to the lower respiratory tract, where real troubles can begin, such as serious pneumonias and other deep-seated infections. It's always easier (and wiser) to treat an upper airway condition *before* it makes its way down the respiratory tree into the lungs.

There are two main types of expectorants: *stimulating* and *relaxing*. Stimulating ones are straightforward; they warm the lungs and help produce more mucus when supply is scant. The relaxing ones include various categories: bronchodilators, antitussives, and demulcents.

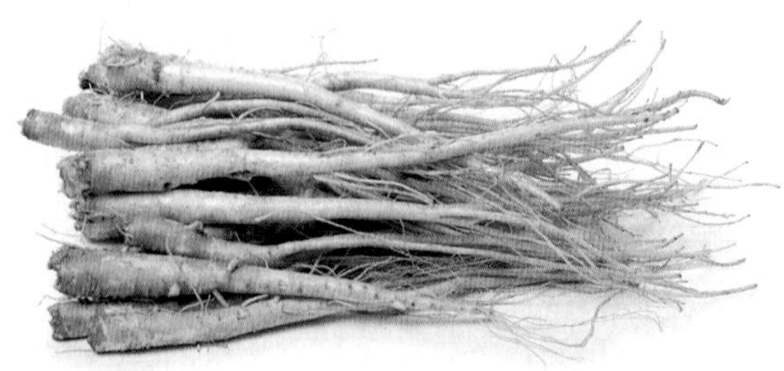

• **Fig. 20.4** Platycodon Jie Geng root is warm, pungent, and stimulating, and yet a versatile expectorant. It excels in helping to loosen and cough up stubborn mucous in both lingering early wind cold and chronic conditions. (iStock.com/Credit: Chengyuzheng.)

TABLE 20.2 **Some Prime Expectorants/Cough Remedies**

Herb	Comments	Warming	Cooling	Demulcent/wet and Soothing	Spasmolytic/ Antitussive	Mucolytic	Astringent and Dry
Tussilago farfara Coltsfoot herb Classic and versatile.	For very thick sputum, sore throat, wheezing, and coughing.		Cools hot phlegm, heat.		Yes	For coughing, and sore throat.	Yes.
Marrubium vulgare White Horehound herb	For very thick sputum, a classic cough syrup addition.		Cools hot, damp phlegm. Pungent.		Yes	For chronic cough, wheezing.	
Eucalyptus globulus leaf Tincture or essential oil	Immune stimulant, antiinfective. For sputum plugs.		Cool for hot phlegm, wind heat.				Yes.
Grindelia robusta Gumweed flower	For viscous phlegm and asthma. Bronchodilator.		Cool, moist, and stimulating.				Yes.
Prunus serotina Wild Cherry bark	Relaxant and bronchodilator. For any type of cough.		Cool and dry.		Relieves coughing and wheezing.		
Verbascum thapsus Mullein leaf	For dry phlegm, hot, weak cough, and deficiency.		Cool, moist, relaxing, and restoring.	Moist, for flu, bronchitis, and asthma.	Broad acting, spasmolytic.	Yes	
Sambucus nigra Elderberry	For full thick sputum and wheezing. Bronchitis.		Cooling, for hot, damp phlegm.			Yes	Dry
Plantago spp. Plantain leaf	For hot phlegm, dry cough. Asthma and wheezing.		Cold, salty, bitter and restoring.				Yes, stops bleeding topically.
Fritillaria thunbergii Zhe Bei Mu Fritillary bulb	For hacky, dry cough, bronchitis, and pneumonia. Antiseptic. Great herb.		Cool and moist, for hot, dry phlegm.		For constant coughing, calming and relaxing.	Yes	
Ophiopogon japonicas Mai Men Dong Dwarf Lilyturf root	For dry, chronic cough and yin deficiency.		Cool, moist, and restoring. For dry phlegm.	Yes	Yes	Yes	
Asclepias tuberosa Pleurisy root	For Lung Wind Heat, tight chest, and fever.		Cold, bitter, and dry.		Relaxing expectorant, bronchodilator.		
Thymus vulgaris Thyme herb	A great drier upper, antiinfective, and bronchodilator.	Warming for cold phlegm.			Antispasmodic for asthma, coughs, and laryngitis.		Yes
Hyssopus officinalis Hyssop herb	For most types of coughs, chronic bronchitis. Bronchodilator.	Warming for cold and damp phlegm.					Yes

(*Continued*)

TABLE 20.2 Some Prime Expectorants/Cough Remedies—cont'd

Herb	Comments	Warming	Cooling	Demulcent/wet and Soothing	Spasmolytic/ Antitussive	Mucolytic	Astringent and Dry
Ligusticum porteri Osha root	Antiinfective, diaphoretic, and pungent. For coughing and wheezing.	Warming dry, and aromatic for cold phlegm.					
Lobelia inflata Lobelia herb	Bronchodilator antiasthmatic. For damp and phlegm, bronchitis.	A little warm, bitter and relaxing.			Spasmodic. For dry hard coughs and wheezing.		Somewhat astringent.
Platycodon grandiflorum Jie Geng Balloonflower root All-purpose, gotta have.	Versatile herb for hot or cold, with or without sputum, acute or chronic. A no-brainer.	Warming	For lung phlegm damp, but also hot phlegm.	Wet and warm, antiinflammatory.		Yes	
Prunus armeniaca Xing Ren Bitter Apricot kernel	In many Chinese Medicine cough syrups.	Warming		Yes	For dry, spasmodic coughing, warm and moist.		
Glycyrrhiza glabra Gan Cao Licorice root	For hot phlegm and dry, cough, antiinfective.			Neutral, moist, and sweet.		Yes	
Trifolium pratense Red Clover flower	Great for bronchitis with cough that won't quit, asthma, croup.			Neutral, sweet, moist, relaxing.	For uncontrollable, spasmodic coughing.		Yes

- *Stimulating expectorants.* These are warming. They irritate the bronchioles and initiate the cough reflex. Some also liquefy thick sputum, making it thinner and more plentiful. Coughing is stimulated, and sputum moves upwards with the help of the tiny hairs lining the respiratory tract (cilia).[10] Botanical examples that warm and dry the lungs are numerous. The three best in the West are *Thymus vulgaris* (Thyme herb), *Angelica archangelica* (Angelica root), and *Inula helenium* (Elecampane root). Not to be sneered at are Hyssop herb, Yerba Santa leaf, Basil herb, and Pinellia Ban Xia (Fermented Pinellia corm). Many of these double as ***bronchodilators*** which widen the air passages, making breathing easier and allowing more room for mucus to ascend. Dilation helps the airway relax.
- *Chinese Medicine viewpoint of warm, stimulating expectorants.* These should be used in a Lung Phlegm Cold condition to warm up the Lungs when they are too cold and moist. There might be early-onset colds or chronic conditions that have gone on for ages (this happens often). There could be coughing, wheezing, or shortness of breath (SOB) on exertion or lying down. **P** Tight or tense. **T** Coat is greasy and white.[11] A great one to use is Platycodon Jie Geng (Balloonflower root) (Fig. 20.4).
- *Relaxing expectorants.* Energetically varied. Some are warming, and some add needed moisture and coolness. In general, they soothe and relax spasms, open the airway, and loosen mucus to promote natural expectoration. Expectorant categories that are relaxing to the respiratory tree include *bronchodilators* and ***antiasthmatics***, which open and increase the diameter of the bronchioles; ***antitussives*** that suppress the cough reflex because of the presence of saponins or cyanogenic glycosides; and *demulcents*, which add moisture and help relax Lung qi.
- *Chinese Medicine viewpoint of relaxing expectorants.* These are needed with tense Lung qi, indicated by a hacking or dry rasping cough, wheezing, and hard sputum with a tight chest. This is a tense, dry condition that requires bronchodilators, antitussives, and demulcents. The chest needs to be opened up and relaxed and this condition shows up as **P** Tight and wiry, denoting tension; **T** Dry, especially in the front (the lung area).[8] Fritillaria Zhe Bei Mu (Sichuan Fritillary root) and Ophiopogon Mai Men Dong (Dwarf Lilyturf root) are winners.
- *Bronchodilators are relaxing expectorants.* There are numerous bronchodilators in Western herbalism. They dilate, making the lumen of the bronchi larger in diameter. Included here are Wild Cherry bark, Cramp bark, Thyme herb, Hyssop herb, Black Cohosh root, Red Clover flower, Coltsfoot herb, Aniseed, Gumweed flower, Elecampane root, and Lobelia herb.
- *Antitussives are relaxing expectorants.* ***Antitussives*** suppress the coughing reflex. Wild Cherry bark is famous (Fig. 20.5). Other good ones are Coltsfoot herb, White Horehound herb, Hops flower, Passionflower, Queen's root, Skunk Cabbage root, Wild Lettuce herb, and Fritillaria Chuan Bei Mu (Sichuan Fritillary bulb).

Demulcents can be relaxing expectorants. Demulcents are good for dry, stubborn, and irritating coughs that need to become

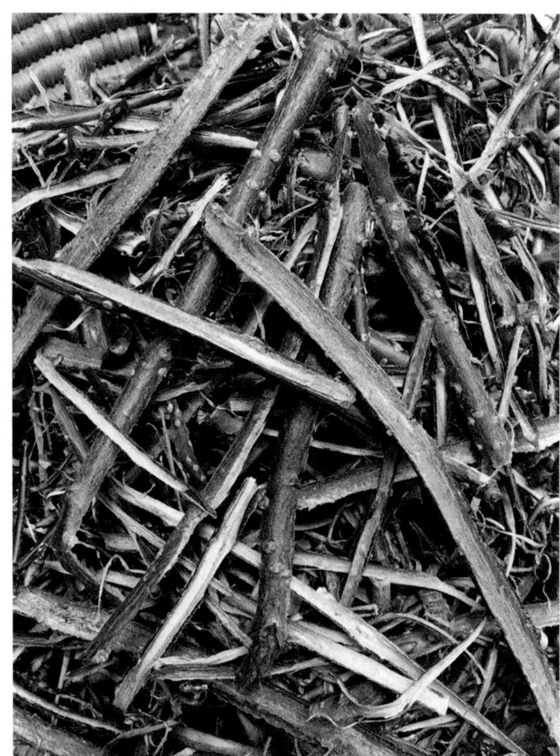

• **Fig. 20.5** *Prunus serotina* (Wild Cherry bark) is a classic Western antitussive and bronchodilator. Notice its identifying raised white lenticels that allow for gas exchange between the atmosphere and the inner bark.

productive and wetter. The types of herbs used in this case are the cooling wet ones, such as Licorice root, Plantain leaf, Irish Moss, Iceland Moss, Mullein leaf, Grindelia flower, Lungwort lichen, Platycodon Jie Geng (Balloonflower root). Many are also expectorants.

Respiratory Antimicrobial Herbs

Antimicrobial herbs for the upper and lower respiratory tract (Table 20.3) are not all that different from general antimicrobials. (Chapter 17). Respiratory antiinfectives are sometimes referred to as *respiratory sedatives*, in the sense that the cold ones sedate or calm heat (not calm the nervous system). This difference was confusing to me for the longest time.

A few respiratory antimicrobials are warming or neutral, but most are cooling. For wind cold early-onset conditions, we want more warming ones. For wind heat conditions, we want them more on the cooling spectrum. Furthermore, some respiratory antimicrobials have affinities/tropisms for various parts of the respiratory tree. Garden Sage loves the throat and makes a good gargle. Andrographis Chuan Xin Lian (Heart-Thread Lotus leaf) goes to hot sinus infections around the eyes, *Usnea* thallus (Old Man's Beard) is specific for strep throats (Fig. 20.6), and Osha root is an upper respiratory herb, for sure.

Diaphoretic Herbs

We sweat all the time, no matter what. Sweating maintains normal body temperature, cools us down, and helps to eliminate toxins. Heat is either lost or conserved, on an as-needed basis, depending on the amount of evaporation occurring through the sweat glands. In early-onset flus and colds, body temperature begins to rise as an inflammatory response to infection. Herbalists are big on promoting sweating when an infection begins in order to lower fever (not necessarily eliminating it) and to push out toxins generated by microorganisms. Promotion of sweating is an important therapeutic principle when treating respiratory infections.

Diaphoretics increase sweating. If we encourage sweating with diaphoretic herbs, we push fluids (blood) toward the skin, the exterior. Herbs that accomplish this task are usually drying, pungent, and spicy; the pungent taste pushes energy outward (Table 20.4). They are often antiinfective, antipyretic, and antiinflammatory as well.[8] Pungent diaphoretic herbs may be warming or cooling. The warm ones are used to banish wind cold. The cooling ones are used to banish wind heat.

- *Arterial stimulant diaphoretics are warm and pungent.* ***Arterial stimulant*** diaphoretic herbs encourage sweating by warming up the exterior. These are used for external wind cold conditions with chills, little sweating, low if any fever, clear nasal discharges, sinusitis, and allergic rhinitis. Warming diaphoretics in this realm include Prickly Ash bark, Ginger root, Peppermint herb, Angelica root, Ledebouriella Fang Feng (Wind Protector root), and Cinnamomum Rou Gui (Cinnamon bark) (Fig. 20.7).[8]
- *Peripheral vasodilator diaphoretics are cool, relaxing and pungent.* These encourage sweating by relaxing and ***vasodilating***, widening the blood vessels/capillaries near the skin (periphery). They are used for external wind heat conditions with fever, few or no chills, swollen red throat or eyes, and yellow-greenish discharges.[8] Some of these are Catnip herb, Yarrow herb, Elderberry flower, Linden flower, Chamomile herb, and Chrysanthemum Ju Hua (Chrysanthemum flower).
- *For best results, diaphoretic herbs are dispensed in a hot tea.* The best delivery of herbs for sweating is with a hot water infusion or decoction, taken every few hours—not a tincture—as in fresh Ginger juice tea (Box 17.2).

Herbs That Drain Lymphatic Fluid

Along with encouragement of sweating comes another therapeutic principle when treating respiratory infections: the promotion of lymphatic drainage. Lymph circulation is part of the immune system. It transports infection-fighting white blood cells to tissues, and filters and catches bacteria through its nodes. Lymph empties into the blood circulation where toxins are filtered and eliminated through the kidneys and bowel. Therefore sponsorship of lymphatic flow and good drainage with the use of ***lymphatic drainer*** herbs is an important aspect of healing respiratory ills. Some prime lymphatic movers are Red Root, Ocotillo bark, Cleavers herb, Calendula flower, Figwort root and herb, and Poke root.

Lymphatic Drainers That Are Liver Decongestants

When the liver is stimulated to do its detoxifying function, it helps the body drain toxins and fluids through the bowel and bladder. Many liver decongestants have a dual function as lymphatic drainers. Some of these double-duty herbs are Figwort root and herb, Calendula flower, Yellow Dock root, Burdock root, Blue Flag root, Poke root, Forsythia Lian Qiao (Forsythia valve), and

TABLE 20.3 Important Respiratory Antimicrobials *(Mostly cooling or cold)*

Herb	Energetics	Comments
Andrographis paniculata Chuan Xin Lian Andrographis herb	Cold, dry, very bitter. Astringent.	Broad-spectrum immunostimulant, antipyretic. For all types of microbes, gastrointestinal bitter. Famous in sinus formulas, Lung phlegm heat, wind heat, and damp heat. Antibiofilm herb.
Lonicera japonica Jin Yin Hua Honeysuckle flower	Cold, dry, sweet, astringent.	Broad-spectrum antiinfective, immunostimulant. For colds, flu, Herpes, early-onset wind heat, and fire toxins.
Forsythia suspensa Lian Qiao Forsythia valve	Cold, bitter, astringent, bit pungent.	Broad-spectrum cold antiinfective, detoxifying, immunostimulant. For colds, flu, measles, and fever.
Usnea spp. Song Luo Old Man's Beard thallus	Cooling, sweet, bit bitter.	Chinese and Western herb. Broad-spectrum antiinfective, immunostimulant, and excellent antifungal. Specific for upper respiratory. Antibiofilm.
Scutellaria baicalensis Huang Qin Baikal Skullcap root	Cold, dry, bitter, astringent, relaxing.	Broad-spectrum, cold antiinfective, immunostimulant, and antitussive. For acute allergies, lung phlegm heat. Antibiofilm.
Ligusticum porteri Osha root	Warm, dry, little bitter, very aromatic.	Upper respiratory tropism. For wind cold, early-onset colds and flu. One of the few warm ones.
Sticta pulmonaria Lungwort thallus	Cooling, moist, dry, bittersweet, astringent, restoring.	Restorative and relaxing, mucostatic (drying), but also moistening for yin deficiencies, Not strictly antiinfective, but a great adjunct. For upper respiratory infections with watery discharge, allergy, fever, headaches, flu, cough. Great for sinus congestion, sinusitis, rhinitis, colds, and flu.
Echinacea angustifolia Echinacea root	Cooling, dry, salty, pungent.	Immunostimulant and detoxifier. For toxic heat and toxicosis, bacterial/viral infections, and immediate allergies. Antibiofilm.
Calendula officinalis Marigold flower	Neutral and a little cooling, dry, salty astringent.	Somewhat antimicrobial, neither warm nor cold. Especially with toxic heat, wind heat, colds and flu with fever. Excels in first aid injuries.
Eucalyptus globulus leaf, tincture, and essential oil	Cooling, pungent, aromatic.	Antimicrobial, wind damp heat, cold/flu onset, sinusitis, rhinitis, diaphoretic, immunostimulant.

Lonicera Jin Yin Hua (Honeysuckle flower) (Table 20.4).[8] Thus, use of liver decongestants can be considered a therapeutic principle in treatment of colds and flus.

Antihistamine Herbs

Histamine is a substance produced by mast cells as part of a local, hyperimmune response to an allergen (such as pollen). The histamine response causes inflammation and the dreaded Type I immediate allergy symptoms: runny, itchy eyes; nasal congestion; sneezing; rhinitis; postnasal drip; and sore, scratchy throat. ***Antihistamines*** are herbs that block histamine. They fix the symptoms. They do not *prevent* the allergy. Addressing allergy prevention is a bit more complicated, because the cause must be found and eliminated. But when a person is suffering from hay fever, the first step is to relieve their misery. Antihistamine herbs that do just that include Xanthium Cang Er Zi (Siberian Cocklebur), Ephedra Ma Huang (Fig. 20.8), Goldenrod herb, Eyebright herb, Ganoderma Ling Zhi (Reishi mushroom), Echinacea root, and Nettle herb (Table 20.4).

About Coughs

A ***cough*** is a reflex, which is the body's way of getting foreign bronchial irritants and excess mucus up and out. A dry, hacky cough irritates and hurts the throat, making it inflamed and sore. But a productive cough brings up stuff like bacteria, viruses, and smoke particles.

Coughing is a symptom. It is caused from something else. The most common reason for an *acute* cough is from a viral or bacterial respiratory infection. Air pollution or a strained or pulled abdominal muscle are other possibilities. Common *chronic* causes are bronchitis, allergies, asthma, gastroesophageal reflux disease (GERD), and postnasal drip.[12] *Red flag:* A cough that doesn't respond to treatment or that produces blood (*hemoptysis*) needs referral. This type of cough could indicate chronic bronchitis, pneumonia, or even cancer. The best way to alleviate a cough is to focus on the underlying cause. Anytime there's a cough on board, the formula must tackle the root and respect and alleviate annoying symptoms. Sometimes, the way to approach this is to

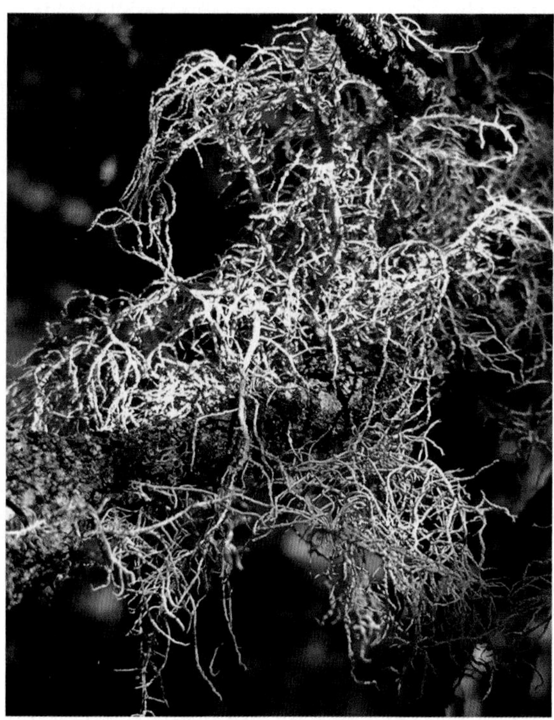

• **Fig. 20.6** *Usnea* spp. (Old Man's Beard thallus) is a respiratory antibiofilm antimicrobial, also specific for strep throat.

have the main formula address the infection (or whatever the cause may be) and then to provide a separate cough syrup, as needed (Box 20.1).

Coughs can be soothed, stimulated, or suppressed. Obviously, if there's infectious mucus to expel, that process needs to be stimulated, not suppressed. That condition calls for an expectorant that is soothing and a bit stimulating. But, if the cough is a nervous, nonproductive, and chronic dry tickle, it serves no purpose. In such cases, *good riddance*. A suppressing antitussive that relaxes and puts an end to that annoying and irritating cough reflex is needed.

About Permanent Prevention of Seasonal Allergies

Recurring immediate allergies such as hay fever are generally a reflection of a deeper underlying problem. The best approach is to first relieve the symptoms, but when they abate, keep digging for answers. There is a reason some suffer from repeated ***hay fever***, seasonal allergies caused from pollens or other environmental allergens year after year. The ultimate answer is to find the cause, and work on that. It is not a quick fix and will take some dedicated time and commitment from client and herbalist. As always, return to root causes. Allergies are just about always associated with digestive functions, including food sensitivities, or weak adrenals and immune function.[13] Establishing good nutrition is paramount.

- *Start with the gut.* Begin the Four-R program about 8 weeks before the usual start of allergy season. If the client is in full allergy mode, begin it anyway.
- *Reminder of the Four-R program protocol* (Chapter 18). The whole program takes about 6 weeks.[14] (1) *Remove.* Identify food sensitivities with a 2-week elimination diet. Reintroduce one removed food at a time and evaluate results. If it's a no-go, that food has to stay out. Remove dairy (absolutely necessary in hay fever), gluten, sugar, soy, salt, and refined carbohydrates. Eat a rainbow veggie diet, because vegetables' bioflavonoid content provides natural antihistamines. Include lots of onions, garlic, ginger, cayenne, horseradish, fermented foods, and pre- and probiotics. (2) *Replace.* After 2 weeks, add in a digestive enzyme supplement. (3) *Reinoculate.* On the third week, add in fermented foods and a probiotic supplement. (4) *Repair.* Continue the herbal gut repair formula for up to 6 months to heal the gut lining. Some herbal choices include purchasing deglycyrrhizinated (DGL) Licorice root lozenges (they heal and soothe the gut). Other possibilities are Turmeric root, Dandelion or Burdock root (healing/bitters), Marshmallow root (soothes gut lining), and Atractylodes Bai Zhu (White Atractylodes root) restores gut.
- *Supplements.* Take these along with the program from the first day. Continue for 4 to 6 months. Purchase freeze-dried Nettle and take 3 to 6 caps a day. It must be freeze dried because that delivery form concentrates active constituents in the plant's stinging hairs and leaves. Include quercetin 500 mg a day, L-glutamine powder 5 to 10 g for 1 month, and fish oil EPA/DHA.
- *The adrenals.* Work on adrenal health by addressing the gut and introducing adrenal restoratives into the overall formula (Chapter 27). Suggestions are Ganoderma Ling Zhi (Reishi Mushroom), Nettle herb, Licorice root, Ashwagandha root, Eleuthero Ci Wu Jia (Siberian ginseng root), Holy Basil herb, Scrophularia Xuan Shen (Black Figwort root), and Rehmannia Shu Di Huang (prepared Rehmannia root).
- *Immune support.* Balance the immune system with adaptogens like Ganoderma Ling Zhi (Reishi mushroom), Astragalus Huang Qi (Astragalus root), *Echinacea* spp., Schisandra Wu Wei Zi (Five Taste berry), Holy Basil herb, and Ashwagandha root.[15]
- *Sample herbal formula for long-term allergy prevention.* Concentrates on gut and adrenal restoratives and immune modulators.
  - *Formula:* 3 parts Licorice root to heal gut; 2 parts White Atractylodes to heal gut; 2 parts Nettle herb, antihistamine/adrenal support; 2 parts Reishi mushroom Ling Zhi or Holy Basil herb for immune/adrenal support; 2 parts Dandelion root or Curcumin root as a bitter; 1 part Ginger root, if there are food sensitivities.
- *Anticipated results.* Seasonal allergies should be eliminated or be a lot milder than usual. Client will have to address gut, adrenal, and immune issues on a long-term basis and with a healthy diet indefinitely. The more years a person suffers with hay fever, the longer it takes to fix. If the program is done faithfully, the next year should be allergy-free.

Common Respiratory Conditions

Laryngitis

- *Definition.* An *itis* inflammation of the ***larynx*** (vocal cords) from irritation, overuse or infection, usually viral. Occurs alone or accompanies a viral infection, cold, or sore throat.

TABLE 20.4 Diaphoretics Lymphatic Drainers Antihistamines

Diaphoretics	Lymphatic Drainers	Antihistamines
For wind cold, use warm arterial stimulants. For wind heat, use cool peripheral vasodilators.	***To eliminate toxins, use fluid movers; lymphatic drainers and liver decongestants.***	***To reduce allergy symptoms from histamine response.***
Zingiber officinale Ginger root Sweet, hot, dry. Arterial stimulant, for wind cold, cold/flu onset.	*Calendula officinalis* Marigold flower For lymphatic congestion, detox, swollen glands. A liver decongestant.	*Euphrasia rostkoviana* Eyebright herb Cool, dry, astringent, antiinflammatory, eye discharges, mucus decongestant.
Angelica archangelica Angelica root Pungent, aromatic, warm, and dry. Arterial stimulant for wind damp cold.	*Galium aparine* Cleavers herb Cold, dry, and salty. Moves lymph, dries damp, dissolves deposits.	*Solidago* spp. Goldenrod herb Bitter, astringent, cool, dry. Stops allergy symptoms of rhinitis, sinus congestion, dries damp, diuretic.
Ledebouriella divaricata Fang Feng Wind Protector root Wet, warm, moist, antiviral, immune and arterial stimulant. For wind cold and wind heat, both.	*Echinacea* spp. Echinacea herb and root Cool, dry, stimulating, dissolving, detoxicant. For swollen lymph glands and sore throat.	*Sticta pulmonaria* Lungwort lichen Cool, moist, dry, salty, and bitter. Clears all kinds of allergic rhinitis, sinusitis, and mucus.
Mentha x *piperita* Peppermint leaf Warm with 2° cooling effect. Vasodilator for both wind cold and wind heat. (No-brainer, if not sure which.)	*Arctium lappa* Burdock root Cool, dry, bitter, pungent, dissolving, kidney detoxicant. For damp heat. A liver decongestant.	*Xanthium sibiricum* Cang Er Zi Siberian Cocklebur One of the best for immediate allergy symptoms, nasal discharge, sinus congestion.
Nepeta cataria Catnip leaf Cool, dry, pungent, aromatic vasodilator for wind heat condition with fever. Good kid herb.	*Scrophularia ningpoensis* Figwort herb and root Clears toxic heat, diuretic, drains water and lymph, liver decongestant.	*Scutellaria baicalensis* Huang Qin Chinese Skullcap root Cold, dry, bitter, antiallergenic. For immune regulation and all inflammation; really helps.
Eupatorium perfoliatum Boneset herb Vasodilator for wind heat fevers, onset cold/flu. Once called sweating weed, used to lower deep pain and fever that goes deep to the bone.	*Phytolacca decandra* Poke root (Medium strength.) Sweet, neutral, pungent, dissolving, diuretic, detoxicant. Dissolves tumors and a liver decongestant.	*Ganoderma lucidum* Ling Zhi Reishi mushroom Broad-spectrum antiallergenic, for all Type I allergies with rhinitis. Also adaptogenic.
Achillea millefolium Yarrow flower Bitter, cool, dry, stimulating. Vasodilator for wind heat. Diaphoretic and diuretic.	*Chimaphila umbellata* Pipsissewa/Wintergreen herb and root Cold, dry, astringent, dissolving, dries damp. Drains water in edema, dissolves deposits.	*Urtica dioica* Nettle herb Cool, dry, salty. Relieves allergy, cough, wheezing, allergic rhinitis. Freeze dried form (not tincture) recommended for allergies.
Chrysanthemum x *morifolium* Ju Hua Chrysanthemum flower Bit bitter, cool, relaxing. Vasodilator for wind heat. Cooling antiinfective and diaphoretic, a classic in Chinese Medicine.	*Rumex crispus* Yellow Dock root Cold, dry, bitter, astringent, dissolving, decongesting, draining detoxicant, diuretic. Drains swollen glands. A broad-spectrum detoxifier and liver decongestant.	*Ephedra sinica* Ma Huang Ephedra stem Warm, very drying. Hard to get, but if you can, it's classic as a nasal decongestant, antiallergenic immune regulator. Also, for spasmodic and asthmatic conditions.
Sambucus nigra Elderberry flower Cool, dry, pungent, aromatic. Vasodilator for wind heat, cold/flu onset with fever.	*Ceanothus americanus* Red Root Bitter, cold, and dry. A lovely lymphatic herb, fluid mover and decongestant.	*Ambrosia artemisiifolia* Common Ragweed herb Antihistamine, dries mucus, hay fever, for immediate allergy symptoms.

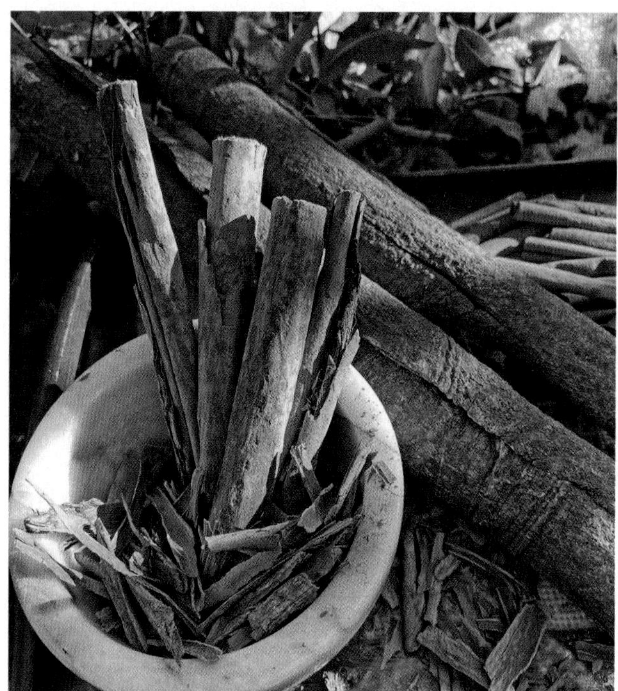

• **Fig. 20.7** Cinnamomum Rou Gui (Cinnamon bark) is a warming diaphoretic that acts as an arterial stimulant. Pictured: *Cinnamomum Cassia* (Chinese or Saigon Cinnamon), larger rolls of bark, and *Cinnamomum zeylanicum* (Ceylon or "True" Cinnamon), smaller rolls, both used medicinally.

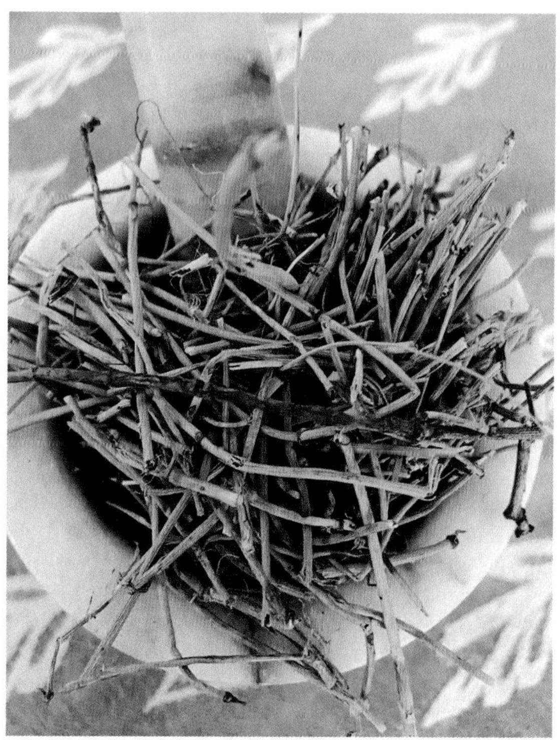

• **Fig. 20.8** Ephedra Ma Huang (Ephedra stem) is a strong antihistamine. It is antiallergenic for immediate allergies like hay fever, a bronchodilator and a nasal decongestant. Because it is so drying and stimulating, do not use with high blood pressure, spontaneous sweating, or insomnia.[8]

• BOX 20.1 Cough Begone and Sore Throat Syrup *Adapted from herbalist Rosemary Gladstar*[13]

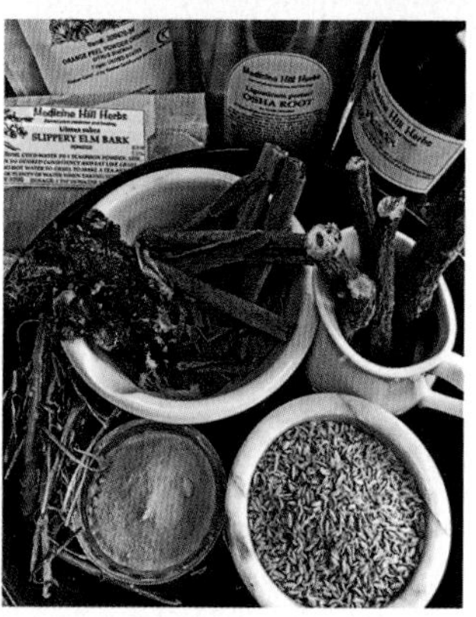

Gathering syrup-making supplies: Dried Osha root, Cinnamon bark, Licorice root sticks, Fennel seed, Orange peel, Wild Cherry bark, and Slippery Elm bark.

Most generic herbal cough syrups contain a little bit of everything. They include an expectorant to bring up phlegm, a demulcent to soothe an inflamed throat, an antitussive to calm the cough (but not stop it short), an antimicrobial, and a nervous relaxant. A nice blend of warming and cooling. A cough syrup should taste good too, as it will be taken often. Have one preprepared to grab right from the fridge.[19,20]

2 tbsp Fennel seed	Demulcent, expectorant, sweet, warm, pungent.
1 tbsp Licorice root	Demulcent, expectorant, synergistic, sweetener.
1 tbsp Valerian root	Spasmolytic, antimicrobial, cool, relieves anxiety and fever.
1 tbsp Wild Cherry bark	Antitussive, relaxant, cool, reduces fever.
1½ tsp Slippery Elm bark. Just enough to thicken but not too gunky.	Demulcent and thickener. Make sure it is finely powdered.
1 tbsp Osha root	Expectorant, relieves pain, antimicrobial, bronchi restorative.
1½ tsp Cinnamon bark	Hot and sweet. Antimicrobial. Opens sinuses, sweet.
3/4 tsp Ginger root	Hot, dry, and sweet. Antimicrobial, protects stomach.
1/4 tsp Orange peel	Stimulant expectorant, protects stomach.
Honey	

Directions. Measure out dried, ground herbs, mix together, weigh 2 oz herb mixture to 1 qt water. The measurements shown here are approximate. Over low heat in a heavy bottom pot, simmer herbs and water until it is reduced by half (1 pint). Strain return liquid to the pot. For each pint of liquid, add 1 cup of honey (or more, if desired). Heat gently and mix until the syrup is well-blended.

Optional. Add 4–8 tbsp brandy and 1–2 tbsp Black Cherry concentrate. Yummy, nurturing, and effective.

Dose. 1 tsp every ½ hour to every 2 hours.

- *Signs and symptoms*. Throat ranges from hoarseness to loss of voice where one can only whisper. Pain when swallowing or speaking, dry throat, dry cough, maybe fever, throat edema, and malaise. If it lasts over 2 weeks, becoming chronic, look for other causes such as smoking, inhaled environmental toxins, chronic sinusitis, and acid reflux. It is a hot, dry condition.
- *General therapeutic principles*. (1) Demulcents to soothe and moisten larynx. (2) Antimicrobials/antiinflammatories to relieve

pain and swelling. (3) Internal and external astringents like Bistort root, Garden Sage leaf, Raspberry leaf, Oak bark, and Yarrow herb to bring down vocal cord edema. (4) External astringent gargles: Garden Sage leaf, Chamomile flower, Coptis Huang Lian (Goldthread root). (5) Cough syrup as needed.
- *Sample formula.*
  - 2 parts Osha root as upper respiratory antimicrobial; 2 parts Echinacea root as antimicrobial, detox; 2 parts Marshmallow root as a cooling demulcent; 1 part Goldenseal or Coptis Huang Lian (Goldthread root) as local antibacterial and astringent.

Sore Throat

A sore throat usually accompanies a viral cold, flu, or upper respiratory inflammation. The *palatine tonsils* (lymphatic tissue on either side of the throat) are sometimes involved. They contain antibodies and are part of the immune system, the first line of defense for the respiratory system. The tonsils trap microorganisms and external pathogens, and they defend against external wind. If they are inflamed or enlarged as in *tonsillitis*, it's a sign the body is attempting to fight an infection.

A *streptococcal* throat infection is a potentially serious bacterial infection. If untreated, it can but may not always go systemic and lead to rheumatic fever, affecting the heart, kidneys, or joints, or cause meningitis or otitis media. It must be treated. On inspection, the throat appears red, sometimes with white or yellow streaks of pus. Red spots are on the soft or hard palate. There can be fever and intense throat pain. Throat cultures can be obtained from an healthcare provider to verify. *Usnea* thallus, the berberines, Juniper berry, and *Echinacea angustifolia* are particularly indicated if you suspect strep throat and must touch the membranes directly.[16]

- *Definition.* A sore, painful ***pharynx*** (the throat) is often accompanied by a cold, flu, or upper respiratory inflammation, called *pharyngitis.*
- *Signs and symptoms.* Pain, scratchiness, or irritation that often worsens when swallowing. There can be neck pain from tonsil enlargement. The most common cause is a viral infection.
- *Allopathic treatment.* If viral, use symptomatic home treatment such as gargles. If bacterial streptococcus, antibiotics are used.
- *General therapeutic principles.* As always, pick and choose wisely. (1) Treat infection with broad-spectrum antimicrobials and antibiofilm herbs. (2) Treat pain with demulcents. (3) Drain toxins with lymphatic drainers and liver decongestants. (4) If there is tonsil involvement (pain and enlargement), use lymphatic drainers to allow organisms to be eliminated and to prevent the tonsils themselves from becoming overwhelmed, enlarged, and infected. (5) Gargles for direct antiseptic and astringent contact with throat tissue (Case History 20.1).

CASE HISTORY 20.1

Case History for Sore Throat and Possible Laryngitis

S. Pete's throat is red and irritated, and it hurts when he swallows. The sides of his neck are tender. He is starting to lose his voice.

O. **P** Superficial. **T** Body red near front, dry. Tonsils slightly enlarged; reports tenderness on palpation. Voice sounds hoarse. No fever or cough.

A. Viral sore throat, enlarged tonsils, impeding laryngitis. External Wind Heat.

P. *Specific therapeutic principles*. (1) Broad-spectrum cooling antimicrobials for heat. (2) Demulcents for pain/dryness. (3) Lymphatic drainage. (4) Internal astringent for laryngitis, vocal cord edema. (5) External astringent gargle.

Herbal Formula and Dose. 4 mL every 2 hours.

Parts	Herbs	Rationale
3	*Usnea* thallus	Cold broad-spectrum and antistrep, just in case.
2	Irish Moss thallus	Cool, demulcent.
2	Osha root	Antiviral for upper respiratory infection.
2	Calendula flower	Upper respiratory antiviral, lymphatic drainage.
2	Yarrow flower	Astringent for laryngitis/restoring.
1	Licorice root	Soothing, antimicrobial, demulcent.

Other Suggestions

Red Flag. If a person is very sick for over 2 weeks with high fever, it could be a streptococcal bacterial infection or tonsillitis. Find out for sure and refer to healthcare provider for lab culture.
- Gargle 3 × day with *Salvia officinalis* (Garden Sage herb) and Coptis Huang Lian (Goldthread root), 1 part each.

Common Cold

Here we must determine stage of infection, whether External Wind Cold, External Wind Heat, or Wind Damp Heat, and treat with appropriate herbs. These Chinese Medicine conditions were laid out in detail in Chapter 17.

- *Definition.* The ***common cold*** is a viral infection and inflammation of the upper respiratory tract. Viral infections will not respond to antibiotics. Colds are caused by many types of viruses that mutate quickly and are too numerous for effective vaccine development. Secondary bacterial infections may occur and progress to bacterial sinusitis, ear infections, or bronchitis. That's why, at the end of the day, some colds are seemingly eradicated with antibiotics.
- *Signs and symptoms.* Rhinitis, headache, chills, sore throat, pain, sneezing, coughing, and sometimes, but not always, fever. Expect full recovery in 7 to 10 days.
- *Allopathic treatment.* Supportive. Tylenol, aspirin, rest, and fluids.
- *General therapeutic principles.* Choose appropriate suspects, depending on condition. Some are givens; some depend on situation. (1) Provide immune support, the earlier the better. (2) Kill viruses with antivirals or broad-spectrum antimicrobials, warming or cooling, as appropriate for condition. (3) If it's wet mucus, expel and dry it up with a drying expectorant/cough remedy. (4) If it's dry sticky mucus, moisturize and expel it with demulcent expectorants. (5) If the picture is Lung Phlegm Cold, use warm, stimulating expectorants. (6) If the picture is Lung Phlegm Heat, use relaxing and cooling demulcent expectorants. (7) Create sweating. If it's a cold condition, use arterial stimulants, and if it's warm, use vasodilators. (8) Drain toxins with lymphatic drainers or liver/gallbladder stimulants. (9) Alleviate pain, as needed, with Passionflower, White Willow bark for headaches, or Boswellia Ru Xiang (Frankincense resin) or Bupleurum Chai Hu (Asian Buplever root) for joint pain. (10) After cold is cleared up and if chronic and frequent, give long-term formula to tonify lungs and enhance immunity (Case History 20.2).

CASE HISTORY 20.2

Case History for Common Cold

Part 1 Common Cold, Day One

S. Elise has had symptoms for 1 day. There is a scratchy throat; white, moist sputum; painful, mostly nonproductive cough; no fever. She is rarely sick.

O. **P** Slippery. **T** Body normal, coat greasy, moist, and white.

A. Early-onset common cold with no fever, Lung Phlegm Cold.

P. *Specific therapeutic principles.* (1) Expel cold, dry damp. (2) Immunostimulants. (3) Antivirals. (4) Warm, pungent arterial stimulant diaphoretics. (5) Expectorants that are warming and stimulating.

Herbal Formula and Dose for Common Cold, Day One. 4 mL every 1–2 hours.

Parts	Herbs	Rationale
3	Osha root	Antimicrobial/warm expectorant/diaphoretic.
3	Angelica root	Warming expectorant/diaphoretic.
2	Honeysuckle Jin Yin Hua	Early-onset antimicrobial/immunostimulant.
2	Forsythia Lian Qiao	Early-onset antimicrobial/immunostimulant.
2	Licorice root	Expectorant/soothing/antimicrobial.

Other Suggestion for Common Cold, Day One

- Elderberry elixir (Box 20.2) 3 mL every 1–2 hours, along with the herbal formula.
- Hot bath with Lavender and Peppermint essential oil to relax and open airway.
- Supplements to increase immunity: Vitamin C 2000 mg or more 3 × day and vitamin D_3 10,000 IU (international units) of a sublingual oil-based solution, zinc lozenges 20 mg sublingual.

Part 2 Common Cold, Day Five

S. Elise felt a little better, so she cut back on the herbs. Now, on day 5, her symptoms have changed. Sputum is sticky and yellow/green, and hard to expectorate. Cough is irritating and scratchy. She has a bad headache and a slight stomachache.

O. **P** Wiry or tense. **T** Body is red, coat dry.

A. Lung Phlegm Heat and Qi Constraint. Common cold, no fever with dry cough.

P. *Specific therapeutic principles.* (1) Overall, expel heat, moisturize lungs, relax Lung qi. (2) Cooling, broad-spectrum antimicrobials. (3) Immunostimulants. (4) Create diaphoresis with vasodilators. (5) Cooling, relaxing, demulcent expectorants. (6) Lymphatic drainage. (7) Relieve headache. (8) Carminative for stomach.

Herbal Formula and Dose for Common Cold, Day Five. 4 mL every 1–2 hours.

Parts	Herbs	Rationale
3	Isatis root	Cold, broad-spectrum antimicrobial.
3	Platycodon Jie Geng	Moist expectorant.
2	*Echinacea* spp.	Immunostimulant/lymph drainer/antimicrobial.
2	Yarrow flower	Vasodilating diaphoretic.
1	White Willow bark	Relieve headache.
1	Citrus Chen Pi	Carminative/liver stimulation.
1	Licorice root	Soothing demulcent/expectorant/protect stomach.

Other Suggestions for Common Cold, Day Five

- Steam to loosen head secretions with Eucalyptus and Tea Tree essential oils.
- Lots of fluids.
- Supplements to increase immunity: Vitamin C 2000 mg 3 × day or make your own pills (Box 20.2), vitamin D_3,10,000 IU a day in an oil-based sublingual solution.

• BOX 20.2 Vitamin C Pills

Courtesy of Rosalee de la Forêt.[21]

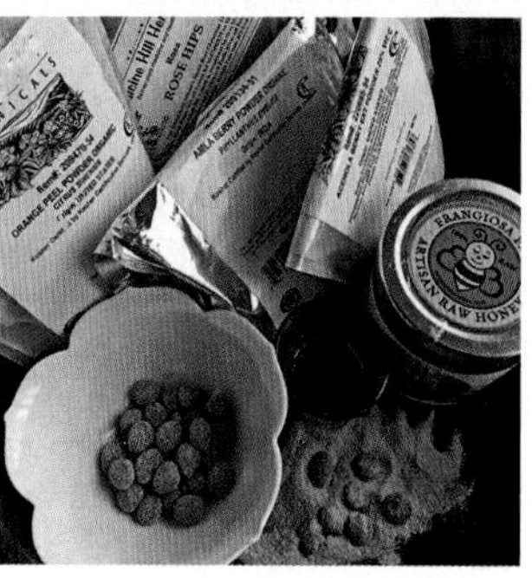

Completed Vitamin C pills and required ingredients.

These tasty, tart pills are easily made by hand and will keep for a very long time. All four herbs are notoriously high in vitamin C and other antioxidants, necessary immune system boosters. The powders may be purchased from Mountain Rose Herbs and other companies.

- *Rosa* spp. (Wild Rose fruit or hips). The fruit of wild roses keeps humans and animals healthy. They were used during World War II in Britain when citrus imports were scarce.
- *Emblica officinalis* (Amla or Indian Gooseberry). One single berry from this Ayurvedic plant contains as much vitamin C as 20 oranges.[22]
- *Malpighia glabra* (Acerola or Barbados cherry). Native to the West Indies, high in vitamin C, other bioflavonoids, and vitamin B complex.
- *Citrus* x *aurantium* var. *sinensis* (Sweet Orange peel). There are substantially more enzymes, flavonoids, and phytonutrients in the peel of the orange than the fruit.

Ingredients

1 tbsp Rose Hip powder
(if grinding your own, remove seeds)

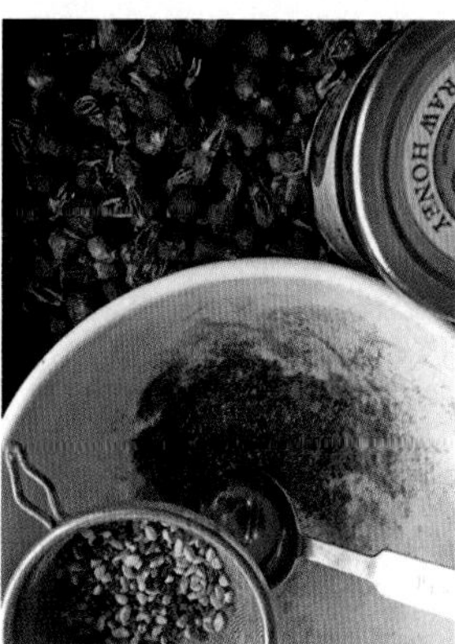

To remove seeds from whole dried Rosehips and obtain a fine powder, stir and coax through a strainer.

1 tbsp Amla berry powder
1 tbsp Acerola powder
Sweet Orange peel powder (optional for rolling)
Honey

Directions

Mix the powdered herbs together, breaking up any clumps. Pour some slightly warmed honey into the powdered mix and stir. Use enough to hold the powders together, not too moist or sticky. Roll into pea-sized balls, and then roll the ball into some extra dried orange powder. (Sweet Orange peel powder is yummy.) Makes about 45 pills. Store in an airtight container. These should last a very long time.

Dose

1–3 balls per day. It is hard to overdose on water-soluble vitamin C. The adverse effect is loose stools. If that happens, decrease dose.

Influenza

- *Definition.* A flu virus is a bigger deal than a cold virus. It is a highly contagious respiratory infection caused by enveloped viruses called ***influenza*** A and B. These can get out of hand, causing death in people who are at high risk—elders and young children; individuals with immune compromised conditions, heart disease, and diabetes; and those on dialysis (Case History 20.3).
- *Reason for flu epidemics and pandemics.* The influenza virus *drifts* (alters its structure very quickly), which is the reason a new flu shot/vaccine must be produced every year. Flu viruses change genetic structure and spread by infecting birds, pigs, and people. The viruses are then carried around the globe each year by train, boat, rail, and plane, hence, another *flu season* with new strains that occur all over the world.
  - Every few years there is a major genetic *shift*, a change to an exceptionally virulent strain, where influenza A exchanges part of its DNA with another virus to which no one has had a chance to become immune. Flu viruses do not only alter DNA; they can also jump species. The Asian flu pandemic of 2004 was a species jump from birds to humans, and the swine flu epidemic of 2009 was a genetic rearrangement that began in pigs but mutated to humans.[17]
- *Signs and symptoms.* Systemic illness with chills, high fever, headache, muscle pain (especially in the back or limbs), extreme fatigue, cough, rhinitis, and malaise. People with the flu are much sicker than those with a cold. The flu can drag on for 1 to 2 weeks, and often cause serious secondary bacterial infections like pneumonia.
- *Allopathic treatment.* Antibiotics, antihistamines, antiviral drugs, and a supportive antiviral flu medication (Tamiflu) that must be given quickly within 2 days of symptom onset.[18] These measures are only marginally effective.
- *General therapeutic principles.* Judiciously select the from these possibilities: (1) Cooling broad-spectrum antiviral/antibacterial herbs, including St. John's Wort and Garlic bulb, which are specifically antiviral. (2) Diaphoretic herbs to decrease fever, including freshly grated Ginger tea. (3) Expectorant herbs for mucus/coughs. (4) Lymphatic drainage herbs to eliminate toxins and circulate infection-fighting white blood cells. (5) Stress control with nervines like Passionflower or Hops flower. (6) Muscle relaxation, headache, and pain control with White Willow bark, Ligusticum Chuan Xiong (Sichuan Lovage root), Lungwort lichen. (7) Support immune function with Andrographis Chuan Xin Lian (Heart-Thread Lotus leaf, Fig. 20.9) or *Echinacea angustifolia*.

CASE HISTORY 20.3

Case History for Influenza

S. Jean came down with chills, 102.3°F, sore throat, painful cough with green sputum, muscle achiness, and fatigue. She has not felt so bad in years. She just wants to sleep.
O. **P** Rapid and wiry. **T** Body red, dry yellowish coat.
A. Wind Heat. Probable flu with high fever.
P. *Specific therapeutic principles.* (1) Expel heat, moisturize lungs. (2) Broad-spectrum antivirals. (3) Cooling, moist expectorants for cough. (4) Lymphatic drainers to expel toxins. (5) Nervines for stress/pain/muscle relaxation. (6) Immune support.

Herbal Formula and Dose for Influenza. 4 mL every 2 hours.

Parts	Herbs	Rationale
3	St. John's Wort	Antiviral.
2	Andrographis Chuan Xin Lian	Antiviral/immune stimulating, antibiofilm, decreases fever.
2	Chrysanthemum Ju Hua	Diaphoretic/reduce fever.
2	Ophiopogon Mai Men Dong	Moist, cool expectorant.
2	Passionflower	Anxiety and relieve muscle pain.
1	Red Root	Lymphatic drainage.
1	Licorice root	Moist, soothing/restorative to throat.

Other Suggestions

- Hot, freshly grated Ginger root tea for diaphoresis.
- Steam with Hyssop essential oil; antiseptic and aromatic to open airway.
- Vitamin C 2000 mg 3 × day or make your own pills (Box 20.2).
- Zinc picolinate 20 mg 2 × day
- Elderberry elixir (Box 20.3).

BOX 20.3 Sensational Fresh Elderberry Elixir

This easy and delicious antiviral elixir is an exemplary remedy to have on hand and quickly bring out for first signs of flu, hacking, and icky colds, sore throats, muscle aches, phlegm, and feeling off and run down. It kills viruses, stops inflammation, and gets the immune system going.

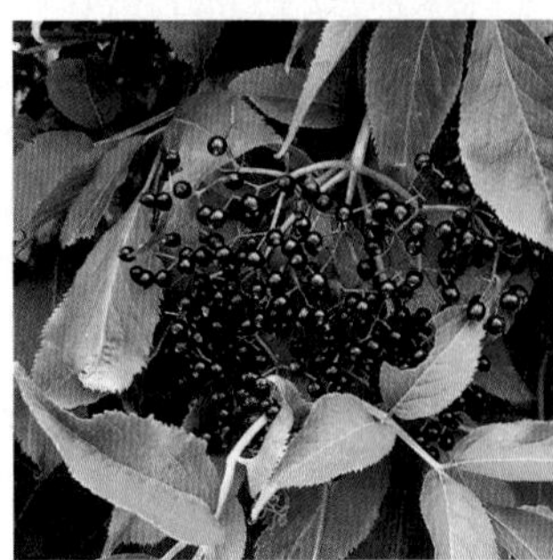

Sambucus nigra fruiting. Dark purple (blue) Elderberries are antiviral, excellent for onset of flu.

Berries, honey, and brandy do the magic when putting up this folk method elixir.

Directions

Fill pint canning jar to the brim with fresh Blue Elderberries. Pour in honey slowly to coat berries. Fill jar with brandy, stirring to release all bubbles. Cover jar with tight-fitting lid. Macerate 4–6 weeks. Strain. Store airtight in cool, dark place.

Dose

3–4 dropper squeezes every 1–2 hours. It works best if taken frequently at first sign of illness.

Prevention

2 dropper squeezes every 4 hours.[23]

Acute and Chronic Sinusitis

- *Definition: Acute **sinusitis*** is an inflammation and infection in the paranasal sinuses. Sinuses are supposed to drain into the nasal cavity. If they get blocked up for any reason, painful pressure builds up, and bacteria breeds in the moist environment. Blockages can easily lead to eye and ear infections. Causes may be hay fever; viral and bacterial infections; thick, nondraining mucus

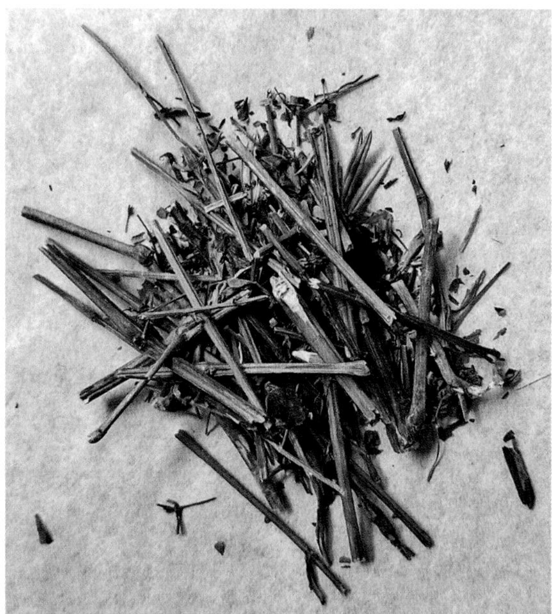

• **Fig. 20.9** Andrographis Chuan Xin Lian (Heart-Thread Lotus leaf) is particularly famous as an immune-stimulating, broad-spectrum, antibiofilm antiinfective for respiratory and intestinal damp heat. It is extremely cold, dry, and bitter, effective for sinus infections and others.

from colds, allergies, pollution, cigarette smoke, nasal, or dental procedures; high-altitude travel; underwater swimming; a deviated septum; or polyps blocking mucus passage to the nose.

- *Signs and symptoms.* Pressure, headache, and pain in the cheeks, teeth, eyes, or brows, depending on which sinuses are affected. Mucus ranging from clear (cold) to yellow or green (hot). Also, headache, malaise, sore throat, possible low-grade fever (99–100°F). If allergies are the cause, the usual histamine effects add to the grief, with runny eyes and rhinitis. Allergic triggers could be from hay fever, molds, pollution, animal hair/fur, and dust.
- *Allopathic treatment.* Antibiotics, antihistamines, steroid decongestant sprays, and allergy testing
- *General therapeutic principles.* (1) Broad-spectrum, cooling antimicrobials for infection. (2) Analgesics to decrease pain and pressure. (3) Lymphatic/fluid draining herbs and astringents to loosen mucus, dry damp. Steams. (4) If allergic, antihistamine herbs. (5) Respiratory restoratives. (6) Neti pot with salt water and Eucalyptus, Tea Tree, or Peppermint essential oil, or a nasal spray with same. (7) Lots of fluids to help loosen and drain mucus.

- *Definition: Chronic sinusitis.* Chronic cases come and go and linger for years with dull pain around eyes, sinuses, temple, possible toothache, or head pressure. Common causes are dysbiosis; depressed immunity; dietary allergens such as soy, dairy, gluten, peanuts, or citrus; and biofilm involvement.
  - *Therapeutic principles.* (1) Find cause. If it's dairy, substitute sheep or goat's milk, nondairy cheese, etc. If dysbiosis, go for fermented foods, Garlic, and Ginger. If allergenic, find allergen and normalize immune system. (2) Use broad-spectrum and antibiofilm antibiotics. (3) Decrease mucus with mucolytics. (4) Use demulcents, if dry. (5) Move fluids with lymphatic drainers, steams, and topical essential oils. (6) Respiratory restoratives are a must (Case History 20.4).

CASE HISTORY 20.4

Case History for Acute Sinusitis and Chronic Sinusitis Flare-Up

Part 1 Acute Sinusitis

Case History for Acute Sinusitis

S. Jim has head pressure, yellow nasal discharge, sore throat, and 100°F temperature. He is not surprised because it's springtime, and the wind is scattering Dandelion puffballs.

O. P Rapid. **T** Body red and dry. Temperature 100.8°F. Throat red on inspection.

A. Acute allergic sinusitis. Head Damp Heat.

P. *Specific therapeutic principles.* (1) Expel Heat. Dry Damp. (2) Cooling antimicrobials for infection. (3) Drain lymph to remove toxins and Damp and relieve pain/pressure. (5) Antihistamines to relieve allergic symptoms. (6) Mucolytics to liquefy secretions. (6) Demulcents to moisten and cool.

Herbal Formula and Dose for Acute Sinusitis. 4–5 mL every 1–2 hours.

Parts	Herbs	Rationale
3	*Xanthium* Cang Er Zi	Dry mucus/antihistamine/decongest sinuses/relieve pain.
2	*Andrographis* Chuan Xin Lian	Cold, sinus specific, antimicrobial, antibiofilm and immune stimulating.
2	Cleavers herb	Drain lymph.
2	Mullein leaf	Moisten, cool sore throat/relieve pain.
2	Elderberry	Relieve fever/dry nasal discharge.

Other Suggestions for Acute Sinusitis

- Sinus nasal spray of Goldenseal root and Myrrh resin (Box 20.4).

Part 2 Chronic Sinusitis Flare-Up

Case History for Chronic Sinusitis Flare-Up

S. Allison, age 36, had a cold, which was followed by her usual chronic sinusitis that has been on and off for 5 years. Experiencing dull pain and pressure around sinuses and nasal discharge. She has a history of allergic rhinitis with antihistamine and nasal steroid use. Lots of dairy in her diet, former smoker. This round of antibiotics did not work.

O. P. Slippery. **T** Coat moist, thick and white.

A. Chronic sinusitis per M.D. Head Wind Damp Cold.

P. *Specific therapeutic principles.* (1) Dry damp, expel cold. (2) Antimicrobials. (3) Lymphatic drainage to drain fluid/toxins. (4) Immunostimulants to support immune system. (5) Antihistamines for allergy and to dry mucus. (6) Respiratory restoratives, as it is a chronic problem.

Herbal Formula and Dose for Chronic Sinusitis Flare-Up. 4 mL every 2 hours.

Parts	Herbs	Rationale
3	*Echinacea angustifolia* root	Detox, immune support, antimicrobial/antibiofilm.
3	Eyebright herb	Antihistamine/antiinflammatory/drying.
2	Andrographis Chuan Xin Lian	Antimicrobial, antibiofilm.
2	Ganoderma Ling Zhi	Broad-spectrum antiallergic/Restorative.
2	Red Root	Drain lymphatics/dry damp.
1	Ginger root	Warming and drying to balance out colder herbs.

Other Suggestions for Chronic Sinusitis Flare-Up.

- Diet: No dairy and add lots of Garlic and Ginger.
- Discontinue antihistamines and steroid nasal spray per healthcare provider.
- Steam with Tea Tree essential oil to relieve pressure/pain/drain sinuses/antimicrobial.
- Sinus spray (Box 20.4)

• BOX 20.4 Nifty Sinus Spray

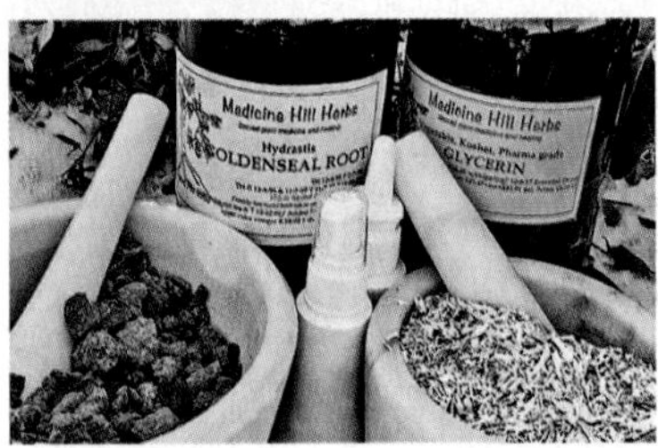

Myrrh resin, berberines Oregon Grape root, dried, and Goldenseal tinctured, with glycerin and nasal spray bottles for sinus spray.

Here's an effective and simple little snort to spray up the nose when there is pain, congestion, and mucus, as in sinusitis.[24]

Ingredients

- 15 drops *Hydrastis canadensis* tincture (Goldenseal or another berberine) for local broad-spectrum antibiotic action.
- 15 drops Myrrh resin tincture to stop discharge and dry up mucous damp.
- 1 tsp vegetable glycerin (no more; it's irritating).
- 2 oz water

Directions

Pour into 2-oz spray bottle for you and clients. Use as needed.

Note: Goldenseal and Myrrh is a classical pair for gum diseases. Spray in mouth for gingivitis and mouth sores. In such cases, leave out the sweet glycerin.

Acute and Chronic Bronchitis

- *Definition: Acute bronchitis* is inflammation of the bronchial tubes (***bronchitis***), usually viral, but sometimes bacterial. Often originates with a cold, flu, or sore throat, and spreads to the lungs. Generally lasts a week, and often confused with asthma or pneumonia.
  - *Signs and symptoms.* Green or yellow sputum, cough, and possible fever, lasting 2 to 3 weeks. Wind Heat.
  - *Allopathic treatment.* Antibiotics, steams, bronchodilators, and antipyretics, as needed.
- *Definition: Chronic bronchitis.* Constant irritation of the bronchi from pollution, smoke, bad nutrition, weak immune system, or infection where the lungs cannot expel the mucus because a deep layer covers the cilia. Coughing doesn't take care of it. This condition can go on for years, becoming chronic.
  - *Signs and symptoms.* Nonproductive cough with white sputum and throat irritation. Lasts 3 months or more, even years. Wind Cold.
  - *Allopathic treatment.* Symptomatically, use antibiotics, steams, bronchodilators, or oxygen, as needed.
- *General therapeutic principles.* Similar to those of acute or chronic. In acute cases, fever is more likely, in which case diaphoresis is necessary. In the chronic variety, there is greater emphasis on Lung yin and qi tonics. (1) Antimicrobials/antiinflammatories, usually antivirals, antibiofilms. (2) Expectorants and demulcents to cool and relax airway. (3) Treat cough with antitussives, stimulating expectorants, depending on type of cough. (4) Treat with diaphoretics if fever is present. (5) Lung tonics (Case History 20.5).

Hay Fever

- *Definition.* Hay fever is a common and annoying seasonal allergy caused by pollens that trigger IgG (Immunoglobulin G) antigen reactions that are not life-threatening reactions. It is considered a Type 1 hypersensitivity response. Other allergies of this type are caused by animal dander, common foods, pollution, dust, chemicals, and many more. In the case of hay fever, the antigens are from airborne pollen present in a wide variety of grasses and trees, not just Ragweed. They won't kill anyone, but they can trigger an asthma attack which *can* kill.
- *Signs and symptoms.* Runny nose (allergic rhinitis), stuffy nose, itchy eyes and nose, headache, and cough.
- *Allopathic treatment.* Symptomatic: antihistamines, steroids, inhalers, nasal sprays, and desensitization injections.
- *General therapeutic principles for immediate hay fever reactions.* (1) Take care of symptoms with antihistamines and antiinflammatories. (2) Provide pain relief, as needed with Bupleurum Chi Hu, Willow bark, or Ligusticum Gao Ben (Chinese Lovage root), specific for vertex headaches. (3) Balance immune system. (4) Remove person from allergen if possible. (5) For long-term prevention, begin Four-R Program (Case History 20.6).

Bronchial Asthma

Asthma is a condition marked by spasms in the bronchi causing narrowing of the airway and difficulty breathing. A chronic allergic reaction can develop over time and involves airway inflammation. It can be controlled but not cured by modern drug therapy. In worst cases, it causes life-threatening respiratory arrest. An *asthma attack* is the tip of the iceberg when an environmental trigger sets off a crisis. Triggers are numerous. They can be from allergens, particularly dust mites; diet (especially dairy, eggs, and nuts); royal jelly; temperature changes; smoking; poor digestion, manifesting as low HCl and acid reflux; viral infections, such as colds or sinusitis; hormonal changes; and of course, stress.[9]

- *Definition.* Bronchial asthma is marked by airway spasms and narrowing with increased swelling and mucus. It usually results from an allergic reaction or other forms of hypersensitivity. Exhaling with wheezing is often more difficult than inhalation.
- *Signs and symptoms.* Coughing, wheezing, shortness of breath, chest tightness, and anxiety.
- *Allopathic treatment.* Rescue inhalers to treat symptoms (Albuterol) and controller inhalers that prevent symptoms (steroids).
- *Herbal approach.* The herbal method is to use *two* formulas, one for symptomatic relief, and the other long-term.
  - *Symptomatic formula.* To have on hand to treat and relax the airway during an acute attack with large, frequent doses. Dose: 4 to 5 mL every 15 minutes to 1 hour. Very often, clients will be using an inhaler prescribed by their healthcare provider to control these frightening episodes.
  - *Long-term formula.* A remedy to treat the underlying issues on a long-term basis when acute period is over.
- *General therapeutic principles for bronchial asthma.* (1) Control bronchospasms with Ephedra Ma Huang (Ephedra stem), Lobelia herb, and/or Grindelia flower. (2) Use expectorant/antitussive/demulcents for cough: Bupleurum Chai Hu (Asian Buplever root), Elecampane root, Licorice root. (3) Control allergenic response with herbs such as Scutellaria Huang Qin (Baikal Skullcap root) or Ayurvedic herbs like *Tylophora asthmatica* (Indian Ipecac leaf) and *Albizia lebbeck* (East Indian Walnut bark, flower, and seed). (4) Control underlying infection with Andrographis Chuan Xin Lian (Heart-Thread Lotus leaf), Ginger root, Yarrow flower, or others. (5) Reduce inflammation with Boswellia Ru Xiang (Frankincense resin), Ginkgo leaf, or Turmeric root.
- *General therapeutic principles for underlying asthma issues.* Cause must be surmised or determined. Each issue (or group) would have its own formula and strategy. Underlying issues are to: (1) Eliminate any sinusitis or infection. (2) Treat digestion by increasing gastric acid with bitter Gentian root or

CASE HISTORY 20.5

Case History for Acute Bronchitis and Chronic Bronchitis

Part 1 Acute Bronchitis

Case History for Acute Bronchitis

S. Mary Jo had a head cold and now it's "in my lungs." Chest feels tight, she has an irritating cough with sticky green sputum, forehead feels hot, and she's chilled. This has been going on for 2 weeks.

O. P Rapid, wiry. **T** Body, red, coat yellow and dry. Temperature 99.5°F.

A. Tense Lung qi with heat. Probable acute bronchitis with fever, dry sticky green sputum.

P. *Specific therapeutic principles.* (1) Relax Lung qi, dispel heat. (2) Cooling antimicrobials. (3) Cool, relaxing expectorants to get out mucus. (4) Vasodilating diaphoretic to bring down fever. (5) Treat cough with cooling expectorants and antitussives. (6) Demulcent to moisten lungs/sputum.

Herbal Formula and Dose for Acute Bronchitis. 5 mL every 1–2 hours.

Parts	Herbs	Rationale
3	*Isatis* Ban Lan Gen	Broad-spectrum antimicrobial, detoxification and cooling.
3	Pleurisy root	Cools lungs/relaxing expectorant/relieves cough.
2	Yarrow flower	Diaphoretic/antimicrobial/expectorant.
2	Coltsfoot or White Horehound	Soothing expectorant/respiratory tonic/ demulcent.
2	Wild Cherry Bark	Relaxing expectorant/antitussive.
1	Licorice root	Soothing/relaxing demulcent/antiseptic.

Other Suggestions for Acute Bronchitis.

- Chest rub: Birch and Peppermint essential oils (in carrier oil). Alternately, use patent medicine Chinese White Flower Oil, which is high in menthols.
- Lots of fluids.
- Stay indoors, if cold or damp, congestion.

Part 2 Chronic Bronchitis

Case History for Chronic Bronchitis

S. Jackie's bronchitis comes and goes, and now it has returned. She has a tight chest, constant cough with white sputum, and fatigue.

O. P Weak. **T** Coat, white and wet. No fever.

A. Lung Phlegm Damp with Lung Qi Deficiency. Chronic Bronchitis.

P. *Specific therapeutic principles.* (1) Dry damp, Tonify Lung qi. (2) Warming antimicrobials. (3) Relieve cough with warming bronchodilators. (4) Restore lung qi. (5) Strengthen immune system.

Herbal Formula and Dose for Chronic Bronchitis. 3–4 mL every 2 hours.

Parts	Herbs	Rationale
4	Elecampane root	Antimicrobial/Tonify Lung Qi/expectorant/ relieve cough.
3	Red Clover blossom/ leaf	Detoxicant/respiratory relaxant/Lung tonic.
2	Thyme herb	Bronchodilator/warming/drying/relaxing.
2	Eleuthero Ci Wu Jia Siberian ginseng	Strengthen immunity/antiinfective.
1	Ginger root	Warming/Dry Damp, synergy to Elecampane.

Other Suggestions for Chronic Bronchitis.

- Chest rub as for acute bronchitis.
- When chronic episode resolved, begin long-term tonic with adaptogens to strengthen immune system and respiratory tonics to strengthen Lung Qi Deficiency.

CASE HISTORY 20.6

Case History for Acute Hay Fever

S. Jodie came back from walking her dog in the park and started sneezing. Her eyes were itchy, nose was stuffy with white mucus, and she had a headache.

O. P Superficial or shallow. **T** Red body, coat moist.

A. Acute allergic rhinitis. Damp heat in the head. Immediate allergy.

P. *Specific therapeutic principles.* (1) Dry damp, clear heat. (2) Treat symptoms with antihistamines, antiinflammatories. (3) Relieve head pain. (4) Immune balance. (5) When episode resolved, investigate long-term gut fix.

Herbal Formula and Dose. 4 mL every 15 min to ½ hour.

Part	Herbs	Rationale
3	*Ambrosia* spp.	Antihistamine, antiinflammatory.
3	Reishi mushroom Ling Zhi	Relieve allergy, immune regulation.
2	Goldenrod herb	Anticatarrhal/antiinflammatory/drying.
2	Eyebright herb	Antihistamine, antiinflammatory.
2	Bupleurum Chi Hu	Pain relief/muscle relaxant.

Other Suggestions

Red Flag. Anaphylactic shock is the result of a severe life-threatening IgE (immunoglobulin E) antigen reaction that blocks airway and breathing and can occur in seconds or minutes. This is not simple hay fever and a different scenario. Common triggers are from peanuts and other foods, bee stings (insect venom), and medications. An automatic ejector of epinephrine (EpiPen) is good to have if person is known to be allergic. Go to a hospital.

- Look for permanent solutions after symptoms abate or begin this approach right now.
- Supplements: Vitamin C 2000 mg 3 × day.

CASE HISTORY 20.7

Case History for Acute Asthma Attack

S. Joe has a history of bronchial asthma brought on by stress. He was anxious about an impeding public speaking engagement and suddenly suffered shortness of breath, wheezing and coughing, and intense anxiety. He began his breathing exercises. His prescription for Albuterol inhaler just ran out.

O. P Rapid and wiry. **T** Normal. In acute respiratory distress. Wheezing heard without stethoscope.

A. Asthma attack. Respiratory distress, anxiety. Lung Qi Constraint.

P. *Specific therapeutic principles.* (1) Relax Lung qi. (2) Control bronchospasms with relaxing expectorants/antitussives/demulcents. (3) Control allergic response. (4) Antimicrobial/antiinflammatories for any underlying infection. (5) Nervines for anxiety.

Herbal Formula and Dose. 4–5 mL every 15 min to 1 hour, as needed.

Part	Herbs	Rationale
4	Grindelia flower	Relaxing expectorant/antispasmodic/ bronchodilator.
4	Lobelia herb	Relaxing expectorant/tonic/ antispasmodic/nervine.
3	Scutellaria Huang Qin Baikal Skullcap	Antimicrobial/antiinflammatory/ antiallergic.
1	Licorice root	Soothing/demulcent/antiallergic/ antiinflammatory.

Other Suggestions

- Support client through deep breathing exercises.
- Relaxing Aniseed or Lavender essential oil. Inhale and apply to brow, sinus area, chest and shoulders.
- If allergic, remove suspected allergens.

Andrographis Chuan Xin Lian (Heart-Thread Lotus leaf) or by decreasing reflux with soothing Meadowsweet herb, Marshmallow root, or Licorice root. Remove offending foods, such as dairy. Use lots of antioxidants, including Green tea. (3) Reduce stress, anxiety, and tension with nervines like Valerian root, Passionflower, or St. John's Wort. (4) Immune balance with adaptogens. (5) Increase antioxidants with Ginkgo leaf, Rosemary leaf, or Turmeric root. (6) Use pulmonary tonics to build and heal tissue. (7) Implement breathing exercises (Case History 20.7).

Summary

A few methods to maintain a healthy respiratory system include good hydration, smoking cessation, breath work, aerobic exercise, and surrounding the environment with green plants.

The respiratory Materia Medica is extensive, and if used wisely, an herbalist could cultivate a friend for life. Expectorants address many types of coughs. Demulcents soothe, moisturize, and decrease inflammation. Spasmolytics stop persistent coughing, and antitussives calm coughs down. Anticatarrhals decrease copious mucus, and bronchodilators widen the airway.

Tonics or restoratives heal and strengthen weak airway tissue in chronic conditions. For immediate allergies, antihistamines lower the inflammatory response and stop symptoms. Diaphoretics cause sweating (a major therapeutic principle for herbalists). Lymphatic drainers eliminate excess fluids, toxins, and dry damp. They must be included in respiratory formulas for those reasons. Topical throat remedies make for good gargles.

Allergies are a common respiratory complaint. Permanent prevention involves returning to gut health with the Four-R program and addressing immune modulation and the adrenals. In Chinese Medicine, the concept of External Wind is basic to the Lungs. Wind can come in with heat, cold, and/or damp on board, and Lungs may be qi and yin deficient.

Review

Fill in the Blanks

(Answers in Appendix B.)

1. Name five herbal categories needed in a good cough syrup: ___, ___, ___, ___, ___.
2. Give five Chinese syndromes common to respiratory conditions. ___, ___, ___, ___, ___.
3. An example of a warming antimicrobial is ___; a cooling antimicrobial is ___; a very cold antimicrobial is ___.
4. Stimulating expectorants are ___ and ___ energetically. Four herbal examples are ___, ___, ___, ___. They are used in energetically ___ conditions.
5. Relaxing expectorants are varied and fall into many categories. These categories include: ___, ___, ___, ___.
6. List five examples of Western respiratory demulcents. ___, ___, ___, ___, ___. List three Chinese demulcents, including pinyin name. ___, ___, ___.
7. In External Wind Damp Heat, the Tongue body could be ___, the coat ___. The pulse is likely ___ and ___.
8. A Lung Yin tonic would be useful for a ___, ___ cough. Two herbal categories to use are ___ and ___.
9. A Lung Qi tonic would be useful for deficient diseases like ___ or ___. Herbal category is ___.
10. List four Therapeutic Principles for a sore throat with rationale. ___, ___, ___, ___.

Critical Concept Questions

(Answers for you to decide.)

1. Why is sweating a therapeutic principle in External Wind Cold conditions?
2. What are the benefits of lymphatic draining herbs and when are they used?
3. Why do you think seasonal allergies are so prevalent?
4. Discuss a protocol for chronic hay fever.
5. Your friend is having an asthma attack. What will you do?
6. Devise the herbs for your own cough syrup.
7. Discuss protocol differences for acute versus chronic bronchitis.
8. Liver decongestants are often included with lymphatic drainers. Why?
9. Why do we say that coughing is a symptom, not really a disease?
10. When should coughs be suppressed and when should they be encouraged?

References

1. Blaha, Michael Joseph. "Five Vaping Facts You Need to Know." Johns Hopkins Medicine. https://www.hopkinsmedicine.org/health/wellness-and-prevention/5-truths-you-need-to-know-about-vaping (accessed July 22, 2019).
2. "CDC: Vitamin E Likely Culprit in Vaping Cases." WebMD. https://www.webmd.com/mental-health/addiction/news/20191111/cdc-vitamin-e-likely-culprit-in-vaping-cases (accessed November 21, 2019).
3. "Vitamin E." National Institutes of Health. https://ods.od.nih.gov/factsheets/VitaminE-HealthProfessional/ (accessed November 21, 2019).
4. Greene, Michelle. "The Best Herbs to Help You Quit Smoking." Flowing Free, Holistic Health and Wellness. https://flowingfree.org/best-herbs-to-help-you-quit-smoking/ (accessed July 22, 2019).
5. "Top 5 Plants for Increasing Oxygen." Lung Institute. https://lunginstitute.com/blog/top-5-plants-for-increasing-oxygen/ (accessed July 22, 2019).
6. Myss, Caroline. *Anatomy of the Spirit* (New York, NY: Three Rivers Press, 1996).
7. "Lung Pattern Differentiation in Chinese Medicine." Sacred Lotus Chinese Medicine. https://www.sacredlotus.com/go/diagnosis-chinese-medicine/get/zang-fu-lung-patterns-tcm (accessed July 23, 2019).
8. Holmes, Peter. *Jade Remedies: A Chinese Herbal Reference for the West* (Boulder, CO: Snow Lotus, 1996).
9. Bone, Kerry and Simon Mills. *Principles and Practice of Phytotherapy* (London, UK: Elsevier, 2013).
10. Hoffman, David. *Medical Herbalism: The Science and Practice of Herbal Medicine* (Rochester, VT: Healing Arts, 2003).
11. Holmes, Peter. *Energetics of Western Herbs* (Boulder, CO: Snow Lotus, 2000).
12. "Cough Symptom Causes." Mayo Clinic. http://www.mayoclinic.org/symptoms/cough/basics/causes/sym-20050846 (accessed January 2019).

13. Lewis, Lisa. "Natural Treatments for Your Seasonal Allergies". Pure Life Clinic. https://purelifeclinic.com/uncategorized/spring-allergies-got-you-down/ (accessed February 8, 2021).
14. Romm, Aviva. "Kick Your Allergies for Good by Healing Your Gut." Facebook blog. https://avivaromm.com/3-steps-to-make-your-allergies-go-away-forever/ (accessed July 25, 2019).
15. Romm, Aviva. *Adrenal Thyroid Revolution* (New York, NY: Harper, 2017).
16. Buhner, Stephen Harrod. *Herbal Antibiotics* (North Adams, MA: Storey, 2012).
17. Buhner, Stephen Harrod. *Herbal Antivirals* (North Adams, MA: Storey, 2013).
18. "What You Should Know About Flu Antiviral Drugs." Centers for Disease Prevention. https://www.cdc.gov/flu/antivirals/whatyou should.htm (accessed January 2019).
19. Gladstar, Rosemary. *Herbal Recipes for Vibrant Health* (North Adams, MA: Storey, 2008).
20. Neverman, Laurie. "Herbal Cold and Cough Care." Common Sense Home. http://commonsensehome.com/cold-and-cough-care/ (accessed July 28, 2019).
21. de la Forêt, Rosalee. "Make Your Own Whole Food Vitamin C Pills with Herbs." https://learningherbs.com/remedies-recipes/whole-food-vitamin-c-pills/ (accessed November 25, 2019).
22. "What is Amla used for?" Gaia Herbs. https://www.gaiaherbs.com/blogs/herbs/amla (accessed November 25, 2019).
23. "How to Make an Elderberry Elixir." Holistic Health Herbalist. https://www.holistichealthherbalist.com/how-to-make-an-elder-berry-elixir/ (accessed July 24, 2019.)
24. Bergner, Paul. Class notes, American Herbalist Guild Symposium. Granby, CO, 2015.

21
Pediatrics

"Love is the best medicine."

—A mother's wisdom.

CHAPTER REVIEW

- Confidence for everybody is key.
- How children's bodies differ from adults. The gut, body composition and hepatic function.
- Chinese Medicine perspective on children.
- About children's herbs and childhood infections.
- Respiratory, eye and ear Materia Medica: Go-to herbs for respiratory, eye, and ear problems (restoratives, antimicrobials, immunostimulants, diaphoretics, expectorants, demulcents, mucolytics, antitussives). Diaphoretics for fever.
    - Common conditions for respiratory, eyes and ears with case histories: Common cold and influenza, acute otitis media (AOM), and chronic otitis media with effusion (OME). Eye infections.
- Digestive system Materia Medica: Carminatives, spasmolytics, antacids, demulcents, carminatives, appetite stimulants, antiemetics, sedatives, antidiarrheals and laxatives.
    - Common digestive system conditions with case histories: Colic, gastritis, constipation, diarrhea.
- Nervous system Materia Medica: Nervines and anxiolytics.
    - Common neurological system conditions with case histories: Insomnia and/or anxiety, and attention deficit hyperactivity disorder (ADHD).
- Skin Materia Medica: Antimicrobials, alteratives, diuretic detoxicants, and lymph drainers.
    - Common skin conditions with case histories: Childhood eczema or contact dermatitis, and cold sores (*Herpes simplex*).
- Safety with children's herbs. Ballpark children's dosages for mild herbs. Calculating children's doses.
- Routes of administration for infants and children. Compliance tips for yucky-tasting tinctures and teas.

KEY TERMS

Acute otitis media (AOM)
Attention deficit hyperactivity disorder (ADHD)
Alteratives
Anxiety
Anxiolytics
Chronic otitis media with effusion (OME)
Clark's rule
Cold sores
Colic
Common cold
Conjunctivitis
Constipation
Diaphoretics
Diarrhea
Diuretic detoxicants
Eczema
Fried's rule
Gastritis
Herpes Simplex Virus 1 (HSV 1)
Influenza
Nervines
Stye
Young's rule

Children respond amazingly well to herbs as long as their parents project confidence. The herbalist's job is to facilitate this situation and make it a win for both. A mother's willingness and success in giving her child herbs depends on her own relationship with health and healing. A trusted parent/herbalist interaction is needed. Along with that, the herbalist needs to have a basic understanding of differences between children and adult physiology and knowledge of a safe Materia Medica and its use. With those tools, a bright future is assured for pediatric herbology.

Herbal administration to kids is a bit different from administration to adults. Digestive systems and livers are immature at first. Dosages for children differ from adult dosages and must be adjusted, and safety issues are a factor. Furthermore, the tricky business of getting a kid to actually ingest a strange, weird-tasting substance is discussed. Time-tested methods from years of experience of mothers and herbalists are included. Last are case histories covering some common childhood illnesses and discussion of the importance of knowing when to refer out and when to recognize the red flags.

Confidence for Everybody Is Key

For most of human history, herbs were the only medicines given to anybody, children included. Herbal medicine has a long track record for safety in treating common childhood-related health concerns. Obviously, not all plants are safe, and strong toxic ones are not suitable for kids or adults. But long lists of botanicals have been used in traditional healing, so use them with confidence, faith, and common sense.

Babies and kids don't have opinions about any philosophy of medicine, allopathic or otherwise. If the parent is confident, the child will accept herbal medicine. If the herbalist is competent and enthusiastic, most parents will give herbal cures a try and end by feeling empowered. A parent is always the first line of defense against their baby's illness. We all know how stressful and scary it is for inexperienced moms and dads to witness their sick child. Happily, a great many childhood illnesses are uncomfortable but self-limiting. Children's bodies are naturally responsive. They recover quickly. Herbalists can play a role in many favorable outcomes.

Try things out on your own children or with a friend's to get a feel. Start with very simple applications, teas, or essential oils. If one formula doesn't work, go for another. Follow the dosage and formulas given later in this chapter and have fun. Confident herbalists and parents make for herbally initiated kids. Help them pass on the tradition.

How Children's Bodies Differ From Those of Adults

Kids are not just miniature people. Babies and children have faster metabolisms than adults. They absorb nutrients differently. Infants have immature livers with less bile and digestive enzymes in the first months of life. This immaturity translates into impaired fat digestion. Kids do not have fully developed gut flora until around 11 or 12 years old. These are just facts; not cause for alarm, but it *does* mean that pediatric herbalism is a bit of a specialty.

The Gut

- *The gut is sterile at birth.* Flora colonization begins during vaginal delivery from contact between mothers' perineal area and infants' mouths and stomachs. In a sterile C-section, this does not happen.[1]
- *Breastfeeding quickly builds up flora.* Hours after birth, an infant's gastric flora reflects mom's flora. Mother's milk introduces *bifidobacteria* that helps digestion, resulting in less colic and greater resistance to infection.[1]
- *Breastfeeding builds baby's immune system.* In addition to nutrients in the form of proteins, fats, and sugars, breast milk passes on the mother's antibodies that she makes when exposed to pathogens. They coat the infant's gut and block entry of infections that could otherwise cause illness.[2] Colostrum, the yellow-colored first milk, contains high levels of white blood cells that fight infection.
- *Weaning helps phytochemical absorption.* On the other hand, when baby weans and starts on food, the microflora changes. Newly introduced bacteria and their enzymes are able to break down plant glycosides and help in the absorption and activation of herbs.
- *Bile and pancreatic enzymes.* Neonates and infants have decreased bile and digestive enzymes in the first few months. Fat absorption is impaired.
- *A child's gut matures by 11 to 12* years old. By that time, the gastrointestinal (GI) tract resembles that of an adult, and absorption is similar.

Body Composition and Hepatic Function

- *Babies have more water and less fat.* At birth, infants have a greater percentage of body water and less body fat than older kids and adults. Therefore water-soluble herbs in teas work really well: Marshmallow and Licorice root, Cleavers herb, Dandelion root, Milky Oat, and California Poppy herb.
- *Infants have larger skin surface relative to body weight.* This means herbs are easily absorbed through the skin. Herbal baths are the ticket. They are easy to administer, and decoctions, infusions, and tinctures can be easily added to bath water.
- *Babies have decreased liver detoxification ability.* Their livers are smaller, and they have less Cytochrome P450 Phase I and II enzymes (Chapter 19). This is why infants are so prone to jaundice; the liver doesn't break down bilirubin efficiently. Young babies have a prolonged herb and drug half-life. Phytochemicals and drugs stay in the body longer. Therefore careful, lower doses are needed.
- *A child's liver matures by 3 years of age.*[3] After this age, we still need to be careful of dosage because of weight and body size, even though they are detoxifying efficiently at this point.

Chinese Medicine Perspective on Children

- *Spleen.* The Chinese Spleen translates as the Western digestive system. A fetus within the amniotic sac (in utero) gets its nourishment from mom and after birth from her breast milk. Digestive functions take a while to establish, and children have many problems in this department. *Spleen deficiency* is common. Carminatives for stomach aches and Spleen tonics are major herbal players.
- *Lung.* External pathogens easily invade children. The lung is the last tissue to develop in utero, and preemies sometimes have respiratory distress because of undeveloped *surfactant* needed to help the alveoli expand. Infant lungs are not mature enough to carry out their defensive function (wei qi). The skin, under control of the Chinese Lung, is an undeveloped barrier. Therefore *Lung deficiency* is common. Lung restoratives (tonics such as Mullein leaf, Red Clover flower, and Astragalus Huang Qi) and gentle skin alteratives (Burdock root, Yellow Dock root, and Dandelion root) are in order.
- *Kidney.* The Kidneys govern growth and development. Because children grow so rapidly, a strain is put on this system. *Kidney deficiency* can be helped with tonics like Goldenrod herb, Dandelion leaf, and Water Plantain leaf.
- *Liver.* At birth, the liver is very active but not fully developed. Infant livers are proportionally larger than adult livers. The liver releases toxins inherited in utero. This can result in

fevers, skin eruptions or hyperactivity, all of which are examples of *Liver excess*. Liver tonics are key: Dandelion root, Artichoke leaf, and Milk Thistle seed.

- *Heart*. The heart is the seat of emotions. Children express emotions loudly and with no filters, and they are highly susceptible to emotional stress. This is *Heart excess*. Nervines are frequently used in herbal pediatrics: Chamomile flower, Melissa herb, and Lavender herb. Heart tonics such as Hawthorn berry are useful.
- *Traditional physical assessment in children*. Pulse and tongue are not easily assessed in children under 3 years old. Some (but not all) Chinese herbalists use the technique of stretching the thumb edge of the second (index) finger and rubbing 40 to 50 times until the vein distends and becomes visible. The color, size, shape, and length are then examined.
  - *Vein distance*. The further up the finger (toward the nail) the vein is felt and seen, the more serious and more internal the problem. If the vein is visible only up to the knuckle (metacarpal phalangeal joint) the problem is external (such as external wind). If the vein is visible up to the next finger joint (proximal interphalangeal joint), there is a low fever. If it extends up to the next joint (distal interphalangeal joint), it is the deepest, most internal, and severe.

About Children's Herbs and Childhood Infections

For beginning herbalists, stick to tried-and-true pediatric herbs (Fig. 21.1). There are plenty of them, and you'll, perhaps, feel on safer ground. In reality, children can be given most of the same herbs as adults, just in lower doses.[1] That said, avoid powerful laxatives like Senna leaf or Rhubarb root, or strong-tasting bitter herbs like Wormwood herb or Goldenseal root. (Most kids will spit them out anyway, even if you get them in.) Anything potentially toxic such as Poke root or Aconite root should absolutely *not* be given.

Most children's illnesses are in the respiratory (viral) and GI areas. In general, kids need herbs with these tropisms, plus gentle nervines for calming and sleep issues. Herbs commonly appearing in children's remedies are Catnip herb for low-grade fevers, respiratory infections, headaches, indigestion, and sleep; Chamomile flower for colic and as a mild sedative; Echinacea root for colds; and Licorice root for lung congestion.[5] Other popular herbs that have historically been safely used for children include Melissa herb for calming and GI spasms; Dill seed, Fennel seed, Aniseed, and Caraway seeds as carminatives for tummy aches and colic; Burdock root and Calendula flower for skin irritations; Elderberry for colds and prevention; Eyebright herb and Chamomile herb for pink eye; and Marshmallow root and Slippery Elm bark to soothe stomachs. There are many more.

Children tend to get infections of the respiratory system, stomach, skin, and eyes. By using the pediatric Materia Medica, apply the same therapeutic principles as for adults:

- *Use antimicrobials*. Kill microorganisms with appropriate herbs, depending on condition. For respiratory, you might use Echinacea root, Calendula flower, Honeysuckle Jin Yin Hua (Honeysuckle flower bud), or Andrographis Chuan Xin Lian (Heart-Thread Lotus leaf). For dermatitis, you might choose Echinacea root, Huang Qin (Baikal Skullcap root), and Nettle herb; or select St. John's Wort for *Herpes* spp.
- *Use diaphoretics*, such as Yarrow flower or Elder flower or Peppermint leaf if fever is present.
- *Use mucolytics to loosen and expel any phlegm*. Try Grindelia flower or White Horehound herb.
- *Use demulcents* to moisturize and cool mucous membranes with Marshmallow root or Slippery Elm bark.
- *Use detoxicants*. Release toxins with Milk Thistle seed for the liver or the docks for the skin.
- *Use immunostimulants*. It is very important to support the immune system; some options are *Echinacea purpurea*, *E. angustifolia* root, or Andrographis Chuan Xin Lian (Heart-Thread Lotus leaf).
- *Use carminatives and relaxing nervines*. Address any other symptoms with digestion-enhancing carminatives, such as Dill seed or Fennel seed, or calming nervines such as Chamomile flower.
- *Fix gut for stomach ailments*. Always consider diet and gut flora.
- *Use alteratives to clear up skin infections*. ***Alteratives*** (sometimes called *depuratives*) improve cellular nutrition and lymphatic drainage through detoxification. Use them internally and externally; some examples are Calendula flower, Nettle herb, or Cleavers herb. You may need to address the diet.

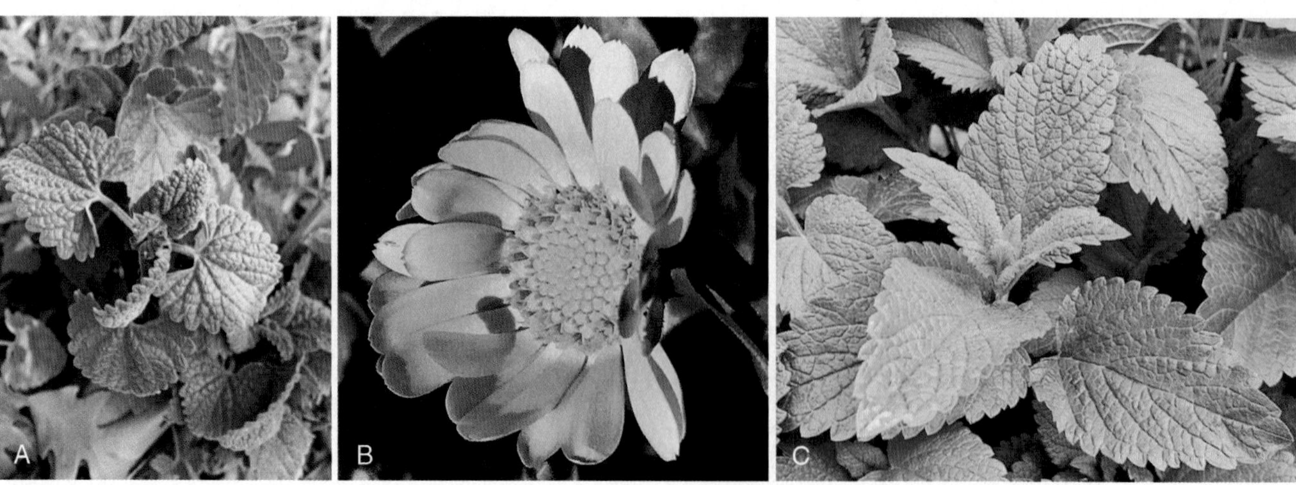

• **Fig. 21.1** Herbs commonly used for children: A, Catnip, hardy late November plant shown, is calming, lowers fever, helps digestion; B, Calendula flower for skin irritations; C, shiny leaves of Lemon Balm/Melissa are uplifting, calming, and antiviral.

Respiratory, Eye, and Ear Materia Medica

Most respiratory infections are viral and spread like wildfire in kids who lack mature immunity, such as those exposed to germs for the first time ever in preschool and kindergarten settings. The child will build up antibodies after recovering from the exposure, not before. Children's respiratory herbs are similar to the adult ones. Just use the milder varieties.

Important immune modulators like Andrographis herb Chuan Lian (Heart-Thread Lotus leaf), *Echinacea* spp. root, and Astragalus root Huang Qi are basic when treating infection. Use antimicrobials, such as Echinacea root, Lonicera Jin Yin Hua (Honeysuckle flower), Forsythia Lian Qiao (Forsythia valve), Andrographis Chuan Lian (Heart-Thread Lotus leaf), Garlic bulb, and Eucalyptus and Tea Tree essential oils. Antitussives include Hops flower, Wild Cherry bark, Licorice root. For allergies, there is Nettle herb and Scutellaria Huang Qin (Baikal Skullcap root).

A major childhood challenge is retained airway secretions, a buildup of mucus caused by a weak cough and impaired cilia. Therefore mucolytics must be used: Aniseed, Fennel seed, Thyme herb, Eyebright herb, Cinnamon bark. Important expectorants include White Horehound herb and Grindelia flower. Demulcents that soothe and cool the lungs are good: Mullein leaf, Slippery Elm bark, or Irish Moss thallus. Spasmolytics are needed to relax the bronchi and bronchioles: Coleus herb, Licorice root, and our friend, Grindelia's milky flower bud. Anticatarrhals to dry upper-respiratory secretions include: Eyebright herb, Peppermint leaf, Elderberry, or Plantain leaf. For lower respiratory tract, use Mullein or Plantain leaf as moisturizers, or strong and bitter Garden Sage leaf to dry up secretions. Honey and Licorice root help the medicine go down; in addition, honey (for children older than 1 year of age) is antimicrobial, and Licorice is antiviral.

Go-To Herbs for Respiratory, Eye, and Ear Problems

These are special choices for use with children but are also used in adult herbalism. They run the gamut with categories already mentioned in Chapter 20: expectorants, demulcents, antitussives, antimicrobials, mucolytics, and antispasmodics (Table 21.1).

Diaphoretics

Children are warm by nature, and they run on the hot side, so generally the cooler vasodilating ***diaphoretics*** are in order. Sweating is a must to bring down a fever and release toxins, because heat can

TABLE 21.1 Children's Favorites for Respiratory, Eye, and Ear Problems

Herbs	Notes
Andrographis paniculata Chuan Lian (Heart-thread Lotus leaf)	Antiinfective and immunostimulant. Clears damp heat and fire toxins.
Astragalus membranaceus Huang Qi (Astragalus root)	Immune-enhancing in chronic stages, not acute.
Calendula officinalis (Calendula flower)	Antiviral and antifungal. In first aid creams. Helps conjunctivitis.
Tussilago farfara (Coltsfoot herb)	Expectorant for coughing and wheezing.
Echinacea spp. (Echinacea root)	Supports immunity, stops infection, detoxes. Does well as a glycerin extract. Helps conjunctivitis.
Sambucus nigra (Elderberry)	Classic for lowering fever and early-onset colds.
Grindelia robusta (Gumweed flower)	Cool, moist expectorant, bronchodilator, draining diuretic, and relaxant. For coughing, wheezing, asthma, and viscous phlegm.
Marrubium vulgaris (White Horehound herb)	No brainer expectorant in a cough syrup.
Hyssopus officinalis (Hyssop herb)	Expectorant. Also, for tummy aches.
Glycyrrhiza glabra or *G. uralensis* Gan Cao Western and Chinese Licorice root are interchangeable.	Multipurpose to soothe airway, expectorant, antimicrobial. Also, for tummy aches. A sweetener. Suck on sweet licorice sticks.
Lonicera japonica Jin Yin Hua (Honeysuckle flower) *Forsythia suspensa* Lian Qiao (Forsythia valve)	The gentle flowers are broad-spectrum antimicrobials for External Wind Heat.
Althaea officinalis (Marshmallow root)	Moist, cool, sweet, soothing demulcent for airway and stomach. Relieves coughing. Cold infusion is best.
Verbascum thapsus (Mullein leaf and flower)	Leaves are a cool, moist, restoring expectorant to lungs or spasmodic asthma. The flowers for ear infections.

(*Continued*)

TABLE 21.1 Children's Favorites for Respiratory, Eye, and Ear Problems—cont'd

Herbs	Notes
Rosa gallica (Rose hips fruit)	Good way to slip in some vitamin C and quite tasty.
Salvia officinalis (Garden Sage leaf)	Cooling. Dries up drippy mucus and mother's milk. Good gargle, if they'll do it.
Mentha spicata (Spearmint leaf) Also use in essential oil form for steams.	Yummy aromatic, promotes sweating, cooling, dispels wind heat, and soothes stomach.
Thymus vulgaris (Thyme herb)	Expectorant, excellent drier-upper.
Usnea spp. (Old Man's Beard thallus)	For wind heat. Strep throat specific.
Prunus serotina (Wild Cherry bark)	Relaxant to relieve wheezing and coughing.
Anemopsis californica (Yerba Mansa root)	Stops discharge, reduces infection. For coughs, bronchitis, and laryngitis.
Euphrasia officinalis (Eyebright herb) *Stellaria media* (Chickweed herb)	Both for conjunctivitis and eye infections.

be transferred from the body core via blood to the skin through vasodilation. Some tried-and-true children's diaphoretics include Yarrow flower, Elderberry flower, Catnip herb, Peppermint herb, and Lemon Balm leaf (Table 21.2).

Fevers

Temperature elevation is a tricky business with no strict rules in children. Children and infants tend to run higher fevers than adults do. Temps can vary by 2°F just from emotional activity, stress, exercise, or being bundled in warm clothing.[6] Usually, a fever is a reaction to an acute viral or bacterial infection and is a sign the body is fighting infection by increasing white blood cells. Fevers can also be caused by dehydration, overexertion, bug bites, and allergic reactions. If a fever is brought down and the child looks and feels better, hooray. If they still look and feel sick, even with a lowered temperature, it's something else. Look elsewhere. Here are some fever guidelines (Box 21.1).

- *High fevers in children are unpredictable.* In kids, a mild head cold could produce a fever of 105°F, whereas something serious, like bacterial pneumonia, might result only in a temperature of 100°F.
- *Fever in infants.* An infant's temperature-control mechanisms are immature. The best thing to do is observe to see how sick the infant seems. Sometimes bringing down a fever helps a child or infant just plain feel better.
- *Infantile seizures.* The dangers of a high fever are dehydration and rarely, but distressingly, infantile seizures. Infantile febrile seizures do *not* lead to epilepsy, nor do they cause permanent brain damage. However, if a seizure occurs, the child will probably have another.[6]

• BOX 21.1 Fever Guidelines in Children

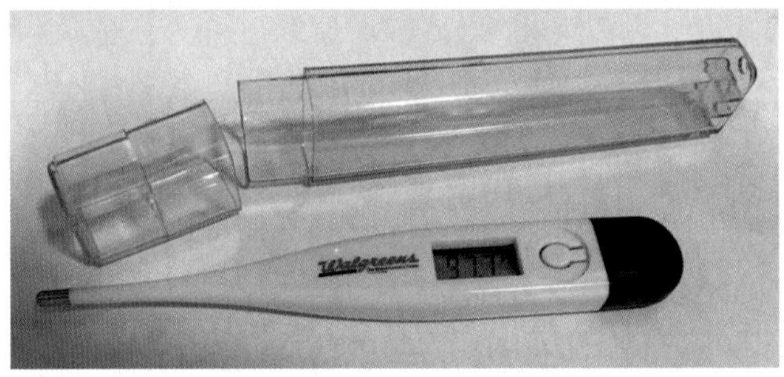

A digital thermometer can be used rectally in infants, or orally in older children.

When to refer out to a pediatrician.[6]

- Fevers in those under 6 months of age.
- Between 6 months and 3 years old, with temperatures of 102°F or higher.
- Over 3 years old with fever of 104°F or higher that does not respond to normal control methods within 4 hours.
- No matter the age, if listless, lethargic, unusually sleepy, in pain, extremely irritable, stiff neck, difficulty breathing, significant decrease in urine output, or if the child just doesn't seem right. Trust your intuition.

Common Conditions for Respiratory, Eye, and Ear Problems

Common Cold and Influenza

Babies and children are especially prone to respiratory infections because the system does not reach full maturity until around 6 years of age. There are many factors involved. The number of alveoli increases with age; kids have a higher basal metabolic rate requiring more oxygen. Infants are nose breathers until they are 3 or 4 months old, and their immune systems, which protect against *outside pernicious influences* (pathogens), are still immature.[8] The best approach to respiratory problems is prevention. Use immune enhancing herbs, such as Echinacea root (Fig. 21.2) or Andrographis Chuan Xin Lian (Heart-Thread Lotus leaf).

TABLE 21.2 Diaphoretic Herbs for Kids

Herbs	Notes
Nepeta cataria Catnip leaf	A primary children's herb. Cool, dry, pungent, aromatic, cool peripheral vasodilator for wind heat conditions with fever.
Achillea millefolium Yarrow flower	Bitter, cool, dry, stimulating diuretic. A peripheral vasodilator for wind heat.
Sambucus nigra Elderberry and flower	Cool, dry, pungent, aromatic peripheral vasodilator for wind heat, cold/flu onset with fever.
Allium sativa Garlic bulb	Diaphoretic, antimicrobial, immunostimulant. Garlic lemonade is great (Box 21.2).
Zingiber officinalis Ginger rhizome	Stimulates circulation, diaphoretic. Good choice for a combined stomachache, nausea. Put in a tea with lots of honey.
Melissa officinalis Lemon Balm leaf	Diaphoretic, antipyretic, and calming.
Tilia cordata Linden flower	Reduces fever, irritability. For external wind heat.
Mentha spp. The Mints	Dispels wind heat, fever, and infection, settles stomach.

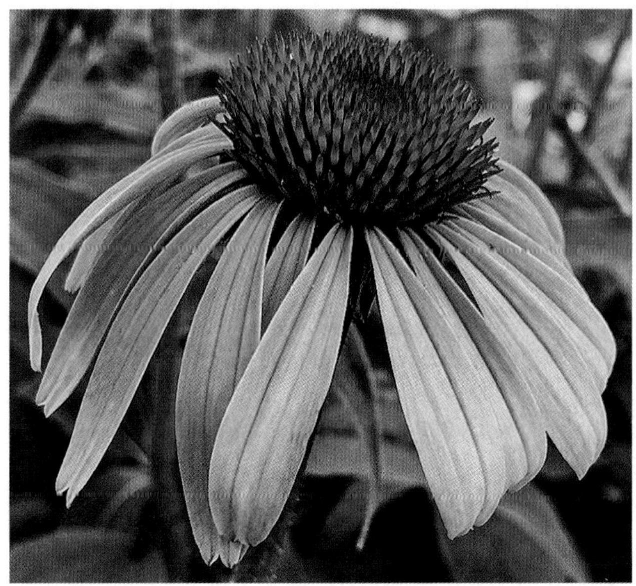

• **Fig. 21.2** *Echinacea purpurea* (Purple Coneflower). The roots and flower cones of this species, and more traditionally, the stronger *E. angustifolia*, are immune-enhancing and effective against local and systemic viral and bacterial infections.

- *Definitions.*
  - *Common cold.* The ***common cold*** is an acute viral infection, causing inflammation of the upper-respiratory tract, the most common infectious disease in children. Benign and self-limiting but can lead to secondary bacterial infections. More than 100 viruses can cause a cold, and in children can lead to acute otitis media (AOM). It is communicable for 2 to 3 days after onset and spreads by airborne droplet, hand-to-hand contact, or touching contaminated objects.
  - *Flu.* ***Influenza*** is a respiratory viral infection caused by influenza type A or B. Sometimes it is difficult to know the difference between a cold and flu, but a flu can be much more serious and even result in death.
- *Signs and symptoms.*
  - *Common cold.* Sore throat, nasal congestion, headache, watery eyes, and fever in kids (rarely in adults).
  - *Influenza.* Muscle pain, high temperature, extreme fatigue, and a severe cough are typical of the flu. As with adults, children can be quite sick. Temp can reach up to 105°F. There are headaches, body aches, vomiting, belly pain, extreme tiredness, and sore throat.
- *Allopathic treatment.* Tylenol, cough syrups, fluids, and rest. Antibiotics, used for bacterial infections, do not cure a cold or a flu because they are viral infections. A yearly flu vaccine is given as a shot or nasally. Tamiflu, an antiviral drug, may help lessen symptoms.
- *General therapeutic principle for colds and flu.* They are very similar. Cover the general therapeutic principles and add in anything else symptomatically. If acute, treat by symptoms. If chronic or recurring, you must use tonics and immunostimulants. Focus on removing stress.
  - (1) Kill viruses with Echinacea root, Calendula flower, or Lonicera Jin Yin Hua (Honeysuckle flower). (2) Diaphoretics: Yarrow flower, Elderberry flower, or Peppermint leaf, if fever present. (3) Loosen and expel any mucus with Grindelia flower bud or White Horehound herb. (4) Moisturize and

CASE HISTORY 21.1

Case History for Common Cold

S. Lisa has no temperature, but seems very uncomfortable, cries and points to head and stomach, cranky and tired. Cries when she eats, clear rhinitis, unproductive cough, stomachache. She is 2½ years old and weighs 28 lb.
O. Index finger vein is pinkish red when rubbed, extending a little past knuckle.
A. Wind Cold turning to Wind Heat. Viral respiratory infection.
P. *Specific therapeutic principles.* (1) Diaphoretics. (2) Antiviral, dispel wind heat. (3) Expectorants. (4) Immunostimulant. (5) Moisturizeld mucous membranes. (6) Treat stomach and headache.

Herbal Formula and Dose.
Adult Dose: 4 mL every 2 hours.
Child's Dose: 0.75 mL every 2 hours per Clark's rule (Box 21.6).

Parts	Herbs	Rationale
3	Lonicera Jin Yin Hua	Clear wind heat/cold, fight virus.
2	*Echinacea angustifolia*	Immune support, fight virus detox.
2	Gumweed flower bud	Decongestant/expectorant.
2	Chamomile flower	Ease stomachache and anxiety/headache.
2	Irish Moss thallus	Protect/moisten mucous membranes.
1	Licorice root	Sweeten, soothe airway/stomach, antimicrobial, expectorant.

Other suggestions

Red Flag. Call a doctor if a fever persists after 3 days, if a cold does not clear up in 3 weeks, or the child develops a rash. Respiratory distress could indicate pneumonia.

- Fluids and rest.
- Avoid dairy because it promotes formation of mucus.
- Garlic lemonade.
- Have child suck on Licorice stick lollipops (Box 21.2).

• BOX 21.2 Garlic Lemonade and Licorice Stick Lollipops

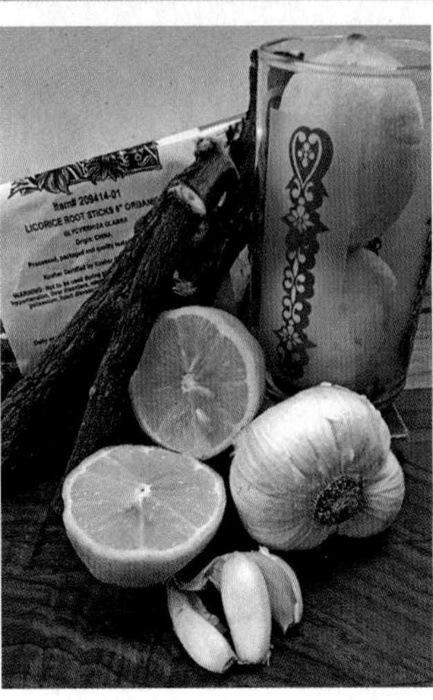

Garlic and lemons for lemonade, and Licorice root sticks for lollipops.

Garlic Lemonade

A yummy way to sweat out a fever. Most kids will merrily comply. Use freely during a cold or flu episode to keep them hydrated.

- **Directions**. Steep 3–4 cloves of chopped raw Garlic in 1 quart of just boiled water. Add lemon and honey to taste if older than 1 year old, or maple syrup if younger. Drink often.

Licorice Stick Lollipops[8]

These are fun to suck on to relieve a sore inflamed throat. Sweet Licorice sticks soothe and moisturize the respiratory mucosa of sick, miserable kids.

- **Directions**. Simmer 2 cups of water, 2 tablespoons honey (children over a year old) or maple syrup (any age), and a few long pieces of whole Licorice root sticks for 5 minutes. Cool sticks and give child one to suck on in am and pm.

cool mucous membranes with Marshmallow root. (5) Release liver toxins with Milk Thistle seed. (6) Immune support. *Echinacea purpurea* or *E. angustifolia* root. (7) Address other symptoms for ear and eye problems. (8) Muscle relaxant for muscle aches, such as Black Cohosh root or Chamomile flower (Case Histories 21.1 and 21.2).

Acute Otitis Media (AOM)

Ear and respiratory infections go hand in hand. Babies and children have short, straight eustachian tubes that provide a direct viral pathway from the throat to the ear, whereas adult tubes are curved, giving them ear infections less frequently. As long as the ear drum is intact, a fresh Garlic and Mullein flower sun oil is used externally (Box 21.3).

- *Definition.* ***Acute otitis media (AOM)*** is a painful middle-ear inflammation and bacterial infection with pus behind the eardrum.
- *Signs and symptoms.* Severe ear pain, sometimes *purulent* (containing or forming pus), discharge from ears, hearing loss, vertigo, tinnitus, and fever. Childhood signs are increased crying, pulling at ear, poor sleep, decreased appetite, and fever.
- *Allopathic treatment.* Antibiotics. If ear drum is bulging, a myringotomy is performed, which involves tube placement and drainage of the tympanic membrane (eardrum).
- *General therapeutic principles.* (1) Antimicrobials to treat infection. (2) Lymphatic drainers to decongest upper-respiratory tract, like Red Root, Echinacea root, and Yellow Dock root. (3) Decongestants to treat mucus, as in Coltsfoot or Plantain leaf. (4) Topical ear oil of Garlic and Mullein flower if eardrum is intact. This treats externally and absorbs through the eardrum (Case History 21.3).

Chronic Otitis Media with Effusion

- *Definition.* ***Chronic otitis media with effusion (OME)*** is a series of recurrent chronic inflammations of the middle ear with fluid and pressure building up, not necessarily pus. It usually has an allergic or viral component. Can occur after AOM, and it often returns. Common allergens are cow's milk (most frequent because it thickens mucus), eggs, wheat, corn, and pet dander.
- *Signs and symptoms.* Nonpurulent, watery fluid behind the middle eardrum that may be either mucoid or *serous* (blood tinged). Does not usually hurt or involve a fever. Because of the pressure, OME could cause mild, temporary hearing loss, which can lead to slow speech and learning development and can cause meningitis.
- *Allopathic treatment.* Oral antibiotics, and antibiotic ear drops, Tylenol, steroids, antihistamines. *Myringotomy*, one of the

CASE HISTORY 21.2

Case History for Influenza

S. Susie is 15 months old, 22 lb. She has runny nose with green secretions, dry hacking cough, temperature of 103.5°F. She refused breakfast (it probably hurts to swallow); her face is flushed, and she is very fussy. Throat was red when inspected with flashlight. She just wants to sleep. Her muscles seem to ache.
O. Index finger vein pink when rubbed, extending to the second joint.
A. Wind Heat. Probable flu and seems quite sick.
P. *Specific therapeutic principles.* (1) Diaphoretics for fever. (2) Cooling antivirals. (3) Settle stomach with carminatives. (4) Help expectorate and stop cough. (5) Moisturize mucous membranes. (6) Stimulate immune system. (7) Muscle and nervous relaxant.

Herbal Formula and Dose.
Adult Dose: 5 mL every 1–2 hours.
Child's Dose: 0.5 mL every 1–2 hours per Fried's rule (Box 21.6).

Parts	Herbs	Rationale
3	Echinacea root or Andrographis Chuan Xin Lian	Cool antiviral/Immune stimulant.
2	Elderberry flower	Diaphoretic to reduce fever, antiviral.
2	Platycodon Jie Geng or White Horehound	Mucolytic, expectorant.
2	Black Cohosh root	Relieve muscle pain and calming.
1	Catnip herb	Cool diaphoretic for fever, calming.
1	Slippery Elm bark	Soothe throat and tummy.
1	Fennel seed	Carminative and expectorant.
1	Licorice root	Sweeten, soothe airway/stomach, antimicrobial. Expectorant.

Other suggestions

Red Flags. Very high fever, seizures, changes in level of consciousness, mental function (could be encephalitis), any respiratory distress manifested as increased breathing rate, gasping, wheezing, nostril-flaring, bluish color.

- Fluids and rest.
- Garlic lemonade and Licorice root stick lollipops (Box 21.2).
- Lavender essential oil, diluted, to belly.
- Cooling bath.

• BOX 21.3 Fresh Garlic and Mullein Flower Sun Oil (A Summer Project)

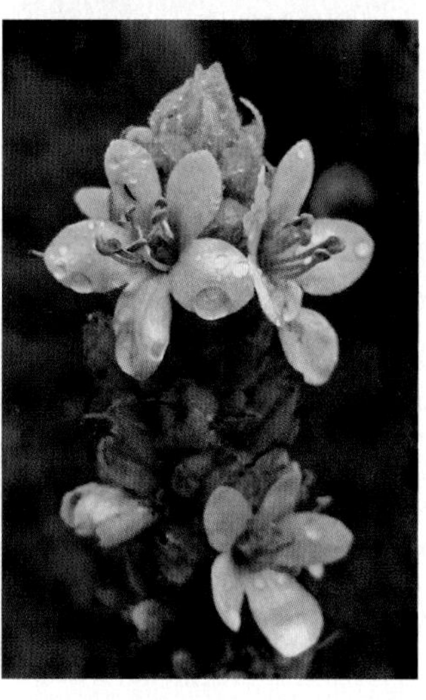

Verbascum thapsus (Mullein flower). The cheerful yellow flowers on the plant's long spike are used for earaches and discharges. You will need to collect a large amount because they are very tiny.

This good outer ear oil can be stashed in the apothecary fridge for use, as needed. Childhood or adult painful ear inflammation and infections respond well. It also softens ear wax (cerumen). The oil absorbs through the tympanic membrane to the middle ear.

Directions

Collect lots of Mullein flowers. Mullein grows everywhere in dry, disturbed ground. Flowers are plentiful in summer and fall, a labor of love to collect, and hard to purchase. Chop fresh Garlic cloves. Mix herbs together, half and half. Pack herbs tightly into an *absolutely dry* ½ pint or smaller Mason jar to very top. Pour in olive oil, so there is no air space between herbs, oil, and underside of lid. Stir with chopstick to expel air bubbles.

Place jar outside in shade on pie tin (it will overflow a bit). Add more oil, as needed. Let it macerate a few weeks, watching as it turns to a lovely yellow green. Strain through knee-high nylon stocking, hooked around top of jar. Squeeze out the oil. Discard oily stocking. Store oil in refrigerator in dark glass Boston round. Change to smaller jar as oil is used up, to decrease air space under lid.

Dose

Safe for children 2 years and older. Use oil at room temperature. Squeeze 3 or 4 drops into ear with pipette. Massage outer ear and around base. *Lightly* place small wad of cotton or tissue at ear opening to catch any excess drips. Repeat every hour, as needed. You'll smell like Italian dressing.

General guidelines

Before use, warm up oil by placing bottle in hot water. Test temperature on wrist. Dose: 3–5 drops in ear every 6 hours. Lightly place a little twist of cotton ball just inside ear opening to soak up drips. (When sleeping, use an old pillowcase.)

Caution: Contraindicated for perforated ear drum (tympanic membrane). Short of visual inspection with an otoscope, signs and symptoms include ear pain that may subside quickly because pressure is released; clear, pus-filled, or bloody drainage; hearing loss; ringing in the ear (tinnitus); spinning sensation (vertigo) with or without nausea or vomiting.

most common reasons for childhood surgery, in which a tube is placed in ear to drain fluid.[6]

- *General therapeutic principles.* (1) Broad-spectrum antivirals. (2) Lymphatic drainers to remove pressure. (3) Immunostimulants. (4) Investigate and remove any allergens, especially cow's milk. In children, goat milk is a good substitute. (4) External ear oil if no perforation (Case History 21.4).

Eye Infections

Kids and babies often get eye infections. Warm compresses and external washes are the best approaches. Application of a wash takes a little practice (Box 21.4).

- *Conjunctivitis (pinkeye).* ***Conjunctivitis*** is a highly contagious viral infection that affects the *conjunctiva*, the thin transparent layer of tissue lining the inner surface of the eyelid and the sclera. It shows up as a swollen, red, and watery eye with an itchy, sticky yellow-green discharge that generally clears up on its own in a week or so.
- *A **stye*** is a bacterially infected, pus-filled oil gland present at the eyelash base. Styes are not contagious but are irritating, itchy, and painful.

CASE HISTORY 21.3

Case History for Acute Otitis Media (AOM)

S. Amelia is 3½ years old and has been tugging and hitting her right ear. "Hurts," she cries. Reports running a fever of 101.1°F. She weighs 32 lb.

O. Temperature 101.3°F when taken by herbalist. Ears reddened on inside.

A. Damp Heat. Probable ear infection. Index finger vein pinkish extending to middle knuckle.

P. *Specific therapeutic principles.* (1) Clear infection with cold, dry antiinfectives. (2) Lymphatic drainage to help drain bacteria. (3) Cool/bring down fever. (4) Stress relief and sleeping help.

Herbal Formula and Dose.
Adult Dose: 5 mL every 1–2 hours.
Child's Dose: 1 mL every 1–2 hours per Clark's Rule (Box 21.6).

Parts	Herbs	Rationale
3	*Echinacea* spp.	Clear infection, damp heat, drain toxins, immunostimulant.
3	Yellow dock root	Lymphatic drainage and detoxify.
2	Elderberry flower	Cool fever, fight infection, immunostimulant.
3	Lemon balm herb	Calm and help sleep, reduces fever.
1	Licorice root	Soothe membranes and improve taste.

Other suggestions

Red Flags for ear infections, acute or chronic, include (1) Severe pain with ear drainage which could mean a perforated ear drum. (2) Hearing loss, severe headache, stiff neck, and/or lethargy could indicate meningitis.[8]

- Cool bath with Lavender essential oil.
- Garlic and Mullein ear oil (Box 21.4). If not tolerated use a warm compress.
- No air travel. Pressure from plane cabin can make AOM worse.
- Cranial sacral and chiropractic work.

CASE HISTORY 21.4

Case History for Chronic Otitis Media with Effusion (OME)

S. Three-year-old and 35 lb. Daniel is finally recovering from an acute cold after 3 weeks. Now he tugs at his ears and cries. They are plugged up and he seems dizzy. No discharge, no fever. Was bottle fed with a soy-based formula and now drinks lots of milk and loves cheese and ice cream.

O. Index finger vein bluish when rubbed. Hard to see.

A. Head Damp. Probable otitis media with effusion (OME).

P. *Specific therapeutic principles.* (1) Use cooling broad-spectrum antivirals. (2) Drain damp with lymphatic drainage and diuretics. (3) Use immunostimulants. (4) Treat pain and anxiety. (5) Apply external ear oil because there is no drainage (indicating intact ear drum).

Herbal Formula and Dose.
Adult Dose: 5 mL every 1–2 hour.
Child's Dose: 1 mL every 1–2 hours per Clark's rule (Box 21.6).

Parts	Herbs	Rationale
3	*Echinacea angustifolia*	Immunomodulating, antiallergic, draining, pain relief.
3	Cleavers herb	Lymphatic drainage. Relieves pressure and pain.
2	Goldenrod herb	Drains fluid, antiinflammatory, and diuretic.
2	Plantain leaf	Decongestant, clears toxic heat from ear, antiallergenic.
2	Chamomile flower	For pain and anxiety.

Other suggestions

- *Diet.* Remove cow's milk from diet. Substitute goat's milk (a hypoallergenic dairy product that supplies vital nutrients and is close in structure to breast milk) and suggest nondairy substitutes as well, like sorbet, nut milks, coconut milk/frozen dessert.
- Decrease other common allergen exposure.
- *Supplements.* Vitamin C for immune support.
- Topical. Garlic bulb and Mullein flower ear oil (Box 21.4) to decrease infection/inflammation.
- Cranial sacral and/or chiropractic body work.

Digestive Materia Medica

Gastric upsets are a frequent occurrence, especially if a child is overwhelmed, nervous, or tired. The gut-brain reaction kicking in. Babies get colicky (Case History 21.5). Tummy problems can be caused by gastritis, constipation, and diarrhea; and by hunger, full bladder, stress, excitement, or food sensitivities. Many digestive herbs double as nervines, the perfect double-duty combination. Some herbal favorites are: Catnip leaf and Chamomile flower for aches and colic; Slippery Elm bark or Psyllium fiber for constipation; Raspberry leaf and Geranium root for diarrhea; and the carminatives, like Fennel seed and Dill seed or Citrus Chen Pi (Ripe Tangerine rind) for indigestion (Stuck Stomach Qi).

Red flags for stomach problems in children include weight loss, growth retardation, GI blood loss, frequent vomiting, chronic diarrhea, constant upper-right or lower abdominal pain, or persistent fever. If any of these are present, a referral is in order. For persistent diarrhea, be aware of dehydration. IV fluids might be needed.

Otherwise, for the vast majority of tummy aches, choose among the herbal categories in this list that will cover most gastric conditions (Table 21.3).

- *Spasmolytics.* Relieve spasms with Chamomile flower, Lemon balm, or Peppermint herb.
- *Antacids.* Meadowsweet herb and Chickweed herb reduce gastric irritation from increased HCl and help build gut flora.
- *Demulcents.* Soothe, coat, and cool down the gut with Slippery Elm bark tea or Licorice root, or a cold infusion of Marshmallow root or Slippery Elm bark.
- *Carminatives.* Stimulate peristalsis and reduce indigestion, burping, gas, and bloating with Peppermint leaf, Dill seed, Fennel seed, or classic Chinese citruses like Citrus Zhi Shi (Bitter Orange peel) or Citrus Chen Pi (Ripe Tangerine peel).
- *Appetite stimulants.* If appetite is an issue, use bitters of citrus peel, Dandelion root and leaf, or Burdock root. Try Fennel seed or Fenugreek seed.
- *Antiemetics.* For nausea, include Peppermint leaf, Chamomile flower, Meadowsweet herb; or for vomiting, give Ginger root.
- *Sedatives.* To calm down anxiety and excitement, turn to Lemon Balm herb, Passionflower herb, Catnip herb, and Meadowsweet herb.
- *Antidiarrheals.* These include astringents such as Cranesbill root or Oregon Grape root (the latter is also antimicrobial). Berberines are classic because they come in direct contact with gut mucous membranes and are also astringent. Raspberry leaf is gentle for young infants.

• BOX 21.4 Application of Eye Washes and Compresses

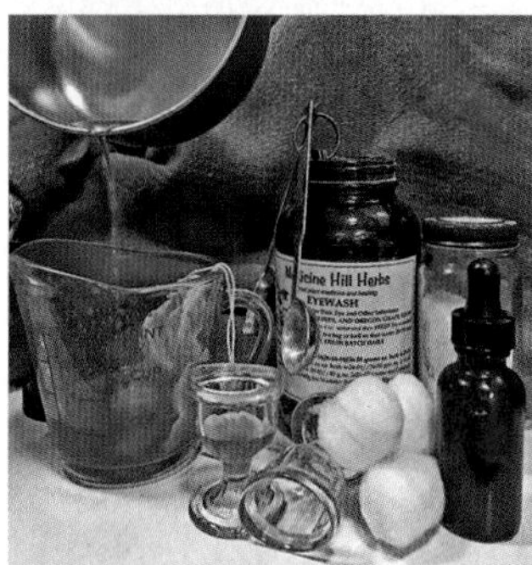

Making an herbal eye wash. Boiling saline solution poured over muslin bag of herbs to steep. Apply with eyecup, dropper, or cotton ball.

Treat eye ailments with washes or compresses. The best herbal bets are antiinflammatory and anti-infectious: Chamomile flower, Goldenseal root, Eyebright, and Chickweed herb. As with all external conditions, treat internally as well. In the case of eye infections, an Echinacea root tincture for the immune system could be part of the program. Cleanliness is essential for eye washes.

A Simple Eye Wash

Clean or sterilize an eye cup and storage container. Boil eye cup and glass storage jar and lid for 5 minutes. Leftover eye wash can be kept and reused from this clean airtight glass jar and will keep safely in the refrigerator for 24 hours. You will be using and applying solution 3 to 6 times a day.

Create a saline solution. A normal saline solution (technically 0.9% sodium chloride to water) is a mixture of water, salt, and a pinch of baking soda that is similar to the salt concentration in blood and tears. It should be the base of eye washes, wound and nasal irrigations, and rehydration drinks.

- Boil 2 cups tap or distilled water in saucepan for 15 minutes take off stove and add 1 tsp fine noniodized salt and a pinch of baking soda.[9]
- Extra finished eye wash can be stored in sterilized jar in refrigerator and reheated as needed, allowing it to cool to room temperature. A tap water solution will remain uncontaminated for 24 hours (distilled water longer). Each day prepare a new solution.

Remove saline solution from stove and steep the herbs

- 2 tbsp Chamomile flower to ½ tsp Goldenseal or Coptis Huang Lian root infused in 2 cups prepared saline solution. Herbs can be put in a muslin bag to steep as shown in illustration. This helps keep out irritating plant particles.
- An alternative to the previous herbal combination is to use Chickweed and/or Eyebright. If the herbs are fresh, use a large handful.
- Steep 10 minutes or until room temperature.
- Strain twice to remove any small particles (especially from the Goldenseal). Rinse eyes with dropper or apply cool compresses 3 to 6 times a day.[4]

Technique. Gently wash eyes with warm water and rub away the dried discharge. Use a *very* clean or sterilized eye cup, a dropper, or a cotton ball soaked in tea and dribbled in the eye. Tilt head back or lay child in your lap and dribble the wash from corner of eye toward ear to prevent contaminating the healthy eye. In the case of a compress, discard after each use. Use a new one for each eye or session.

Keep it clean. Pink eye and other infections are highly contagious from kid to kid, kid to adult, and adult to adult. Discard any tissue that touches infection, so it doesn't spread to the other eye or from person to person. Using personal towels and pillowcases is important. Wash them daily. Wash your own hands before and after treatment. Discourage child from rubbing eyes. (Good luck with that one.)

A Compress

This is soothing and can bring down swelling, although the eye is closed so the medicine does not get in direct contact with the conjunctiva. A child might be more compliant with this method. Soak a clean cloth in the herbal infusion (the same as the one made for the wash) and place over eye. Keep it warm. Another compress idea is a conveniently prepackaged black tea or Chamomile tea bag that is wet, wrung out, and used as a compress, which is both astringent and antiseptic.

- *Laxatives*. Stimulate bile flow with Yellow dock or Burdock root. Slippery Elm bark and Psyllium fiber bulks and softens stool for easier passage.

Common Digestive System Conditions

Colic, Gastritis, Constipation, Diarrhea

The four conditions listed here are the most common GI complaints in kids (Case History 21.5). Whatever the case, please check the *red flags* in the case histories presented later because sometimes any one of these conditions can be serious.

- *Colic*. Vigorous crying that persists for long periods despite all efforts at consolation is known as ***colic***[6] (also called gripe). It is severe, often with fluctuating pain in the abdomen caused by intestinal gas or obstruction for 3 or more hours per day for 3 or more days per week. Colic can send any sane parent slightly mad with frustration and fatigue. No one in the family gets enough sleep, and crankiness is the norm.
- *Gastritis*. An old-fashioned tummy ache is known as ***gastritis***, inflammation of the stomach lining. It is another problem

• BOX 21.5 Slippery Elm Gruel and Rehydration Drink for Diarrhea

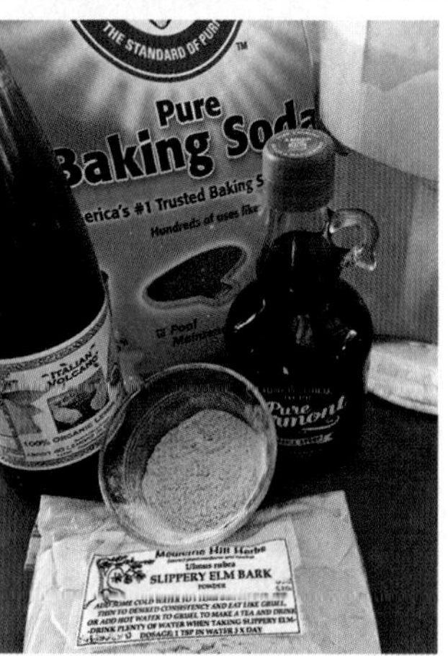

Slippery Elm bark, finely powdered in bowl for gruel, and some rehydration drink ingredients: Filtered water, lemon juice (fresh lemons best), maple syrup, and baking soda.

Slippery Elm Gruel

This is a bland herbal food that heals the gut and absorbs water. It bulks up the stool to stop watery diarrhea.[6] (This gruel also treats constipation, because it softens stool and helps movement.)

- **Directions**. Mix *very* finely ground Slippery Elm bark into a paste with dilute apple juice, apple sauce, or water.
- **Dose.** Ages 3 to 6, 1 tsp each day; ages 7 to 12, 3 tsp each day.

Re-Hydration Drink

This drink balances electrolytes, adds fluids, and vitamin C that helps immunity. Water and electrolytes (sodium Na + and potassium K +) are lost in sweating, diarrhea, and/or fever.

4 cups water (1 quart)	Rehydrate with water.
2 tbsp fresh lemon	A source of vitamin C adds acidity.
2 tsp Morton's Lite Salt	Contains and replaces sodium and potassium.
2 tbsp maple syrup (or to taste)	For energy and flavor.
Pinch of baking soda	Alkaline, to neutralize the pH.

- **Directions**. Mix ingredients together.
- **Dose**. Drink 1 cup 3 times a day.

CASE HISTORY 21.5

Case Histories for Common Gastrointestinal (GI) Conditions *(Colic, Gastritis, Constipation, Diarrhea)*

Part 1 Colic

S. Jerry is 3 months old. Even when dry, fed, and rocked, he doubles up and cries inconsolably every evening starting around 8:00 pm. He was recently weaned off breast milk. He sucks the bottle vigorously for about 30 seconds and pulls off the nipple. This has been going on 3 times a week for 4 weeks and lasts about 3 hours. His parents are at wit's end.

O. Tense abdomen, distress.

A. Stagnant Stomach Qi. Infantile colic.

P. *Specific therapeutic principles.* Gripe water. (1) Remove spasms and inflammation with carminatives. (2) Calm with nervines. (3) Cool with demulcent.

Herbal Formula for Gripe Water.
(A classic colic formula.)
Adult Dose: 5 mL every ½ hour.
Child's Dose: 0.1 mL every ½ hour per Fried's rule, for babies under 24 months old (Box 21.6).

Parts	Herbs	Rationale
1	Chamomile flower	Reduce spasms, calm anxiety.
1	Catnip leaf	Nervine for colic.
1	Fennel seed	Carminative.
1	Licorice root	Soothes stomach, demulcent.

Other suggestions for colic

- Introduce *Lactobacillus acidophilus* into bottle to balance flora, because he is now off breast milk.
- Lavender oil bath and drop or two of diluted essential oil on stomach.
- For parents. Avoid feeling frustrated, guilty, or inadequate about being a good parent and remain confident of your relationship with your newborn.

Part 2 Gastritis

S. Lily was running around in glee during her 8th birthday party. She ate two helpings of ice cream and cake. The guests have gone home, and she now has pain, nausea, stomach cramping, gas, and bloating. She is balled up on the couch crying. She weighs 63 lb.

O. T Greasy, white coating.

A. Food stagnation. Stress and overeating. Stomachache with gas. Birthday party syndrome.

P. *Specific therapeutic principles.* (1) Carminatives to stimulate peristalsis, eliminate gas and nausea. (2) Nervines to calm anxiety. (3) Spasmolytics to relieve cramping.

Herbal Formula and Dose for Gastritis.
Adult Dose: 4 mL every ½ h.
Child's Dose: 1.7 mL every ½ h per Clark's rule (Box 21.6).

Parts	Herbs	Rationale
1	Aniseed	Carminative.
1	Peppermint leaf	Antispasmodic, relieves gas.
1	Fennel seed	Carminative, soothe stomach.
1	Chamomile flower	Calms stress, harmonizes digestion.

Other suggestions for gastritis

- Have child suck on Licorice root sticks (Box 21.2).
- Apply Chamomile essential oil, diluted in carrier oil, topically to stomach.
- Drink Peppermint tea.

Part 3 Constipation

S. Timmy is 2½ years old, weighs 31 lb. He has been eating mainly bananas and cheese, and not drinking much. Has not had a bowel movement for 4 days and complains of stomach cramps. His last stool was hard and dry.

O. Dry, hard stools; no bowel movement in 4 days. Index finger red.

A. Constipation with heat. Finger vein reddish, extending between first and second knuckle.

P. *Specific therapeutic principles.* (1) Increase bile flow. (2) Moisten and cool gut. (3) Relieve cramping.

Herbal Formula and Dose for Constipation.
Adult Dose: 4 mL every 1 hour.
Child's Dose: 0.8 mL every 1 hour per Clark's rule (Box 21.6).

Parts	Herbs	Rationale
3	Yellow Dock or Dandelion root	Increase bile flow.
2	Licorice root	Restore gut, demulcent, soothing.
2	Peppermint leaf or Chamomile flower	Relieve cramping.
2	Chickweed herb	Cool, moist, and softening.

Other suggestions for constipation

Red Flags: Constipation is a symptom, not a disease. Beware a vomiting infant who won't nurse, bloody stools, severe pain when passing stool, and chronic or persistent constipation. Serious complications include fecal impaction, painful tears around the skin (anal fissures), intestinal protrusion out of the anus (rectal prolapse).

It is necessary to ascertain causes, such as dehydration, high carb and low fruit and vegetable diet, bed rest, lack of exercise, potty training stress, cow milk allergy.

- Back off constipating foods like bananas (especially unripe), white rice and flour, dairy.
- Encourage fluids like herbal tea, diluted juice, prune juice, soups, and high fiber foods such as peas, beans, apricots, prunes, pear.
- *Lactobacillus acidophilus* or *bifidum* to restore flora, as well as fermented foods.
- Licorice root tea to soothe, moisten, and restore gut.
- Bulking laxatives such as Psyllium fiber or 10 drops of flaxseed oil 2 times a day in food to lube gut.

Part 4 Diarrhea

S. Jenny has had frequent loose watery stools for 2 days, abdominal cramps that come and go, some vomiting. There is no fever. She is 4 years old and weighs 40 lb.

O. Watery stools for 2 days. **P** Rapid. **T** Body red, coat slightly dry.

A. Diarrhea. Spleen Damp Heat.

P. *Specific therapeutic principles.* (1) Astringent antidiarrheals. (2) Broad-spectrum antiinfectives, berberines. (3) Carminatives for cramping. (4) Avoid dehydration. Use Rehydration drink (Box 21.5). (4) Immune support.

Herbal Formula and Dose for Diarrhea.
Adult Dose: 5 mL every 2 hours.
Child's Dose: 1.3 mL every 2 hours per Clark's rule (Box 21.6).

Parts	Herbs	Rationale
2	Bilberry leaf	Astringent and sweet for compliance.
1	Cranesbill root	Astringent, antidiarrheal.
2	Coptis Huang Lian or *Echinacea* root	Antimicrobial/drying, immune support.
1	Slippery Elm bark	Heal and soothe gut.

(Continued)

CASE HISTORY 21.5 (cont'd)

Other suggestions for diarrhea

Red Flags. Dehydration, persistent cramping, and bloody stools, going on for more than 2 weeks.[6] Serious reasons for diarrhea are from: reactions to medications, irritable bowel disease, hepatitis, cystic fibrosis, and fistula. Diarrhea is often caused by an infection, such as a virus, bacteria, fungus, or plasmodium. Can be spread from other kids, or contaminated food or water. Also, food sensitivities from newly introduced foods can do it, such as lactose intolerance, citrus fruits, wheat, sugar, and dairy. The *priority is to keep the child hydrated.*

- *Diet.* Keep hydrated. (Fever is a good indicator of dehydration.) Frequent sips of water; ingesting too much at one time will cause vomiting. Lots of clear liquids like diluted apple juice, herbal teas, and rehydration drink (Box 21.5). Not too much food. Intestines must rest and heal. Dry toast, pureed rice, bananas, dry cereal, and mashed potatoes without butter. No sugar, because it feeds bad bacteria. Avoid protein for 48 hours.
- *Rehydration drink.* Yum. Balances electrolytes.
- *Slippery Elm Gruel.* Bulks, heals, and absorbs water.
- Detect and eliminate any food sensitivities.
- Rice water is a worldwide classic: Cook rice or barley and sip the water.
- *Lactobacillus acidophilus* or *bifidum* and fermented foods to restore flora.

TABLE 21.3 Gastrointestinal Herbs for Kids

HERB	NOTES
Nepeta cataria (Catnip leaf)	Versatile gut and nervous relaxant and diaphoretic. For agitated babies with colic.
Matricaria recutita (Chamomile flower)	For stomach aches and colic with crying and anxiety. Settles stomach and nerves.
Geranium maculatum (Cranesbill root)	Astringent for diarrhea.
Foeniculum vulgaris (Fennel seed) *Anethum graveolens* (Dill seed)	Carminatives for tummy aches, overeating, Stuck Stomach Qi.
Melissa officinalis (Lemon Balm leaf)	Helps digestion and clears heat. For fever, allergies, nervous tension, colic, and anxiety.
Rubus idaeus (Raspberry leaf)	Lovely, mild astringent for infant diarrhea.
Zingiber officinalis (Ginger root)	Stomach relaxant for nausea and colic.
Ulmus fulva (Slippery Elm bark) *Plantago psyllium* (Psyllium husk fiber)	Helps constipation by bulking up stool. Also coats and soothes gut.
Filipendula ulmaria (Meadowsweet herb)	Builds gut flora and antacid.
Achillea millefolium (Yarrow flower)	Spasmolytic for gastrointestinal spasms, wind heat/cold.
Chondrus crispus (Irish Moss thallus)	Moist, antiinflammatory and nourishing.
Citrus reticulata Chen Pi (Ripe Tangerine peel)	Digestive aid, regulates Stomach qi.

caused by overeating, ingesting too many sweets, emotional excitement and stress, or the need for an excuse to avoid problems at school.

- *Constipation*. A decrease in the number and consistency of bowel movements or pain and difficulty passing stools is known as ***constipation***. A child who goes 2 or 3 days without a movement is constipated.[6] The causes run the gamut from potty training stress or not drinking enough water to refusing veggies and fibrous foods.
- *Diarrhea*. Frequent or watery stools, ***diarrhea***,[8] often comes from infections, food sensitivities, and stress.

Nervous System Materia Medica

We all get stress, kids included. ***Nervines*** that calm the nervous system and ***anxiolytics*** (herbs that treat anxiety) are the ticket (Table 21.4). When parents are stressed and anxious, a child quickly picks up on it. Stress decreases immune function and leads to more respiratory infections. Infant sleep problems are among the most common conditions seen by pediatricians.[1] If you can help a parent get their child to sleep, you'll have a convert for life (Case History 21.6). Another very common problem is attention deficit hyperactivity syndrome (ADHD).

TABLE 21.4 Kid-Specific Nervines

HERB	NOTES
Withania somnifera Ashwagandha root	For a stressed, underweight child.
Zizyphus spinosa Suan Zao Ren Sour Jujube seed	Calming nervous tonic for sleep with anxiety.
Matricaria recutita Chamomile flower	Classic nervine. For nervousness, stomach aches, irritability, restlessness, sleeplessness, allergy, and skin wounds.
Eschscholzia californica California Poppy herb	Sleeplessness and anxiety.
Nepeta cataria Catnip herb	Stress, sleep problems, stomach aches, colic, irritable bowel syndrome.
Hyssopus officinalis Hyssop herb and essential oil	For spasms, pain, and wheezing.
Lavandula angustifolia Lavender flower and essential oil	Relaxant for anxiety, sleeplessness, agitation, and stomach aches. Use in tincture and essential oil form.
Melissa officinalis Lemon Balm leaf	Cooling and relaxing. For fever, anxiety, allergy, depression, and fussy teething children.
Tilia cordata Linden flower	For headaches, migraines, tense painful conditions.
Leonurus cardiaca Motherwort herb	Calms anxiety, for the heart.
Bacopa monnieri Bacopa or Water Hyssop herb	Ayurvedic. All around brain tonic and nervous relaxant, specific for ADHD and anxiety.

Common Nervous System Conditions

Insomnia and/or Anxiety

Anxiety refers to a state of excessive uneasiness and apprehension, sometimes with compulsive behavior or panic attacks. Anxiety may or may not be chronic. Sleep problems are common complaints. Babies, toddlers, and school-age kids don't necessarily sleep through the night. Lack of sleep can lead to concentration and learning problems.

There are many fail-safe childhood nervous system remedies for sleep, anxiety, and stress. Chamomile flower is the supreme goddess of them all. Also, honor Passionflower, Lemon Balm herb, California Poppy, and Lavender herb and essential oil. For pain, use Catnip leaf or a Lavender essential oil bath. Don't forget the nervous system. The Ayurvedic tonic, *Bacopa monnieri* (Water Hyssop, all parts used medicinally) and Chinese Medicine's Ziziphus Suan Zao Ren (Sour Jujube seed) are for matters of the Heart, or shen disturbances, which include sleeplessness, anxiety, and worry.

CASE HISTORY 21.6

Case History for Insomnia and/or Anxiety

S. Alex is 18 months old, weighs 27 lb, and doesn't yet sleep through the night. He wakes frequently, cries, responds to his mother singing softly, goes back to sleep, but awakens 10 minutes later. Mom is exhausted. He is on solid foods, with a little breast feeding still being done for comfort.

O. Agitated and cries constantly. No apparent stomach distress. Cries too much when finger is rubbed.

A. Heart Yin Deficiency. Difficulty staying asleep.

P. *Specific therapeutic principles.* (1) The best approach to anxiety and sleep disturbances is to find the cause, be it colic, teething, nightmares, pain, indigestion from eating spicy meals too close to bedtime, or in older children, underlying stress or worry. (2) Nervines/antianxiety herbs to calm NS and help sleep. (3) Nervous system tonics.

Herbal Formula and Dose for Insomnia and/or Anxiety.
Adult Dose for insomnia: 4 mL at bedtime; then 2 mL every 15 min as needed up to 2 hours, then STOP.
Child's Dose for insomnia: 0.5 mL at bedtime and then 0.2 mL every 15 min as needed up to 2 hours, then STOP. Per Fried's rule (Box 21.6). (Same frequency as adult schedule in 5 mL of expressed breast milk.)

Parts	Herbs	Rationale
1	Chamomile flower	Anxiety and sleep and possible stomachache.
1	Ziziphus Suan Zao Ren	Heart yin deficiency, and anxiety.
1	Passionflower herb	Nervine and anxiolytic.
1	Lemon Balm herb	Nervine/anxiolytic.
1	Ashwagandha root	Adaptogen/nervous system tonic.

Other Suggestions for insomnia and/or anxiety

- Warm milk before bedtime, high in the amino acid, tryptophan, which stabilizes moods and helps sleep. Similar foods are bananas, cottage cheese, dates, peanuts, and turkey.
- Herbal bath with Lavender essential oil.
- Small evening meal and light snack of a complex carbohydrate at bedtime like toast or crackers.
- Regular sleep schedule and a bedtime ritual, bath, and story, etc.

Attention Deficit Hyperactivity Disorder (ADHD)

- *Definition.* ***Attention deficit hyperactivity disorder (ADHD)*** is a chronic condition marked by persistent inattention, hyperactivity, and sometimes impulsivity (Case History 21.7). It is the most commonly diagnosed mental disorder of children, more frequently in boys than in girls.[7] Diagnosis of ADHD is open to subjective interpretation and cultural influences.
  - Causes (based on studies done over the years) include stress response, food intolerances and additives, allergies and sleep disorders, abnormal glucose tolerance, environmental exposures to substances heavy metals, oxidative stress caused by an abnormally high level of omega-3 breakdown, mineral deficiencies (particularly zinc), and leaky gut. These factors are worth considering when you obtain a thorough health history.
- *Signs and symptoms.* There are no biological markers. ADHD is diagnosed behaviorally. The *attention deficit* part includes

CASE HISTORY 21.7

Case History for Attention Deficit Hyperactivity Disorder (ADHD)

S. John is 15 years old. He has always been a handful. He was diagnosed with ADHD at age 11 years old and has been on Ritalin ever since. His mother is seeking an alternative. He has had poor concentration, inattention, clashes with teachers, truancy, impulsiveness, inability to complete tasks or do his homework. He is not aggressive or angry. Diet includes lots of soda pop, junk food, and sugar. There is slight abdominal distention and occasional constipation and trouble sleeping.

O. P Wiry and rapid. **T** Red tip, thin yellow coat. Observed restlessness and inattention.

A. Spleen Qi and Heart Yin Deficiency with heat. ADHD per physician's diagnosis with indigestion and probable leaky gut, nerve excess.

P. *Specific therapeutic principles.* Two formulas. *Daytime:* formula to restore nervous system and help with sugar cravings. *Night time:* formula with nervines to help anxiety and insomnia. (1) Nervous system tonics/adaptogens. (2) Adrenal tonics. (3) Increase microcirculation to brain. (4) Heal the gut with help for sugar cravings and Spleen tonics. (4) Relaxing nervines and anxiolytics.

Daytime Herbal Formula and Dose for ADHD.
Adult Dose for John: 8 mL 2 × day in morning and lunchtime.

Part	Herbs	Rationale
2	Bacopa leaf	Helps concentration.
2	Ginkgo leaf	Helps concentration/microcirculation.
2	Schisandra Wu Wei Zi	Adaptogen/liver detox/cognition.
2	Withania root	Nerve tonic and adaptogen.
2	Gymnema leaf	Helps with sugar cravings.
2	Licorice root	Spleen Qi deficiency, adrenal and liver support, constipation.

Evening Formula and Dose for ADHD.
Adult Dose for John: 8 mL before dinner, and 1 hour before bedtime.

Parts	Herbs	Rationale
2	Hops flower	Sleep and relieves anxiety.
2	Skullcap herb	Calm Heart, nervine.
1	Zizyphus Suan Zao Ren	Calm Heart, help sleep.
1	Bacopa leaf	Cognition and sedative.

Other suggestions

- *Diet:* The *Ben Feingold Diet for ADHD*[11] is an allergen elimination diet that has had a great track record for helping many kids with ADHD. *Remove* food additives such as artificial flavors, dyes, and preservatives, and allergenic foods such as refined sugar, corn, wheat, milk, oranges, eggs, and chocolate. *Replace* the above with high protein foods and complex carbohydrates that help make neurotransmitters and promote calmness and alertness, such as grass-fed, free-range poultry and beef, vegetables, fruit, and foods with essential fatty acids. *Reinoculate* gut flora with fermented foods and pre- and probiotics. The diet takes work, but anything's possible with intention and determination.
- *Supplements:* Essential fatty acids in supplement and diet form. Essential fatty acids also help treat constipation. Pycnogenol (French Maritime Pine bark extract), Grape seed extract, as well as Turmeric root, Rosemary leaf, and Green tea leaves as antioxidants for oxidative stress.
- Bedtime tea. Long-term nerve tonics at bedtime. Milky Oat berry, Lemon Balm tea.
- Assess for environmental toxins.
- Exercise, fresh air, love, and kindness.

neither sustaining nor paying attention, ignoring details, being disorganized, not listening or not following through on tasks, being easily distracted, and being forgetful. The *hyperactivity/impulsivity* part of the diagnosis involves symptoms such as fidgeting, running around, and leaving seat inappropriately; excessive talking; blurting out; not waiting for a turn; and being constantly in motion. For definitive diagnoses, six or more items in each category must be present for 6 months or more. These symptoms, of course, are subjective opinions and often arrived at by an overworked teacher.

- For all diagnoses of ADHD, herbalists need be very discerning and consider the whole child, and his or her needs versus parents' and teachers' expectations. Help parents make an honest assessment without judgment about how they might be contributing to this social and cultural problem (if true) and how to reach a solution. There is often a bit of denial going on.

- *Allopathic treatment.* For 50 years, the drug of choice has been the stimulant Ritalin, a Schedule II drug with a high potential for abuse. Some of the many side effects include rebound exacerbation of symptoms (the drug making the situation worse), dependence, withdrawal, depression, anxiety, insomnia, anorexia, and liver dysfunction. We have indeed created a doped-up, drug-dependent generation.
- *General therapeutic principles.* Take a good health history and choose herbs depending on condition. (1) Support the nervous system with tonics and herbs to help cognition and brain microcirculation, such as *Bacopa monnieri* leaf and seed capsules (a proven Ayurvedic nerve tonic for helping concentration in ADHD kids), Gotu Kola leaf, Schisandra Wu Wei Zi (Five Taste berry), Rosemary leaf, or Ginkgo leaf. (2) Support the adrenal system with adaptogens, nerve tonics like Ashwagandha root, Eleuthero Ci Wu Jia (Siberian ginseng root), and Licorice root. (3) Help digestion and leaky gut with Meadowsweet herb, Chamomile herb, Citrus Chen Pi (Ripe Tangerine peel), and fermented foods. (4) Liver tonics: Dandelion root or Milk Thistle seed. (5) Nervines at night; using nervines in the daytime can make matters worse. Try Lemon Balm leaf, Ziziphus Suan Zao Ren (Sour Jujube seed), and Skullcap herb.

Skin Materia Medica

Babies get diaper rash and atopic dermatitis. Children 2 to 5 years old get eczema, viral warts (*Human papilloma virus*, also called HPV), and impetigo (usually from *Staphylococcus aureus*). Teenagers get *Acne vulgaris* (Chapter 25). Often, this is because their usual avenues of detoxification (the liver, the bowel, and the bladder) are overloaded. Hence, skin eruptions occur in the body's attempt to eliminate the waste. The skin is considered a detoxifying organ, too, sometimes called the *third kidney* (Chapter 25).

Herbal categories that address detoxification through the kidneys are important in clearing up the skin. These herbs work by increasing diuresis (urination). They are sometimes called the ***diuretic detoxicants***: Burdock root, Nettle herb, Celery seed, Parsley leaf, and Dandelion leaf. *Lymphatic drainers* also channel water through the kidneys and help the child to pee out toxins. *Antimicrobials* are generally included because so many skin problems have a primary or secondary infectious component (Table 21.5).

In Chinese Medicine, the Lungs rule the exterior of the body and manifest in the body hair. It is interesting that respiratory problems are the most common problems found in kids, with skin

TABLE 21.5 Skin Care for the Kiddies

HERB	NOTES
Hypericum perforatum St. John's Wort	Nervous system trophorestorative and relaxant for nerve injury (shingles), and antiviral. For *herpes simplex* (cold sores), bruises, sprains, depression, and anxiety.
Matricaria recutita Chamomile flower	Clears damp heat, reduces swelling, analgesic, helps nerve pain, antiallergic. Use in skin eruptions and dermatitis.
Lavandula angustifolia Lavender flower and essential oil	Repairs skin, cooling, antiinfective. Excellent for burns, bites, wounds, itching, eczema, hives, and accompanying anxiety.
Calendula officinalis Marigold flower	Major first aid remedy for use in salves. Clears toxic heat, reduces infection, detoxicant and skin healer. For all types of cuts, bruises, bites, sprains, slow healing, torn skin, and *herpes simplex* (cold sores).
Trifolium pratense Red Clover flower	Tissue repair and detoxifies. For sores, burns, eye inflammations, bites, eczema, impetigo, herpes, and ringworm.
Urtica dioica Nettle herb	Detoxes and restores. For infantile eczema.
Plantago major Plantain leaf	Tissue repair. Clears toxic heat in eczema, dermatitis, boils, burns. Use fresh for topical first aid compress for bleeding.
Galium aparine Cleavers herb	Lymphatic drainer, dissolves deposits, and skin eruptions. For burns, sunburns, fresh wounds, and eczema.
Arctium lappa Burdock root	Hair, skin, and scalp. Diuretic detoxicant for chronic skin/scalp infections, rashes, eczema.
Apium graveolens Celery seed	Diuretic detoxicant. Dries damp.
Taraxacum officinale Dandelion leaf and root	Diuretic detoxicant, drains lymph. For eczema.
Andrographis paniculata Chuan Xin Lian Heart-thread Lotus leaf	Clears damp heat, broad-spectrum antimicrobial for all skin infections.

ailments way up on the list. The high incidence of respiratory infections accompanied by eczema confirms this.[10] Most skin problems are *damp heat*. There is heat because of inflammation and emotional stress, and damp because of insufficient flushing of waste and toxins, water retention, and a humid or moist environment. Thus the therapeutic intention is to *clear damp heat*.

Some prime skin herbs are the antiviral St. John's Wort; antimicrobial and skin healing Calendula flower; the alteratives Red Clover flower and Nettle herb; diuretic detoxicants such as Burdock root; and lymph draining Cleavers herb. To clear damp heat, we need cool, drying herbs like Andrographis Chuan Xin Lian (Heart-Thread Lotus leaf) and Scutellaria Huang Qin (Baikal Skullcap root).

Common Skin Conditions

Childhood Eczema or Contact Dermatitis

- *Definition. **Eczema*** is a skin inflammation and is also known as dermatitis or contact dermatitis (Case History 21.8). It can be caused by direct contact with soaps or chemicals, or it can originate from inside sources caused by toxicity and food sensitivities, especially cow's milk. Many kids with childhood eczema go on to have allergies and asthma later in life because of its allergenic connection. *Cradle cap* is called seborrheic eczema, where oil cakes up on the scalp, causing thick greasy scales and redness. *Diaper rash* is also a type of eczema, caused by friction, wetness, and prolonged exposure to feces and urine in the diaper.
- *Signs and symptoms.* Severe itching, peeling, weepy, or sometimes thickened dry skin. Scratching can lead to bleeding and infection.
- *Allopathic treatment.* Eliminate known allergens; treat inflammation; apply wet dressings, topical steroids, or tars. Antibiotics are used for secondary infections.
- *General therapeutic principles.* Pick and choose appropriate therapeutic principles, depending on cause, signs, and symptoms. (1) Find cause. Rule out external irritants. Detect any dietary food allergens, such as cow's milk (common in kids), cheese, soy, eggs, nuts, peanut butter, and sugar. (2) Use alteratives such as Cleavers herb for lymph drainage or Nettle herb or Red Clover flower for the blood. (3) Use antimicrobials if infectious component. (4) Choose liver stimulants such as Burdock root or

CASE HISTORY 21.8

Case History for Childhood Eczema or Contact Dermatitis

S. Allison is 13 months old and weighs 24 lb. Her mom gave her a bath with Melaleuca essential oil for the first time. She now has a dry, red rash all over her buttocks. She is crying and anxious.
O. Rubbing/scratching buttocks. Face red. Finger vein dark pink, extending a little above knuckle.
A. Contact dermatitis, probably from newly added Tea Tree oil to bath. Heat and inflammation.
P. *Specific therapeutic principles.* (1) Discontinue Tea Tree oil from bath. (2) Alteratives. (3) Lymphatic movers. (4) Calm anxiety with nervines.

Herbal Formula and Dose.
Adult Dose: 6 mL three times daily.
Child's Dose: 0.5 mL three times daily, per Fried's rule (Box 21.6).

Parts	Herbs	Rationale
2	Cleavers herb	Alterative, lymph tonic, antiinflammatory, diuretic.
2	Nettle herb	Alterative, lymph drainer, diuretic.
1	Red Clover flower	Alterative and detoxification.
2	Passionflower herb	Nervine for anxiety.

Other suggestions

- *Bath:* Oatmeal bath for itching. Wrap 1 cup ground oatmeal powder in a washcloth or bag. Swish in bath water under running water. Squeeze and rub on her skin. Keep nails short to stop breaking open lesions, which can cause bleeding and infection.
- *Treatment for dry rash:* Keep it moist. Plain, unscented, antiallergenic lotion after bath is helpful.
- Dress in soft cotton clothing, absolutely free of soap residue.
- Topical cream: Chickweed herb, Chamomile flower, and Calendula flower for healing and to retain moisture.
- If asthma is present, add Grindelia flower and Lobelia herb to herbal formula.
- With food sensitivities, add Atractylodes Bai Zhu (White Atractylodes root) or Codonopsis Dang Shen (Downy Bellflower root) to herbal formula, and of course, remove offending food.
- With diaper rash, use Calendula flower and Chamomile flower added to bath water, followed by a Calendula flower and Lavender essential oil cream applied to buttocks afterward, which is helpful.
- With cradle cap, rub an herbal cream on the scalp. Use 50 mL of a plain unscented cream and mix with 2 capsules of a gamma linolenic acid (GLA) oil, such as Borage, Evening Primrose, or Black currant seed. Pierce capsules with a sterile needle and squeeze into the cream. Mix and apply.[6]

Coptis Huang Lian (Goldthread root) and Oregon Grape root to detoxify and help digestion. (5) Incorporate antiinflammatories to help alteratives work. (6) Use nervines to help with any stress/anxiety. (7) Use mild diuretics such as Dandelion root or Nettle herb to eliminate toxins. (8) Consider astringents to dry up wet, weepy secretions. If dry, keep lesions moist. (9) Provide topical creams or emollients. (10) Treat externally and internally.

Cold Sores (Herpes simplex)

- *Definition.* ***Cold sores*** are tiny, fluid-filled blisters on and around the lips. They are not caused from colds but may occur with colds. The ***herpes simplex virus 1 (HSV 1)*** is the culprit (Case History 21.9). Once in the body, the virus remains dormant in the nervous system. It can be reactivated by fever (causing sores sometimes called *fever blisters*), other physical or emotional stress, excessive sunlight exposure, and some foods or drugs.
- *Signs and symptoms.* Contagious, small, red, burning, itching fluid-filled blisters around the edges of the lips or nose. They eventually crust over and disappear, indicating the infectious stage is gone.
- *Allopathic treatment.* Topical xylocaine, Tylenol, Campho-Phenique, and the antibiotic generic acyclovir in pills or ointment form.
- *General therapeutic principles.* (1) Use antivirals. (2) Cool and decrease inflammation. (3) Stimulate immunity. (4) Use astringents to close blisters. (5) Use nervines for stress. (6) apply topical antiviral cream.

CASE HISTORY 21.9

Case History for Cold Sores (Herpes simplex)

S. Annie is 8 years old and weighs 59 lb and just got over a "cold." On the edge of her left upper lip, she has a painful "cold sore," which has red edges and tiny fluid-filled blisters that hurt and burn. She keeps touching it and fussing.
O. **P** Rapid and wiry. **T** Red and moist. Reddish, fluid-filled blisters around upper lip.
A. Skin Damp Heat/Fire Toxins. Cold sore.
P. *Specific therapeutic principles.* (1) Cooling antivirals. (2) Decrease inflammation. (3) Dry damp. (3) Relaxing nervine for anxiety.

Herbal Formula and Dose.
Adult Dose: 6 mL 3 times daily.
Child's Dose: 2.4 mL 3 times daily per Clark's rule (Box 21.6).

Parts	Herbs	Rationale
3	Lonicera Jin Yin Hua	Antiviral/immunostimulant, for Fire toxins, astringent (dries damp).
3	Andrographis Chuan Xin Lian	Clear Fire toxins, immunostimulant, astringing.
2	Licorice root	Detoxifying, soothing, alterative.
2	Lemon Balm leaf	Nervine to calm anxiety and also antiviral.

Other suggestions.[6]

- *Diet:* Very simple foods. Good hydration, water, herbal teas, soups, and diluted juices. Avoid sugars and caffeinated beverages, including teas, dairy, and grains, which aggravate virus. Cleansing alkaline diet with lots of veggies. Citrus slows down healing.
- *Topically.* Fresh Grindelia flower tincture to lip or a paste made from ground Oregon Grape root and water—or a cream with St. John's Wort, Calendula flower, Chamomile flower, and Lemon Balm.
- *Prevention.* Cold sores are contagious. Minimize contact. Keep hands clean and eat Garlic to help immunity.
- *Stress control.* Rest, quiet time, Lavender flower and Lemon Balm tea.
- *Restrict direct sun exposure.* It's a trigger; sun makes it worse and may have caused it in the first place.

Safety with Children's Herbs

As a general rule, a child can be given the same herb that you would give an adult but at lower doses.[5] Naturally there are qualifications. You wouldn't give a child a strong laxative, very strong-tasting herbs, or anything potentially toxic. As true in pregnancy and lactation, there are very few good studies on this topic. It seems that women and children have been left behind in the research department. Herbal decisions are typically based on traditional use, anecdotal comments, existing studies, and knowledge of phytochemical constituents found in the plants (Table 21.6). Many widely used pediatric herbs are known to be safe because of long historical use. Let common sense prevail.

Ballpark Children's Dosages for Mild Herbs

Obviously, children's doses need to be smaller than those for adults. Infants up to 1 year of age and sometimes kids up to 6 years of age absorb herbs differently than adults do because of erratic transit times and lower levels of digestive enzymes. Hence, the bioavailability of herbs could be compromised. Furthermore, lots of children get tummy aches with constipation or diarrhea. Constipation decreases transit time; diarrhea speeds it up. Either way, there is no consistency. So be careful and conservative with doses, particularly with children younger than 3 years of age.

Begin on the lower end of dosage range and watch a child's reaction. It is important that an herbalist maintain good communication with the parent. Have caregivers check for signs that symptoms are easing. Ask parents to observe how the child is feeling and reacting. Children are sensitive. They get sick quickly and get well quickly. It is always best to consider each child individually, their weight, the severity of the condition, and their overall health.

In general, children respond very quickly to small doses. More frequent smaller doses, rather than less frequent higher doses, are the rule. If there is no response after a couple of doses in acute conditions, then increase the dose. For a chronic condition, if there is no positive change after a week, increase the dose. If the herbs are medium strength, such as Lobelia herb or Pasqueflower herb, rather than mild herbs like Catnip herb, the dose must be smaller. Test out a small amount and see how they do. Use tried-and-true pediatric herbs on the very young. They are in the mild category.

Calculating Children's Doses

There are a variety of ways to calculate a child's dose. Two traditional methods are ***Clark's rule*** that goes by weight, and ***Young's rule*** that goes by age in years (Box 21.6). Clark's weight-based method makes more sense, because the so-called normal growth and development charts hardly apply these days, what with childhood obesity being so common. Weights of different children of the same age vary widely. If a kid is an *average* weight, according to the standard growth chart, the calculated dosage between the two methods will be close. If they are not, the answer will be skewed. So go by Clark's rule, which goes by weight, to be safe. ***Fried's rule*** is for infants younger than 24 months old. Fried's rule uses the age in months, rather than in years.

• BOX 21.6 Children's Dosage Calculations

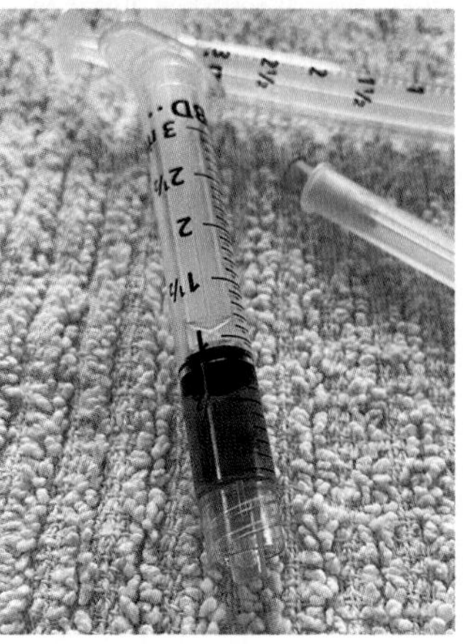

A 3 mL syringe holding 0.9 mL of tincture. The closed needle is twisted off.

Tip. To measure out children's dosages in fractions of a milliliter, such as a 0.7 mL dose, invest in some syringes which are calibrated in tenths and available in pharmacies. Twist off the covered needle and dispose properly in a sharps container. Fill the syringe to desired tenth of a mL dose, and gently push the tincture into the back of the child's mouth.

Clark's Rule[12] (weight-based)

Divide weight of the child in pounds by 150 = fraction of adult dose.
Then multiply fraction by adult dose.
Adult Dose × (Child's weight in pounds ÷ 150) = Child's Dose
Example: Adult dose is 3 mL. Child weighs 35 lb.
35 ÷ 150 = 0.2333 = fraction of adult dose. Then: 0.2333 × 3 mL = 0.699. Round up to 0.7 mL (child's dose)

YOUNG'S RULE (age-based)

Child's age in years divided by age plus 12 = fraction of adult dose.
Then multiply fraction by adult dose.
Adult Dose × Child's age ÷ (Age + 12) = Child's Dose
Example: Adult dose is 3 mL and child is 3 years old.
3 ÷ 15 = 0.2 = (fraction of adult dose). Then, 0.2 × 3 mL = 0.6 mL (child's dose)

FRIED'S RULE[13] (Infants up to 24 months)

Age in months divided by 150 = fraction of adult dose.
Then multiply fraction by adult dose to get child's dose.
(Age in months ÷ 150) × adult dose = child's dose
Example: Child is 4 months old. Adult's dose is 5 mL.
4 months ÷ 150 = 0.266 (fraction of adult dose). Then: 0.266 × 5 mL = 0.13 mL (child's dose)

Routes of Administration for Infants and Children

- *Nursing*. Controversial. Old-school herbalism says most herbs will pass through the breast milk if the mother ingests them first. Very few studies have been conducted. We don't know how much a mother must take or what amount actually transfers to baby, if any. According to Santich and Bone, "It is unlikely that a therapeutic dose taken by the mother will have any effect on the infant."[1]
- *Expressed breast milk*. A better method is to blend 5 mL of expressed milk with the infant's therapeutic herbal dose. Draw into a syringe and apply with steady pressure to the back of the infant's throat. Or the baby can suck the medicated milk off the caregiver's finger.
- *Herbal baths*. This approach is a good method of administration for neonates and infants. Transdermal absorption works well because of a baby's large surface area and thin skin. Anything taken orally can go in the bath water, including essential oils. Add herbal tea to the bathwater; alternatively, you could place herbs in a muslin tea bag or sock, soak bag in warm water, and squeeze liquid into tub. Then drop the whole bag in the bath.
- *Orally in cups, measuring spoons, or syringes*. Children can be given decoctions, infusions, and tinctures, just like adults. Tinctures

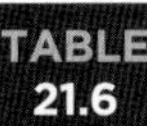

TABLE 21.6 Safety Information on Common Children's Herbs[1]

HERB	SAFETY INFORMATION
Angelica Dong Quai Astragalus Huang Qi Black Haw root Boswellia resin Burdock root Calendula flower Chamomile flower Cleavers herb Codonopsis Dang Shen Couch Grass herb Cramp bark Elderberry and flower Eyebright herb Fenugreek seed Globe Artichoke leaf Goldenrod herb Grindelia flower Gymnema herb Hawthorn leaf, flower and berry Hops flower Lavender herb Lemon Balm leaf Marshmallow herb Milk Thistle seed Mullein leaf Myrrh resin Nettle leaf and root Passionflower herb Prickly Ash bark Saw Palmetto berry Shepherd's Purse herb Eleuthero Ci Wu Jia (Siberian ginseng root) Turmeric root White Horehound herb Wild Cherry bark	No specific information available but adverse effects not expected. This long list has been used for centuries by Wise-Women and Men. 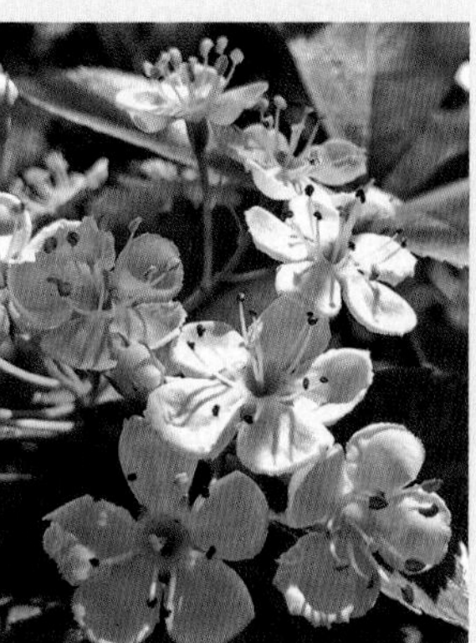 *Crataegus oxycantha* (Hawthorn berry) is a gentle heart tonic, also used for insomnia and anxiety. The gorgeous white flowers and the leaves are often used alone or in combination with the berries. 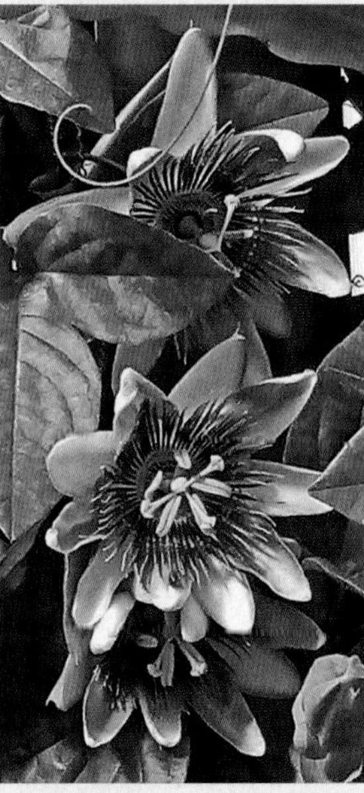 *Passiflora incarnata* (Passionflower herb) is a nervine that calms the mind and relieves anxiety.
Black Walnut hull Bupleurum Chai Hu Celery seed Creosote/Chaparral leaf Chastetree berry Elecampane root Feverfew herb Horsetail herb Jamaican Dogwood root bark Motherwort herb Pasqueflower root and herb Rosemary herb Thyme herb Wild Lettuce leaf	No safety information available, for these examples, but this group of herbs is frequently used for children. 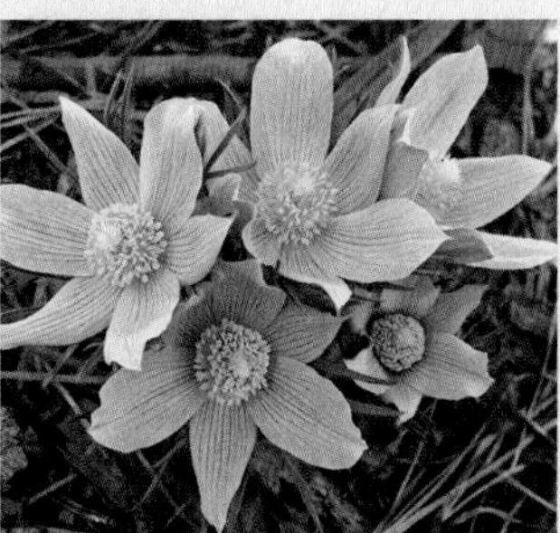 *Anemone pulsatilla* (Pasqueflower root and herb) is a nervine that lifts depression, helps pain and has traditionally been used for skin eruptions associated with infections.[1]

(*Continued*)

TABLE 21.6 **Safety Information on Common Children's Herbs[1]—cont'd**

HERB	SAFETY INFORMATION
Cranberry berry Garden Sage leaf Raspberry leaf Rehmannia Shu Di Huang Skullcap herb	No adverse effects expected within recommended dosage. Eclectics used Skullcap herb for teething. Raspberry leaf is totally safe in pregnancy.
Ashwagandha root	Used in Ayurvedic medicine for failure to thrive children.
Asparagus (Shatavari root)	Used in Southeast Asia as a nutritive tonic.
Barberry root and other berberines	Used for diarrhea and *giardiasis.* Contraindicated in neonatal jaundice.
Bearberry leaf	Not recommended for under 12 years of age.
Bilberry fruit	Safe for infants with acute diarrhea.
Black Cohosh root	Used by Eclectic physicians for fever.
Blue Flag rhizome	Used for infantile eczema. Adverse effects not expected within dose range.
California Poppy herb and root	Traditionally used as sedative and analgesic, no adverse effect expected.
Cascara bark Senna leaf or pod	Stimulant laxatives should not be used in children under 10 years old. Senna has caused rash and skin blisters and sloughing.
Corn silk	Used by Eclectic physicians for bladder disorders.
Echinacea root and herb	Used for otitis media and upper respiratory infections in children ages 2 to 11 years old. No adverse effects expected.
Fennel seed	Rare cases of allergic reactions. Otherwise used in infants.
Garlic bulb	Mild gastrointestinal discomfort possible. Not for children under 3 years old.
Gentian root	May react to bitter taste.
Ginger root	May react to pungent taste.
Ginkgo leaf	No side effects in infants from 2 to 7 months. Poisoning reported with seed ingestion.
Kava root	Traditionally used in Polynesia for fretting, debility, and stomach disorders.
Licorice root	Monitor excessive candy intake and flavoring in herbal medicines.
Peppermint leaf and essential oil	Leaf safe. Avoid essential oil to nasal area or chest of babies and young children because of risk of laryngeal and bronchospasm.
Schisandra Wu Wei Zi (Five Taste berry)	Used to treat infantile diarrhea.
Valerian root	Not for children under 3 years old.
Wormwood herb	No safety information, but best avoided in children. Quite strong and bitter.

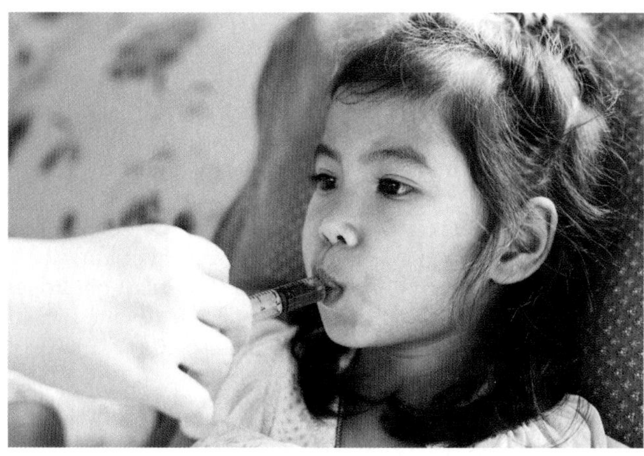

• **Fig. 21.3** Mother giving medicine to her sick child with a calibrated syringe. (iStock.com/Credit: Sasiistock.)

may be mixed in a little fruit juice or mother's milk. Babies and children can be given teas or tinctures in droppers or syringes (Fig. 21.3). Teas are a nice, gentle way to introduce herbs.

- *Glycerites* are nice and sweet and help with compliance in kids of all ages.
- *Suppositories*. These absorb directly into the bloodstream through the rectal mucosa, bypassing the gut and the liver, which have absorption uncertainties. This method also avoids the taste issue. Use same dose as for other forms of delivery.
- *Essential oils*. Diffusing oils into a sickroom is certainly an option when respiratory infections are the problem, as they so frequently are. Essential oils may also be applied to the skin when diluted in a carrier oil such as olive or grape seed.
- *Topical applications*. These come in handy for diaper rash, eczema, or ear infections.
- *Tablets*. Not the best method for children. Kids younger than 8 or 9 years old usually can't swallow pills. And the pills taste terrible when crushed. It's a rare child who will comply with that ruse.
- *Alcohol*. Controversial. It is true that children clear ethanol less efficiently than adults, and the age at which this changes is variable. However, there is very little ethanol in a child's tincture dose, and most kids tolerate it just fine. (There's probably more alcohol in mouthwash and cough syrups.) However, if it's an issue, use glycerites or tea. Contrary to popular herbal lore, dropping the tiny ethanol dose in just-boiled water is ineffective to eliminate alcohol because the water is not hot enough to effectively evaporate off all the ethanol.

Compliance Tips for Yucky-Tasting Tinctures and Teas

- *Dilution*. Dilute the tincture but not too much. If the dose is 5 mL of tincture, double the dilution with fruit juice or water to 10 mL. This mixture can be swallowed at one go, making minimal contact time with the tongue, but is not overly diluted.
- *Teas*. Try brewing the tea in organic apple juice instead of water. Sweeten with maple syrup, rice bran syrup, barley malt syrup, or honey (but not for children less than 1 year old).
- *Ice*. Have the child suck on ice first. Ice will temporarily numb the mucous membranes and deaden the taste buds and olfactory nerve.
- *Chilled water*. Mixing the dose with cold or chilled water can reduce taste intensity.
- *Water or juice chaser*. Swallow the dose all at once and follow with about 50 mL of nice-tasting or neutralizing liquid.
- *Gelatin capsules*. This method is a bit of trouble, but it works if the child will swallow pills. Use a dropper to fill a gel cap with the dose and have the child swallow it. If taken within the hour and with no procrastination, there is no gooey mess caused by the herb dissolving the gel cap.
- *Herbal popsicles*. This technique is a fun one for sick kids and will cheer them up. Make a strong tea and triple the dose. Dilute tea down with equal amount of a favorite juice and freeze each dose in the form of an ice cube or popsicle. The ice is soothing to raw throats.
- *Jell-O herbal cubes*. Pour gelatin into an ice cube tray. Put one herb dose in each cube.
- *Glycerites*. Although weaker than alcoholic tinctures, they taste better. Many health food stores sell tinctures with glycerin as the menstruum or half and half with alcohol. You can also make your own.
- *Camouflage*. Cover flavors with nut butters, apple sauce, berry syrups, yogurt, or jelly, or blend in a smoothie. It sometimes works.

Summary

Many of the herbs used for children are the same as those for adults but in smaller doses. In the early years, children's GI system, livers, and lungs are immature. They need mild, gentle herbs. The majority of health problems herbalists see with kids involve lung infections, tummy aches, and accompanying emotional disturbances, such as sleep challenges and anxiety. Skin outbreaks are also common. For this reason, sample Materia Medicas and case histories are given in those areas.

For respiratory infections, we use immune builders, antimicrobials, and diaphoretics to sweat out a fever; mucolytics to break up phlegm; and antitussives to calm coughs. For eye infections, use antimicrobials, especially the berberines; for ear infections, antimicrobials and lymphatic drainers. For stomach ailments, such as gastritis and colic, use the relaxants and carminatives; for constipation, choose the cholagogues; and for diarrhea, use astringents. For anxiety or ADHD, turn to the standard nervines and nerve tonics. In the skin department, look to alteratives.

Very few studies have been conducted on herbal safety in children. Usage is based on traditional use, anecdotal reports, and a little research. Many plants that have been used safely over time have never been investigated. Dosage calculations are based on Clark's rule that goes by weight, Young's rule that goes by age, and Fried's rule that is used for infants under 2 years old. Methods of administration include teas, baths, steams, and topical essential oils. Inventive compliance tips gained from trial and error were enumerated.

Review

Fill in the Blanks

(Answers in Appendix B.)

1. Adult dose is 4 mL. What is a 4-year-old, 42-pound child's dose per Clark's rule? ___ mL. Per Young's rule? ___ mL.
2. The baby is 13 months old. If adult dose is 5 mL, give the infant's dose. ___.
3. Name the four most common body systems that affect children: ___, ___, ___, ___.
4. What are three benefits of breast milk? ___, ___, ___.
5. A child's liver matures by age ___. The gut matures by age ___.
6. Name four children's herbs for sleep, anxiety and stress: ___, ___, ___, ___.
7. Which herbal classification is useful for fever? ___. Name three herbs in this category: ___, ___, ___.
8. Name four causes of constipation in children: ___, ___, ___, ___.
9. What are four tips for administering herbs to kids? ___, ___, ___, ___.
10. Name four red flags in cases of diarrhea: ___, ___, ___, ___.

Critical Concept Questions

(Answers for you to decide.)

1. Do you feel secure about administering herbs to children?
2. What are the implications of liver detoxification in infant dosing?
3. Discuss whether you would choose Young's rule or Clark's rule to calculate dosage for a 40-pound, 3½-year-old child.
4. The same 3½-year-old, 40-pound child is to receive Elderberry tincture for his cold, 3 times a day. The adult dose is 5 mL. How much is the child's dose in mL per Clark's rule? ___ mL. How much is the dose per Young's rule? ___ mL.
5. Would you choose to use Clark's dosage or Young's dosage and why?
6. What are some reasons for caution with dosages for children under 3 years old, besides their small size?
7. Why do you think ADHD is so prevalent in our society?
8. Discuss when and when not to bring down a fever.
9. Why is *Vitex Agnus-castus* included in a teenage acne formula?
10. Why would Slippery Elm gruel work for both constipation and diarrhea?

References

1. Santich, Rob and Kerry Bone. *Phytotherapy Essentials: Healthy Children* (Queensland, Australia: Phytotherapy Press, 2008).
2. "Breastfeeding and Immunity." Australian Breastfeeding Association. https://www.n.au/bfinfo/breastfeeding-and-immunity (accessed August 3, 2019).
3. Beath, SV. "Hepatic Function and Physiology in the Newborn." PubMed. https://www.ncbi.nlm.nih.gov/pubmed/15001122 (accessed August 2, 2019).
4. Romm, Aviva. *Naturally Healthy Babies and Children* (Berkeley, CA: Celestial Arts, 2000).
5. "Herbs for Kids: What's Safe, What's Not." WebMD. https://www.webmd.com/balance/features/herbs-for-kids-feature#1 (accessed August 2, 2019).
6. Zand, Janet, et al. *Smart Medicine for a Healthier Child* (New York, NY: Avery, 1994).
7. Shiel, William C. Jr. "Medical Definition of ADD (attention deficit disorder)." MedicineNet. http://www.medicinenet.com/script/main/art.asp?articlekey = 2138 (accessed August 2, 2019).
8. Hoffman, David. *Medical Herbalism: Science and Practice of Herbal Medicine* (Rochester, VT: Healing Arts, 2003).
9. "Everything You Need to Know About Making and Using Homemade Saline Solution." Healthline. https://www.healthline.com/health/make-your-own-saline-solution#how-to-use-it (accessed December 5, 2019).
10. Rohland, Katherine. Afterthird. "Treating Pediatric Eczema with Acupuncture & Chinese Medicine." https://www.afterthird.com/treating-pediatric-eczema-with-acupuncture-chinese-medicine/ (accessed February 13, 2021).
11. "What is the Feingold Program?" The Feingold Association of the United States. http://feingold.org/about-the-program/what-is-the-feingold-program/ (accessed August 1, 2019).
12. "Clark's Rule and Young's Rule." Pharmacy Tech Study. https://www.pharmacy-tech-study.com/dosecalculation.html (accessed August 12, 2019).
13. "Pediatric Dosage Rules." Austin Community College. https://www.austincc.edu/rxsucces/ped5.html (accessed August 12, 2019).

22

The Cardiovascular System

"There is no greater love than healing the heart, for the heart is the spark of the soul."

—Message from Hawthorn tree, heard while collecting berries.

CHAPTER REVIEW

- Maintaining cardiovascular health. Coronary artery disease (CAD), risk factors, cholesterol and the fractionated/advanced lipid panel. Lifestyle fixes.
- The heart chakra, unconditional love.
- Chinese Medicine perspective: The Heart and major syndromes.
- Cardiac Materia Medica: Cardiac herbs worth honorable mention. Restoratives/tonics (general restoratives, arterial stimulants, venous decongestants, and capillary stimulants). Anticoagulants, antilipemics, and arterial relaxants.
- Common cardiovascular conditions with case histories: Hypertension, hyperlipidemia, congestive heart failure, angina pectoris, post myocardial infarction, and varicose veins.

KEY TERMS

Advanced lipid panel
Angina pectoris
Anticoagulants
Antilipemics
Atherosclerosis
Cholesterol
Congestive heart failure (CHF)
Coronary artery disease (CAD)
Fractionated/advanced lipid panel
Heart attack
Insulin resistance
Leptin resistance
Myocardial infarction (MI)
Plaque
Thrombus/thrombosis
Varicose veins
Vasodilation

The heart sings and hums as its miraculous pump keeps us alive, circulating oxygen-rich blood to every cell and accepting it back for another round. The heart is accompanied by its transportation network: arterial and venous blood vessels and capillaries (cardiovascular). An herbalist's task is to keep the system healthy. Lifestyle, diet, exercise, and spiritual and emotional health have a huge impact. Prevention is the best medicine and then come herbs, but if you're not getting anywhere, refer the client to a good cardiologist and work together.

Esoterically, the heart is the fourth chakra, the place of healing and unconditional love. The best heart tonics are love, kindness, caring, and service. Mind-body connection is heart connected. The opposite of unconditional love is hatred, resentment, loneliness, and bitterness (the Heart's taste in Chinese medicine). In the East, the Heart houses the shen or spirit. Mental, emotional, and spiritual conditions are affairs of the heart and, as such, are intertwined with its health. *All you need is love* is a truth.

Our cardiovascular Materia Medica covers the physical heart and blood vessels. Chapter 23 covers its shen aspects. A few herbal highlights are restorative Hawthorn berry used in the East, West, and Ayurvedic systems; the heart stimulant Lily of the Valley herb; the venous decongestant Horse Chestnut seed; Ginkgo leaf for microcirculation; and Salvia Dan Shen (Cinnabar Sage root) and Ligusticum Chuan Xiong (Sichuan Lovage root) used as multipurpose antilipemics, coronary restoratives, vasodilators, and anticoagulants.

Maintaining Cardiovascular Health

Coronary artery disease (CAD) is the leading cause of death in the United States and worldwide.[1] CAD refers to a full or partial blockage of one or more of the coronary arteries that supply blood to the heart. A waxy substance called ***plaque*** can build up inside the coronary arteries, creating *atherosclerosis*. Blockage deprives the heart muscle of oxygen that is critical for contraction. If attacked, the heart stops beating, and death results. All of the measures discussed are ultimately to prevent this from occurring, an honorable job and responsibility for any herbalist.

Coronary Artery Disease (CAD) Risk Factors

Multiple related factors cause CAD, some widely touted, some not so much. Common, well-accepted risks include smoking, hypertension, high cholesterol, diabetes, obesity, and family history. Under-the-radar aspects involve insulin and leptin resistance (Chapter 27), gluten sensitivity, dysbiosis, and diets high in saturated and trans fats.[2] Insulin and leptin resistance and an abnormal waist-to-hip ratio are also predictors of CAD risk.

- *Insulin resistance.* This leads to type 2 diabetes mellitus (DM2), hypertension, and CAD. The pancreatic hormone insulin regulates blood glucose levels. If the pancreas is overworked from a long-term high-carb/high-sugar intake, cell receptor sites become resistant to the insulin trying to hook onto them. Blood insulin levels rise higher and higher in the body's attempt to push enough glucose into the cells for energy production (Chapter 27). This situation is known as ***insulin resistance***, precursor to type 2 diabetes (metabolic syndrome).
  - *Sequel to insulin resistance.* If things go unchecked, the pancreas eventually wears out to the point where it can't keep up with insulin demand, goes on strike, and decreases insulin production. Blood glucose levels then rise as insulin levels decrease. Metabolic syndrome has officially arrived. The good news is that diet, herbs, and regular exercise can be major players in preventing and/or reversing insulin resistance.
- *Leptin resistance.* ***Leptin resistance*** is linked to insulin resistance and hypertension. Our friend, leptin, is the appetite-control hormone made in fat cells that signals the body when we are full and can stop eating. Hunger decreases; weight loss occurs. All is well.
  - *Leptin problems.* Troubles arise when the body gets into an inflammatory state and leptin loses its effectiveness. This state is often caused by a diet high in sugar (particularly fructose), grains, and processed foods. As sugar metabolizes in fat cells, the fat releases surges in leptin. Over time, if exposed to too much leptin, the body becomes resistant. Leptin stops working and weight is gained, just as in insulin resistance. For related syndromes of leptin and insulin resistance, with resultant high blood pressure (BP), the answer is to prevent surges in insulin and leptin. This is done with a whole-food diet low in simple sugar and carbohydrates.
- *Air and noise pollution.* Surprisingly (or not), toxic air and constant loud noises increase BP. Don't live in a smoggy city close to an airport if you can avoid it.
- *Apple shape.* The so-called apple-shaped female body that has lost its waistline, instead of the larger-hipped pear shape, indicates a higher risk of CAD, diabetes, and in some cases, cancer. Extra fat in the waist, arms, and breasts with very little body fat stored in the lower body are indicators.

Cholesterol and the Advanced Lipid Blood Panel

Cholesterol is a sterol made by the liver and found in most body tissues. It is not inherently bad, a myth that has been perpetrated by Big Pharma to sell more statin drugs, (e.g., Lipitor, Crestor, Mevacor), which have significant side effects and do not always work. Cholesterol is necessary and used by the body in manufacturing cell membranes, sex hormones, vitamin D, and for immune health. (Very low levels are unsafe and can indicate cancer, and a total cholesterol count is irrelevant, unless over 400.) When cholesterol oxidizes by contacting free radicals, toxins, and other inflammatory particles in the blood, it becomes dangerous. Once oxidized, cholesterol particles can damage the delicate endothelial lining of arteries and cause clogged arteries and coronary heart disease.[4] That's why a toxin-free, antiinflammatory diet is so important.

- *The fractionated or advanced lipid analysis panel.* The ***advanced lipid panel*** provides very important lipid blood measurements, which are highly reliable indicators of CAD risk. This test is a newer and much better indicator of CAD than what has been done in the past (Box 22.1). Request it if available, and follow along with this explanation. This blood test differentiates cholesterol *particle size*. It breaks down all the cholesterol subtypes or subpopulations in the two broad categories of high-density lipoproteins (HDLs), traditionally considered the good kind, and low-density lipoproteins (LDLs), traditionally considered the bad type of cholesterol. Here's how the test works.
  - *Low density lipoproteins (LDLs)* at high levels are considered high risk. However, some people with high blood levels of the so-called *bad* LDL never do develop heart disease, and some people with even normal LDL levels do. It turns out that LDLs come in two sizes: large and small particles (and subdivisions within the two). The large buoyant particles of LDL called lipoprotein B are harmless, but the small heavy LDL particles are inflammatory, especially the genetically induced *lipoprotein A* or *Lp(a)*.[3] This inherited particle resists all medications, including the overprescribed statins, and is the most predictive of risk. That is why, in some people, statins don't help at all. And they should definitely not be indiscriminately prescribed, particularly for people with high Lp(a) blood levels. The cholesterol and statin myths are just that. The true culprits are the inflammatory agents that caused the damage in the first place.
- *High density lipoproteins (HDLs).* High levels of HDL are associated with a lower risk of CAD because HDLs take up

• BOX 22.1 The Advanced Lipid Analysis, Risk Factors, and Its Relationship to Statin Drug Effectiveness

The advanced, fractionated cholesterol blood panel is the best indicator of coronary artery disease and tells whether statin drugs can help the situation or make matters worse. Not all LDL particles are necessarily bad, and some HDL particles are not so good. Furthermore, high triglycerides are pretty bad across the board.

- *LDLs, the generally bad LDL particle.* Lipoprotein A also known as Lp(a) is a small, dense and heavy LDL protein that is inflammatory and resists all medications, including the overprescribed statins. The higher the Lp(a) value, the higher the coronary artery risk. It is the leading cause of familial heart disease.
- *HDLs, the generally good HDL particle.* Apolipoprotein A (ApoA) is the most prevalent good protein in HDL, compared with Apolipoprotein B (ApoB). The ratio between ApoB to ApoA should be low. The higher the ApoA in the blood, the lower the coronary artery risk.[5]
- *Triglycerides.* High triglycerides indicate coronary artery risk. A high triglyceride to HDL ratio indicates a high risk of heart disease.

any extra cholesterol in the tissues and direct it back to the liver for excretion through the bile. There are advanced panel tests for two sizes of high-density HDL particles, traditionally considered good. But even among the good guys, some are better than others. Apolipoprotein A (ApoA) is the most prevalent good protein in HDL. High levels are a very good thing. The other particle, Apolipoprotein B (ApoB), is a heavy, not-so-good HDL. The advanced panel measures the *ratio of ApoB to ApoA*. It is an even better indicator of coronary artery risk than a high Lp(a). The ratio should be low.[4]

- *Triglycerides*. These are the most common kinds of fat molecules in the body and are produced by the liver, used for energy or stored as fat. Elevated levels are associated with a high CAD risk. The fractionated panel tests the *triglyceride to HDL ratio*. A high ratio is dangerous. The culprits causing high triglycerides are consumption of large amounts of simple carbohydrates and sugar.

Lifestyle Fix for Coronary Artery Disease

The factors in this list are all good measures for herbalists to suggest when devising a heart-healthy regime for prevention or when a cardiac event has occurred.[4] Another is routine preparation and consumption of a heart-healthy tea (Box 22.2).

- *Real food*. Have clients dramatically reduce dietary sugar and processed fructose (sugary drinks, sweet junky food) since high sugar intake is the main culprit that causes dyfunctional HDL.[4] Reduce unhealthy, artery-clogging trans fats. Replace processed foods with whole plants and healthy fats, such as avocado and virgin coconut oil. Include soaked raw nuts and grass-fed sources of meat. These foods will favorably address hypertension, insulin and leptin resistance, elevated uric acid levels, and cardiac health.
- *Vegetables high in NO_3 (nitrate)*. The body converts NO_3 to NO (nitric acid). Nitric acid dilates blood vessels and helps prevent clots. Sunlight exposure helps its absorption. Vegetables with high levels of nitric acid include radishes, kale, celery, mustard greens, spinach, cabbage, eggplant, leeks, scallions, string beans, and carrots. (Sounds like the makings of a good soup or salad.)
- *Omega-3 fatty acids (FAs)*. Use omega-3 fatty acids in food and other forms of supplementation. Good sources can be found in nontoxic sea oils and cold-water marine fish (salmon, tuna, sardines). Research indicates that plant-based FAs (Flax seed oil and Evening Primrose oil) are less effective than animal sources because the conversion rate of plant-based alpha-linolenic acid (ALA) omega-3 fats to the animal-based docosahexaenoic acid (DHA) is clinically insignificant. Many people are unable to convert plant FAs into the type the body needs and uses; thus animal based DHA becomes essential, even though wild sources of DHA come from more limited resources. However, if your client is vegan and does not indulge in animal sources, plant-based ALA sources are better than not using any. Supplement with 1000 mg or more per day.
- *Vitamin D_3*. Vitamin D_3 stops vessel stiffness and helps blood vessels relax, which in turn decreases BP. Low levels of D_3 further lead to insulin resistance, elevated cholesterol and triglycerides, obesity, and high BP. Vitamin D levels can be checked through blood testing and are commonly ordered by doctors these days.
- *Coenzyme Q_{10}*. An antioxidant found all over the body and abundant in heart muscle, coenzyme Q_{10} increases HDL levels, especially the good protein in HDL, ApoA. It builds energy and heart tissue and helps prevent CAD.
- *Nattokinase*. This is an enzyme extracted from a Japanese food called Natto, made from boiled and then fermented soybeans. Natto works as a natural clot buster and blood thinner and also decreases brain plaque in dementia. It is the most important supplement to take if the client has elevated bad Lp(a) that is resistant to statin drugs.[4] Take Natto on an empty stomach 30 minutes before meals, or between meals, because food inhibits its absorption.
- *Red yeast rice*. This is a product of rice fermented with a yeast, *Monascus purpureus*. It has a bright reddish-purple color. The original statin drug was formulated from red yeast rice, and this supplement is used to lower Lp(a), the worst of the LDLs.
- *Weight control and regular exercise*. Healthy diet and regular exercise help weight control. One feeds the other (no pun intended). Exercise about 30 minutes per day. Get up and move around frequently for emotional, spiritual, and psychological health and deliciously sound sleep. Walk as much as possible. Park the car far from the store.
- *No smoking*. Stay off recreational tobacco, a worthwhile challenge.
- *Sunlight exposure*. It's always good to go outside. The UV-B spectrum in sunlight converts cholesterol in the skin into vitamin D_3, another good use of cholesterol.
- *Calm outlook*. Love and kindness, deep breathing, yoga, meditation, music, family, good friends and relationships, community, service, and living with joy in your heart are all factors that lead to a long, happy, and healthy life. For real.

• BOX 22.2 Healthy Heart Tea

Chrysanthemum Flower, Hawthorn Berry, and Green Tea

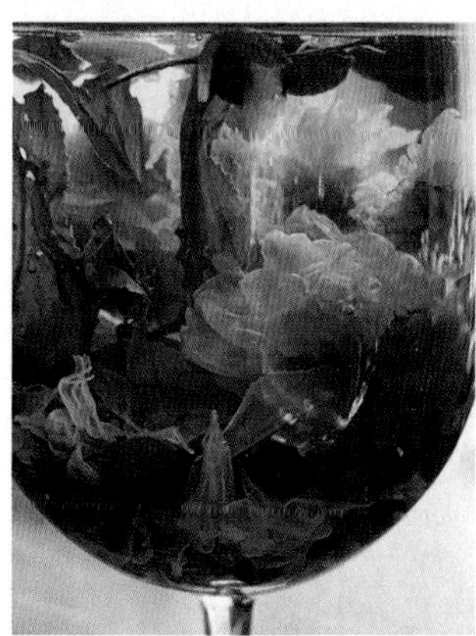

Chrysanthemum Ju Hua, Hawthorn berry, and Green Tea leaf make a heart-healthy tea. Just one look at this beautiful tea is enough to lift and heal the heart.

A lovely tonic tea, suitable any time, to maintain a peaceful, healthy heart and helpful for hypertension, coronary artery disease, and high cholesterol.

- 10 g *Chrysanthemum x morifolium* Ju Hua (Chrysanthemum flower)
- 10 g *Camellia sinensis* (Black or caffeine-free Green tea)
- 30 g *Crataegus* spp. (Hawthorn berry)

Directions

Place dried herbs in 8-oz cup. Pour in boiling water and let steep. Strain and drink freely.[6] Make it a part of a healthy ritual.

The Heart Chakra, Unconditional Love

Energetically and metaphysically, the heart is the fourth chakra, residing right behind the sternum (Fig. 22.1). It refers to unconditional love and healing. It is the middle chakra, number four out of seven. It is considered the bridge between the physical and the spiritual body, so it mediates body and spirit. As such, many issues related to love reside here. In its highest form, love is unconditional and pure, with an endless capacity to forgive and respond to prayer. This applies to self and to others. When heart chakra energy is low, we have feelings such as jealousy, bitterness, and anger and an inability to forgive ourselves and others.[7]

The heart's challenge is to deal with loaded issues such as grief, anger, hatred, trust, loneliness, fear, jealousy, betrayal, and absence of commitment to relationships. Metaphysically, aspects of CAD, heart failure, heart attacks, breast and lung cancer, and upper back and shoulder problems are spiritually connected to heart.

Because the heart chakra is the place of unconditional love, it is where healing energy resides. When an herbalist heals from this center, no harm can ever be intentionally caused. This space holds no blame, no judgments, no opinions, and no prejudice. We may think we live here all the time, but what happens if a client pushes one of our buttons? These triggers could be philosophical; related to sexual orientation, addiction, race, money, or political views; related to how the client smells or dresses; or based on whether they instill fear. I have never met anyone (myself included) who is totally without baggage in this regard. If some thought or negative feeling gets in our way, and we cannot approach a client unconditionally, the ethical action is to refer the client out. The heart chakra will let you know.

Chinese Medicine Perspective: The Heart and Major Syndromes

- *The Heart houses the shen or spirit.* Mental, emotional, and spiritual conditions are intertwined with Heart health. The Heart's positive emotion is joy, with its opposite being sadness or depression. Although we are grouping mental health issues such as anxiety, insomnia, depression, and addictions with the Western nervous system (Chapter 23), they would be included under the Heart if viewed from a Chinese Medicine perspective.
- *The Heart reflects the Western nervous system.* Problems like stroke, multiple sclerosis, or Parkinson's disease relate to the Heart.
- *The Heart governs the blood and rules the blood vessels.* The Heart is responsible for a smooth blood flow. Poor circulation means deficient Heart qi. Bleeding disorders can be found here. The cardiac Materia Medica includes herbs that address coagulation and also those that move blood and increase circulation.
- *The Heart influences the complexion.* Good circulation makes skin rosy and lustrous. Poor circulation makes a person pale or chalky.
- *Stagnant Heart blood.* This condition makes the complexion bluish-purple.
- *From a Five-Element standpoint, the Heart opens to the tongue.* The tongue body should be pale, red/pink. The tip reflects the Heart. If it's bright red, there's heat. If very pale, there is deficiency. Purple or purple spots indicate cold or Blood Stagnation.
- *The Heart controls sweat.* The Heart controls sweat and body fluids through heat.
- *Nourishment.* As in the West, nourishment is transported through the blood.

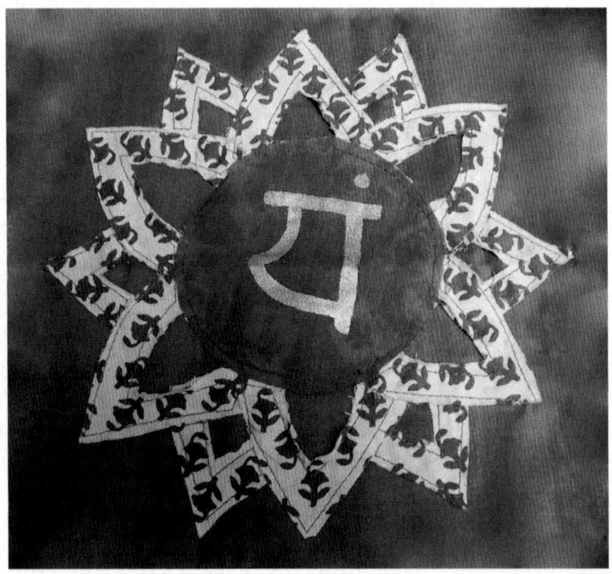

• **Fig. 22.1** The Heart Chakra is the bridge between the physical and the spiritual, and represents the place of unconditional love and healing.

Chinese Medicine Major Heart Syndromes

- *Heart Qi Deficiency.* A weak heart or pump without enough qi results in ***congestive heart failure (CHF)***. The main signs are palpitations, arrhythmias, anxiety, shortness of breath, sweating, memory problems, and fatigue. **Pulse (P)** Weak on left side under herbalist's index finger, the heart point. **Tongue (T)** Normal or pale. The solution is to tonify Heart qi with herbs such as Salvia Dan Shen (Cinnabar Sage root) or Ligusticum Chuan Xiong (Sichuan Lovage root). Western equivalents are heart restoratives: Hawthorn berry, Ginkgo leaf, Lily of the Valley herb, and Night Blooming Cereus stem and flower.
- *Heart Blood Stagnation.* This problem resembles angina. Symptoms include cyanosis of lips and nails and cold hands. **P** Choppy or rough, like sand through a straw. **T** Purple or with purple spots. The Heart needs warming, and qi needs to move. Ginkgo Yin Xing Ye (Ginkgo leaf), Ligusticum Chuan Xiong (Sichuan Lovage root), and Hawthorn berry all help coronary circulation.
- *Heart Yang Deficiency.* If Heart yang is too weak, blood is not circulating effectively through the coronary arteries. This can cause a myocardial infarction (MI), a heart attack. Symptoms include cold, clammy hands, pale face, sweating without exertion, shortness of breath, and signs of cold. There is chest pain and edema in men and nausea, anxiety or flulike symptoms in women (often with no chest pain). **P** Slow, deep, and weak. **T** Pale, wet, and swollen. To treat, tonify, and warm Heart yang with herbs that promote coronary circulation, use Salvia Dan Shen (Cinnabar Sage root), Ligusticum Chuan Xiong (Sichuan Lovage), and Carthamus Hong Hua (Safflower).

- *Venous Blood Stagnation.* When blood flows sluggishly through the veins and wants to clot, it can manifest as varicose veins, phlebitis, hemorrhoids, and leg cramping at night. **P** Wiry. **T** Sublingual veins enlarged and purplish. Use venous decongestants such as Red Root, Witch Hazel herb, Horse Chestnut seed, and Calendula flower.[8]

Cardiac Materia Medica

Many tried-and-true cardiac herbs overlap in multiple categories. They are the "must haves" in your cardiac apothecary. Pay attention to ones that are multipurpose and fit many situations. Some of these are Hawthorn berry, Ligusticum Chuan Xiong (Sichuan Lovage root), and Salvia Dan Shen (Cinnabar Sage root).

Cardiac Herbs Worth Honorable Mention

This list includes very valuable herbs for use in cardiac formulations.

- *Convallaria majalis* (Lily of the Valley herb) (Fig. 22.2). This is an arterial neurocardiac stimulant and restorative containing more than 40 cardiac glycosides[9] that increase the force of contractions and decrease heart rate, exactly what's needed in CHF, Heart Yang Deficiency. The herb tonifies the heart and serves as a draining diuretic to reduce ankle edema. Lily of the Valley is a safe, medium-strength herb that works like digitoxin and digoxin in the very toxic (don't use it) Foxglove. Use Lily of the Valley herb in formula with others such as Hawthorn berry and Ginkgo leaf. In addition, its sweet smell lifts the spirits and helps depression.
- *Hamamelis virginiana* (Witch Hazel leaf). A cool, drying astringent, this plant has a tropism to capillaries and blood vessels. It restores, vasoconstricts, and tightens blood vessel walls. Use for varicose veins, phlebitis, and hemorrhoids in venous Blood Stagnation. It helps hemorrhages anywhere. It also helps stop menstrual cramps from congestive dysmenorrhea.
- *Olea europaea* (Olive leaf). These antioxidant leaves are antihypertensive, antispasmodic, vasodilating, antiarrhythmic, antihyperlipidemic, and hypoglycemic. They are a good addition to a high BP formula with or without elevated fat and glucose levels. Leaves are also antimicrobial for viral, fungal, and bacterial infections. This is a natural ingredient to include in many cardiac formulas.
- *Salvia miltiorrhiza* Dan Shen (Cinnabar Sage root) (Fig. 22.3). This bitter, cool, dry salvia is very different from Western *Salvia officinalis* (Garden Sage leaf). Dan Shen functions as a cardiac tonic, vasodilator, antilipemic, and anticoagulant. Therefore it increases circulation through the coronary arteries and carries away the sludge caused in Heart Qi Stagnation. Furthermore, it restores and protects the liver. Use it preventatively and after a MI. This is a Chinese herb you should have on hand.
- *Ligusticum wallichii* Chuan Xiong (Sichuan Lovage root). Another ligusticum, Sichuan Lovage is a cardiovascular restorative and tonic. It is a capillary stimulant, vasodilator, antilipemic, and anticoagulant. Use it in hypotensive formulas with Olive leaf and Dan Shen, perhaps, for Heart Blood and Qi Stagnation. Furthermore, it is estrogenic and used in women's formulas involving PMS, where its analgesic qualities come into play. The root is contraindicated during pregnancy or heavy menstrual bleeding because it stimulates the uterus.[9]

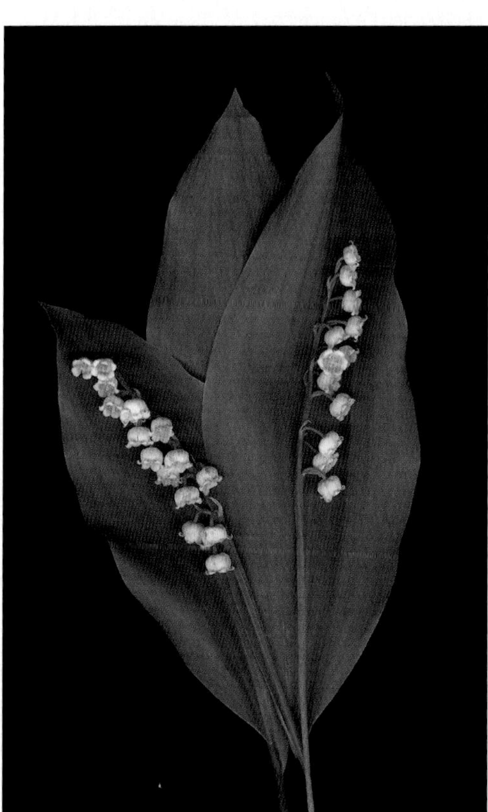

• **Fig. 22.2** *Convallaria majalis* (Lily of the Valley herb) contains cardiac glycosides, good for congestive heart failure. (Copyright Lang/Tucker Photography. Photographs loaned with permission, from *The Botanical Series* are copywritten by Jennifer Anne Tucker and Gerald Lang from the Studio at Hill Crystal Farm. www.jennifer-tucker.com.)

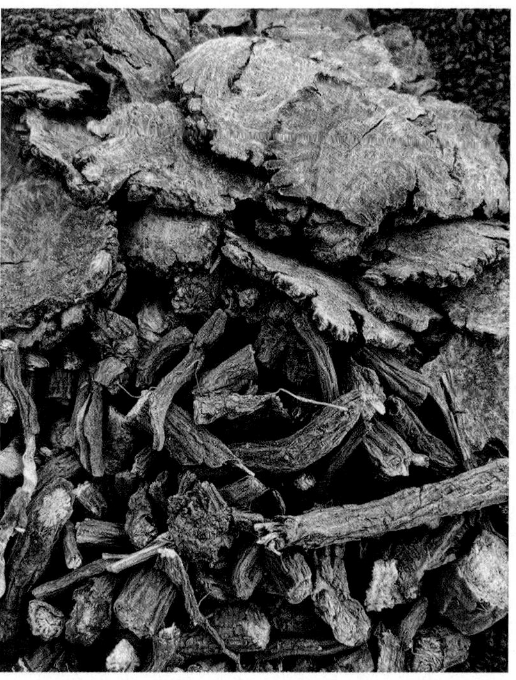

• **Fig. 22.3** Salvia Dan Shen (Cinnabar Sage root), bottom, and Ligusticum Chuan Xiong (Sichuan Lovage root), top, are multipurpose antilipemics, coronary restoratives, vasodilators, and anticoagulants.

Cardiac Restoratives

Some restoratives are general heart tonics; some work on arteries; others work on veins, and still others apply to capillaries. Use what's appropriate, depending on condition.[10]

- *General multipurpose restoratives.* These work with chronic stress and fatigue to tonify and build up the heart, help it to function well, and relieve palpitations. *Crataegus* spp. (Hawthorn berry) is perhaps the most famous in the East and West. Other general tonics include Salvia Dan Shen (Cinnabar Sage root), Ginkgo leaf, beloved Motherwort herb, Garlic bulb, Linden flower, and even Yarrow herb. Think of these when you need to beef up the sick or elderly or both (Table 22.1).
- *Arterial stimulants/restoratives.* These are used when the pump is not strong and arterial blood flow needs a little oomph. The person might have cold hands and feet, CHF, and Heart Qi Deficiency. These are slow-acting systemic herbs (could take 3 months to kick in). Here we have Lily of the Valley herb, Prickly Ash bark, Cinnamon bark, or Ginger root. All are warming (Table 22.2).
- *Venous decongestant/restoratives.* Most in this group are dry, cool astringents that firm up and tone the veins and increase venous circulation and capillary perfusion (Table 22.3). They help blood return by going upward against gravity on the circulatory system's journey back to the heart. Slow moving blood in the veins is known as Venous Blood Stasis/Stagnation. To aid

TABLE 22.1 General Cardiac Restoratives/Tonics
(Build cardiac function and relieve palpitations)

Herb	Notes
Salvia miltiorrhiza Dan Shen (Cinnabar Sage root)	General cardiovascular restorative/tonic, vasodilator, antilipemic, and anticoagulant. This is a must-have Chinese herb.
Crataegus spp. (Hawthorn berry)	Famous and fabulous cardiovascular restorative and tonic. Antilipemic, anticoagulant, and antihypertensive. For Heart Yin Deficiency.
Ligusticum wallichii Chuan Xiong (Sichuan Lovage root)	General cardiovascular restorative/tonic, capillary stimulant, vasodilator, antilipemic, and anticoagulant.
Ginkgo biloba (Ginkgo leaf)	General cardiovascular restorative, and antilipemic. For systemic capillary circulation, particularly to coronary arteries and brain.
Leonurus cardiac (Motherwort herb)	General heart qi restorative/tonic. For Heart Qi Deficiency with palpitations from anxiety, and stress. A woman's friend in menopause with hot flashes and worry.
Coleus forskohlii (Coleus root)	General cardiovascular restorative/tonic.
Allium sativum (Garlic bulb)	General cardiovascular restorative/tonic. For Heart Qi and Blood Stagnation. Balances blood pressure. A superfood.

TABLE 22.2 Arterial Stimulants/Restoratives
(Strengthen the heart pump)

Herb	Notes
Convallaria majalis (Lily of the Valley herb)	Arterial stimulant, restorative, cardiac glycoside, and draining diuretic. Excellent for CHF, Heart Qi and Yang Deficiency. Use in formula, not as a simple. Medium strength.
Xanthoxylum americanum (Prickly Ash bark)	Arterial stimulant and restorative. Helps peripheral circulation, particularly good in chronic arthritis.
Capsicum annuum (Cayenne pepper)	Pungent, hot, dry arterial stimulant, and restorative. Creates sweating, strengthens systemic and heart circulation. For Heart Blood and Qi Stagnation. Use in small amounts.
Cinnamomum spp. (Cinnamon bark and twig)	Warming, restorative arterial stimulant that increases circulation. For Heart Yang Deficiency. Also helps balance glucose.
Angelica sinensis Dang Qui (Angelica root or Dong Quai root)	Coronary restorative, antilipemic, anticoagulant, and vasodilator. Also, estrogenic.
Allium sativum (Garlic bulb)	Hot, dry arterial stimulant, restorative, anticoagulant, and antilipemic. For Heart Yang Deficiency, Blood and Qi Stagnation.

TABLE 22.3 Venous Decongestants/Restoratives
(Cool astringents that tone veins and increase venous return)

Herb	Notes
Aesculus hippocastanum (Horse Chestnut seed)	Venous decongestant for blood stagnation, varicose veins, hemorrhoids, and thrombosis. Venous restorative, astringent, and anticoagulant. Also, for uterine blood congestion with cramps.
Collinsonia canadensis (Stone root)	Venous decongestant for blood stagnation with varicosities. For leg cramps, hemorrhoids, constipation. Also, for liver and pelvic blood congestion, mucous congestion. Anticoagulant for bleeding.
Hamamelis virginiana (Witch Hazel herb)	For varicose veins, phlebitis, hemorrhoids in venous blood stagnation. Also, for congestive dysmenorrhea (menstrual cramps).
Cupressus sempervirens (Cyprus tip)	Astringent, toning, hemostatic, for blood congestion, varicose veins, hemorrhoids, phlebitis, menstrual cramps, heavy periods.
Calendula officinalis (Marigold flower)	Astringes veins. Helps hemorrhoids and phlebitis in venous blood stagnation.
Quercus alba (White Oak bark)	For hemorrhoids, swelling, dermatitis. Use freshly crushed as a styptic for bleeding, itching, bites, and stings.
Achillea millefolium (Yarrow herb)	A venous decongestant for Venous Blood Stagnation in varicose veins. Also, its astringency lessens heavy uterine bleeding and diarrhea.

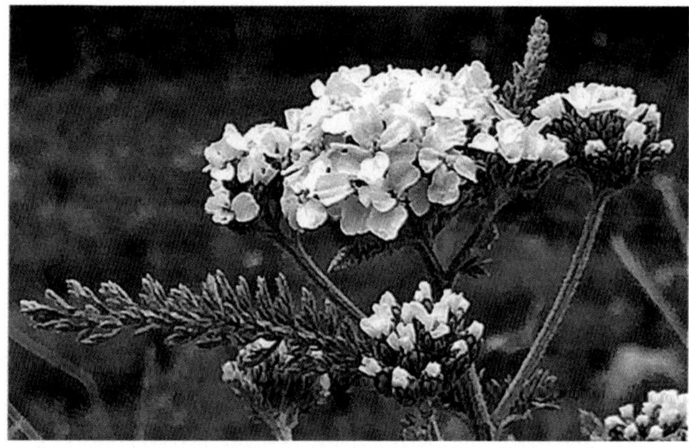

• **Fig. 22.4** *Achillea millefolium* (Yarrow herb) is a circulatory and venous decongestant making it useful for varicose veins.

venous return, try Horse Chestnut, Red Root, Yarrow herb (Fig. 22.4), or Calendula flower. Bioflavonoids tone and strengthen veins and capillaries. Colorful berries and many venous decongestant herbs contain this antioxidant. Hawthorn berry, *Vaccinium* spp. (Bilberry) berry and leaf, and Green tea leaf all work in this manner.

- *Capillary stimulants/restoratives*. These restore microcirculation, be it in the eyes, heart, pelvis, brain, or under the skin (a bruise). Anything that works on a capillary level helps both venous and arterial circulation because capillaries connect the two types of vessels. To help microcirculation to the eyes, use *Vaccinium* spp. (Bilberry) leaf and berry (Fig. 22.5) and Ginkgo leaf. Call on Ligusticum Chuan Xiong (Sichuan Lovage root), Hawthorn berry, and Calendula flower, which all work on the heart. For blood pooling in the uterus and qi and blood stagnation (menstrual cramps), Calendula flower, Yarrow flower, and Witch Hazel herb are specific. To bring blood to the brain, use Ginkgo leaf, Gotu kola herb, and Rosemary leaf (Table 22.4).

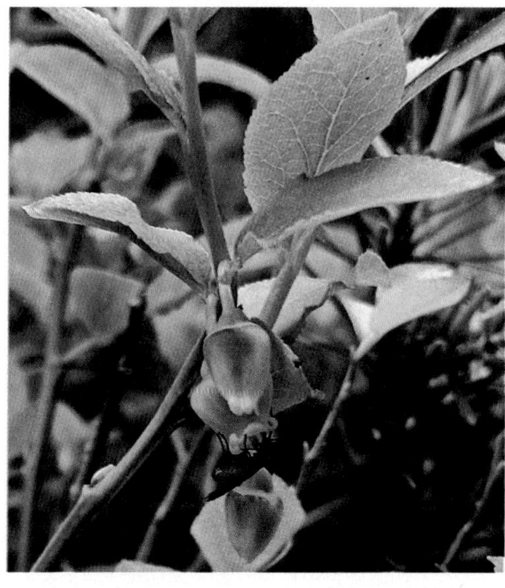

• **Fig. 22.5** *Vaccinium* spp. (Bilberry, Huckleberry, Whortleberry, Grouseberry), one of three Colorado mountain species, is high in antioxidants that tone and strengthen veins and capillaries.

Anticoagulants

Anticoagulants increase clotting time and decrease blood clots. By thinning the blood, they prevent bleeding and clotting in all the wrong places: coronary arteries, veins, microcirculation or capillaries, uterus, urine, and gut, wherever. A ***thrombus*** is a blood clot in the vascular system that blocks or impedes blood flow. A clot in the coronary arteries causes a heart attack; a clot in the vessels of the brain creates a stroke. To work with these issues, select herbs with the correct anticoagulant tropism. Ligusticum Chuan Xiong (Sichuan Lovage) root, Hawthorn berry, and Gingko leaf all lessen coronary clotting (Table 22.5). Witch Hazel leaf or White Oak bark help varicose veins (venous decongestants). Yellow Sweet Clover, Lady's Mantle, and Shepherd's Purse (Fig. 22.6) herbs help heavy menstrual clots with dysmenorrhea (obviously, this use is out of the coronary realm, but it illustrates the point).

In Chapter 8, we discussed the coumarin controversy and the fact that certain herbs, such as the clovers and some grasses containing coumarins were not anticoagulants, particularly the legume plants of the Fabaceae/Pea family, such as *Melilotus officinalis* (Yellow Sweet Clover herb); however, when they were newly mowed in the fields they fermented (spoiled), changing their chemical structure into dicoumarol, which did in fact cause coagulation and bleeding in grazing animals.

However, another study published in 2017 found that fresh, unspoiled Yellow Sweet Clover herb does contain coumarin, and yes, it does have anticoagulant properties.[11] So the takeaway is to

TABLE 22.4 Capillary Stimulants/Restoratives *(Increase microcirculation)*

Herb	Notes
Ligusticum wallichii Chuan Xiong (Sichuan Lovage root)	Capillary stimulant, restorative, vasodilator, antilipemic, and anticoagulant for Heart Blood and Qi Stagnation.
Ginkgo biloba (Ginkgo leaf)	Absolutely indicated for capillary circulation anywhere, especially the brain. A must-have.
Crataegus spp. (Hawthorn berry)	This herb is a no-brainer, cardiac-wise. Restores capillaries and helps circulation.
Vaccinium myrtillus (Bilberry leaf)	Helps microcirculation, strengthens the capillaries in Venous Blood Stagnation.
Xanthoxylum americanum (Prickly Ash bark)	One of best all-around blood movers, capillary circulators, for peripheral circulation.

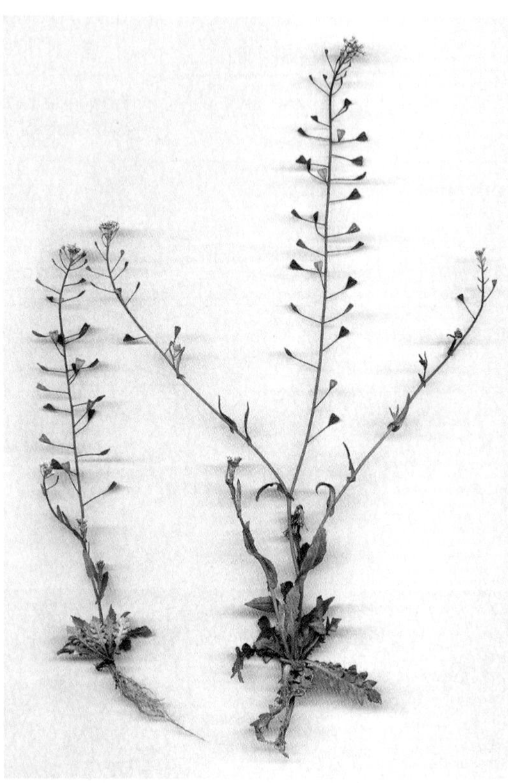

• **Fig. 22.6** *Capsella bursa-pastoris* (Shepherd's Purse herb) with its uterine tropism is an anticoagulant that breaks up heavy menstrual clots. Note its distinctive triangular seed pods. (Copyright Lang/Tucker Photography. Photographs loaned with permission, from *The Botanical Series* are copywritten by Jennifer Anne Tucker and Gerald Lang from the Studio at Hill Crystal Farm. www.jennifer-tucker.com.)

TABLE 22.5 Anticoagulants

Herbs	Notes
Ginkgo biloba Yin Xing Ye (Ginkgo leaf)	Anticoagulant for coronary clots and thrombosis. Restorative, and increases microcirculation.
Crataegus spp. (Hawthorn berry)	Anticoagulant for clots. Heart restorative, antilipemic, and vasodilator.
Melilotus officinalis (Yellow Sweet Clover herb)	Reduces blood stasis (clots or thrombus). For congestive dysmenorrhea.
Ligusticum wallichii Chuan Xiong (Sichuan Lovage root)	Coronary anticoagulant, vasodilator, antilipemic, and restorative.
Carthamus tinctorius Hong Hua (Safflower flower)	Anticoagulant for coronary thrombosis, uterine clots, and antilipemic. Classic for hypertension.
Convallaria majalis (Lily of the Valley herb)	Softens all deposits, antitumoral, draining diuretic. Restores heart and stimulates contractions in congestive heart failure.
Salvia miltiorrhiza Dan Shen (Cinnabar Sage root)	For all types of blood stasis: coronary clots, fibroids, endometriosis, and dysmenorrhea.

be careful with these plants and assume that they may have anticoagulant properties after all. This is another example of how evolving research is constantly changing beliefs and information about our healing plants.

Antilipemics

Antilipemics are herbs that lower cholesterol levels in the coronary arteries. As noted earlier, cholesterol is not necessarily bad. The body uses it to make hormones and vitamin D, and to aid digestion, protect nerves, and produce all cell membranes. Statin drugs happen to block liver enzymes responsible for making all kinds of cholesterol. They come with numerous nasty side effects: liver dysfunction, increased risk of diabetes, nerve damage, muscle weakness, and more. Wise herbalists use botanicals that raise HDL, rather than indiscriminately lowering any and all cholesterol.

Some of the best botanicals to reduce bad LDL and increase healthy HDL are our friends: *Curcuma longa* (Turmeric root), *Cynara scolymus* (Globe Artichoke), *Crataegus* spp. (Hawthorn berry), and high doses of the berberines. Garlic bulb capsules help blood quality, whereas Gotu kola herb manages unstable plaque. Green tea reduces cholesterol and triglycerides, increases HDL, and decreases platelet clumping (Table 22.6).[2] Clumped blood cells lead to clots.

Arterial Relaxants/Vasodilators

Arterial relaxants dilate or widen the systemic arteries (***vasodilation***) throughout the body and lower BP. When the tubes or vessels are dilated or when their size increases, the pressure in them drops, and more blood flows. Also, more oxygen will reach the cells, with more nutrients delivered and waste removed. Hence, this category is used for treating hypertension, enhancing oxygenation, and improving circulation flow when called for. Many arterial relaxants are also coronary vasodilators, which increase blood flow/oxygenation systemically and to the heart muscle directly. This improved flow helps prevent angina and heart attacks. *Prunella vulgaris* (Selfheal spike) (Fig. 22.7), Chrysanthemum Ju Hua (Chrysanthemum flower), Valerian root, Skullcap herb, and Lily of the Valley herb are examples. Be patient. They act over the long term, requiring a few months to make a difference. Notice that many of these are also nervine relaxers (Table 22.7).

TABLE 22.6 Antilipemics
(A star * means very important)

Herb	Notes
**Curcuma longa* (Turmeric root)	Dissolves fatty deposits, helps circulation in Heart Blood Stagnation. Number one herb in this department.
***All berberines** Roots of Goldenseal, Oregon Grape, Barberry, Coptis Huang Lian, Corydalis Yan Hu Suo, and Phellodendron Huang Bai bark	Antilipemic. These plants contain the berberine alkaloid. Number two herbs.
**Cynara scolymus* (Globe artichoke leaf)	Dissolves deposits in hyperlipidemia. Rich in saponins shunting fat to the gastrointestinal tract. Renowned liver herb. Number three herb.
Gymnema sylvestre (Gymnema herb)	Saponin-rich. Reduces sweet taste and cravings in diabetes types I and II.
Camellia sinensis (Green Tea leaf)	Drink many cups a day. Reduces triglycerides and increases HDL.
Crataegus spp. (Hawthorn berry)	Antilipemic, restorative, anticoagulant, hypotensive, and a vasodilator.
Allium sativum (Garlic clove)	Best form is allium-releasing tablets, providing 12 mg allicin per day. (If using fresh, take 6–12 g of bulb.)
Cinnamomum cassia (Cinnamon bark)	Antilipemic and antihypertensive. Lowers blood sugar and helps dysbiosis. Use liberally in food.
Ligusticum wallichii Chuan Xiong (Sichuan lovage)	Antilipemic, vasodilator, coronary restorative, hypotensive. Heart Blood and Qi Stagnation.
Centella asiatica (Gotu Kola herb)	Antilipemic and also helps venous circulation.
Ginkgo biloba Yin Zing Ye (Ginkgo leaf) Used in Western and Chinese medicine.	Antilipemic, coronary restorative, vasodilator, and capillary restorative. For Heart Blood and Qi Stagnation.
Salvia miltiorrhiza Dan Shen (Cinnabar Sage root)	Antilipemic, coronary restorative, vasodilator, anticoagulant, Heart Blood and Qi Stagnation.
Convallaria majalis (Lily of the Valley herb)	For Heart Qi and Yang Deficiency, angina, and palpitations.

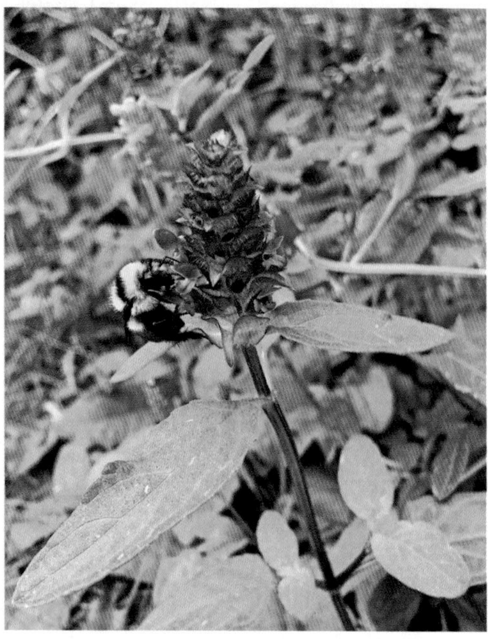

• **Fig. 22.7** *Prunella vulgaris* Xia Ku Cao (Selfheal Spike) is a vasodilator for hypertension.

Common Cardiovascular Conditions

Hypertension

High BP is risky and should always be screened. Don't take a client's word for their BP level; take it yourself and know the parameters (Table 22.8). Herbalists should own a stethoscope and a regular adult and large size BP cuff. Hypertension increases chances of heart disease, leading to heart attacks, heart failure, stroke, kidney disease, eye damage, and foggy brain (e.g., dementias and Alzheimer's). These are good reasons to check BP often and to obtain a baseline pressure. When Western medicine can offer no known cause and no symptoms are present, the disorder is called *essential* or *primary hypertension* (Case History 22.1). But high BP doesn't just come out of nowhere. Look carefully and find the reason.

Hyperlipidemia

- *Definition.* Abnormally high concentration of certain cholesterol factions and triglycerides in the blood, which can lead to fatty buildups, called plaques, on the vessel linings of the coronary arteries (***atherosclerosis***), blood clots (***thrombosis***), and ultimately CAD, heart attacks, and strokes (Case History 22.2).

TABLE 22.7 Arterial Relaxants/Vasodilators

Herb	Notes
Ligusticum wallichii Chuan Xiong (Sichuan Lovage root)	Coronary vasodilator, anticoagulant, antilipemic, and restorative. Important for hypertension.
Salvia miltiorrhiza Dan Shen (Cinnabar Sage root)	Vasodilator, coronary restorative, capillary stimulant, antilipemic, and anticoagulant.
Viscum album (European Mistletoe herb)	For hypertension with Liver Yang Rising (headache, dizziness, tinnitus), palpitations, and also stops uterine bleeding. A diuretic.
Crataegus spp. (Hawthorn berry)	Coronary vasodilator, restorative, antilipemic, and anticoagulant. For Heart Yin Deficiency with congestive heart failure, hypertension, and palpations.
Tilia cordata (Linden flower)	Vasodilator, anticoagulant, and antilipemic. For hypertension with Liver Yang Rising, neurocardiac component, and angina.
Coleus forskohlii (Coleus root)	Ayurvedic peripheral vasodilator with antiplatelet activity. Works quickly.
Olea europaea (Olive leaf)	Antihypertensive, antispasmodic, vasodilator, and antiarrhythmic. Need fairly high dose.
Prunella vulgaris Xi Ku Cao (Selfheal spike) Same species used in Western and Chinese herbalism.	Cooling vasodilator, hemostatic, relaxant, hypotensive for Liver Yang Rising (headache, dizziness, tinnitus). Also, a detoxicant/antiinfective.
Scutellaria lateriflora (Skullcap herb)	Spasmolytic. For hypertension with a nervous component; anxiety, restlessness, sleep loss.
Chrysanthemum x morifolium Ju Hua (Chrysanthemum flower)	Peripheral vasodilator and coronary relaxant for Liver Yang Rising/hypertension with headache, dizziness, and tinnitus. Also antimicrobial for Wind Heat.
Passiflora incarnata (Passionflower herb)	Neurocardiac relaxant. For stress-related hypertension with anxiety, restless sleep, and palpitations.
Essential Oils Chamomile, Bergamot, Lavender, Lemon Balm, Marjoram, Motherwort, Neroli, Rose, Ylang Ylang	These essential oils are arterial relaxants and vasodilators that help with hypertension.

(*Continued*)

TABLE 22.7 Arterial Relaxants/Vasodilators—cont'd

Herb	Notes
Gastrodia elata Tian Ma (Celestial Hemp corm)	Hypotensive and cardiac and nervous relaxant. For essential hypertension, Liver Yang Rising, and Liver Wind with headache, dizziness, and tinnitus.
Uncaria rhynchophylla Gou Teng (Gambir Vine twig)	Peripheral vasodilator, cardiac and nervous relaxant. For Liver Yang Rising and Liver Wind with dizziness, tinnitus.
Leonurus cardiaca (Motherwort herb)	Relaxing, calming. Primarily for Heart Qi Deficiency, congestive heart failure or angina with palpitations. Classic in menopausal anxiety with palpitations.
Carthamus tinctorius Hong Hua (Safflower flower)	Vasodilator, coronary restorative, antilipemic, and anticoagulant. For chronic hypertension, heart and cerebral microcirculation.

TABLE 22.8 Blood Pressure Parameters

Systolic	Diastolic	Category
<120	<80	Normal
120–139	80–89	Prehypertension
140–159	90–99	Stage I Hypertension
160 or higher	100 or higher	Stage II Hypertension[12]

- *Risk factors.* These include cigarette smoking and having hypertension, insulin and leptin resistance, gluten sensitivity, dysbiosis, diabetes types 1 or 2, and a diet high in saturated and trans fats.[2]
- *Labs.* The best test is a fractionated/advanced lipid panel (Box 22.1).
- *Signs and symptoms.* There really are none. Other than an abnormal lab test, you won't know it's there unless it manifests as angina, heart attack, or stroke. If some of the risk factors are present, you'll have a clue. After all, we treat people, not lab results.
- *Allopathic treatment.* Statins to lower cholesterol. Low-fat diet, exercise, not smoking. A note on statins: they are abused and misused.
- *General therapeutic principles.* Most people with hyperlipidemia will have other factors that need attention. Create a formula based on those. (1) Decrease fatty deposits with antilipemics. (2) Decrease any blood clots with anticoagulants. (3) Antihypertensives as needed. (4) Hypoglycemics as needed. (5) Diet, supplements, and lifestyle changes.

Congestive Heart Failure (CHF)

- *Definition.* In *Congestive Heart Failure (CHF)*, the heart cannot supply enough blood to body because of weak, inadequate pumping action. Fluid eventually backs up to the lungs, causing shortness of breath, coughing, fatigue, and fluid retention, especially edema in feet/ankles with retention of fluid and sodium (Case History 22.3).

CASE HISTORY 22.1

Case History for Essential Hypertension

S. Alex is 49, just divorced, has a blood pressure (BP) reading of 172/95. He has palpitations and anxiety. Sometimes he gets dizzy. He is quick to anger. There are no arrhythmias and his ECG is normal. Has been unresponsive to meds prescribed by his healthcare provider. Maintains a junk food diet.

O. P Forceful, strong, rapid. **T** Red, thin yellow coat. BP 172/95. Pulse rate 93.

A. Liver Yang Rising with tinnitus and dizziness. Essential hypertension with nervous component.

P. *Specific therapeutic principles.* (1) Clear heat, sedate yang. (2) Vasodilators. (3) Nervous system relaxants. (4) Diuretics to remove excess fluids. (5) Cardiac restoratives. (6) Look for other causes and treat as indicated.

Herbal Formula and Dose. 6 mL 3 × day for 3 months minimum; monitor BP weekly.

Part	Herbs	Rationale
2	Gastrodia Tian Ma	Vasodilator specific to Liver Yang Rising.
2	Uncaria Gou Teng	Vasodilator specific to Liver Yang Rising, cooling.
2	Ginkgo herb	Palpitations.
2	Passionflower	Nervous sedative/decrease palpitations.
2	Ziziphus Suan Zao Ren	Cooling neurocardiac sedative.
1	Dandelion leaf	Draining diuretic to decrease fluid volume, cooling.
1	Hawthorn berry	Cardiac restorative, antilipemic, anticoagulant.

Other Suggestions

Red Flags. Refer out if you do not get results after 3 months, or if blood pressure (BP) is very high, for example, 180/120, or with confusion or other neurological symptoms, nosebleed, fatigue, blurred vision, chest pain, or abnormal heartbeat.

- *Diet.* More fruits, veggies, cruciferous, marine fish. Nitrate-based veggies. Cooking lessons?
- *Supplements.* EPA/DHA 2000 mg per day. Vitamin D_3.
- Exercise program.
- Meditation or stress reduction techniques, and psychotherapy as needed.
- Monitor BP weekly and if no improvement in a few months, refer out.

CASE HISTORY 22.2

Case History for Hyperlipidemia

S. Melissa is 35, has elevated LDLs, a high Lp(a). Reports her blood pressure (BP) is 150/90 and she frequents fast food places. Says she has a lot of bloating and burping. She is overweight, never exercises. Her father died of an myocardial infarction (MI) at 59 years old. She has a stressful, fast-paced job.

O. P Forceful, rapid. **T** Body red. Coat greasy and yellow. BP 155/92.

A. Damp heat. Elevated statin-resistant cholesterol, hypertension, probable dysbiosis and stress.

P. *Specific therapeutic principles.* (1) Antilipemics. (2) Antihypertensives. (3) Normalize gut flora with cool bitters. (4) Stress control. (5) Dry damp.

Sample Formula and Dose. 8 mL 3 × day.

Part	Herbs	Rationale
3	Turmeric root	Antilipemic, bitter to heal gut.
2	Hawthorn berry	Lowers LDL, tonic, antihypertensive/anticoagulant.
2	Salvia Dan Shen	Cardiovascular tonic/vasodilator/antilipemic/anticoagulant.
2	Passionflower herb	Nervine for stress and BP.
2	Poria Fu Ling	Dry damp, restore Spleen.
1	Cinnamon bark	Antilipemic, hypoglycemic, and tastes good.
1	Globe Artichoke leaf	Antilipemic and liver cleansing.

Other Suggestions

- *Diet.* Green tea, 3 cups per day. Lots of Garlic. Paleo diet. Probiotics/prebiotics. Start cooking lessons perhaps. All these help any insulin or leptin resistance.
- *Supplements.* Red yeast rice, nattokinase, specific for high Lp(a). Coenzyme Q_{10}, EPA/DHA, nitric acid, Garlic, vitamin D_3, probiotics, blue-green algae, Turmeric capsules.
- *Lifestyle.* Begin exercise program, yoga?
- Monitor BP.

CASE HISTORY 22.3

Case History for Congestive Heart Failure (CHF)

S. Fred is 82. When he moved to Denver from New Jersey to be with his grandkids, he began having shortness of breath, and his ankles swelled up. He was diagnosed with CHF, begun on Digitalis. Now, 8 months later, he is stable and would like to begin herbal treatment. He is on the beta blocker Atenolol and a diuretic for hypertension. He is nervous.

O. P Weak. **T** Normal. BP 134/90 maintained with Atenolol and diuretic. Ankles become swollen when sitting.

A. Heart Qi Deficiency. Stable CHF.

P. *Specific therapeutic principles.* (1) Use arterial stimulant herbs that contain milder cardiac glycosides than the very toxic strong herb, Foxglove, from which Digitalis is derived. Cardiac glycosides increase the force of heart contractions and decrease heart rate, both needed in CHF. Lily of the Valley herb and/or Coleus root[14] are the safest to use. (2) Diuretic herbs like Dandelion leaf/root or Goldenrod herb or Poria Fu Ling. (3) Restoratives like Hawthorn berry, Salvia Dan Shen. (4) Decrease stress with nervines.

Sample Formula and Dose. 6 mL 3 × day.

Part	Herbs	Rationale
3	Lily of the Valley herb	Tonifies heart qi, cardiac glycoside, diuretic.
2	Coleus root	Cardiac glycoside, restorative, antihypertensive.
2	Hawthorn berry	Cardiac restorative, increases circulation.
2	Poria Fu Ling	Diuretic, helps edema, restores Spleen.
2	Mistletoe twig	Astringent, helps edema.
2	Linden flower	Calm heart, decrease stress.

Other Suggestions

Red Flag: For acute episodes with difficulty breathing, refer to a hospital emergency room. When stable, may be able to wean off meds with herbal intervention, as shown in earlier case history. Cooperation with the doctor is needed. *Never* administer Lily of the Valley concurrently with Digitalis. Client should be completely off the drug for about 4 days, before starting Lily of the Valley. If on Digitalis, drug levels should be drawn periodically.

- *Diet:* Mediterranean or Paleo, healthy fat, and reduced salt.
- Exercise as tolerated.
- *Supplements.* Fish Oil 1000 mg per day, coenzyme Q_{10}, vitamin D_3.
- Monitor blood pressure, edema, breathing, and weight. A 3-lb weight gain in 1 day or 5 lb in a week is a danger sign.
- Assess gastrointestinal history for possible dysbiosis.

- *Signs and symptoms.* Shortness of breath, coughing, wheezing, pallor, arrhythmias, and fluid retention with edema in feet and ankles.
- *From Chinese Medicine perspective.* A weak heart pump results in Heart Qi Deficiency, or lack of energy.
- *Allopathic treatment.* Digitalis to increase myocardial contractility, vasodilators, diuresis, oxygen, and bed rest.
- *General therapeutic principles.* (1) Use arterial stimulants/cardiac glycosides like Lily of the Valley herb to increase contractility. (2) Use diuretics like Dandelion leaf or Poria Fu Ling to decrease fluids. (3) Decrease stress with nervines. (4) Choose cardiac restoratives.

Angina Pectoris

- *Definition. **Angina pectoris*** is temporary chest pain on exertion and/or stress when the heart muscle is not getting enough oxygen (Case History 22.4). This condition is caused by a partial blockage in the coronary arteries from fatty plaque or a blood clot. It is not a heart attack, but it's close and is a warning. It may also be caused by arrhythmias, anemia, and valve damage, and it can be triggered by exercise, stress, extreme temperature changes, alcohol, smoking, overeating,[13] or any activity requiring more oxygen than the heart can deliver.
- *Signs and symptoms.* Chest tightness and pain and/or pain radiating down arm, jaw, abdomen, or back. Sometimes the pain feels like and mimics indigestion. The hallmark of angina is that the pain is activated by triggers and subsides when they are removed.
- *Allopathic treatment.* Rest and sublingual nitroglycerin as needed. Nitroglycerin relaxes the coronary arteries and reduces the heart's workload.

CASE HISTORY 22.4

Case History for Angina Pectoris

S. Marc has been getting chest pain whenever he runs or gets stressed. He was diagnosed with angina after a scare and a hospital stay. A myocardial infarction was ruled out. Cardiac catheterization showed beginnings of atherosclerosis. His blood pressure (BP) is elevated. He was sent home with a statin, two BP meds, and nitroglycerin as needed for chest pain. He had a cursory nutritional consult. He mainly eats in restaurants, and he smokes a pack a day.
O. **P** Choppy. **T** Purple spots. BP 180/90.
A. Heart Blood Stagnation. Angina pectoris, per healthcare provider. Hypertension.
P. *Specific therapeutic principles*. Remove stasis, get blood moving. (1) Arterial stimulants/restoratives. (2) Antihypertensives. (3) Antilipemics. (4) Nervine for stress.

Sample Formula and Dose. 6 mL 3 × day.

Part	Herbs	Rationale
4	Hawthorn berry	Restorative, antilipemic, arterial stimulant.
3	Turmeric root	Antilipemic.
2	Salvia Dan Shen	Antilipemic, anticoagulant, restorative, vasodilator.
2	Lily of the Valley herb	Arterial stimulant/restorative.
2	Passionflower herb	Nervine/antihypertensive.

Other Suggestions

- *Diet*. Heart healthy diet with simple recipes.
- *Supplements*. Coenzyme Q10, EPA/DHA, vitamin D_3.

CASE HISTORY 22.5

Case History for Post Myocardial Infarction (MI)

S. Joseph was rushed to the emergency room after experiencing stabbing chest pain at work. He was diagnosed with an MI and started on all the usual hospital meds and IVs. Now he is home and back to work. He is on Coumadin, a statin, an antihypertensive, diuretic, and antianxiety medications. One MI is enough. He is only 41 years old. Can he get on some herbs? His dietary and exercise habits are marginal.
O. **P** Tight, wiry. **T** Purplish.
A. Post MI. Heart Yang Deficiency. Hypertension, hyperlipidemia, anxiety.
P. *Specific therapeutic principles*. (1) Cardiac restoratives like Ligusticum Chuan Xiong, Salvia Dan Shen, and Hawthorn berry. (2) Anticoagulant herbs in conjunction with coagulation labs: Ginkgo leaf, Salvia Dan Shen, Lily of the Valley herb. (3) Antihypertensives like Ligusticum Chuan Xiong or Coleus root. (4) Antilipemics such as Turmeric root or Artichoke leaf. (5) Stress control.

Sample Formula and Dose. 6 mL 3 × day.

Part	Herbs	Rationale
4	Sichuan Lovage Chuan Xiong	Vasodilator, restorative, anticoagulant, antilipemic.
4	Salvia Dan Shen	Heart restorative, relaxant, anticoagulant, antilipemic.
2	Turmeric root	Antilipemic.
2	Hawthorn berry	Restore heart, decrease cholesterol, dilate arteries.
2	Passionflower	Stress and anxiety, hypertension.

Other Suggestions

Red Flags For any chest pain, refer quickly to a hospital emergency room. Herbalists cannot legally adjust prescription meds, but client can be weaned down under a doctor's supervision. Caution combining anticoagulant herbs if client is on Coumadin. Client will require an INR (blood clotting ratio) level drawn periodically to monitor and maintain therapeutic drug levels.

- *Diet*. Antiinflammatory and supplement suggestions stated earlier.
- Check for dysbiosis and diabetes risk.
- Exercise program.
- *Work with healthcare provider on labs*. The mild anticoagulant herbs in formula are fine as long as clotting blood levels are monitored (red flag). It would be nice if the prescribed Coumadin dose could be eventually weaned down and discontinued as herbal amounts are adjusted. Also monitor lipid levels and blood pressure.

- *General therapeutic principles*. Be proactive. It is very important to investigate dietary and lifestyle habits to prevent a future heart attack. (1) If LDL level is high, use antilipemics. (2) If the client has clots, use anticoagulants. (3) If the client has hypertension, use antihypertensives. (4) Use major cardiac restoratives for all. (5) Choose arterial stimulants to increase contractility. (6) Use relaxing nervines as needed.

Myocardial Infarction (MI)

- *Definition. A **heart attack**, or **myocardial infarction** (MI)* refers to reduced blood flow to one or more of the coronary arteries (*infarction*), resulting in lack of oxygen (*ischemia*) and ultimate cell death *(necrosis)* to the portion of the heart muscle supplied by that artery. This event is the unfortunate result of CAD.
- *Signs and symptoms*.
  - In *men*, crushing substernal chest pain that may radiate to the left arm, jaw, neck, or shoulder blades; nausea; fatigue; shortness of breath; and restlessness.
  - In *women*, symptoms are often much less dramatic than in men, and frequently with no signature chest pain. Diagnosis and treatment are often missed. There may be nausea, vomiting, fatigue, acid reflux, possible neck pain, flulike symptoms, or anxiety. These are very vague and sadly often ignored because women tend to write them off, insisting they feel merely run down or have a cold. Be aware of the differences and trust your intuition if something just doesn't feel right.
- *Allopathic treatment*. Diagnosed by elevated cardiac enzymes in the blood and abnormal ECG, or abnormal cardiac catheterization showing coronary clots. An MI is treated with oxygen; IV Heparin to thin the blood; and later, oral Coumadin and/or aspirin to thin clots; antiarrhythmics; and statins to keep lipids normal.
- *General therapeutic principles*. Once a person is home from the hospital and stabilized, an herbalist can do a lot to help prevent another episode and regain cardiac health (Case History 22.5). The client and/or herbalist must work with the person's doctor because of the prescribed drugs.

CASE HISTORY 22.6

Case History for Varicose Veins

S. Mary Jo works at the checkout in a supermarket. Her veins around her medial knees are large, soft, bluish, and snakelike. They do not hurt.
O. P Wiry, weak on right under Spleen pulse. **T** Sublingual veins enlarged and purplish.
A. Venous Blood Stagnation. Spleen Qi weakness. Varicose veins.
P. *Specific therapeutic principles.* (1) Astringents to decrease vein diameter. (2) Restoratives to tone and strengthen connective tissue vessels. (3) Antiinflammatories to ease discomfort. (4) Bioflavonoids to strengthen vessel walls. (5) Increase circulation, stop stasis, move blood. (6) External lotion/compresses (Box 22.3).

Sample Formula and Dose. 5 mL 3 × day.

Part	Herbs	Rationale
3	Horse Chestnut seed	Tones vein walls, antiinflammatory/breaks clots.
3	Yarrow, Marigold, or Red Root	Vascular astringent and tonic.
3	Ginkgo leaf or Gotu Kola herb	Heals connective tissue, circulatory stimulant.
2	Hawthorn or Bilberry or both	Bioflavonoid, vein tonic.
1	Prickly Ash bark	Move blood/circulation.

Other Suggestions

- Varicose vein liniment (Box 22.3).
- Wiggle feet and move them around as much as possible when at work.
- Elevate feet/legs when possible and try compression stockings.

Varicose Veins

- *Definition.* ***Varicose veins***, a type of peripheral vascular disease (PVD), refer to a weakening and widening of the venous walls in the lower legs (Case History 22.6). The valves do not assist blood return to the heart adequately, and the venous walls are fragile. If the blood slows down enough, clots will form (thrombosis/stagnation). This condition often occurs with overweight individuals, in cases of CHF, during pregnancy, and in individuals with occupations involving a lot standing, such as on hard, concrete floors for long periods.
- *Signs and symptoms.* Tortuous lower leg veins that can bulge prominently in the ankles, legs, and inner knees and that are more visible when standing. May be sensitive, painful, and sometimes become inflamed.
- *Allopathic treatment.* Decrease standing, elevate legs, wear compression stockings, engage in more exercise, or have removed surgically with stripping and ligation. Injections of a salt solution into the veins and laser therapy are sometimes done.
- *Chinese view.* Because the Spleen holds the blood, sagging and weak varicose veins are considered a Spleen qi weakness with the production of damp.[9]
- *General therapeutic principles.* (1) Use astringents to decrease vein diameter. (2) Select restoratives to tone and strengthen connective tissue vessels. (3) Use antiinflammatories to ease discomfort. (4) Use bioflavonoids to strengthen vessel walls. (5) Increase circulation/stop stasis. (6) Apply external liniment or lotion/compresses (Box 22.3).

• BOX 22.3 Varicose Vein Liniment

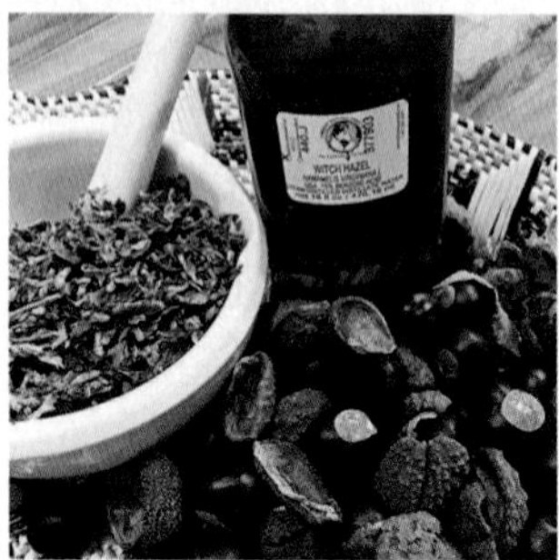

Commercial Witch Hazel extract, *Aesculus hippocastanum* (Horse Chestnut seed), and *Sarothamnus scoparius* (Scotch Broom tops) or the root of other Broom species make an astringent liniment that tightens and tones the veins.

This easy liniment involves making a maceration of dried herbs and soaking them in store-bought distilled Witch Hazel extract.[15] The astringency of the herbs and the tannins in the barks tighten the vessels. Calendula and Horse Chestnut contain flavonoids and saponins that stimulate venous circulation.[9] The remedy addresses Chinese Venous Blood Stagnation.

2 parts	Calendula flower	Astringing, softening, dissolving, stimulates venous return.
2 parts	Horse Chestnut seed	Restores veins, astringes, reduces venous Blood Stagnation.
2 parts	Comfrey root	Astringing, restoring to connective tissue (veins).
1 part	Butcher's Broom root	Reduces venous Blood Stagnation, restores veins.
1 part	Witch Hazel bark	Highly astringent tannin content, venous vasoconstrictor.
To cover	Witch Hazel extract	Perfect astringing, shrinking medium to soak up all the herbs.

Instructions. Place herbs in quart jar and cover them with Witch Hazel extract. Macerate for 4 weeks, strain and rebottle.

Administration. For compress, soak a small cloth in the liniment, wring out, and place over varicosities. Alternately, pour a little liniment into hand and gently rub over veins 3 × day.

Summary

In addition to the traditional cardiovascular disease risk factors such as family history, hypertension, and smoking, we also considered insulin resistance and leptin resistance. A major dietary remedy for cardiac risk is to reduce dietary sugar and processed fructose.

From the Chinese Medicine perspective, the Heart reflects physical heart, vascular problems, and spiritual issues. Because the Heart houses the shen or spirit (emotional and psychological center), mental illness and emotional troubles are part of its domain. Some common physical cardiac syndromes include Heart Qi Deficiency (comparable to CHF), Heart Blood Stagnation (similar to angina), Heart Yang Deficiency (often seen as a heart attack), and Venous Blood Stagnation (varicose veins or sluggish peripheral blood flow).

The cardiac Materia Medica includes general restoratives and herbs with a unique affinity to veins, arteries, and capillaries. The fact that many single cardiac botanicals have multiple actions makes it very convenient and easy to use them for more than one purpose in formulas. Always refer a client with a cardiac emergency to a hospital. Case histories included are for the stable heart situations an herbalist is likely to encounter.

Review

Fill in the Blanks

(Answers in Appendix B.)

1. Two types of foods most important to avoid in insulin and leptin resistance are ___, ___, ___.
2. Six risk factors in heart disease are ___, ___, ___. ___, ___, ___.
3. Two very important findings in a lipid panel are ___ and ___.
4. Four categories of herbal heart restoratives are ___, ___, ___, ___.
5. Another name for anticoagulant herbs is ___. Two Chinese Medicine examples are ___, ___ and three Western examples are ___, ___, ___.
6. Herbs that relax the heart help treat ___. Three herbs are ___, ___, ___.
7. Name four therapeutic principles for treating Venous Stagnation: ___, ___, ___, ___.
8. Client has fatigue, coughing, shortness of breath, and weak, empty pulse. Likely Western diagnosis is ___ and Chinese medicine syndrome is ___.
9. What category of herbs would you choose for high LDL? ___. Name four herbs. ___, ___, ___, ___.
10. Capillary stimulant herbs ___ heart rate and ___ force of contractions.

Critical Concept Questions

(Answers for you to decide.)

1. Discuss the mind-body aspects of heart disease.
2. A client brings in their lipid blood panel. How do you interpret all those numbers in terms of CAD risk?
3. If your client is taking statins, what would you tell them?
4. Your client has hyperlipidemia. Give diet recommendations.
5. John did not know that his BP was 182/90 before you took it. He feels fine and doesn't see why it's a problem. What would you tell him?
6. You can have only four herbs. Which ones would you choose for your cardiac apothecary and why?
7. What is the difference between angina and a heart attack?
8. Describe the many virtues of Hawthorn berry.
9. Name four Chinese cardiac herbs with common name, botanical name, and pinyin name. Give their actions.
10. What does "*The Heart houses the shen*" mean?

References

1. "Heart Disease Facts." Centers for Disease Control and Prevention. https://www.cdc.gov/heartdisease/facts.htm (accessed August 13, 2019).
2. Bone, Kerry and Simon Mills. *Principles and Practice of Phytotherapy* (London, UK: Elsevier, 2013).
3. Sinatra, Stephen. "VAP Test is Back for Testing Particle Size." Heart MD Institute. https://heartmdinstitute.com/heart-health/vap-test-cholesterol-particle-size/ (accessed August 13, 2019).
4. Wolfson, Jack. *The Paleo Cardiologist* (New York: Morgan James, 2015).
5. "Apo-A1" Lab Tests Online. https://labtestsonline.org/understanding/analytes/apoa/tab/test/ (accessed August 13, 2019).
6. Xiao-Fan, Zong and Gary Liscum. *Chinese Medicinal Teas* (Boulder, CO: Blue Poppy, 1996).
7. Myss, Caroline. *Anatomy of the Spirit* (New York, NY: Three Rivers, 1996).
8. "Heart Pattern Differentiation in Chinese Medicine." Sacred Lotus Chinese Medicine. https://www.sacredlotus.com/go/diagnosis-chinese-medicine/get/zang-fu-heart-patterns-tcm (accessed August 13, 2019).
9. Holmes, Peter. *Energetics of Western Herbs* (Boulder, CO: Snow Lotus, 2006).
10. Holmes, Peter. Class notes. Denver, CO; 1997.
11. Hashim, Farah J. et al. "Separation, Characterization, and Anticoagulant Activity of Coumarin and its Derivatives Extracted from Melilotus officinalis." http://www.biotech-asia.org/vol14no1/separation-characterization-and-anticoagulant-activity-of-coumarin-and-its-derivatives-extracted-from-melilotus-officinalis/ (accessed December 1, 2019).
12. "Blood Pressure Chart: What Your Reading Means." Mayo Clinic. https://www.mayoclinic.org/diseases-conditions/high-blood-pressure/in-depth/blood-pressure/art-20050982 (accessed August 13, 2019).
13. Hoffman, David. *Medical Herbalism: The Science and Practice of Herbal Medicine* (Rochester, VT: Healing Arts, 2003).
14. Alfs, Matthew. *300 Herbs: Their Indications and Contraindications* (New Brighton, MN: Old Theology Book House, 2003).
15. Gladstar, Rosemary. *Herbal Recipes for Vibrant Health* (North Adams, MA: Storey, 2008).

23 The Neurological System

"If you think it's all in your head, it's probably all in your gut."

—Rachel Lord, herbalist

CHAPTER REVIEW

- The mind-body connection.
- The sixth chakra, the intuitive.
- The gut-brain axis/connection and leaky brain: The enteric nervous system, the vagus nerve, neurotransmitters, and gut-brain recap.
- Maintaining a healthy brain and nervous system.
- Chinese Medicine perspective: The neurological system, shen, and major syndromes.
- Nervous system Materia Medica: Nervous system herbs worth honorable mention. Nutritive restoratives and antidepressants, trophorestoratives and adaptogens, relaxants (including anxiolytics, spasmolytics, hypnotics, analgesics, and anticonvulsants), and stimulants.
- Common neurological conditions with case histories: Anxiety and panic attacks, depression with anxiety and insomnia, peripheral neuropathy, tension headaches, migraine headaches, and neurological autoimmune diseases (highlighting Parkinson's).

KEY TERMS

Adaptogens
Analgesics
Anticonvulsants
Anxiolytics
Blood-brain barrier (BBB)
Enteric nervous system (ENS)
Gut-brain axis
Headache
Hypnotics
Leaky brain
Leaky gut
Mind-body connection
Neurogastroenterology
Neuropathy
Neurotransmitters
Nervine(s)
Psychoneuroimmunology
Pulse dosing
Spasmolytics/antispasmodics
Stimulants
Vagus nerve

Physically, the nervous system (NS) is a specialized collection of cells called neurons. The *central nervous system* (CNS) consists of the brain and spinal cord. *The peripheral nervous system* (PNS) consists of the peripheral nerves that branch out from the brain and cord to every cell. This miraculous communications network sends chemical messages (***neurotransmitters***) released at the end of nerve fibers in response to the arrival of an electrical nerve impulse. These messages travel place to place and cell to cell, telling us to take another breath, to keep the heart beating, and to contract smooth muscles without conscious thought.

The NS is also the ultimate seat of the mind-body connection, how our thoughts and emotions influence physical health. On the emotional and spiritual level, we transcend to a connectedness of physiological and psychological factors. Our thoughts, beliefs, and emotions affect physical health and vice versa. This powerful understanding allows us free will about our life and our health.

The Chinese intuited the mind-body connection long before modern science identified nerves. The Western concept of the nervous system actually encompasses all the Chinese Medicine organ systems. The joyful Heart is the place where the shen (spirit), psyche, and emotions reside. Excessive thoughts and worry belong to the Spleen. The physical brain is an extension of the bone marrow, which is the Kidney's body part, and thus receives its nourishment. Even the Liver, associated with anger and unpredictable wind, has its own neurological syndromes.

The Mind-Body Connection

The ***mind-body connection*** refers to how our thoughts, feelings, beliefs, and attitudes can positively or negatively affect our biological functioning. From a scientific standpoint, emotions are chemicals that can have desirable or harmful effects on health. The only way we can truly heal is by attending to deep-seated belief patterns and emotional and spiritual issues, along with physical body concerns. Among many who have famously explored and practiced these ideas are endocrinologist and holistic thinker Deepak Chopra, M.D.; the late inspirational teacher Louise Hay; medical intuitive Carolyn Myss; and holistic women's health practitioner Christiane Northrop, M.D.

The nervous, endocrine, and immune systems share a common chemical language that allow constant communication between the mind and body through hormones and neurotransmitters.[1] ***Psychoneuroimmunology*** is a growing field that studies and acknowledges the interaction between the brain, the nervous system, the immune system, and how they affect each other. We can literally laugh ourselves well or cry ourselves sick. As odd as that might seem, we frequently set ourselves up for physical *dis-ease* because of the biochemical effect suppressed emotions and undealt-with issues have on our immune and endocrine systems.[2] Healing tools used for this nonphysical, emotional, and spiritual work include meditation, stress reduction, visualization, yoga, biofeedback, psychotherapy, medical intuitive work, and prayer. Herbalists are reminded to respect this holistic viewpoint and its healing potential when working out therapeutic strategies.

The Sixth Chakra, the Intuitive

Energetically and metaphysically, the brain and nervous system are part of the sixth chakra (Fig. 23.1), located in the center of the forehead between the eyebrows. Also associated with this chakra are the eyes, ear, nose, and the sinuses. Those types of physical issues reside here.

The sixth chakra connects the mental to the emotional. It is esoterically known as the *third eye*, the place of intuitive sight and wisdom where we learn to distinguish between false truths, fear, and illusion (what we believe or wish to be true) versus *the truth*. False truths are a result of fears, personal experiences, and memories that can distort the facts. The intuitive center activates the link between mind and psyche that leads to wisdom. A mantra for the sixth chakra is "I see." It helps us become conscious, to detach from subjective perceptions, and to see the truth and symbolic meanings in a situation, as painful as that might be.

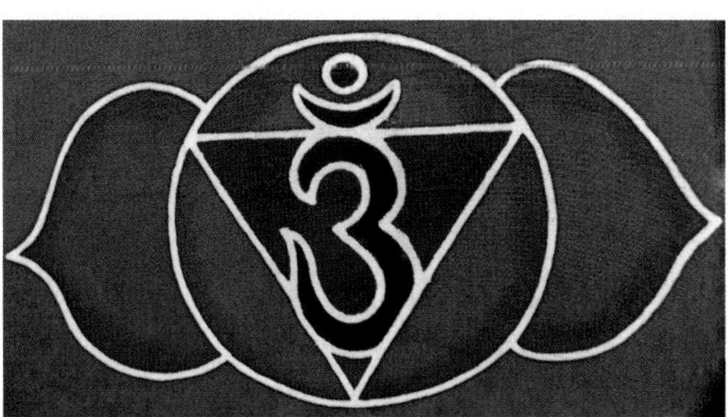

• **Fig. 23.1** The Sixth Chakra, the third eye, is the place of intuitive sight and wisdom.

The challenge is to look within and separate and detach from our fears, external counsel, and our shadow side, and to see clearly. Clarity of mind is the essence of wisdom.[3]

The Gut-Brain Axis and Leaky Brain

The concept of the ***gut-brain axis*** explains the interaction between a healthy microbiome and mental and neurological health. The axis is a communication network that enables a bidirectional association between the brain and the gastrointestinal (GI) tract.[4] It refers to the physical connections (nerves) and the chemical connections (neurotransmitters) running between the two and how they affect health and emotions.

We have already discussed the implications of intestinal permeability or ***leaky gut*** (Chapter 18). When that exists there is also permeability in brain tissue, ***leaky brain***, where cell junctions around the capillaries of the ***blood-brain barrier (BBB)*** become too large, allowing harmful bacteria and toxins to leak into the brain causing chronic inflammation. The technical name for leaky brain is the *blood brain barrier hyperpermeability syndrome*.

Inflammation caused from leaky brain can result in eating disorders and obesity, as well as disturbances in cognitive function, including intuitive decision making. Other neurological diseases can occur, such as dementia, autism, seizures, Alzheimer's, Parkinson's, multiple sclerosis (MS); attention deficient disorder (ADD); and amyotrophic lateral sclerosis (ALS), which is also known as Lou Gehrig's disease. These problems would be a lot less likely if the gut was taken care of in the first place.

Enteric Nervous System

When it comes to mental and neurological well-being, appreciate the fact that we have two brains and must treat both. The obvious one is the brain in the head. The other is the older, primitive brain embedded in the wall of the gut, called the ***enteric nervous system*** (ENS). The ENS is composed of two layers of gut tissue running from esophagus to anus. It's a meshlike system of neurons that governs the function of the GI tract. The ENS sends out signaling neurotransmitters, just as brain neurons do.[4]

The ENS explains many things that have been long intuited regarding the mind-body-gut connections. It involves the field of ***neurogastroenterology***, the study of the gut and brain, and their interaction as related to mental/neurological illnesses. We feel emotions on a gut level when we're nervous. We can make ourselves sick when we are stressed. Do these emotions originate in the brain or the gut? We used to assume it was all in our head and that emotions began there.

Vagus Nerve

The gut-brain communication pathway is a two-way street occurring via the neurotransmitters traveling from gut to brain and from brain to gut. These chemicals pass back and forth via the long wandering pair of the tenth cranial nerves, the ***vagus nerve***. (There are really two, but they are usually referred to as a single nerve, *the vagus*.) The majority of neurotransmitters travel from the gut to the brain, not the reverse.[4] Gut conditions like irritable bowel syndrome (IBS) or Crohn's disease originate in the gut but go up to the brain, leading to their connection to mental health problems, such as anxiety and depression. However, nervous *butterflies* originate in the brain's autonomic sympathetic nervous system (SNS), the fight-or-flight area, and travel down to the gut, causing us to have nausea and diarrhea and run to the bathroom because we're so stressed out.

Neurotransmitters

Many gut-produced neurotransmitters are of the same class as those produced in the brain: dopamine, serotonin, glutamate, norepinephrine, and nitric oxide. For instance, dopamine is considered a feel-good neurotransmitter, and serotonin prevents depression, regulates sleep, appetite, and body temperature. Implications of this chemical communication show how emotions, mental illness, and gut health are microbiome, gut-related phenomena. Microbiome integrity influences the type of brain neurotransmitters produced. The takeaway for mental illness is to always treat the gut.

Gut-Brain Recap

- *Structures of the gut-brain axis.* These include the brain and spinal cord (CNS); the involuntary autonomic nervous system (ANS) comprising the sympathetic, parasympathetic and enteric nervous systems; and the hypothalamic-pituitary-adrenal axis (HPA) (Chapter 27).
- *The ENS is the primitive nervous system, the second brain.* The enteric nervous system in the gut wall emerged in first vertebrates more than 500 million years ago. It may have been the original brain and contains millions of neurons. One theory is that it served as a survival warning system about bad or poisonous food.
- *Vagal connection and the second brain.* The ENS is the body's second brain that connects to the vagus nerve, the longest of the 12 paired cranial nerves. It physically connects the gut to the brain, carrying chemical messages back and forth and in doing so influences mood: happiness and joy, anxiety, or depression. In fact, about 90% of vagus fibers carry information from the gut to the brain, not the reverse.[5]
- *Leaky gut equals leaky brain.* A key concept is that gut flora influences the brain for better or worse. The blood brain barrier (BBB) is a selective, semipermeable membrane formed by endothelial cells that line the brain capillaries. It allows some nutrients and drugs to enter and protects the brain from an influx of harmful microbes, chemicals, and cancer cells.
- *If the gut flora is healthy, the BBB is intact.* However, if the gut leaks, so does the brain. Cell junctions around the capillaries of the BBB become too large, allowing bacteria and toxins to leak into the brain tissue, causing chronic inflammation.[6]
- *The autoimmune connection in leaky brain.* Many of the neurological conditions previously listed are considered autoimmune diseases where the tissue attacks itself, an epidemic in our society. Therefore calming an overactive immune system must be part of the treatment. Recall the Gut and Psychology Syndrome (GAPS) protocol (Chapter 16).

Maintaining a Healthy Brain and Nervous System

- *Herbalist's alert.* Keep the gut healthy, because leaky gut equals leaky brain. For any mental health or neurological problem we must first treat the gut with proper diet, fermented foods, and bitters. Health begins at gut level, no matter which body system is involved.
- *Brainy diet.* Prevent or lessen instances of brain fog, dementia, and mental illness with a brain-happy diet. The usual mantra applies: eat antiinflammatory foods with real, whole, unprocessed foods. Include colorful antioxidant- and antiinflammatory-rich fruits and veggies, some slow-burning (probably gluten-free) complex carbs, healthy fats, omega-3 eggs, lean range-fed animal protein, and a little dark chocolate.
- *Eliminate* simple sugar, high-fructose corn syrup, additives, and preservatives, all of which poison the nervous system and brain, and disrupt biochemistry.
- *Supplements.* Include vitamin D_3, omega-3 fatty acids, probiotics, and the B vitamins: especially methyl MTHF folate (activated, bioavailable B_{12}, not plain folic acid) and B_6. Deficiency of B_{12} has been linked to Alzheimer's.
- *Good-quality sleep.* It turns out that 8 hours for adults and more for children and teens are essential to function well. During sleep, neurons regenerate, emotions sort themselves out, problems are solved, and the brain becomes more elastic. We must not just sleep, but sleep well. This means going through dream cycles and making sure there is no sleep apnea. Undiagnosed sleep apnea is common and has been associated with memory loss, depression, attention deficits, Alzheimer's, diabetes, heart disease, and obesity.
- *Investigate heavy metals and hidden food sensitivities.* Mercury is often present in those with dementia. This condition can be checked through a blood test or hair analysis. If present, detoxification is in order (Chapter 19), and removal of gluten or lactose may be indicated in the case of food sensitivities.
- *Brain games.* Reading, games, chess, crossword puzzles, and other types of stimulating mental activity all help.
- *Dry heat sauna.* This helps brain detoxification. In Finland, where most homes have a sauna, it was found that regularly sweating it out reduced risk of dementia, Alzheimer's, and cardiovascular events. The skin is the largest organ in the body, and its sweat glands expel toxins, including heavy metals such as cadmium, mercury, and lead. Dry sauna heat also improves circulation and mitochondrial function, and it kills microbes.

Chinese Medicine Perspective: The Nervous System and Major Syndromes

The Kidneys are an extension of the marrow (correspondences) and enter into the neuro picture because they nourish the brain, spinal cord, and cerebral spinal fluid. However, Chinese Medicine does not recognize a nervous system per se. No single Chinese organ system is responsible for the care, maintenance, and functioning of what is called the nervous system in the West. There is no neat translation. After all, if you think about it, the Western nervous system travels all over the body to every cell, tissue, gland, and organ. Each case needs to be treated individually. This list describes how emotional and mental problems are related to the Chinese Heart, Spleen, or Liver.

- *Heart and emotions.* Emotions lead to heat. The tip of the tongue is the Heart area, and thus a red-tipped tongue is a good reliable indicator of emotional stress. The Heart is responsible for the shen or spirit. This affects mood, anxiety, depression, memory, and schizophrenia. Possible syndromes are Heart Fire, Heart Yin or Yang Deficiency, and Phlegm Misting the Heart. Herbs would be selected to cool and moisten the Heart yin. We could use nervous system anxiolytics, antidepressants, and restoratives as needed.
- *Spleen and emotions.* The Spleen is the seat of thought, exaggerated into excessive thinking and worry. Inability to concentrate and obsessive internal debating and overthinking, called obsessive compulsive disorder (OCD) in the West, come

under Spleen jurisdiction. Possible syndromes are Spleen Qi or Spleen Yang Deficiency with or without damp. Restore the Spleen with Codonopsis Dang Shen (Downy Bellflower root) or Atractylodes Bai Zhu (White Atractylodes root).

- *Liver and emotions.* Because Liver's emotion is anger, the hot, angry person with tinnitus is placed under the syndrome Liver Yang Rising. In this case, the Liver yang requires sedation, perhaps with Skullcap herb or Valerian root. Liver wind relates to symptoms that are rapid and unpredictable, such as shaking, tremors, spasms, seizures, or bipolar symptoms; for those, we decrease Liver wind with notables like Uncaria Gou Teng (Gambir Vine twig) and Gastrodia Tian Ma (Celestial Hemp corm).

Nervous System Excesses and Deficiencies Related to the Kidneys

In Chinese Medicine, nervous system deficiencies and excesses are sometimes related to the Kidneys. They may represent deficiencies, the overall "blahs," such as exhaustion, depression, despair, lack of initiative, or apathy, brain depletion, poor memory (senior moments), absentmindedness, and emptiness. Or they may relate to excess conditions such as stress, anxiety, being riled up and hyper, manic behaviors, bipolar symptoms, and attention deficit hyperactivity disorder.

- *Kidney yang and the SNS.* Overstimulation of the nervous system is the stress response of the SNS. In Chinese Medicine, it has been likened to Kidney Yin Deficiency manifesting as heat, particularly in the Liver. (To a Westerner, it may appear as excess Kidney yang, but that is unlikely because almost no such thing exists in classic texts. There is really a vacuity or not enough cooling yin, resulting in heat.) If there is undue stress and anxiety, the nervous system needs relaxants: Valerian root or Hops flower; and restoration with trophorestoratives, such as Polygonum He Shou Wu (Flowery Knotweed herb) and Milky Oat tops. **Pulse (P)** Rapid. **Tongue (T)** Red.
- *Kidney yin and the PNS.* The relaxation response of the PNS has been compared with Kidney yin and coolness. The ability to relax should be honored. However, if there is depression and lethargy, antidepressant restoratives and nervous system and adrenal tonics are needed to boost Kidney yang, qi, or essence, like Schisandra Wu Wei Zi (Five Taste berry) or Rhodiola root or Ashwagandha root. **P** Slow, thin, and weak. **T** Normal or red body with patchy or absent coat, possible cracks.
- *Nervous system degenerative conditions point to the Kidney,* its marrow, and its decline of yin and essence. Parkinson's or Alzheimer's are examples of degenerative Kidney conditions. The indication is to tonify Kidney yin with Artichoke leaf or Asparagus Tian Men Dong (Asparagus root). Syndromes can include Kidney yin, yang, qi or essence deficiencies. **P** Weak and thin. **T** Body pale. Coat dry, scant, and patchy.

Nervous System Materia Medica

Nervine is a general catch-all Western term for any herb that affects the nervous system, whether restoratives, uppers, or downers. Nervines can either warm things up or relax and cool things down. The term is not much help when you are trying to be specific. It is best to use designations like nervous system restoratives, relaxants, or stimulants, because they are much more descriptive. Within those categories, further breakdown is made, depending on where you look and who you read. As usual, many nervous system herbs fit into more than one category.

Neuro Herbs Worth Honorable Mention

- *Avena sativa* (Milky Oat tops). This is a nervous system superfood (Fig. 23.2). Oat straw or stem is adequate medicine; however, the milky oat stage of the tops occurs after flowering but before the seed hardens and becomes the oat grain we eat as oatmeal. In this stage the unripe seed is milky inside and available only about 1 to 2 weeks out of the year. It is high in nutrients, such as magnesium and vitamins, and is used for chronic depression/anxiety and a deficiency of Kidney essence. Best used long-term in tea (decoct for an hour) or as a tincture. Milky Oat tops combine well with Rhodiola root or Skullcap herb. This is a great herb for children and elders.
- *Polygonum multiflorum* He Shou Wu (Flowery Knotweed root) (Fig. 23.3). This is a nervous system super-restorative, named

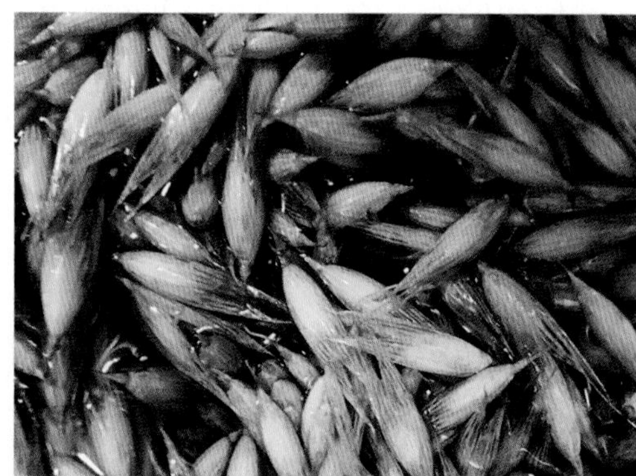

• **Fig. 23.2** *Avena sativa* (Milky Oat tops), fresh, in alcohol beginning the maceration process. Being sweet, warm, and moist, it tonifies and restores the nervous system, making it fitting for many neuroendocrine deficiencies.

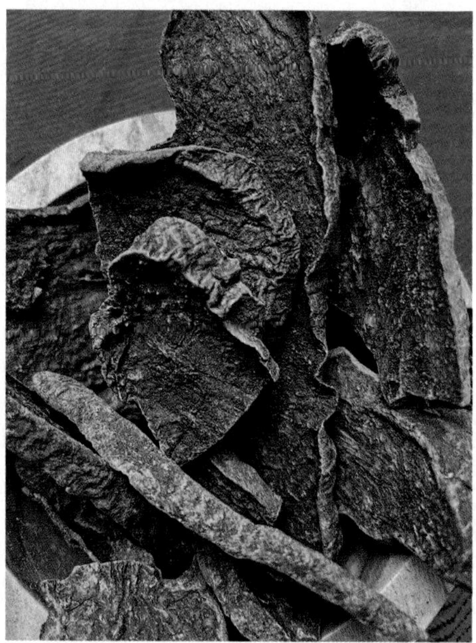

• **Fig. 23.3** *Polygonum multiflorum* He Shou Wu (Flowery Knotweed root) is a first rate nervous system trophorestorative.

after black-haired Mr. He, whose hair reportedly turned from gray to black after repeated use of his namesake plant, He Shou Wu. It is a superlative Chinese CNS nerve and brain trophorestorative, like Western Milky Oat tops. Combine it with St. John's Wort for chronic depression. A go-to remedy for nervous stress and breakdown, Alzheimer's, MS, and premature aging. Tonifies qi, blood, and Kidney Essence Deficiency.

- *Panax quinquefolius* Xi Yang Shen (American ginseng root). The perfect urban tonic (Fig. 23.4). The word *shen* in pinyin means gods, deity, or spirit. It is used to describe the *Panax* genus. Ginsengs are venerated, high-cost roots that take many years to mature. They are broad-spectrum, superlative neuroendocrine restorative remedies for deficiency syndromes, a true adaptogen in every sense. Ginseng root comes in prepared (red) and unprepared (white) forms. American ginseng root was used by Native Americans, later imported to China, and highly sought after there. American ginseng is considered less stimulating and more moistening than the very warming Eastern Ren Shen. Use cultivated (Fig. 23.5) (farm-grown, not wild, as it's endangered) American ginseng in formula with other adaptogens for chronic fatigue, depression, poor concentration, insomnia, low libido, and to restore adrenals, energy, and sex drive.
- *Centella asiatica* Ji Xue Cao (Gotu Kola leaf, Asiatic Pennywort) (Fig. 23.6). A well-known Ayurvedic, East Asian, and now Western herb, it is used in India as a skin detoxifier for boils, psoriasis, wound healing, and as a connective tissue restorative.[7] In China and the West, it is best known as a brain and nervous stimulant and adrenocortical restorative, a lot like Milky Oats. Use for both purposes. Gotu Kola leaf helps nerves regenerate and is used for nerve and brain deficiency, memory loss, chronic mental and physical fatigue.

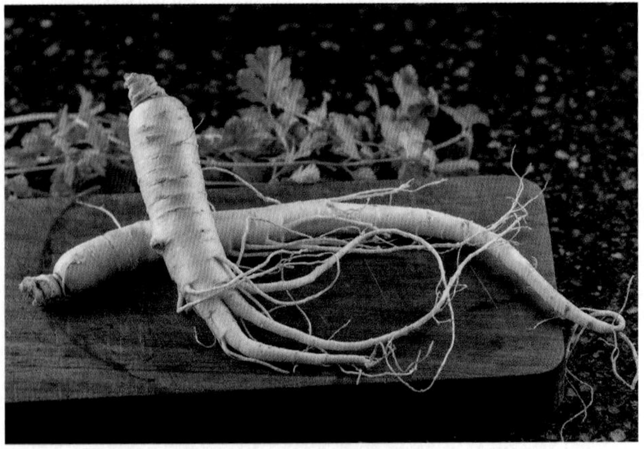

• **Fig. 23.4** *Panax quinquefolius* Xi Yang Shen (American ginseng root). shown in its fresh, unprepared form. This ginseng is a bit less stimulating and more yin than the Chinese and Korean varieties. (iStock.com/4kodiak.)

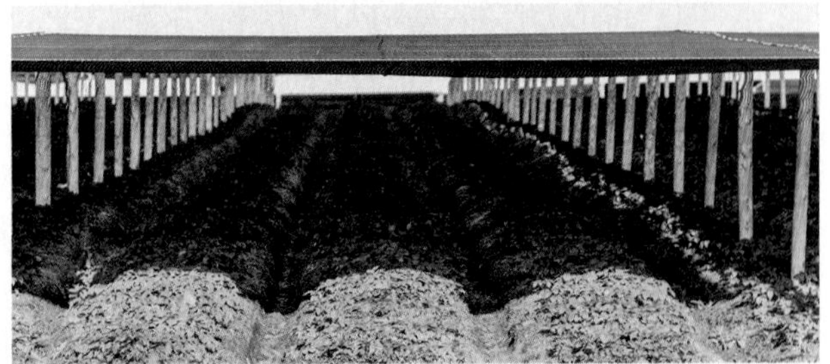

• **Fig. 23.5** Rows of valuable cultivated ginseng growing under shade in a late Wisconsin summer. Wild *Panax* spp. is an endangered plant. (/iStock.com/Michael-Tatman).

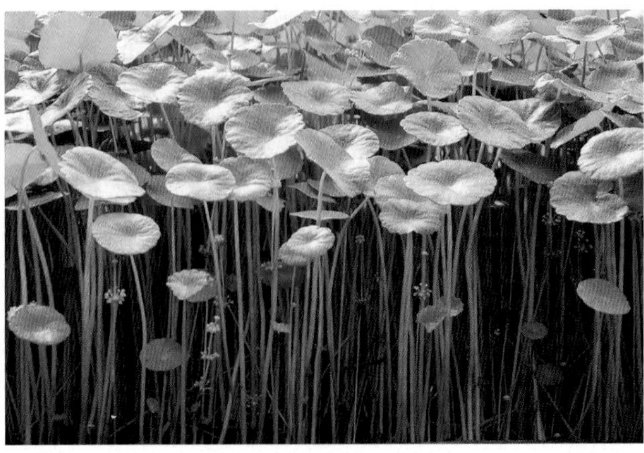

• **Fig. 23.6** *Centella asiatica* Ji Xue Cao (Gotu Kola leaf, Asiatic Pennywort) is used as a brain and nervous system stimulant and restorative for fatigue, nerve regeneration, and many other neuro deficiencies. (/iStock.com/Piyathet).

Nutritive Restoratives and Antidepressants

Nervous system nutritive restoratives treat deficiencies like mental fog, decreased concentration, Parkinson's, and Alzheimer's. Mental depression is a deficient condition, and deficiencies need to be strengthened, nourished, and restored. Basil leaf, Ginkgo leaf, Rosemary leaf, Garden Sage leaf (adrenal tonic), Skullcap herb, Thyme leaf, and Polygonum He Shou Wu (Flowery Knotweed root) all achieve this action. Included under restoratives are the highly nourishing nervous system superfoods, such as Flower pollen, Milky Oat tops, microalgae, green tea, and shitake mushrooms, all important when taken as food and/or a supplement (Tables 23.1 and 23.2).

Trophorestoratives and Adaptogens

Major trophorestoratives and/or ***adaptogens*** have a specific affinity for the neuroendocrine/HPA axis, so their influence is widely spread and goes deep by protecting cells from oxidative stress, decreasing damage from stressors, helping mental fatigue, enhancing learning and memory, and relieving emotional disorders.[8] These herbs tonify qi, blood, and essence, and are used to treat weak or deficient conditions, such as depression or fatigue, that have gone on for long periods of time. Trophorestoratives also balance hormonal secretions and enhance the immune system (Table 23.3).

Patience is needed to see their effects. They are subtle, important, and precious. The trophorestoratives are safe but effective and should be used with chronic, longstanding conditions, especially when anxiety is pronounced.[8] They are long-term tonics, our super friends and relations: Panax Xi Yang Shen (American ginseng root), Schisandra Wu Wei Zi (Five Taste berry), Eleuthero Ci Wu Jia (Eleuthero/Siberian ginseng root), and Ashwagandha root. Rhodiola root is an adaptogen that has a marked and fast-acting antidepressant action (Fig. 23.7).

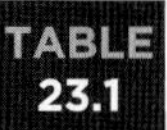

TABLE 23.1 Nutritive Nervous System Restoratives

Herb	Notes
Ocimum basilicum Basil leaf	NS restorative with mental exhaustion, memory loss, and nervous depression with yang deficiency.
Ginkgo biloba Ginkgo leaf	Ayurvedic. Restores brain and nerves, helps focus. For Kidney Essence Deficiency with absent mindedness, poor memory, depression, insomnia, and senility.
Centella asiatica Ji Xue Cao Gotu Kola leaf (Combine with Ginkgo, Schisandra Wu Wei Zi, and Polygonum He Shou Wu for memory loss/premature aging.)	Nerve and brain builder. For memory loss, mental and physical fatigue, depression, and chronic stress. Treats Kidney Essence Deficiency.
Polygonum multiflorum He Shou Wu Flowery Knotweed root Also called Fo Ti, meaning Black haired Mr. He. Therefore helps with early graying.	CNS restorative, helps concentration, premature aging, tonifies qi, blood, essence. For nervous stress/breakdown, Alzheimer's, multiple sclerosis, Kidney Essence Deficiency. Combine with St. John's Wort for chronic depression.
Ligustrum japonicum Nu Zhen Zi Glossy Privet berry	Restores nerves/brain if worn out and absentminded. For Kidney Essence Deficiency and also helps vision.
Rosmarinus officinale Rosemary leaf	Nervous system stimulant, restores brain, helps concentration, memory loss, and depression. Shakespeare's Ophelia said, "There's rosemary, that's for remembrance."
Salvia officinale Garden Sage leaf	Bitter, cool, and dry, tones the adrenals. Versatile, for stress, fatigue, and debility. Medium strength. Use long term in formula. Contraindicated in pregnancy and nursing.
Scutellaria lateriflora Skullcap herb	Restores nerve cells, mild sedative, and spasmolytic. For neuralgia (nerve pain), longstanding stress, and depression.
Hypericum perforatum St. John's Wort	For stress, depression, and anxiety. (Takes 4–8 weeks to act.) Combine with Melissa and Skullcap. For neuralgia, viral infections (especially *Herpes*), muscle tension, spinal pain, spasms, Kidney Essence Deficiency.
Thymus vulgaris Thyme leaf	Nerve/adrenal restorative with qi deficiency (nervous exhaustion), in addition to its respiratory uses.
Pollen spp. Flower Pollen	Superfood. Restores brain and nerves, strengthens mind, regenerates cells. For chronic depression, degenerative mental and neuro conditions. Broad-spectrum nutritive.
Avena sativa Oat Straw and Milky Oat tops	Superfood. Milky oat stage best. For chronic depression/anxiety. Combines well with Rhodiola or Skullcap. Decoct for an hour as a simple. Use long term.
Chlorella spp. and *Spirulina* spp. Microalgae	Superfood. Nourishes blood, qi and essence. For chronic fatigue, weakness, dementias, anxiety, and depression.
Sesamum indicum Black Sesame seed	Superfood. For nervous system deficiency/exhaustion. Very nourishing. Eat them.

Nervous System Relaxants

Nervous system relaxants are a large group with many overlapping actions and body system tropisms. Some are general relaxants for any body system, and others have affinities to particular ones (Table 23.4).

Most nervines are quite general and have multiple functions and subclasses. Relaxing nervines can help with anxiety and irritability (***anxiolytics***), calm smooth-muscle spasms (***spasmolytics*** or ***antispasmodics***), help with sleep (***hypnotics***), relieve pain (***analgesics***), and reduce seizures (***anticonvulsants***). Representatives from various nervous system relaxant subclasses include the analgesics: Jamaican Dogwood root bark, Bupleurum Chai Hu, Kava root, Corydalis Yan Hu Suo (Corydalis corm), and Skullcap herb (nerve pain). Some spasmolytics are Black Cohosh root and Skullcap herb. Anticonvulsants, which treat internal wind, include Lobelia herb, Jamaican Dogwood root, Valerian root, Uncaria Gou Teng (Gambir Vine twig), Gastrodia Tian Ma (Celestial Hemp corm), and Passionflower and Hops flower (Table 23.5).

Energetically, nervous system relaxants are cooling and both bitter and sweet, or a combination of the two tastes (bittersweet). The person could have fatigue, nervous tension, depression, vague

TABLE 23.2 Antidepressants
(These are nerve restoratives/tonics, especially indicated for depression)

Herb	Notes
Turnera diffusa Damiana leaf	Nerve tonic and brain stimulant. Relieves depression, anxiety, debility, and chronic fatigue. Considered a yang tonic for impotence; increases testosterone and progesterone.
Scutellaria lateriflora Skullcap herb	Nerve tonic and antidepressant. For chronic depression, fatigue, sleep loss, stress-related conditions in general, including pain and spasms.
Schisandra chinensis Wu Wei Zi Five Taste berry	Nerve tonic and antidepressant. Adaptogen.
Hypericum perforatum St. John's Wort	Nerve tonic/antidepressant. Stress and anxiety. (Takes 4 to 8 weeks to act.) For mental/nervous tension and neuralgia. Well-studied plant.
Bacopa monnieri Indian Pennywort, Water Hyssop Entire plant used medicinally.	Renowned Ayurvedic nerve tonic. Antidepressant, anxiolytic, helps memory, focus, and cognition.
Lavandula angustifolia Lavender flower	For anxiety and depression. Uplifting, especially the essential oil.
Melissa officinalis Lemon Balm herb	Important nervous system restorative. For depression in excess and deficiency conditions, fatigue, and insomnia.
Rhodiola rosea Rhodiola root	Adaptogen that doubles for chronic depression, anxiety, insomnia, and brain restorative.
Curcuma longa Turmeric root	Highly antiinflammatory to brain tissue. Essential in helping depression.[9]
Crocus sativus Saffron flower styles and stigmas	Antiinflammatory to brain. Proven better than Prozac. Exorbitantly expensive.

TABLE 23.3 Nervous System Trophorestoratives and Adaptogens
(They work on the HPA axis, adrenal tonics)

Herb	Notes
Panax quinquefolium Xi Yang Shen American ginseng root	Central nervous system (CNS) restorative helps digestion. Use with chronic fatigue, depression, poor concentration, insomnia, and Heart Blood Deficiency. Less stimulating than Ren Shen.
Panax ginseng Ren Shen Asian red ginseng root	Broad-spectrum neuroendocrine restorative. For deficiencies of qi, blood, and essence. A botanical superstar if you can afford it.
Rhodiola rosea Rhodiola root	Cooling, astringent, and sour, restores nerves, relieves acute and chronic/stress and anxiety, and helps insomnia. Good in chronic depression and schizophrenia.
Eleutherococcus senticosus Ci Wu Jia Eleuthero/Siberian ginseng root	CNS restorative for deficiencies of qi, blood, and essence with insomnia, memory and concentration loss, and chronic stress.
Astragalus membranaceus Huang Qi Astragalus root	Energy and qi tonic. Helps in stress with adrenal burnout.
Schisandra chinensis Wu Wei Zi Five Taste berry	Tonifies blood, qi, and essence. For Kidney Yang Deficiency with forgetfulness, fatigue, bad sleep, depression, and chronic stress.
Withania somnifera Ashwagandha root, Indian ginseng	Important Ayurvedic adaptogen for stress, improves learning and memory, reduces anxiety and depression.

feelings of anxiety, poor sleep, feelings of being generally stressed-out even if they don't know why, and vague aches and pains.[13] These herbs work well in combination. Some of the most popular are St. John's Wort, Chamomile flower, Lavender flower, Passionflower herb, Lemon Balm leaf, and Wild Lettuce leaf. Heart Blood Deficiency and Heart Yin Deficiency go here. Most of these also double as cardiac relaxants.

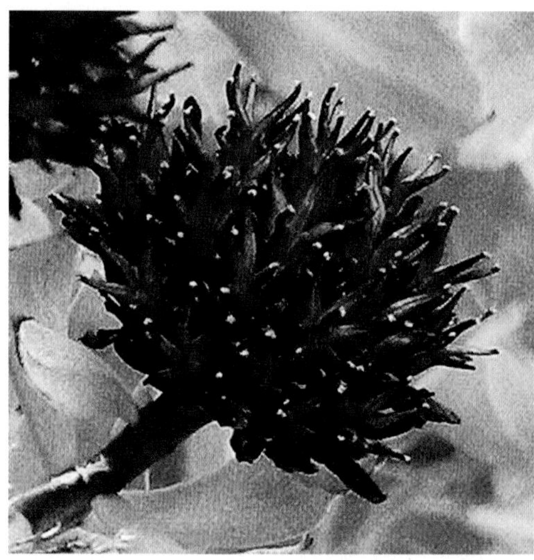

• **Fig. 23.7** *Rhodiola integrifolia* (King's Crown) flowering in the Colorado Rockies. The species *R. rosea* is sold commercially as an adaptogen and fast-acting antidepressant.

Hypnotics are herbs that cause drowsiness, depress the CNS, and inhibit motor function. They induce a healing state of sleep. They are *not* related to hypnotism or the sedative-hypnotic classification of Western drugs. Examples of herbal hypnotics are Kava root, Passionflower herb, Wild Lettuce leaf, Jamaican Dogwood root bark, and Valerian root.

There are also nervous system relaxants for over-the-top hyper situations that treat excess with heat and that are cooling, relaxing. and sedating. They are for anxiety disorders, agitation, seizures, and hyperactivity, all states that warrant calming down and cooling. The person is stressed, anxious, sleepless, overworked, or in chronic physical and emotional stress. How many of these folks do you know? Herbs include Wild Lettuce leaf, Melilot herb, and Hops flower.

Relaxing nervines come in varying strengths. Here is a subjective synopsis of their relative potencies (Table 23.5):[10]

- *Mild.* Hyssop herb, Lavender flower, Red Clover flower, Lemon Balm leaf, Cramp bark, Black Haw bark, Black Horehound herb, California Poppy root and herb, and Wild Lettuce leaf (Fig. 23.8).
- *Moderate.* Black Cohosh root, St. John's Wort, Motherwort herb, Lobelia herb, Chamomile flower, Pasqueflower flower and leaf, Skullcap herb, Linden flower, Damiana herb, Vervain herb.
- *Strong.* Hops flower, Passionflower herb, Jamaican Dogwood root bark, Corydalis Yan Hu Suo, and Valerian root.

Nervous System Analgesics and Pain

Pain is a demanding problem. Back pain is one of the top reasons people initially seek allopathic help. Herbal analgesics tend to work with mild to moderate pain, especially if the pain is linked to

TABLE 23.4 Nervines with Body System Tropisms[10]

Respiratory All antispasmodic	Cardiac All relaxing, except Cramp bark	Digestive First four are relaxing; others are antispasmodic	Reproductive First three are relaxing; others are antispasmodic
Antispasmodic	**Relaxing**	**Relaxing**	**Relaxing**
Grindelia spp. Gumweed bud	*Melissa officinalis* Lemon Balm	*Matricaria recutita* Chamomile flower	*Anemone pulsatilla* Pasqueflower herb
Lobelia inflata Lobelia herb	*Actaea racemosa* Black Cohosh root	*Humulus lupulus* Hops flower	*Scutellaria lateriflora* Skullcap herb
Prunus serotina Wild Cherry bark	*Lavandula angustifolia* Lavender flower	*Melissa officinalis* Lemon balm herb	*Valeriana officinalis* Valerian root
Lactuca virosa Wild Lettuce leaf	*Leonurus cardiaca* Motherwort herb	*Valeriana officinalis* Valerian root	**Antispasmodic**
Lactuca serriola Prickly Lettuce leaf	*Valeriana officinalis* Valerian root	**Antispasmodic**	*Paeonia lactiflora* Bai Shao Yao White Peony root
Tussilago farfara Coltsfoot herb	*Ligusticum walichii* Chuan Xiong Sichuan Lovage root	*Viburnum opulus* Cramp bark	*Viburnum opulus* Cramp bark
Marrubium vulgare White Horehound herb	*Crataegus oxyacantha* Hawthorn berry	*Foeniculum vulgare* Fennel seed	*Bupleurum chinensis* Chai Hu Buplever root
Verbascum thapsus Mullein leaf	**Antispasmodic**	*Mentha* x *piperita* Peppermint leaf	*Actaea racemosa* Black Cohosh root
	Viburnum opulus Cramp bark	*Dioscorea villosa* Wild Yam root	

TABLE 23.5 Nervous System Relaxants

Herb	Notes
Scutellaria lateriflora Skullcap herb	Relaxant, spasmolytic, analgesic, hypotensive that also restores nerves. For stress, restlessness, anxiety, chronic longstanding depression, and especially nerve pain.
Lavandula angustifolia Lavender flower	Relaxing for any nerve excess like agitation, anxiety, irritability, and stress in general. Sedating for the nervous and cardiac systems. The essential oil is stimulating for depression.
Valerian officinalis Valerian root Could have paradoxical (opposite) results than intended. Use with deficiencies (cool) conditions only, not with excess (heat). The fresh root (versus the dried root) is less likely to have this effect.	Calming, antispasmodic, and anticonvulsant in deficiency conditions. For anxiety, insomnia, and worry from exhaustion, not from overstimulation. High doses can have an unintended stimulating effect in excess conditions.[11] Freshly dug *Valerian officinalis* root runners. It calms the mind, relieves anxiety, and clears internal wind. Choose Valerian for insomnia due to emotional unrest, hypertension from suppressed anger, vertigo, and nervous irritability.
Humulus lupulus Hops flower	Cold, dry, analgesic, and hypnotic. For nerve excess with internal wind (tremors, twitches, abdominal spasms), insomnia, and anxiety.
Melissa officinalis Lemon Balm leaf	Cooling, calming, anxiolytic, and antidepressive. For insomnia, stress in general.
Melilotus officinalis Yellow Clover herb	Cold, relaxing, calming, and anxiolytic. For anxiety and all stressful situations.
Lobelia inflata Lobelia root and herb	Relaxing, for nervous and cardiac tension, pain, spasms, and acute stress. Medium strength for short-term use. Large doses stimulate vomiting.
Gastrodia Tian Ma Celestial Hemp corm	Spasmolytic, and anticonvulsant. For internal wind, cerebral palsy, cramps, and hypertension from Liver Yang Rising.
Uncaria macrophylla Gou Teng Gambir Vine twig	Spasmolytic (especially motor muscles), anticonvulsant, and hypotensive. For internal wind, irritability, stroke, and insomnia.
Matricaria recutita Chamomile flower	General nervous system relaxant, analgesic, and antispasmodic. For any stressful condition, insomnia, neuralgia, and depression. Also relaxes gastrointestinal and cardiac systems. Very safe for children.

inflammation or visceral or vascular spasm (Table 23.6). If pain is very severe, then unfortunately, strong prescription pharmaceuticals are best for the job, including the synthetic opioids derived from the latex of the Opium Poppy, and the alkaloid, cocaine, derived from Coca leaf. These drugs give relief but are highly addictive and must be discontinued (the sooner, the better). There is an opioid crisis in the United States. Various cultivars of *Cannabis* spp. have been successfully used medically (where legal) for pain relief, muscle spasms, seizures, and insomnia, when accompanied by a healthcare provider's prescription and purchased at specially licensed venues. Another controversial herb, also for pain and opioid withdrawal, is *Mitragyna speciosa* (Kratom leaf), which is in limbo regarding U.S. Food and Drug Administration approval.

Traditionally, weaker botanicals are most often used in clinical herbalism. Tried-and-true allies are the salicylate sources from Willow bark, Birch bark, Aspen bark, and Meadowsweet herb; and some mild nonaddictive plants from the Poppy family, such as California Poppy herb and Corydalis Yan Hu Suo (Corydalis corm). Westerners use Jamaican Dogwood bark or Valerian root. As always, when treating pain, its cause needs to be addressed to adequately approach the problem. Chinese Medicine is especially skilled at this (Chapter 24).

- *Pulse dosing.* For symptomatic relief of acute pain, frequent dosing of an analgesic formula is necessary. This method is referred to as ***pulse dosing***. A good general regimen for administration is 3 to 5 mL every 1/2 to 1 hour for a few hours, as needed. This regimen can always be titrated up or down, and client should be aware that they can safely experiment with dosage schedules (within limits) for their own individual needs. Pulse dosing is also used for insomnia, acute infection, bleeding, and bringing on labor (Appendix A).

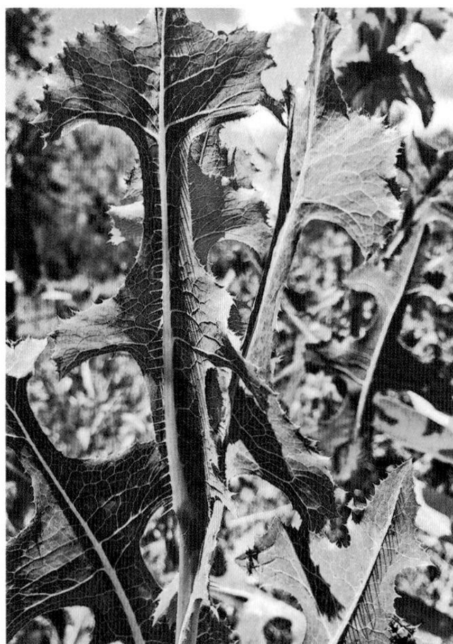

• **Fig. 23.8** *Lactuca serriola* (Prickly Lettuce) has tell-tale prickly spines on the underside rib of the leaf and bleeds a milky-white latex sap. It is a gentle nervous system relaxant and hypnotic that can help with sleep. *L. virosa* (Wild Lettuce) has smoother leaves and the same medicinal actions.

- *Combining herbal analgesics and analgesic drugs.* Care must be taken when combining analgesic herbals with strong prescription pain meds or sedatives. One or the other has to be weaned down, whereas the other gradually increased.
- *Children.* Go very easy with this process, and use mild analgesics such as California Poppy herb or Lemon Balm leaf.
- *Depression.* Combining antidepressive drugs with analgesic herbs could depress the nervous system too much. Be vigilant and selective in these cases. Often, when the depression lifts, the pain is relieved and vice versa.

Nervous System Stimulants

Stimulants get us going, create movement, and warm us up (Table 23.7). Some contain caffeine, and some don't. Stimulants treat depression and deficiency and often pair as nerve restoratives; examples are Panax Xi Yang Shen (American ginseng root) or Ginkgo leaf. Stimulants that give the mind focus and help us pay attention include Rosemary leaf, Basil leaf, Skullcap herb, Garden Sage leaf, Ginkgo leaf, and Polygonum He Shu Wu (Flowery Knotweed root).

Those that provide quick mind stimulation are the caffeine-loaded herbs like Coffee bean, Tea leaf, Cocoa leaf, and Maté leaf, all of which can be overused and abused and have been linked to elevated blood pressure, gastric upset, and anxiety. But nervous stimulants are not all one way, and these plants have their benefits. Newer research credits coffee with helping in the treatment of chronic diseases, including cancer, metabolic syndrome, heart disease, Parkinson's, and Alzheimer's.[12] Green tea is filled with healthy antioxidants.

Common Neurological Conditions

Anxiety and Panic Attacks

- *Definition.* Feelings of apprehension, exaggerated feelings, stress often below a conscious level, repressed thoughts or memory, and post-traumatic stress disorder (PTSD), all signal various degrees of anxiety (Case History 23.1).
- *Signs and symptoms.* Mild to acute panic state with tachycardia, hypertension (sometimes), sweating, palpitations, intense stress, and inability to respond appropriately and make decisions. Client could have chest pain that mimics a heart attack but isn't.
- *Allopathic treatment.* Rule out heart attack; use of sedatives, tranquilizers, antihypertensives, psychotherapy, and relaxation techniques.
- *General therapeutic principles.* (1) Anxiolytics/neuro-cardiac sedatives to calm the spirit. (2) Nervous system/adrenal tonics to restore nerves and help with any depression. (3) Spasmolytics as needed. (4) Hypnotic formula at night as needed. (5) Treat any other problems.

Depression

- *Definition.* Persistent sadness or clinical depression that lasts longer than 2 weeks and is uncomplicated by recent grief, substance abuse, or mental disorder.[11] This type of depression is different and goes beyond externally related *reality depression,* something that would normally affect anyone, such as a death in the family. Herbal treatment should be reserved for mild to moderate depression only. If depression is severe and the person is perhaps suicidal, herbalists can augment and support but are not equipped to treat. Chinese Medicine views depression as a shen disturbance of the Heart (Case History 23.2).
- *Signs and symptoms.* Feelings of doom, loss of interest or pleasure in daily activities. No ambition; feeling lethargic; experiencing fatigue, insomnia, loss of appetite or constant eating, or suicidal thoughts. May be accompanied by anxiety.
- *Allopathic Treatment.* Antidepressant meds and psychotherapy.
- *General therapeutic principles.* Treatment depends on what accompanies the depression, be it anxiety, insomnia, and/or lethargy. (1) Always use antidepressant, nervine tonic herbs: St John's Wort, Damiana herb, Skullcap herb, Schisandra Wu Wei Zi (Five Taste berry), Bacopa plant, or Rhodiola root. (2) Decrease brain inflammation with Turmeric root. (3) Adrenal restoratives for sure, including Sage leaf, Schisandra Wu Wei Zi (Five Taste berry), Rhodiola root, Ashwagandha root, or Polygonum He Shu Wu (Flowery Knotweed root). (4) If anxiety is a factor, choose anxiolytics: Valerian root, Passionflower herb. (5) Hypnotics for sleep if needed but only at bedtime. In fact, a separate bedtime formula is a useful solution. (6) Consider a brain-blood circulator such as Ginkgo leaf if thinking is foggy.

Neuritis and Peripheral Neuropathy

- *Definition.* ***Neuropathy*** refers to damaged or diseased nerves. Peripheral neuropathy is when nerves that carry messages to and from the brain and spinal cord to the extremities are damaged or diseased. Damage can impair sensation, movement, or organ function, depending on type of nerve affected. A leading cause of peripheral neuropathy is type 1 diabetes. Other causes are

TABLE 23.6 Analgesics
(Pulse Dose for Pain: 3–5 mL every 1/2 to 1 hour)

Herb	Notes
Corydalis turtschaninovii Yan Hu Suo *Corydalis* corm Best in Chinese medicine; medium-strength.	Major nonaddictive Poppy family Chinese nervous sedative, analgesic, hypnotic, and coronary vasodilator. Many uses for abdomen, joints, muscles, postpartum, headaches, dysmenorrhea, and neuralgia with pain, anxiety, and insomnia.
Piscidia erythrina Jamaican Dogwood root bark Best in the West, strong.	Major pain herb in Western herbalism. Cool and astringent, spasmolytic, antiinflammatory, anxiolytic, and antitussive. For internal wind.
Salix alba White Willow bark	Heat-clearing, analgesic because it contains salicin, tannins, and acids. Antiinflammatory, analgesic, and antiseptic. Used for headaches and urinary tract infections.
Betula alba Birch leaf and bark in tincture and essential oil form.	Contains tannins and salicylic acid. For joint pain, fever, and inflammation.
Populus tremuloides Poplar/Quaking Aspen bark	Antiinflammatory, heat-clearing, mild salicin-containing analgesic.
Piper methysticum Kava root	Hypnotic analgesic, for muscle tension, neuralgia, insomnia. Urinary tropism.
Eschscholzia californica California Poppy herb	Cool, bitter, mild analgesic and sedative. Poppy family herb for pain, anxiety, insomnia, and spasms.
Bupleurum chinensis Chai Hu Asian Buplever root	Nervous sedative, analgesic, and spasmolytic. Especially protective of the liver.
Lavandula angustifolia Lavender flower and essential oil	Relieves pain for nerve excess with insomnia, anxiety, and palpitations (all riled up). For myalgia, neuralgia, colic, and gastrointestinal (GI) spasms.
Valeriana officinalis Valerian root	For pain in general, with anxiety and sleep loss, tension headaches, and migraines. May have opposite effect in high doses and excess conditions.
Lactuca virosa Wild Lettuce leaf	Cold, bitter, and calming. For pain, insomnia, and spasms.
Dioscorea villosa Wild Yam root	Has tropism for GI pain and uterus. For ovulation pain and menstrual cramps, acute arthritis with hot joints, and fibromyalgia.
Actaea racemosa Black Cohosh root	Cool, dry, and possibly estrogenic. For muscle pain, spasms, myalgia; menstrual, prostatic, and arthritic pain; and seizures.
Cannabis spp. Marijuana leaf and bud (Illegal in some locations.)	Analgesic, antiemetic, spasmolytic, antiinflammatory, and endocannabinoid modulating.[13] For nerve and muscle pain, insomnia, and stopping some seizures.

trauma; severe cold; nerve compression (as in carpel tunnel or sciatica); autoimmune diseases, such as arthritis; toxic exposure; or infections like West Nile virus, Lyme disease, or shingles (Case History 23.3).

- *Signs and symptoms*. Often burning pain, numbness, or tingling, muscle weakness, abnormal or exaggerated sensations, acute sensitivity to touch. It's no fun. Affected nerves can be motor or sensory.
- *Allopathic treatment*. Choices are not great. Addressing underlying cause is the best bet. Transcutaneous electrical nerve stimulation (TENS) units could be used for pain. Anticonvulsants like Gabapentin, capsaicin in hot peppers that modifies peripheral pain receptors, and antidepressants are used.
- *General therapeutic principles*. Go with internal and external remedies and try to ascertain and fix root problem. (1) Main intention is to nourish the nerves with tonics, such as St John's Wort or Garden Sage leaf. (2) Nervous system relaxants such as Skullcap herb. (3) Antispasmodics to decrease muscle spasm. (4) Antiinflammatories. (5) Adaptogens to help with stress.[11]

Tension Headaches

- *Definition*. A ***headache*** (HA) is a symptom characterized by continuous pain over various parts of the head (Case History 23.4). There are many types, the most common being a tension headache, which has pain bilaterally, often with

TABLE 23.7 Nervous System Stimulants

Herbs	Notes
Turnera diffusa Damiana herb	Nerve stimulant, warming. Helps chronic fatigue. Nerve/brain deficiencies. Mental dullness. Kidney Essence Deficiency.
Panax ginseng Ren Shen Asian Red Ginseng root	Adaptogenic and restorative. Sympathetic nervous system, cardiovascular, and adrenal stimulant.
Ocimum basilicum Basil herb	Sympathetic nervous system stimulant, restorative, warm and dry. For deficiencies, chronic depression, migraines, and adrenal fatigue.
Cinnamomum camphora Camphor resin	Stimulates brain and heart, spasmolytic, and analgesic. For Heart and Kidney Yang Deficiency, depression, memory loss. Used in essential oil form and as a smelling salt to arouse consciousness.
Theobroma cacao Cacao nut/Chocolate	Contains caffeine and many antioxidants, particularly dark chocolate that does not have a lot of milk and sugar.
Coffea arabica Coffee bean	Caffeine content varies, depending on brand. A highly sprayed crop. Best is organic dark roast, freshly ground, with no cream or sugar. May protect against cancer, metabolic syndrome, heart disease and Parkinson's in moderate amounts.
Camellia sinensis (Tea) Green tea leaves are wilted, steamed, and dried. Black tea leaves are crushed or rolled and allowed to oxidize before being dried. They are the same plant.	Although both green and black *Camellia sinensis* contain some caffeine, green tea is linked to brain-friendly antioxidants that improve mood, vigilance, reaction time, and memory.[14] Black, less so.
Ilex paraguariensis Yerba Maté leaf and twig	A tropical caffeinated South American plant similar to Black tea.

muscle contractions in the head and posterior neck regions. There is no nausea or vomiting. Anyone can get an HA once in a while. They become a problem when frequent and recurring. Causes are numerous, ranging from dehydration to a brain tumor. A discerning herbalist tries to find the reason.

- *Chinese Medicine remedies.* There are many kinds of headaches and many syndromes that all boil down to finding and treating the pain and the cause, as is done in the West. Type of pain and location is important. For instance, if sharp, it's blood stagnation; if a chronic, dull ache, it could be a Kidney deficiency; if there is a sense of heaviness or swelling like the head feels like it might split open, it's damp. If it's on the sides or top of the head (vertex), it's Liver-Gallbladder organ meridian related. If relieved by warmth or pressure, it's a qi deficiency.[15] And so on. One needs to be accurate at assessment to deduce the syndrome (Boxes 23.2 and 23.3).
- *Signs and symptoms.* Mild to moderate, diffuse, dull ache in the head. Sometimes feels like a *band around the head or forehead.*
- *Allopathic treatments.* Nonsteroidal antiinflammatory drugs (NSAIDs) including aspirin; other analgesics like Tylenol. Quit smoking; seek biofeedback. Possibly, MRI may be needed.
- *General therapeutic principles.* Obviously, when there is pain involved, deal with that first. (1) Analgesics, such as Corydalis Yan Hu Suo (Asian Corydalis corm), Jamaican Dogwood root, and the natural aspirin White Willow bark. (2) Antispasmodics, including Cramp bark, Lobelia herb, Hops flower. (3) The bigger picture is to search and fix the cause, the root. HA causes are numerous. For instance, if it's from stress, use anxiolytics such as Skullcap herb or Kava root. If there is eye strain, use some high-dose Bilberry berry. If there are hormonal considerations related to the menstrual cycle, Chaste Tree berry would be called for. If it's caused by decreased blood to the brain, choose Ginkgo leaf. If it's sinusitis, clear the infection with Andrographis Chuan Xin Lian (Heart-Thread Lotus leaf). Sometimes it's from a food trigger, such as red wine containing sulfites, other alcohol, artificial sweeteners, or caffeine. PMS with hormone imbalances can be a culprit. Often Chasteberry will balance this out (Case History 23.4).

Migraine Headaches

- *Definition.* Recurrent throbbing headaches on one or both sides of the head and often accompanied by nausea and disturbed vision (Case History 23.5). Triggers vary: stress, fatigue, insomnia, food sensitivity, hormonal changes right before or after menses, strong smells, sounds, and light exposure. Figuring out and treating the cause is the best route. Have client keep a migraine diary to compare headache onset and occurrence with foods or other triggers. Migraine cause is unknown and hotly debated in allopathic circles.

CASE HISTORY 23.1

Case History for Anxiety and Panic Attacks

S. Alice seems to get stressed for no reason, especially in social situations when out with her husband. She feels she is being judged. She becomes sweaty, mouth is dry, heart races, and blood pressure is elevated. She has trouble sleeping.

O. P Rapid and thin. **T** Coat dry, red tip.

A. Heart Yin Deficiency. Anxiety attacks.

P. *Specific therapeutic principles.* (1) Anxiolytics/neuro-cardiac sedatives to calm the spirit. (2) Heart tonics for palpitations. (3) Nerve-adrenal tonics. (3) Antihypertensives. (4) Demulcents to build yin.

#1 Herbal Formula and Dose.
5 mL 3 × a day, plus a separate before bed sleep formula.

Part	Herbs	Rationale
3	Skullcap herb	Anxiolytic, calms the shen, antihypertensive.
3	Kava root	Anxiolytic, calms the shen, helps sleep.
3	Schisandra We Wei Zi	Adrenal-nerve tonic.
2	Hawthorn berry	Palpitations, antihypertensive, Heart tonic.
1	Marshmallow root	Moisture, builds yin.

#2 Herbal Formula for Sleep and Dose.
4 mL 1 hour before bed, 4 mL at bedtime, and every 15 minutes for 2 hours, as needed.

Part	Herbs	Rationale
1	Valerian root	Nervous relaxant.
1	Passionflower herb	Calms mind, stops spasms.
1	Zizyphus Suan Zao Ren	Relaxant, calms shen.

Other Suggestions

- Breathing exercises when feel panic attack coming on.
- Yoga.
- Lavender essential oil bath.
- Psychotherapy to get at root of panic attacks.
- Tea for nervous stress (Box 23.1).

• BOX 23.1 Tea For Nervous Stress

It's always nice to have a calming blend up in the cabinet. This one is mellow and relaxing, a good sleep aid.

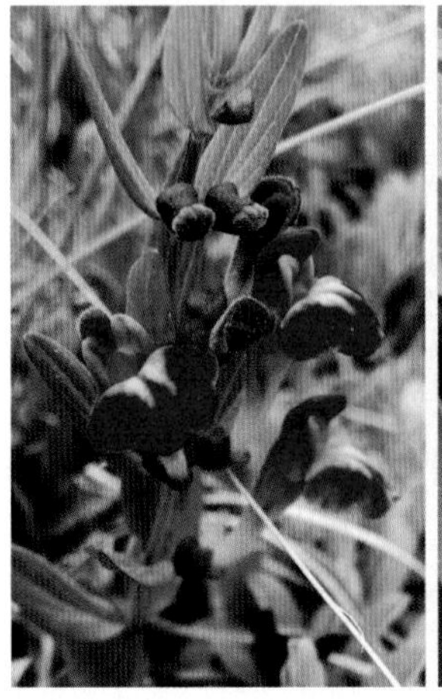

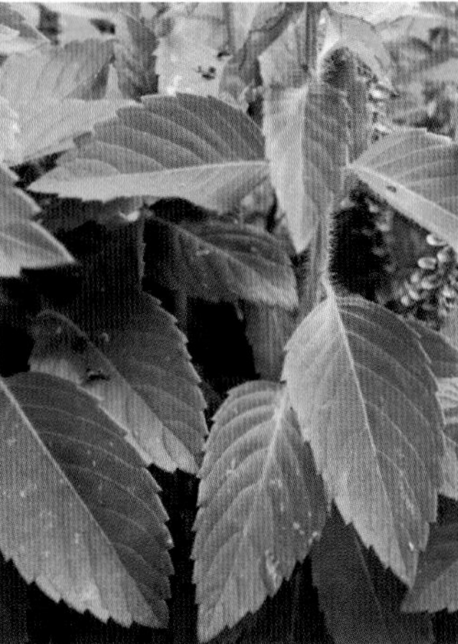

Scutellaria brittonii (Skullcap herb), a Colorado native, and *Ocimum tenuiflorum* (Tulsi, Holy Basil leaf), a summer garden favorite. These calming nervines are part of our stress-reducing tea.

Ingredients

3 parts	Lemon Balm leaf	Use the largest quantity of relaxing, lemony Lemon Balm.
2 parts	Chamomile flower	Gentle nervous and stomach relaxant.
1 part	Holy Basil leaf	Relaxant and antiinflammatory.
1 part	Skullcap herb	Relaxant, restores nerves, stops spasms.
½ part	Valerian root	Strongest acting and strongest tasting, smallest proportion.

Directions. Measure out a quantity of dried herbs; mix up and store blend in a closed glass jar or tin.

To brew. Steep 1 tbsp per cup in just boiled water for 20 min. Strain and enjoy any time it's needed.

- *Chinese Medicine.* Migraines are frequently attributed to Liver qi and blood obstruction/stagnation in the head. Therefore herbs that move Liver qi and blood are used.
- *Signs and symptoms.* Not nice. Throbbing, pulsating, severe pain on one or both sides of the head, worse with activity. Can last for hours or days. There is often nausea, vomiting, and sensitivity to light and noise. Many people do best in a dark, quiet environment. Sometimes, but not always, a migraine is preceded by a visual phenomenon called an *aura,* which appears as color or flashing light, blind spots, or distortion.
- *Allopathic treatment.* Many health care providers don't know how to handle migraines. Pain management, avoiding triggers, diet modification, relaxation techniques, and referral for acupuncture are sometimes effective.
- *General therapeutic principles.* Two formulas, one during an acute attack and one for prevention.
    - *Part 1, Acute.* (1) Strong analgesics. (2) Antiinflammatories: Ginger root, Boswellia resin. (3) Liver support.
    - *Part 2, Prevention.* Long-term formula.[10] Feverfew herb is very specific for headaches and migraines preventatively. It is relaxing, analgesic, and antiinflammatory, takes 4 to 6 months to kick in, but is proven effective in the long term. (1) Nervine tonics for stress, such as St. John's Wort or Ashwagandha root. (2) Both Eastern and Western traditions always address the Liver: Globe Artichoke leaf, Milk Thistle seed, or Bupleurum Chi Hu (Asian Buplever root). (3) Spasmolytics: Cramp bark or Chamomile flower. (4) Decrease inflammation with Ginger root, Turmeric root, and Boswellia resin. (5) Possibly choose anticoagulants like Ginger root and Turmeric root. (6) Spleen tonics, such as Codonopsis Dang Shen (Downy Bellflower root) or White Atractylodes Bai Zhu. (7) Menstrual migraines need hormonal herbs, such as Black Cohosh root or Wild Yam root. (8) Perfuse brain with Ginkgo leaf. (9) Attend to gut health. If a trigger food has been identified, remove it.

CASE HISTORY 23.2

Case History for Depression with Anxiety and Insomnia

S. Cassandra reported depression going on 2 years after her mom died and requested an herbal treatment (no drugs). She cries frequently, can't concentrate, has anxiety, palpitations, and difficulty sleeping.
O. P Thready, weak. **T** Red, no coating.
A. Heart and Kidney Yin Deficiency, Shen imbalance. Depression, anxiety, and insomnia.
P. *Specific therapeutic principles.* (1) Antidepressants/nerve tonics. (2) Nerve/adrenal tonics to restore Heart shen. (3) Nervous system relaxants for anxiety. (4) Increase brain capillary blood circulation. (5) Restore Kidney yin. (6) Separate sleep formula.

#1 Herbal Formula and Dose.
6 mg 3 × a day. Last dose before dinner.

Part	Herbs	Rational
3	Polygonum He Shou Wu	Nerve/adrenal tonic for chronic depression.
3	Turmeric root	Decreases brain inflammation.
2	St. John's Wort	Depression, nerve tonic, anxiety palpitations.
2	Passionflower herb	Decreases anxiety.
1	Ginkgo Leaf	Microcirculation to brain for focus.
1	Licorice root	Adrenal restorative, addresses Yin Deficiency.

#2 Herbal Formula for Sleep and Dose.
4 mL 1 hour before bed, 4 mL at bedtime and every 15 mins × 2 hours as needed.

Part	Herbs	Rational
3	Passionflower herb or Zizyphus Suan Zao Ren	Hypnotic, sleep, balances shen.
3	Valerian root	Hypnotic, muscle relaxant, antispasmodic.
2	Motherwort herb	Anxiolytic, palpitations.

Other Suggestions

Red Flags. Must seek professional help if person appears suicidal, or if depression is severe.

- *Important.* Herbalists must bring down brain inflammation and improve gut-brain connection. This means concentrating on microbiome health, antiinflammatory diet, and including *Curcuma longa* in the formula, specific for brain inflammation.
- *Supplements:* Omega-3 fatty acids, vitamin D_3, folic acid in the form of methyl folate, and possibly SAMe. This last is a synthesized form of S-adenosylmethionine, a compound made in the body that helps depression.
- *Treat holistically.* Including diet, lifestyle, exercise. It is a challenge to get a depressed person to accomplish any of these things. They need lots of support.
- Psychotherapy referral, if needed.
- Yoga.
- Before bed: Milky Oat tops tea, Lavender essential oil bath.
- *Yoga asana (legs up the wall).* If clients can't get to sleep or waken in the middle of the night and can't get back to sleep, tell them to get out of bed, lie on their back on the floor, wiggle in close to a wall so buttocks touch it, and raise legs up against the wall for a few minutes and breathe. This inverted pose is extremely helpful.

CASE HISTORY 23.3

Case History for Neuritis

S. Joey overtwisted his back and hip while doing yoga. He has a nasty burning pain in his left buttock radiating down his left leg. It is numb and tingly.
O. P Wiry and rapid. **T** Purplish, if chronic.
A. Acute blood stasis. Sciatic nerve compression from a piriformis muscle spasm.
P. *Specific therapeutic principles.* (1) Move qi and blood. (2) Relieve pain. (3) Antispasmodics. (4) Nerve tonics. (5) Bring down inflammation.

Herbal Formula and Dose.
Pulse dose for nerve pain, 3-5 mL every 1/2 to 1 hour.

Part	Herbs	Rationale
3	Jamaican Dogwood root	Relieve nerve pain, antispasmodic, antiinflammatory.
3	Bupleurum Chai Hu	Antispasmodic, analgesic, move qi, clear Liver stagnation.
3	Valerian root	Antispasmodic, analgesic, move qi.
3	Turmeric root	Move blood, decrease inflammation.
2	Astragalus Huang Qi	Dry damp, adaptogen, nerve tonic.

Other Suggestions

- *Topical.* St. John's Wort and Peppermint essential oil or Cayenne pepper (capsicum) ointment to relieve inflammation.
- *Manual therapies.* Massage and/or chiropractic, to relieve nerve compression, the root problem. Piriformis muscle stretch.

Neurological Autoimmune (AI) Diseases

- *Definition.* There is an epidemic of autoimmune (AI) diseases these days, in which the body attacks its own healthy cells, building up antibodies against them. Why? At their core, they are all similar in that the immune response is caused by systemic inflammation instigated by leaky gut. This condition encourages the body to attack itself. Nearly any body cell can be affected. In rheumatoid arthritis, it's the joints; in type 1 diabetes, the pancreas; in Hashimoto's thyroiditis, the thyroid gland; in psoriasis, the skin; in celiac disease, the gut reacts against gluten; in chronic fatigue, it's the mitochondria, etc. AI diseases are overwhelming, confusing, and scary.
- *Common autoimmune neurological diseases.* In multiple sclerosis (MS), the myelin sheath of nerve cells is attacked, affecting movement and vision. In Parkinson's disease (Case History 23.6), it's the brain, where the neurotransmitter dopamine is depressed, causing tremors, weakness, and movement problems. In Alzheimer's disease, beta-amyloid plaques build up in the brain affecting memory and mental functions. In Amyotrophic lateral sclerosis (ALS), the muscles are attacked, causing progressive weakness, loss of movement, and eventually affecting the diaphragm muscle and ability to breathe.
- *Common signs and symptoms of AI diseases.* Very vague and diffuse and can go on for years: fatigue, muscle pain or weakness, heat or cold intolerance, brain fog, or GI symptoms.

CASE HISTORY 23.4

Case History for Tension Headaches (HA)

S. Joan frequently gets a dull pain in both temples and the back of her neck every day since she began a new job 6 months ago. As a single mom, she has been under much stress and is nervous about succeeding at work. The situation is becoming chronic.

O. P Fast, superficial, and light. **T** Thin coat.

A. Chronic tension HA related to stress and muscle tension.

P. *Specific therapeutic principles.* (1) Anxiolytics for stress and anxiety. (2) Analgesics for pain. (3) Spasmolytics and muscle relaxants that help circulation. (4) Nervous restoratives.

Herbal Formula and Pulse Dose.
6 mL every 15–30 min, as needed

Part	Herbs	Rationale
3	Corydalis Yan Hu Suo	Analgesic, spasmolytic, moves qi and blood, nerve tonic.
3	Cramp bark	Spasmolytic, relaxing, moves blood for circulation.
3	White Willow bark	Analgesic, antiinflammatory.
2	Eleutherococcus Ci Wu Jia	Nerve trophorestorative for chronic stress.

Suggestions

Red Flags. HA with a fever, stiff neck, mental confusion, seizures, double vision, weakness, numbness, or speaking difficulties could indicate a brain injury and is a medical emergency.

- *Essential oil.* Lavender, Birch, Marjoram, or Chamomile: 1 or 2 drops on the temples.
- *Acupuncture.* Effective for chronic tension headaches.
- Relaxation in form of breath work, yoga, meditation, and time out.

• BOX 23.2 Type of Headache Pain

Related to Chinese Medicine Syndromes

In Chinese Medicine a description of the type or *kind* of pain a person experiences can give clues as to which syndrome is involved. A good history and careful questioning are in order. A lot of headaches imply heat to the head (yang), so bringing heat down to the feet with a hot footbath and a cool head cloth is one hydrotherapy approach.

- If it feels better with warmth or pressure, it's yin or a qi deficiency.
- If it feels better without pressure, it's yang.
- If it comes and goes, it's liver wind.
- If it feels dull and achy, it's a kidney deficiency.
- If it's sharp, it's blood stagnation.
- If it feels like the head is swelling and heavy, there is dampness.[15]

Symptoms are more specific, depending on which tissue is attacked. Some are obvious, like diabetes affecting insulin and blood sugar, or classic hypothyroid symptoms indicating Hashimoto's thyroiditis. Other symptoms are Butterfly rash (lupus); vision disturbances (MS); severe short-term memory loss with decreased ability to handle body functions (Alzheimer's); muscle or joint pain, weakness, tremors (Parkinson's).

• BOX 23.3 Location of Headaches in Chinese Medicine

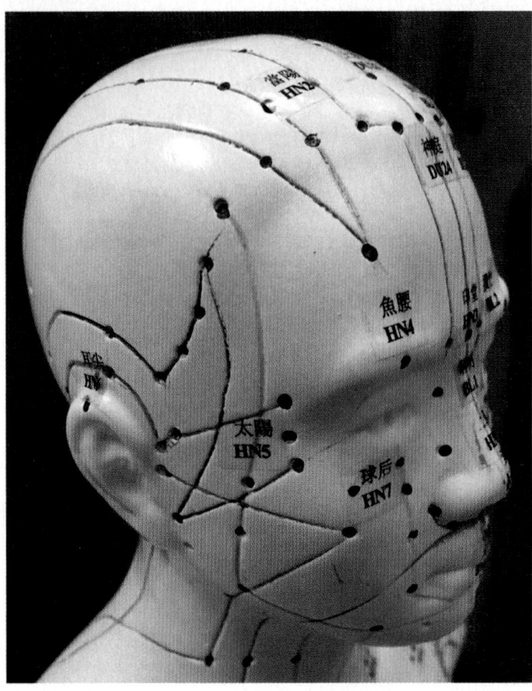

Meridians carry qi through different areas of the head. They give a clue as to the type of headache and which herbs to use in treatment.

In Chinese Medicine, there are perhaps 10 types of headaches. They frequently apply to location: Where on the head or face does it hurt, and which meridian passes through that area? Pain along a meridian indicates a blockage of qi. For instance, pain along the sides (temples) or top (vertex) of the head is related to Liver and Gallbladder. Pain in the front of the face is caused from a blockage of qi in the stomach and large intestine.

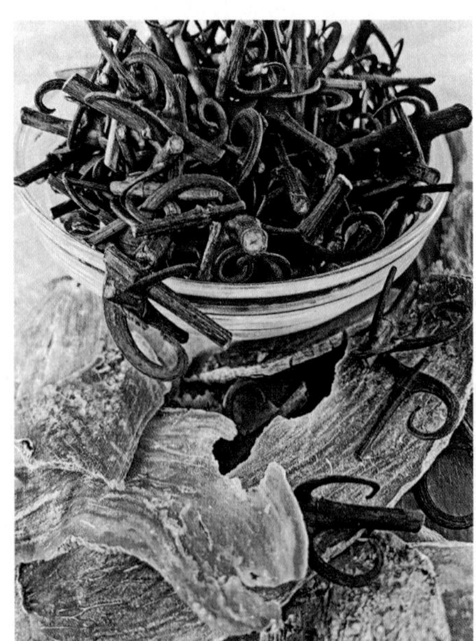

• **Fig. 23.9** Uncaria Gou Teng (Gambir Vine twig and thorn) and Gastrodia Tian Ma (Celestial Hemp corm) are a Chinese combination often used for internal wind such as the spasms of Parkinson's disease or with seizures.

CASE HISTORY 23.5

Case History for Migraine Headache (HA)

Part 1

S. Louise has had debilitating migraines for years. Presently, there is distended, pulsating pain on her left temple, over eyes, and at top of head. She applies a cold compress and lies in a dark, absolutely quiet room. The only triggers she can identify are gluten, which she has now removed from her diet, and the fact that she has a lot of stress in her life.

O. P Superficial, wiry and fast. **T** Red tip, purplish edges.

A. Liver Qi Stagnation. Active migraine HA, probably from acute stress.

P. *Specific therapeutic principles.* First deal with pain: (1) Use analgesics for pain and qi stagnation. (2) Soothe liver. (3) Antiinflammatories.
Part 2. When episode resolved, begin long-term prevention: (1) Use relaxing nerve tonics. (2) Use liver restoratives. (3) Use Stomach/Spleen tonics.

Formula #1 Acute Migraine Attack - Pulse Dose.
6 mL every 15 min to 1/2 hour as needed.
Catch early, start immediately, at first aura or prodromal symptom.

Part	Herbs	Rationale
4	Corydalis Yan Hu Suo	Analgesic, spasmolytic, move qi and blood.
3	Jamaican Dogwood root	Analgesic, spasmolytic, anxiolytic, move qi.
3	Boswellia resin or Ginger root	Antiinflammatory, analgesic.
2	Valerian root	Analgesic, relaxant.

Suggestions for Migraine Headache

- *Topical essential oils.* Lavender, Peppermint, Basil over temples.
- *Essential oil compresses.* Cold head/neck/forehead compresses: 2 drops Peppermint, 1 drop Ginger, 1 drop Marjoram at first sign of migraine.

Part 2

Preventative Nerve, Spleen, and Liver tonic
Dose 5 mg 3 × day between meals

Part	Herbs	Rationale
3	Feverfew herb	Analgesic, antiinflammatory, migraine prophylactic. (Takes 4–6 months to kick in. Use long-term.)
2	Artichoke leaf	Nerve and liver tonic.
2	Dandelion root	Liver restorative, stimulant, and gut health.
2	Codonopsis Dang Shen	Spleen/digestive tonic.
2	Oregon Grape root	Berberine for leaky gut, liver stimulant.
1	Ginger root	Heal gut, decrease inflammation.

Suggestions for Preventative measures

- *Diet.* Heal gut. Four-R program; identify any food allergens other than gluten, which she knows about. Antiinflammatory diet. Eliminate caffeine, alcohol, and cigarettes (and any suspected personal triggers, such as chocolate and peanuts) for 2 months and use migraine diary to monitor changes in symptoms. Fermented foods and bitters.
- *Stress reduction.* Yoga, meditation, or other methods.

CASE HISTORY 23.6

Case History for Parkinson's

S. Lacy is 52 years old. It began with a right-hand tremor. Then developed stiff gait, slow movement, worsening balance. Neurologist gave a diagnosis of Parkinson's.

O. P Thin. **T** Pale, quivering and dry.

A. Parkinson's, an autoimmune disease caused by decreased dopamine. Liver yin has become weak, causing tremors or wind.[16]

P. *Specific therapeutic principles.* Cause is from decrease of the neurotransmitter dopamine, which is converted from the amino acid l-dopa. (1) Replace dopamine with *Macuna pruriens* (Velvet bean). This herb is proven to contain l-dopa. The drug, Levodopa (or l-dopa) is the precursor to dopamine, and a class of medications that is the Western gold standard treatment for Parkinson's.[17] (2) Nourish the nervous system, kidney yin, and liver. (3) Sedate internal wind and tremors. (4) Nervous system restoratives. (5) Adaptogens.

Formula and Dose.
5 mL 3 × day.

Part	Herbs	Rationale
4	Velvet bean	Dopamine replacement.
2	Ashwagandha root	Nerve tonic, adaptogen.
2	Uncaria Gou Teng	Liver wind, spasmolytic, nervous relaxant.
2	Gastrodia Tian Ma	Liver wind, spasmolytic, nervous relaxant.
2	Gotu Kola herb	Central nervous system/ adrenal restorative.
1	Shatavari root/Asparagus root	Tonify yin and liver.
1	Triphala	Helps elimination, circulation, and inflammation. See suggestions.

Suggestions

Many of these factors listed are best identified with functional medicine testing, but basics can be addressed with good assessment and herbs. Autoimmune diseases are a challenge and take a long time to reverse.

- *Fix leaky gut and inflammation.* Paleo diet and Four-R program or GAPS protocol. Carbs, white-sugar-heavy diets, and unhealthy saturated fats create inflammation and are a set-up for small intestinal bacterial overgrowth (SIBO) that cause leaky gut.
- *Triphala.* This is a three-herb Ayurvedic herbal combination of fruits (available in bulk as one herb called Triphala). The three fruits are *Emblica officinalis* (Indian gooseberry or amalaki or amla), *Terminalia chebula* (Chebulic myrobalan or Haritaki), and *Terminalia bellirica* (Belleric Myrobalan or Bibhitaki). Each fruit acts on a different dosha, and the synergistic combination has been used in India for over 1000 years for inflammation and many chronic diseases, even cancer.[18]

- *Allopathic treatment.* Western medicine has very little to offer, and there is no cure. Immunosuppressant drugs, corticosteroids, intravenous immunoglobulin therapy, and symptomatic treatments are used.
- *General therapeutic principles.* The overall functional medicine Four-R approach, which may not eliminate the AI disease totally but can lead to remissions the client can live with. The main triggers are food sensitivities, leaky gut, toxins, stress, and infections. (1) Antiinflammatory gut fix. Because nearly 80%

of the immune system is in the gut, identify inflammation to fix or eliminate the triggers. This is done with diet and herbs. (2) Herbal bitters and berberines help reduce gut inflammation. (3) Use any herbs specific for the AI disease in question. (4) Symptomatic herbs, such as Gastrodia Tian Ma and Uncaria Gou Teng for spasms (Fig. 23.9), and shaking in Liver wind, used in Parkinson's. (5) Nerve tonics.

Summary

The nervous system was investigated on the physical level and as an aspect of the mind-body and gut-brain connection. The nervous system is a communications network sending chemical messages in the form of neurotransmitters throughout the body. Emotionally and spiritually, our thoughts, beliefs, and emotions affect our physical health. When leaky gut is present, so too is leaky brain, both factors adversely affecting neurological health.

In Chinese Medicine, the mind-body connection affects every organ system. The spirit, psyche, and emotions reside in the Heart. Thoughts and worry are Spleen functions. The brain is an extension of the bone marrow, the Kidney's body part. The Liver is concerned with wind, a manifestation of abnormal movement, shakes, and spasms.

Nervines are a general catch-all Western term for any herb that addresses the nervous system. The nervous system Materia Medica includes restoratives, trophorestoratives, adaptogens, stimulants, spasmolytics, hypnotics, analgesics, and anticonvulsants.

Of particular relevance today are the numerous autoimmune diseases. Our example in the neurobiology realm is Parkinson's. However, the basic treatments presented are the same for any autoimmune condition in any body system. *Heal thy gut.*

Review

Fill in the Blanks

(Answers in Appendix B.)

1. Name four things one can do to improve neurological health: ___, ___, ___, ___.
2. Name four neurotransmitters appearing in the brain and the gut: ___, ___, ___, ___.
3. What are four actions of hypnotics? ___, ___, ___, ___?
4. Name four hypnotic herbs: ___, ___, ___, ___.
5. Name five nervous system restorative herbs: ___, ___, ___, ___, ___. Relaxants include five categories of Western herbal descriptions. These are ___, ___, ___, ___, ___.
6. A strong Western analgesic herb is ___. A well-known Chinese analgesic herb is ___.
7. Name five stimulant herbs that do not contain caffeine: ___, ___, ___, ___, ___.
8. Chinese medicine views depression as what? ___.
9. Which antiviral herb is specific for shingles? ___.
10. Name five nervines that are relaxing to the stomach: ___, ___, ___, ___, ___.

Critical Concept Questions

(Answers for you to decide.)

1. What is the mind-body connection?
2. What is the gut-brain connection?
3. How does Chinese medicine view the nervous system?
4. A client would like to get off their doctor-prescribed opioids for pain. What do you suggest?
5. Why are autoimmune diseases so prevalent in our society?
6. Why are antidepressant herbs so often nerve tonics as well?
7. Would you advise your client to get a shingles vaccine? Why or why not?
8. Name various herbs you might use for depression? When should an herbalist not attempt to treat depression?
9. How would the tongue appear if a person has emotional stress?
10. Describe a typical Pulse and Tongue for Parkinson's disease and give rationale.

References

1. Weinberg, Jennifer. "Mind-Body Connection: Understanding the Psycho-Emotional Roots of Disease." The Chopra Center. http://www.chopra.com/articles/mind-body-connection-understanding-the-psycho-emotional-roots-of-disease (accessed November 29, 2019).
2. Northrup, Christiane. *Women's Body, Women's Wisdom* (New York, NY: Bantam, 2002).
3. Myss, Caroline. *Anatomy of the Spirit* (New York, NY: Three Rivers, 1996).
4. Mayer, Emeran A. "Gut Feelings: The Emerging Biology of Gut–Brain Connection." U.S. National Library of Medicine, National Institutes of Health. https://www.ncbi.nlm.nih.gov/pmc/articles/PMC3845678/ (accessed November 30, 2019).
5. Breit, Sigrid, et al. "Vagus Nerve as Modulator of the Gut–Brain Axis in Psychiatric and Inflammatory Disorders." Frontiers in Psychiatry. https://www.frontiersin.org/articles/10.3389/fpsyt.2018.00044/full (accessed November 29, 2019).
6. Figeley, Melanie "Do You Have a Leaky Brain?" Biotics Research NW Inc. https://www.bioticsnw.com/blogs/news/do-you-have-a-leaky-brain (accessed November 29, 2019).
7. Holmes, Peter. *Energetics of Western Herbs* (Boulder, CO: Snow Lotus, 2006).
8. Yance, Donald. *Adaptogens in Medical Herbalism* (Rochester, VT: Healing Arts, 2013).
9. Goel, Ajay. "Can Curcumin Solve Depression?" Natural Medicine Journal. https://www.naturalmedicinejournal.com/journal/2014-11/can-curcumin-solve-depression. (accessed February 18, 2021).
10. Hoffman, David. *Medical Herbalism: The Science and Practice of Herbal Medicine* (Rochester, VT: Healing Arts, 2003).
11. Bone, Kerry and Simon Mills. *Principles and Practice of Phytotherapy* (London, UK: Elsevier, 2013).
12. "Black Coffee in the Morning and Green Tea in the Afternoon May Provide Valuable Health Benefits." Mercola, Take Control of Your Health. https://articles.mercola.com/sites/articles/archive/2016/01/18/black-coffee-green-tea-health-benefits.aspx (accessed August 12, 2019).

13. Russo, Ethan B. "Cannabinoids in the Management of Difficult to Treat Pain." U.S. National Library of Medicine, National Institutes of Health. https://www.ncbi.nlm.nih.gov/pmc/articles/PMC2503660/ (accessed December 1, 2019).
14. Gunnars, Chris. "Ten Evidence-Based Benefits of Green Tea." Healthline. https://www.healthline.com/nutrition/top-10-evidence-based-health-benefits-of-green-tea (accessed August 10, 2019).
15. Tierra, Michael. *The Way of Chinese Herbs* (New York, NY: Pocket Books, 1998).
16. Dharmananda, Subhuti. "Parkinson's Disease: Possible Treatment with Chinese Medicine." Institute for Traditional Medicine. http://www.itmonline.org/arts/parkinsons.htm (accessed August 12, 2019).
17. Pulikkalpura, Haridas, et. al. "Levodopa in *Macuna pruriens* and its Degradation." Scientific Reports. https://www.nature.com/articles/srep11078 (accessed August 12, 2019).
18. Kubala, Jillian. "What is Triphala?" Healthline. https://www.healthline.com/nutrition/triphala#section1 (accessed August 9, 2019).

24 The Muscular-Skeletal System

"The doctor of the future will give no medicine but will interest his patients in the care of the human frame, in diet, and in the cause and prevention of disease."

—Thomas Edison, Inventor

CHAPTER REVIEW

- Overview of the muscular-skeletal system.
- Pain, inflammation, and analgesia: Inflammation. Pain, inflammation, and external applications. Nonsteroidal antiinflammatory drugs.
- Cannabis and the endocannabinoid system.
- The overrated alkaline diet pH test.
- Chinese Medicine perspective: The muscular-skeletal system and major syndromes.
- Muscular-skeletal Materia Medica: Muscular-skeletal herbs worth honorable mention. Restoratives (tonics). Warming arterial stimulants. Relaxants (analgesics, salicylates, antiinflammatories, spasmolytics, antipyretics, and rubefacients for topical applications).
- Common muscular-skeletal conditions with case histories: Soft-tissue damage (sprains and strains), osteoporosis and fracture, acute and chronic rheumatoid arthritis, osteoarthritis, gout, and fibromyalgia.

KEY TERMS

Analgesics
Arthritis
Bi syndrome
Bone
Cartilage
Contusion
Cupping
Endocannabinoid (ECB) system
Fascia
Fibromyalgia syndrome (FMS)
Gout
Hydrotherapy
Inflammation
Ligament
Moxibustion
Muscle
Myalgia
Neuralgia
Nonsteroidal antiinflammatory drugs (NSAIDs)
Osteoarthritis (OA)
Osteoporosis
Phytocannabinoids
Pulse dosing
Rheumatoid arthritis
RICE
Rubefacients
Salicylates
Sinews
Spasm
Sprain
Sterols
Strain
Tendon
Tui na

Humans have always contended with muscle aches, bone pain, and structural injuries. Egyptian mummies and ancient skeletal remains have been unearthed showing signs of degenerative discs and arthritis. Bones and muscles give us our form, support our weight, allow us to move, and hold us together; they get plenty of wear, tear, and abuse. Joint disorders and back problems are primary reasons people visit their doctor, because the first thing bringing them to a healthcare provider's door is pain.

Pain, inflammation, and analgesia are primary topics, and alleviating discomfort with nonaddictive herbs is a worthwhile skill for any herbalist. The endocannabinoid system and its role in pain relief is explained. Nonsteroidal antiinflammatory drugs (NSAIDs) are explained, and their dangerous side effects are an important concept. External and internal herbal applications are explored in depth.

Overview of the Muscular-Skeletal System

The muscular-skeletal (M-S) system is made up of various forms of fibrous connective tissue: muscles, tendons, ligaments, cartilage, fascia, and bone. Connective tissue binds and supports, and it ranges in density from liquid (blood) to bone, the hardest tissue in the body. ***Muscles*** contract and relax, move joints, pump blood, and support vessels and hollow organs. ***Bone*** supports the body and give it shape and structure. ***Tendons*** connect and bind muscles to bones. ***Ligaments*** connect one bone to another. ***Cartilage*** is flexible tissue found on the articulating surfaces of joints. ***Fascia*** comprise thin fibrous sheets that enclose and separate muscles and organs like a stocking and winds continuously throughout the body.

The internal environment and health have a lot to do with the state of our muscles and bones. Pain, of course, is a chief concern and must always be addressed. But pain is a symptom, a sign that something is wrong. We must always find the cause of injury and promote healing. Along with providing antiinflammatory herbs and analgesia, herbalists heal from the inside out, because systemic factors play a huge role in chronic muscular-skeletal degenerative diseases. Rheumatoid arthritis, lupus, and fibromyalgia have autoimmune causes.

Diuretics, alteratives, digestive aids, liver restoratives, and stimulants are often key therapeutic herbal categories because of the systemic nature of chronic M-S problems. Fixing leaky gut and dysbiosis is paramount because they contribute to chronic inflammation. Circulation and elimination must be improved. Lifestyle, exercise, and hydration are factors, as are the manual therapies and structural analysis. The M-S system must be looked at holistically. As Chinese Medicine has always understood, we must treat the root along with the branch.

Pain, Inflammation, and Analgesia

Pain and its sidekick, inflammation, take first priority when treating muscular and skeletal injury. These symptoms are present in muscle strain; joint, back, knee, and neck pain; arthritis; and nerve compression in sciatica and repetitive stress injuries like carpel tunnel. Bodywork of all types help immensely—massage, myofascial release, reflexology, chiropractic and osteopathic adjustments. Internal and external herbals are important accompaniments.

Inflammation

Inflammation is a localized physical condition in which part of the body becomes reddened, swollen, hot, and painful, especially as a reaction to injury or infection. Back strains, shoulder pulls, and knee twists all become inflamed. This inflammation can happen externally to all types of M-S tissue: muscles (myositis), joints (arthritis), bursa (bursitis), fascia (fasciitis), and internally to bones (osteomyelitis). Inflammation is a defense mechanism that attempts to localize and eradicate the irritant and repair the surrounding tissue. Without inflammation, wounds would never heal.

We have discussed pathological, chronic internal inflammation (Chapter 16) as a contributor to many diseases, such as irritable bowel disease (IBD) and heart disease, but here we are concerned with M-S inflammation, sometimes acute, as from immediate injury from sprains and strains, and sometimes chronic, as with arthritis or persistent lower back pain. Acute injury treatment focuses on cooling off and bringing down this hot condition. Chronic injuries will need some warming up. In all cases, pain relief and antiinflammatory measures come first, although other important systemic measures are part of the herbal solution.

Pain, Inflammation, and External Applications

- *Inflammation signs and symptoms.* There is pain caused by inflammatory cytokines and neutrophils (white blood cells), pressure from swelling, and redness as the capillaries fill up with blood. There is heat because blood brings warmth. There is swelling because immune cells and fluids rush to the site.
- *RICE.* This is an acronym (***RICE***) for a first-aid protocol for sprains, strains, and trauma injury. ***R*** stands for rest. Give it a chance to heal and don't insist on running back to the gym. ***I*** stands for ice because it's a hot condition. Ice brings down pain and swelling. ***C*** stands for compression in the form of an Ace wrap or bandage to help squeeze fluid away from area. ***E*** stands for elevation. Raise injured extremities above heart level. Let gravity return fluids to circulation.
- *Chinese Medicine treatments.* In Chinese Medicine, blood and qi stagnation are prime reasons for pain. When qi and blood flow smoothly, pain is relieved. Acupuncture is a revered way to alleviate pain by freeing up the smooth flow of qi through the meridians. ***Moxibustion*** involves using a smoking stick of *Artemisia vulgaris* (Mugwort herb), called *moxa*, near the skin to warm the blood, stimulate circulation, and relieve stagnation. ***Cupping*** involves using glass cups placed on the skin under a vacuum, which sucks up the tissue, draws out toxins, and increases flow of qi and blood. Cupping is used on large surfaces, such as the back or thighs, and placed along meridians of the back. ***Tui na*** is a traditional form of Chinese massage combining massage, acupressure, and other forms of body manipulation.
- *External herbal treatments.* This method includes compresses and liniments. Make your own compress by soaking a cloth in hot herbal tea, wringing out it out, and applying to area. There are many prepared, over-the-counter (OTC) remedies out there, including adhesive bandages infused with Cayenne pepper, Ginger root, or Mustard seed. Chinese patent formulas can be convenient and helpful (Box 24.1).
- *Heat and cold.* Heat increases blood flow and flexibility, whereas cold tends to numb nerves and decrease swelling. The decision whether to use warmth or cold depends on the condition. Acute hot injuries like a just-sprained ankle need cooling, whereas cold long-term situations, such as chronic back or arthritic pain, feel better with warmth. Herbs and essential oils can easily be added to compresses or foot baths. Lavender, Peppermint, Clary Sage, Roman Chamomile, Juniper, and Eucalyptus essential oils all help muscle pain and inflammation.
- *Hydrotherapy.* The therapeutic use of water in various forms and temperatures is called ***hydrotherapy***. Saunas, steam baths, Native American sweat lodges, Russian banyas, therapy pools, whirlpools, hot tubs with their jets, hydrocollator packs (moist heat silica gel packs) are possibilities. All cultures have some type. Physical therapists and massage therapists routinely use hydrotherapies. Saunas are traditional to help fibromyalgia and muscle aches through detoxification and muscle relaxation. In general, wet heat penetrates tissues more deeply than dry heat does.

• BOX 24.1 External Chinese Patent Pain Remedies

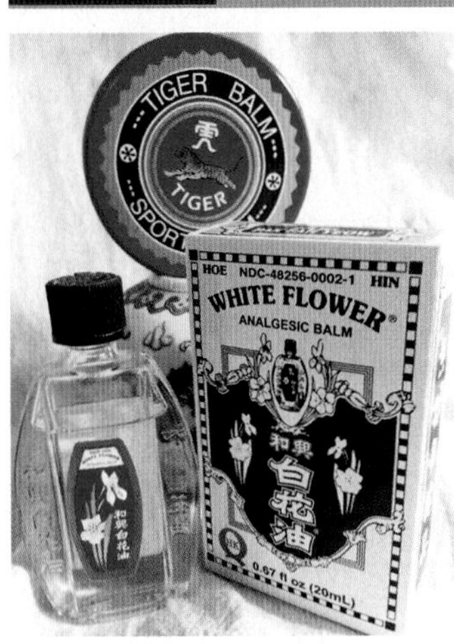

External Chinese patent remedies are often beautifully packaged. They relieve pain by moving blood and Liver qi.

Patent pain remedies are available at Chinese pharmacies, and some are now even sold in health food stores and regular supermarkets. They are very handy to use on clients or to suggest for purchase.

- **Kwan Loong oil**. An antiinflammatory blend. Main ingredients include the analgesic methyl salicylate (found in aspirin) and aromatic menthol from Peppermint herb, acting as a rubefacient or counterirritant. Provides a wonderful tingly feeling.
- **Tiger Balm**. Camphor and menthol, again rubefacients, give Tiger Balm a confusing hot-one-minute-and-cold-the-next effect to move qi and blood and relieve pain at least temporarily.
- **White Flower Analgesic Balm**. White Flower is another camphor-menthol and methyl salicylate balm and feels wonderful when rubbed on sore muscles; it also opens the airway and helps breathing when rubbed on the chest during a cold or flu.
- **Dit da Jow liniment**. This liniment was formulated as a first-aid treatment for the bangs and bruises from martial arts and provides relief from M-S trauma. Dit da Jow is pinyin meaning *hit liniment*. Many versions of this effective brew are available. Dit da Jow heals tissues and bruising and removes pain and inflammation by moving qi and blood and extinguishing wind. Dit da Jow formulas are warm, spicy, damp resolving, and exterior releasing (Box 24.4).

• BOX 24.2 Sports Massage Oil

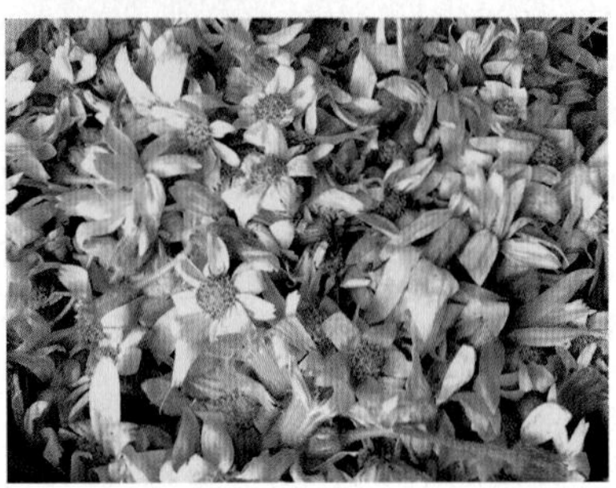

Arnica cordifolia (Heart-leaf arnica) flowers, wilted and drying. Arnica is an excellent herb to include in external remedies for many soft tissue injuries and bruises.

This blend is nice to have on hand for muscle aches and pains and for use as an alternative to NSAIDs. This preparation calls for the quick, accelerated version of making an herbal oil. Start with dry herbs, put them in a blender with an olive oil carrier, and afterward add a few drops of essential oils.

Ingredients

2 parts	St. John's Wort	Antiinflammatory, relieves nerve pain and swelling.
1 part	Hops flower	Relieves stress and pain.
1 part	Arnica flower or Comfrey root	Antiinflammatory, restorative.
1 part	White Oak bark	Blood circulation, moves qi.
1 part	Mullein leaf	Reduces swelling, relieves pain.
4 drops	Wintergreen or Peppermint essential oil	Relieves pain and inflammation.

Directions

Blend herbs by weight. Moisten with 95% alcohol. Let stand 20 minutes to 1 hour to break down cell walls. Put herbs in blender. Cover with olive oil. Blend on high until mixture becomes warm. Strain. Add essential oils. Rub onto sore muscles as needed.

Nonsteroidal Antiinflammatory Drugs

Nonsteroidal antiinflammatory drugs (NSAIDs), the most commonly used painkillers on the market, are the mainstays to treat M-S pain, but they are also riddled with nasty side effects. Many are available OTC without a prescription. Just walk into your corner drugstore and pick from countless products lining an entire aisle. They stop pain and inflammation by blocking cyclooxygenase (COX) enzymes, which in turn inhibit production of prostaglandins, part of the inflammatory cascade. They are also prescribed by doctors, just in higher doses.

NSAIDs include aspirin compounds, such as Bayer and Bufferin; ibuprofen compounds, such as Motrin and Advil; and naproxen sodium compounds, such as Aleve. NSAIDs are antiinflammatory, analgesic, and antipyretic (reduce fevers). NSAIDs are commonly used for back and muscle pain, injuries, dental pain, PMS, and all types of inflammation, including arthritis, tendonitis, and bursitis. Tylenol is *not* an NSAID; it comes from the compound acetaminophen that stops pain and lowers fever but does nothing for inflammation.

The problem with NSAIDs is that, yes, they help pain and inflammation temporarily, but chronic use causes high risk for gastrointestinal (GI) bleeds, ulcers, internal bleeding, heart disease, and kidney failure. Reye's syndrome has occurred in children as a result of being treated with aspirin. People pop NSAIDs like candy, but eventually it has a rebound effect and doesn't work as well as it did initially.[1] Taking more and more accomplishes less and less. Herbalists can do better by making their own healing oils and liniments (Box 24.2).

Cannabis and the Endocannabinoid System

It has long been claimed that *Cannabis* spp. (Marijuana bud) helps relieve pain (Fig. 24.1). The proof is now in. It happens via the ***endocannabinoid (ECB) system***, named after *Cannabis sativa*, the plant leading to its discovery. The ECB system is a biochemical signaling system that helps maintain normal cerebral and physiological functions.[2] This neurotransmitter system communicates between the central nervous system, the immune system, and connective tissue (including bones, muscles, fascia, and tendons), and it regulates pain, damage, and inflammation caused by injury. It also controls mood, appetite, and cellular life and death cycles. It does this via chemical neurotransmitters that are produced in the fat cells of all mammals.

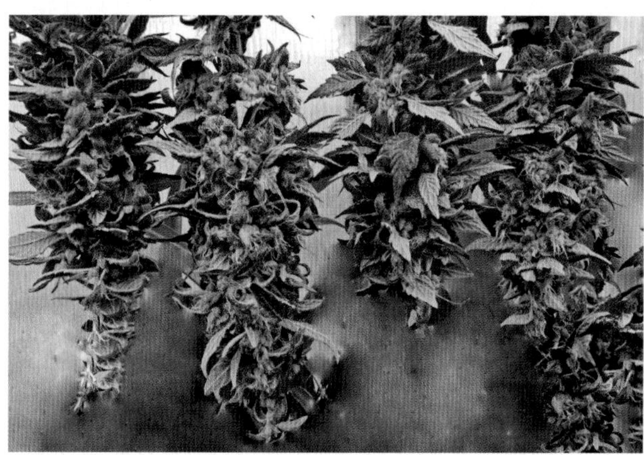

• **Fig. 24.1** *Cannabis* spp. buds hanging to dry.

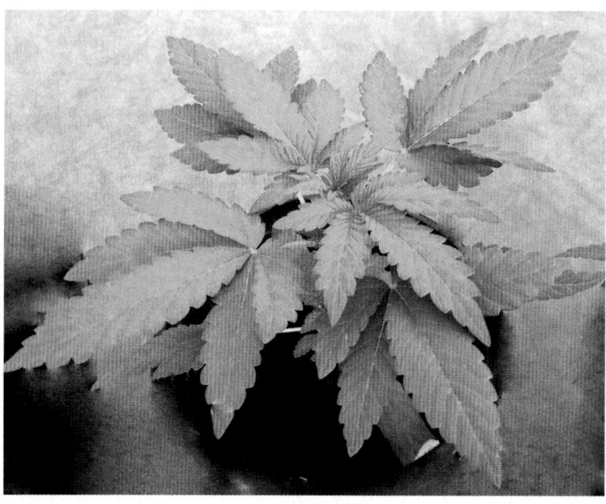

• **Fig. 24.2** Young *Cannabis* spp. plant showing its serrated compound leaves.

Endocannabinoids naturally produced in the body hook on to various nervous system receptor sites, such as CB1 and CB2, among others. In the case of pain, they send messages that act as a dimmer switch to prevent excessive nerve-firing by other neurotransmitters. The result is turned-down pain signals. Endocannabinoids prevent the release of proinflammatory substances (histamine, kinins, leukotrienes, prostaglandins) and are thus, antiinflammatory. Pain and damage caused by injury is minimized.[3]

This bridge between the body's organs and the nervous system, as seen in the ECB system, is a classic example of the mind-body connection. When a postsynaptic neuron is activated, cannabinoids released from the nerve cell travel backward, attaching to the cannabinoid receptors on the presynaptic neuron. The pain response is decreased by limiting the amount of neurotransmitter being released. Some research suggests that deficiencies in the ECB system are found in conditions associated with pain and inflammation in fibromyalgia, migraines, and irritable bowel disease. This deficiency could be helped or alleviated with medical cannabis[2] and other plants, because the ECB system controls inflammatory complications, energy balance, intestinal permeability, immunity, and development of obesity.

The first external substance discovered to supply ECB neurotransmitter chemicals was CBD (*cannabidiol*) in *Cannabis sativa*, hence the name *cannabinoid*. The CBD portion of cannabis is not psychoactive or intoxicating, but the THC (*tetrahydrocannabinol*) portion *is* psychoactive. Medically used cannabis is an extract that has varying ratios of CBD to THC. Cannabis plants (Fig. 24.2) can be cultivated or cloned to be high in one active ingredient or another. Improved strains that are specific for different conditions are constantly being developed. In fact, THC and CBD are a tiny fraction of 120 or so chemicals and alkaloids present in the herb. As we know, plant synergy has a lot to do with actions and safety.

Phytocannabinoids are plant substances that stimulate and attach to various cannabinoid receptor sites in humans (Fig. 24.3). *Theobroma cacao* (Dark Chocolate), *Echinacea* spp., *Humulus* spp. (Hops strobiles), *Helichrysum italicum* essential oil, *Piper nigrum* (Black Peppercorn), *Ruta graveolens* (Rue herb), and even broccoli are all phytocannabinoids. *Cannabis sativa* is obviously another. More phytocannabinoids are being identified. Peppercorns and helichrysum have historically been included in pain formulas. Now we know another reason why.

There are records of cannabis being used with great medicinal success 4000 years ago in Mesopotamia and in ancient India, Egypt, Persia, and China. Unlike opioids, cannabis is not physiologically addictive. The chief temporary side effects are dizziness, dry mouth, increased appetite, and drowsiness. Unfortunately, its legal status in the United States as of 2019 remains in limbo. Well into the 20th century, cannabis was included in the U.S. Pharmacopeia. It was removed from it in 1942. Presently in the United States, the federal

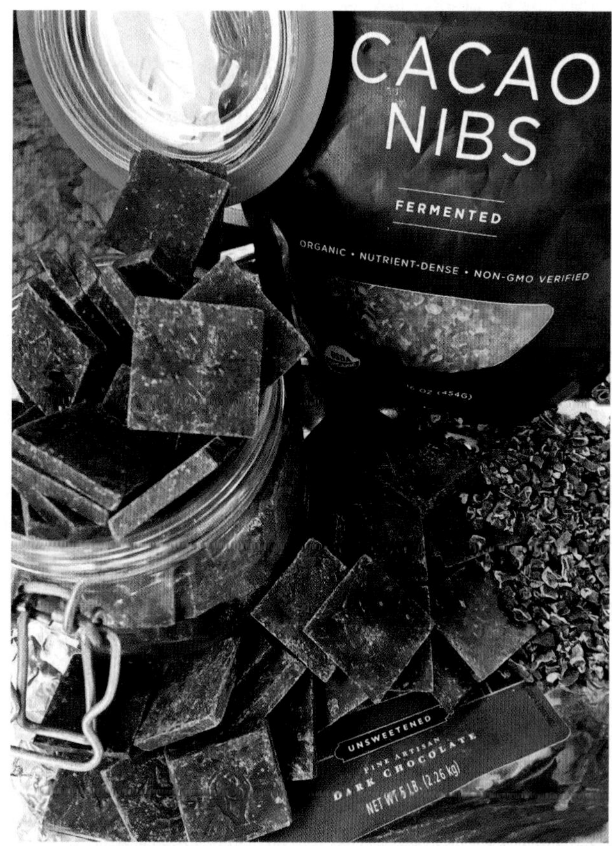

• **Fig. 24.3** *Theobroma cacao* (Dark Chocolate) in baking squares and fermented cacao nibs. Chocolate is a phytocannabinoid that attaches to cannabinoid receptor sites.

Drug Enforcement Administration (DEA) classifies it as a Schedule I controlled substance, meaning it has a "high potential for abuse and no currently accepted medical use."[2] This statement is untrue and merely a matter of political debate.

Hemp is the fiber of the cannabis plant that comes from the stem and is traditionally used to make rope, stout fabrics, fiberboard, and paper. It happens to be high in CBD and low in THC. The cannabis *bud*, on the other hand is higher in THC. Hemp is used as a source of CBD oil. Hemp's legal status as a cash crop in the United States is in flux, as is that of the bud.

Cannabis has been legalized in many states in both recreational and medical capacities and is now used for pain relief, in calming of muscle spasms, in treating asthma, for control of nausea and vomiting in chemotherapy, in cancer treatment, as a sleep aid, in posttraumatic stress disorder (PTSD), and for childhood and adult epilepsy, where antiseizure drugs have all but failed. There is hope for future federal legalization, and the only thing that can be depended on is change. Cannabis is another of our herbal allies. Stay tuned.

The Overrated Alkaline Diet pH Test

This diet is a regimen that has been embraced by herbalists and naturopaths since the 1920s and is frequently used in arthritis cures. The problem is that one of its goals is for the client to produce alkaline urine as proof it is working, which is a very hard thing to do. The diet is still popular today, so herbalists need to know of it. Urine pH kits and strips can be purchased at health food stores, so pH can be monitored.

An *alkaline diet* is a cleansing and detoxifying regimen that is rich in fresh fruits and vegetables and low in proteins and processed foods. Any diet that accomplishes this goal reduces inflammation and oxidative stress and will improve arthritis symptoms. So far, so good. The body is always making and eliminating acids in the form of acid metabolites and products of digestion. Arthritic joint problems are a classic outcome of a failure to do this.[4]

Alkaline foods are rich in calcium, potassium, and sodium. When they are digested, they leave an alkaline residue. Examples are fresh fruits and veggies of a rainbow-colored diet. Alkalinity cuts down on inflammation. Acid foods do the opposite. When acids are digested in the body, they leave an acidic residue. Acidic foods consist of coffee, tea, grains, processed foods, and proteins that are high in sulfur (meat, eggs, and cheese). An overly acidic diet contributes to inflammation, oxidative stress, leaky gut, and dysbiosis, all the factors leading to chronic inflammation and autoimmune diseases.[4]

The kidneys and lungs are responsible for maintaining acid-base (pH) balance and normally do an excellent job of keeping the urine slightly acid. Average urine pH is an acidic 6 (Seven is neutral and over seven is alkaline) (Chapter 26). One way to make urine a little less acid for a while is to eat prodigious amounts of fruits and vegetables. Consuming acidic foods (and other factors like dehydration, diarrhea, diabetes, and respiratory problems) will all swing the urine pH in the acid direction. When concentrating on detoxification, many practitioners and their clients become quite obsessive about creating alkaline urine by following an incredibly strict diet. They monitor urine with pH test strips in hope of moving the scale in an alkaline direction. This goal is exceedingly difficult to accomplish and could drive anyone nuts, creating unnecessary stress.

Clinical pearl: If acute arthritis with inadequate detoxification is a factor, a strict alkaline regime (without pH testing) can be healing for a limited time. A one- or two-day veggie juice fast wouldn't hurt, but when acute arthritis symptoms calm down and become chronic, it is far better to eat a well-balanced diet that includes moderate protein. Follow a Mediterranean or Paleo diet and all should be well.

Chinese Medicine Perspective: The Muscular-Skeletal System and Major Syndromes

General Principles

- *Pain.* Pain is caused by an obstruction of qi, blood, and/or wind penetrating muscles, ligaments, tendons, or another affected region. Most types of pain are caused by blood and qi stagnation. Energy needs to flow easily through the meridians and in the right direction. If qi becomes blocked, there is pain. The same goes for blood. If blood circulation is restricted or slowed down in a muscle or elsewhere, the person will feel pain. Therapeutic massage aims at increasing circulation for this reason. *Wind* denotes spasms and pain that move around. Spasms frequently accompany muscle pain; thus antispasmodics would be required.
- *Moving qi and blood for pain relief.* Any good pain formula must include herbs that move qi and blood. Qi and blood are closely related. Blood is said to be a denser form of qi, just moister or more yin.[5] Both need to be moved and circulated for pain relief. We move qi with Cinnamomum Gui Zhi (Cinnamon twig), White Willow bark, or Frankincense resin; we move blood with Ligusticum Chuan Xiong (Sichuan Lovage root), Black Cohosh root, or Red root. Most of these herbs move both qi and blood.
- *Bi syndromes.* Pronounced like bumble *bee*, ***Bi syndromes*** imply painful obstructions. *Obstruction* includes a group of M-S symptoms associated with pain, arthritis, trauma, swelling, spasms, stiffness, and decreased range of motion, and it sometimes affected by the weather. The syndromes involved are Wind Damp Heat and Wind Damp Cold. *Wind* is moving pain. *Damp* implies a dull heavy achy pain with swelling and numbness. The syndromes manifest as fixed or migrating pain, soreness, aches, and spasms; numbness or heaviness of muscles, tendons, and joints; swelling and burning pain; and lower back or knee pain.[6] These symptoms cover the gamut from hot to cold.
- *Herbs for Bi syndromes.* They are chosen based on the source and type of pain. The herbs must always dispel wind and damp. Other than that, choosing is based on whether the situation is hot or cold.
  - If there is heat and inflammation caused by prolonged stagnation, the herbs must clear heat with cooling botanicals, ranging from strong Gentiana Qin Jiao (Gentian root), Anemarrhena Zhi Mu (Know Mother root), classic Siegesbeckia Xi Xian Cao (Hairy Siegesbeckia herb), or Wild Yam root to mild Meadowsweet herb or Celery seed.
  - If the pain is caused by cold, we warm things up with warm, pungent arterial stimulants that increase circulation, such as Cinnamomum Gui Zhi (Cassia Cinnamon twig), Angelica Du Ho (Hairy Angelica root), Coix Ye Ye Ren (Job's Tears seed), Jamaican Sarsaparilla root, Prickly Ash bark, Juniper berry, or very hot and strong Cayenne pepper.
- *Liver and Kidney as related to muscular-skeletal tissue.* According to the correspondences, the Liver rules the ***sinews*** (tendons and ligaments), and the Kidneys rule the bone. If there is weakness or chronic problems with the tendons, ligaments, bones, legs, knees, or lower back, these organs are depleted.

Syndromes

- *Wind Damp Cold Bi.* The key words here are long-term chronic, referring to pain that is fixed, stiff, aggravated by damp and cold weather, and relieved by warmth. Examples are chronic arthritis and other muscular-skeletal pain, including tendonitis, bursitis, and carpel tunnel. Wind Damp Cold Bi needs pungent, warming qi and blood movers. **Pulse (P)** Wiry, tight or soggy. **Tongue (T)** Normal.
- *Wind Damp Heat Bi.* The key words here are acute onset, something like that of chronic gout, which can flare up and become acute. Symptoms include inflammation and acute arthritic joint or other pain that is burning, red, and swollen; involves decreased movement; and is warm to touch and relieved by cold. Conditions in this category include acute tendonitis and bursitis. Wind Damp Heat Bi needs cooling qi-moving and blood-moving herbs. **P** Rapid or slippery. **T** Body red with thin or thick yellow coat.
- *Liver and/or Kidney Depletion.* This syndrome involves pains in joints and muscles that are aggravated by overstrain or stress and alleviated by rest. Soreness and weakness in the knees and lower back, listlessness, and low-grade fever are typical. The fix is tonic herbs: Eucommia Du Zhong, Comfrey root, or Acanthopanax Wu Jia Pi. **P** Thin. **T** Body red or pink with scanty or thin, white coat.

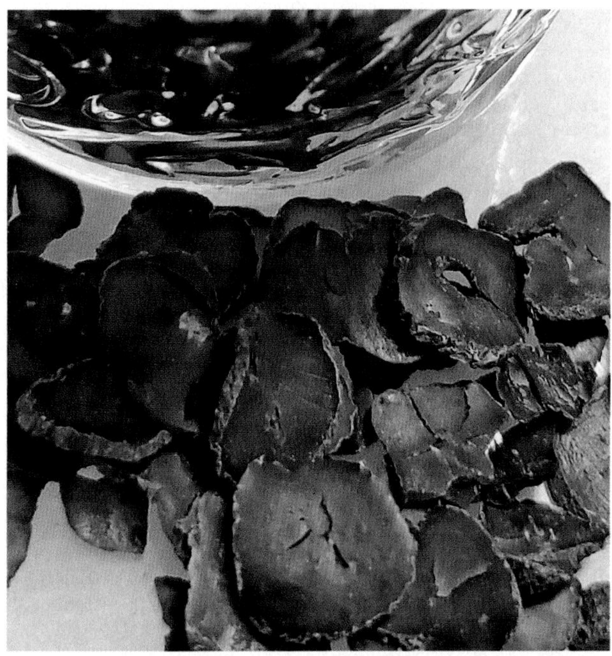

• **Fig. 24.4** Corydalis Zhi Hu Suo (vinegar prepared Asian Corydalis corm), an analgesic for pain anywhere in body, including the skeletal muscles.

Muscular-Skeletal Materia Medica

Main categories are muscular-sketetal restoratives, stimulants, relaxants, and/or sedatives. Additional sections have been included for analgesics, spasmolytics, and topical applications. These designations should facilitate success when searching for herbs to include in a formula. Within each main category are various subcategories that encompass Western descriptive terms.

- *Restoratives.* These are for weak deficiency conditions and include the Chinese syndrome Liver and Kidney Depletion. They are the tonics, the tissue builders.
- *Stimulants.* The warmer-uppers for chronic Wind Damp Cold Obstruction, including analgesics, antiinflammatories, and spasmolytics.
- *Relaxants and or sedatives.* The cooler-downers that relieve pain; analgesics, antiinflammatories, antispasmodics/spasmolytics (same thing), antipyretics for Wind Damp Heat Obstruction.

Muscular-Skeletal Herbs Worth Honorable Mention

- ***Piscidia erythrina*** (Jamaican Dogwood bark). *The* Western analgesic for pain, spasm, neuralgia, anxiety, and inflammation. It is pungent, astringent, calming, and relaxing to move qi and blood and relieve pain. Its relaxing, antispasmodic qualities make it great for uncontrolled coughing. Mix this with its Eastern equivalent, Corydalis Yan Hu Suo and include together in pain formulas.
- ***Corydalis turtschaninovii*** Yan Hu Suo (Asian Corydalis corm) (Fig. 24.4). A classic Chinese analgesic from the Poppy family, yet nontoxic and nonaddictive. Yan Hu Suo circulates qi and blood. It is used for general pain anytime, anywhere in the body, including muscles. It is a vasodilator, making it hypotensive. For chronic pain, combine with other herbs having a tropism to target area.[6]
- ***Siegesbeckia pubescens*** Xi Xian Cao (Hairy Siegesbeckia herb). A must-have multipurpose herb for any kind of muscle and nerve pain, hot or cold, acute or chronic. This includes Wind Damp Cold Bi and Wind Damp Heat Bi, and it is a first choice for arthritis. It is cool, bitter, and good for heat but also pungent and qi moving, making it effective for cold. It is analgesic, antiinflammatory, and restorative.[7] Additional virtues: it is vasodilating for hypertension and helps stress and tension. The fact that it contains salicylic acid doesn't hurt. Use with Jamaican Dogwood root bark.
- ***Stephania tetrandra*** Hun Fang Ji (Stephania root). A cold one, bitter cold, dry, and pungent. It is one of the best for hot, acute M-S pain, Wind Damp Heat Bi, acute arthritis, and fibromyalgia. It is spasmolytic, analgesic, antiinflammatory, and also diuretic, making it helpful for edema. It vasodilates in hypertension, especially combined with Ligusticum Chuan Xiong (Sichuan Lovage root) or Passionflower herb.
- ***Eucommia ulmoides*** Du Zhong (Eucommia bark). Sweet, warm, and dry restorative yang tonic. Very important M-S and connective tissue healer for Liver and Kidney depletion, bones, ligament, tendons, muscles, and osteoporosis. The silver white stretchy substance holding the bark together looks like connective tissue and contains a small amount of latex. Good quality Du Zhong is judged in China by how elastic this springy rubbery material is. This resemblance to human connective tissue corresponds nicely to the Doctrine of Signatures, as shown in Fig. 24.5. A very slight chance exists that those with multiple food allergies, chemical sensitivities, or a known latex allergy might have a bad reaction.[8] Eucommia Du Zhong is detoxifying and diuretic, needed actions in chronic connective tissue degeneration. Combine with fresh, young Horsetail herb, a nice Western equivalent.

Muscular-Skeletal Restoratives

M-S connective tissue restoratives and tonics tend to be warming and dry and contain alkaloids, glycosides, essential oils, and organic acids (Table 24.1).[7] They are indicated for cold, long-standing chronic M-S issues where the tissue has deteriorated over time. Restoratives are also used in acute trauma with tissue damage to sinews, muscle, or bone. Arthritis erodes and wears down cartilage in knees, shoulders, and hip joints, and intervertebral discs degenerate. ***Sprains*** are a stretching or tearing of a ligament. ***Strains*** are when muscles or their tendons are pulled or overstretched. Fractures are broken bones. All of these situations call for reparative restoratives. The Chinese refer to problems of worn-out and damaged tissue as Liver and Kidney depletion, because Liver rules the sinews and Kidney rules the bones.

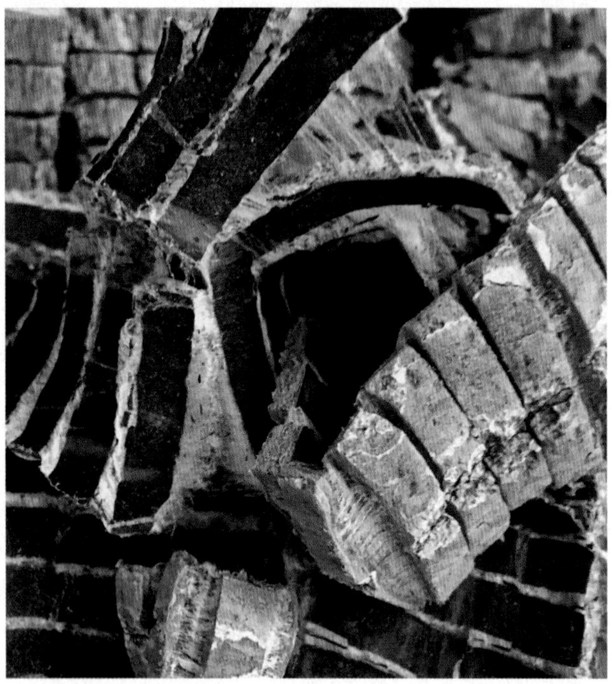

• **Fig. 24.5** Stretchy Eucommia Du Zhong (Eucommia bark) is a connective tissue restorative for acute and chronic muscle, tendon, ligament, and bone injury and degeneration.

Many restorative herbs double as detoxicants. This dual action is convenient because detoxification is an important therapeutic principle in tissue repair when toxins have formed because of the inflammatory process caused by lactic acid buildup that happens in muscle overuse, in tissue breakdown, or from underlying metabolic toxicosis. Many restoratives happen to have a diuretic and alterative action also. Alteratives help the body eliminate waste, and diuretics are needed to flush out those wastes through the kidneys. It's always lovely and elegant to use one herb for multiple purposes.

Warming Arterial Stimulants

These are the ones for cold, chronic situations, Wind Damp Cold Obstruction (Table 24.2). They are warm, bitter, and pungent. Some are diaphoretic, relieve external wind, and are often used in respiratory infections. These qualities also make them analgesic, antiinflammatory, muscle relaxing, and/or spasmolytic.[7] Arterial stimulation is needed to move qi and blood, increase circulation and warm up the area, and thereby relieve chronic muscle pain, radiating nerve pain (***neuralgia***), and bruising (***contusions***). Bruises form when blunt force causes capillaries under the skin to tear and bleed, leaving a discoloration under the skin.

TABLE 24.1 Connective Tissue Restoratives and Tonics

Herb	Notes
Eucommia ulmoides Du Zhong Eucommia bark	For Wind Damp Cold Bi. Classic restorative, detoxicant, and diuretic.
Eleutherococcus senticosus Ci Wu Jia Eleuthero root, Siberian Ginseng	For Wind Damp Cold Bi. Restorative and detoxicant. Adaptogen.
Equisetum arvense Horsetail herb	For Wind Damp Cold Bi. Restorative and detoxicant.
Symphytum officinalis Comfrey root	For Wind Damp Cold Bi. Bone restorative and detoxicant.
Urtica dioica Nettle herb	For Wind Damp Cold Bi. Restorative and detoxicant. Vitamin and mineral dense.
Juglans regia Walnut hull and leaf	For liver and kidney deficiency with lower back, knee, or leg weakness. Builds bone; rich in minerals for osteoporosis. Also, a skin detoxicant for parasites.
Vaccinium myrtillus Bilberry berry	For connective tissue with toxicosis.
Taraxacum officinalis Dandelion root	Heat clearing detoxicant and diuretic. For Liver and Kidney deficiency.
Serenoa serrulata Saw Palmetto berry	Specific for restoring striated muscle tissue, builds bulk. Also has male reproductive tropism to shrink prostate.

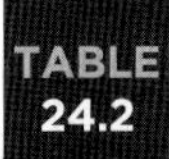

Warm Arterial Stimulants for Chronic Conditions
(Moves qi and blood. For Wind Damp Cold Bi. These are antiinflammatories, circulatory stimulants, and analgesics for nerve pain)

Herb	Notes
Zanthoxylum americanum Prickly Ash bark	Number one Western herb for Wind Damp Cold Bi. Tingly, bitter, salty, diaphoretic, moves blood. Helps neuralgia.
Angelica pubescens Du Ho Hairy Angelica root	For Wind Damp Cold Bi, circulatory stimulant, and spasmolytic. Helps nerve pain.
Cinnamomum cassia Gui Zhi Cinnamon twig	For Wind Damp Cold Bi, warming, spasmolytic, arterial stimulant that moves qi and blood. Helps nerve pain.
Caulophyllum thalictroides Blue Cohosh root	For Wind Damp Cold Bi. Detoxifying diuretic, specific to fingers and toes. Helps nerve pain. Also, a uterine stimulant and brings on labor.
Ledebouriella divaricata Fang Feng Wind Protector root	For Wind Damp Cold Bi. Warming stimulant, antiinflammatory, analgesic, and spasmolytic. Wind protecting refers to the wind of rheumatic pain and the external wind of influenza.[7]
Smilax officinalis Jamaican Sarsaparilla root	For Wind Damp Cold Bi. Pungent, circulates qi and blood. Steroidal saponin content makes it antiinflammatory. Also detoxifies skin, specific for psoriasis. Helps nerve pain.
Dioscorea villosa Wild Yam root	For Wind Damp Cold Bi with skin outbreaks. Antispasmodic. Helps nerve pain.
Zingiber officinalis Gan Jiang Dried Ginger root	Peripheral circulatory stimulant, qi and blood mover. For muscle aches and pains, regardless of origin, and helps nerve pain.
Ligusticum wallichii Chuan Xiong Sichuan Lovage root	Moves qi and blood. Vasodilator, and arterial stimulant.
Siegesbeckia pubescens Xi Xian Cao Hairy Siegesbeckia herb	For any kind of muscle and nerve pain, hot or cold, acute or chronic. Important arthritic herb.
Juniperus communis Juniper berry	For Wind Damp Cold Bi, diuretic, and detoxicant. For nerve, muscle, and joint pain.
Capsicum annuum Cayenne pepper	Hot arterial stimulant for Wind Damp Cold Bi. Use in small amounts in ointments, liniments as a counterirritant.

Indications for blood-moving arterial stimulants are limited range of motion; painful joints and muscles; bruising; and chronic versions of rheumatoid arthritis, osteoarthritis, tendonitis, bursitis, torticollis (stiff neck), and carpal tunnel syndrome (*myalgia*, muscle pain, in this case caused by nerve compression).

Herbs appropriate to use as warming arterial stimulants include Ledebouriella Fang Feng (Wind Protector root), Cassia Gui Zhi (Cinnamon twig), Juniper berry, and Prickly Ash bark. In the Western tradition, warming arterial stimulants appear in descriptive categories such as antiarthritics or muscle relaxants, useful in cold M-S ailments.

Relaxants

The relaxants and/or sedatives are frequently cooling herbs that treat acute, hot painful, inflammatory conditions (Table 24.3). Acute situations include flare-ups of rheumatoid or osteoarthritis, gout, tendinitis, bursitis, osteomyelitis, and lupus. The Chinese syndrome is Wind Damp Heat Obstruction/Bi. Energetically, M-S relaxers are bitter, pungent, and cool.

In Western descriptive terms, relaxants fall into various categories. Just about all of them are *analgesic* and *antiinflammatory*, such as Jamaican Dogwood root bark, Wild Yam root, and Celery seed. Some are quite cold *antipyretics*, like Wormwood herb, or Gentiana Qin Jiao (Gentian root). Others are *antispasmodics*, such as Valerian root and Black Cohosh root. Most of these herbs fall into many of these relaxant or sedative categories. For this reason, it is just as easy to call them all relaxants.

Analgesics

Analgesics relieve the symptom of pain (Table 24.4). The only way to truly relieve pain (and not just mask it) is to fix the underlying problem. However, all self-respecting herbalists should have a good internal formula (Box 24.3) and external pain remedy (Box 24.4) ready to recommend. Some analgesics are warm, and some are cold. Select appropriately. Some herbs, like Celery seed, have an alterative and diuretic action that creates analgesia by eliminating excess fluids that cause painful swelling, tissue compression, and edema. *Boswellia serrata* (Frankincense resin) is particularly

TABLE 24.3 Relaxants for Acute Conditions
(Cold, bitter, and pungent for Wind Damp Heat Bi)

Herb	Notes
Actaea racemosa Black Cohosh root	Important for Wind Damp Heat Bi, analgesic, antiinflammatory, and spasmolytic. For any type of muscle tension or nerve pain, especially with heat.
Siegesbeckia pubescens Xi Xian Cao Hairy Siegesbeckia herb	Versatile for hot or cold pain, antiinflammatory. For neuralgia and muscle tension.
Apium graveolens Celery seed	Cooling, antiinflammatory diuretic for edema, and detoxicant. Include in formulas for Wind Damp Heat Bi, Liver and Kidney depletion.
Bupleurum chinense Chai Hu Asian Buplever root	For any pain, spasms anywhere. Cool, bitter, very dry. Antiinfective, restores liver. Moves qi.
Harpagophytum procumbens Devil's Claw root	Bitter, cold analgesic. Best for heat, fibromyalgia, and myalgia. Alterative detoxicant.
Uncaria tomentosa Cats Claw root bark	For Wind Damp Heat Bi, antiinflammatory. For arthritis, fibromyalgia, joint pain, and leaky gut.
Filipendula ulmaria Meadowsweet herb, Queen of the Meadow	For Wind Damp Heat Bi, analgesic, neuralgic, antiinflammatory. Also, restores connective tissue and balances gut flora. A salicylate.
Stephania tetrandra Han Fang Ji Stephania root	Classic for heat. Striated muscle relaxant.
Yucca spp. Yucca root	Contains saponins. Antiinflammatory.

indicated to relieve pain and inflammation, whereas another species, *B. carterii* Ru Xiang, is an important Chinese Medicine wound healer/vulnerary/antihemorrhagic used in first-aid formulas and for analgesia in rheumatic pain or Wind Damp Obstruction.[7]

When dosing symptomatically for acute pain, the only way to get results with the nonaddictive mild- to medium-strength herbs used in this text is to employ frequent ***pulse dosing*** at 3 to 5 mL every ½ to 1 hour (Appendix A). An acute pain formula might contain an analgesic or two for the chief herb, an antiinflammatory, a vulnerary, a spasmolytic, and herbs to move qi and blood. Dit da Jow liniment (Box 24.4) is a good example. Pulse dosing does not apply to prevention formulas or to those meant to build and strengthen connective tissue. which would be given on a schedule of 3 times per day.

Salicylates are a group of phenols contained naturally in some plants (Chapter 8). These compounds include salicin (which does not demonstrate the antiplatelet effect seen with aspirin), methyl salicylate, and salicylic acid. Salicylate-rich herbs have been used with good results for pain and inflammation, particularly in arthritis.

The plants contain varying amounts of salicylates, are slower acting than aspirin, but work for mild to moderate pain. Salicylate botanicals include the inner barks of many trees, such as White Willow, Cottonwood, Birch, Aspen, Black Haw, and Cramp bark (these last two are typically used for menstrual cramps).[9] Others are Wintergreen, Pipsissewa, Meadowsweet herb (Figs. 24.6 and 24.7), and Poplar leaf buds (Balm of Gilead). All are antiinflammatory, analgesic, antipyretic, and antiseptic.

The active chemical in aspirin is acetylsalicylic acid (ASA). This chemical has an extra acetyl group that gives it blood-thinning properties.[10] Aspirin famously irritates the stomach and can cause bleeding ulcers because of this antiplatelet activity. Fortunately for the herbalist, salicylate-containing plants differ chemically and do not have this acetyl group, so they do not have this danger. Enteric-coated aspirin is used therapeutically by cardiologists as a preventative blood thinner. It is coated to prevent it dissolving in the stomach, which allows it to bypass intact to the small intestine and prevent gastric irritation.

Phytosterols, meaning plant ***sterols*** (Chapter 8), are antiinflammatory saponins, a group of chemicals occurring naturally in some botanicals. Phytosterols have various actions. In the muscular-skeletal realm, phytosterols act as saponin *steroids* that bring down inflammation. (Steroids are used in Western medicine for their antiinflammatory actions.) Some important antiinflammatory phytosterols used for the Bi syndromes of arthritis are Wild Yam root, Bupleurum Chai Hu (Asian Buplever root), and Jamaican Sarsaparilla root.[10]

Other plant sterols, such as Saw Palmetto berry and Pygeum bark, contribute to sexual and hormonal balance. Some act as adaptogens, such as the ginsengs and Licorice root. Some lower cholesterol, and Horse chestnut seed and Rehmannia Shu Di Huang (prepared Rehmannia root) are useful sterol-containing adrenal tonics and antiinflammatories used for autoimmune diseases.

Spasmolytics

One way to remove pain is to ease muscle spasms using spasmolytic herbs (Table 24.5). A muscle ***spasm*** is an abnormal, involuntary contraction of a skeletal muscle that can cause a great deal of pain. There are three types of muscle tissue: striated, smooth, and cardiac. *Striated* muscles are the skeletal muscles under voluntary control. *Smooth* muscles are involuntary and outside of conscious control (except with conscious practice), and they reside inside

TABLE 24.4 Analgesics
(Many are important antiinflammatories)

Herb	Notes
Corydalis turtschaninovii Yan Hu Suo (Corydalis corm)	Number one general Eastern analgesic for hot or cold conditions.
Piscidia erythrina (Jamaican Dogwood bark)	Number one general Western analgesic for pain, spasm, neuralgia, anxiety, inflammation.
Siegesbeckia pubescens Xi Xian Cao (Hairy Siegesbeckia herb)	For pain and any type of arthritis, hot or cold.
Salix alba (White Willow bark)	Salicylic acid content. For general pain including neuralgia, and antiinflammatory.
Boswellia serrata (Frankincense resin)	Classic resin. This species is a warming analgesic, antiinflammatory, spasmolytic, and slightly hemostatic.
Commiphora myrrha Mo Yao (Myrrh resin)	Classic resin. Warming, analgesic, moves qi and blood. For pain, swelling in wound care. Hemostatic.
Stephania tetrandra Han Fang Ji (Stephania root)	Bitter, cold, analgesic, skeletal and smooth muscle relaxant, and diuretic. For Wind Damp Heat Bi.
Essential oils Birch Wintergreen	Use topically. Salicylic acid content. For muscle pain.
Antiinflammatory triad *Zingiber officinale* (Ginger root)	Ginger, a circulatory stimulant, qi mover.
Curcuma longa (Turmeric root)	Turmeric, for pain, swelling, inflammation, and vulnerary.
Boswellia serrata (Frankincense resin)	Frankincense, for pain and inflammation.
Qi and blood movers *Zanthoxylum americanum* (Prickly Ash bark) *Ligusticum wallichii* Chuan Xiong (Sichuan Lovage root) *Boswellia serrata* and *B. carterii* Ru Xiang (Frankincense resin) *Commiphora myrrha* Mo Yao (Myrrh resin) *Pseudoginseng notoginseng* San Qi (Pseudoginseng root) *Citrus reticulata* Chen Pi and Qing Pi (Green and Ripe Tangerine peel) *Bupleurum chinense* Chai Hu (Asian Buplever root) *Angelica sinensis* Dang Qui (Dong Quai root)	
Salicylate-containing herbs *Salix alba* (White Willow bark) *Betula* spp. (Birch bark) *Populus* spp. (Aspen and Cottonwood bark) Poplar leaf bud (Balm-of-Gilead) topical *Filipendula ulmaria* (Meadowsweet herb) *Viburnum* spp. (Black Haw and Cramp bark) *Siegesbeckia pubescens* Xi Xian Cao (Hairy Siegesbeckia herb) *Chimaphila umbellata or Pyrola umbellate* (Pipsissewa or Wintergreen herb and root)	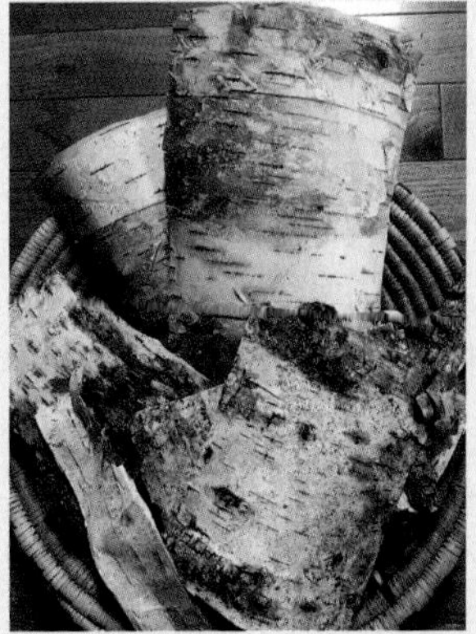 Beautiful *Betula alba* and spp. (Birch bark) reduces pain due to its antiinflammatory and antipyretic action. Its salicylic acid content makes it useful for joint inflammation/pain and fever.

(Continued)

TABLE 24.4 Analgesics (Many are important antiinflammatories)—cont'd

Herb	Notes
Phytosterol antiinflammatories	
Aesculus hippocastanum (Horse chestnut seed)	For inflammation with swelling.
Smilax spp. (Jamaican Sarsaparilla root)	Chronic arthritis.
Rehmannia Shu Di Huang (Prepared Rehmannia root)	Adrenal tonic and antiinflammatory in autoimmune diseases, rheumatoid arthritis.
Dioscorea villosa (Wild Yam root)	Antispasmodic, antiinflammatory.
Actaea racemosa (Black Cohosh root)	Small joint osteoarthritis
Chimaphila umbellata or *Pyrola umbellata* (Pipsissewa or Wintergreen herb and root, Rheumatism weed)	Saponin antiinflammatory, diuretic, detoxicant, vulnerary, salicylate.

• BOX 24.3 Frankincense and Myrrh Pain Balls

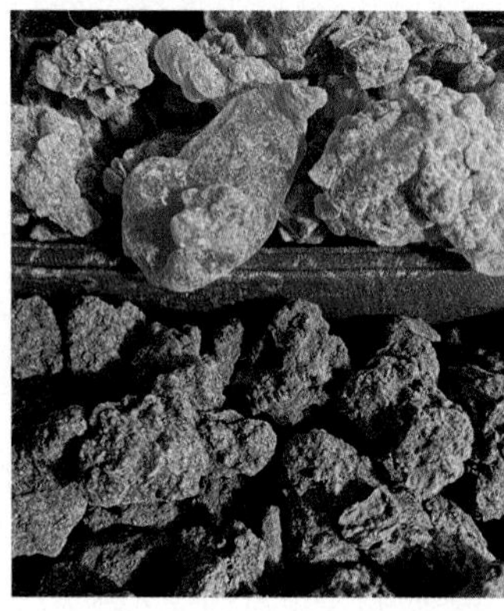

Boswellia serrata (Frankincense resin, top) and Commiphora Mo Yao (Myrrh resin, bottom) are prized for analgesia and wound healing.

Most types of pain are caused by qi and blood stagnation, so remedies involve herbs that move qi and blood. There are countless excellent internal and external pain combinations in the literature. These balls are an example, best used for chronic pain. Frankincense and Myrrh resins are pain-relieving classics.

Pain Balls

Ingredients

- *Boswellia serrata* (Frankincense resin). Analgesic, antiinflammatory, hemostatic.
- Commiphora Mo Yao (Myrrh resin). Analgesic, anticontusion.
- Corydalis Yan Hu Suo (Asian Corydalis corm). Warming, analgesic, nervous sedative.
- Angelica Dang Gui (Dong Quai root). Warming, analgesic, antiinflammatory.
- Ligusticum Chuan Xiong. (Sichuan Lovage root). Analgesic and sedative.

Directions. Grind equal parts of these herbs. Mix with warm honey and roll them into little balls (that contain 6–9 g of the mixture).
Dose. Take 1 pill 2 × day with a little water.

organs and blood vessel linings. *Cardiac* muscle is specialized involuntary heart muscle with its own conduction system and has a different set of relaxing herbals (Chapter 22).

Most spasmolytics (antispasmodics or muscle relaxants) affect both smooth and striated muscles. However, they may have tropisms to a specific area. For instance, Wild Yam root is often indicated in menstrual cramps/spasm of the smooth muscle of the uterus, but it will work for skeletal problems. Black Cohosh root works well for either. Lobelia herb is specific for relieving bronchial asthma, but there is no protocol against using it for a back spasm. It is probably best to select an herb that is traditionally used for the area intended.

Topical Applications—Rubefacients

Rubefacients (sometimes known as counterirritants) are hot, pungent herbs used topically in compresses, baths, liniments, and creams (Table 24.6). They increase blood flow to the skin and relieve congestion, pain, and irritation. Use in sprains, strains, muscle aches, and pains caused by overdoing it, the weekend warrior syndrome. They make wonderful topical remedies, feel fabulous, and are easy for herbalists to concoct. Those that come in essential oil form, such as Peppermint, Wintergreen, and Camphor, are usually applied with a carrier oil or a few drops added neat to liniments.

Rubefacients range from warming to very hot. Hot ones such as Mustard seed or Cayenne pepper can redden, blister, and irritate the skin, so care is needed with people who are sensitive to such substances. Capsicum, the pungent chemical in Cayenne pepper, stimulates and then blocks transmission of the pain neurotransmitter, substance P.[11] Ginger root and Cinnamon bark are medium heat. Some rubefacients are cooler and contain menthol, like Mint or Wintergreen essential oils. Menthols have an alternating heating and cooling effect on the skin, moving qi and blood. Camphor is a resin derived from the wood of *Cinnamomum camphora* (Camphor tree). OTC Bengay ointment contains camphor and menthol, as does Chinese Tiger Balm.

Rubefacients are contraindicated in people with delicate skin, babies, young children, and elders, and on damaged or open skin. Use caution in clients with very fair complexions and red hair, and people with sensitivity to heat. If using in essential oil form, mix with a carrier oil. In general, rubefacients bring blood to the skin surface and relieve pain.

Common Muscular-Skeletal Conditions

Soft-Tissue Damage: Sprains and Strains

- *Definition*. A ***sprain*** is a stretching or tearing of a ligament that may be complete or partial (Case History 24.1).

• BOX 24.4 Dit Da Jow Liniment

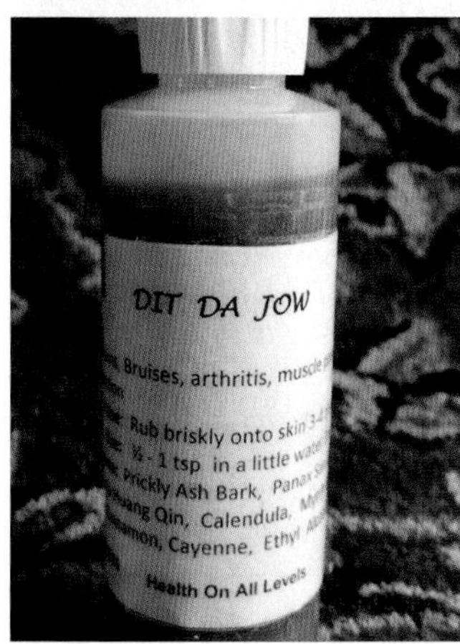

This particular Dit Da Jow liniment uses a combination of Western and Chinese herbs.

Dit Da Jow, Hit Liniment

There are numerous versions of Chinese hit liniments out there, called "hit" because they are traditionally used in martial arts training to ease the many strains, sprains, bangs, and bruises that so often occur. Many of these blends are secret and remain so in their martial arts lineages. This blend is public and does all the right things. It moves qi and blood, is analgesic, antiinflammatory, and antimicrobial; it also repairs tissue and resolves bruises. Ideal for the acute traumas of everyday life.

Ingredients. Equal parts 1:8 40%

Use 95% Ethyl alcohol. (1:8 40%) Ingestible alcohol allows liniment to be taken internally and rubbed on externally.

Panax notoginseng San Qi Pseudoginseng root	Analgesic, vulnerary, anticontusion, anticoagulant.
Hyssopus officinalis (Hyssop herb)	Antiseptic and astringent. Repairs tissue.
Cinnamomum cassia Rou Gui Cinnamon bark	Moves qi and blood, analgesic.
Commiphora myrrha Mo Yao Myrrh resin	Vulnerary, antimicrobial, moves qi and blood.
Calendula officinalis (Marigold flower)	Vulnerary, antiinfective, detoxicant.
Capsicum annuum (Cayenne pepper)	Arterial stimulant, moves qi and blood, vulnerary.
Zanthoxylum americanum Prickly Ash bark	Warm arterial stimulant, neuromuscular pain.
Scutellaria baicalensis Huang Qin Baikal Skullcap root	Broad-spectrum cold antibacterial.

Directions. For sprains, strains, bruises, arthritis, muscle pain, and inflammation.

External use. Not for open sores. Rub briskly onto affected part 3 to 4 × daily—or every ½–1 hour as needed for acute pain. If a joint is injured, apply liniment entirely around it, not just where it hurts.

Internal use. ½–1 tsp in a little water 3 × daily. Or pulse dose, 3–5 mL every ½–1 hour, only for a few hours, as needed for acute pain.

Sprained ankles are some of the most common sports or recreational injuries in the United States. Knees are second and wrists are third. Sprains occur from trauma, falls, slips, twists, sudden blows, overexertion, and sports injuries. They are graded in severity from a little pull to a full tear requiring surgical repair.

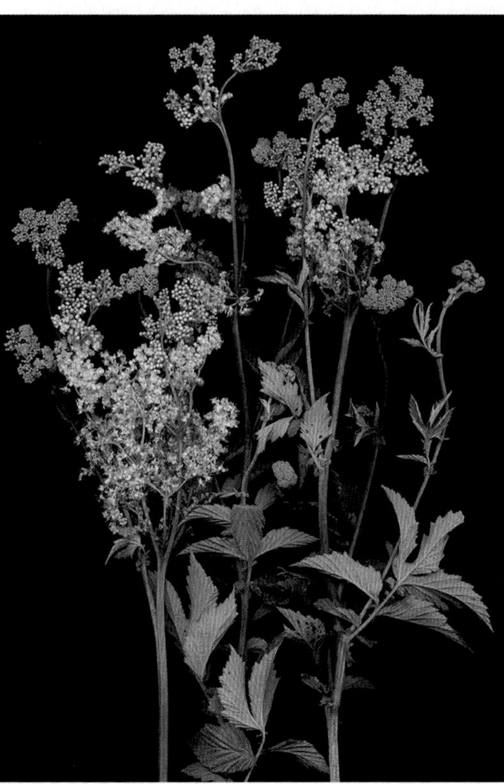

• **Fig. 24.6** *Filipendula ulmaria* (Meadowsweet herb), a salicylate-containing herb that works like aspirin, decreases inflammation and pain but without the drug's side effects. (Photographs loaned with permission from **THE BOTANICAL SERIES** are copywritten by Jennifer Anne Tucker and Gerald Lang from the Studio at Hill Crystal Farm. http://www.jennifer-tucker.com)

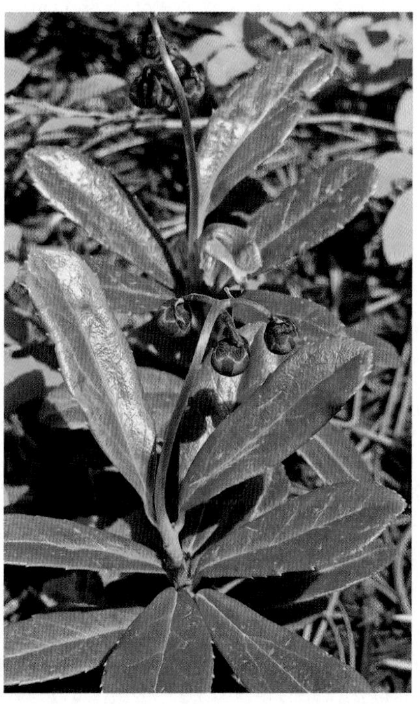

• **Fig. 24.7** *Chimaphila umbellata* (Wintergreen, Pipsissewa, Prince's Pine herb) contains salicylates and saponins, and is antiinflammatory, diuretic, detoxicant, and vulnerary.

TABLE 24.5 Spasmolytics
(Includes herbs for skeletal and smooth muscle; A star * means one of the big three)

Herbs	Notes
*Piscidia erythrina** Jamaican Dogwood bark	One of the big three. For skeletal and smooth muscle.
*Bupleurum chinensis** Chai Hu Bupleurum	One of the big three. Cooling, spasmolytic, antiinflammatory, clears heat. For skeletal and smooth. Also, a Liver restorative and sedative.
*Stephania tetrandra** Han Fang Ji Stephania root	One of the big three. Cold, bitter, antiinflammatory, analgesic, draining diuretic, and hypotensive. Excellent for striated and smooth. For Wind Damp Heat Bi.
Ledebouriella divaricata Fang Feng Wind Protector root	Warm, sweet and moist for Wind Damp Cold Bi. Fang Feng treats the wind of rheumatic pain and the wind of influenza onset.
Actaea racemosa Black Cohosh root	Skeletal and smooth.
Humulus lupulus Hops flower	Skeletal and smooth.
Matricaria recutita Chamomile flower	Skeletal and smooth.
Lobelia inflata Lobelia herb	Skeletal and smooth, particularly respiratory for asthma.
Valerian officinalis Valerian root	Skeletal.

TABLE 24.6 Rubefacients
(External applications)

Herb	Notes
Capsicum annuum Cayenne pepper	Very hot, pungent and aromatic. A little goes a long way. For Wind Damp Cold Bi, sprains, strains, bruises, and sore muscles.
Zingiber officinale Ginger root	Very pungent, hot, and dry. Add a little in a liniment.
Cochlearia armoracia Horseradish root	Very pungent and hot. For painful Wind Damp Cold Bi, arthritis, and insect stings. One whiff opens the airway.
Brassica spp. Mustard seed	Very hot. Go easy on Mustard. Can burn skin.
Mentha x *piperita* Peppermint essential oil	Spasmolytic, antiinflammatory. Menthol content makes it warming and then cooling.
Rosmarinus officinalis Rosemary essential oil	Pungent, warm, and dry.
Gaultheria procumbens Wintergreen herb from eastern United States *Chimaphila umbellata* Pipsissewa, Wintergreen herb, root, and essential oil	Cold and dry. Both plants contain analgesic salicylic acid and have identical uses. The creeping evergreen groundcover *Gaultheria procumbens* grows in the northeastern Americas and *Chimaphila umbellata* is a tiny evergreen plant that grows throughout the cool temperate northern hemisphere.
Cinnamomum camphora Camphor resin and essential oil	Warm and then cooling, analgesic, and antiinflammatory. Partners with menthol in Tiger Balm.

CASE HISTORY 24.1

Case History for Sprain

S. Jerry came down hard on his right lateral ankle while playing basketball. The ankle is red, swollen, painful, bruised, and hard to move. He limped off the court. There was no deformity or appearance of bones sticking out. Coach sent him to hospital emergency room (ER). X-ray showed no fracture.
O. **P** Rapid. **T** Red. Appears red, swollen, and bruised.
A. Wind Damp Heat, qi and blood stasis. Sprained ankle.
P. *Specific therapeutic principles*. (1) RICE. (2) Analgesics. (3) Antiinflammatories. (4) Relaxing nervine for stress. (5) Diuretic for swelling. (6) M-S restorative.

Sample Formula and Dose.
Pulse dose 5 mL every ½–1 hour. Taper down as indicated.

Parts	Herbs	Rationale
3	Panax San Qi	Edema, bruising; antiinflammatory, analgesic, moves qi and blood.
3	Jamaican Dogwood bark	Analgesic, blood mover.
3	Eucommia Du Zhong	Heals ligament; restorative and diuretic.
3	Valerian root	Calming, analgesic.

Other Suggestions

Red Flags. If in doubt, send client to an ER to rule out fractures with x-ray. Ascertain amount of ligament tearing shown on MRI. Signs of fracture: inability to bear weight, take any steps, or move area at all; area looks crooked or has lumps. Other red flags are numbness (nerve damage), red streaks (sepsis), or repeated injury of same place.

- RICE. For first 24–48 hours. This is basic first aid, be it herbal or allopathic. Use Dit Da Jow liniment in between ice applications (Box 24.4).
- Exercise: perform range of motion as tolerated.
- After acute period, follow-up with herbal formula aimed more at restoratives.

- *Definition*. A ***strain*** is a torn muscle or tendon that may be partial or complete. If it is partial, it will heal on its own, given enough rest. If the tendon is completely detached, it requires suturing. Strains are caused from repetitive motion or overuse of a muscle. Common sites of strains are the back and hamstrings.
- *Signs and symptoms*.
  - *Sprains*. Pain, swelling, bruising, and varying degrees of loss of motion.
  - *Strains*. Swelling, cramping, inflammation, and some loss of muscle function and weakness, which are signs of heat and inflammation but affect different body parts.
- *Allopathic treatment*. Not very different for sprains and strains. RICE (rest, ice, compression, and elevation). Gradual increase of exercise; physical therapy; NSAIDs. Surgical repair of tendon or ligament if needed. Sprains can take from 3 weeks to a year to heal.
- *General therapeutic principles*. (1) RICE first 24 to 48 hours and Dit da Jow liniment. (2) Analgesics. (3) Antiinflammatories. (4) Diuretics. (5) Restoratives. (6) Nerve relaxant for stress.

Osteoporosis and Fracture

- *Definition*. ***Osteoporosis*** means porous bone, where calcium is lost more quickly than it is replaced (Case History 24.2).

CASE HISTORY 24.2

Case History for Osteoporosis and Fracture

S. Jody is 65, postmenopausal. She fell and broke her wrist last year, and now she slipped off a curb and fractured her hip, requiring a hip replacement. She does not want to go on Fosamax. She has not had a period in 10 years, her skin is dry, and she still gets hot flashes and is quite nervous.
O. **P** Thready. **T** Red with thin coat.
A. Kidney Yin Deficiency (Chapter 28). Liver and Kidney depletion. Osteoporosis per bone density test. Hip fracture.
P. *Specific therapeutic principles*. In Chinese Medicine, the Kidneys rule the bones. The woman is postmenopausal and shows signs of heat (dry skin, hot flashes, red tongue). (1) Strengthen Kidney yin with demulcents for dryness. (2) Repair and build bone tissue with restoratives and mineral-rich herbs. Comfrey root is classic. (3) Adrenal support for stress. (4) Dietary and supplemental calcium, vitamin D_3, vitamin K_2, magnesium.

Sample Formula and Dose. 4–5 mL 3 × daily between meals.

Parts	Herbs	Rationale
3	Comfrey root	Bone, connective tissue restorative.
2	Rehmannia Shu Di Huang (prepared)	Kidney yin, moisture, night sweats, adrenals.
2	Eucommia Du Zhong	Connective tissue repair.
2	Chickweed herb	Moisturizing, clear heat, hot flashes.
1	Licorice root	Moisture, adrenal support.
1	Horsetail herb	Mineral-rich restorative.
1	Nettle herb	Trace minerals.

Other Suggestions

- *Diet*. Dietary calcium. Sources are dairy, canned fish with bones, such as sardines; sesame seeds; almonds; dark green, leafy veggies: wheat grass, kale, broccoli, watercress, spinach, collards, arugula, mustard greens, and beet greens.
  - Avoid foods that interfere with calcium absorption: Red meats, soft drinks, processed foods, excessive amounts of alcohol and caffeine.[13]
- *Supplements*.
  - Calcium (Ca+) is the major bone mineral. Calcium citrate is an absorbable form. There is debate over which compound is most bioavailable.
  - Magnesium (Mg+) aids calcium absorption and helps relax signs of wind: spasms, twitching, leg cramps, restless legs, charley horse. Any of these are signs of Mg+ deficiency.
  - Vitamin D_3 (not D_2) is necessary for Ca+ absorption from the diet and promotes bone deposition.
  - Vitamin K_2 makes coronary artery walls resistant to binding to Ca+ and promotes moving it into bone.[14]
- *Weight-bearing exercise 3× wk*. Physical therapy for hip fracture. Long-term approach is to increase bone density by walking, running, hiking, aerobics, dancing, and climbing stairs.
- *Smoking*. Risk factor in osteoporosis. Don't start; if client smokes, help client quit.
- *Sunlight exposure*. Vitamin D is made in the skin with the aid of ultraviolet (UV) rays from the sun. In turn, vitamin D_3 is necessary for calcium absorption. The exact amount of time needed for adequate UV exposure varies greatly, depending on skin type, location, latitude, season, and time of day. Without actually testing UV exposure, it's impossible to know how much anyone is getting.[15]
- *Tea*. Oat straw and Milky Oat tops mixed with Licorice root to provide minerals and moisture. Drink 1 cup daily.

Bone is the body's hardest connective tissue, constantly remodeling; building up and breaking down throughout a lifetime. Normally, old worn-out bone cells (osteoclasts) are removed from the skeleton (resorption) at the same rate at which new bone is formed from baby bone cells (osteoblasts). If breakdown overtakes formation, bone is weakened, and fractures occur easily in the hips, spine, and wrist, which is very common in menopausal women because of decreased estrogen. Other risk factors are smoking, lack of weight-bearing exercise, and a thin build. Osteoporosis is diagnosed by bone density tests. Early bone density loss is called *osteopenia* before it progresses into full-blown osteoporosis.

- *Signs and symptoms.* Commonly frequent bone fractures and loss of height.
- *Allopathic treatment.* The drug Fosamax, which can cause esophageal bleeding and cancer. Yes, it does harden bone, but it makes bone brittle and inflexible and has been cited in causing delayed healing in jaw injuries, such as after a tooth extraction, and in causing hip fractures. In fact, doctors advise going off Fosamax after 10 years of continual use because of all this.[12]
- *General therapeutic principles.* (1) Mineral-rich Oat straw and milky tops, Horsetail herb, and Nettle herb are traditional for long-term osteoporosis treatment. (2) Restore and build bone tissue and increase density. (3) Increase Kidney yin. (4) Treat any other problems.

Rheumatology versus Arthritis

The medical specialty, *rheumatology*, treats more than 100 different connective-tissue diseases. Many affect the joints, muscles, and ligaments, and others affect blood vessels or skin. Some are systemic; others are local. Well-known M-S rheumatic problems are osteoarthritis, tendonitis, bursitis, gout, spondylitis, and even growing pains. Some rheumatic diseases are autoimmune, such as rheumatoid arthritis, lupus, scleroderma, sarcoidosis, and fibromyalgia. ***Arthritis*** simply means inflammation of the joints and is a category of diseases within the large rheumatology specialty. Joint diseases are just a fraction of rheumatoid diseases.

The problem is that in Western herbology there is a whole section of herbs called *antirheumatics*. This is unfortunate and confusing. That heading really includes plants with various actions that help arthritis indirectly and in different ways by being antiinflammatory, analgesic, alterative, antispasmodic, and/or diuretic. Please erase that vague herbal classification from your mind. Examples in this list are: Celery seed, Yarrow herb, Mugwort herb, Blue and Black Cohosh root, Yellow Dock root, Wild Yam root, and Blue Flag root.

For the record, we can be thankful for Chinese Medicine, because it does not even bother with the names of the various rheumatic diseases. Wind Damp Heat Bi or Wind Damp Cold Bi are fine designations that say it all. Therapeutic principles are based on what is observed and reported, plus any knowledge you might have about the disease.

Acute and Chronic Rheumatoid Arthritis (RA)

- *Definition.* ***Rheumatoid arthritis (RA)*** is a chronic systemic autoimmune inflammatory disease that attacks peripheral joints and surrounding muscles, tendons, and ligaments, especially the hands, feet, ankles, and knees. The cartilage is destroyed, and joints fuse together. It's a crippling lifelong disease (Case History 24.3). In children, it's called juvenile RA. In RA, inflammation is systemic and can affect other tissues, such as skin, lungs, heart, liver, spleen, or eyes.
- *Signs and symptoms.* Tender, warm, and swollen joints; stiffness worse in the morning and after inactivity; fatigue; fever; and weight loss. There are often symmetrical bony nodules over finger joints, elbows, or feet. Symptoms fluctuate. There can be flare-ups and remissions. Flare-ups are acute and hot, whereas periods of relative calm are chronic and cold and require separate formulas, depending on the stage.
- *Allopathic treatment.* Antiinflammatories, immunosuppressive drugs, physical therapy, moist heat during acute episodes, and surgery.
- *General therapeutic principles.* Choose treatment depending on presentation. In acute situations, concentrate on bringing down inflammation, pain, and stress. When chronic, use more tonics; particularly for connective tissue and immune support.[13] Also, treat infection. A few studies give infection as an underlying cause.[4] (1) RA is autoimmune and inflammatory. Always treat for dysbiosis, leaky gut especially in chronic stages. (2) Analgesics. (3) Antiinflammatories; add in a salicylate herb. (4) Qi and blood movers. (5) Alteratives. (6) Diuretics. (7) Antispasmodics if needed. (8) Relaxing nervines for stress and sleep, as needed. (9) Connective tissue restoratives and immune modulation.

Osteoarthritis (OA)

- *Definition.* ***Osteoarthritis (OA)*** is damage to weight-bearing joints caused by mechanical stress on a joint that progresses to wearing down of articular cartilage, joint fusion, and immobility, especially the knees and hips but also fingers and the back. It is the most common joint disorder and reason for disability in those over 60 years of age (Case History 24.4). Hip and knee replacements are common. Evidence links OA to insulin resistance and cardiovascular disease.[4]
- *Signs and symptoms.* Joint pain, usually worse later in day or after long periods of inactivity, stiffness, swelling, warmth, creaking, and decreased range of motion.
- *Allopathic treatment.* NSAIDs, steroids, exercise. Surgery, such as hip and knee replacements.
- *General therapeutic principles.* (1) Alteratives. (2) Antiinflammatories, especially Frankincense resin, Turmeric root, Ginger root, or Bupleurum Chai Hu (Asian Buplever root). (3) Salicylate herbs: White Willow bark or Meadowsweet herb. (4) Antispasmodics. (5) Circulatory and microcirculatory stimulants: Prickly Ash bark or Ginkgo leaf. (6) Diuretics. (7) Carminatives as needed. (8) Bitters as needed. (9) Detoxifying/alkalizing herbs. Main ones are Celery seed, which increases excretion of acidic metabolites in urine, and Dandelion leaf.[4] (8) If pain from nerve entrapment, St. John's Wort.

Gout

- *Definition.* ***Gout*** is a type of arthritis and the most painful form of them all (Case history 24.5). May cause kidney stone formation and failure. Fluctuates from acute to chronic and back. Hard urate nodules or lumps called *tophi* can develop under the skin, under the ear rim, and around joints, causing crippling deformities. Tophi sometimes ooze a white, chalky liquid. Gout is caused by an inability of the kidneys to break down purines into uric acid and eliminate it through the

CASE HISTORY 24.3

Case Histories for Acute Rheumatoid Arthritis (RA) and Chronic RA

Part 1

Case History for Acute RA

S. Sandra was diagnosed with RA when she was 34 and has been living with it for 20 years. She complains of burning pain that is worse in the morning and spasms. Her fingers have large nodules and are hard to move. Her knees are red and swollen and won't bend. Anything cool helps. She is burping and bloated, has a "bit" of indigestion. Appears quite stressed.

O. **P** Rapid, slippery and weak on right wrist (Spleen side). **T** Red.

A. Wind Damp Heat Bi. Spleen Qi Deficiency.

P. *Specific therapeutic principles.* (1) Reduce pain and include a salicylate and saponin. (2) Antiinflammatories. (3) Antispasmodics. (4) Relaxing nervine for stress. (5) Immune support. (6) Tonify Spleen and dry damp with astringents, diuretics.

Sample Formula and Dose for Acute RA.

Pulse dose 4 mL every hour.

Parts	Herbs	Rationale
3	Stephania Han Fang Ji	Cold, analgesic, antispasmodic, antiinflammatory.
3	Meadowsweet herb	Antiinflammatory, salicylate, gut-regulating.
2	Poria Fu Ling	Tonify Spleen, dry damp.
2	Valerian root	Antispasmodic, analgesic, helps sleep and stress.
1	Celery seed	Cool, alterative, antiinflammatory, diuretic.
1	Wild Yam root	Antiinflammatory, antispasmodic, saponin.
1	Atractylodes Bai Zhu	Tonify Spleen. Astringent, draining diuretic.

Other Suggestions for Acute Rheumatoid Arthritis

- *Diet.* Cleansing, mainly veggie-based, and some fruit during the acute stage. Veggie smoothies.
- *Topical.* No rubefacients, as these are too hot and can aggravate symptoms.[13] Instead, use ice, cooling poultices, compresses, or ice gel packs. Kwan Loong oil, or Birch or Wintergreen essential oil.

Part 2

Case History for Chronic RA

S. After 3 weeks, Sandra's burning pain has subsided. Finger pain has shifted to a dull ache. She is stiff with a dull ache all over, and because it is a cold winter day, she knows it will be rough. She can't wait to find her heating pad. And yes, she is still bloated.

O. **P** Weak on right. **T** Normal.

A. Wind Damp Cold Bi. Spleen Qi Deficiency. Chronic rheumatoid arthritis.

P. *Specific therapeutic principles.* During chronic stages, must work on the gut and address any underlying infection. (1) Warming arterial stimulants for pain. (2) Antiinflammatories. (3) Alteratives for detoxification. (4) Diuretics. (5) Connective tissue tonic. (6) Immune support. (7) Gut rebuilding.

Sample Formula and Dose for Chronic RA.

4–5 mL 3 × day.

Parts	Herbs	Rationale
2	*Boswellia serrata* resin	Antiinflammatory, a qi and blood mover.
2	Jamaican Sarsaparilla root	Arterial stimulant, alterative, saponin.
2	Blue Cohosh	Antiinflammatory specific to fingers, diuretic.
2	Prickly Ash bark	Arterial stimulant, move qi and blood, analgesic.
2	Eucommia Du Zhong	Connective tissue restorative, detoxification.
2	Atractylodes Bai Zhu	Restore gut/Spleen, draining diuretic.
2	Turmeric rhizome	Antiinflammatory, gut bitter, antiinfective.
1	Glycyrrhiza Zhi Gan Cao Honey Fried Licorice	Restores Spleen, cools heat.

Other Suggestions for Chronic RA

- *Diet.* Concentrate on autoimmunity. Fix leaky gut and inflammation: Four-R program or Gut and Psychology Syndrome (GAPS) protocol. No carbs and white sugar. Eat healthy fats. Sometimes the nightshades aggravate RA (tomatoes, potatoes, peppers, eggplant). Test this out as part of elimination diet. Meat/bone stock to restore joints.
- *Supplements.* EPA/DHA 1000–2000 mg a day or Flax seed oil 1–2 tbsp daily.
- *External treatment.* Warmth. Hot pack or heating pad. Liniments like White Flower oil or Tiger Balm, or whatever works for her.

CASE HISTORY 24.4

Case History for Chronic Osteoarthritis

S. Jim was an avid golfer who was having increasingly incapacitating bilateral knee pain relieved by rest. An MRI showed cartilage degeneration. He has a lot of gas and bloating. Loves sweets, meat, and bread.

O. **P** Thready, weak on right. **T** Body pink. Coat, thin, yellowish, greasy.

A. Liver and Kidney Depletion. Wind Cold Bi. Spleen Qi Deficiency.

P. *Specific therapeutic principles.* Must heal the gut. (1) Analgesics. (2) Antiinflammatories. (3) Alteratives. (4) Diuretic. (5) Alkalinize joints with Celery seed or Dandelion leaf.

Sample Formula and Dose. 5 mL 3 × day.

Parts	Herbs	Rationale
3	*Boswellia serrata* resin	Antiinflammatory, moves qi and blood.
3	Meadowsweet herb	Gut healing and salicylate.
2	Nettle leaf	Alterative, antiinflammatory specific for OA.
2	Celery seed	Alterative, diuretic, antiinflammatory, alkalinizing.
2	Comfrey root	Tonic, build connective tissue.
2	Turmeric root	Antiinflammatory, digestive bitter, insulin resistance.

Other Suggestions

- *Diet.* Antiinflammatory fruit and vegetable-based diet. Begin Four-R program. Dark red foods and blueberries, sources of flavonoids. See whether nightshades bother him (tomatoes, potatoes, eggplant, peppers).[11]
- *Supplements.* Pycnogenol (Pine bark extract) for pain relief.
- *Exercise.* Range of motion, gentle aerobics, strength training, swimming.

CASE HISTORY 24.5

Case History for Gout

S. John has burning, excruciating pain in his right great toe. It is red, swollen, stiff, and so tender he cannot stand to wear socks. He does love his beer.

O. **P** Slippery and rapid. **T** Red, body with yellow coat.

A. Wind Damp Heat Bi

P. *Specific therapeutic principles.* (1) Key herbs are large doses of Celery seed with Dandelion leaf to inhibit uric acid. (2) Antiinflammatories like *Boswellia serrata* (no salicylates. See note under "Other Suggestions"). (3) Alteratives, especially Sarsaparilla root. (4) Diuretics to eliminate uric acid through the kidneys. (5) Cholagogues because uric acid is also excreted in the bile.

Sample Formula and Dose. Pulse Dose 5 mL every ½–1 hour. Taper frequency and dose as indicated.

Parts	Herbs	Rationale
4	Celery seed	Inhibits uric acid; diuretic, alterative.
3	Dandelion root	Inhibits uric acid; cholagogue and diuretic.
3	Sarsaparilla root	Alterative.
3	*Boswellia serrata* resin	Antiinflammatory.

Other Suggestions

Note: Salicylates are contraindicated in gout. They inhibit uric acid excretion.[4]

- *Diet.* Antiinflammatory. Time-honored consumption of ½ lb of cherries a day is classic for gout and other arthritic diseases because of high antioxidant (anthocyanidin) content that reduces oxidative stress and builds collagen. An option to all those fresh or frozen cherries (which are expensive, a lot to eat, and not always in season) is Black Cherry concentrate made into juice and taken daily. Other deep red and blue fruits, like Hawthorn berry and blueberries.
    - Avoid high-purine foods, red meats, organ meats like liver, all shellfish, alcohol, asparagus, mushrooms, and legumes.[4]
- *Hydration.* Lots of water to flush out uric acid crystals from kidney. An 8-oz glass of water every 2 hours.
- *Pain.* Even the weight of a sheet can cause pain. Protect gouty foot with a protective box or plastic laundry basket turned on its side. Apply cool pack wrapped in a soft towel.
- *Supplements.* Antiinflammatory EPA/DHA essential fatty acids 12,000 mg 3 × day. *Magnesium* is a very alkaline mineral and deficiency can lead to gout: 500 mg a day, best taken at night.

urine. Purines are chemicals with a high content in seafood, organ meats, legumes, anchovies, beer, and other alcoholic beverages. King Henry VIII of England had gout, and it didn't make him or anyone near him very happy. So did Leonardo Da Vinci and Benjamin Franklin.

- *Signs and symptoms.* Swelling and intense burning pain, stiffness, redness, and swelling in the joints, particularly the big toe, although it can also occur in other joints. Feels like the foot is on fire. Risk factors include high purine diet; obesity; overconsumption of alcohol, which interferes with uric acid excretion; and lead exposure.[13]
- *Allopathic treatment.* NSAIDs, steroids, Colchicine, and allopurinol to decrease uric acid production, thereby helping pain.

CASE HISTORY 24.6

Case History for Fibromyalgia

S. Shelia has been diagnosed with fibromyalgia. She has diffused, dull, chronic pain on her hips, neck, shoulder, and back. It moves around. She is anxious, depressed, and exhausted. Cannot sleep. Stomach has gas, belching, bloating, and alternating constipation and diarrhea. Right now, it's the diarrhea stage. Has gotten minimal relief from her healthcare provider.

O. **P** Slippery on right, tense on left. **T** Greasy, red coat.

A. Wind Damp Heat. Liver Invading Spleen. Shen Disturbance. Fibromyalgia with chronic fatigue, anxiety, and depression.

P. *Specific therapeutic principles.* Two formulas: one for day and one for sleep. (1) Analgesics and antiinflammatories move qi and blood. (2) Adrenal support. (3) Immune support. (4) Nerve tonic. (5) Antidiarrheals and gut restoratives. (6) Separate sleep formula. (7) Four-R Program.

Part 1

Daytime Sample Formula and Dose.

6 mL 3 × day between meals.

Equal Parts	Herbs	Rationale
1	Bupleurum Chai Hu	Analgesic, muscle relaxant, move qi and blood.
1	Jamaican Dogwood root	Analgesic, antiinflammatory, spasmolytic.
1	Hops flower	Antianxiety, muscle relaxant, nerve tonic.
1	St. John's Wort	Nerve tonic, depression.
1	Turmeric rhizome	Antiinflammatory, bitter for gut, antidiarrheal.
1	Calamus root	Diarrhea, gastrointestinal restorative, bloating.
1	Rhodiola root	Depression, energy, tonic, immune support.
1	*Boswellia serrata* resin	Antiinflammatory.
1	Ginger root	Digestion, move qi and blood.
1	Echinacea root	Immune support.

Part 2

Nighttime Formula for Sleep.

Dose: 4 mL at bedtime; then 2 mL every 15 min as needed, up to 2 hours, then STOP

Equal parts	Herb	Rationale
1	Zizyphus Suan Zao Ren	Sleep and anxiety, worry.
1	Skullcap herb	Stress, sleep, anxiety, nerve tonic, muscle relaxant.
1	Valerian root	Stress, anxiety, sleep, muscle relaxant.

Other Suggestions

- *Diet.* Although the herbal formula will be based on symptom relief, if gut problems are in the picture (as in case history), the Four-R Program is a go: healthy alkaline, antiinflammatory diet; identifying and eliminating food sensitivities; removing pathogens; adding pre- and probiotics; repairing gut lining. Bitters and fermented foods (Chapter 18).
- *Supplements.* Fish oil EPA/DHA 2000 mg, D_3 5000 IU a day.[16] 5-HTP for depression. Magnesium 500 mg a day to help relax muscles best taken at night.
- *Lifestyle.* Daily exercise, yoga, meditation to help pain.
- *Body work.* Acupuncture, massage, reflexology, myofascial release.

- *General therapeutic principles.* (1) Diuretics to flush urates from kidneys. (2) Antiinflammatories. (Salicylates can make gout worse.) (3) Herbs to inhibit uric acid. (4) Alteratives to release toxins. (5) Cholagogues to excrete uric acid from the bile.

Fibromyalgia Syndrome

Definition. ***Fibromyalgia syndrome (FMS)*** is a rheumatic disease with a large group of symptoms: widespread muscular-skeletal pain with trigger points, sleep disturbances, and GI and emotional problems (Case History 24.6). FMS has been linked to increased amounts of neurotransmitter substance P (for pain) in cerebral spinal fluid, chronic fatigue syndrome, adrenal depletion, and viral-induced changes in cytokines,[4] or inflammatory markers. It is not yet an official autoimmune disease, but it sure looks like one. Treat accordingly.

- *Signs and symptoms.* Overlap of many *diseases*. Chronic diffuse and migratory muscle pain on specific spots (trigger points), usually on the back of the head, neck, shoulders, trunk, back, hips, thighs, or knees. Eighteen fibromyalgia pain points are identified in medical texts, showing typical locations. FMS involves chronic fatigue, irritable bowel, anxiety, depression, and brain fog. Diagnosed with a pain index of trigger point areas.
- *Allopathic treatment.* A bagful of pills. Analgesics, muscle relaxants, NSAIDs, antidepressants, sleeping pills, anticonvulsants, and antipsychotics. Stress management, hydrotherapy, acupuncture, and massage. FMS wasn't even recognized as genuine until the 1990s and was originally treated as a mental illness. It occurs more in folks with other rheumatic diseases and is more prevalent among women.
- *General therapeutic principles.* (1) Nervine tonics: St. John's Wort, Bacopa (all parts), Skullcap herb. (2) Adrenal support with Astragalus Huang Qi, Licorice root, Eleutherococcus Ci Wu Jia (Siberian ginseng root), Rhodiola root, Ashwagandha root, or Rehmannia Shu Di Huang (Prepared Rehmannia root). (3) Immune modulation: Echinacea root. (4) Anxiolytics, hypnotics, and antidepressants: Zizyphus Suan Zao Ren, Kava root, Valerian root, Passionflower herb, or Rhodiola root. (5) Antiinflammatories, analgesics, antispasmodics such as *Boswellia serrata* resin, Turmeric rhizome, and Bupleurum Chai Hu.

Summary

The muscular-skeletal system includes connective tissue: bone, muscles, tendons, ligaments, and fascia. Pain is a chief reason a person visits an allopathic healthcare provider. Herbalists have many tools and opportunities to keep folks off addictive narcotics and NSAIDs which can cause ulcers, GI bleeds, heart disease, and kidney failure. A wise herbalist addresses pain symptomatically but focuses on the root of the problem. Alteratives are used to dredge up toxins, and diuretics flush them out. Chronic inflammation is present in many M-S conditions and often requires a leaky gut fix.

RICE (rest, ice, compression, and elevation) is a basic first-aid procedure. External remedies can range from a bag of frozen peas to compresses, creams, and liniments. Manual therapies like massage, reflexology, tui na, osteopathy, and hydrotherapy are useful tools, as is moxa and cupping. The ECB system is a way the body manages pain. Phytocannabinoids are plants that hook on to its receptor sites and include *Cannabis* spp., Hops flower, and Echinacea root. Rubefacients are forms of topical analgesia that bring blood to the skin surface. Plants containing salicylates and sterols help reduce pain.

In Chinese Medicine, pain is caused by a blockage of qi and blood which must be moved to free up energy flow and give relief. Bi means painful obstruction and Bi syndromes involve pain, inflammation, and arthritic symptoms that are either acute (hot) or chronic (cold).

Review

Fill in the Blanks

(Answers in Appendix B.)

1. In what disease are salicylates contraindicated? ___.
2. Name five types of connective tissue: ___, ___, ___, ___, ___.
3. Four types of foods that interfere with calcium absorption are ___, ___, ___, ___.
4. Two M-S conditions that are autoimmune are ___, ___.
5. The Kidneys rule the ___, and the Liver rules the ___.
6. Name five excellent dietary sources of calcium: ___, ___, ___, ___, ___.
7. Give two Chinese Medicine and two Western herbs for Wind Damp Cold Bi. ___, ___, ___, ___.
8. Give two Chinese Medicine and two Western herbs for Wind Damp Heat Bi. ___, ___, ___, ___.
9. Give two Chinese Medicine and two Western M-S tonics or restoratives. ___, ___, ___, ___.
10. Name four external Chinese Medicine techniques for M-S pain: ___, ___, ___, ___.

Critical Concept Questions

(Answers for you to decide.)

1. What is a Bi syndrome? List two examples.
2. How does our state of health affect M-S conditions?
3. What does "Pain is a symptom" mean?
4. What is the difference between Tylenol and aspirin?
5. How do qi- and blood-moving herbs help pain?
6. A 53-year-old woman complains of bilateral knee pain after running. This pain has been going on for the previous 6 months, whereas before there was no problem. It is relieved by rest and ice. **P** Thready. **T** Red. What is it? Therapeutic principles? Herbs?
7. Would you use medicinal *Cannabis sativa* in your practice, assuming it is legal in your location and you could obtain it? Why or why not?
8. Give a few options for external approaches to a just-sprained ankle.
9. A client asks how much sunlight they need to get enough vitamin D. Your answer?
10. What does menopause have to do with bones? What about Fosamax?

References

1. "Common Pain Relievers Are Causing Heart Attacks." Mercola. https://articles.mercola.com/sites/articles/archive/2017/05/24/common-pain-relievers-heart-attack-risk.aspx (accessed December 2, 2019).
2. Yearsley, Connor. "The Use of Medical Cannabis Preparations to Treat Epilepsy." HerbalGram: The Journal of the American Botanical Council. Aug-Oct 2017.
3. Sulak, Dustin. "Introduction to the Endocannabinoid System." NORML. http://norml.org/library/item/introduction-to-the-endo-cannabinoid-system (accessed August 16, 2019).
4. Bone, Kerry and Simon Mills. *Principles and Practice of Phytotherapy* (London, UK: Elsevier, 2013).
5. "Relationship of Qi and Blood-Vital Substances in TCM." Sacred Lotus Chinese Medicine. https://www.sacredlotus.com/go/foundations-chinese-medicine/get/relationship-of-qi-blood-in-tcm (accessed August 16, 2019).
6. Marcus, Alon. "Bi Syndromes." Integrative Health Medicine. http://www.integrativehealthmedicine.com/bi-syndrome.htm (accessed August 16, 2019).
7. Holmes, Peter. *Jade Remedies: A Chinese Herbal Reference for the West* (Boulder, CO: Snow Lotus, 1996).
8. Flaws, Bob. "Cortex Eucommiae Ulmoides Du Zhong and Latex Allergy." Acupuncture Today. https://www.acupuncturetoday.com/mpacms/at/article.php?id = 27967 (accessed December 3, 2019).
9. Marciano, Marissa. "Salicylates." The Naturopathic Herbalist. https://thenaturopathicherbalist.com/plant-constituents/salicylates/ (accessed August 18, 2019).
10. Ganora, Lisa. *Herbal Constituents: Foundations of Phytochemistry* (Louisville, CO: Herbalchem Press, 2009).
11. Murray, Michael. *Encyclopedia of Nutritional Supplements* (Rocklin, CA: Prima, 1996).
12. "Osteoporosis Drugs, Risk of Bone Problems in Jaw and Thigh?" Mayo Clinic. https://www.mayoclinic.org/diseases-conditions/osteo-porosis/expert-answers/osteoporosis-drug-risks/faq-20058121 (accessed August 18, 2019).
13. Hoffman, David. *Medical Herbalism: The Science and Practice of Herbal Medicine* (Rochester, VT: Healing Arts, 2003).
14. "Reduce Your Risk of Arterial Stiffness." *Life Extension Magazine.* March-April 2018.
15. "How Much Sunshine Does It Take to Make Enough Vitamin D? Perhaps More Than You Think." Mercola. https://articles.mercola.com/sites/articles/archive/2009/10/29/how-much-sunshine-does-it-take-to-make-enough-vitamin-d-perhaps-more-than-you-think.aspx (accessed August 18, 2019).
16. Axe, Josh. "Natural Fibromyalgia Treatment Options Including Diet and Supplementation." Dr. Axe. https://draxe.com/health/natural-fibromyalgia-treatment/ (accessed August 18, 2019).

25 The Integumentary System

"Nettle is good for washing old rotten stinking sores."

—Nicholas Culpeper, English botanist, herbalist, astrologist, and physician (1616–1654)

CHAPTER REVIEW

- Overview of the skin: The skin as the third kidney; detoxification, functions, assessment, and types of skin applications.
- Skin health and care.
- Chinese Medicine perspective: The skin and major syndromes, featuring hives, eczema, and shingles.
- Skin Materia Medica: Skin herbs worth honorable mention. Vulneraries (first-aid herbs, soft tissue restoratives, astringents, antipruritics, bruise remedies, antiinflammatories, antimicrobials, and styptics). Alteratives (lymphatic drainers, diuretics, and liver stimulants).
- Considerations for treating the skin.
- Common integumentary conditions with case histories: Minor skin trauma, acute eczema, psoriasis, shingles, acne, and athlete's foot.

KEY TERMS

Abrasion
Acne vulgaris
Alteratives
Anhidrosis
Antiseptics
Athlete's foot
Eczema
Emollient
Hematoma
Herpes
Hyperhidrosis
Hypohidrosis
Integument
Laceration
Pruritus
Psoriasis
Puncture wound
Shingles
Styptics
Urticaria
Vulnerary

Our outer layer, the ***integument***, is better known as the skin. It includes the hair, nails, skin glands, and nerves. The skin is the largest organ in the body, covering about 10 square feet in adults (if laid out flat), and weighing approximately 10 pounds. Skin disorders are common reasons for a doctor's visit. Although rarely life threatening, they can create genuine embarrassment or emotional, physical, and mental anguish.

The skin is out there and mirrors our internal health and well-being. People experience their self-image through their skin, and it communicates who we are to the world. In Chinese Medicine, the Lungs rule the exterior of the body (skin) and manifest in the body hair. Skin is also related to Liver, Blood, and Heart shen in certain ways.

The integumentary Materia Medica revisits many old herbal friends and acquaintances, with some new ones joining the scene. Selected skin cases were reviewed in pediatrics (Chapter 21). Therapeutic principles do not change much for adults, but stronger botanicals could be indicated. Frequently the same standbys apply: the flowers of Chamomile, Red Clover, and Calendula; and of course, Burdock root and seed and Yellow Dock root.

Overview of the Skin

A common consensus among present-day herbalists is that skin diseases are among the most complicated and inconsistent to treat. There is little agreement on any particular herb or regimen for a given problem. A this-for-that approach doesn't work. Results are unpredictable and unreliable, no matter what is tried. A skin condition may appear to be all cleared up, only to return again and be worse. Each case must be taken individually, and an herbalist must doggedly return to the basics of digestive and liver health. Chinese Medicine always advises to treat what you see. Address the syndrome, not the disease. If an immunological or allergic problem exists, this approach is even more important.

Skin as the Third Kidney and Detoxification

Internal and external skin problems test an herbalist's holistic skills. If there is external trauma with bruising or open wounds, the focus is to avoid infection; restore and heal the cells; treat any bites, stings, or poison ivy; or remove offending chemicals the skin has touched. These irritants obviously come from the outside environment.

Treatment of chronic skin problems with internal causes involves more than rubbing on a salve. Topical creams soothe symptoms, but internal detoxification is needed. The Eclectics espoused this and so do Chinese Medicine practitioners. If the body cannot eliminate poisons adequately through the bowel or bladder, they will manifest on the skin. They have to go somewhere.

For this reason, the skin has historically been seen as *the third kidney*. The fix is to use alteratives and herbs that stimulate, push, and coax eliminatory functions, and call on help from the kidneys, colon, liver, and lymphatics. Red Clover flower and Yellow Dock root change the internal environment, and Cleavers herb moves lymph. Nettle herb provides nourishment and removes toxins through its diuretic action, and Burdock root works on the kidneys and liver. For stubborn chronic skin outbreaks and autoimmune or allergic reactions, an herbalist must obtain a thorough health history and assessment to get to the root cause.

The liver's role on skin is basic. If Phase I and Phase II detoxification pathways are out of sync (Chapter 19), where do the toxins go? They build up in the body, causing oxidation and inflammation in susceptible places. Allergies follow. Metabolic overload and failure of adequate liver detoxification often show up as chronic skin problems, such as acne, rosacea, eczema, or psoriasis. Liver stimulants and detoxification herbs are part of the skin fix: Dandelion root, Artichoke leaf, Turmeric root, and the very strong Poke root. Liver herbs work robustly on the skin, so use them conservatively in small amounts.

Then there's the gut. When dysbiosis occurs, the skin suffers. Chronic skin problems such as psoriasis, cutaneous lupus, and autoimmune skin diseases are frequently a sign of an unbalanced microbiome and probable food sensitivities. If we eat too much sugar, the face can yell loudly. Our beloved Four-R program would be the solution.

Skin Functions

Like any other organ, the skin has many responsibilities.

- *The skin is a protector.* It contains us. It seals in the good and keeps out the bad. It is our shell, a protective barrier against the exterior. It is our boundary between sun and radiation exposure, microorganisms, excess moisture and to a certain extent, cold weather. It keeps internal organs from drying out. Too much moisture causes wrinkly, waterlogged skin.
- *The skin has an immune function.* The skin is the first line of defense and acts as a shield that blocks microorganisms from entering. Burns are very dangerous because they make openings in the epidermis, dermis, and subcutaneous layers (depending on depth), allowing microbes and potentially severe infection to move in.
- *The skin is an endocrine gland.* Endocrine glands produce and release hormones into the blood. The skin produces vitamin D_2 with the help of ultraviolet rays of sunlight. It also is the site of vitamin D_3 synthesis.
- *The skin is an exocrine gland.* Exocrine glands produce and excrete substances by way of ducts. The skin has two types. Sweat glands (*sudoriferous*) rise out of the second skin layer (*dermis*), and oil glands (*sebaceous*) occur next to the hair follicles and keep the skin and hair moist.
- *The skin regulates body temperature.* The skin cools us down through sweating, bringing blood to the surface, and eliminating heat. It warms us up through vasoconstriction, which helps to retain heat. In Chinese Medicine, copious sweating or lack of it is a Lung problem because the Lungs rule the exterior (sweat glands and body hair). Everyone needs to sweat, or they would become dangerously overheated.
  - *Decreased sweat.* No sweating, or the inability to sweat, is called ***anhidrosis***. Not enough sweat is called ***hypohidrosis***. Yarrow flower and Chrysanthemum Ju Hua are diaphoretics that help us sweat.
  - *Profuse sweating.* ***Hyperhidrosis*** is the opposite and, besides being embarrassing, can cause skin infections and rashes. Garden Sage herb, an astringent, is a classic remedy to stop excessive sweating. Astragalus Huang Qi is indicated for either hyper- or hypohidrosis because it regulates water balance on the endocrine level. Jade Windscreen formula containing Astragalus Huang Qi along with Atractylodes Bai Zhu (White Atractylodes root) and Ledebouriella Fang Feng (Wind Protector root, Siler) is one solution for spontaneous sweating (see Box 25.2).
- *The skin is a sense organ.* Different types of cutaneous nerve endings detect pain, touch, pressure, and temperature. Such nerve endings are necessary to provide environmental information so that appropriate reactions to stimuli are possible. This function is an important safety issue.
- *The skin is a detoxifier.* Skin is constantly sloughing off the outer layer (epidermis) and removing harmful pathogens in the process. Toxins are eliminated through sweat and exercise, although sweat's primary function is to regulate temperature. Sweat lodges, saunas, and Russian banyas are traditional sweating methods to ward off pathogens, those nasty external pernicious influences.

Skin Assessment

Skin assessment includes observing factors such as color, complexion, radiance, or dullness. Nails and hair are extensions of the skin.

- *Complexion.* The skin speaks volumes about our health. Melanocytes (pigment-producing skin cells) in the epidermis produce the pigment melanin that give skin its color or lack thereof. Skin of any shade should have an inner glow. Paleness of the face, nails, and the conjunctiva, indicate anemia. Very red skin indicates too much blood flow or anger, Liver Yang Rising.
  - *Lack of oxygen.* Lack of oxygen in white skin casts a blue or purplish hue (cyanosis). It is harder to assess decreased oxygen (hypoxemia) in people with darker pigments. Generally, there is a lack of vitality and glow, and the skin looks gray. Decreased oxygen can be evaluated in any skin shade by checking out paleness versus redness in the oral mucosa inside the cheek and on the conjunctiva (mucous membrane inside and below the lower eyelids). This is a good assessment tool to remember.

- *Hair.* Hair and nails are dead cells made of keratin, both continuations of skin. Hair extends from living hair follicles. Healthy hair is shiny and strong. Harsh chemicals and dyes damage hair. Hair should be elastic and shed minimally. Hair sheds most in the fall and winter and grows fastest in the summer. Bald spots, thinning hair, or clumps coming out when brushed indicate excessive loss caused from chemotherapy, malnutrition, and severe illness. Hair should not be dry and brittle, so it needs essential fatty acids in the diet and minimal electric dryer exposure and chemicals to retain its moisture and sheen.
- *Nails.* These extend from nail beds and should look translucent, shiny, and firm. They can reflect the interior and may indicate an underlying systemic disease. Or sometimes a nail deformity may be a sign of trauma. Nail examination is only one part of a thorough assessment. Western medicine, Chinese Medicine, and Ayurveda all have systems of nail analysis. A few indicators follow.
  - *Western allopathic medicine. Clubbing* indicates lack of oxygen from lung or cardiac problems and/or inflammatory bowel diseases. *Spoon shape* (concave) nails are related to iron deficiency. *Pitting* is common in psoriasis. A *thickening or yellow discoloration*, sometimes curled, is often seen in elders with poor circulation and in fungal infections. *Pale* nails are a sign of anemia. *White spots* point to mineral deficiency, especially of zinc. *Red puffy cuticles* are a sign of infection. Deep *horizontal ridges* called Beau's lines may indicate trauma to the nail bed or malnutrition or serious disease. *Vertical ridges* can be from stress, psoriasis, rheumatoid arthritis, or aging.[1]
  - *Chinese Medicine.* Pale nails are considered a blood deficiency. Moons (lunulae) should appear on every finger and take up one-fifth of each nail, which is a sign of heat and high vitality. Absence of or very small moons indicate cold and mucus.
  - *Ayurveda.* Moons represent fire *(agni)* in the body. Small or absent lunula mean weak digestion or lack of fire, with toxin buildup or circulation problems. If there are no moons or extremely small moons, warming digestive Ginger tea is recommended.[2]
- *Chinese Medicine facial skin assessment.* A bright shiny face means qi deficiency or a cold condition. Facial redness is a sign of heat, and if the whole face is red, it's excess heat. Paleness with no shine is a blood deficiency. *Blackness* under the eyes indicates either not enough sleep or Kidney yin, yang, or qi deficiency. A red-tipped nose indicates Spleen problems, often seen in alcoholics. A bright yellow skin tone can indicate damp heat (or jaundice). Pale yellow is a sign of damp cold caused by deficiency.[3]

Skin Applications

- *Internally.* Internal remedies should be used along with the externals to assure more complete healing within and without the body. Tinctures, infusions, and decoctions are examples of internal remedies.
- *Baths.* The skin absorbs herbs through the bath water, a pleasant approach. The simple act of being submerged can soothe itching and inflammation. Medicated bath salts can be dissolved under the faucet. A knotted sock or stocking filled with herbs function as a tea bag, an infusion. Essential oils, herbal tinctures, or extracts may be added to baths.
- *Colloidal oatmeal bath.* This is an effective, old-fashioned remedy for itching. It relieves dry, itchy, irritated skin in eczema, bites, psoriasis, and diaper rash. Colloidal oatmeal refers to any very finely ground, powdered, unflavored natural oatmeal, such as Bob's Red Mill Organic Rolled Oats. When added to water, the powder forms a suspension and turns the water milky and silky, not clumpy. Use 1 cup meal to a tub of water. For baby baths, use ⅓ cup. Adding some Chamomile or Calendula flower doesn't hurt, and you may put the whole mixture in a muslin bag or stocking instead of directly in the water for greater ease in cleaning up. Works well; takes a little doing.
- *Fomentations or compresses.* This is simply a cloth or piece of gauze dipped into a strong herbal tea or tincture and wrung out. It is usually applied warm and changed often. A bit more aesthetic and cleaner than a poultice when a pot, heat source, and a cloth are handy.
- *Poultices.* This is a messier variation of a compress but works well outdoors when you can quickly wildcraft a healing herb. The herb is crushed and applied directly to wound, wrapped to hold in place, and changed often. The substance (whatever it is) comes in direct contact with the skin. Raw honey, Aloe Vera juice or gel, wide Plantain leaf, or Yarrow herb all make nice poultices. Good in the woods for outdoor first aid, and to impress friends.
- *Lotions, salves, ointments, and creams.* Lotions are water- or oil-based liquids. Salves and ointments are semisolid lipid-based preparations. Creams are suspensions of oil in water (Chapter 6). Lotions absorb well and cool as they evaporate. Salves are protective and stay on the skin for a fairly long time. Creams are protective but care should be taken not to insulate the skin too much, which could cause overheating.[4] Lotions, creams, ointments, and salves are ***emollients*** that soften, moisten, and soothe skin. Keep a vulnerary salve in the fridge and in the car's first-aid kit.
- *Powders.* A powder is a finely ground herb put directly on a wound, like Cayenne pepper which is used as a first-aid styptic. Powders are messy and impractical, and really don't work very well. They may wash away before the bleeding even stops; if not, the wound still has to be cleaned, which washes away the herb anyway and restarts the bleed.[5]
- *Plasters.* These are protective dressings of cloth or other material that are infused with an herb or covered with an herbal paste. Mustard plasters are used for coughs, colds, and rheumatic pain. Chinese Medicine patent stick-on analgesic plasters are often infused with Camphor, Wintergreen, Cayenne, or Ginger. They are convenient and provide soothing warmth for a fairly long time. It would be a good thing to stick some patent plasters in a first-aid kit to cover situations involving muscle pulls and achy backs.
- *Steams.* A facial steam is a great way to achieve deep pore cleansing (Box 25.1). Aromatic oils, such as those in Peppermint leaf or Chamomile flower, are released by the heat and absorbed through the skin. In addition to feeling wonderful, a steam adds an antiseptic quality and softens blemishes, such as pimples and acne, so they can come to a head and pop on their own to prevent scarring. Add any herbs or essential oils, depending on condition: Tea Tree for an infection or Lavender for a burn.

Skin Health and Care

- *Sunburn.* Sun damage is dangerous and carcinogenic. At the least, it causes premature wrinkling and spotting. Severe and repeated exposures create burning, blistering, and peeling,

• BOX 25.1 Cleansing Facial Steam[6]

by Rosemary Gladstar

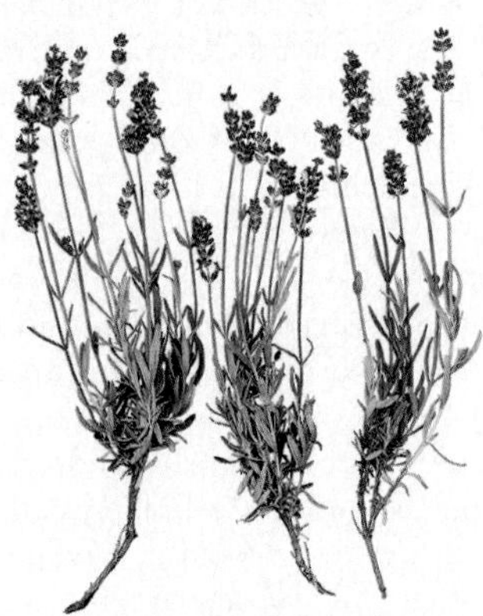

Lovely flowering *Lavandula angustifolia* herb is cooling, calming, astringing, and an antiinfective vulnerary. (Copyright Lang/Tucker Photography. Photographs loaned with permission from *The Botanical Series* are copywritten by Jennifer Anne Tucker and Gerald Lang from the Studio at Hill Crystal Farm. www.jennifer-tucker.com)

Aromatic steams open the pores and help blemishes such as whiteheads, blackheads, and acne come to a head. Normal skin does well with a lot of Comfrey, a moisturizing, mucilaginous herb; and if skin is on the oily side, more drying astringents are added such as Witch Hazel leaf or Garden Sage leaf. Steams call for dried, raw herbs, but 2–3 drops of essential oil could be substituted for any of the dried botanicals.

Steam for Dry to Normal Skin

3 parts	Comfrey root or leaf	Exceptionally good moisturizing vulnerary. The chief herb.
2 parts	Chamomile flower	Cooling vulnerary, antiinflammatory, and nervous relaxant.
2 parts	Rose petal	Both drying and moisturizing and helps repair tissue.
2 parts	Calendula flower	Clears damp heat, vulnerary, astringent, absorbs exudates.
1 part	Lavender flower	Cooling, calming, astringing, and antiinfective vulnerary.

Steam for Oily Skin

2 parts	Calendula flower	Dry, astringing, vulnerary, detoxicant, antiinflammatory.
1 part	Witch Hazel leaf	Dry, astringing, vulnerary, antiinflammatory.
1 part	Garden Sage leaf	Cool, dry, antiseptic vulnerary.
¼ part	Rosemary leaf	Warm, drying, aromatic, vulnerary, mildly antiinfective.

Directions (for either formula)

Weigh out and mix herbs together. Bring 2–3 qt of water to a boil and drop in about a handful of the mixture. Turn down to a simmer with lid on for 2 min. Remove from heat, place pot on hotplate, and cover head with a towel. Allow steam to waft up in the face. Come up for air when necessary.

which can lead to skin aging and melanoma (skin cancer). Encourage stylish wide brimmed hats for women, cute head gear for babies, and brimmed hats and caps for men. In the past, cowboy hats were worn for sun protection, not style. For sunburns, use a cool bath, adding 1 cup vinegar to soothe skin or baking soda for itching and inflammation. Aloe Vera gel and Lavender essential oil work wonders. Sunscreen with a sun protection factor (SPF) around 50 is recommended. It blocks about 98% of harmful ultraviolet-B (UVB) rays, which play a major role in skin cancer.[7]

- *Hydration.* Very important for skin and whole-body health. Drinking adequate warm water and warm beverages keeps the skin moist. Natural herbal moisturizers containing Rose water, Calendula flower, Red Clover flower, or Mullein leaf are lovely and therapeutic. Sesame oil rubbed on the body before bathing is an Ayurvedic approach to keep in moisture. Oily sebaceous glands seal in moisture.
- *Itching.* Itchy skin is a symptom called ***pruritus***. It is caused by allergic reactions to histamine and by inflammation, dryness, or other skin damage. Itching is common with hives, eczema, and bug bites. Calendula flower, Comfrey root, Chickweed herb in a cream are soothing, moisturizing, and antiitch. In Chinese Medicine, pruritus is often referred to as wind in the skin.
- *Thickness.* Depends on age and location. The yang sides of the body (back, outer legs, and outer arms) have thicker skin; the yin side (front, belly, face, inner arms, and inner legs) has thinner skin. Skin is thickest on the heels, which endure maximum pressure in walking and need protection. Skin is thinnest on delicate eyelids. Older people have thinner skin than younger; men have thicker skin than women. Babies have soft, translucent, brand-new skin.
- *Nourishment.* Healthy skin, hair, and nails require a diet rich in omega-3 fatty acids from foods such as walnuts, flaxseeds, almonds, salmon, soy, navy beans, and kidney beans, which gives skin that fresh, moisture-rich glow. Green leafy veggies and a Mediterranean diet help inside and out.
- *Dry skin brushing.* The epidermal surface layer of the skin is constantly shedding and regenerating. It is renewed every 2 to 4 weeks, and we lose 1.5 pounds of skin a year.[8] Brushing with a dry washcloth, natural bristle brush, or luffa sponge is a way to help slough off dead epidermal cells. Dry brushing exfoliates, stimulates blood and lymphatic circulation, aids in detoxification, and offers stress relief and invigoration. Brush before bathing, stroking gently toward the heart to stimulate circulation, as done in Swedish massage.

Chinese Medicine Perspective: the Skin and Major Syndromes

- *The Lungs rule the skin and body hair.* The Lungs are the most superficial organ of the body and connect to the outside, as does the skin. Therefore, skin problems are Lung related. Glossy, smooth, supple skin and a shiny complexion reflect Lung and skin health. In this dual connection, Houttuynia Yu Xing Cao (Fishwort herb) is a commonly used herb for treating both pneumonia and skin eczema (Fig. 25.1).
- *Profuse spontaneous sweating or no sweat.* The pores on the surface of the skin are qi gates in charge of body breathing.[9] This is a Lung function, another kind of breathing called wei qi. It is in charge of opening and closing the sweat pores (glands) on the skin, the doors of qi. If wei qi is deficient, the pores open and we sweat too much, a sign of lung qi deficiency. If wei qi stagnates, we don't sweat enough. Another more common reason for dryness is yin deficiency. Harmonious wei qi

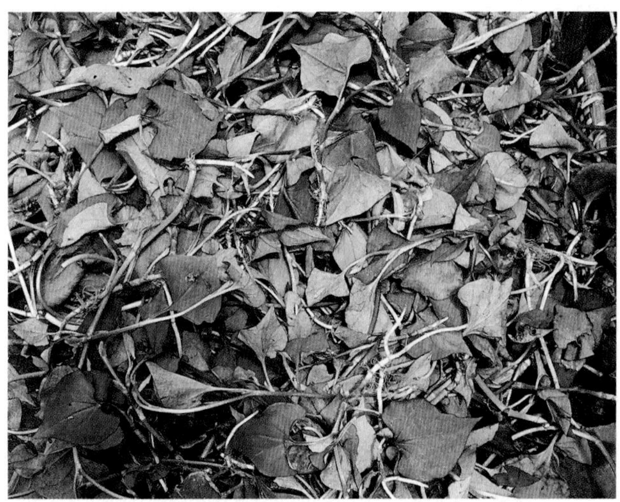

• **Fig. 25.1** Houttuynia Yu Xing Cao (Heart-shaped Fishwort herb) ready to go in a fresh tincture. The herb can be used as an antiinflammatory detoxicant for acute eczema, swellings, insect bites, and psoriasis. It is also antiinfective, expectorant, and antitussive; a true skin and respiratory ally.

moistens the body hair and the skin. From a Lung standpoint, wei qi is also part of the immune system, protecting the body from external pathogens.

Chinese Medicine Major Skin Syndromes

Some typical scenarios involve the skin, described in this list in terms of their Western disease counterpart. Treatment depends on assessment. These syndromes apply to many skin conditions, not just the ones given.

Hives in Chinese Medicine

Hives (***urticaria***) are a rash of pale or red welts on the skin that itch intensely, sometimes with dangerous swelling, caused by an allergic reaction, typically to specific foods.

- *Wind Cold.* Wind denotes a sudden onset or rapid disappearance of lesions. It also alludes to itching and emotional stress. Western interpretation is acute allergy-induced hives. This involves severe itching, pale wheals, chills, and no thirst. **Pulse (P)** Superficial and soft (indicating external wind). **Tongue (T)** Normal color, thin white coat. Fix: Ledebouriella Fang Feng (Wind Protector root) or Schizonepeta Jing Jie (Japanese Catnip herb). *Nepeta cataria* (Western Catnip herb) also remedies hives.
- *Wind Heat.* Hives that appear suddenly (wind) with heat. The wheals are red and itchy, and there is fever and thirst. **P** Superficial, rapid. **T** Red in front with thin yellow coat. Fix: Antiviral, wind- and heat-clearing herbs. Sometimes the standard patent formula Yin Chiao, which has these actions, is used (Box 17.1).
- *Defensive Qi Deficiency.* Chronic hives that often recur because of an underactive, low immune system (wei qi). **P** Weak on the right (lung side). **T** Normal or pale. Fix: Jade Windscreen formula with Ledebouriella Fang Feng, which is used for Lung infections to strengthen and stabilize the exterior. It is also useful for hives and allergic dermatitis and is known to protect the wei qi (Box 25.2).[10]

• **BOX 25.2 Jade Windscreen Formula (Yu Ping Feng San)**

A versatile combination of only three herbs that act as a barrier from external wind.

The main classical actions of Jade Windscreen are to protect and stabilize the immune system (wei qi), disperse external wind and pathogens, and to stop spontaneous sweating from qi deficiency. In modern times, it is used for food or seasonal allergies and hives, spontaneous sweating, immunodeficiency, environmental sensitivities, as well as more traditional protection from external wind, such as coughs, colds, bronchitis, viral infections, and more. (For this reason Jade Windscreen could also have just as appropriately appeared under Respiratory (Chapter 20).[11] The name *Jade* indicates how highly valued this trio is in Chinese Medicine.

Parts	Herb	Rationale
2	Ledebouriella Fang Feng (Wind Protector root, Siler)	Stabilizes the exterior (wei qi) immune system. Antiviral. Expels hot or cold wind, and for arthritic Bi syndromes, which are also wind.
2	Atractylodes Bai Zhu (White Atractylodes rhizome).	Dries damp in spontaneous sweating, supports Spleen qi.
1	Astragalus Huang Qi (Astragalus root)	Dries damp, supports Spleen, adaptogen.

Eczema in Chinese Medicine

Eczema refers to small blisters or pustules that can later become chronic, with crusty or dry itchy patches. When there are red raised papules that weep and ooze, it is a sign of damp heat. Later in the crusty stage, it's damp heat with dryness. Syndromes follow from acute to old, chronic, and dried-up eczema.

- *Wind Damp Heat.* Sudden onset, severe itching, burning. Eruptions with unclear borders. **P** Superficial, wiry, rapid. **T** Red body, yellow, thick sticky coat. Fix: Yin Chiao, a classic Lung formula for early-onset colds or flu (Box 17.1).
- *Toxic Heat.* Eczema, skin ulcers, eruptions, pustules, with fever or thirst. This is a step beyond damp heat. Here, there is infection and pus. **P** Fine and rapid. **T** Red body, possible yellow coating. Use cooling, detoxifying herbs.
- *Wind Damp Heat with Dryness.* Eczema that is starting to dry up and calm down. There is less inflammation, less itching. **P** Superficial and rapid (heat), and thin on the left (for dryness). **T** Red body with possible cracks, or dry and thick (dryness), yellow and sticky coat. Fix: Jade Windscreen Formula (Box 25.2), starring Ledebouriella Fang Feng. Then add something moist and soothing to counteract the dryness of the Jade Windscreen, such as Plantain leaf or Asparagus root.
- *Damp combining with wind dryness caused by blood deficiency.* Chronic symptoms or repeat attacks, and thick and rough skin with pigmentation. **P** Thready or weak, especially on the left. **T** Slightly red with white coat. Fix: Build blood and moisture with Angelica Dang Gui (Dong Quai root) and Glycyrrhiza Gan Cao (Licorice root), or both.

Shingles in Chinese Medicine

Shingles are painful viral skin blisters that follow nerve pathways on one side of the body. Syndromes range from horribly acute pain and burning and proceed to end stages when lesions dry up. Nerve pain should ease but sometimes goes on for years.

- *Wind Heat.* Fever, malaise, and papular eruptions with prickly, burning pain and heat; restlessness; thirst. **P** Superficial, wiry, rapid. **T** Red body, thin yellow coat. Fix: Viral lung infection, heat clearing Yin Chiao with the flowers Lonicera Jin Yin Hua (Honeysuckle) and Forsythia Lian Qiao.
- *Qi and Blood Stagnation.* Later stage of shingles when it's going away (thank heavens). Dry, crusty red or brown spots, nerve pain. **P** Wiry. **T** Slightly purple body, thin white coat. Fix: Main herbs are Bupleurum Chai Hu (Asian Buplever root) that restores the liver and Angelica Dang Gui (Dong Quai) to move blood and qi.

Skin Materia Medica

The skin Materia Medica ranges across the board. Some herbs treat symptoms, whereas others address underlying causes. Categories include *vulneraries* used for tissue healing in wound trauma; ***antiseptics*** applied locally to wounds to clear infection; *hemostatics* to stop any bleeding; *antimicrobials* for varied skin infections; ***alteratives*** that restore proper functioning through detoxification and waste elimination; *lymphatic drainers* to encourage cleansing, reduce edema, help immune function; *diuretics* to move out toxic wastes and dry damp; *antiinflammatories; analgesics; antipruritics* for any itching; and *anticontusion* remedies.

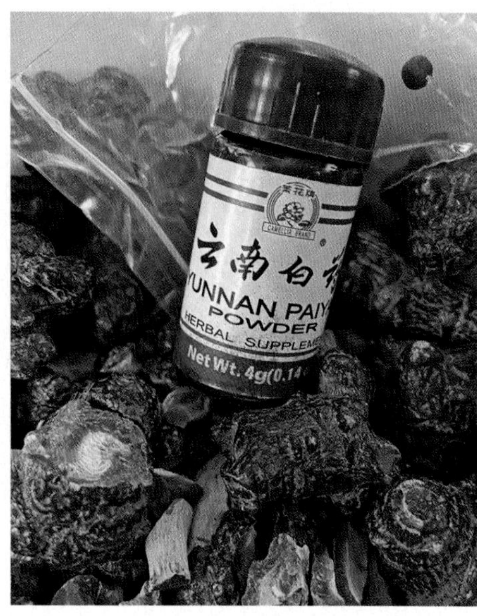

• **Fig. 25.2** *Panax notoginseng* San Qi (Notoginseng root) is a revered Chinese herb that moves qi and blood and is used for acute injuries. It is a key ingredient in Yunnan Baiyao powder with its vulnerary, analgesic, and hemostatic attributes. The patent comes with a little red pill to be used for emergency hemorrhage.

Skin Herbs Worth Honorable Mention

- *Panax notoginseng* San Qi (Notoginseng, Pseudoginseng, or Tienchi ginseng root). This qi-moving and blood-moving, rock-hard root is the most highly valued Chinese herb for tissue trauma, the gold standard. It is featured in Dit da Jow liniment (Box 24.4) and is specially indicated for traumatic injuries accompanied by bleeding, and followed by pain, bruising, swelling, and infection. San Qi contains more than 200 identified constituents that provide vulnerary, antioxidant, analgesic, hemostatic, immunostimulant, and hypotensive (vasodilation) properties all at once.
  - Notoginseng appears in another famous (and secret) Chinese Medicine patent trauma remedy called Yunnan Baiyao, historically used in World War II and carried by Viet Cong soldiers in the Vietnam War (Fig. 25.2). The little red pill included with the powder is an emergency treatment for hemorrhage. Use in tinctures, liniments, and balms. Pair with Western Calendula flower.
- *Smilax officinalis* (Jamaican Sarsaparilla root). This root is frequently used and is a respected Western detoxicant alterative for chronic skin conditions, such as psoriasis, which is a form of arthritis, and genital herpes. It is also notable as an arterial stimulant in chronic rheumatoid arthritis of Wind Damp Bi as discussed in Chapter 24. It contains many types of saponins, giving it a hormonal, antiinflammatory action. Exemplary as a chronic rheumatic skin and chronic arthritis remedy because both problems respond well to detoxification.
- *Boswellia serrata* (Frankincense resin). Dry, astringent, warm, and stimulating Middle Eastern Frankincense oleoresin has been burned as incense ceremonially and medicinally in Egyptian, Greek, and Hebrew medicine and is one of the most highly valued herbs in Ayurveda. *B. serrata* is foremost an antiinflammatory and inhibits many inflammatory cascade enzymes such as 5-lipoxygenase. It has been shown to be antiarthritic, antiinflammatory, antihyperlipidemic, antiatherosclerotic, analgesic, and hepato-protective.[12] In addition to chronic inflammatory disease, it has been traditionally used as a vulnerary. But for its antiinflammatory effect, this is the species to use (according to firsthand advice from more than one herbalist).
  - *Boswellia carterii* Ru Xiang (another Frankincense species) was incorporated into Chinese Medicine where its main action is as a vulnerary in trauma, for pain, and to stop bleeding. It is a great remedy for sores that do not exhibit draining pus, and for ulcers, wounds, swollen gums, and Wind Damp Bi syndromes. Its analgesic effect is also applied to menstrual and arthritic pain.[13] *B. carterii* is used spectacularly in essential oil form to stop tumor growth of the breasts, pancreas, and bladder.
- *Commiphora myrrha* Mo Yao (Myrrh resin). For acute and chronic sores, ulcers, and nonhealing wounds that contain puslike boils, abscesses, carbuncles, and toxic heat stages of eczema.[13] Use for acute trauma as a first-aid medicine to reduce pain and swelling and to treat chronic nonhealing infectious wounds because it is antibacterial, antiviral, and antifungal. It is antiinflammatory, analgesic, and anticontusion, and it excels as a mouthwash for gingivitis (inflamed and infected gums).
- *Honey.* Raw and unfiltered honey from the Manuka bush in New Zealand is considered the best kind of honey because of its high antibacterial action produced by a unique compound in the Manuka flower. It is also very expensive. Any honey derived from wild unsprayed flower pollen is better than no honey. Honey is antimicrobial and antiinflammatory, and it prevents scarring, controls odor, absorbs moisture (hygroscopic), and lasts forever without spoiling, because most pathogens can't survive in it.[5] For bed sores, burns, and other wounds, apply directly to gauze bandage to avoid the sticky factor. It is a good medium in which to infuse other herbs or essential oils such as Lavender or Tea Tree for burns and wound healing. When infused with Osha root and Garlic clove, honey may be taken internally for a sore throat and cough.

Vulneraries, the Wound Healers

Vulneraries are herbs that heal general skin lesions and soft-tissue injuries. Soft-tissue injuries refer to open trauma wounds such as ***lacerations*** (a deep cut or tear), ***abrasions*** (superficial scrapes), ***hematomas*** (bruising or localized swelling of clotted or partially clotted blood and caused by a break in the wall of a blood vessel that makes a black-and-blue mark), and ***puncture wounds*** (caused by splinters, thorns, or foreign objects that pierce the skin). Vulneraries that heal soft-tissue injuries could be in an herbalist's basic first-aid kit (Table 25.1).

Vulneraries are also used for healing lesions from various conditions, such as acne, shingles, eczema, boils, and skin eruptions of all kinds. Vulneraries can be applied externally through liniments, salves, soft and hard plasters, poultices, and compresses. They are used internally through decoction or tincture.

Vulneraries can have many actions. They are tissue repairing and can be antiseptic and/or antimicrobial, antiinflammatory, *emollient* (a demulcent used on the skin), and analgesic; they can also reduce swelling (*edema*). Bruising calls for Arnica flower and/or Panax San Qi (Notoginseng root). To reduce itching, consider Witch Hazel leaf, Calendula flower (Fig. 25.3), or Chickweed herb. Good astringents to reduce discharge and sepsis include Wild Geranium root and Witch Hazel leaf. For inflammation, use Boswellia resin, Chamomile flower, Calendula flower, and Plantain leaf. For strong broad-spectrum antimicrobial vulneraries, single out Frankincense and Myrrh resins, Creosote (Chaparral leaf), and Turmeric root. Bleeding wounds call for hemostatics or ***styptics***, such as Panax San Qi, Yarrow flower, and Shepherd's Purse herb (Table 25.2).

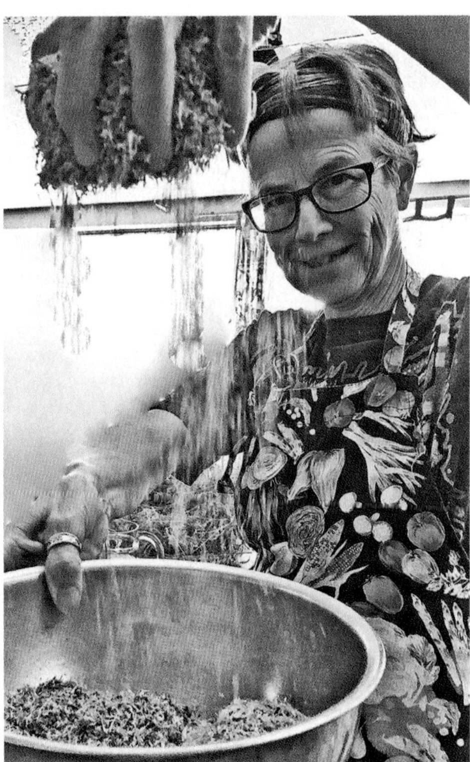

• **Fig. 25.3** Lisa sifting through *Calendula officinalis* flower, a classic skin vulnerary. Lisa Ganora, Director of Colorado School of Clinical Herbalism, Lafayette, CO.

Alteratives

This category is variously called alteratives, depuratives, blood cleansers, and blood purifiers. ***Alteratives*** work from the inside out and help the body eliminate toxins (Table 25.3). They do this in diverse ways by cleansing through the liver, kidneys, and/or lymph. Some are antibacterial (Echinacea root). Blue Flag rhizome, Yellow Dock root, Dandelion root, and Poke root stimulate the liver. Burdock root and Knotgrass herb work chiefly through the kidneys. Some move lymph (Fig. 25.4) (Cleavers herb and Red Root), which activates lymphocytes and macrophages and helps drain bacteria and toxins, returning them to the bloodstream so that elimination can take place.

Because many chronic skin diseases such as eczema, psoriasis, or herpes are in part caused by toxic overload, alteratives are needed as a part of those formulations. The Eclectics used them extensively with good results. They take a long time to work their magic. Ideally, include one or two that affects more than one avenue of elimination. For instance, combine a lymphatic drainer with a diuretic or combine a liver and lymphatic stimulant, all depending on individual case. If the problem is glaringly liver related, then use two liver alteratives (Fig. 25.5).

In the Chinese Medicine system, skin outbreaks call for alteratives (although not called that). They are herbs that clear heat, damp heat, or toxic heat; one example is Lonicera Jin Yin Hua (Honeysuckle flower).

Indications for alteratives include:

1. Skin diseases traditionally associated with toxemia or metabolic overload.
2. Many cases of eczema and hives.
3. Many other skin diseases, if accompanied by wider acting botanicals addressing underlying problems, like gut and liver health.
4. Joint and other connective-tissue diseases.

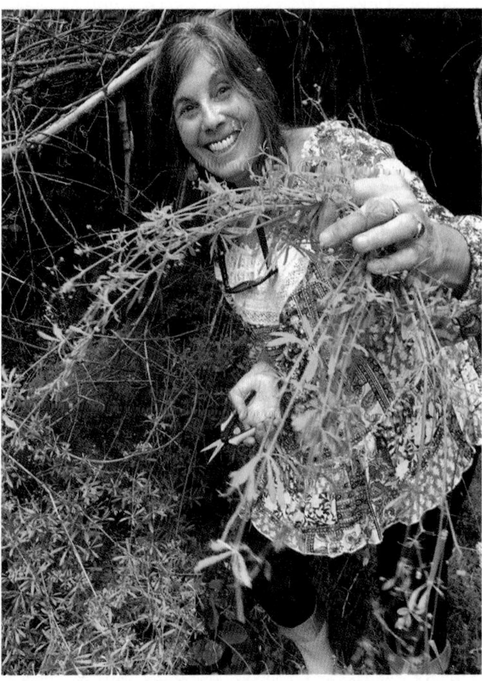

• **Fig. 25.4** Rachel Lord collecting *Galium aparine* (Cleavers herb), an alterative, kidney diuretic/detoxicant, and lymphatic drainer.

TABLE 25.1 Basic First Aid for Wounds[5]

Herbs		First Aid Steps
Step #1 Antiseptics to irrigate dirty wounds. • Normal saline (1 tsp. salt to 1 qt. boiled water) • *Salvia officinalis* (Garden Sage herb) • *Achillea millefolium* (Yarrow herb) • *Monarda* spp. (Bee Balm herb) • *Propolis* (Bee glue). Resinous, waterproof mixture made by bees to seal up the hive. Antimicrobial, antiseptic, and antioxidant. A waterproof band-aid.	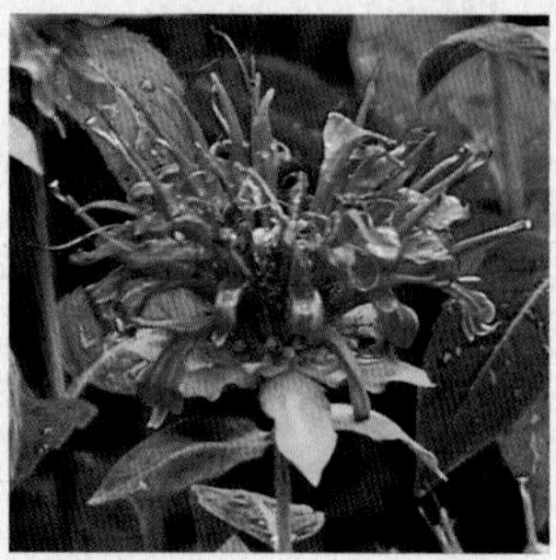 Bright purple Bee Balm herb makes a good antiseptic tea to irrigate dirty wounds.	**Step #1 Clean wound.** 1. Clean wound (wash or irrigate). Get rid of all debris before applying a vulnerary. 2. Normal saline works as an irrigant. Have at least a gallon ready to pour over wounds. 3. If using herbs to irrigate, make a light infusion, strain, cool to room temperature, and gently clean wound. 4. Cover wound with either an herbal vulnerary cream or an essential oil; do not need both. 5. Alternately, cover with a high alcohol 80% Propolis tincture. Acts as an exceptionally effective antimicrobial vulnerary.[5]
Step #2 Hemostatics or styptics. • *Larrea* spp. (Creosote, Chaparral leaf) • *Achillea millefolium* (Yarrow flower) • *Plantago* spp. (Plantain leaf) • *Capsella bursa* (Shepherd's Purse herb) • *Hamamelis virginica* (Witch Hazel leaf) • *Geranium* spp. (Cranesbill root) • *Quercus* spp. (Oak bark)	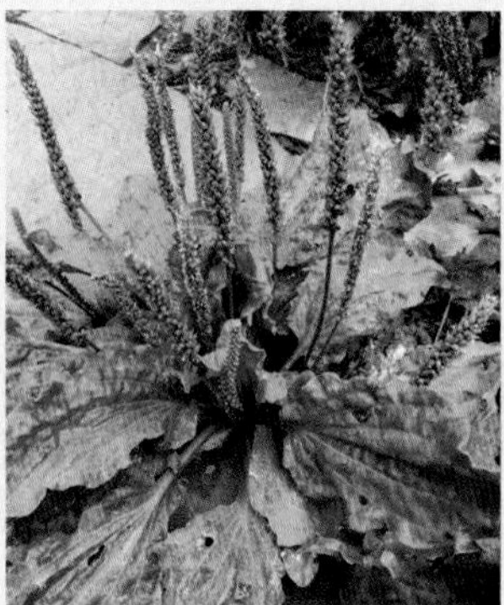 Plantain leaf is a great first aid herb because of its styptic and vulnerary actions.	**Step #2 Stop bleeding.** 1. If bleeding is severe, apply pressure. 2. If not, irrigate first, apply pressure to stop bleeding, then allow clot to form. Otherwise, a clotted dirty wound will still need to be cleaned. And then while cleaning, the clot will break and start bleeding all over again. (This clinical pearl comes from practical experience.)
Step #3 Vulnerary essential oils.[20] Lavender, Chamomile (all types), Geranium, Myrrh, Frankincense, Hyssop, Patchouli, Rose, Spearmint, Thuja, Rose, Spearmint, Juniper.		**Step #3 Use healing essential oils.** These essential oils double as vulneraries and antiseptics. After wound is cleaned and bleeding is under control, apply oils neat or mix in a carrier medium like olive or grapeseed oil or honey. Test on noninjured area to evaluate skin sensitivity.

There is such a thing as a *healing crisis* that once upon a time was sought after in traditional homeopathic and naturopathic circles. It refers to a dramatic detoxification reaction with temporary worsening of skin symptoms and eruptions, often brought on by fasting and heroic cleanses. It used to be considered a positive sign of healing, a sign of the toxins coming out. However, healing is not a crisis, and if this exacerbation occurs, too much has happened too quickly, and otherwise healthy skin has become inflamed and damaged. One herb known to accomplish a healing crisis was Burdock root.[15] So do not provoke the situation and instead combine Burdock root with other alteratives to balance out the effect.

Considerations for Treating the Skin

Therapeutic principles and herbal choices for skin management depend on suspected cause. This should be determined initially, if possible. Without expecting herbalists to be full-fledged dermatologists, a few good questions, awareness of the possibilities, and deductive reasoning can help. Here are some possible causes.

- *Microbe-induced eruptions*. Sometimes skin eruptions are from microorganisms. They may come from interior infections or from outside sources. Fungi cause athlete's foot and yeast infections. Bacterial infections often arise from *Staphylococcus aureus* and *Streptococcus pneumoniae*. Viruses cause warts,

TABLE 25.2 General Vulneraries (Wound healers)

Herbal Vulneraries	Notes
Larrea spp. Creosote, Chaparral leaf	Hemostatic, antiinflammatory, broad-spectrum antimicrobial for tissue repair.
Achillea millefolium Yarrow herb	Hemostatic, antiinflammatory. Convenient, outdoor, field first-aid herb.
Panax notoginseng San Qi Notoginseng or Pseudoginseng root	Most valued vulnerary in Chinese medicine. First choice for bleeding, followed by pain, bruising, and swelling.
Boswellia serrata Ru Xiang Frankincense resin	Hemostatic, strong antibacterial, antiviral, antifungal, antiinflammatory, and antiseptic. For edema, and wounds with pus.
Commiphora myrrha Mo Yao Myrrh resin	Hemostatic. For wound healing with pain, swelling, pus, bruising, and inflammation. Great for skin and mouth ulcers, loose teeth.
Calendula officinalis Pot Marigold flower	Antiinflammatory, mild antiinfective, prevents scarring, detoxicant, lymphatic drainer. For burns, bites, cuts, diaper rash.
Plantago spp. Plantain leaf	Hemostatic, draws out infection, antimicrobial, clears toxic heat. For pain, contusions, and bleeding. Great outdoor field herb.
Arnica spp. Arnica flower Medium strength.	Classic externally for bruises. Used in sprains, strains. Not for sensitive or broken skin.[20] Said to be toxic internally.
Symphytum officinalis Comfrey leaf For proliferation and remodeling stages of healing.	Comfrey is such a quick wound healer it should not be used without other strong antimicrobials if there is infection. Otherwise infection can seal in under the healed skin. Use in later stages of healing, i.e., proliferation and remodeling.[5]
Curcuma longa Turmeric rhizome	Has pronounced antiinflammatory effect on the skin.[15] Broad-spectrum antimicrobial.
Antiitching for pruritus *Stellaria media* (Chickweed herb) *Hamamelis virginica* (Witch Hazel leaf) *Calendula officinalis* (Marigold flower) *Hypericum perforatum* (St. John's Wort) *Avena sativa* (Colloidal oatmeal bath) Apple cider vinegar (organic)	Chickweed herb is exemplary for soothing and cooling. Use for chickenpox lesions, eczema, poison ivy, and bug bites; all itch. Over the counter, double-distilled T.N. Dickinson's Witch Hazel extract with 14% alcohol is tried and true for itchy rashes, and bites. It has been around since the mid-1800s.
Emollients for dryness *Plantago* spp. (Plantain leaf) *Aloe vera* (Aloe gel) *Stellaria media* (Chickweed herb) *Calendula officinalis* (Marigold flower) *Matricaria recutita* (Chamomile flower)	Emollients contain mucilage, moisten, and soothe. Indicated for dry stages of skin lesions, especially eczema and psoriasis and for dry, aging skin.
Strong skin antimicrobials *Commiphora myrrha* Mo Yao (Myrrh resin) *Scutellaria* Huang Qin (Baikal Skullcap root) *Larrea* spp. (Chaparral leaf) *Curcuma longa* (Turmeric rhizome)	These are cooling, broad-spectrum antimicrobials that have an affinity for skin lesions. Damp Heat and Toxic Use for damp heat and toxic heat.

shingles, and herpes. Parasites cause body and head lice. If the exact organism is unknown, choose one or two broad-spectrum antimicrobial herbs.

- *Hampered elimination*. Skin rashes from hampered elimination arise from insufficient detoxification through the kidney, liver, colon, and lymphatics. The toxins exit through the skin when other avenues are overloaded. Toxic exposure from fertilizers, pollution, food sensitivities, heavy metals, and errors of metabolism all cause internal toxic buildup. These causes are best determined through a good health history. Herbal choices

TABLE 25.3 Alteratives
(Traditionally called blood cleansers; clear Damp Heat)

Herb	Notes
Galium aparine Cleavers herb	Kidney diuretic/detoxicant and lymphatic drainer. For skin eruptions, Skin Damp Heat, and Toxic Heat.
Urtica dioica Nettle herb	Kidney, diuretic/detoxicant. General for all skin eruptions to eliminate metabolic waste.
Solidago spp. Goldenrod herb	Kidney, diuretic/detoxicant, antiallergenic and antiinflammatory. For chronic skin conditions, dermatitis, eczema, and acne.
Arctium lappa Burdock root	Kidney and liver detoxicant, diuretic, antiinflammatory, helps immune function. For damp and toxic heat. Skin-specific for burns, sores, and ulcers.
Taraxacum officinalis Dandelion root	Liver stimulant and kidney diuretic, antiinflammatory, detoxicant. For Skin Damp Heat, Toxic Heat, boils, and abscesses.
Berberis aquifolium Oregon Grape root, Mountain Holly	Liver detoxifier. For herpes, acne, and skin specific scaly eruptions, like psoriasis.
Smilax officinalis Jamaican Sarsaparilla root	Liver stimulant. Exceptional general alterative for any chronic skin eruption, such as eczema, psoriasis, or acne. Excels in chronic rheumatoid arthritis.
Iris versicolor Blue Flag rhizome Medium-strength, use with other herbs.	Liver stimulant. For Skin Damp Heat. Use with Dandelion root.
Phytolacca decandra Poke root Medium-strength; stronger than Blue Flag. Use in small quantities with other herbs. Can be toxic.	Liver stimulant, deep and strong systemic detoxicant. For eczema with chronic dryness, painful swollen hard glands, especially breast lumps; used in a poultice. Combine with a diuretic.[5]
Rumex crispus Yellow Dock root	Well-rounded detoxicant works through kidneys, liver, and lymph. Support with other alteratives. For psoriasis.
Scrophularia nodosa Figwort root and herb	Liver and lymph alterative, vulnerary, antiinflammatory, and antifungal.
Ceanothus americanus Red Root	Lymphatic drainer, stops bleeding, immune stimulant. Damp Heat with liver and lymph stagnation. Combines nicely with Burdock root.
Chimaphila umbellata Pipsissewa/Wintergreen herb, root and essential oil from the northern hemisphere. *Gaultheria procumbens* Wintergreen herb from northeastern North Americas.	Lymphatic drainer, detoxicant, and a salicylate. For Skin Damp Heat. Both botanicals, commonly called Wintergreen, are interchangeable in usage.
Echinacea angustifolia Echinacea root	Lymphatic drainer, detoxicant, immunostimulant, antiviral, and antibacterial.
Calendula officinalis Pot Marigold flower	Lymphatic drainer. Skin Damp Heat and toxic heat. Antiinflammatory.
Juglans regia Walnut leaf and hull	Lymphatic drainer, antiparasitic, dries damp. For eczema, ringworm, and herpes.
Viola tricolor Heartsease, Wild Pansy herb	Lymphatic mover, helps immunity, vulnerary. For allergic eczema, herpes, psoriasis, Wind Damp Heat. Skin-specific.
Equisetum arvense Horsetail herb	General alterative and connective tissue trophorestorative and clears damp heat. For toxicosis in all skin rashes, chronic eczema, arthritis, and osteoporosis.
Trifolium pratense Red Clover flower	General alterative. For Skin Damp and Toxic Heat, chronic skin conditions. Combines nicely with Cleavers.

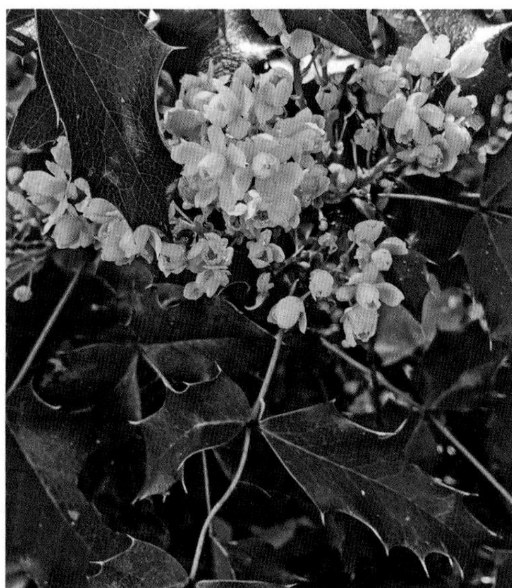

• **Fig. 25.5** *Berberis aquifolium* (Oregon Grape root, Mountain Holly) flowering. The root is a detoxifying alterative, with a tropism to the liver. Use for herpes, acne, and skin-specific scaly eruptions, like psoriasis.

call for alteratives, lymphatic drainers, and diuretics. Of course, a good look at the microbiome and liver never hurts.

- *Timing.* When and how quickly the outbreak occurred is a factor.
  - *Immediate.* If something erupts quickly, as in hives, a likely suspect is some type of allergic reaction. Symptoms range from hives and itching to totally emergent anaphylactic shock status. Type I immediate allergies from ingestion of antigenic foods (strawberries, peanuts, corn, wheat, milk, shellfish, or eggs) come on fast, as can physical triggers from heat, cold, or exercise. To treat acute hives, include antiallergic herbs that clear heat, inflammation, and itching. For chronic hives, use alteratives, immunomodulators, and antiallergics. Miscellaneous outbreaks of hives occur from all kinds of medication reactions, especially antibiotics. Oh, and did I mention that allergies have a gut-liver relationship?
  - *Delayed skin reactions.* These reactions often involve allergic eczema or contact dermatitis, maybe taking a few hours to occur. An example is an itchy skin rash after coming in contact with an allergen such as mold, dyes, cosmetics, perfumes, and soaps. Don't forget about insect bites, ticks, or poison ivy if the client is an outdoor type. These reactions can occur right away or even the next day. On the other hand, the plaques of psoriasis, the most common autoimmune skin disease out there, has a gradual onset.
- *Stress.* Anxiety and stress cause many existing skin conditions to become worse or to recur. Flare-ups of shingles or adult acne are stress related. Unconscious scratching caused by stress may result in reddened, raised, and inflamed areas. Remember, even herbs can cause skin reactions. Most skin conditions will require a sedating nervine in the mix.
- *Trauma.* This term refers to first-aid issues: bites, cuts, abrasions, and such. Treatment depends on where it happened. If in town, the herbalist can be conservative and err on the side of caution because medical help is accessible. If camping or out in the woods, more heroics might be necessary. This text covers the small stuff, minor skin trauma (Case History 25.1). Your intentions are to stop bleeding and prevent infection. Herbal categories include hemostatics (or almost any astringent for bleeding), antimicrobials, antiinflammatories, vulneraries, and analgesics.

CASE HISTORY 25.1

Case History for Road Rash

S. Jack scraped up his knee when he fell off his mountain bike riding very fast around a curve. He was wearing shorts. The wound covers his entire knee, which is raw, red, bleeding, and filled with dirt and gravel.
O. **P** Rapid. **T** Normal. Raw, dirty wound.
A. Trauma-induced scrape or road rash.
P. *Specific therapeutic principles.* (1) Irrigate and clean off dirt and gravel with normal saline using a gauze pad. (2) Cover a new large sterile gauze pad (or two) liberally with a first aid salve containing hemostatic, tissue healer, and antibiotic herbs. (3) Apply to knee and wrap with paper tape or elasticized bandage to hold gauze in place. (4) Change dressing daily. If gauze becomes dried up and stuck to the wound, dribble some normal saline over it to loosen without disturbing clot. (5) Internal formula: use same type of herbs as in salve, plus something for anxiety and pain.

Herbal First-Aid Salve.

This salve should obviously be pre-made in your first aid kit or pack.
Apply externally to wound. Change dressing daily, if wet, and/or more often, as needed.

Parts	Herbs	Rationale
2	Calendula flower	Antimicrobial, antiinflammatory, tissue repair.
2	Myrrh resin	Stops bleeding, pain, swelling, antimicrobial.
1	Yarrow herb	Stops bleeding, heals tissue.
1	Chaparral leaf	Hemorrhagic, antiinflammatory, antimicrobial, tissue repair.

Internal Herbal Formula and Dose. 5 mL 3 × daily

Parts	Herbs	Rationale
3	Calendula flower	Antimicrobial, antiinflammatory, vulnerary.
2	Panax San Qi	Bleeding, pain, bruising, swelling.
2	Prickly Ash bark	Move qi and Blood, analgesic.
2	Passionflower herb	For pain and anxiety.

Other Suggestions

Change dressing daily or when needed. May need to wet bandage before removing so scab isn't pulled off. Apply salve to bandage and secure.

Common Skin Conditions

Minor Skin Trauma

- *Definition.* Minor skin trauma refers to simple first aid for minor cuts, abrasions, puncture wounds of the everyday type (Case History 25.1) that are not spurting or bleeding profusely, not life threatening, and don't require sutures unless you have experience and comfort with butterfly bandages or Steri-strips (sterile pieces of medical tape used to close wounds and help edges grow back together). The moment skin is broken, even for a second, microbes are already entering. Preventing infection is key. Anything more serious requires a first-aid course or a hospital emergency department visit.

- *Stages of wound healing.* (1) *Hemostasis.* When injury occurs and a wound bleeds, the clotting phase (coagulation) begins. Platelets and clotting factors stabilize and form platelet plugs. This stage might need help. Yarrow herb or Wild Geranium root are hemostatic. (2) *Healthy inflammation.* This occurs within minutes or hours to neutralize toxins and prevent infection. White blood cells and macrophages clean up the area, and fluid rushes in. Skin looks pale or slightly reddened, does not grow or spread, and feels warm but shows no pus, with a light uniform swelling. Myrrh resin or Oak or Willow bark are helpful in this stage. (3) *Proliferation* is next if all goes well, lasting a few days to a few weeks. The wound meshes together and closes, taking on the original growth pattern and shape. Vulneraries, Plantain, and Comfrey leaf help proliferation. (4) *Remodeling.* After the tissue is regrown and closed, original tissue is slowly replaced to regain full strength and function. This process takes months to years or may never occur. If scar tissue has formed, remodeling remains incomplete. Scar tissue is not the original. It has no blood supply and is weaker than the unscarred area around it. It is prone to injury and reinfection.[5] Scar tissue is a common site of cellulitis with dangerous staph or strep infections under the skin. Comfrey leaf, Calendula flower, and Aloe gel help remodeling.
- *Overall therapeutic principles.* Minor skin trauma involves more consciousness and awareness than just slapping on a Band-Aid. There are many considerations.
  - (1) *Clean it up.* Even if nothing else is done, the wound needs to be clean. Sometimes just the act of allowing fresh bleeding cleans out debris. *Irrigate* (clean it) by slowly pouring normal saline (1 teaspoon noniodized salt to 1 quart water) over it. Normal saline is a 0.9% solution of salt and water. It is isotonic, the same tonicity as tissue fluids and blood, so cell fluid volume stays constant and water does not leak in or out. An alternative to normal saline is a weak herbal tea with Nettle herb, Plantain leaf, or Yarrow herb. Or just tap water with or without mild soap (castile is excellent). If outdoors, a natural running stream will do in a pinch, but the wound will need recleaning when the person gets home. If a wound has been opened and uncovered for more than 20 minutes, do not use herbs, because they could make it worse. Infection is too likely. Clean, bandage, cover, and watch. If it is healing well in a day or two and no infection present, then add the herbals.[5]
  - (2) *Stop bleeding.* Spurting, bright red blood implies an arterial bleed. This is not minor, and further help is needed. Apply pressure immediately. No butterflies unless you are confident and experienced. If the wound just oozes or bleeds dark red, it indicates a venous bleed and can usually be handled. Wash it up before applying pressure. If pressure is applied to a dirty wound, it will still need to be cleaned later. This could break the clot and reopen the wound, causing it to again bleed, bringing you back to square one. If that situation happens, apply more gauze to the clean wound. Hold gauze on with pressure to stop or ease bleeding and add another gauze pad if needed, without removing the first.
  - (3) *Apply dressing.* This step is when a vulnerary might be used. If using a first-aid salve (that ideally contains a styptic, a tissue healer, and an antibacterial), apply salve to the Band-Aid or gauze pad (not to wound) and tape the whole thing down or wrap it up, using enough pressure to hold gauze in place and stop any bleeding but not tight enough to block circulation. The pressure helps clot formation, and the medicated ointment stops the gauze from sticking to the wound and breaking the clot the next time the dressing is changed. If out in the woods with no cream, use an herbal poultice. Pick some Plantain leaf or Coltsfoot leaf or Yarrow herb, or any of the countless other astringent plants. After cleaning wound, crush the leaves and place over area. Then wrap with gauze and a bandana (or whatever is available) to hold it together. (Do not chew or spit on leaves; the human mouth is filled with bacteria.) This method eliminates use of the popularized but ill-advised spit poultice.
  - (4) *Change dressing as needed.* Minimally, change daily or if and when it gets wet or blood soaked or smelly. Watch for signs of infection, which can be detected through foul smell, pus, and an extremely angry, large reddened area that has gone beyond the normal pink-around-the-edge look that indicates healthy inflammation. Add stronger antibiotics, such as Chaparral leaf or Myrrh resin, or both.

Eczema

- *Definition.* ***Eczema*** is referred to as dermatitis or atopic dermatitis; both terms mean the same thing (Case History 25.2). It's a superficial skin inflammation. An allergic component is common. Eczema may be caused by outside exogenous sources, most often from direct contact with dyes, solvents, metals (often nickel), soaps, or leather-tanning chemicals, and it often occurs in people with history of hay fever and allergies. You must detect and remove the source if possible. Endogenous inside sources include food allergies and sensitivities (often milk and milk products), stress, and toxicity.
- *Signs and symptoms.* Acute stage presents with toxic heat, including redness, itching, peeling, weepy skin, sometimes pustules. Later it dries up, becomes chronic, and looks like scratched-up, scaly, thickened dry skin, a little darker than surrounding tissue. Scratching can lead to bleeding and infection. Eczema comes and goes, from acute to chronic and back, depending on triggers, which are often from stress, heat, mechanical irritation, and dietary factors. Lesions are commonly on elbows, back of knees, ankles, feet, and face.
- *Allopathic treatment.* Eliminate known allergens and treat inflammation; use topical steroids, wet dressings, and antibiotics for secondary infection.
- *General therapeutic principles.* There are many, depending on cause. (1) If external, remove allergens. (2) If related to food sensitivity, remove wheat or dairy first, using elimination diet with Four-R Program. (3) Alteratives are basic, classic long-term remedies. Choose those that work on lymphatic, kidney, and then liver levels.[4] Try Red Clover flower, Cleavers herb, and Jamaican Sarsaparilla root. If necessary, go to stronger liver herbs like Burdock root or Blue Flag rhizome to support detoxification and digestion. Liver herbs are the last choice because they may be too strong for eczema and make it worse.[4] (4) Use antiinflammatories. (5) Use immunomodulators like Echinacea root. (6) Topically, use vulneraries, antiinflammatories, antipruritics, antimicrobials, astringents if draining and weeping, and moist and cooling emollients for soothing.

CASE HISTORY 25.2

Case History for Acute Eczema

S. Elise has had a skin rash for the last 5 years that comes and goes with frequent flare-ups. Presently, it has flared up with weeping raised papules on her stomach and hips and behind her elbows and knees. They burn and itch like crazy. She tries not to scratch. She does not think it's from touching anything. She has been under a lot of stress lately. Her favorite foods are cheese and ice cream.
O. **P** Fine and rapid. **T** Red body.
A. Toxic Heat. Acute eczema with pustules, oozing, and itching.
P. *Specific therapeutic principles.* (1) Cooling antibacterials. (2) Antiinflammatories. (3) Alteratives for kidney and lymphatics. (4) Calming nervine. (5) Digestive restorative. (6) External cream: antipruritic, antiinflammatory, antimicrobial, and astringent.

Herbal Formula and Dose. 5 mL 3 × daily

Parts	Herbs	Rationale
3	Chaparral leaf	Antibacterial.
2	Nettle herb	Kidney detox, diuretic, lymphatic drainer, antiallergic.
2	Echinacea root	Antibacterial and immune modulation.
2	Passionflower herb	Calming, antianxiety.
1	Licorice root	Antiinflammatory, gut healing, soothing.

External Herbal Salve. Apply 3 × daily and after bath

Parts	Herbs	Rationale
2	Myrrh resin	Antiseptic, antiinflammatory, astringent for pus, analgesic.
2	Turmeric rhizome	Strong skin antiinflammatory and antibacterial.
1	Chickweed herb	Emollient and antipruritic.
1	Calendula flower	Antiinflammatory, antiseptic, vulnerary, prevents scarring.

Other Suggestions

Strategy. When acute phase is gone, change formula and begin long-term alteratives, Spleen tonics, and bitters. Concentrate on Four-R program.

- *Diet.* Elimination diet: Remove dairy first. Cleansing vegetable and meat broth based. No sugar.
- Nettle tea 3 × daily.
- Daily bath with colloidal oatmeal.
- *Supplements.* Essential fatty acids EPA/DHA 2000 mg a day.

CASE HISTORY 25.3

Case History for Psoriasis

S. Ed has psoriasis, as diagnosed by his dermatologist. It has been unresponsive to all over-the-counter medications over the years. At the consultation, his chest, elbows, and knees have thick silvery scaly patches outlined in red that are difficult to scrape off. It is actually better than usual. His blood pressure is 180/100, and he appears very stressed and sweating.
O. **P** Fast. **T** Red body, dry sticky coat.
A. Heat with dryness. Chronic psoriasis with hypertension and anxiety.
P. *Specific therapeutic principles.* (1) Clear heat and detox with alteratives for liver first, then kidney and lymph. (2) Diuretics to clear damp. (3) Antiinflammatories. (4) Nervine relaxant for anxiety. (5) Hypotensives. (6) External cream: cooling, soothing, and antiinflammatory.

Herbal Formula and Dose. 6 mL 3 × daily

Parts	Herbs	Rationale
4	Jamaican Sarsaparilla root	Alterative, liver detoxification.
3	Yellow Dock root	Alterative, liver detoxicant and diuretic.
2	Cleavers herb	Lymphatic drainage, antiinflammatory, diuretic.
2	Passionflower herb	Stress, anxiety, and hypotensive.
2	Valerian root	Hypotensive, anxiolytic.
1	Licorice root	To add a little cooling moisture.

Cooling External Herbal Salve. Apply 3 × daily

Parts	Herbs	Rationale
1	Chickweed herb	Cooling emollient, antiinflammatory.
1	Calendula flower	Cooling emollient, antibacterial, vulnerary.
1	Boswellia resin	Clears heat, infection, and inflammation.
3–4 drops	Thuja or Cajeput essential oil	Antiinflammatory, antimicrobial.

Other Suggestions

- *Stress management.* Very important; yoga, meditation, massage, or whatever works.
- *Diet.* Mediterranean diet. Limit coffee, alcohol, and red meat. Lots of green veggies with rice, chicken, eggs, and fish.
- *Acupuncture.* For stress and anxiety.
- *Psychotherapy*, as needed.
- *Sunlight exposure.* Known to help.
- *Supplements.* Flax seed oil or EPA/DHA. Of some help may be Planetary Herbals' *Triphala* blend that provides gentle detoxification of the gastrointestinal tract and liver and the *Guggul* blend for antiinflammatory, detoxifying, qi- and blood-moving properties.[17]

Psoriasis

- *Definition.* ***Psoriasis*** refers to nasty, slow-developing, noncontagious, raised plaques caused from abnormally fast turnover of skin cells that do not shed, an autoimmune condition (Case History 25.3). Normally, skin cell life cycle is about 28 days, going from new epidermal tissue to sloughing and shedding. In psoriasis, the process takes 3 or 4 days. There are many forms. One is a type of arthritis where skin and joints are affected. In another, the nails (part of the skin) are affected, change color, and have small pinprick pitting holes.
- *Signs and symptoms.* Red skin with silvery scaly patches, usually on the joints of the elbows, knees, and feet; on the lower back; or on the scalp. They often crack and bleed. It is not an infection but may become so if opened. Itching is rare. It looks a lot like eczema, except psoriasis is usually well-defined and rarely itches, whereas eczema tends to cause a generalized rash and to be accompanied by intense itching.[19] Skin biopsy is diagnostic.
- *Cause.* Psoriasis is autoimmune. It has periods of remission and flare-ups, caused by triggers such as stress, skin trauma, tattoos,

cold and dry weather, and medications. It is very difficult to manage, much less cure. Psoriasis is very disfiguring and just having it is stressful, which, of course, triggers it further.

- *Allopathic treatment.* Hit or miss. Over the counter (OTC) creams with salicylic acid and coal tar, retinoid, and vitamin D_3. Coal tar and salicylic acid shampoos. Light therapy. Steroids, cortisone cream, and biologics, such as Humira. Biologics are genetically engineered proteins derived from human antibody cells. They block inflammatory TNF alpha.[14] Steroids and biologics depress the immune system, and a side effect is increased chance of infection.
- *General therapeutic principles.* As with any autoimmune disease, holistic measures are required, and an individualized program needs be designed. No herbs are specific. (1) Alteratives, the stronger hepatic ones should be included.[4] Burdock root and Figwort root to address detoxification and gut. (2) Alteratives working on lymphatic and kidney level. (3) Calming nervines. (4) Address gut health if needed. (5) External creams: emollients to help moisten and help scale removal, antiinflammatories, and antimicrobials.

Shingles

- *Definition.* ***Shingles*** is a herpes viral infection that causes a painful rash, which follows and affects a nerve ganglion on one side (Case History 25.4). It is caused by *Varicella-zoster virus* (VZV), the same virus that causes chickenpox. ***Herpes*** is a genus of viruses that comes in many forms and causes many diseases. All forms of herpes can go dormant. Once in the body, they're there for life and can pop up under stress. *Herpes simplex 1* (HSV1) causes cold sores on the face, lips, or mouth. *Herpes simplex 2* (HSV2) (and sometimes HSV1) causes sexually transmitted genital herpes; *Varicella-zoster virus* (VZV) causes chickenpox, goes into a latent stage in the nerves, and can later cause shingles *(Herpes zoster)*.[16] Shingles are no joke. In addition to being incredibly painful, they can lead to serious eye damage, bacterial infections, and Guillain-Barré syndrome. Sometimes the burning nerve pain becomes chronic and is known as *postherpetic neuralgia*. Shingles must be treated ASAP.
- *Signs and symptoms.* Burning, tingling, and severe pain along an affected nerve branch on one side of the body only, following a dermatome. Highly contagious, pus-filled blisters that look like chickenpox may erupt. Causes of outbreaks are all kinds of stressors, such as illness, pain, surgery, and spinal cord trauma. In rare cases, persistent deep nerve pain (neuralgia) can exist for years after the blisters heal.
- *Allopathic treatment.* Acyclovir, cortisone. Pain relief includes Tylenol, NSAIDs like ibuprofen, numbing agents such as lidocaine, topical capsaicin (Cayenne pepper), antidepressants, and anticonvulsants.
- *General therapeutic principles.* (1) Antivirals: St. John's Wort is specific. (2) Nerve tonics for traumatized tissue. (3) Nerve relaxants for pain and emotional stress. (4) Antispasmodics for muscle tension and pain. (5) Topicals: plasters and antiviral essential oils, such as Bergamot and Melaleuca.

CASE HISTORY 25.4

Case History for Shingles

S. Charles is 83 years old. His wife suddenly died, and he had a severe case of flu, which is now resolved. Suddenly, he broke out with whitish pustules down the left side of his neck onto his shoulder. They are horribly painful, burning, and itchy.

O. P Wiry, rapid. **T** Red body, thin yellow coat. White pustules observed down the left side of neck and onto shoulder.

A. Toxic Damp Heat. Shingles.

P. *Specific therapeutic principles.* (1) Antivirals. (2) Antiinflammatories. (3) Nervines and nerve relaxants. (4) External plasters and essential oils. (5) Drain damp, clear heat. (6) Support immune system.

Herbal Formula and Dose. 6 mg 3 × daily

Part	Herbs	Rationale
4	St. John's Wort	Antiviral, nerve tonic, antiinflammatory, antispasmodic.
3	Andrographis Chuan Xin Lian	Clear damp heat/viral infection.
3	Jamaican Dogwood or Corydalis Yan Hu Suo and/or Valerian root	Pain and spasms.
2	Skullcap herb	Nerve relaxant/antispasmodic.
1	Echinacea root	Immune support, antiviral.

Suggestions

Red Flag. If no improvement after a few days, refer out to a healthcare provider. Can have long-lasting complications, such as vision loss if it's in the eyes, or painful and chronic postherpetic neuralgia.

- *External treatment.* External salve of St. John's Wort and Calendula flower or essential oils of Lavender or Tea Tree, or Ravensara. Antiinflammatory.
- *Bath.* Colloidal oatmeal bath and/or plasters for pain and inflammation. This is traditional.
- Oat Straw or Milky Oat tops. Infusion 3 × daily as a nerve tonic.

Acne Vulgaris

- *Definition.* ***Acne vulgaris*** is an inflammatory skin condition involving oversecretion of sebum (oil) from the sebaceous glands into the hair (Case History 25.5). Hair follicles contain bacteria and join with lipase in the skin, creating a plug in the dilated follicle. What results is unsightly inflammation and often secondary infection. Acne can be a source of embarrassment, low self-esteem, and at worst, depression for a teenager or an adult, especially if all over the face, back, neck, or chest. It is often caused by genetics and by androgens (testosterone) that stimulate sebaceous gland growth. Production of this hormone peaks in puberty in both boys and girls. In adults, it can persist into the mid-20s and even into the 50s.
- *Signs and symptoms.* Eruptions on the face, neck, back, and chest in various forms. Blackheads are sebum (oil) plugs in a hair follicle that is blackened by oxidation; whiteheads are whitish elevations of sebum in blocked skin pores; papules are raised, red, solid, and inflamed pimples. Any of these can cause scarring if chronic. Acne becomes infectious when normal skin bacteria gets inside the lesions, which often happens.
- *Allopathic treatment.* Dismal choices. Cortisone creams, routine antibiotics (Tetracycline), estrogen therapy for girls (to counteract androgens), Retin-A to reduce sebum production (a dangerous idea that can cause birth defects), and huge doses of vitamin A, which can be toxic.
- *General therapeutic principles.* (1) Alteratives are the core treatment, especially hepatics like Burdock root or Yellow dock

CASE HISTORY 25.5

Case History for Acne Vulgaris

S. Kelly has been plagued with unsightly raised red pimples and whiteheads all over her face and neck ever since she got her period at age 11. She is now 29 years old. Pimples are worse just before her menses. She has tried every over-the-counter cream she could find, even stopped eating chocolate (which was hard). She was on Tetracycline for 3 years, to no avail.
O. **P** Rapid, wiry. **T** Thick white coat, teeth marks.
A. Skin Damp Heat. Persistent infectious acne.
P. *Specific therapeutic principles.* (1) All types of alteratives, including those for liver. (2) Clear heat and inflammation with cold, antiinfectious herbs. (3) Balance pituitary. (4) Topicals.

Herbal Formula and Dose. 5 mL 3 × daily for at least 3 months.

Part	Herbs	Rationale
3	Scutellaria Huang Qin	Clear damp heat, antimicrobial/astringent.
3	Burdock root	Liver and kidney alterative, diuretic, skin damp heat.
3	Chastetree berry	Balance hormones on pituitary level.
2	Cleavers herb	Lymphatic drainage/diuretic/detoxicant.
1	Echinacea root	Stop infection, detox, immune support.

Other Suggestions

- *Hygiene.* Keep hair and hands off the face. Wash face and hair often. No synthetic cosmetics/chemicals. Don't squeeze pimples.
- *Topical wash.* Witch Hazel leaf and strong Calendula infusion mixed 1:1. Tea Tree essential oil to pimples 3–4 × daily.
- *Nettle leaf infusion.* 3 cups 3 × daily.
- *Diet.* Very clean diet does wonders. Alkaline diet, meaning lots of fresh green veggies, lean meat, legumes, whole grains, and potatoes. Fermented foods are also recommended. Cut out alcohol, sodas, sugar, refined sugar, fried foods, and dairy.
- *Supplements.* Calcium/Magnesium that calms nervous system and helps stop sugar cravings; take minerals at night. Vitamin E 400 IU every day. Selenium 200 mcg PM, zinc 50 mg PM; all for normal skin function. If stimulated by menses, add vitamin B_6 for hormone balance.[15]
- *Digestion.* Balanced probiotic to counteract long dose of antibiotics, plus fermented foods. Dark leafy, bitter leaves and veggies.

root. (2) Other liver stimulants, such as Dandelion root or Blue Flag rhizome. (3) Cooling antimicrobials/antiinflammatories for secondary infection. (4) Detox/lymphatic drainers and diuretics to help elimination through kidneys like Cleavers herb or Red Root. (5) Nervines for anxiety as needed. (6) Hormone balance, Chastetree berry. (7) Topically, astringents and antimicrobials. See Pimple Juice in Box 25.3.

Athlete's Foot

- *Definition.* ***Athlete's foot*** *(Tinea pedis; pedis* means foot) is the most common kind of human fungal infection and occurs between the toes and on soles of the feet (Case History 25.6). *Tinea* spp. includes many types of fungi that cause conditions such as athlete's foot, ringworm, and jock itch. Athlete's foot spreads in warm, humid environments like swimming pools, from walking barefoot in locker rooms and showers, and from sharing wet towels. Sweaty feet make matters worse. It is highly contagious through direct and indirect contact and can be chronic and relapsing.

• BOX 25.3 Pimple Juice and Face Mud for Acne[6]

by Rosemary Gladstar

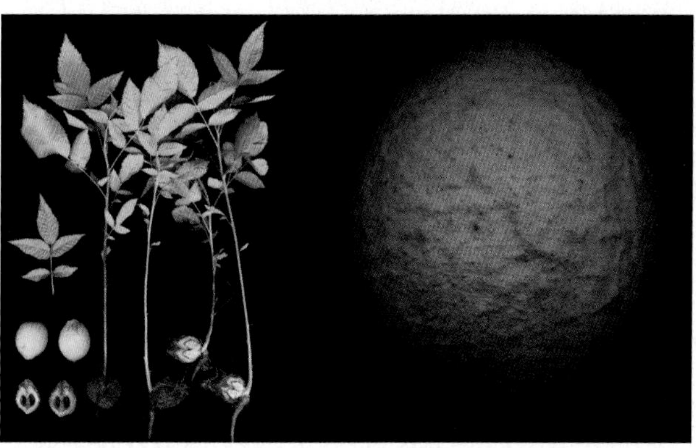

Antifungal Black Walnut tree sprouts and hull. (Copyright Lang/Tucker Photography. Photographs loaned with permission from *The Botanical Series* are copywritten by Jennifer Anne Tucker and Gerald Lang from the Studio at Hill Crystal Farm. www.jennifer-tucker.com.)

This astringent and antimicrobial blend works nicely to use topically over acne pimples. It can also be made into a face mud, as an overnight plaster.

Pimple Juice

Ingredients		
½ oz	Black Walnut hull	Astringent.
½ oz	Coptis Huang Lian or Goldenseal root	Astringent and antimicrobial.
½ oz	Echinacea root	Antimicrobial and detoxifying.
½ oz	Myrrh resin	Tissue repair, stops swelling, antiinflammatory.
1 pint	Isopropyl (rubbing) alcohol or Ethyl (grain) alcohol.	Isopropyl alcohol is toxic internally, but often used externally. Ethyl alcohol can be ingested.

Directions

Grind herbs into a powder and mix. Put in jar. Pour in rubbing alcohol, just covering herbs. Shake daily for 2–3 weeks. Strain or press and bottle. Add 2 drops Tea Tree essential oil to the finished juice. Apply to blemishes with cotton ball, as needed.

Face Mud for Acne

Ingredients	
Green, red, or white cosmetic clay	A carrier clay base is astringent and closes pores.
Pimple juice (recipe above)	Antimicrobial, astringent, antiinflammatory, and healing.
2 drops Tea Tree essential oil	Antifungal, antimicrobial.

Directions

Mix clay and Pimple Juice into a thick paste. Blend in essential oil. Store with tight-fitting lid or it will dry out. Apply mud overnight to areas with acne.

CASE HISTORY 25.6

Case History for Athlete's Foot

S. Jerry is on a basketball team and repeatedly gets athlete's foot. His feet have thick scales and angry redness and cracks between his toes. His feet itch and burn.
O. **P** Superficial and slippery. **T** Red sticky coat.
A. Wind Damp Heat. Athlete's foot.
P. *Specific therapeutic principles.* (1) Support immune function. (2) Antifungals. (3) Clear damp and heat with dry, cooling antimicrobials. (4) Topical antiinflammatory bath with apple cider vinegar (ACV) for itching and apply Tea Tree essential oil regularly. (5) Foot hygiene.

Herbal Formula and Dose. 5 mL 3 × daily for at least 4 weeks, even if cleared up.

Parts	Herbs	Rationale
4	*Echinacea angustifolia* root	Immune function and antiinfective.
3	Scutellaria Huang Qin	Clear damp heat and inflammation, antimicrobial.
3	Black Walnut hull	Antifungal.
2	Pau d'arco bark	Antifungal, metabolic toxicosis.

Other Suggestions

- *Foot hygiene.* Wash feet often. Wash socks and infected tennis shoes with bleach in separate machine load. Keep feet dry, toenails short, using a separate nail clipper for infected toenails. Change white cotton socks often, avoid tight-fitting footwear, and wear waterproof sandals in common areas. Let shoes dry out between use or alternate pairs.
- *Foot baths.* Soak feet in saltwater or diluted ACV to help dry up blisters.
- *Tea Tree essential oil.* 50% solution applied to feet.
- *Antifungal salve* (Box 25.4).

- *Signs and symptoms.* Scaling, redness, and thickening of the soles and between toes. Becomes red, itchy, peeling, and stinging or cracked and raw. Often occurs in people with weakened immune systems. Can cause secondary bacterial infections.
- *Allopathic treatment.* Topical antifungals. Antibiotics if infected. Keeping feet dry and wearing shoes.
- *General therapeutic principles.* (1) Improve immune function per internal tincture. (2) Clear itching if present (wind). (3) Clear heat with antibacterials and antifungals. (4) Clear damp. (5) External antifungal salve or essential oils of Tea Tree, Oregano, Thyme, Orange, or Lemon.[15]

• BOX 25.4 Antifungal Salve[18]

by Rosemary Gladstar

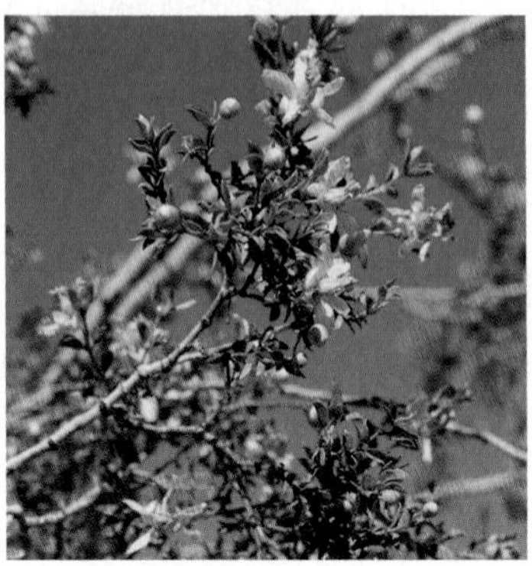

Strong smelling *Larrea tridentata* (Creosote/Chaparral leaf) is a key herb in this basic salve for many types of fungal infections. (/iStock.com/Jared Quentin.).

A useful antifungal emollient salve. This includes infections such as athlete's foot, nail fungus, jock itch, ringworm, and *Candida.* Will require frequent applications over a few weeks.

Ingredients

2 parts	*Larrea* spp. (Creosote, Chaparral leaf)	Antifungal.
2 parts	*Juglans nigra* (Black Walnut hull)	Antifungal.
1 part	Goldenseal or Coptis Huang Lian	Antifungal, and broad-spectrum antimicrobial.
1 part	*Commiphora myrrha* (Myrrh resin)	Antifungal.
1 part	*Echinacea angustifolia* root	Balance immune function and detoxification.
	Olive oil and beeswax	1 oz melted beeswax per 1 cup herbal oil.

Directions for accelerated oil made into a salve

Weigh out and grind herbs. Moisten with 95% ethyl alcohol to break down cell walls. Let stand 20 minutes to 1 hour. Put herbs in blender and cover with olive oil. Blend on high until warm. May have to let motor cool down intermittently. Strain. To each cup of herbal oil, start with 1 oz melted beeswax. Test for firmness by placing a little dollop in freezer to cool. Adjust thickness. For harder salve, add more wax; for thinner salve, add oil. Pour into jars or tins and let harden.

Dose

Apply to lesions 3 × daily up to 1 month, even if lesions have cleared up. Do not double dip. Remove enough for one application and discard applicator after use. Fungi are contagious.

Summary

Skin functions range from temperature regulation to immune protection. Problems must be treated internally and externally. Assessments of complexion, hair, and nails reveal multitudes about whole body health and can indicate internal problems. Healthy skin requires good hydration, a diet rich in essential fatty acids, and protection from harmful UV rays. Topical skin remedies take the form of baths, compresses, poultices, creams, lotions, and salves. Herbalists would do well to keep one or two basic preparations on hand. A pain relief liniment and a first aid wound healer are decent choices.

In Chinese Medicine, the Lungs are the most exterior organ and rule the skin and body hair. Sweating is a Lung function, another kind of breathing called wei qi. If this energy is deficient, we sweat excessively (hyperhidrosis), a major sign of Lung Qi Deficiency. From a skin standpoint, wind refers to itching, acute hives, and spontaneous sweating.

Two main categories of the skin Materia Medica are vulneraries and alteratives that work on an internal detoxifying level. Common skin situations confronting herbalists include first-aid measures for cuts and scrapes, itchy stress-related eczema, autoimmune psoriasis where cells proliferate quickly and wildly, painful burning shingles that follow nerve pathways, embarrassing acne, and the locker-room hazard, athlete's foot.

Review

Fill in the Blanks

(Answers in Appendix B.)

1. Give six functions of the skin ___, ___, ___, ___, ___, ___.
2. The Lungs rule the ___ and ___.
3. Nail clubbing indicates ___. Pale nails indicate ___ and ___ in Chinese Medicine. Pitting indicates ___. Thickening and yellowing indicates ___ and ___.
4. An example of skin endocrine function is ___. An example of skin exocrine function is ___.
5. Typical Pulse and Tongue for acute eczema. **P**___. **T** ___.
6. Give two herbal examples of lymphatic alteratives: ___, ___. Kidney alteratives ___, ___ Liver alteratives ___, ___.
7. What are five properties of honey? ___, ___, ___, ___, ___.
8. Name and define three types of open trauma wounds: ___, ___, ___.
9. Three antipruritic herbs (common and botanical name) are ___, ___, ___.
10. Syndrome for a chronic, dry, whitish, itchy lesion ___. Syndrome for an acute, inflamed, itchy lesion ___. Syndrome for painful boil with pus ___.

Critical Concept Questions

(Answers for you to decide.)

1. What does healthy skin look like?
2. What can be learned from a nail assessment? Give some examples.
3. How does the skin affect psychological and emotional health?
4. Discuss the ins and outs of stopping wound bleeding and applying vulneraries. When should irrigation be done? When should vulneraries be used?
5. Give therapeutic principles for acute and chronic eczema.
6. What are shingles? How would you recognize it? What are serious complications?
7. Discuss the virtues of Panax San Qi.
8. Discuss the many kinds of *Herpes* spp.
9. Which herbs and supplies would you put in a first-aid kit?
10. Name some first aid herbs you might find on a hike.

References

1. Flint, Margi. *The Practicing Herbalist: Meeting with Clients, Reading the Body* (Marblehead, MA: Earthsong, 2013).
2. "What Your Fingernails Are Trying to Tell You About Your Health." Organic Olivia. https://www.organicolivia.com/2016/01/what-your-fingernails-are-trying-to-tell-you-about-your-health/ (accessed August 19, 2019).
3. Schoenbart, Bill, and Ellen Shefi. "Traditional Chinese Medicine Diagnosis." How Stuff Works. https://health.howstuffworks.wellness/natural-medicine/chinese/traditional-chinese-medicine-diagnosis.htm (accessed August 19, 2019).
4. Hoffman, David. *Medical Herbalism: The Science and Practice of Herbal Medicine* (Rochester, VT: Healing Arts, 2003).
5. Coffman, Sam. *The Herbal Medic,* Volume 1 (San Antonio, TX: The Human Path, 2014).
6. Gladstar, Rosemary. *Herbal Healing for Women* (New York, NY: Simon and Schuster, 2017).
7. "Does a High SPF Protect My Skin Better?" Skin Cancer Foundation. https://www.skincancer.org/skin-cancer-information/ask-the-experts/does-a-higher-spf-sunscreen-always-protect-your-skin-better (accessed August 19, 2019).
8. "In One Lifespan, How Many Times Does a Human's Skin Peel Off?" Quora. https://www.quora.com/In-one-life-span-how-many-times-does-a-human%E2%80%99s-skin-peel-off (accessed August 19, 2019).
9. Shen, Jin'ao. "The Lung Network: Views from the Past." Institute for Traditional Medicine. http://www.itmonline.org/5organs/lung.htm (accessed August 20, 2019).
10. Dharmananda, Subhuti. "The Jade Screen." Institute for Traditional Medicine. http://www.itmonline.org/arts/jadescreen.htm (accessed August 20, 2019).
11. "Jade Windscreen Formula." Eastern Currents. (accessed August 20, 2019).
12. Siddiqui, MZ. "Boswellia Serrata, A Potential Antiinflammatory Agent: An Overview." U.S. National Library of Medicine, National Institutes of Health. *Indian J Pharm Sci.* 2011;73(3):255–261. https://www.ncbi.nlm.nih.gov/pmc/articles/PMC3309643/ (accessed December 13, 2019).
13. Holmes, Peter. *Jade Remedies: A Chinese Herbal Reference for the West* (Boulder, CO: Snow Lotus, 1996).
14. Nordqvist, Christian. "Humira (Adalimumab) and its Uses." Medical News Today. https://www.medicalnewstoday.com/articles/humira (accessed August 21, 2019).
15. Bone, Kerry and Simon Mills *Principles and Practice of Phytotherapy* (London, UK: Elsevier, 2013: Churchill Livingstone, 2013).
16. Boskey, Elizabeth. "Herpes Zoster Virus Overview." Verywell Health. https://www.verywell.com/what-is-herpes-zoster-3132938 (accessed August 22, 2019).
17. Tierra, Michael. "Treatment of a Particularly Difficult Case of Psoriasis." East West School of Planetary Herbology https://planetherbs.com/research-center/case-studies/treatment-of-a-difficult-case-of-psoriasis/ (accessed August 22, 2019).
18. Gladstar, Rosemary. *Herbal Recipes for Vibrant Health* (North Adams, MA: Storey, 2008).
19. "What is Psoriasis?" Explore Health. https://www.health.com/condition/psoriasis/psoriasis (accessed August 22, 2019).
20. Holmes, Peter. *Energetics of Western Herbs* (Boulder, CO: Snow Lotus, 2000).

26

The Urinary System

"Everything on the earth has a purpose, every disease an herb to cure it, and every person a mission. This is the Indian theory of existence."

—Mourning Dove, Native American author (1884–1936)

CHAPTER REVIEW

- Overview of the urinary system and kidney functions.
- Maintaining healthy kidneys.
- Urine assessment.
- Chinese Medicine perspective: The Kidneys and major Lin syndromes.
- Urinary Materia Medica: Urinary herbs worth honorable mention. Restoratives, stimulants (diuretics), relaxants (antispasmodics, analgesics, antilithics), and sedatives (antimicrobials).
- Common urinary conditions with case histories: cystitis, acute urinary tract infections (UTIs), chronic recurrent cystitis, interstitial cystitis, renal stones or calculi, and urinary incontinence.

KEY TERMS

Angiotensin converting enzyme (ACE 2)
Antilithics
Cystitis
Diuretics
Draining diuretic
Dysuria
Electrolytes
Enuresis
Hematuria
Incontinence
Lin syndrome
Potential of hydrogen/pH
Proteinuria
Pyelonephritis
Renal calculi
Renin-angiotensin-aldosterone (RAA) pathway
Urea
Urethritis
Urinary tract infection (UTI)

The kidneys are an extremely complicated body system. Anatomically, the urinary system (also called the renal or urogenital system) is made up of only four structures: the kidneys, ureters, bladder, and urethra. That's it. Physiologically, kidneys do far more than make urine, although that is certainly a most obvious and important function. Kidneys are vital organs of detoxification, water balance, blood pressure, acid-base electrolyte balance, and more. We can't live without them for longer than a week, give or take. Beyond that time frame, a person must be on dialysis or get a transplant to stay alive.

Keeping the kidneys healthy is important to our well-being. We usually make urine unconsciously and urinate easily and painlessly; except when we don't. Normal adult output is around 1.5 to 2 liters a day (1 liter is close to a quart), depending on the weather and body's hydration. Urine characteristics tell a lot about overall health. This chapter will explore these parameters.

In Chinese Medicine, Kidneys affect whole body and, in that sense, are the most holistic of organ systems. In Chinese Medicine, the Kidneys make urine, as in Western medicine, and are involved on the physical level with the ills that function entails. This chapter deals with that aspect. Chapters 27 and 28 involve other Chinese Medicine Kidney functions. Physical Kidney conditions are known as Lin syndromes. They include urinary tract infections (UTIs), other infections, and calculi (stones).

Overview of the Urinary System

Kidney Functions

- *The kidneys excrete metabolic waste and chemicals.* Kidneys make urine, which in itself is a complicated process, and in doing so, eliminates toxins. This process involves many back-and-forth exchanges between the bloodstream and the microscopic kidney tubules, where the product is fine-tuned and adjusted, eventually exiting as urine. Urine is named after ***urea***, which is the product of protein metabolism. Some of the normal waste products in urine include creatinine, uric acid, blood urea nitrogen (BUN), and products from the breakdown of hemoglobin in red blood cells (RBC). Urobilin from RBC breakdown makes urine yellow. A blood chemistry test fractions out these urinary waste products, which are indicators of renal function, in addition to providing parameters on liver function and electrolyte levels.

- *The kidneys adjust fluid volume—water balance.* It is important that the body maintains the right amount of physiological fluids in their proper compartments, both within the cells (intracellular fluid, ICF) and outside the cells (extracellular fluid, ECF). The body loses water through the kidneys, skin, lungs, and colon. In health, the amount of water taken in (input) should equal the amount lost (output). Kidneys are constantly adjusting urine output to maintain this equilibrium so body tissues stay properly hydrated.
- *The kidneys adjust electrolyte balance.* ***Electrolytes*** are compounds that separate into ions in solution and conduct an electrical charge, such as sodium ($Na+$), potassium ($K+$), calcium ($Ca+$), and chloride (Cl^-).[1] The kidneys retain proper electrolyte levels in the blood and excrete any excess in the urine. They maintain fluid balance by working with $Na+$, the main ion in ECF. Sodium (salt) has an osmotic pull that attracts water and adjusts fluid volumes inside and outside the cells. Potassium is a major electrolyte in the intracellular fluid, and correct $K+$ blood levels are crucial to maintaining nerve impulses that enable skeletal and cardiac muscles to contract.
- *The kidneys regulate pH balance.* The kidneys are one of many systems in the body that help regulate ***pH, potential of hydrogen***, known as acid-base balance. This measurement is shown on a logarithmic scale of 1 to 14, in which 1 is the most acid, 7 is neutral, and 14 is the most alkaline (or base). The kidneys take on the job of long-term pH regulation by resorbing (eliminating) hydrogen ($H+$) in the urine.[1] If the pH of the blood is not kept within the tiny and slightly alkaline range of 7.35 to 7.45 on the pH scale, it can be fatal. A shift in either direction by three-tenths of a point can cause cardiac arrest.
- *The kidneys regulate and maintain healthy blood pressure.* This is essential to assure proper heart function. For this to happen the kidneys do everything in their power to make it so by initiating a complex pathway. As you will see, this is no small undertaking.
  - *The* ***renin-angiotensin-aldosterone (RAA) pathway***. (1) When blood pressure drops too low, specialized kidney cells called the juxtaglomerular (JG) apparatus secrete the enzyme *renin* into the blood. (2) Renin stimulates the liver to release angiotensin I. (3) Angiotensin I is then converted into *angiotensin II* by the nudging of another protein called the ***angiotensin converting enzyme (ACE 2)***. ACE 2 is made by capillary endothelium all over the body, especially the cilia of the lungs, of course the kidneys, the cardiovascular and GI systems. It is found on cell surfaces (membranes) in all these organ systems. (4) Angiotensin II is an extremely strong vasopressor that constricts blood vessels, causing BP to rise. (5) Angiotensin II also stimulates the adrenal glands on top of the kidneys to release the hormone *aldosterone*. (6) Aldosterone increases sodium ($Na+$) in the blood. Where $Na+$ goes, water follows. Additional water increases blood volume, and further raises BP. (7) If this weren't enough, angiotensin II also stimulates the release of antidiuretic hormone (ADH) from the posterior pituitary in the skull, which decreases urination causing further water retention.[2]
  - *Kidney-based drugs can regulate blood pressure in case it gets too high.* As you may have deduced, the downside of the powerful vasoconstrictor, angiotensin II, is that in susceptible folks, BP can get too high. Should this happen, a classification of antihypertensive drugs can be used that work on the kidney level. They are the ACE 2 receptor inhibitors and blockers that control BP by decreasing or blocking angiotensin production.
  - *Herbs and foods that act as ACE inhibitors. Allium sativa* (Garlic bulb), Salvia Dan Shen (Cinnabar Sage root), Andrographis Chuan Xin Lian (Heart-Thread Lotus leaf), *Crataegus* spp. (Hawthorn berry), Pueraria Ge Gen (Kudzu root) and East Indian *Hibiscus sabdariffa* (Hibiscus flower) have been found to have BP regulating and ACE inhibiting actions.[3] High antioxidant foods that also inhibit and regulate ACE 2 receptors include pomegranate juice, beet juice, apple juice, kiwis, blueberries, and dark chocolate.
- *The kidneys stimulate production of red blood cells (RBCs).* When the kidneys do not get enough oxygen, they produce the hormone erythropoietin (EPO). This stimulates RBC production in the bone marrow.

Maintaining Healthy Kidneys

- *Hydration.* The body is 50% to 70% water. The kidneys deal with water directly. They carry away toxins in urine and balance fluid volume, which helps to adjust BP. Serious dehydration can cause seizures and kidney failure, and without water, we die in 3 to 4 days. There are varying words of wisdom on how much water we need to drink daily. Perhaps a half-gallon is average. Generally, once a person feels thirsty, she or he is already dehydrated. If dehydrated, the kidneys conserve water and urine gets darker and more concentrated; if overly hydrated, we pee more.
- *What to drink.* People should stay hydrated to flush the kidneys with pure, preferably unchlorinated, spring water. Foods with high water content, like melons, oranges, and herbal teas, count. Fresh lemon and lime juices help decrease kidney stone occurrence.
  - *Liquid chlorophyll.* In the morning, people should rehydrate with alkalizing and antioxidant chlorophyll, available in health food stores (Fig. 26.1). Dilute it with water. It is delicious and refreshing, especially the mint-flavored kind. Chlorophyll is cleansing and filled with iron, fights odors, and kills bacteria. Nettle herb, another dark green plant, is also kidney friendly for similar reasons.
  - *Cranberry juice* (unsweetened). Sour cranberry juice is a good kidney drink because it stops bacteria from adhering to mucous membrane surfaces and hence is recommended for individuals with urinary tract infections (UTIs).
- *What not to drink.* Caffeinated coffee and, to a lesser extent, tea with caffeine are irritating to kidney tubules. Alcohol and caffeinated drinks, including soda pop, are dehydrating because they cause diuresis. Additionally, many types of soda pop, such

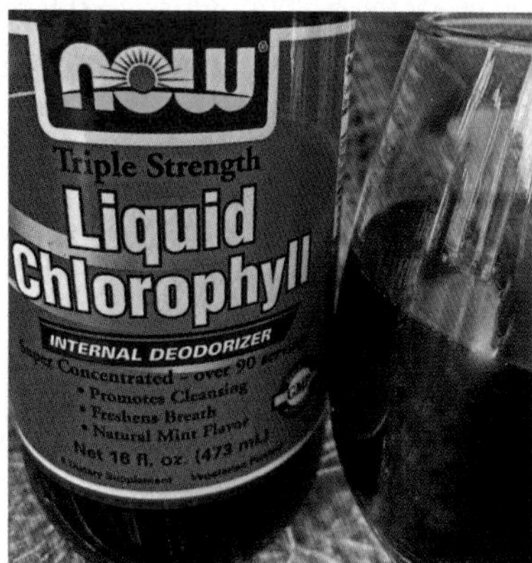

• **Fig. 26.1** Liquid chlorophyll is cleansing, alkalizing, and antioxidant, excellent to help maintain healthy kidneys.

as colas, contain phosphates to give them a crisp, tangy taste. However, phosphates leach calcium out of bones and certainly don't help people with osteoporosis.

- *What to eat.* Green leafy veggies are kidney foods, especially parsley (Box 26.1). A clean diet with three or four servings of veggies and some fruit each day works wonders. Kidney-loving foods include antioxidant rich garlic, onions, cabbage, kale, green tea, olive oil, berries, nuts, and seeds.
- *What not to eat.* If kidneys are healthy, there should be no problem with good-quality protein. But a high-protein diet can strain compromised kidneys because they are involved in metabolizing protein into urea. If the kidneys are failing, a low-protein diet is recommended. Added salt can also put extra stress on compromised kidneys, because their job is to eliminate salt and fluids as needed.
- *Chinese Medicine recommendations.* In addition to healthy dark leafy veggies, the correspondences associate the Kidneys with the color black. Therefore black foods such as black rice, black lentils, black beans, black garlic (it's a thing), and blackberries are recommended.
- *Exercise.* Along with the clean foods mentioned earlier, aerobic exercise and strength training have been found to contribute highly to kidney health.
- *Maintain normal BP, glucose levels, and cardiac health.* Major contributors to kidney failure include diabetes, hypertension, and heart failure. Of these three, type 1 diabetes and hypertension are tops. All those to-do measures counteract those conditions.

Urine Assessment

A simple visual inspection of urine is easy and can tell the herbalist a lot. Normal urine appears in various shades of yellow, is clear and not cloudy, has no visible blood, no suspended particles, and smells like ammonia if there is dehydration. A simple dipstick that can be purchased in pharmacies will show pH and presence of microscopic blood. Determination of bacteria, sediments known as *casts*, crystals, protein, white and red blood cells, and other parameters require microscopic examination and is carried out in a urine analysis (UA).

- *Color.* Urine color ranges from light pale yellow to deep amber. If a person is well-hydrated, urine is light yellow. It gets less dilute, darker and darker, and more odiferous as dehydration occurs, where the kidneys make less urine to conserve water. If urine is pink or reddish, it could indicate blood caused by the red pigment hemoglobin in red blood cells or prior ingestion of beets or rhubarb. Certain medications that are metabolized through the urine make pee appear a frightening bright orange. Orangey urine could also be caused by eating a lot of carrots or by the laxative herb *Cascara sagrada*.
- *Smell.* Normal urine smells like urea, its namesake. When proteins are broken down, highly toxic ammonia is formed. The liver converts the ammonia into urea, which is then excreted by the kidneys, hence that distinct smell. The more dilute the urine, the less smelly; the less diluted, the stronger. That's normal. A sweet fruity smell can indicate high blood sugar, a sign of type 1 diabetes. Bacteria can cause a nasty odor. And here's an odd one: eating asparagus changes urine's smell into a sulfurlike odor. But only about a quarter of the population appears to have the gene that allows them to smell those chemicals.[4] Everyone's pee achieves this alchemy and changes odor from ingestion of asparagus; it's just a privileged few who can detect it.

• BOX 26.1 Happy Kidney Tea with Parsley

Petroselinum crispum **(Parsley leaf, root, and seed)**

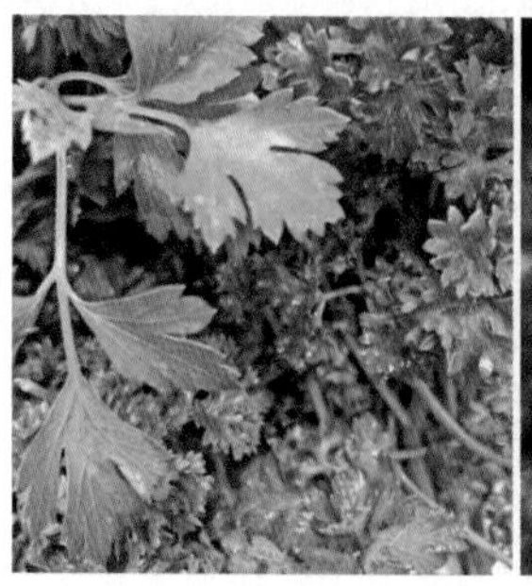
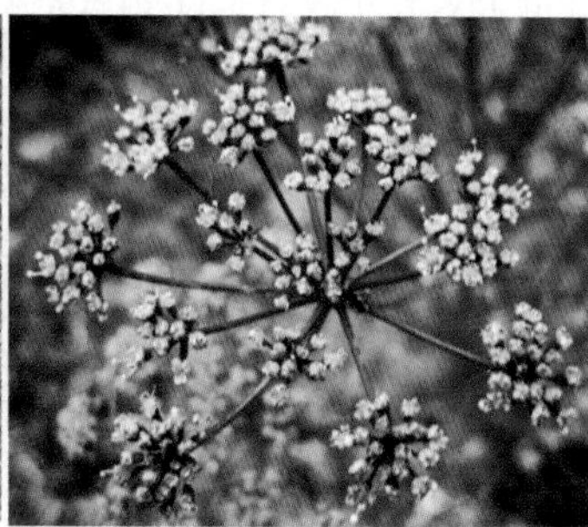

Parsley, flat leaf Italian and curly leaf, and Parsley seeding. The whole plant, root, leaf, and seed is nutritive and healing for a variety of kidney woes.

Nutrient-dense Parsley from the carrot family is a lot more than a pretty garnish to be daintily put aside on the plate. The leaves are an excellent source of iron, vitamins K and C and folate. The flavonoid, apigenin, is anticarcinogenic, antiinflammatory, and antioxidant.

Parsley leaf, root, and seed have long been used for the kidneys. The leaf contains cleansing chlorophyll, the seeds are filled with kidney-loving essential oils, and the root dissolves stones.

Ingredients for Happy Kidney Tea with Parsley

3 parts	Parsley root	Draining diuretic, dissolves stones.
2 parts	Parsley leaf	Cleansing chlorophyll.
2 parts	Bearberry leaf	Antibacterial to kidneys.
1 part	Parsley seed	Essential oil content is diuretic and antispasmodic.
1 part	Marshmallow root	Coats and soothes the urinary mucosa.
1 part	Licorice root	Soothes urinary mucosa and sweetens formula.

Directions

Pour freshly boiled water over 2 tsp of tea. Steep for 3 to 5 minutes. strain and drink. Add honey or lemon to taste.

- *Clarity*. Normal urine should be clear. Cloudy urine can indicate infection, excess protein, sediment, or kidney stones.
- *Urine pH*. Normal urine is slightly acidic, ranging between 5.5 and 6.5. Remember the alkaline diet, often recommended for arthritis? Urine tries very hard to stay acidic, no matter what is consumed. If the kidneys can't acidify urine, something is very wrong.
- *Hematuria*. Urine should not contain blood. If a dipstick test is positive for blood, there could be an irritating UTI, passage of a stone, prostatitis, kidney damage, or even cancer.[5] If blood is detected visually in the toilet, it indicates quite a lot of bleeding. Blood cannot always be seen by the naked eye.
- ***Proteinuria***. Protein in the urine can only be detected microscopically. A small amount is not a problem. Larger amounts could indicate diabetes, hypertension, or kidney disease.
- *Bacteria*. Normal urine is usually sterile, meaning no microorganisms present, although often there is a little bacteria present with no noticeable infection. Bacteria indicates an infection somewhere in the urinary tract; it could be in the bladder or higher up in the kidneys. Herbalists use broad-spectrum urinary antibacterials, such as Uva ursi leaf or Juniper berry to treat these issues.

Chinese Medicine Perspective: The Kidneys and Major Lin Syndromes

- *The physiological Kidney in Chinese Medicine*. This part of the Chinese Medicine Kidney is closest to Western medicine and includes the function of the kidneys in regulating urination, water balance, electrolyte balance, and homeostasis. This chapter deals with the physical urinary system.
- *The Kidney Organ System in Chinese Medicine*. The Kidney system appears all over the Western spectrum. It appears prominently in neurological, respiratory, endocrine, and reproductive areas, and it does not translate neatly into Western boxes. Kidneys are paramount to the endocrine system, especially the adrenal glands.[6] They deal with breathing and circulate the qi, so lung-wise deficiencies relate to shortness of breath or asthma. Kidneys involve the nervous system by nourishing the brain, spinal cord, and cerebral spinal fluid. They manifest in the head hair, so they deal with hair growth or baldness. They are in the skeletal area because Kidneys govern the bones, marrow, and teeth, and they are the seat of lower back and knee joint pain because the meridian travels right through lower back. Because Kidneys store the jing, or essence, they govern the life cycle of birth, growth, and reproduction. They determine graceful aging and longevity.
- *Correspondences*. Kidneys open to the ears, govern the bones (marrow) and teeth, and manifest in the head hair. Kidney emotion is fear; the positive side being willpower and/or courage. The element is water, and the color is dark blue or black.

Chinese Medicine Major Kidney Lin Syndrome

- *Lin syndrome in general*. ***Lin syndrome*** a general term for physical urinary disorders involving frequency, dribbling, and painful issues. There are various kinds of Lin syndromes that describe the nature of urine and symptoms. They deal with heat (infection), passing of blood (***hematuria***), painful urination (***dysuria***), kidney stones, greasy urine, and chronically weak deficiencies, like dribbling and incontinence. Western diagnoses name these things acute or chronic UTIs, kidney stones or calcifications, incontinence, and bed-wetting.
- *Re Lin (damp heat)*. This syndrome is all too common. It is an acute UTI with painful, frequent, burning, and urgent urination. **Pulse (P)** Rapid, slippery or wiry. **Tongue (T)** Red or yellow body, sticky coat.
- *Xue Lin (passing blood)*. Damp heat with hematuria. Painful burning urination with blood. **P** Rapid, thready, or soggy. **T** Red or yellow body with sticky coat.
- *Shi Lin (stones or calcification)*. Kidney stones. Dysuria, urgency, dribbling, sudden interruption of flow with severe prickling pain that radiates to the abdomen during urination, and dark yellow, turbid urine with blood and or calculi (stones). **P** Rapid, wiry. **T** Red or yellow body, sticky coat.
- *Gao Lin (greasy)*. Caused by damp heat, involves dark yellow urine with a cloudy or greasy appearance. There is dysuria, difficult urination (hard to start flow), and dribbling. **P** Rapid or soggy (wet). **T** Red or yellow body, sticky coat.
- *Lao Lin (chronic because of Kidney and Spleen deficiencies)*. Recurring frequency, dribbling or incontinence, indicating weakness. **P** Thready, weak, or rapid. **T** Normal, pale or red with thin white coat.

Urinary Materia Medica

These fit into the categories of restoratives, stimulants (diuretics), relaxants (antispasmodics and analgesics), and sedatives that are also antimicrobials. The herbs are a Western and Chinese mix.

Urinary Herbs Worth Honorable Mention

- *Solidago* spp. (Goldenrod herb) (Fig. 26.2). One of the very best all-around kidney trophorestoratives (and there aren't that many); cool, drying, bitter, and astringent. Indispensable for use in acute and long-term kidney conditions. Goldenrod has a strong downward energy, a draining diuretic that clears edema and stimulates the kidneys. Its cool, bitter, antiseptic,

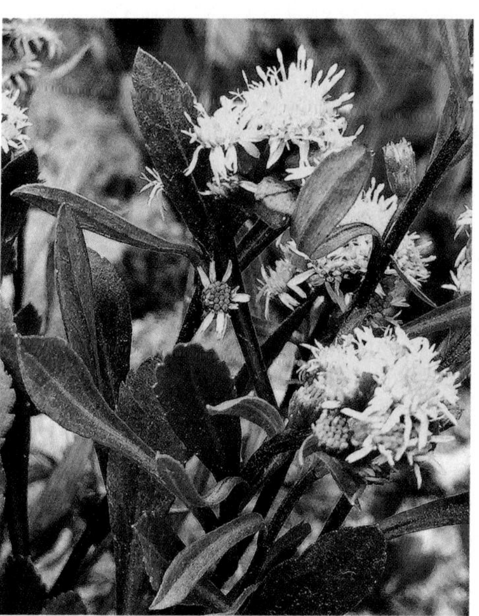

• **Fig. 26.2** *Solidago* spp. (Goldenrod herb) is indispensable in acute and long-term kidney conditions. This kidney trophorestorative acts as an antimicrobial, draining diuretic, and antilithic.

and antiinflammatory actions qualify it for acute and chronic Kidney damp heat infections. If the UTI is chronic and cold, combine with a warming diuretic, such as Lovage root or Horseradish root.[7] Goldenrod is also exemplary for upper respiratory allergies in allergic rhinitis, and it is an important vulnerary for skin and toxicosis. Just about any variety will do. It grows everywhere and is a no-brainer for any apothecary. In fact, there are more than 100 species just in North America alone, and *Solidago* spp. range from sea level to alpine locations.

- *Elymus repens* (Couch grass root). This plant is an extremely versatile Western herb for urinary pain, urgency, Damp and Toxic Damp Heat because it draws pus. It is a strong, draining diuretic and a demulcent filled with saponin mucilages to cool heat and irritation for acute and chronic UTIs. Couch Grass has a detoxicant alterative effect because it drains lymph.[6]
- *Dianthus superbus* Qu Mai (Proud Pink herb). Bitter, cold, and dry. A lot like Western Goldenrod in that it's useful for acute UTIs and skin. It is antibacterial, antiinflammatory, antiseptic, stimulant, and diuretic. Alkaloid content makes it excellent for acute bladder damp heat infections. Especially good for dysuria because of its soothing saponin content. Also a vulnerary for Skin Damp Heat, it is a cleansing herb for eczema and metabolic toxicosis.
- *Alisma orientalis* Zi Xie (Water Plantain root). This cooling herb is another strong and well-known potent draining diuretic that is antimicrobial to boot for UTIs with hematuria, scanty urine, and dysuria. For any damp condition that needs drying out.[8]
- *Poria cocos* Fu Ling (Hoelen fungus). A classic Chinese herb for drying damp (Box 26.2). Known as a renal stimulant, it is a draining diuretic for any kind of edema or diarrhea, scanty urine, and water retention. It has a neutral temperature, making it ideal for hot or cold conditions alike. Poria also tonifies the Spleen, so it doubles as a digestive restorative with diarrhea and indigestion. Extremely useful herb.

• BOX 26.2 Dry Damp with Poria Fu Ling

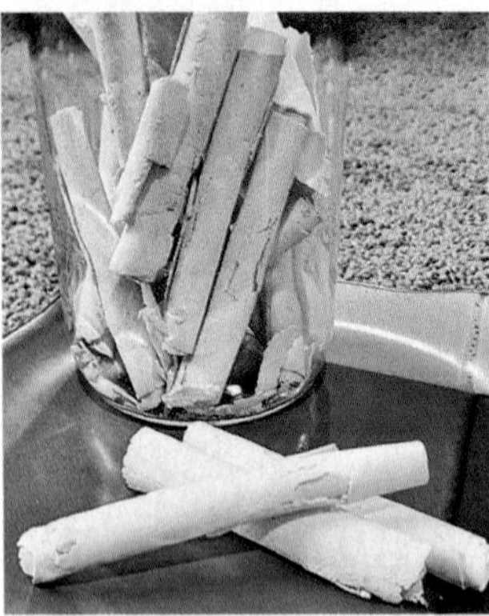

Curly Poria Fu Ling (Hoelen fungus) is a draining diuretic, useful for any type of dampness.

Poria Fu Ling (Hoelen fungus) is a curious fungus that grows on the lower trunks of conifer trees and under the ground. It is a perennial white or pinkish fungus, commercially available in various shapes (curly, flat and cubed) although shape has no bearing on its properties. (I like the curly one; it's more fun.) It can be found in central and coastal China on dry hillsides and in Japan and North America. It is a favorite of many herbalists, East and West.

Its primary use is as a bland, drying, and draining diuretic, useful for any dampness, such as edema, mucus accumulation, or diarrhea. It is gentle, but effective and safe for children. It can be found in many Chinese Medicine formulas, not used on its own.[7] Think of Fu Ling whenever anything needs drying out. It has the added bonus of restoring the Spleen, in Spleen Qi Deficiency, and of being a mild nervous relaxant.

Urinary Restoratives

Urinary restoratives are used for any chronic urinary problem where the bladder and kidneys are weakened or deficient, as in dribbling, incontinence, chronic UTIs that won't quit or ***enuresis*** (involuntary urination or bed-wetting). Urinary restoratives tend to be astringent and tone the smooth muscles of the urinary tract. They also help in UTIs where there is residual urine left in the bladder after voiding.[11] Bladder restoratives help flush the bladder completely and not leave any bacteria-filled urine behind (Table 26.1, Box 26.3).

Urinary Stimulants, the Diuretics

Diuretics are urinary stimulants that increase secretion and elimination of urine from the body. In doing so, waste products are

TABLE 26.1 Urinary Restoratives

Herb	Notes
Solidago spp. Goldenrod herb	One of the few Western trophorestoratives with a kidney affinity for acute and chronic infections. Dissolves stones, antiinfective, draining diuretic. Also used for skin and lymph.
Cuscuta chinensis Tu Si Zi Asian Dodder seed	Chinese Kidney astringent restorative specified with chronic incontinence and enuresis. For Kidney Yang Deficiency.[8]
Piper methysticum Kava root	Detoxicant, draining diuretic tones and restores muscles in incontinence and benign prostatic hypertrophy (BPH). Also used for anxiety and depression.
Eupatorium purpureum Gravel root	Dissolves stones and restores and strengthens and disinfects urinary and reproductive systems.
Coix lachryma-jobi Yi Yi Ren Job's Tears seed	Chinese kidney restorative, demulcent, diuretic. Also, for diarrhea, beautifies skin.
Serenoa serrulata Saw Palmetto berry	Urinary, reproductive, respiratory, and digestive and nutritive tonic.[7] Strengthens bladder tone. For leakage, incontinence, BPH. Androgenic.
Equisetum arvense Horsetail herb	Kidney, lungs, connective tissue, bones, and skin restorative.
Galium aparine Cleavers herb	Kidney restorative, antiinflammatory, diuretic, cooling for heat.
Elymus repens Couch grass root	Restorative, antimicrobial, demulcent, draining diuretic.

• BOX 26.3 Tea to Restore the Kidneys[9]

A preventative tonic tea for kidney health and restoration and for people prone to urinary tract infections

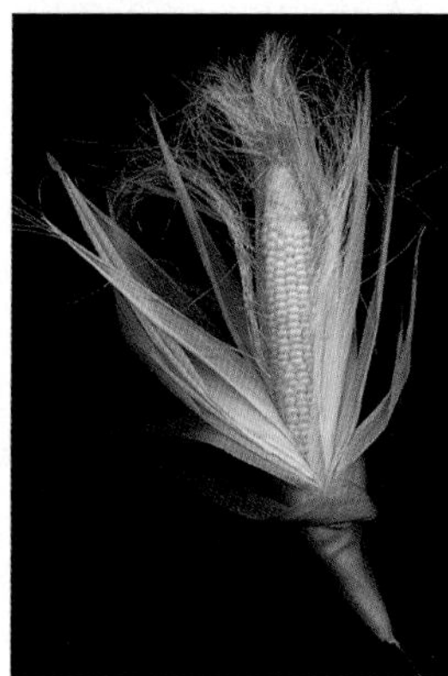

Zea mays, fresh off the cob Cornsilk style is a versatile remedy for acute and chronic urinary infections, a diuretic and restorative. This native North and Central American plant was passed on to European colonists and pioneers for food and medicine. It was even introduced to China.[7] (Copyright Lang/Tucker Photography. Photographs loaned with permission from THE BOTANICAL SERIES are copywritten by Jennifer Anne Tucker and Gerald Lang from the Studio at Hill Crystal Farm. www.jennifer-tucker.com)

Ingredients

Parts	Herb	Rationale
1	*Galium aparine* (Cleavers herb)	Kidney restorative, detoxifier, lymphatic mover.
1	*Althea officinalis* (Marshmallow root)	Mild demulcent. For irritation and pain.
1	*Ocimum tenuiflorum* (Tulsi/Holy Basil herb)	Ayurveda restorative/kidney adaptogen.
1	*Taraxacum officinalis* (Dandelion leaf)	Gentle diuretic, high in potassium.
1	*Urtica dioica* (Nettle herb)	Kidney restorative, diuretic, flushes uric acid to prevent stones.
½	*Zea mays* (Cornsilk, fresh off the cob)	Mild diuretic, soothing demulcent, restorative.

Directions

Parts are measured by weight. Mix dry herbs together. If using fresh Cornsilk, increase amount to 1 part and add to tea. Use 1–2 tbsp per cup and drink a cup a day.

Note: Marshmallow root can be taken alone for a urinary tract soother. If so, use a cold infusion, 2 tbsp herb to 1 qt water. Let sit in fridge overnight.

excreted, and the detoxification process is enhanced. Any circulatory stimulant is a diuretic in that it increases blood flow, resulting in greater blood circulation through the renal arteries, and thus, more urine production. Caffeine-containing herbs such as Coffee bean and Black tea leaf also do this. So-called ***draining diuretics*** are a stronger designation and are indicated in generalized edema anywhere in the body, including in ankles and lower legs, as seen in congestive heart failure (CHF) and renal failure. Examples: Alisma Zi Xie (Water Plantain root) or Couch grass root.

Kidney herbs tend to double as diuretics; they dry damp. They regulate water balance and promote lymphatic drainage, increasing the volume of urine. Celery seed and Uva ursi leaf are both antiinflammatory and diuretic. Gravel root (Fig. 26.3) and Stone root are ***antilithics*** (break down mineral deposits in stones) and are diuretic. Uva ursi and fresh Yarrow are antimicrobial, astringent, and diuretic. Cornsilk is demulcent and diuretic and soothes, coats, and cools the mucous membranes, taking down pain and

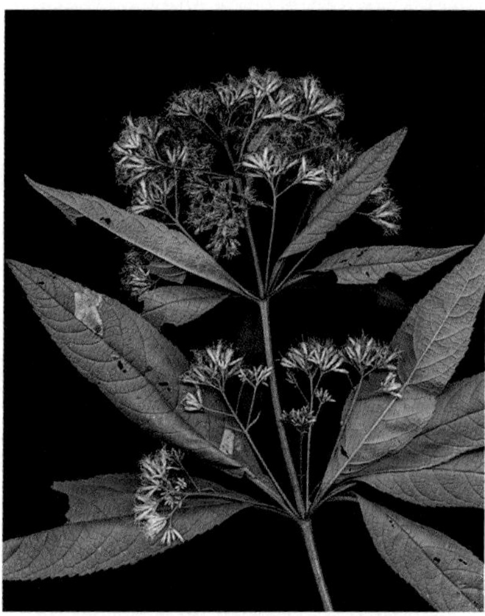

• **Fig. 26.3** *Eupatorium purpureum* (Gravel root), so named because its antilithic and diuretic actions help dissolve and eliminate gravel and stones so they pass into the urine. Its astringency makes it useful for incontinence. (Copyright Lang/Tucker Photography. Photographs loaned with permission from THE BOTANICAL SERIES are copywritten by Jennifer Anne Tucker and Gerald Lang from the Studio at Hill Crystal Farm. www.jennifer-tucker.com)

inflammation. It is helpful to select your diuretic with its other action(s) in mind (Table 26.2).

Diuretics are indicated in most kidney problems where flushing out the urine is a good idea. This is true for UTIs, kidney stones, hematuria, dysuria, benign prostatic hyperplasia (BPH), renal failure with *oliguria* (abnormally small amount of urine), and *anuria* (failure to produce any urine). Naturally, diuretics are important in skin conditions, rheumatoid arthritis, and any foot and ankle edema, such as occurs with a sprained ankle, congestive heart failure, and renal failure. For the last two, draining diuretics are needed, although those clients will likely be hospitalized. Selection would be based on a diuretic's tropism to various body systems, such as Lily of the Valley herb for the heart, Celery seed for the skin and muscles, Dandelion leaf (best when used fresh) for liver and digestive areas.

Urinary Relaxants: Spasmolytics, Analgesics, and Antilithics

Urinary relaxants are *spasmolytics* that have a tropism to the smooth muscles of the urinary tract (Table 26.3). These would be called on especially for pain or dysuria, renal colic. This occurs in UTIs or prostatitis. They also are used in dribbling, discharges, and incontinence caused by weakness and muscle spasms.

Relaxants also include analgesics, many of which work by relaxing muscle spasms. Some analgesics are general and useful for pain anywhere in the body, such as Corydalis Yan Hu Suo (Asian Corydalis corm) or Jamaican Dogwood bark. Willow bark is specific for the bladder pain of UTIs, although it is also used for headaches and inflammation.

Another category of urinary relaxants are the antilithics (Table 26.4) that break up stones and dissolve hardened calcium or uric acid oxalates. Urinary stones cause incredible pain and spasm when they pass into the narrow ureters, and once broken up and dissolved, there is blessed relief. Stone breakers are dissolving, diuretic, and detoxifying. They tend to prevent stone formation

TABLE 26.2 Urinary Stimulants
(Diuretics, and may double as demulcents, antimicrobials, and/or antilithics)

Herb	Notes
Demulcent diuretics	
Zea mays (Cornsilk) *Althea officinalis* (Marshmallow leaf) *Elymus repens* (Couch grass root) *Hydrangea arborescens* (Hydrangea root)	All are diuretics and demulcents. Demulcents bring down inflammation and soothe the urinary mucous membranes lining the ureters and bladder. They are needed when there is pain on urination (dysuria).
Antimicrobial diuretics	
Achillea millefolium (Fresh Yarrow herb)	Yarrow is best tinctured fresh for antimicrobial effect.[10]
Arctostaphylos uva ursi (Uva ursi leaf)	Uva ursi, classic acute urinary tract infections (UTIs) antimicrobial.
Juniperus communis (Juniper berry)	Juniper for chronic UTIs; may irritate/overstimulate kids.
Elymus repens (Couch grass root)	Couch grass is a strong draining diuretic.
Barosma betulina (Buchu leaf)	Buchu is warming, used for chronic UTIs, and antispasmodic.
Dianthus superbus Qu Mai (Proud Pink herb)	Dianthus Qu Mai is diuretic and alterative.
Alisma orientalis Zi Xie (Water Plantain root)	Alisma Zi Xie, a very strong draining diuretic.
Antilithic diuretics	
Apium graveolens (Celery seed)	Celery, a detoxicant for stones and sand.
Juniperus communis (Juniper berry)	Juniper, for stones, use as draining diuretic, and to address chronic UTIs.
Hydrangea arborescens (Hydrangea root)	Hydrangea for stones, diuresis, demulcent.
Zea mays (Cornsilk style)	Cornsilk clears damp, demulcent for dysuria.
Draining diuretics	
Strong stimulants drain damp. For edema in ankles, legs, or anywhere.	
Solidago spp. (Goldenrod herb)	Goldenrod, strong diuretic, restorative.
Taraxacum officinale (Dandelion leaf)	Taraxacum leaf, any water congestion, hypertension.
Poria coccus Fu Ling (Hoelen fungus)	Poria, strong general use draining diuretic.
Cytisus scoparius (Scotch Broom tops)	Broom with Couch grass for CHF, any edema.
Apium graveolens (Celery seed)	Celery, for stones, alterative detoxicant.
Juniperus communis (Juniper berry)	Juniper, strong draining diuretic, stones.
Petroselinum crispum (Parsley seed)	Parsley for BPH, spasmolytic for dysuria.
Alisma orientalis Zi Xie (Water Plantain root)	Alisma Zi Xie for acute UTIs, anything damp.
Elymus repens (Couch grass root)	Couch grass, strong diuretic and demulcent.
Hydrangea arborescens (Hydrangea root)	Hydrangea is antilithic, antispasmodic, demulcent.
Piper methysticum (Kava root)	Kava, first rate analgesic, relaxant, restorative.
Cooling diuretics for infection with fever	
Alisma plantago Ze Xie (Water plantain root)	Ze Xie, draining diuretic and for acute UTIs.
Eupatorium purpureum (Gravel root)	Gravel root for stones, Damp Heat UTIs.
Galium aparine (Cleavers herb)	Cleavers: cool, diuretic, detoxicant.
Apium graveolens (Celery seed)	Celery: cooling, acute UTIs, antilithic, detox.

TABLE 26.3 Urinary Relaxants
(Spasmolytics and analgesics)

Herbs	Notes
Salix alba White Willow bark	Any type of pain, analgesic, antiinflammatory. Clears heat.
Viburnum opulus Cramp bark	Smooth and skeletal muscle relaxant and spasmolytic for dysuria, and incontinence.
Piper methysticum Kava root	Strong spasmolytic, analgesic, draining diuretic, and restorative. For dribbling, incontinence, and depression with anxiety.[7]
Daucus carota Wild Carrot seed and herb	Urinary relaxant for dysuria, stones, draining diuretic.
Petroselinum crispum Parsley seed	Strong spasmolytic for dysuria, a draining diuretic. Uterine stimulant; not for pregnancy.
Dioscorea villosa Wild Yam root	Spasmolytic, analgesic, and antiinflammatory.
Humulus lupulus Hops flower	Strong spasmolytic, antiinflammatory, dissolves stones, detoxicant diuretic.
Lobelia inflata Lobelia herb	Spasmolytic analgesic. For dysuria, incontinence, stress, and nervous tension.
Hydrangea arborescens Hydrangea root	Spasmolytic, dissolves deposits for stones, demulcent, and draining diuretic.
Barosma betulina Buchu leaf	Good for spasms, dysuria, urgency, incontinence, and chronic UTIs.
Piscidia erythrina Jamaican Dogwood root bark	Antispasmodic, analgesic, antiinflammatory. For pain of any type.
Corydalis turtschaninovii Yan Hu Suo Asian Corydalis corm	General analgesic, muscle relaxant, antispasmodic. For stress and anxiety.
Hypericum perforatum St. John's Wort	Antispasmodic, specifically for spastic bladder, incontinence, and other areas. Depression, anxiety, stress. Astringent.
Verbascum thapsus Mullein root (not leaf)	Clinical pearl: the root is great for enuresis in the elderly, postpartum, and perimenopausal women. Antispasmodic, strong astringent.

TABLE 26.4 Antilithics
(Break up and dissolve stones, many are diuretics)

Herbs	Notes
Eupatorium purpureum Gravel root	Spasmolytic. Noted for breaking up uric acid stones and gravel (its common namesake). Restorative, diuretic and astringent.
Collinsonia canadensis Stone root	Antilithic, diuretic for edema, and incontinence.
Galium aparine Cleavers herb	For all types of deposits: tropism to kidneys, lymph, and skin. For kidney stones, swollen glands, and breast tumors.
Crataeva nurvala Crataeva stem and root bark	This Ayurvedic herb works so well, they consider it their *drug of choice* for kidney and bladder problems, especially stones.[12] Antilithic, diuretic, antiinflammatory, demulcent. Also used for prostatitis.
Hydrangea arborescens Hydrangea root	Breaks up stones, draining diuretic, and superb demulcent like Cornsilk and Couch grass root.
Rubia tinctorum Madder root	Detoxifies and astringes. For hard kidney and gallstone deposits, incontinence, discharges.
Apium graveolens Celery seed	Dissolves stones, draining diuretic, detoxifying, clears heat in acute urinary tract infections (UTIs).
Parietaria officinalis Pellitory of the Wall herb	Old European remedy for stones. Works for UTIs, bladder irritation, gallstones.
Zea mays Cornsilk style	Breaks up stones, diuretic, so clears damp and a soothing demulcent for pain and dysuria.
Polygonum aviculare Knotgrass root	Antilithic, astringent for incontinence, discharges, diarrhea, and bleeding.
Equisetum arvense Horsetail herb	Dissolves deposits, restores bladder and connective tissue, astringent for incontinence.
Urtica dioica Nettle herb	Dissolves hard deposits for urinary and gallstones, draining diuretic.
Arctium lappa Burdock root	Detoxifier, diuretic. Dissolves hard deposits, moves lymph. Also, for eczema, psoriasis, gout, and arthritis.

and weaken and slowly dissolve existing stones. Mineral deposits imply a damp, weak, and deficient condition with irritation and scanty urine and possible physical obstruction.

Antilithics work for hardenings other than urinary stones, such as calcium bone spurs, atherosclerosis, gouty deposits, and gallstones.[6] Their diuretic action is needed to help the dissolved stones or gravel pass out in the urine to dry up damp.

Urinary Sedatives: The Antimicrobials for Damp Heat

These are the antimicrobial herbs that treat infections, bladder Damp Heat Lin syndromes (Table 26.5). There is painful, burning, urgent, frequent cloudy urination, and the client experiences thirst, nausea, or backache. These herbs tend to be antimicrobial,

TABLE 26.5 Urinary Antimicrobials ***(For acute and/or chronic Kidney Damp Heat/Re Lin/infection)***

Herb	Notes
Arctostaphylos uva ursi Bearberry, Kinnikinnick leaf	Western classic for Re Lin/Kidney damp heat/acute UTIs, dysuria, incontinence, stones with infection. Terpene content. Heath family. Penetrates biofilms.
Vaccinium myrtillus Bilberry leaf and fruit (Dried fruit is best for UTIs)	For Re Lin/Kidney damp heat/acute UTIs. Like Cranberry, Bilberry stops bacterial adhesion to bladder walls. Heath family. Leaves are hypoglycemic. Both leaf and fruit restore and strengthen capillaries in the eyes, gums, and elsewhere.
Equisetum arvense Horsetail herb	Clears damp heat, UTIs and a strong astringent. Restorative for kidneys, lungs, connective tissue, and skin.[7]
Dianthus superbus Qu Mai Proud Pink herb	Antibacterial, antiinflammatory, antiseptic, stimulant, diuretic. For acute UTIs, Damp Heat and skin.
Alisma orientalis Zi Xie Water Plantain root	Strong draining diuretic that is antimicrobial. For Re Lin/Kidney damp heat/acute UTIs.
Elymus repens Couch grass root	Strong draining diuretic, and demulcent. For Toxic Damp Heat (draws pus), and Re Lin/Kidney damp heat/acute UTIs.
Akebia quinata Mu Tong Akebia stem	Antiinflammatory, antiseptic, draining diuretic, and analgesic. For Re Lin/ Kidney damp heat/acute UTIs.
Solidago spp. Goldenrod herb	Draining diuretic and detoxicant. For both acute and chronic damp heat, but for chronic UTIs, add a warming herb.
Echinacea angustifolia Echinacea root	Immunostimulant and detoxicant. For acute or chronic UTIs, especially with mucus in urine. Penetrates biofilms.
Agathosma betulina Buchu leaf	Warming spasmolytic with a terpene content. For chronic UTIs, incontinence and dysuria.
Juniperus communis Juniper berry	Detoxicant, draining diuretic. For stones and chronic UTIs. Contraindicated in acute kidney inflammation; it may overstimulate and irritate bladder.
Piper methysticum Kava root	A warming, detoxicant, diuretic. For chronic UTIs combine with Juniper berry. Also, for incontinence and bed-wetting.

antiseptic, antiinflammatory, and spasmolytic. Uva ursi leaf and Dianthus Qu Mai (Proud Pink herb) are examples. Some in this antimicrobial category are on the warmer side and are therefore used for cooler chronic urinary infections. Examples here are Juniper berry or Kava root.

Common Urinary Conditions

Urinary Infections: Acute and Chronic

Urinary tract infections (UTIs) involve the bladder and urethra and are known as *cystitis*. Most urinary infections are Lin Damp Heat syndromes and can be effectively treated with herbs (Case History 26.1). Urinary infections and/or inflammations generally come from an outside source and ascend into the urethra (***urethritis***), up to the bladder (***cystitis***), to the ureter (*ureteritis*), to kidney level (***pyelonephritis***). Pyelonephritis is much more serious than an infection of the bladder. Sometimes the infection begins at kidney level. If kidney infections are not aggressively treated, they could lead to kidney failure. This is the time to be careful and refer to a healthcare provider.

- *Allopathic treatment*. Broad-spectrum antibiotics, or the one that had worked in the past. Repeat culture and increase fluids.

CASE HISTORY 26.1

Case History for Cystitis, Acute Urinary Tract Infection (UTI)

S. Tonya has burning pain on urination; her urine is a little pinkish and appears cloudy. She feels urgency or a need to go often but does not produce much urine.
O. **P** Rapid. **T** Red with sticky coat.
A. Lin Damp Heat. Cystitis or acute UTI.
P. *Specific therapeutic principles*. (1) Antimicrobials. (2) Antiinflammatory demulcents. (3) Antispasmodics and analgesics. (4) Astringents for hematuria. (5) Diuretic to flush kidneys.

Herbal Formula and Dose. Pulse dose 5 mL every 1–2 hours.

Parts	Herbs	Rationale
3	Uva ursi or Dianthus Qu Mai	Antimicrobial, antiinflammatory, diuretic.
3	Goldenrod herb	Draining diuretic, clear damp heat, restorative, astringent.
2	Kava root	Spasmolytic, antiinflammatory.
2	Cornsilk style	Demulcent, antiinflammatory.
2	White Willow bark	Analgesic, antimicrobial.

Other Suggestions

- *General advice*. Women should void after sex. After urination, wipe from front to back so that urethra does not become contaminated with feces. Teach girls and daughters to do same.
- *Urination*. Empty bladder completely. This means that after it seems empty, wait a few seconds and try again once or twice. This empties any normal residual urine so that bacteria can't hang around.
- *Hydration*. Lots of pure water is essential to help flush bladder.
- *Cranberry juice*. Unsweetened or very diluted sour cranberries help prevent bacteria from adhering to bladder mucosa and urethra mucous membranes. Sugar feeds bacteria.
- *Clear Streams Tea* (Box 26.4).

• BOX 26.4 Clear Streams Tea

by Amanda McCabe Crawford

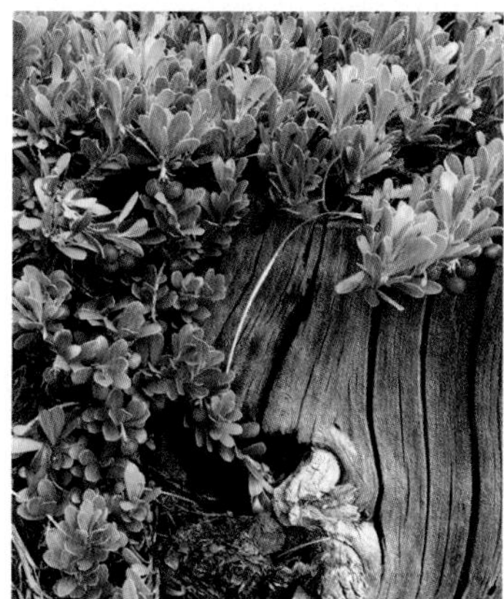

Arctostaphylos uva ursi leaf with its bright red fall berries beloved by bears. Use leaf as an antibiofilm/antibacterial in acute cystitis/Lin Damp Heat. Its high tannin content makes it very drying, so combine with a soothing demulcent such as Licorice root or Cornsilk style.

This tea is for an acute urinary tract infection (UTI) with burning urgency, pain, and misery. Drink the tea and include lots of water and unsweetened cranberry juice.

3 parts	*Arctostaphylos uva ursi* (Bearberry, Kinnikinnick leaf)	Clears urinary Damp Heat, antimicrobial.
3 parts	*Althea officinalis* (Marshmallow root)	Urinary demulcent, soothing, and analgesic.
1 part	*Passiflora incarnata* (Passionflower)	Spasmolytic and analgesic.
1 part	*Viburnum opulus* (Cramp bark)	Spasmolytic, analgesic.

Directions: Mix up dry herbs. Use ½ oz herbs mixed up in proportion to 3½ cups water. Remove from heat. Steep 20 minutes and strain. 1 cup 3 × day. Store in fridge. One day's worth.

- *Definition of acute UTI.* Cystitis is when the bladder or urethra, or both, become infected with bacteria. Normally the walls are smooth and glassy, but in cystitis the bacteria are able to adhere. Cystitis is more prevalent in women and girls than in men and boys, because in females the urethra is shorter and closer to the rectum and more easily contaminated when wiping. It also occurs after the use of irritating soaps and douches, and often from bladder pressure and hormonal changes in pregnancy. Most UTIs result from ascending infection by gram-negative bacteria, 80% from *Escherichia coli*, but sometimes from *Staphylococcus saprophyticus*, *Klebsiella pneumoniae*, or *Proteus mirabilis*. Most recurrent infections result from the same organism.[6] Acute infections are also frequent after antibiotic use, during stress when immunity is lowered, and in people with diabetes.
  - *Signs and symptoms of an acute UTI.* Frequency, urgency, dysuria, cramps or spasms of the bladder, dark urine, itching, and frequent nighttime urination. There may be fever, lower abdominal pain, nausea or vomiting, and hematuria. Urine is often cloudy or bloody and has a bad smell. Diagnosed by a midstream urine sample that shows increased white blood cells (WBC) that indicate an infection and from a high bacteria count. A urine culture and sensitivity test show the exact organism involved, and which antibiotic will treat it.
  - *General therapeutic principles for an acute UTI.* (1) Urinary-specific antimicrobials that are high in terpenes and excreted through the bladder, the site of infection. Of note are Uva ursi leaf, Buchu leaf, and sometimes fresh Yarrow herb.[11] Bilberry leaves stop bacterial adhesion to the bladder walls, as do Cranberries. Note that Bilberries, Cranberries, and Uva ursi are all in the Heath family. (2) Antiinflammatory demulcents to soothe pain. (3) If hematuria is present, use astringents. (4) Diuretics to flush bladder. (5) Antispasmodics and analgesics as needed. (6) When acute infection is resolved, begin a preventative, restorative formula.
- *Definition of chronic recurrent cystitis.* Sometimes UTIs become chronic and are known as *recurrent cystitis* (Case History 26.2). Chronic cystitis is more serious than acute cystitis because there are more opportunities for bacteria to travel upward to the kidneys. Chronic infections are hard to

CASE HISTORY 26.2

Case History for Chronic Recurrent Cystitis

S. Sally is 25 years old and has had chronic urinary tract infections (UTIs) since high school. She takes antibiotics, and infection goes away for a while but always comes back. She is between episodes. When pressed, she admits they occur in times of stress.

O. **P**. Weak, especially on right, the Kidney yang side. Tight. **T** Normal.

A. Lin syndrome. Kidney Qi Deficiency. Recurrent UTIs with stress and anxiety.

P. *Specific therapeutic principles.* (1) Tonics. (2) Prophylactic antimicrobials. (3) Demulcents to control inflammation. (4) Immune support. (5) Diuretics to keep kidneys flushed. (6) Nervines for stress.

Herbal Formula and Dose. 5 mL 3 × day for 3–4 months.

Part	Herbs	Rationale
3	Goldenrod herb	Trophorestorative, antiinfective, draining diurotic.
3	Juniper berry	Draining diuretic, antimicrobial for chronic UTIs.
3	Skullcap herb	Nervous system relaxant.
2	Couch grass root	Restorative, antimicrobial, demulcent, diuretic.
2	Echinacea root	Immune support, detoxicant.

Other Suggestions

- *Diet.* Lots of dark green veggies, fruit, and walnuts to tonify Kidney qi.
- *What not to drink.* Alcohol and caffeinated drinks, including soda pop, are dehydrating because they cause diuresis. Soda pop contains phosphate, which can contribute to kidney stones.
- *Morning kidney flush with liquid chlorophyll.* One teaspoon liquid chlorophyll to 8 oz water every morning before breakfast.
- *Good hydration.* This must become a way of life. Three quarts per day. Include 16 oz unsweetened cranberry juice daily or cranberry extract.
- *After sex.* Urinate ASAP.
- *Stress management.* Yoga, exercise, meditation, barefoot walking on the earth.
- *For acute flareup.* Use usual therapeutic principles for treating Lin Damp Heat. Then revert back to preventative measures for a few months.
- *Supplements.* Probiotics to restore flora lost from recurrent antibiotic treatments.
- *Tea to restore the kidneys* (Box 26.3).

eradicate, because bacteria tend to stick to the urinary tract walls and become dormant, and then resistant to another round of antibiotics.[8]

- *Therapeutic principles for recurrent cystitis.* Herbal treatment involves 3 to 4 months (or more) of preventative herbs including: (1) Tonics. (2) Prophylactic antimicrobials. (3) Demulcents to control inflammation. (4) Immune support with Echinacea root or Licorice root. (5) Diuretics to flush kidneys. (6) If acute flare-up recurs, revert back to the usual therapeutic principles described earlier for treating acute Lin Damp Heat and when resolved return to the preventative measures for a few months.

- *Definition of interstitial cystitis.* This is a persistent, difficult-to-treat urinary irritation with *no* obvious signs of infection (Case History 26.3). Sometimes it begins after a UTI. Signs and symptoms are similar to a UTI, except no bacteria are present when urine is cultured, and antibiotics do not help. It can flare up during sex, exercise, stress, and during menses. It may be autoimmune.
- *Therapeutic principles for interstitial cystitis.* (1) Kidney tonics. (2) Demulcents. (3) Spasmolytics and analgesics. (4) Immune modulators. (5) Begin autoimmune protocol.

CASE HISTORY 26.3

Case History for Interstitial Cystitis

S. For the past 5 years, Madeline has been getting chronic bladder pressure, frequency, urgency, and burning dysuria. Her urine never shows any bacteria, although she has constant pain. Now it happens during intercourse, too. Antibiotics do not help. She has tried them often. There is anxiety and depression. She reports frequent belching, burping, and indigestion. She loves cheese.
O. **P** Rapid. and weak on right, the Spleen side. **T** Pale, yellow sticky coat.
A. Lin syndrome with Spleen Qi Deficiency. Interstitial cystitis with indigestion/probable dysbiosis.
P. *Specific therapeutic principles.* (1) Kidney restoratives. (2) Draining diuretics. (3) Spasmolytics and analgesics. (4) Demulcents for pain and dysuria. (5) Treat anxiety and depression. (6) Autoimmune Four-R Protocol incorporating the Gut and Psychology Syndrome (GAPS) diet.

Herbal Formula and Dose. 5 mL 3 × day.

Parts	Herbs	Rationale
3	Goldenrod herb	Kidney trophorestorative, draining diuretic.
3	Kava root	Anxiety and depression, diuretic, tones muscles, spasmolytic.
2	White Willow bark	Clear heat, analgesic, antiinflammatory.
2	Couch grass root	Demulcent, draining diuretic, detoxicant, drains lymph.
2	White Atractylodes Bai Zhu	Spleen tonic.

Other Suggestions

- *Diet.* Cranberry juice, Four-R program for possible autoimmune-gut connection, but take it slow. Consider GAPS diet (Chapters 16 and 18).
- *Supplements.* Probiotics for gut, vitamin B complex for nervous tension, anxiety.
- *Urinary lifestyle measures.* Good hydration, void and good hygiene post sex.
- *Stress management.* Yoga, meditation, acupuncture, or massage.

Kidney Stones or Renal Calculi

- *Definition.* ***Renal calculi*** or kidney stones are hardened mineral formations anywhere in the urinary tract (Case History 26.4). Size ranges from a grain of sand to as large as a golf ball. They usually develop in the renal pelvis or calyces of the kidneys. Most stones are made of calcium oxalate or calcium phosphate; a few from uric acid. Normal urine contains uric acid and calcium in solution, which passes right through. When and if they harden and crystalize in the kidneys, they pick up more and more solid matter, forming into gravel and then stones. If a large piece breaks off and passes into the ureter, it creates exceedingly painful spasms.
- *Signs and symptoms.* None, until stone moves from kidney into the ureters. Then intensely horrible *flank* pain in lower back over the involved kidney and on the sides radiating into the groin. Pain comes in waves. Could be nausea, vomiting, sweating, hematuria, and sometimes infection. Most pass from kidneys by peristalsis down to the bladder, taking

CASE HISTORY 26.4

Case History for Kidney Stones or Renal Calculi

S. Jerry complains of intense flank pain radiating to genital area, on and off, that comes and goes. He has hematuria and nausea. No fever. He thinks he has a urinary tract infection (UTI). Urine is dark and pinkish.
O. **P** Wiry and thready. **T** Dusky, thick coat.
A. Lin Syndrome. Probable renal calculi.
P. *Therapeutic principles.* (1) Antilithics. (2) Antispasmodics to decrease pain. (3) Analgesics. (4) Demulcents.

Herbal Formula and Dose. 5 mL every ½ to 1 hour.

Parts	Herbs	Rationale
3	Crataeva root bark	Antilithic.
3	Cramp bark	Antispasmodic.
3	Corydalis Yan Hu Suo	Analgesic.
2	Stone root	Antilithic, diuretic.
2	Cornsilk style	Demulcent, antispasmodic, diuretic.

Other Suggestions

Note: If possible, have client strain urine and save stones to be analyzed. Diet therapy may be based on type of mineral content.

- *Superhydration.* Essential to dilute urine to help stone passage. Should be making at least 3 pt of urine per day. Urine should be light yellow. This is even more important if there is a calculi history. No soda pop; it contains phosphates.
- *Diet.* Fresh whole foods. An alkaline diet with lots of vegetables and reduced meat and sugar is indicated. No processed foods, which contain loads of salt. Salt increases calcium and oxalate in the urine. No sugar. Sugar interferes with calcium and magnesium absorption.
- *Stone content analysis.* (Done in a lab per healthcare provider's order.)
  - *Stones with calcium oxalate salts.* Restrict high oxalate foods, such as spinach, rhubarb, beets, parsley, strawberries, nuts, pepper, and chocolate.
  - *Stones with uric acid.* Restrict protein because protein increases uric acid levels.
  - *Stones with calcium phosphate.* These often form if infections are present. Work on protocols for recurrent cystitis, as needed. Do *not* restrict dietary calcium. It is needed for general health and this measure does not help, although it is used in old school thinking.

minutes to days, and the pain is then gone. Diagnosed by ultrasound or CT scan, stones or gravel in urine.
- *Allopathic treatment*. Pain meds and smooth muscle relaxants. If stone is not resolved on its own, surgical removal, lithotripsy which uses ultrasound shock waves aimed at stone to break it up. Diet adjustments based on content of stones are used but not always effective.
- *General therapeutic principles*. Given time, herbs work well to dissolve stones or prevent more. (1) Antilithics such as Gravel root, Stone root, or Couch grass root. (2) Antispasmodics. (3) Antiinflammatories. (4) Demulcents, which usually double as antiinflammatories. (5) Analgesic herbs like Jamaican Dogwood bark or Corydalis Yan Hu Suo. (6) If repeated urinary infections are part of history, work on decreasing these.

Urinary Incontinence

- *Definition*. ***Incontinence*** is lack of voluntary control over urination (Case History 26.5). There are a few major causes in adults, and if these can be determined, it is most helpful.
  - *Stress incontinence or qi deficiency*. This is the most common type, a connective tissue deficiency where the pelvic floor muscles become weakened. It is caused by multiple pregnancies and births, menopause, being overweight, and from prostatitis. Urine leaks when there is pressure on the bladder from coughing, sneezing, laughing, exercising, or lifting something heavy.
  - *Neurogenic bladder incontinence: spastic or atonic*. Neurogenic bladder may be from muscle spasms when the bladder is empty, but it feels like the need to go (*spastic*), or it may be from no muscle tone whatsoever (*atonic*), where the bladder is full, but there is no awareness of it being so.
  - *Estrogen deficiency incontinence*. Common in menopause, from a thin urethra and mucosa that lead to decreased blood flow, decreased contraction, itching, dryness, prolapse, and incontinence.
- *Signs and symptoms*.
  - *Stress incontinence* causes leakage with coughing, straining, lifting, abdominal pressure.
  - *Neurogenic bladder*. If spastic, it feels like an intense need to urinate, even when the bladder is empty or nearly so. There is no distention. If atonic, it's the opposite. The bladder is distended and full, but there is no feeling or urge to void. Leakage occurs on exertion (Fig. 26.4).
  - *Estrogen deficiency*. Here there is pain, itching frequency, and irritation when estrogen is low, around menopause, or with a total hysterectomy.
- *Allopathic treatment*. Medications, surgery, or exercises.
- *General therapeutic principles*. (1) *Stress incontinence*. Strengthen connective tissue with Horsetail herb, Nettle herb, Eucommia Du Zhong. It is also important to strengthen pelvic floor muscles (the trigone) with Mullein root and physical exercises. (2) *Spastic:* Use smooth muscles relaxants and spasmolytics with a tropism for urinary tract, such as Kava root, Wild Carrot root, Parsley seed, Wild Yam root, or St. John's Wort.[7] Astringents are also indicated. If there is spastic *enuresis*, or nighttime incontinence, Mullein root (not leaf) works wonders, especially

CASE HISTORY 26.5

Case History for Incontinence

S. Every time Louise laughs, coughs, or lifts a heavy package, she "pees a little in her pants." She is 50 lb overweight and has had five children. She is quite stressed.
O. **P** Weak. **T** Pale.
A. Kidney Qi Deficiency. Stress incontinence.
P. *Specific therapeutic principles*. (1) Strengthen connective tissue. (2) Decrease stress with nervous relaxants.

Herbal Formula and Dose. 5 mL 3 × day.

Parts	Herbs	Rationale
3	Eucommia Du Zhong	Connective tissue strengthener.
3	Horsetail herb	Connective tissue strengthener, and astringent.
3	St. John's Wort	Calming, spasmolytic, and astringent.
2	Mullein root	Strengthens trigone muscle in pelvic floor.
2	Nettle herb	Connective tissue strengthener, and astringent.
1	Passionflower	Calming, and spasmolytic.

Other Suggestions

- ***Diet***. Work on achieving a healthy weight with a pure foods, clean Mediterranean or Paleo diet. Avoid bladder irritants, such as caffeine, alcohol, and acidic foods. Eat more fiber, which can prevent constipation and straining.
- *Kegel exercise and Pilates*. Kegels are pelvic floor exercises where the muscles are tightened and relaxed repeatedly. One method is to sit on toilet and hold urine stream, let a little out, repeat. Or tighten and relax pelvic muscles when standing up, sitting down, in the grocery line, wherever. *Pilates* to strengthen abdominals and pelvic muscles; bouncing on a mini trampoline.
- *Lifestyle*. Don't smoke—or seek help to quit.

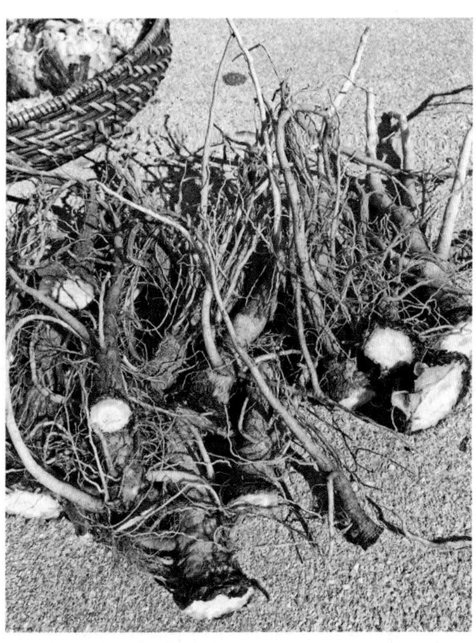

• **Fig. 26.4** *Verbascum thapsus* (Mullein root) specifically strengthens the trigone sphincter, the same muscle targeted in Kegel exercises. The root works well to remedy incontinence.

for elders. (3) *Atonic*: Use neuromuscular restoratives such as Buchu leaf, Fennel seed, or Prickly Ash bark. (4) *For estrogen deficiency*: Increase estrogen with Black Cohosh root, Fennel seed or root, or Ligusticum Chuan Xiong (Sichuan Lovage root) and use urinary demulcents, such as Marshmallow root, Couch grass root, or Cornsilk style.

Summary

Kidneys make urine, and through this process waste is removed, and pH, electrolytes, and water volume are balanced. Electrolytes are charged elements that are essential to the body in very correct amounts. Water must be in its designated compartments in and out of the cells and in the right amounts. The kidneys regulate and maintain blood pressure through the renin-angiotensin-aldosterone (RAA) pathway and also make red blood cells.

Normal urine is light yellow, has an acceptable odor, and does not look murky or have sediment or pinkish signs of blood. Being kind to the kidneys includes staying well hydrated and consuming a diet filled with greens, fruits, and veggies. In Chinese Medicine, the Kidney organ system is basic to whole body well-being, but the physical kidneys are addressed in the form of Lin syndromes—bladder and kidney infections, stones, and incontinence—the same as in the West.

The urinary Materia Medica includes restoratives, stimulating diuretics, relaxants in the form of antispasmodics and analgesics, stone-dissolving antilithics, and the sedating antimicrobials. Common Lin conditions include acute and recurrent bladder infections; the elusive interstitial cystitis, which is probably autoimmune and not really an infection at all; and calculi that are most easily treated when small.

Review

Fill in the Blanks

(Answers in Appendix B.)

1. Name five functions of the Western kidneys: ___, ___, ___, ___, ___.
2. Kidneys open to the ___, govern the ___, and manifest on the ___. Emotion is ___. Element is ___, and color is ___.
3. Name three Chinese urinary antimicrobials: ___, ___, ___. Name three Western antimicrobials: ___, ___, ___.
4. UTIs are ___ syndromes. Acute UTIs are what temperature? ___. Chronic UTIs are what temperature? ___.
5. Five Western antilithics are: ___, ___, ___, ___, ___.
6. Name five types of urinary incontinence and what they mean: ___, ___, ___, ___, ___.
7. Two functions of urinary restoratives are ___ and ___. Name two Chinese restoratives: ___, ___ and three Western restoratives: ___, ___, ___.
8. Name three antimicrobial Western diuretics: ___, ___, ___. Name two Chinese antimicrobial diuretics: ___, ___.
9. Identify four causes of bladder connective tissue deficiency or stress incontinence: ___, ___, ___, ___.
10. Name four Lin syndromes and Western counterparts: ___, ___, ___, ___.

Critical Concept Questions

(Answers for you to decide.)

1. Why is it said the kidneys are the most complicated of all body systems? The most holistic?
2. Explain how the kidneys regulate blood pressure. What are ACE inhibitors?
3. Why is it hard to fit the Chinese Medicine Kidney Organ System into Western medicine?
4. What are Kegel exercises? How are they done? Why and when?
5. What is the difference between a diuretic and a draining diuretic? Name two of each.
6. Why is liquid chlorophyll beneficial to the kidneys?
7. How can we keep the kidneys healthy?
8. A client reports all the symptoms of a UTI, but repeated tests show no bacteria in her urine. Your answer?
9. What herbs would be best for urinary damp heat and why?
10. If you could pick only three herbs for your kidney apothecary, what would they be?

References

1. Taylor, James and Barbara Cohen. *Memmler's Structure and Function of the Human Body* (Philadelphia, PA: Lippincott, 2013).
2. Cohen, Barbara. *Memmler's The Human Body in Health and Disease, 12th Edition*. (Baltimore, MD: Lippincott, 2013).
3. Disi, Sarah et. al. "Anti-hypertensive Herbs and their Mechanisms of Action: Part I." U.S. National Library of Medicine, National Institutes of Health. Frontiers of Pharmacology. https://www.ncbi.nlm.nih.gov/pmc/articles/PMC4717468/ (accessed March 1, 2021).
4. O'Neil, Carolyn. "Why Your Pee Smells Funny After Eating Asparagus." WebMD. https://www.webmd.com/food-recipes/features/why-pee-smells-funny-eat-asparagus (accessed December 15, 2019).
5. Simerville, Jeff A., William C. Maxted, and John J. Pahira. "Urinalysis: A Comprehensive Review." American Family Physician. https://www.aafp.org/afp/2005/0315/p1153.html (accessed August 24, 2019).
6. Tierra, Michael. "Integrating the Traditional Chinese Understanding of the Kidneys Into Western Herbalism." East West School of Planetary Herbology. https://planetherbs.com/research-center/theory-articles/integrating-the-traditional-chinese-understanding-of-the-kidneys-into-western-herbalism/ (accessed August 24, 2019).
7. Holmes, Peter. *Energetics of Western Herbs* (Boulder, CO: Snow Lotus, 2000).
8. Holmes, Peter. *Jade Remedies: A Chinese Herbal Reference for the West* (Boulder, CO: Snow Lotus, 1996).
9. "Herbal Care for the Urinary Tract and Kidneys." (adapted). Adiantum School of Plant Medicine. http://www.adiantumschool.com/single-post/2016/08/05/Herbal-Care-for-the-Urinary-Tract-and-Kidneys (accessed August 24, 2019).
10. Hoffman, David. *Medical Herbalism: The Science and Practice of Herbal Medicine* (Rochester, VT: Healing Arts, 2003).
11. Bone, Kerry and Simon Mills. *Principles and Practice of Phytotherapy* (London, UK: Elsevier, 2013).
12. "Crataeva: Crataeva nurvala." Institute for Traditional Medicine. http://www.itmonline.org/ayurreview/ayurcrat.htm (accessed August 24, 2019).

27 The Endocrine System

"The throat chakra acts as a bridge between the intelligence of the heart and the intelligence of the mind. When your throat chakra is strong and free of blockages your heart and head will work together in harmony."

—***Kalashatra Govinda***[1]

CHAPTER REVIEW

- Overview of the endocrine system. The neuroendocrine system; the HPA axis; adaptogens and their relationship to the HPA axis.
- The adrenals and stress.
- The thyroid. The hypothyroid epidemic, and what's with iodine?
- Keeping the thyroid and adrenals healthy.
- The pancreas. Diabetes mellitus type 1. The hypoglycemic, insulin resistance, and diabetes mellitus type 2 spectrum.
- The endocrine chakras.
- Chinese Medicine perspective. The endocrine system and major syndromes.
- Endocrine Materia Medica. Endocrine herbs worth honorable mention.
  - Adrenals: Neuro-endocrine restoratives, yin and yang tonics, primary, secondary, and companion adaptogens.
  - Thyroid: Endocrine restoratives, yin and yang tonics, superfoods, liver supportives, and sea vegetables.
  - Pancreas: Hypoglycemics, bitters, liver restoratives, antioxidants, microvascular stabilizers, and dark green nutritive herbs.
- Common endocrine conditions with case histories: Adrenal fatigue, Hashimoto's thyroiditis, hyperthyroidism, and insulin resistance type II.

KEY TERMS

Adaptogens
Adrenal fatigue/burnout
Cortisol
Diabetes mellitus type 1 and 2 (DM1 and DM2)
Endocrine system
Epinephrine
Ghrelin
Glucagon
Goitrogens
Halogens
Hashimoto's thyroiditis
Hemoglobin A1c (HgA1c)
Hormones
Hypothalamic-pituitary-adrenal axis (HPA axis)
Hypothalamic-pituitary-thyroid axis (HPT axis)
Insulin
Insulin resistance
Leptin
Leptin resistance
Negative feedback
Neuroendocrine system

The ***endocrine system*** consists of an assortment of glands that are stimulated to produce chemicals that regulate the body. Known as hormones, these chemicals are communicators, making the body hum and keeping things in balance. If the thyroid gland needs removal because of a tumor or cancer, then hormone replacement drugs would need to be taken for life. As a nurse, I've seen first-hand the havoc that can occur from the loss of just a single one of these tiny groups of specialized cells.

A takeaway from the study of the endocrine system is how chronic stress negatively affects chronic health issues in Western societies, such as hypothyroidism, digestive ills, blood sugar imbalances, autoimmune disorders, and reproductive problems. We will investigate the adrenals, thyroid, and pancreas. Chapter 28 covers reproductive glands and hormones. Relevant syndromes in Chinese Medicine are matched with Western endocrine diseases. The entire chakra energy system also coordinates with the endocrine.

Overview of the Endocrine System

Endocrine glands comprise a network of ductless glands that produce ***hormones***, which are chemical messengers that regulate all types of body functions from stress, energy, growth, and development to metabolism, immunity, sexual function, and many others. Endocrine hormones are secreted directly into the bloodstream and carried through the blood to their target organs.

For instance, the thyroid gland makes T3 and T4, which deal with metabolic activity and the body's ability to produce and consume energy. Those hormones are carried to every cell in the body. The adrenals, located over each kidney, secrete the stress hormones adrenaline and cortisol (among others). The pancreatic islet cells secrete insulin and glucagon involved in blood sugar regulation. They are regulated and controlled by a ***negative feedback*** loop: when a hormone level gets too high, the brakes are set, and production decreases until the next time it is needed; when levels get too low, more hormone is produced and circulated.

The Neuroendocrine System

The interaction between the nervous and the endocrine systems is known as the ***neuroendocrine system***. They are the two main body controllers and work together. The *neuro* portion of the endocrine refers to the *hypothalamus*, a tiny part of the brain which could be considered a rapid-relay station linking the nervous system to the endocrine glands via the pituitary. The hypothalamus acts as a collecting center for information regarding the internal well-being and homeostasis of the body.[2]

The hypothalamus is located right below the pituitary gland and behind the *third eye* (right between the eyebrows). This mission control center receives and regulates signals from all over the body through the autonomic nervous system (ANS). The ANS regulates involuntary vital signs like breathing, heart rate, blood pressure (BP), and stress response signals.

The Hypothalamic-Pituitary-Adrenal Axis (HPA Axis)

The ***hypothalamic-pituitary-adrenal axis (HPA axis)*** is an interactive system linking the hypothalamus to the pea-sized pituitary gland and then to the adrenals. The hypothalamus also has other pathways. After it sends either nervous signals and/or hormones to the pituitary, instead of messaging the adrenals, the pituitary can connect to the parathyroid glands, the thyroid gland, or the ovaries or testes. It all depends on which hormone it releases. Even the pancreas is involved, because it has been recognized that a subgroup of hypothalamic neurons and neurons elsewhere in the brain have the capacity to sense glucose and influence the secretion of anti-insulin hormones and hepatic glucose production.[3]

Adaptogens and Their Relationship to the HPA Axis

The herbal takeaway, as far as the HPA axis goes, is that whenever an herb is designated a neuroendocrine stimulator, it balances the entire hormonal pathway from the brain to the adrenals. True ***adaptogens*** meet this criterion. Adaptogens, such as Schisandra Wu Wei Zi (Five Taste berry) and Ashwagandha root regulate and normalize stress responses, blood glucose levels, and cardiovascular, immune, and nervous system functions, e.g., stress, and can have enormously positive effects on chronic and autoimmune diseases, premature aging, and our health (Chapter16).[2] This effect is particularly true when combined with optimal nutrition, exercise, and rest. That's why adaptogens are so precious and revered. They smooth out the highs and lows of neuroendocrine imbalances and decrease elevated cortisol, the classic sign of prolonged stress.

The Adrenals and Stress

The two adrenals are little triangle-shaped glands that sit on top of each kidney and have an enormous amount to do with stress. There are two parts. The adrenal medulla is the inside portion and secretes *adrenaline* (also called ***epinephrine***); the outside covering, the adrenal cortex portion, secretes the glucocorticoid hormones, one being *cortisol*, when stimulated by adrenocorticotropic hormone (ACTH) from the pituitary.

Short-acting epinephrine is considered the survival fight-or-flight hormone that deals with immediate stress and processes fear or danger. This action happens when you get a *rush*, run from a threat, are thrilled by something new and exciting, ride a roller coaster, or look down over the edge of a high mountain. Alertness, heart rate, BP, and oxygen intake increase because of signals from the hypothalamus' regulation of the ANS.[4] Runners experience so-called *adrenaline highs* and are able to get a last burst of energy to complete a race. In the hospital, nurses who thrive on trauma and excitement in the emergency room or intensive care unit (like me at one time) refer to being *adrenaline junkies*.

Sometimes, this stress becomes chronic, and the body never quits being in this constantly wired state. Prolonged stress that lasts for weeks, months, or years, can be detrimental and turn into anxiety and illness. Fight-and-flight epinephrine has been used up and is long gone, and the body then switches to cortisol from the adrenal cortex to maintain the habitually stressful state. ***Cortisol*** is a vital steroid hormone that acts to help stop inflammation and to regulate the immune system, libido, reproduction, and production of thyroid hormones.[4] Its bad reputation as a *stress hormone* occurs when stress is continual, and cortisol is called on to maintain an unhealthy high-alert state in place of epinephrine. Cortisol blood levels soar, and trouble begins. For instance, ultrahigh sustained cortisol levels can make thyroid hormones less available to cells and can also reduce the liver's ability to clear used-up estrogen from the system.[4] The former leads to hypothyroidism; the latter leads to estrogen dominance with premenstrual syndrome (PMS) problems, good examples of the results of unending stress and the interconnectedness of the various body systems.

Cortisol blood levels are normally highest in the morning when we rise and lowest in the evening and night when we rest and sleep, a typical biorhythm cycle. But if a perpetual pattern of high alert and chronic anxiety ensues, and the person (typically a female) never stops running and busily doing activities, rarely relaxes, has little time or ability to sleep, cortisol levels can become alarmingly skewed. Cortisol might be low in the morning (lazy Mary), when we are supposed to rise and shine without the help of stimulants. Blood levels can slump in the late afternoon, necessitating a caffeine frenzy in the midafternoon (the 4 p.m. cortisol and glucose slump). Levels could also peak at night (the night owl scenario) when some people work late, can't sleep, or lie in bed worrying till dawn.

Eventually, as we never *turn off*, cortisol production runs out of steam and goes from high to low. This result is the so-called overdrive, *adrenal fatigue/burnout* stage that is rarely recognized by allopathic medicine. Interestingly, the World Health Organization officially included adrenal burnout as an *occupational phenomenon* (workplace stress) in its revision of the International Classification of Diseases in May 2019.[5]

Symptoms of adrenal burnout include energy depletion and exhaustion, brain fog, digestive problems, blood sugar fluctuations, salt and fat cravings especially in late afternoon, food sensitivities, depression, and anxiety. Sex drive goes out the window, immunity is lowered, and frequent colds and skin outbreaks occur. PMS or menopausal symptoms peak as hormones go berserk. Autoimmune syndromes kick in, most notably Hashimoto's thyroiditis and insulin resistance. Time to hit the *pause* button.

The Thyroid

The thyroid is a butterfly-shaped gland located in the front of the neck at the base. Its main functions are to regulate metabolism, growth, and development. It is like a thermostat that increases or decreases the amount of energy (adenosine triphosphate or ATP) called on to carry out many functions, such as how efficiently calories are burned and whether weight can be lost. It regulates mood and memory, body temperature, skin health, and in women, hormones governing menstrual cycles, PMS, or even the tendency for breast lump formation.

Just as the HPA axis regulates adrenal activity, the ***hypothalamic–pituitary–thyroid axis (HPT axis)*** regulates thyroid activity. It triggers the hypothalamus to stimulate the pituitary gland to release thyroid stimulating hormone (TSH), which in turn causes the thyroid gland to produce larger or smaller quantities of T3 and T4, based on negative feedback. Thus a well-working pituitary becomes part of the puzzle when balancing out the thyroid, an example of the neuroendocrine connection.

The Hypothyroid Epidemic

Hypothyroidism is the most prevalent type of thyroid disease in the United States, and for years the synthetic thyroid hormone Synthroid has been one of the most frequently prescribed medications. There is a nonautoimmune type (*hypothyroidism*) and an autoimmune type called ***Hashimoto's thyroiditis***. In countries where iodine is deficient in the diet and for other reasons, nonautoimmune hypothyroidism heads the list; but in the United States and in most developed Western countries where there is no dietary iodine deficiency, the situation is reversed.

In the Hashimoto's epidemic, antibodies attack the thyroid cells for similar reasons that other autoimmune diseases occur. These reasons are all the items repeatedly alluded to in this text: a standard American diet (SAD), toxic overload, inflammation, dysbiosis and leaky gut, food sensitivities, hidden infections with immune disruptions, insulin resistance, chronic stress, and lack of sleep. Isn't it interesting that an herbalist's tools of the trade boil down to a few basic principles and fixes, no matter which body system is involved?

The symptoms of hypothyroidism and Hashimoto's are the same, and the list is long. They are what would be expected to occur if thyroid functions are down and there is an internal energy crisis. Fatigue is the primary symptom, followed by cold intolerance (putting on jackets even in warm weather); lack of sweating with dry skin; constipation; hair loss; weight gain; anxiety, depression, and insomnia; low immunity; and hormone imbalances with PMS, low sex drive, irregular periods, breast tenderness, or postpartum depression.[4] There are more symptoms but that's enough to get the idea.

What's With Iodine?

The thyroid gland uses iodine found in many foods and converts it into thyroid hormones. Thyroid cells are the only cells in the body that can absorb iodine. Too much or too little iodine can cause a *goiter*, where the thyroid becomes enlarged and can become cancerous. The thyroid combines dietary iodine and the amino acid tyrosine to make the hormones T3 and T4. These are then used to control metabolism by converting glucose and oxygen into energy ATP. Inactive T4 must be converted to the active form, T3, with the help of selenium, zinc, and iron. The question becomes, how much iodine do we need in our diet, and should it be supplemented for a healthy thyroid? Generally, the amount of iodine in food and herbal sources is totally adequate. Before iodine is supplemented, the herbalist must be very sure that it is needed.

Sometimes supplemental iodine is a hindrance. An iodine *excess*—iodine-induced hypothyroidism—has been recognized as a trigger to Hashimoto's autoimmune hypothyroidism following acute or chronic iodine exposure, and in those cases a *low* iodine diet has been helpful in normalizing function.[6]

Keeping the Thyroid and Adrenals Healthy

- *Iodine in the correct amount.* In countries where iodine is deficient, lack of iodine is a leading cause of hypothyroidism. However, excess iodine can also do the opposite; it can *cause* the same symptoms as hypothyroidism.[6] It is best to get iodine from foods and from natural sea salt that already contains iodine and other trace minerals. Salt mined in the Midwest has neither, so it usually has iodine added (iodized salt). High iodine-containing foods include animals that live in the sea: shellfish such as shrimp, crab, and lobster; tuna, herring, sardines; and any of the sea vegetables, such as dulse, kelp, or nori. Eat more sushi and live longer.
- *Foods high in B vitamins.* Necessary for adrenal and thyroid health, vitamin B_{12} helps activate T4 to T3. B vitamins support adrenal function also. Include wheat germ, range-fed beef and liver, eggs, beans, lentils, seeds and nuts of sunflower, sesame, cashew, or almond in the diet to ensure a good vitamin B supply.
- *Thyroid and adrenal foods.* Embrace an antiinflammatory diet, because chronic inflammation is a culprit for both glands. The thyroid and the adrenals thrive on green superfoods, fish, eggs, legumes, and nuts. Omega-3 fatty acids are in many of these foods and are necessary additions Maintaining blood sugar balance is a must, as is a healthy intestinal flora. Eliminate gluten, dairy, eggs, soy, and corn if food sensitivities are an issue.
- *Caffeine.* This stimulant must either go or be consumed in moderation, as far as adrenal health is concerned. When adrenal fatigue creeps up, the body wants to remain on the go, and speedy caffeine becomes a self-medicating crutch. However, over time, as it stimulates and spikes more and more cortisol production, it has diminishing returns. This effect applies to coffee, black tea, and caffeinated soft drinks. Caffeine withdrawal, if any, usually results in fatigue, headaches, and maybe constipation and lasts for only about 3 days. Staying well-hydrated and substituting herbal teas and water with lemon are alternatives, as is taking some Magnesium, 300 to 800 mg, to keep the bowels moving. Staying caffeine-free for at least 3 weeks is sufficient to help the body adjust. Then evaluate symptoms and energy level to determine whether caffeine can be reintroduced with consciousness and moderation.
- *Selenium, zinc, and iron.* These trace minerals are needed to convert T4 into usable T3. Brazil nuts are jam-packed with selenium; shellfish (especially oysters), nuts, and seeds are

high in zinc; iron sources include beans, lentils, dark leafy greens, and even dark chocolate. Three cheers for cacao.

- *Halogens and dry saunas.* The ***halogens*** are a group of elements on the periodic table that include fluorine, chlorine, bromine, and yes, iodine. Being chemically similar, halogens compete with iodine for binding sites. Halogens are often found in fluoridated drinking water and toothpaste, chlorinated swimming pools, brominated soft drinks, and pesticides, and in baked goods made with bleached, brominated white flour that is grown in contaminated soil. Halogens even appear in nonstick cooking pan coatings, bleach, flame retardants, and plastics.[4] For this reason, treated waters and these other products are best avoided, especially in light of the hypothyroid epidemic.
  - One symptom of hypothyroidism can be lack of sweating. Dry saunas encourage sweating and help excretion of harmful halogens.
- *Goitrogens.* Substances that *may* disrupt the production of thyroid hormones by interfering with iodine uptake in the thyroid gland are called ***goitrogens***. Common goitrogens are raw cruciferous vegetables, such as cabbage, Brussels sprouts, broccoli, cauliflower, and kale. However, these foods are filled with cancer-preventing antioxidants and help maintain *good* estrogen. Only if there is a problem, such as a goiter, might these foods become a drawback. In that case, if they are eaten lightly steamed rather than raw, the goitrogenic properties of cruciferous veggies are reduced.[7]

The Pancreas

The pancreas, located deep in the mid-abdomen, is another endocrine gland with two major functions. It is both an *exocrine* gland and an *endocrine* gland. Exocrine glands have *ducts*, and in the pancreas's case, they empty digestive enzymes into the gastrointestinal (GI) system.

The *ductless* component of the pancreas is the endocrine gland function that regulates how the body uses glucose, and its relationship to insulin. ***Insulin*** is the hormone, made in specialized pancreatic beta cells, that drives glucose-rich carbohydrates from digested food in the bloodstream onto receptor sites in the cells so that glucose can then be used as a raw material in the manufacture of the energy molecule ATP.

Another beta cell hormone is ***glucagon***, which raises blood sugar levels if they fall too low, thereby turning off insulin. Insulin lowers blood sugar when it drives glucose into the cells. It is crucial to have the correct amount of glucose in both places. Therefore glucagon and insulin work together in opposition to make up the pancreas's negative feedback loop. When one goes up, the other comes down.

Diabetes Mellitus Type 1

- ***Diabetes mellitus type 1 (DM1).*** This is an *autoimmune*, and often inherited, disease where the body attacks its own beta cells. In diabetes mellitus type 1 the pancreas produces very little or no insulin at all. The word *mellitus* means *sweet*, referring to the fact that if left untreated, there is sugar in the urine, giving it a sweet taste on analysis. But this word is frequently omitted from the designation. DM1 is caused by hereditary or environmental triggers and occurs at any age, but it frequently affects children and young adults. Insulin injections or an insulin pump are needed for life, and currently there is no cure. Stem cell implants are a promising solution. If very high glucose blood levels are not controlled, the brain is affected, leading to mental confusion, diabetic coma, and eventual death. Serious long-term DM1 complications are numerous, including retinopathy (resulting in blindness), peripheral neuropathy (resulting in amputations), kidney failure, and serious immune impairments. The sooner a cure evolves, the better.
- *Treatment of DM1.* A healthy antiinflammatory diet is imperative, and carbohydrate intake must be calculated and coordinated with insulin needs. Food intake, exercise, emotional stress, and illness are all factors that affect and contribute to balancing blood sugar levels. As with any autoimmune situation, diet, exercise, and stress reduction are necessary treatment strategies. *Gymnema sylvestre* (Gurmar, Gymnema leaf) (Fig. 27.1) has been shown to lower insulin requirements by blocking sugar binding sites and hence, not allowing the sugar molecules to accumulate in the body.[8] Foot reflexology has similar effects because of its relaxation potential.
- *Glycemic index.* This index is a dietary guide that ranks carbohydrate foods based on how quickly they are burned in the body to provoke an insulin response. Chemically simple carbohydrates, like white bread or candy, require very little digestion and are quickly absorbed and so have a high glycemic index. These foods cause rapid fluctuations in glucose levels, stress out the pancreas, and lead to DM1 and insulin resistance (see next section). Chemically complex carbs such as whole grains—like barley, quinoa, rice, or millet—and vegetables such as sweet potatoes, squash, and beans take longer to digest than the simple ones.[9] Complex carbohydrates are the way to go.
- *Magnesium-rich foods.* Because magnesium helps promote insulin production, foods high in this element are a good idea. These include spinach, tofu, almonds, broccoli, lentils, pumpkin and sunflower seeds.
- *Omega-3-rich supplements and foods.* EPA/DHA capsules and marine fish, walnuts, pumpkin seeds, ground golden flax seeds that bring down inflammation are important additions.
- *Other supplements.* The trace element chromium and alpha lipoic acid (ALA) help insulin transport glucose into the cells. Coenzyme Q10 helps cardiac functioning.

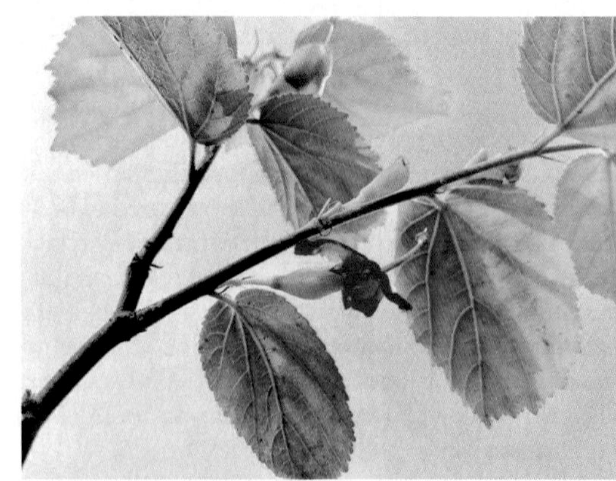

• **Fig. 27.1** *Gymnema sylvestre* (Gymnema leaf/Gurmar) is an Ayurvedic herb that temporarily masks the sweet taste. In Sanskrit, *Gurmar* means *destroyer of sugar*. Therefore Gurmar is indicated for use in DM1 and DM2. (/iStock/Subrata Dutta)

The Hypoglycemia, Insulin Resistance, and Diabetes Mellitus Type 2 Spectrum

Because of poor lifestyle choices, blood sugar problems (*dysglycemia*) typically occur on a gradual continuum, not overnight. Fatigue, depression, hypoglycemia, and food cravings are at one end of the spectrum. Insulin resistance/metabolic syndrome is in the middle. Prediabetes and adult-onset type 2 diabetes are at the other end.

Normally blood sugar levels stay at 80 to 120 mg per deciliter. Insulin produced in the pancreatic islet cells moves sugar in the food we eat (glucose) from the bloodstream to the cells. When blood glucose levels fall too low, glucagon slows down insulin production to maintain a normal range. High blood sugar is called *hyperglycemia*, and low blood sugar is *hypoglycemia*.

- *Hypoglycemia*. Because of a SAD diet, stress, lack of exercise, and constant blood sugar fluctuations and demands over the years (as seen in frequent yo-yo weight-loss dieting), the pancreas can become overworked and begins to work at a fast pace to regulate the quickly fluctuating high and low glucose levels. The negative feedback loop can't keep up with demand, and low blood sugar becomes frequent.
  - *Symptoms and warnings of low blood sugar* include forgetting to eat right, with jittery, shakiness, irritability, fatigue, exhaustion, anxiety, and not thinking straight. A common but temporary fix when this happens is to grab a quick dose of a fatty, simple carbohydrate like a donut or candy bar to right all these wrongs by quickly spiking blood sugar. But these simple carbs are speedily digested and absorbed, and it is not long before another glucose dip occurs. The person becomes ravenously hungry, satisfies their fat and carb cravings, and the cycle repeats, which is an excellent time to begin dietary changes to normalize the hypoglycemia.
- *Insulin resistance and metabolic syndrome*. The next step on the dysglycemia continuum is when cell receptor sites become resistant to receiving insulin that is trying to hook on, known as ***insulin resistance***. The pancreas produces more and more insulin in an attempt to keep blood sugar levels normal. (A blood test done at this point shows normal glucose, but elevated insulin.) So called *metabolic syndrome* occurs as triglycerides, fasting blood sugar, and BP rise, with increased risk of heart attack and stroke. Cholesterol levels get skewed, waistline disappears, and weight gain is common with the help of leptin resistance (Chapter 22).[10]
- *Leptin resistance, ghrelin, and weight gain.* ***Leptin*** is the appetite-control hormone made in fat cells that signals fullness when told to do so by the hypothalamus. Leptin helps to decrease hunger and regulate weight. It signals we are satiated and to quit eating. However, as inflammation increases because of the chronically elevated insulin levels of insulin resistance, leptin is adversely affected and hooks onto cells less efficiently in what is known as ***leptin resistance***. To make matters worse, the hormone ***ghrelin*** secreted from the stomach lining when the stomach is empty crosses the blood-brain barrier into the hypothalamus, sending signals of hunger.[11] We then eat more than necessary and gain more weight, a losing battle.
  - *Apple shape*. In insulin resistance, the body's abdominal shape goes from that of a pear to that of an apple, with loss of a waistline and development of a big gut. Hip circumference becomes smaller than waist circumference. If prolonged stress with adrenal depletion is in the picture, cortisol comes into play, causing sweet cravings and even more weight gain.
- *Treatment of insulin resistance*. Physiologically, insulin resistance has to do with the pancreas, the gut, and the liver. The pancreas's involvement was just described; gut dysbiosis *must* be addressed; and the liver, which stores extra glucose as glycogen and converts it back to glucose when needed, has to function optimally and not be compromised or bogged down in toxic overload. As usual, a toxin-free, antiinflammatory diet is critical. Supplementation is the same as that described previously with DM1.
- ***Diabetes mellitus type 2 (DM2)***. Insulin resistance and metabolic syndrome merge into DM2 nonautoimmune- and noninsulin-dependent diabetes, often still called insulin resistance and/or metabolic syndrome. DM2 is rampant in the West because of poor lifestyle choices, but it is reversible with diet, herbs, supplements, and lifestyle changes if caught early enough. If not, the pancreas goes on strike and produces less and less insulin. Glucose blood levels go from low to high, from *hypo*glycemia to *hyper*glycemia. DM2 has officially arrived. This condition leads to hypertension, coronary artery disease, inflammation, dysbiosis, kidney disease, and possibly insulin dependence.

The Endocrine Chakras

The chakra system, the endocrine system, and the nervous system are intricately related (Fig. 27.2). As we ascend each spinning energetic ball, from the first at the root to the seventh at the crown, an endocrine gland is associated with each. The glands are located in the physical vicinity of their associated chakra.

Our metaphysical chakras (consciousness) are understood to communicate with the physical body through the nervous system and the endocrine system (neuroendocrine). This communication is yet another awesome example of the mind-body connection. Each chakra is associated with an endocrine gland and a physical nerve bundle called a *plexus*.[12] When the chakra system was first intuited, no one knew we had endocrine glands or physical nerve bundles.

All the chakras have physical, mental, and spiritual associations and challenges. Our task on the physical plane is to keep the chakras open and in balance to achieve physical and mental health, and ultimately, spiritual enlightenment. This formidable challenge is approached through meditation, yoga, and various spiritual practices throughout many lifetimes. Often, healing on the physical level cannot occur unless core issues associated with the related chakras are resolved. Herbalists must be aware of this to help healing occur on all levels.

- *First chakra: adrenals/root*. The root chakra is located at the base of the spine near the adrenals and is our connection to Earth, our tribe, our survival. It is associated with fears of not having what we need, physical survival (fight or flight), abandonment. Sacred truth: All is One. Mantra: I Have.
- *Second chakra: ovaries/testes/generative*. The reproductive, the creative, and the relationship chakra is located in the pelvis, holding the testes and ovaries. It relates to our need to procreate, for sexual and platonic relationships, and our relationships with morality and money. Primary fears are loss of control, being dominated by others, rape, addictions, impotence, betrayal, and loss of power of the physical body. Sacred Truth: Honor One Another. Mantra: I Feel.

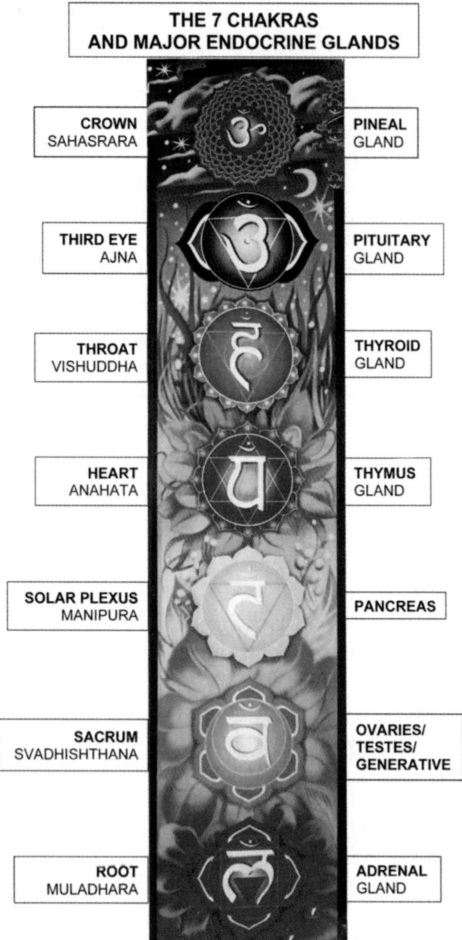

• **Fig. 27.2** Each of the 7 metaphysical chakras are related to an endocrine gland which connect through the spinal cord. This illustrates our neuroendocrine communication between the mental, spiritual, and physical bodies, representing the mind-body connection.

- *Third chakra: pancreas/solar plexus.* The solar plexus is the seat of personal power and the emotional center, located in the gut, the stomach/pancreas. It is associated with self-esteem, respect, and finding our inner power and strength. Primary fears are rejection, criticism, and fears related to our looks. Sacred Truth: Honor Oneself. Mantra: I Can.
- *Fourth chakra: thymus/heart.* Located behind the heart, the thymus gland is associated with immunity. Being the fourth, middle chakra, it bridges the physical body below and the spiritual body above. It is the place of healing and love in its purest form, which is unconditional and without judgment. It includes love for oneself, ability to forgive and have compassion. Fears are loneliness and inability to commit to another or to follow one's heart. Sacred Truth: Love Is Divine Power. Mantra: I Love.
- *Fifth chakra: thyroid/throat.* The throat chakra, which houses the thyroid gland, bridges the intelligence of the heart below and the intelligence of the mind above. It represents the power of will, speaking our truth, having a voice, and making choices with its consequence of spiritual karma. Fears relate to willpower, not being allowed a choice, and the ability to give up our power when need be. Sacred Truth: Surrender of Personal Will to Divine Will. Mantra: I Speak.
- *Sixth chakra: pituitary/third eye.* The pituitary is located behind the third eye, between the eyebrows, the intuitive. It relates to the power of the mind and separation of truth from illusion and fear, seeking wisdom, and being open to and using the intuition. Fears are an unwillingness to look within and to see the shadows. Sacred Truth: Seek Only The Truth. Mantra: I See.
- *Seventh chakra: pineal/crown.* The pineal gland is located above the pituitary, in the center of the brain; the chakra is at the crown or top of the head. This chakra is our spiritual connector to cosmic consciousness, spiritual awakening, the divine light, the energy of grace and prana, and the power of prayer. Fears relate to spiritual abandonment, loss of identity, and connection with others. Sacred Truth: Live in The Present Moment. Mantra: I Know.[13]

Chinese Medicine Perspective: The Endocrine System and Major Syndromes

- *The multifaceted Kidney organ system in Chinese Medicine.* We have already discussed how the Chinese Kidneys influence the entire body (Chapters 23 and 26). There is no endocrine system and no nervous system in Chinese Medicine per se, yet the Kidneys are assigned roles in both areas. The Chinese Kidneys are responsible for growth and development and relate to nervous system excesses and deficiencies. Physical Kidney conditions are the Lin syndromes.
- *The Chinese Kidneys and the endocrine system.* The endocrine system is the home of Kidney jing or essence, one of the vital substances. The Kidneys relate to any Western system where *hormones* are key players. Because the role of hormones was not known in ancient China, hormonal concerns were assigned to the Kidneys, and today translate into the Western understanding of the endocrine and reproductive (Chapter 28) systems.
- *The Kidneys and the thyroid gland.* Thyroid function has a lot to do with yin-yang imbalances. Energy, or its lack, is very much related to the Kidneys. Hypothyroidism follows a deficiency pattern, a lack of Kidney qi and yang, whereas hyperthyroidism follows an active, hot Liver fire pattern.
- *The Kidneys and the adrenal gland.* The Chinese Medicine concept of Kidney yin prominently involves the secretion of the glucocorticoid hormone, cortisol, from the adrenal cortex. Cortisol is a hormone that can help or hinder how we deal with stress, and when it builds up over the long term, it hinders. Kidney yang involves epinephrine and norepinephrine, which trigger the immediate active stress response (fight or flight) secretions from the adrenal medulla.[14] A gradual loss of adrenal function is understood to contribute to a decline in health.
- *The Kidneys and the pancreas.* DM1 has three Chinese Medicine syndromes, depending on symptoms and progression of the illness. Insulin resistance is considered to be Spleen Qi Deficiency with Phlegm Dampness.
- *The Chinese Kidneys and the ANS.* One way to translate Chinese Medicine thinking into a Western concept (arguably, not totally accurate) is to use the ANS as an example. The ANS is composed of the *sympathetic* nervous system (SNS),

which is responsible for managing immediate stress responses, and the *parasympathetic* nervous system (PNS), which is long-term and helps us relax.

- Kidney yang represents the quickly reactive, the SNS, with its stress secretions of epinephrine (adrenaline) and norepinephrine from the adrenal medulla.
- Kidney yin represents the passive or receptive, the parasympathetic, relating to the secretion of corticosteroids (cortisol) from the adrenal cortex. A clinical pearl when treating adrenal fatigue is to use both yin and yang tonics.[14]

Chinese Medicine Major Endocrine Syndromes

- *Kidney Yang Deficiency.* The key symptom of adrenal fatigue (burnout) is extreme exhaustion and represents a lack of energy. Because the Kidneys store energy (qi), this syndrome is also seen as a deficiency of Kidney qi, a lack of the energetic Kidney yang. Fix: Kidney yang tonics are needed. **Pulse (P)** Deep and weak. **Tongue (T)** Pale, swollen, and wet.
  - Other symptoms of Kidney Yang Deficiency include soreness of the back, cold knees, weak legs, impotence, dizziness, vertigo, loose stools, aversion to cold or feeling cold, edema and abundant clear urination, nocturnal emission, and in women scanty menstrual flow and amenorrhea, flushed complexion, nervousness, anxiety, insomnia, dryness, and chronic signs of inflammation and wasting.
- *Kidney Yin Deficiency.* Deficient kidney yin is another aspect of adrenal burnout or fatigue and represents the cortisol side. This deficiency is a state of extreme exhaustion, where even cortisol levels have hit rock bottom. **P** Wiry, rapid, or thready. **T** Reddish, little or no coat. Here yin tonics are in order.
  - Other symptoms of Kidney Yin Deficiency include achy lower back, weakness of the legs and knees, tinnitus, warmth in the soles and palms, constipation, night sweats, insomnia, dry throat, nocturnal emission, and in women, scanty menstrual flow and amenorrhea.
- *Kidney Qi Deficiency.* Often referred to as hypothyroidism and Hashimoto's thyroiditis. It is a lack of energy (qi), so it is addressed with qi and yang tonics, just as in adrenal exhaustion. **P** Slow, weak, and deep. **T** Pale with a white coat.
- *Kidney Qi and Yin Deficiency.* In Chinese Medicine, hyperthyroidism is considered to be hot and fiery overactivity, where prolonged overstimulation results in qi (energy) and yin (moisture) deficiencies.[15] **P** Rapid, thin, and weak. **T** Very red with patchy or no coat and possible cracks. Treatment is to clear heat, possibly with Milky Oat berry, and to tonify qi and yin.
- *Xiao Ke syndromes.* This refers to a group of syndromes involving DM1, where the pancreas is no longer producing insulin. The main symptoms (when untreated) are thirst with excessive drinking, hunger with excessive appetite, profuse urination, lassitude. Treatment and diagnosis depend on which type presents.
- *Spleen Qi Deficiency with Phlegm Dampness.* This syndrome lines up best with insulin resistance, metabolic syndrome or DM2, where the pancreas produces some insulin, but not enough. From the Chinese standpoint, the fix is to use Spleen (stomach) tonics, boost qi with qi tonics, and in most cases dry damp.

Endocrine Materia Medica

Endocrine Herbs Worth Honorable Mention

- *Anemarrhena asphodeloides* Zhi Mu (Know Mother root). This lily family herb blooms only at night and is frequently used as a women's botanical (knows the mother), although it is often useful for men. It is wonderfully moisturizing and cooling and works on the HPA axis, making it a prime adrenal herb. It is a yin tonic that pairs with Rehmannia Shu Di Huang (Prepared Rehmannia root) and Black Figwort root. This herb is exactly what's needed for menopausal hot flashes. Anemarrhena could have had special mention under reproduction.
- *Rehmannia glutinosa* Shu Di Huang (Prepared Rehmannia root). This Chinese Medicine herb comes in prepared and unprepared forms. The prepared form used here provides sensational adrenal, HPA, and liver restorative effects, and it provides blood sugar stabilization both in hyper- and hypoglycemia. It is traditionally washed in millet wine, steamed on a willow frame in a porcelain vessel, and then dried and resteamed and redried *nine* times, until it looks inky, black, and shiny as lacquer with the consistency of leather.[25] No joke. Shu Di Huang is sweet, oily and moist, and it is considered a yin tonic. In my opinion, it is a very useful endocrine herb. The only concern is that for some, it can be too rich *(cloying)* and may disturb digestion, causing damp, so it is contraindicated in Spleen Qi Deficiency.
- *Lepidium meyenii* (Maca root). Maca is an ancient adaptogenic superfood grown in the Andes and sometimes called *Peruvian ginseng,* although not a panax or true ginseng. This root vegetable is a staple of the Inca that provides energy and stamina when climbing mountains and herding llamas and alpacas. Maca is a nutty, butterscotch tasting root, rich in protein, fiber, calcium, magnesium, and amino acids. It helps balance the HPA axis in adrenal fatigue by reducing cortisol levels. It also helps libido, fertility, hormonal balance, and mood.[16] Use Maca in a smoothie (Box 27.1) or give clients 1 teaspoon of the powder in warm water daily. It could be tinctured, but I've never tried it in that form.
- *Gymnema sylvestre* (Gurmar, Gymnema leaf). Its Hindu name, Gurmar, means *destroyer of sugar.* When a few drops of tincture are placed on the tongue or when some of the leaves are chewed, the sweet taste buds are temporarily anaesthetized for about 2 hours because of the presence of gymnemic acid. This is a fun thing to try out and see for yourself. Furthermore, Gymnema has been shown to raise insulin levels and seems to repair damaged beta cells (at least in rats). In insulin-dependent humans with DM1, the herb actually *lowered* insulin requirements by about 50%.[18] These are very exciting findings for this Ayurvedic herb.
- *Olea europaea* (Olive leaf) (Fig. 27.3). This antioxidant, antiinflammatory leaf is hypoglycemic, lowers cholesterol, lowers BP, and is even cancer protective because of its oleuropein content. One of the key components of the healthy Mediterranean diet is olive oil. Studies have shown that Olive leaf extract (1:2 or 1:3 50%) slows down the entire glucose pathway. Specifically, it decelerates digestion of starches into simple sugars, slows glucose absorption into the bloodstream, and decreases glucose uptake into tissues from the blood.[19] These actions translate into lowered blood glucose and HgA1c levels. Another reason to include olive oil in the diet.
- *Ocimum sanctum and O. tenuiflorum* (Tulsi, Holy Basil leaf). The plant's common name, Tulsi, means *the incomparable one.* It is a staple Ayurvedic medicinal plant that has been used in India and other cultures for thousands of years. It is closely

• BOX 27.1 Hormone Balancing Maca, Cinnamon Smoothie

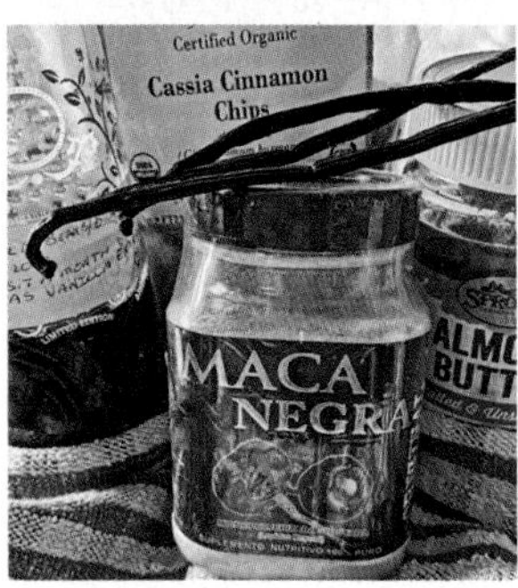

Ingredients in this nutritious and delicious hormone-balancing smoothie include ground Maca root, almond butter, Cinnamon chips, and vanilla bean.

Lepidium meyenii (Maca root) is an earthy Peruvian superfood in the Mustard family that looks like a turnip. It is an endocrine and immune restorative (companion adaptogen) with a rich, pleasing flavor. This smoothie could serve as a quick, easy, and filling morning drink, when too busy to make breakfast, a candidate for the adrenal fatigue, on-the-go client. It is gluten-free and contains healthy fats and protein.[17] Extra protein powder could be added to help stay full longer. Could add a banana or cocoa powder, or mix Maca root with spinach and avocado for a green drink.

Ingredients

1–2 tbsp Maca powder	Chief herb.
2 tbsp almond butter	Protein rich and healthy fat.
2 tbsp ground flaxseed	Moisturizing, gives fiber and helps digestion.
½ tsp ground cinnamon	Adds sweetness, flavor, and helps normalize blood sugar.
1 tsp vanilla extract	Added flavor.
1½ cups nut milk	Fat and protein.
2 pitted dates	Yumminess.
Approximately 10 ice cubes	Water and coolness.

Instructions

Blend it all together until smooth. Add more or fewer flavors, as needed.

related to *O. basilicum* (Sweet Basil leaf) of the Mint family but tastes a lot stronger. It contains the volatile oil eugenol (present in Clove) and ursolic acid (in Rosemary). Holy Basil has been attributed to many uses, which makes sense because of its adaptogenic properties. Research gives it high marks in lowering cortisol in adrenal fatigue and helping stress-induced depression, balancing insulin and glucose metabolism, protecting the liver, normalizing BP, and helping in drug and nicotine withdrawal.[2]

Adrenal Herbs

Neuroendocrine restoratives are needed in adrenal burnout or extreme fatigue (Table 27.1). These translate into yin and yang

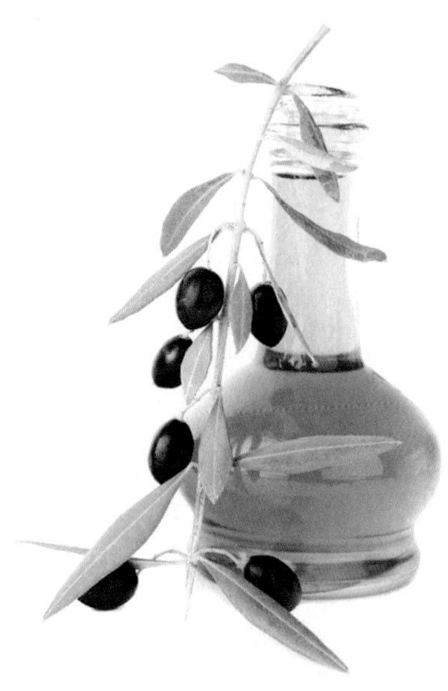

• **Fig. 27.3** *Olea europaea* (Olive leaf and oil). The tinctured hypoglycemic leaf is used to slow down glucose absorption and raise HgA1c levels. The pressed oil from the fruit is a staple in a healthy Mediterranean diet. (/iStock/Anna_Om)

TABLE 27.1 Adrenal Herbs
(Neuroendocrine restoratives, adaptogenic yin or yang tonics)

Herb	Notes
Panax ginseng Ren Shen Asian ginseng root	Stimulates HPA axis. Classic Chinese prototype adaptogen and qi tonic.
Eleutherococcus senticosus Ci Wu Jia Siberian ginseng root	Adaptogenic, stimulates the HPA axis. For loss of energy and immune deficiency. Kidney yin and qi tonic. From Russia and not a true ginseng, although it has that common name.
Schisandra chinensis Wu Wei Zi Schisandra berry, Five Taste berry	Stimulates HPA axis. Adaptogen. For Kidney qi, yin, and yang deficiency. Astringent, warm, and dry. Excellent for adrenal fatigue.
Rhodiola rosea Rhodiola root	Stimulates HPA axis. For adrenal fatigue, reduces cortisol, increases energy and concentration, antidepressant, and cardioprotective.

(*Continued*)

TABLE 27.1 Adrenal Herbs *(Neuroendocrine restoratives, adaptogenic yin or yang tonics)*—cont'd

Herb	Notes
Withania somnifera Ashwagandha, Winter Cherry root	Stimulates HPA axis. Well-balanced, combines well with other adaptogens. Means *strong as a horse*, called Indian ginseng.
Panax quinquefolius Xi Yang Shen American ginseng root	Stimulates HPA axis. This and Asian ginseng are spectacular herbs, qi tonics.
Polygonum multiflorum He Shou Wu Flowery Knotweed root, Fo-Ti	Nervous system trophorestorative helps essence (qi). Also, antidepressant and for chronic stress.
Rehmannia glutinosa Shu Di Huang Prepared Rehmannia root	Kidney yin tonic; sweet and oily-rich quality could produce nausea, being a little cloying, but less so when mixed in formula; add some Ginger root to counteract. Balances parasympathetic nervous system (PNS).
Astragalus membranaceus Huang qi Astragalus root	Kidney yin and qi tonic, sweet, warm, and dry, adrenal and liver restorative. Balances PNS.
Glycyrrhiza uralensis Gan Cao Licorice root (Interchangeable with Western *G. glabra)*	Sweet, moist, restoring yin tonic. For adrenals, liver protective. Also, restores the gut. Caution in hypertension with water retention. *Not* for continual use as a simple.
Ganoderma lucidum Ling Zhi Reishi mushroom	Kidney yin, qi tonic, and liver tropho-restorative, immune regulator, antiallergenic. PNS balance.
Anemarrhena asphodeloides Zhi Mu Know Mother root	Yin tonic. Cool, moist, restores adrenals, clears empty heat in hot flashes. Balances PNS.
Cervus nippon Lu Rong Velvet Deer antler	Kidney yang tonic. Balances sympathetic nervous system (SNS). Use for adrenal fatigue and helps libido and fertility.
Eucommia ulmoides Du Zhong Eucommia bark	Kidney yang tonic, balances SNS. Also, a connective tissue, and muscular-skeletal restorative.
Dioscorea opposita Shan Yao Mountain Yam root	Kidney yang tonic and mild qi tonic, balances SNS. Helps to make adenosine triphosphate and build hormones (essence)[25]
Cuscuta chinensis Tu Si Zi Asian Dodder seed	Kidney yang tonic to balance the SNS and adrenals. Also, a urinary restorative for weakness and discharges.
Ocimum sanctum, and *O. tenuiflorum* Tulsi, Holy Basil leaf	Ayurvedic tonic that normalizes cortisol, helps stress-induced depression, balances glucose metabolism.

tonics, the adaptogens. Ideally, adaptogens work on the HPA axis. The ones that do this superbly are the *primary adaptogens*. Primary adaptogens have all been well-researched and proven beyond doubt to address the HPA axis. These include Schisandra Wu Wei Zi (Five Taste berry), Ayurvedic Ashwagandha root, Eleuthero Ci Wu Jia (Siberian ginseng root), and Rhodiola root.[2] Primary adaptogens also include the classic ginsengs, such as Panax Ren Shen (Asian ginseng root) and Panax Xi Yang Shen (American ginseng root), although they are very costly and might not be economical to use freely.

Other adaptogens are sometimes called *secondary adaptogens* because they are not 100% proven to address the HPA axis. However, tradition and many well-known herbalists have always classified them as bona fide adaptogens, being in the neuroendocrine category. These include notables such as Astragalus Huang Qi (Astragalus root), Ganoderma Ling Zhi (Reishi mushroom), Licorice root, Rehmannia Shu Di Huang (prepared Rehmannia root), Holy Basil herb (Tulsi), Milky Oat seed, and others.[2] They are especially effective when combined with the must-have primary list.

• BOX 27.2 Rooibos Tea

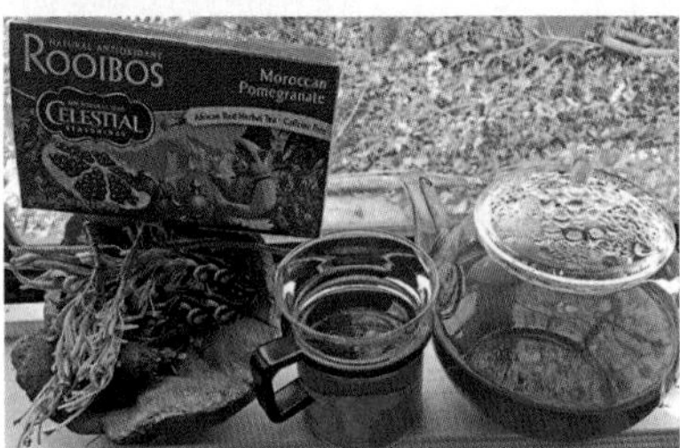

Aspalathus linearis (African Red Bush/Rooibos leaf) makes a beautiful red brew.

A sweet and nutty noncaffeinated tea for adrenal fatigue

Rooibos tea (pronounced ROY-boss), is a traditional, noncaffeinated, antiinflammatory, South African tea that brews up into a beautiful, bright reddish-brown color with a sweet, fruity taste. It is traditionally consumed to improve appetite, calm digestion, and reduce nervous tension and anxiety. It is filled with antioxidants, more so than green tea. Other proven benefits include antiviral, antiallergenic, cholesterol-reducing, and immune-modulating properties. The plant is cut by hand and then bruised to encourage oxidation, which develops the rich color and flavor. As it oxidizes, Rooibos becomes redder and sweeter.[23]

Preparation

8 oz boiling water per heaping teaspoon loose leaves. Steep at least 5 minutes. Drink plain or add plant-based milk, honey to taste.

• BOX 27.3 Microalgae

A neuroendocrine superfood

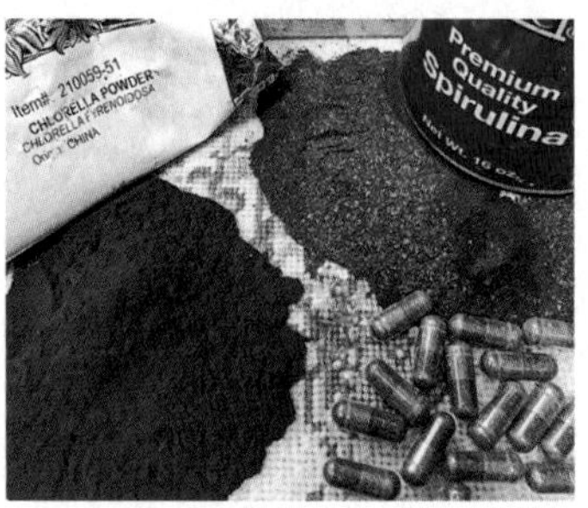

Chlorella spp. and *Spirulina* spp. (Microalgae) can be purchased in bulk and encapsulated for economy. These nutrient-dense foods contain vitamins, minerals, chlorophyll and essential fatty acids.

- Excellent restorative for neuroendocrine and immune functions.
- For all endocrine deficiencies, including adrenal fatigue, hypothyroidism, low blood sugar, chronic anxiety, and depression.
- It tonifies Kidney yin, qi, and essence.

Microalgae are microscopic, salty-tasting water plants that live in colonies. They are one of the most nourishing foods on the planet, containing high amounts of protein, omega-3 fatty acids, and cleansing chlorophyll. They contain the nucleic acids RNA and DNA, all eight essential amino acids; the macrominerals calcium, potassium, phosphorous, and magnesium; numerous trace minerals, including iodine, iron, zinc, copper, titanium, and cobalt; the entire vitamin B complex, vitamin C, and vitamin K. If you could have only one single food if stranded on a desert island, microalgae would be a wise choice.

Microalgae were the earliest forms of plant life, originating billions of years ago, the beginning of all life on planet Earth. They live in saltwater marine sources and in freshwater lakes and ponds. *Spirulina* spp. is a blue-green alga that grows in fresh and salt water and *Chlorella* spp. is a freshwater green alga. These two are the main forms of edible microalgae.[24] Various cultures worldwide have used them as food, with good reason.

Preparation

Sold without prescription in tablets, powders, granules, and tinctures. You can also fill your own capsules with the bulk powder, as shown. May be taken internally and used topically as gargles and mouth washes.

Dose

For maintenance and prevention 2–5 g per day. For treatment: 5–10 g per day.

Adaptogen companions consist of plants that focus on the immune, nervous, and hormonal systems. They are often foods, herbs, and beverages consumed frequently in various cultures, such as Rooibos tea from Africa (Box 27.2), Maca root from Peru, green tea from China, Rose Hips and Elderberry from the West, and Grape seed and skin from the Mediterranean. It is difficult to refrain from expounding on the enormously long list of superior foods and herbs, so I'll just add microalgae (Box 27.3), Polygonum He Shou Wu (Flowery Knotweed root), Nettle herb, Ginger root, Saw Palmetto berry, and Bee Pollen.

It is definitely best to mix and match all types of adaptogens and to include adaptogenic companion foods when addressing the many things adaptogens help, including loss of energy, adrenal fatigue, and compromised immunity. They are to be considered long-term therapeutics, requiring a good 3 months for results.

From the Chinese Medicine standpoint, herbs for adrenal fatigue are those that tonify both Kidney yin and Kidney yang. Moist, cooling tonics are on the yin side and could be considered to help the PNS. These botanicals include Asparagus Tian Men Dong (Asparagus root), or Solomon's Seal, and Comfrey root.

Drying and warming Kidney yang herbs are on the SNS side and include botanicals such as Eucommia Du Zhong (Eucommia bark) or Rosemary leaf.

Thyroid Herbs

Endocrine restoratives are needed that have a tropism to the thyroid (Table 27.2). Artichoke leaf, Saw Palmetto berry, Coleus root, and the adaptogenic Ashwagandha root are all valuable thyroid allies, particularly for *hypo*thyroidism. For *hyper*thyroidism, Bugleweed herb (Fig. 27.4) and Motherwort herb stand out and are two of the few in this category. These two Mint family plants have been traditionally used to reduce cardiac symptoms such as hypertension, palpitations, and irritability,[24] which often accompany hyperthyroidism.

A very promising herb, *Nigella sativa* (Black seed, Black Cumin), native to the Mediterranean and Southwest Asia and long used around the world, has now been shown to cut down on thyroid antibodies present in Hashimoto's disease and to normalize blood flow to the thyroid.[21] *Nigella sativa* is certainly an herb to try.

Thyroid *superfoods* are filled with trace minerals and vitamins needed by that gland. Watercress herb that grows in cold running water has an amazing range of minerals and trace minerals, especially iron and iodine. Milky Oat berry is an archetypal nutritive restorer for neuroendocrine deficiencies of all kinds; it tonifies the thyroid, adrenals, and pancreas. Maca root is another.

Liver herbs should be considered in formulas for thyroid imbalance because the liver converts T4 to bioavailable T3. Therefore *liver-supportive* herbs such as Dandelion root, Oregon Grape root, or Burdock root are used. They also happen to be *cholagogues* that will help any constipation problem that is frequently present in hypothyroidism (Chapter 19).

TABLE 27.2 Thyroid Balancers

Herb	Notes
Cynara scolymus Artichoke leaf	For hypothyroidism. Major endocrine/thyroid restorative. Restores liver and pancreas and lowers cholesterol.
Withania somnifera Ashwagandha root or Winter Cherry root	For hypothyroidism. Thyroid/adrenal/hepatic support. Decreases stress, helps sleep, increases T3 and T4.
Coleus forskohlii Coleus root	For hypothyroidism. Makes thyroid hormones T3 and T4 more sensitive to thyroid stimulating hormone (TSH) from pituitary. Also an impressive cardiac restorative and a quick acting vasodilator for high blood pressure.
Eleutherococcus senticosus Ci Wu Jia Siberian Ginseng root	For hypothyroidism. Thyroid and adrenal support/endocrine restorative.
Turnera diffusa Damiana leaf	For hypothyroidism. Kidney yang tonic. Bitter, pungent, neuroendocrine restorative.
Lycopus virginicus Bugleweed herb	For hyperthyroidism. Heart relaxer and thyroid inhibitor.
Leonurus cardiaca Motherwort herb	For hyperthyroidism, helps the cardiac hypertensive, palpitation aspects.
Arctium lappa Burdock root	Liver support. Liver converts T4 to T3.
Mahonia aquifolium Oregon Grape root	Liver support. Liver converts T4 to T3.
Taraxacum officinale Dandelion root	Liver support. Liver converts T4 to T3.
Chondrus crispus Irish Moss thallus	Iodine-rich sea veggie. A type of red algae or seaweed. Almost identical to Iceland moss. A little sweet and bitter. Caution in Hashimoto's because it could cause rebound *hyper*thyroidism. This effect will normalize if herb is discontinued.
Cetraria islandica Iceland Moss lichen	Moist, cool, and salty; bitter and nutritive lichen. Iodine rich, for chronic weakness. Caution in Hashimoto's as it could cause rebound hyperthyroidism.
Laminaria spp. Kelp thallus	Sea veggie. Neuroendocrine restorative, containing iodine and trace minerals. All seaweeds do this. Caution in Hashimoto's, same reason as with above iodine rich herbs.
Fucus vesiculosus Bladderwrack thallus	Sea veggie. Thyroid restorative and stimulator, containing iodine and trace minerals. Caution in Hashimoto's same as above.
Thyroid superfoods	
Lepidium meyenii (Maca root)	Maca, across the board hormonal superfood.
Avena sativa (Milky Oat berry)	Milky Oat, highly nutritive.
Pollen (Flower pollen)	Pollen, remarkably nutrient rich, systemic.
Nasturtium officinalis (Watercress herb)	Watercress works on hypothalamic-pituitary-thyroid (HPT) axis. Iron and iodine rich, for thyroid, adrenals, and pancreas, important detoxicant.
Spirulina spp. and *Chlorella* spp. Microalgae	Algae, filled with iodine, other trace minerals, and vitamins to support thyroid function.

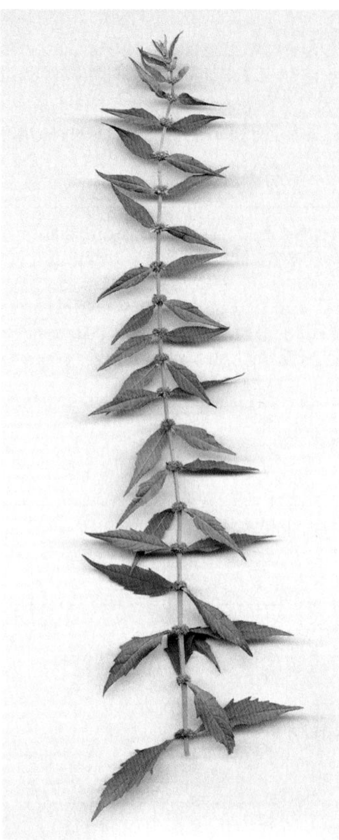

• **Fig. 27.4** *Lycopus virginicus* (Bugleweed herb) is a thyroid inhibitor and cardiac relaxant, an ally for treating hyperthyroidism often accompanied by palpitations and anxiety. Copyright Tucker/Lang Photography. Photographs loaned with permission from *The Botanical Series* are copywritten by Jennifer Anne Tucker and Gerald Lang from the Studio at Hill Crystal Farm. www.jennifer-tucker.com

Iodine-rich sea vegetables work well to maintain healthy thyroids. But they should be used discriminatively and included only in *some* formulas involving hypothyroidism. Their use could backfire in some folks with autoimmune Hashimoto's thyroidits (discussed earlier). Start slowly with sea veggies to determine whether or not there is improvement. Examples that wash up on the Atlantic and Pacific shores in profusion include *Fucus vesiculosus* (Bladderwrack), which has air-filled bladders that can be popped like bubble wrap, and long strands of *Laminaria* spp. (Kelp thallus) illustrated in Fig. 27.5.

Pancreatic Herbs

Herbs that help lower blood sugar are called *hypoglycemics* (Table 27.3). The opposite of these are substances that increase blood sugar, *hyperglycemics.* (It is possible that black coffee may do this in some individuals

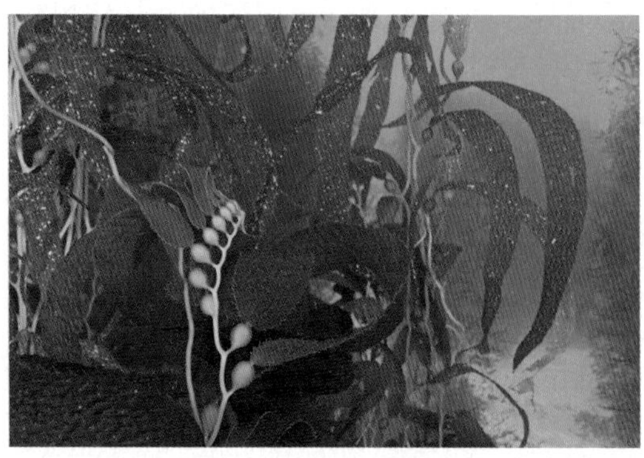

• **Fig. 27.5** *Laminaria* spp. (Kelp thallus) with its long green fronds in its natural habitat, under the sea. This iodine-rich sea veggie is intended for careful use in hypothyroidism and as a heavy metal chelator. (/iStock/KGrif)

TABLE 27.3 Blood Sugar Regulators

Herb	Notes
Gymnema sylvestre Gymnema leaf	For diabetes type 1 (DM1), insulin resistance, and diabetes type 2 (DM2). Lowers Hemoglobin A1c (HgA1c), repairs beta cells, decreases insulin requirements in DM1.
Momordica charantia Bitter Melon fruit	Important bitter to lower glucose and HgA1c.
Curcuma longa Turmeric root	Important bitter to lower glucose and HgA1c.
All berberines Oregon Grape root, Goldenseal root, Barberry root, Bayberry root, Coptis Huang Lian and Phellodendron Huang Bai (Siberian Cork Tree bark).	This category of bitters all help glycemic control.
Olea europaea Olive leaf	Normalizes HgA1c. Antioxidant, lowers blood pressure and cholesterol, hypoglycemic, neuro and cancer protective.

(Continued)

TABLE 27.3 Blood Sugar Regulators—cont'd

Herb	Notes
Trigonella foenum-graecum Fenugreek seed	Hypoglycemic, lowers cholesterol. Helps normalize insulin sensitivity and a renowned digestive aid.
Cynara scolymus Artichoke leaf	Hypoglycemic, major neuroendocrine detoxicant. Tropism to and restorative for liver (regarding glycogen storage). Also, for pancreas and thyroid.
Silybum marianum Milk Thistle seed, St. Mary's Thistle seed	Liver restorative, proven to lower HgA1c, and insulin resistance.
Cinnamomum cassia Rou Gui Cinnamon bark Other Cinnamon species are effective.	Decreases HgA1c, improves insulin sensitivity. Eat ½ tsp (equivalent to 1 g) per day in food.
Eleutherococcus senticosus Ci Wu Jia Siberian ginseng root	Helps stabilize blood sugar levels.
Ocimum sanctum/O. tenuiflorum Tulsi, Holy Basil leaf	Stabilizes glucose and blood sugar metabolism, regulates cholesterol, and lowers blood pressure.
Antioxidants and microvascular stabilizers *Vaccinium myrtillus* (Bilberry leaf) *Ginkgo biloba* (Ginkgo leaf) *Pinus maritima* (Pine bark extract) *Vitis vinifera* (Grape seed extract)	These all help prevent and treat diabetic complications involving the microcirculation, which can lead to retinopathy and peripheral neuropathy.
Dark greens and nutritious herbs *Medicago sativa* (alfalfa herb) *Urtica dioica* (Nettle herb) *Nasturtium officinale* (Watercress leaf)	Hypoglycemic. Supports pancreas and high or low blood sugar. Contains many vitamins, minerals, and organic acids.

whose blood sugar is super-sensitive to caffeine.) Most often, herbalists are concerned with lowering blood sugar levels. If a person becomes hypoglycemic, as frequently happens in the early stage of insulin resistance, the best fix is with foods. Reach for a good protein, such as a hard-boiled egg, or a healthy carbohydrate, such as an apple or orange, rather than a Danish and coffee.

Bitters are extremely important in lowering and normalizing blood sugar in insulin resistance. The bitter taste is antiinflammatory, hypoglycemic, and enhances fat metabolism. *Momordica charantia* (Bitter Melon) and *Curcuma longa* (Turmeric root) are famous for this.

Others, not quite as bitter but superb nevertheless, are hypoglycemic: Ayurvedic *Gymnema sylvestre* that masks the sweet taste on the tongue and *Vaccinium myrtillus* (Bilberry leaf). *Opuntia* spp. (Prickly Pear cactus, Nopal) is a versatile and useful tart cactus native to Latin America and the arid American Southwest. The fruit, flowers, and leaf pads are traditionally used for food and medicine (Box 27.4). The pad pulp is known for treating insulin resistance and DM2 because of its high inulin content and ability to lower the glycemic index of any food eaten with it when taken before meals, and also because of its high pectin content that lowers LDL cholesterol. The mucilaginous inner pads and flowers are a superb internal mucosal vulnerary for upper airway (infections), digestive (ulcers and gastroesophageal reflux disease), and the genitourinary tract (urinary tract infections, stones, and gout). And the Aloe Vera-like mucilaginous pad gel acts as an external first-aid vulnerary when rubbed onto the skin or used as a poultice to heal burns, contusions, and minor abrasions. Even the fruit, which is high in vitamin C, flavonoids, and minerals, can be cooked down into medicinal syrup bases, jams, liquors, or used as a hangover cure.[20]

In summary, herbalists are looking for herbs that improve insulin sensitivity. Botanicals that restore the liver are important to include because the liver plays an important role in glucose metabolism. ***Hemoglobin A1c (HgA1c)*** is an important blood test marker that reflects average glucose levels over a 2- to 3-month period and so provides a long-term trend in diabetes risk. The famous liver restorative, Milk Thistle seed, has been cited in many

• BOX 27.4 Prickly Pear Cactus Pad Preparation

For insulin resistance and diabetes type 2

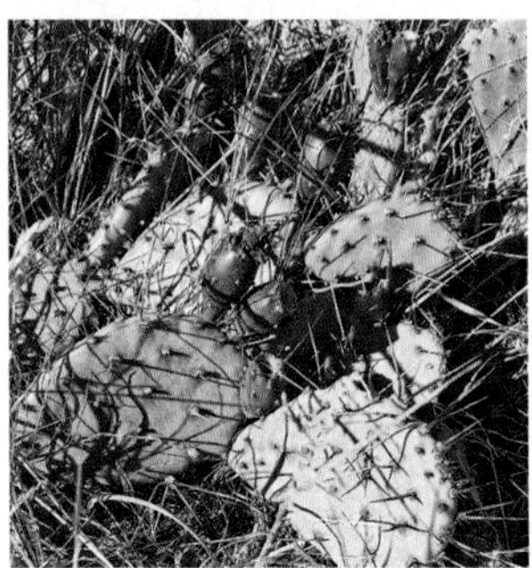

Opuntia spp. (Prickly Pear cactus, Nopal). The high inulin content of the pad's pulp can treat insulin resistance and also lower the glycemic index of foods when the two are eaten close together.

If you happen to live in the American Southwest, you might want to be hardcore and take on the herbalist's Prickly Pear challenge. First the thorns. Use thick gloves. The best way to harvest is with the pad still attached to the plant. Pick one that is sticking out by itself away from the others. The long spines and the fine, human-hair-thick barbed thorns at their base (called glochids) are then *carefully* scraped or sanded off between two large flat rocks that fit well into your hands. Know that glochids can be felt, if not always seen. When clear of nasties, cut off the pad.[26] An alternate traditional method is to sear the spines off using a gas flame torch or open fire.

The pad is then cut open like a bagel (longitudinally) and the pulp from the center is scraped out into a bowl. Repeat. This mucilaginous gel will keep for 2–3 weeks in the refrigerator.

Internal insulin resistance use

Make a pulp slurry (folk method). Mix several ounces of hard-earned pulp with several ounces of water. Blend and drink 1–2 oz before meals.

External vulnerary use

Make an infusion of the pad pulp and flowers (the redder the better, according to Michael Moore).[22] Make into a salve or compress and apply to wounds 3 × a day. Or mix the cactus gel with Aloe vera gel, honey, or other dried or fresh herbs and apply as a poultice to the skin.[26]

If you're hungry from all this work

Cut the dethorned pads into slices like a bell pepper and fry them up (skin and all) into a scramble with mushrooms, onions, and eggs.

studies to normalize HgA1c.[18] Others are Cinnamon bark, Olive leaf, and Gymnema leaf (Table 27.3).

Diabetes can damage blood vessels and capillaries and decrease circulation, leading to nerve damage and complications of blindness (diabetic retinopathy) and to foot and lower limb amputations (as a result of peripheral neuropathy). *Antioxidants* and *microvascular stabilizers* help prevent and repair these damaged capillaries. Consider herbs such as Bilberry leaf, Ginkgo leaf, Pine bark extract, and Grape seed extract. These also help repair cerebral vessels that are damaged in strokes.

Nutritious green superfoods are another category for prevention of insulin resistance. These foods are similar to ones used for any other neuroendocrine conditions: Nettle leaf, Alfalfa leaf, Maca root, and others.

Common Endocrine Conditions

Adrenal Fatigue or Adrenal Burnout

- *Definition. Adrenal fatigue/burnout* is a collection of chronic signs and symptoms that result when adrenal glands function suboptimally. Characterized by extreme stress, fatigue, and nervous exhaustion (Case History 27.1). Can be diagnosed by a saliva test that checks for circulating cortisol levels. In early stages, they are significantly elevated and later become extremely low.
- *Signs and symptoms.* Fatigue not relieved by sleep. Person is too wired to fall asleep or relax and has difficulty rising in the morning and gets midafternoon fatigue. Other symptoms include brain fog, depression, low thyroid, hypoglycemia, insulin resistance, lowered immune function, low sex drive, and muscle pain. Person may look and act relatively normal but has a general sense of unwellness, tiredness, or *gray* feelings. Typically, person consumes large amounts of caffeine and sugar in an attempt to get more energy.
- *Causes.* May start after a chronic respiratory infection, pneumonia, major stressful life event, and long-term inflammatory diet.

CASE HISTORY 27.1

Case History for Adrenal Fatigue

S. Yvonne is a 35-year-old single mom who is juggling two kids in junior high and a full-time job. She is up half the night doing laundry, answering email, getting a head start on work. She has a hard time waking up, drinks 5 cups of coffee throughout the day. She is exhausted, can't think straight, and feels understandably depressed. Lots of burping, bloating, abdominal cramping, and she leans toward fast foods to save time.

O. **P** Slow, soft, and deep. **T** Pale with a white coat. Probably very high cortisol levels.

A. Kidney Yang Deficiency. Approaching adrenal fatigue. (Could change to a yin deficiency in a few years if no health changes are made.)

P. *Specific therapeutic principles.* (1) Kidney yin and yang tonics. (2) Hypothalamic-pituitary-adrenal (HPA) axis adaptogens. (3) Support liver. (4) Antidepressants. (5) Berberines for gut. (6) Relaxing nervine.

Herbal Formula and Dose. 6 mL 3 × day between meals.

Parts	Herbs	Rationale
4	Rhodiola root	Adaptogen, HPA axis balancer, antidepressant.
3	Schisandra Wu Wei Zi	Stimulates HPA axis, tonifies kidney yin, yang, qi.
2	Holy Basil herb	Normalizes cortisol, decreases stress-induced depression, balances glucose metabolism.
2	Lemon Balm herb	Antidepressant, relaxing nervine.
2	Codonopsis Dang Shen	Mild adaptogen, restore gut, yin tonic.
1	Oregon Grape root	Liver support and bitters for gut.

Other Suggestions

- *Diet.* Antiinflammatory; no fast food. Less caffeine. Peppermint tea, which will help stomach and still give some energy.
- Consider Four-R program.
- *Supplements.* EPA/DHA, vitamin B complex.
- *Teas.* Adrenal Support Adaptogenic Tea (Box 27.5) in daytime. Chamomile tea at night.
- *Stress management.* Suggestions such as yoga, music, bubble bath.
- Have thyroid levels checked, as high cortisol decreases thyroid hormones.

• BOX 27.5 Adrenal Support Adaptogenic Tea

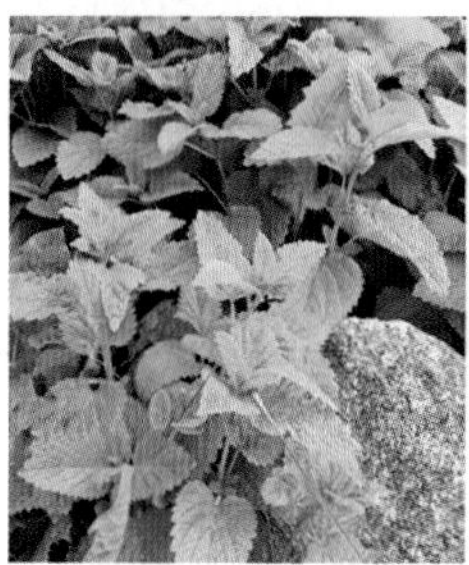
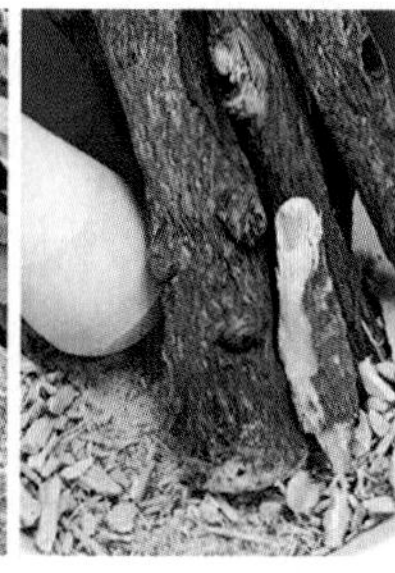
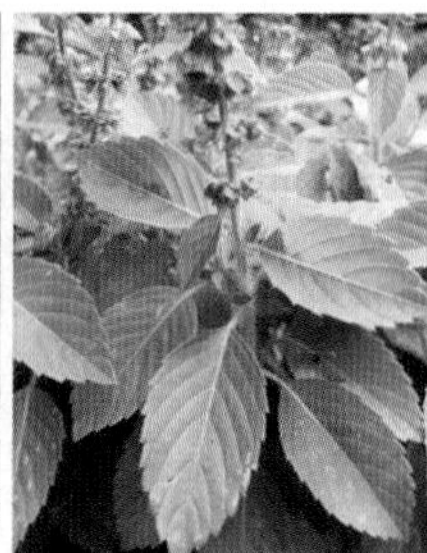

Melissa officinalis (Lemon Balm herb), Glycyrrhiza glabra (Licorice root), and *Ocimum tenuiflorum* (Tulsi/Holy Basil herb) are some of the gentle adrenal balancers in this tea.

This tea contains a lovely blend of adaptogens to heal adrenal fatigue, help depression, and lift the spirts. It is appropriate for the needed long-term use in this condition.

¼ cup, ground	Eleuthero Ci Wu Jia	Yin and qi tonic that supports the HPA axis.
¼ cup	Schisandra Wu Wei Xi	For Kidney qi, yin, and yang deficiency.
¼ cup	Holy Basil leaf	Lowers cortisol, decreases stress-induced depression.
2 tbsp	Ashwagandha root	Stimulates HPA axis.
2 tbsp	Lemon Balm herb	Lifts the shen (spirit) and calming.
1 tsp	Licorice root	Sweet balancer, yin tonic.

Instructions: Mix up dried herbs. Use 1 tbsp plus 1½ tsp per 2 cups of water. Simmer in 2 cups plus a little more cold water, covered, for 20–30 minutes. Let stand for 20 minutes. Strain and serve.

- *Allopathic*. Not recognized in allopathic medicine by most doctors.
- *Recovery*. Can take 2 years or more and usually requires a change in diet, improving lifestyle, herbs, nutritional supplements, detoxification procedures, and attention to emotional and spiritual health.
- *Chinese Medicine perspective*. Starts with a Kidney Yang Deficiency (high cortisol levels) and proceeds to a Kidney Yin Deficiency (low cortisol levels). Fix is to tonify both Kidney yin and yang with adaptogens.
- *General therapeutic principles*. (1) Tonify Kidney yin and yang with adrenal adaptogens, especially Rhodiola root, Ashwagandha root, and Eleuthero Ci Wu Jia (Siberian ginseng root). (2) Choose relaxing nervines such as Skullcap herb or Chamomile flower. (3) Support liver. (4) Include relaxing nervines. (5) Consider dysbiosis and/or hypothyroidism.

CASE HISTORY 27.2

Case History for Hashimoto's Thyroiditis

S. Annise has been on Synthroid for 5 years. She has gained weight and is tired, sluggish; hair is thinning; is often constipated; has little energy and is stressed. Would like to get herbal supplementation. Her cholesterol and triglycerides are elevated.
O. **P** Slow, weak, deep. **T** Pale with white coating.
A. Kidney Yang and Qi Deficiency. Hypothyroidism.
P. *Specific therapeutic principles.* (1) May have to supplement (not eliminate) hormone replacement therapy, at least at first. (2) Nourish and restore thyroid with qi and yang tonics such as Gotu Kola herb and Siberian Ginseng root. (3) Treat chronic constipation with hepatic laxatives that increase bile flow like Yellow Dock root, Oregon Grape root, Blue Flag rhizome, and Cascara Sagrada root. (4) Prevent/treat coronary artery plaque with heart tonics like Hawthorn berry and Ginkgo leaf. (5) Mild relaxing nervines for stress or insomnia like Milky Oat berry or Passionflower.

Herbal Formula and Dose. 8 mL 3 × day between meals.

Parts	Herbs	Rationale
4	Gotu Kola or Artichoke leaf	Restore thyroid.
2	Eleuthero Ci Wu Jia	Thyroid restorative.
2	Lemon Balm herb	Calm anxiety.
2	Yellow Dock root	Constipation and liver support.
2	Hawthorn berry	Decrease plaque and triglycerides.

Suggestions

- *Diet.* Use autoimmune protocol and possible Gut and Psychology Syndrome (GAPS) diet (Chapter 16). Fix gut, as needed with Four-R program (Chapter 18). Eliminate gluten, dairy, and sugar and introduce sea veggies in cooking. Sea salt, but iodine has a narrow therapeutic index, so use carefully.
- *Supplements.*
  - Selenium methionine. 200 mcg at night. This is supplement number one; it reduces thyroid antibodies and anxiety. In cases of iodine excess, when the thyroid gland processes iodine from foods we eat, it causes release of the free radical, hydrogen peroxide. Selenium reduces this free radical, cutting down on oxidative damage to the thyroid.[4]
  - Magnesium at night to bowel tolerance. Helps bowel movements and promotes restful sleep.
  - B-Complex vitamins in morning for stress and energy.
  - Iodine. Be careful. Try supplementation with iodine-rich Kelp tablets or Spirulina blue-green algae to see if seaweed helps or hinders. If things improve, consider adding a sea veggie to formula. Too much seaweed may affect the thyroid stimulating hormone and thyroid antibody levels, so be sure to monitor. Iodine has a narrow therapeutic index. Doses that are too low lead to iodine deficiency, but doses that are too high can cause or make Hashimoto's thyroiditis worse.[27]
- Oat straw and Passionflower tea 3 × per day as a nerve tonic.

Hashimoto's Thyroiditis

- *Definition*. Hashimoto's thyroiditis is epidemic. It is an autoimmune (AI) disease where the immune system attacks the thyroid gland, with a resultant decrease of thyroid hormones (Case History 27.2). It is the most common cause of hypothyroidism, up to 95%. *Myxedema* is also hypothyroidism, an advanced underactive thyroid, where the thyroid does not make enough hormones; it is very rare. Myxedema is *not* autoimmune.
- *Signs and symptoms*. Fatigue, lethargy, cold intolerance, constipation, weight gain, stress, depression, heavy menses, puffiness, hair loss, and coarse, dry skin. Hormone imbalance

with estrogen dominance (Chapter 28). Diagnosed by a thyroid hormone blood panel and the presence of antibodies.

- *Allopathic treatment*. Synthroid (levothyroxine), synthetic T4. It is a top brand-name drug prescribed in the United States and is produced from genetically modified yeast that has a molecular folding structure quite different from the natural hormone. Another, often better-tolerated, option is a natural desiccated thyroid like Armour, which is derived from thyroid glands of pigs and is considered bioidentical to the hormones produced by the thyroid gland. It contains T1, T2, T3, and T4, unlike Synthroid, which contains only T4.
- *Chinese Medicine perspective*. Most often, qi and yang tonics are used.
- *General therapeutic principles*. (1) Heal the gut, because Hashimoto's thyroiditis is an AI problem. (2) Use thyroid restoratives such as Artichoke leaf, Saw Palmetto berry, or Milky Oat berry. (3) Provide Liver support. The liver is the primary organ in which T4 is converted to active form of T3. (4) Choose thyroid stimulators, which make thyroid hormones more sensitive to TSH,[18] such as Ashwagandha root, and *Coleus forskohlii* (Coleus) herb, Burdock root, Dandelion root, or Oregon Grape root. (5) Choose sea veggies, such as Iceland Moss or Bladderwrack thallus, with *caution* and in moderation. (6) Treat other symptoms, such as constipation or estrogen dominance.

Hyperthyroidism

- *Definition*. A hyperactive thyroid is known as *Graves' disease*. There is overactivity and overproduction of thyroxine caused by a large number of thyroid antibodies that stimulate the gland (*autoimmune component*) (Case History 27.3). Causes range from leaky gut, goiter, inflammation and infection, to autoimmune factors. It is not nearly as prevalent in the United States as hypothyroidism.
- *Signs and symptoms*. Restlessness, irritability, flushing and heat, weight loss with increased appetite, tremors, racing heart, hypertension, increased sweating, soft nails, amenorrhea, insomnia, hot and moist diarrhea, and bulging eyes (exophthalmos).

CASE HISTORY 27.3

Case History for Hyperthyroidism

S. Meredith is always on the go. She is anxious, her blood pressure (BP) is 160/90, she complains of palpitations and frequent burning diarrhea and has lost 45 lb in 2 years. She is on a beta blocker for BP and takes radioactive iodine. She might have to have a thyroidectomy but hopes to avoid this with herbals.

O. **P** Rapid, irregular. **T** Very red with yellow coating.

A. Liver fire pattern. Hyperthyroidism.

P. *Specific therapeutic principles*. Cool down Liver fire. The body is generating too much heat. (1) Hypothyroid herbs. (2) Antihypertensives. (3) Cooling nervines for stress (4) Astringents and cooling herbs for diarrhea. (5) Immunomodulation.

Herbal Formula and Dose. 4 mL 3 × day between meals.

Parts	Herbs	Rationale
3	Bugleweed herb	To bring down T4, relieves palpitations.
2	Echinacea root	Immunomodulation.
2	Motherwort herb	Nerve relaxant and antihypertensive.
2	Lemon balm	Antianxiety, cooling.
2	Scutellaria Huang Qin	Cool fire, antiinflammatory.
2	Cranesbill root	Stop chronic diarrhea.
1	Bupleurum Chai Hu	Restores liver, hypotensive, cooling, decrease stress.

Other Suggestions

- *Diet*. Consider autoimmune protocol and Gut and Psychology Syndrome (GAPS) diet. Fix gut, as needed with Four-R program (Chapters 16 and 18).
- *Stress management*. Rest, yoga, and meditation to help calm down. Oat Straw tea 3 × day for neuroendocrine calming.
- *Supplements*. L-carnitine 1000 mg 2–4 × daily and a vitamin B complex to help nerves.

CASE HISTORY 27.4

Case History for Insulin Resistance

S. Lois is 45 years old, has lost her pretty waistline, and just can't seem to lose weight, no matter what she tries, which was never a problem in the past. She loves pasta and sweets. Has noticed a lot of gas and bloating. Her insulin, total cholesterol, and triglyceride levels are elevated for the first time. Her healthcare provider wants to put her on Glucophage, a statin, and Mylanta. She is understandably stressed.

O. **P** Wiry and weak. **T** Pale with teeth marks.

A. Spleen Qi Deficiency with Phlegm Damp. Insulin and leptin resistance, dysbiosis, and stress.

P. *Specific therapeutic principles*. (1) Hypoglycemics. (2) Heal gut and dysbiosis. Restore Spleen with gut restoratives. (3) Dry damp with diuretics. (4) Help stress/balance adrenals. (5) Help cholesterol and triglycerides with antilipemics. (6) Restore liver.

Herbal Formula and Dose. 5 mL 3 × day between meals, in a little water.

Parts	Herbs	Rationale
3	Fenugreek seed	Hypoglycemic, lowers triglycerides and total cholesterol, raises HDL.
3	Gymnema sylvestre herb	Hypoglycemic, decreases desire for sweet taste.
2	Salvia Dan Shen or Ligusticum Chuan Xiong	Decreases cholesterol, normalizes blood pressure (BP); vasodilator, anticoagulant.
2	Passionflower herb	Relaxing nervine for stress.
2	Atractylodes Bai Zhu White Atractylodes root	Restore gut, dysbiosis.
1	Poria Fu Ling Hoelen fungus	Drains excess fluid to lower BP, help insulin resistance.
1	Licorice root	Blends other herbs, heal gut, help adrenals.

Other Suggestions

- *Diet*. Antiinflammatory. Four-R program. Bitter foods in diet.
- *Supplements*. EPA/DHA, Chromium, Zinc, Magnesium, B vitamins.
- Exercise program.
- Stress management, as needed.

- *Allopathic treatment.* Radioactive iodine therapy to slow down and shrink thyroid, beta blockers to decrease BP, and surgery to remove most of the thyroid.
- *Chinese Medicine perspective.* Thyroid hyperactivity is thought to begin as a hot fire condition, so cooling herbs are in order.
- *Therapeutic principles.* May have to supplement herbs in addition to allopathic therapy. (1) Consider two traditional herbs for hyperthyroidism, Bugleweed herb and Motherwort herb. Another option: Ligusticum Chuan Xiong (Sichuan Lovage root). (2) Modify hyperactivity with strong nervines such as Passionflower herb or Hops flower. (3) Treat other symptoms like insomnia with *nervines/hypnotics*, such as Kava root or Hops flower. If diarrhea, use astringents, like White Oak bark or Wild Geranium herb. For inflammation and heat (cool fire), use Gardenia Zhi Zi (Gardenia pod) or Scutellaria Huang Qin (Baikal Skullcap root).

Diabetes Mellitus Type 1 and Insulin Resistance

- *Definition.* DM1 is the inability of the pancreas to produce any or enough insulin, resulting in blood sugar imbalances. Can cause hypertension, heart disease, diabetic retinopathy, peripheral neuropathy, kidney failure, limb amputations, decreased immunity, and mental confusion.
  - *DM1,* child onset. Pancreas stops producing any or enough insulin to regulate glucose.
  - *DM2,* adult onset. Variously called *syndrome X, insulin resistance,* or *metabolic syndrome.* The pancreas produces inadequate amounts of insulin (Case History 27.4). May be reversed with diet, herbs, supplements, and lifestyle changes.
- *Signs and symptoms.*
  - DM1: Hunger, thirst, polyuria. Weight gain, elevated blood insulin or glucose levels, triglycerides (TGLs), and cholesterol.
  - DM2: Apple shape. Midriff weight gain; waistline expands, becoming larger than hip circumference. Associated with hypertension, coronary artery disease, inflammation, dysbiosis, kidney disease, poor diet, lack of exercise, and weight gain.
- *Allopathic.*
  - DM1: Insulin injections or insulin pump for life. Low glycemic food calculations.
  - DM2: Oral antihyperglycemics, such as Glucophage. Could progress to need for insulin injections. Diet and exercise.
- *General therapeutic principles.* (1) Decrease glucose levels with hypoglycemic herbs. (2) Decrease cholesterol and TGLs with antihyperlipidemic/antilipemic herbs. (3) Decrease BP with antihypertensives. (4) Normalize gut with GI restoratives. (5) Must detoxify and restore liver with liver restoratives and stimulants, like Bitter Melon or Blessed Thistle herb.
- *Diet.* Mediterranean, small amount complex carbohydrates, high in veggies. Drinks such as herbal teas and sparkling water (can be sweetened with stevia). Garlic and onions lower glucose, cholesterol, and BP.
- *Supplements.* EPA/DHA, Chromium, Zinc, Manganese, Vanadium, Magnesium, B vitamins, Pycnogenol (Pine bark extract).

Summary

Endocrine glands produce hormones, chemical messaging substances, and deliver them directly into the bloodstream. The neuroendocrine system includes the hypothalamus that links the ANS to various endocrine glands via the pituitary. These include the adrenals (the HPA axis) and the thyroid (the HPT axis). Primary adaptogens, secondary adaptogens, and companion superfoods are crucial endocrine allies.

The Chinese Medicine Kidneys are associated with the nervous and endocrine systems because they are linked with life force, essence, and energy. Many endocrine conditions are deficiencies, with a decrease of Kidney yin, yang, or qi. Therefore, tonics are used in cases like adrenal fatigue and hypothyroidism.

Stress hormones include fast-acting epinephrine produced during immediate fight-or-flight stress situations and long-lasting cortisol made during prolonged, unproductive stress. Elevated cortisol can result in adrenal fatigue, which causes many chronic health problems.

Autoimmune endocrine disorders include Hashimoto's thyroiditis, hyperthyroidism, and diabetes type 1. Unlike insulin dependent diabetes where insulin injections are a lifetime requirement, insulin resistance can be reversible with proper lifestyle changes.

Review

Fill in the Blanks

(Answers in Appendix B.)

1. Cortisol is made in the ___, and adrenaline is made in the ___. They are known as the ___ hormones.
2. Give three other names for metabolic syndrome. ___, ___, ___.
3. Three examples of goitrogens are ___, ___, ___.
4. What is Hemoglobin A1c (HgA1c)? ___.
5. Give botanical names for two kinds of microalgae. ___, ___.
6. In Chinese Medicine, hypothyroidism is known as what syndrome? ___. Pulse is ___, Tongue is ___.
7. Name four herbs that lower HgA1c. Give botanical and common name. ___, ___, ___, ___.
8. Name five super foods for the adrenals: ___, ___, ___, ___, ___.
9. Name four halogens: ___, ___, ___, ___. Name three environmental sources: ___, ___, ___.
10. Give a yin, yang, and qi tonic, with botanical, common, and pinyin names. ___, ___, ___.

Critical Concept Questions

(Answers for you to decide.)

1. What is the neuroendocrine system?
2. Client asks, "Should I take iodine? And which is better, sea salt or regular? Why?"
3. What are adaptogens? What types are there? Give some examples.
4. Define microalgae. What are its benefits? Who should take it?
5. What does the Chinese Kidney have to do with the neuroendocrine system and disorders?

6. What is Hashimoto's thyroiditis? Why is it so epidemic in the United States? How is it related to the adrenals?

7. What are some of the leading causes of the current autoimmune epidemic?

8. A client can't seem to lose weight, and she has lost her waistline. What would you suspect? What would you suggest?

9. What are some of the benefits of bitter herbs and foods?

10. What are the halogens? What relationship do they have on our health?

References

1. Govinda, Kalashatra. *A Handbook of Chakra Healing: Spiritual Practice for Health, Harmony, and Inner Peace* (Old Saybrook, CT: Konecky and Konecky, 2002).
2. Yance, Donald R. *Adaptogens in Medical Herbalism* (Rochester, VT: Healing Arts, 2013).
3. Burdakov, Denis, et. al. "Glucose-Sensing Neurons of the Hypothalamus." U.S. National Library of Medicine, National Institutes of Health. https://www.ncbi.nlm.nih.gov/pmc/articles/PMC1569598/ (accessed August 27, 2919).
4. Romm, Aviva. *Adrenal Thyroid Revolution* (New York, NY: Harper Collins, 2017).
5. "Burn-out an 'occupational phenomenon': International Classification of Diseases." World Health Organization. https://www.who.int/mental_health/evidence/burn-out/en/ (accessed December 21, 2019).
6. Katagari, Ryoko, et. al. "Effect of excess iodine intake on thyroid diseases in different population: A systematic review and meta-analysis including observational studies." U.S. National Library of Medicine, National Institutes of Health. https://www.ncbi.nlm.nih.gov/pmc/articles/PMC5345857/ (accessed December 14, 2019).
7. Meyers, Amy. "Do Cruciferous Vegetables Cause Hashimoto's?" https://www.amymyersmd.com/2017/03/cruciferous-vegetables-cause-hashimotos/ (accessed August 27, 2019).
8. Kanetkar, Parijat, et. al. "Gymnema sylvestre: A Memoir." U.S. National Library of Medicine, National Institutes of Health. https://www.ncbi.nlm.nih.gov/pmc/articles/PMC2170951/ (accessed December 21, 2019).
9. Weil, Andrew. "Diabetes, Type 1." https://www.drweil.com/health-wellness/body-mind-spirit/diabetes/diabetes-type-1/ (accessed August 27, 2019).
10. "Insulin Resistance Syndrome." Green Mountain Natural Health. https://www.greenmountainhealth.com/conditions/insulin-resistance-syndrome/ (accessed December 21, 2019).
11. Kollias, Helen. Precision Nutrition. "Leptin, Ghrelin, and Weight Loss." https://www.precisionnutrition.com/leptin-ghrelin-weight-loss (accessed August 27, 2019).
12. Pope, Timothy. "Chakras and the Endocrine System." https://www.timothypope.co.uk/chakras-endocrine-system/ (accessed August 27, 2017).
13. Myss, Caroline. *Anatomy of the Spirit* (New York: Three Rivers Press, 1996).
14. Tierra, Michael. "Integrating the Traditional Chinese Understanding of the Kidneys Into Western Herbalism." East West School of Planetary Herbology. https://planetherbs.com/research-center/theory-articles/integrating-the-traditional-chinese-understanding-of-the-kidneys-into-western-herbalism/ (accessed August 27, 2019).
15. Chen, John. "Treatment of Hyperthyroidism." Acupuncture Today. https://www.acupuncturetoday.com/mpacms/at/article.php?id=32299 (accessed August 27, 2019).
16. Myers, Amy. "The Five Best Adaptogens to Combat Stress and Adrenal Fatigue." Amy Meyers, MD. https://www.amymyersmd.com/2018/08/adaptogens-stress-adrenal-fatigue/ (accessed August 29, 2019).
17. Wallflower Kitchen. http://wallflowerkitchen.com/hormone-balancing-almond-maca-cinnamon-smoothie/ (accessed August 29, 2019).
18. Bone, Kerry, and Simon Mills. *Principles and Practice of Phytotherapy* (London, UK: Elsevier, 2013).
19. Schwingshackl, L. et al. U.S. National Library of Medicine, National Institutes of Health. "Olive Oil in the Prevention and Management of Type 2 Diabetes Mellitus: A Systematic Review and Meta-Analysis of Cohort Studies and Intervention Trials." https://www.ncbi.nlm.nih.gov/pmc/articles/PMC5436092/ (accessed August 29, 2019).
20. Coffman, Sam. *The Herbal Medic* (San Antonio: The Human Path, 2014).
21. Farhangi, Mahdieh et al. PMC, U.S. National Library of Medicine, National Institutes of Health. "The effects of Nigella sativa on Thyroid Function, Serum Vascular Endothelial Growth Factor (VEGF) – 1, Nesfatin-1 and Anthropometric Features in Patients With Hashimoto's Thyroiditis: A Randomized Controlled Trial." https://www.ncbi.nlm.nih.gov/pmc/articles/PMC5112739/ (accessed September 15, 2019).
22. Moore, Michael. *Medicinal Plants of the Desert and Canyon West* (New Mexico: Museum of New Mexico Press, 1989).
23. 'The Tao of Tea." WebMD Archives. https://www.webmd.com/food-recipes/features/tao-of-tea#1 (accessed August 29, 2019).
24. Holmes, Peter. *Energetics of Western Herbs* (Boulder, CO: Snow Lotus Press, 2006).
25. Holmes, Peter. *Jade Remedies: A Chinese Herbal Reference for the West* (Boulder, CO: Snow Lotus, 1996).
26. Kane, Charles W. *Medicinal Plants of the American Southwest* (Tucson, AZ: Lincoln Town Press, 2011).
27. Wentz, Izabella. *Hashimoto's Protocol* (New York, NY: Harper Collins, 2017).

28 The Reproductive System

"The joy of menopause is the world's best kept secret."

—Susun Weed, herbalist

CHAPTER REVIEW

- The second chakra, partnerships.
- Maintaining reproductive health in women and men.
- The sacred moon cycle.
- Estrogen: Benefits and functions. Estrogen dominance and estrogen insufficiency.
- Progesterone: Main progesterone functions, excess, and deficiency.
- Hormone replacement therapy and bioidentical hormones.
- Prolactin.
- Testosterone and male hormone facts.
- Chinese Medicine perspective: Reproduction and major syndromes.
- Reproductive Materia Medica: Reproductive herbs worth honorable mention. Restoratives and tonics for men and women, phytoestrogens, and progesteronics. Bleeding (anticoagulants and emmenagogues). Uterine pain (venous decongestants, arterial stimulants, and spasmolytics). Male-oriented yang tonics and miscellaneous categories.
- Common reproductive conditions with case histories: Phase dosing. Dysmenorrhea, dysfunctional uterine bleeding, premenstrual syndrome, fibrocystic breasts, uterine fibroids, perimenopause, benign prostatic hypertrophy, and infertility in women and men.

KEY TERMS

Amenorrhea
Androgen
Benign prostatic hypertrophy (BPH)
Corpus luteum
Dysfunctional uterine bleeding (DUB)
Dysmenorrhea
Dysplasia
Emmenagogues
Estrogen
Estrogen dominance
Fibrocystic breasts
Follicle stimulating hormone (FSH)
Gonads
Hemostatics
Hypothalamic-pituitary-gonadal (HPG) axis
Lignins
Luteinizing hormone (LH)
Menarche
Menopause
Menorrhagia
Menstrual cycle
Menstruation
Ovulation
Phase dosing
Phytoestrogens
Progesterone
Prolactin
Pulse dosing
Selective estrogen receptor modulators (SERMs)
Testosterone
Uterine fibroids
Xenoestrogen

Male and female reproduction involves the sex hormones estrogen, progesterone, and testosterone. They are steroids derived from the cholesterol molecule and are major players in reproductive health. Female reproduction is complicated and changeable as a woman journeys through her life. When one problem is solved, another can appear. Herbalists need an excellent grasp of the menstrual cycle, the function of each hormone, and the results of imbalances. Most reproductive fixes involve juggling these hormones.

In men, matters are frequently simpler, and a vast quantity of male reproductive challenges can be helped by improving health habits and incorporating lifestyle changes. These include concerns such as poor diet involving too much sugar and bad quality fats, hypertension, and high blood sugar (all insulin resistance related). Another consideration is cutting down on excessive alcohol and smoking.[1]

The Chinese Kidneys govern jing and essence and are involved in the life cycle from conception to death. An expression of Kidney essence is in the progression of women traveling through the *Triple Goddess* triad of the maiden, mother, and wise woman; and for men, journeying through the triad of youth, the warrior or father, and finally attaining the status of wise man or sage.

The Second Chakra, Partnerships

The reproductive organs are associated with the second generative chakra located in the pelvic area (Fig. 28.1). It relates to our need for relationship. It is sometimes called the *partnership* chakra.[2] When children start making friends outside the home, this chakra kicks in. It has to do with control of our external lives or fear of losing that control. It includes relationships that are sexual and platonic and how we relate to money, power, ethics, honor, blame, and guilt.

The second chakra easily becomes unbalanced when loss of control is real or feared. Creation of a new life happens at second chakra level, as does infertility or abortion. Creativity includes conception and giving birth but manifests in other areas such as when reinventing our lives, cooking a good meal, playing music, and painting a wall or a canvas. All these activities bring out the *creative*. Sexual inequalities, such as fear, rape, or incest, are second chakra issues, in these cases, sex not being a fair exchange of yin and yang energy.

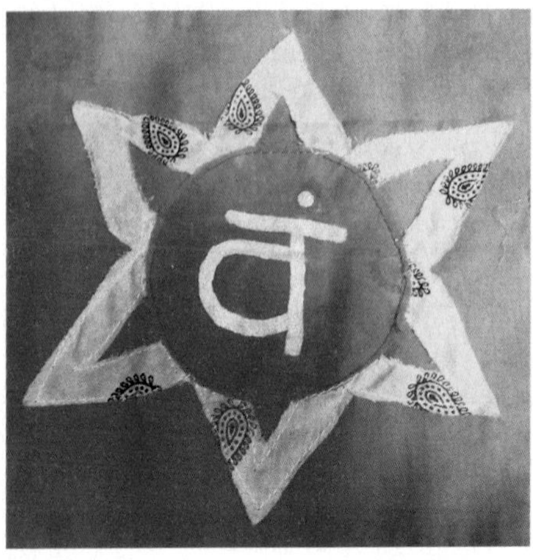

• **Fig. 28.1** The Second Chakra, the creative, resides in the pelvic area and represents platonic and sexual partnerships, and even our relationship to power and money. It involves loss of control and may manifest on the physical level with many types of reproductive problems.

On the physical level, an askew partnership chakra can lead to prostate or ovarian cancer, or chronic lower back pain (our physical support system). Reproductive issues include hot flashes, fibroids, infertility, and menopausal or erectile dysfunction. Rape, addiction, financial loss, frigidity, and abandonment by parents, primary partners, or professional colleagues are all issues that challenge a healthy second chakra.

On the plus side, ability to survive financially, psychically, and physically; to protect ourselves; and to take risks and/or to recover from any loss of close family members, partners, occupation, or bodily health denote a healthy partnership chakra.[2] The mind-body connection involves all seven chakras. Healing needs to happen emotionally, spiritually, and physically.

Maintaining Reproductive Health in Women and Men

- *Keep the microbiome balanced.* The microflora balances hormones and plays a role in the regulation of circulating estrogen levels.[3] If dysbiosis is present, unfriendly bacteria produce an enzyme called *glucuronidase*, which reactivates and recirculates old, used-up estrogen. As it accumulates each month, the liver is strained.
- *Minimize xenoestrogen exposure.* **Xenoestrogens** are industrial compounds in the environment that mimic human estrogen molecules and hook on to estrogen receptor sites in the body, displacing human estrogen. They are found everywhere, including in fertilizers, pesticide residues, artificial food additives, plastic water bottles, commercially raised meat and dairy, and even makeup. Environmental xenoestrogen exposure taxes the liver's deconjugation capacities, leading to estrogen dominance and the dangers therein.
    - *Note.* The industrial compounds that mimic human estrogen are also similar in structure to male androgens and thyroid hormones, and they attach to those receptor sites as well. They are endocrine disruptors affecting thyroid function, metabolism, and insulin and glucose homeostasis.
- *Maintain liver health.* Estrogen is produced in the ovaries each month and broken down (*deconjugated*) by the liver after use and eliminated through the bowel. Unfortunately, the liver can be easily overloaded with toxins from constant xenoestrogen exposure and from a woman ingesting synthetic estrogenic drugs for a large portion of her life in the form of birth control pills (BCP) and/or hormone replacement therapy (HRT). In such cases the liver's estrogen-deconjugating task becomes one job too many. Hence, liver health *and* liver herbs are an important part of most premenstrual syndrome (PMS) and menopausal formulas.
    - *Diindolylmethane (DIM) and liver deconjugation.* Estrogen can be broken down by the liver through various pathways into good and bad metabolites. *Good* estrogen molecules go through the *2-hydroxy* pathway and are antioxidant, protecting the heart and brain, and in men, creating a healthy balance of estrogen to testosterone. *Bad* estrogen molecules go through the *16-hydroxy* and *4-hydroxy* pathways that increase the risk of estrogen dominance and estrogen-responsive cancers in men and women (breast, uterine, endometrial, ovarian, and prostate).[4] Natural compounds that encourage good metabolite production are called *indoles*. They contain DIM, found in cruciferous veggies, and increase the 2-hydroxy to 16-hydroxy ratio. *Clinical pearl:* Eat more DIMs; high levels are found in broccoli, cauliflower, Brussels sprouts, cabbage, and kale.
- *Maintain a balanced immune system.* A women's immune system is stronger than a man's, probably because nature is all about reproduction. She is made for bearing children, child rearing, and carrying on the species. The female sex chromosomes are *XX*. A male's are *XY*. Her second *X* chromosome carries more antibodies and more immune cells than a man's single *X* chromosome. Because her immune system is stronger, it can also overreact, going haywire more easily. It can get hyperactive with allergies or turn on itself, as happens in autoimmunity. Women get, amazingly, 80% of all autoimmune diseases, including hypothyroidism.[5] Testosterone, the dominant male hormone, actually depresses the immune system.

- Immune and autoimmune health depend on colorful whole foods and veggies, a fiber-filled antiinflammatory, anti-SAD diet. This healthy diet approach also implies decreasing alcohol consumption.
- *Manage stress and resolve emotional issues.* Chronic stress strains the adrenals and thyroid, which in turn burdens sex hormones and the gut and contributes to insulin resistance. Address second chakra issues by banishing negativity and using positive imagery.
- *Supplements.* Vitamin D_3 is an essential vitamin to help calcium absorption, and also for gene and hormone regulation and optimum health. Blood levels are easily obtainable. Essential omega 3 fatty acids like EPA (eicosapentaenoic acid) and DHA (docosahexaenoic acid) lower the risk of inflammation and heart disease.

The Sacred Moon Cycle

The wisdom of a woman's cyclic nature is profound, her bleeding the most basic earthly cycle she has. It follows moon phases, tides that ebb and flow with the moon's pull, and the changing seasons (Fig. 28.2). When left to the forces of nature, ovulation and conception most often occur at the time of a full moon; blood flows during the dark, new moon. In many cultures still, a woman's cycle is sacred, as is her connection to the archetypal feminine.[6] These truths are worth remembering for ourselves and our clients when plagued with problems and things going awry in this complicated process.

The ***menstrual cycle*** is the hormonal process a woman's body goes through each month to prepare for a possible pregnancy. Figure 28.3 illustrates the 28-day menstrual cycle in a linear clinical format, frequently seen in traditional text books. It shows the phases, the rise and fall of hormone levels and the uterine lining (*endometrium*) thickening and shedding. On the other hand, Fig. 28.2 depicts the moon cycle in a circular presentation, emphasizing our metaphysical relationship to the moon phases, and cyclic changes in our moods. The first half is a woman's outward yang time, and the second half a yin, going within time.

Each cycle lasts on average 28 days and is divided into two halves. The first half (days 1–14) is the *follicular phase*. It is the time between menses and ovulation when the endometrial lining thickens, and an egg grows inside its *follicle* (egg sac) residing within the ovaries. Energetically, women are ripening an egg. It is the time of increased drive, preparing to give birth to someone or something; acting on ideas; starting new projects; being out in the world and feeling upbeat, enthusiastic, extroverted, social, and loving. It is an outward, exterior *yang* time.

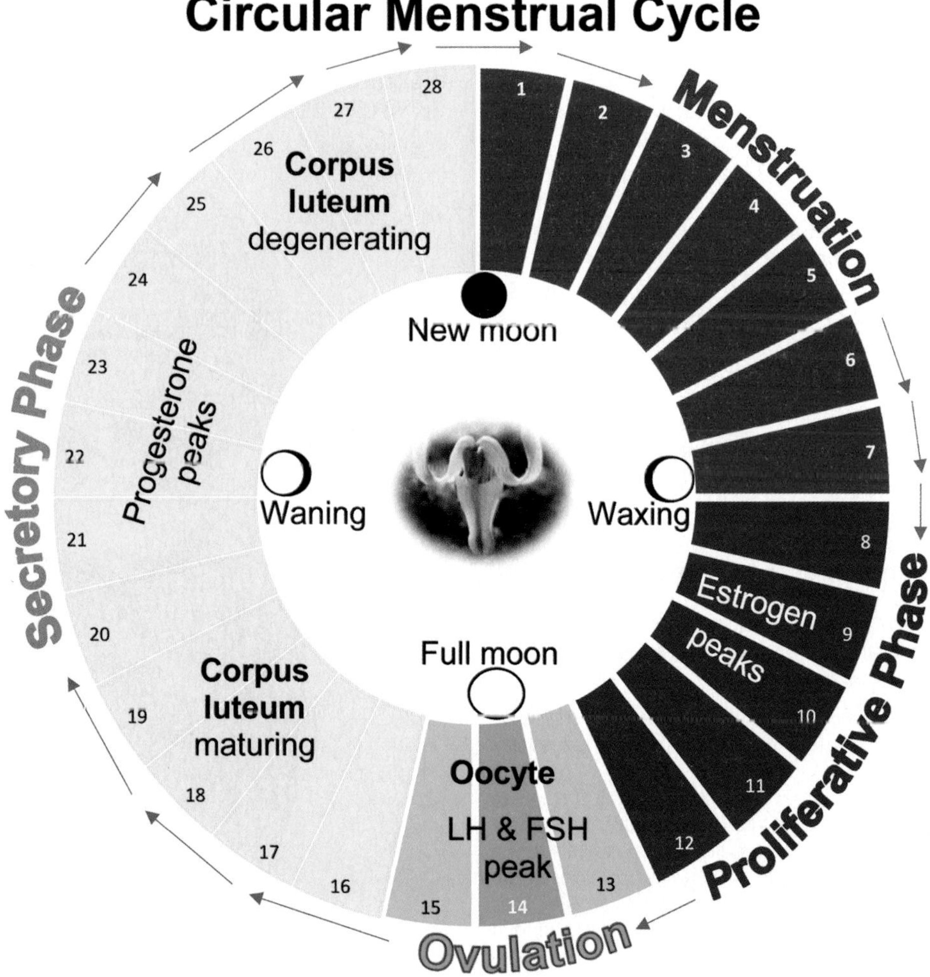

• **Fig. 28.2** If allowed to follow a natural flow, in contact with nature and away from modern day stresses, a woman's menstrual cycle tends to sync up with the phases of the moon. The chart shows this sacred relationship to the natural world, our bodies, our hormones, and our emotions. Day 1-14 is a naturally outward, extroverted time, and day 14-28 is a going within, intuitive time. Chart created by Joan Zinn.

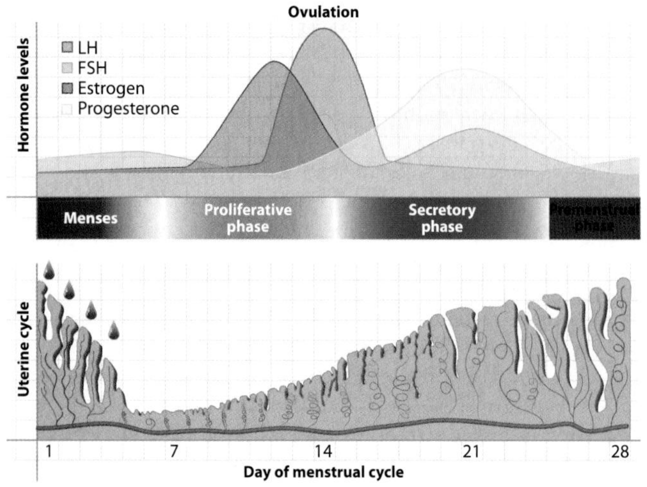

• **Fig. 28.3** Linear menstrual chart showing the phases of the cycle, the formation and shedding of the endometrium lining, and its relationship to the ebb and flow of the female hormones. (/istock/ttsz)

Ovulation occurs at mid-cycle (about day 14) when the egg pops out of its sac and starts its journey down a fallopian tube in preparation for fertilization. Ovulation is the time when a woman is fertile and sexual desire peaks, at full moon. Follicle stimulating hormone (FSH) and also luteinizing hormone (LH) are at their highest and changes occur with basal body temperature, consistency of cervical mucus and position and texture of the cervix (Box 28.1).

The second half of the menstrual cycle (days 14–21) is the *luteal phase*. This lasts from ovulation to the onset of menstruation when the endometrial lining sheds. The second half is premenstrual time, a more reflective going-within spell, when the female body is preparing for possible conception as the released egg travels up through one of her fallopian tubes to the uterus for a possible meet-up with a sperm. This lunar time is when a woman can be most in tune with her intuition and can work her magic. Her inner knowing tells her what isn't working in her life. She feels more withdrawn and less receptive to love and relationships.[6] This second half of the cycle is called the luteal phase because the emptied egg sac remnant changes into a yellow body called the ***corpus luteum***, a temporary gland that produces large amounts of progesterone. This is an inward, interior, *yin* time.

Finally, when hormones are at their lowest ebb, the *menstrual phase* occurs. Women bleed, have less energy, and rightfully should slow down. In some religions and cultures, women isolate themselves or gather together in groups during their menses, the new moon.

From the standpoint of the mind-body connection, problems often begin when the inner guidance system and natural flow of the cycle is ignored. Physical and menstrual troubles appear, especially PMS. It is easy to overlook the moon cycles and our connection with nature when the busy lifestyles of Western societies take over. Menstruation is often brushed aside unheeded. It is frequently considered taboo in modern cultures and sometimes called a *curse*.[6]

One encouraging Wise-Woman trend is to celebrate and honor our daughters when their bleeding begins at ***menarche***, helping them to shift joyfully from their maiden to mother stage. When menopause is eventually reached and bleeding stops, another transition takes place. Children have flown away, and women leave their earlier, younger worries behind, hopefully evolving from mother to crone or Wise-Woman. They become mentors, examples of a sagely lived feminine. Many herbal grandmothers are gracing this phase. These three stages are often depicted as the Triple Goddess Triad of Maiden, Mother, and Crone (Fig. 28.4).

• BOX 28.1 A Woman's Fertile Time

A woman can become pregnant only during a few days in each menstrual cycle. This 5-day window of opportunity (or signal to take preventative measures) occurs midcycle around ovulation: 2 days before, 1 day during, and 2 days after the egg leaves its sac and begins traveling up a fallopian tube to meet a sperm. Sperm live for 5 days. Eggs can be fertilized up to 24 hours after ovulation.[17] There are three basic signs signaling fertile time. (Cramps don't count, and ovulation times can vary, so it is best to keep records.)

- *Cervical mucus changes.* Goes from dry, sticky, and crumbly to creamy, to clear and elastic, like raw egg white being stretched between two fingers. That's fertile mucus.
- *Basal body temperature elevates.* Temperature goes from 0.15°C to 0.5°C, higher during fertile time lasting for 3 days (0°C = 32°F). Changes are very slight, so a special basal thermometer is used that is more accurate than a regular one. It measures changes up to 0.1°F. Take oral basal temperature first thing in morning before rising and compare to numbers at other times in the cycle. A temperature that rises and stays up for 3 days straight provides proof an egg has been released.
- *Cervix changes position and texture.* When a finger is inserted, the cervix is high up in the vagina, and texture changes from feeling like a hard rubber ball to the softness of lips.[17]

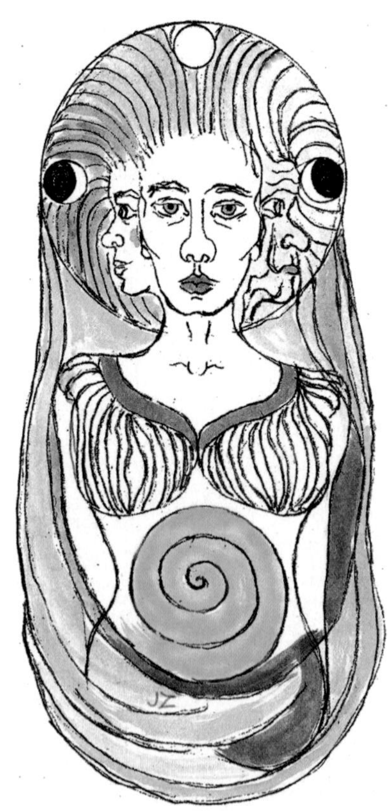

• **Fig. 28.4** The Maiden, the Mother, and the Wise-Woman Triad, depicting the three faces and stages of a woman's life from puberty (maiden) to mother (childbearing years) to Wise-Woman (menopause and beyond). Original art, copyright, Joan Zinn.

Estrogen

Estrogen is classically a female reproductive sex hormone that peaks during the first half of the cycle and is highest just before ovulation. Its primary and traditional function is to stimulate development of female characteristics—breasts, underarm hair, and pubic hair—and to regulate the menstrual cycle. Like all sex hormones, it is stimulated by the ***hypothalamic-pituitary-gonadal (HPG) axis***. Please, do not confuse this pathway with the hypothalamic-pituitary-adrenal (HPA) pathway which connects the brain to the adrenal glands located on top of the kidneys. When reproduction is involved, the hormonal pathway/axis ultimately leads to the ovaries and testes (***gonads***).

In the hypothalamic-pituitary-gonadal (HPG) axis, the hypothalamus in the brain releases gonadotropin-releasing hormone (GnRH) that tells the pituitary to release follicle stimulating hormone (FSH), which signals the ovaries to produce estrogen, which in turn stimulates growth of a mature egg inside. During fertile years, the highest estrogen levels are at mid cycle and indicate ovulation; the lowest levels are during menses.

Estrogen is produced in the ovaries, in fat cells, in the adrenal glands, and in the male testes. In men, it helps sperm mature and maintains libido. Estrogen is really a group of three hormones.

- *Estradiol (E2).* Most common type of estrogen in childbearing age, the fertile years. It is produced in the adrenals, ovaries, and placenta, and it is the kind that can cause estrogen dominance, increased menstrual problems, abnormal cell growth, and possibly fibroids and cancer.
- *Estriol (E3).* The dominant type of estrogen during pregnancy. Because estrogen stimulates cell growth, E3 helps the uterus and lining grow, helps fetal maturation, and regulates hormones.
- *Estrone (E1).* A little estrone is made in the adrenals during and after menopause, when production in the ovaries has stopped. It is the weakest type, but as they get older, women are grateful it's there. (A good reason never to have ovaries surgically removed unless absolutely necessary.)

Benefits and Functions of Estrogen

In proper amounts, estrogen has multiple benefits and functions. Its good effects keep us healthy and sane.

- *Estrogen receptor sites.* These sites are found mainly in the ovaries but are on other body locations as well. Estrogen receptor sites exist on fat cells, breast tissue, skin, muscles, lung cells, and in the gut. They are even found in the mitochondria of liver cells.
- *Estrogen increases lean body mass.* This action is one reason why weight gain can become problematic after menopause. Another reason is insulin and leptin resistance.
- *Cholesterol.* Estrogen maintains healthy cholesterol levels.
- *Estrogen is antiinflammatory.* In reproduction, the highest estrogen levels occur just before ovulation and in pregnancy, which are times of lowest inflammation. (Mother Nature demands successful reproduction so the species may continue.)
  - Lowest estrogen levels occur during the second half of the menstrual cycle and during menses, childbirth, early postpartum period, and menopause. During low-level estrogen periods, inflammation is at its highest. And we now know that PMS, postpartum depression, and menopausal problems are caused by inflammation. Consequently, to avoid these ills, it is especially important for women to habitually consume an antiinflammatory Mediterranean or Paleo diet.
- *Estrogen modulates and enhances the immune system.* The Mother protects women from infections during her vulnerable fertile times of ovulation and pregnancy. Autoimmune diseases (immunity gone overboard) are more frequent in women than in men because of estrogen's influence.
- *Estrogen maintains bone density* in both women and men. It inhibits bone resorption, providing more calcium for strong bones.
- *Estrogen and mood.* Estrogen dominance can cause anxiety, anger, and mood changes. During PMS, a woman can be overly emotional, irritated, anxious, and touchy.
- *Estrogen, serotonin receptors, and depression.* Serotonin is a hormone that helps stop depression, and its receptor sites are estrogen dependent. Postpartum, menopause, and luteal phases are times of lowered estrogen when depression often increases.
- *Estrogen and the skin.* Estrogen keeps the skin and vagina moist. It is quite yin.
- *Estrogen and the endocannabinoid system (ECS).* The ECS is partially regulated by estrogen. Endogenous endocannabinoids are highest at ovulation when estrogen peaks. These help with stress and anxiety and also help regulate menses and fertility.
- *Estrogen, the thyroid, and adrenals.* Estrogen helps regulate the thyroid and adrenals. Proper estrogen levels help energy and help maintain a healthy thyroid.
- *Estrogen in men.* All men have a small amount of estrogen that helps their bone health. Surprisingly, new studies show that abnormally low levels contribute to increased belly fat and decreased sexual desire,[7] just as in low testosterone.

Estrogen Dominance

Too much of a good thing can be problematic. ***Estrogen dominance*** is epidemic, a common hormonal imbalance in women of childbearing age, usually a result of not enough progesterone to counteract it.[8] Xenoestrogen (environmental) exposure is a major cause, occurring via our food supply, water, personal care products, and clothing. Logical herbal therapeutic principles for estrogen dominance are to (1) Counteract estrogen by adding progesteronic herbs; (2) Decongest the liver because it has the formidable job of deconjugating used-up estrogen every month and detoxifying all those endocrine disrupters, the xenoestrogens; (3) Decrease heavy flow and clots, which inevitably appear, with antihemorrhagics. Estrogen dominance results in numerous health problems.

- *Periods and PMS.* Because estrogen builds up tissue, too much results in an overly thick uterine lining *(endometrium)*, with heavy and irregular periods and mood swings.
- *Influences cell growth.* Estrogen dominance exacerbates growth of uterine fibroids and fibrocystic breasts. The worst-case scenario can cause abnormal cervical cells (***dysplasia***), leading to estrogen-dependent cancers of the breast, ovaries, and uterus. Because estrogen hooks onto fat cells, fat gain occurs on the abdomen and on the front of the thighs.[8]
- *Decreased libido.* Estrogen maintains healthy desire.
- *In men.* Estrogen dominance is sometimes caused by a relative decrease in testosterone, and results in abdominal weight gain, fatigue, feeling more emotional, prostate problems, diminished sex drive, enlarged breasts (*gynecomastia*), poor erections, and infertility.

Estrogen Insufficiency

Estrogen deficiency is the flip side of estrogen dominance. It produces symptoms that look a lot like menopause and normally (but

TABLE 28.1 **Phytoestrogenic Foods**

ESTROGENIC ISOFLAVONE FOODS *Soybeans and soy products*	ESTROGENIC LIGNIN FOODS *Undigestible plant fiber*
Soy and soy products are the richest dietary source of *isoflavones*, the most predominant ones being *daidzein* and *genistein.* Soy foods are considered selective estrogen receptor modulators (SERMs), and breast cancer protective as evidenced by lower breast cancer rates in East Asian countries, where soy is predominant in the diet. SERM foods decrease hot flashes.	Flax seeds are a major dietary source of lignins. ***Lignins*** are a weak form of phytoestrogens, so they bind to and take up room on estrogen receptors and decrease the growth of breast cancer. Flax seed oil also provides omega-3 fatty acids, protein, and fiber. Studies show that breast cancer survivors with higher lignin levels in their blood survive longer.[9] Foods other than flax also contain lignins but in smaller amounts.
Soybeans and edamame (soybeans harvested when young and soft)	Golden Flax seed, very high in lignins
Soymilk	Sesame seed
Tofu and fermented tempeh	Whole grains
Miso, fermented soybean paste	Legumes
Soy flour, full fat	Fruits
Soy sprouts	Vegetables

not always) occurs during that transitional time. Women experience trouble sleeping, headaches, decreased libido, irregular periods, cramps, mood swings, dry skin, and hot flashes. In men, sexual desire decreases, and there is fat around the middle. Use phytoestrogenic foods (Table 28.1), phytoestrogenic herbs, demulcents for dryness, spasmolytics for cramps, and treat any other symptoms.

Progesterone

Progesterone is named for *progestation*, the precursor to pregnancy. Progesterone hormone peaks in the second half of the cycle, after the egg has developed in the first half under the influence of ***follicle stimulating hormone (FSH)*** and estrogen. High FSH from the follicular phase triggers ***luteinizing hormone (LH)*** to surge from the pituitary and stimulate ovulation, which is when the egg in the follicle bursts out. Progesterone levels increase as FSH decreases. The endometrial lining of the uterus gets very thick in preparation for potential implantation. If implantation does not happen, progesterone and estrogen levels drop, and with both hormones at their lowest, the uterine lining sheds during ***menstruation***. After 2 to 7 days of bleeding, the cycle repeats every 21 to 35 days, give or take.

Progesterone, like estrogen, is regulated by the HPG axis. Because estrogen dominance is usually a result of not enough counteracting progesterone, it follows that a progesterone deficiency would make the situation even worse, and it does.

Main Progesterone Functions, Excess, and Deficiency

Like estrogen, its other half, progesterone, has a lot of functions. The two hormones rise and fall by negative feedback mechanisms. It can be hard to keep their roles straight, so a handy little cheat sheet is provided in Table 28.2.

- *Progesterone maintains pregnancy.* Because it is the progestation hormone, it supports the placenta and fetal development. Blood levels go way up in pregnancy, and reduced amounts can cause miscarriage.
- *Progesterone balances estrogen.* Because progesterone counterbalances estrogen, estrogen dominance can be caused by a deficiency of progesterone. Unopposed estrogen irritates the nervous system. One herbal possibility for progesterone deficiency is using laboratory-produced progesterone cream. It can be purchased over the counter (OTC) as a 2% topical cream like Progest and applied to the yin inner arms, thighs, or abdomen, starting 1 or 2 days before ovulation to help moderately depressive, *dark* mood changes in PMS.[6] Higher doses must be obtained by a healthcare provider's prescription.
  - *Progesterone imbalances and menses.* Progesterone excess is the other side of the coin from estrogen excess. Estrogen excess builds up thick uterine tissue, creating frequent periods and heavy bleeding. Estrogen deficiency and excess progesterone create long cycles, breast tenderness and lumps, infertility, and PMS with dysfunctional bleeding patterns. Progesterone deficiency produces a shorter luteal phase and shorter periods.
- *Progesterone releases water.* Progesterone acts as a diuretic. Low levels can cause water retention, bloating, and weight gain. When menses occurs, progesterone levels drop, and bloating disappears.
- *Progesterone raises body temperature.* Higher body temperature promotes metabolism, so low progesterone makes individuals feel tired and sluggish.
- *Progesterone and emotions.* Progesterone is calming and relaxing to the nervous system; it is the *going-within* hormone. It also helps sleep and so can help with insomnia. Progesterone can be antidepressive, but *too much* is overly calming, making people feel weepy and emotional, leading to depression. As in everything, balance is critical.
- *Ovulation and anovulation.* A good surge of LH at mid-cycle causes an egg to release and the corpus luteum to produce progesterone. If ovulation does not occur (*anovulation*), no progesterone is produced in the corpus luteum, and there is no period. If there is infrequent ovulation, there are missed periods. Anovulation is temporary and normal after childbirth,

TABLE 28.2 Comparison of Estrogen to Progesterone and Their Effects

Estrogen	Progesterone
Peaks and function. First half of cycle, follicular phase. Triggered by follicle stimulation hormone (FSH). Proliferates endometrium. High in pregnancy; improves vascularization in the uterus and placenta.	***Peaks and function.*** Second half of cycle, luteal phase. Triggered by luteinizing hormone (LH). Ovulation occurs and corpus luteum forms. Thickens endometrium lining to prepare for implantation and maintains pregnancy.
Produced. In ovary, and a little in the adrenals. Stored in fat cells.	***Produced.*** In corpus luteum, and a little in the adrenals.
Fat. Increases synthesis.	***Fat.*** Helps use fat for energy.
Bones. Maintains density. Osteoporosis occurs in menopause when levels decrease.	***Bones.*** Stimulates osteoblasts that increase bone formation.
Moisture. Increases vaginal secretions, keeps skin moist and supple. Increases bloating from salt and fluid retention.	***Moisture.*** Natural diuretic. No bloating unless there is a deficiency.
Menses. Excess causes short cycles, heavy flow. Deficiency has long cycles, scanty flow.	***Menses.*** Excess increases temperature, appetite, weight gain, length of flow. Deficiency creates long cycles.
Cramping. Stimulates uterine cramps.	***Cramping.*** Quiets uterine muscular activity.
Mood. Excess increases anxiety, anger, irritability, extroversion, hyperactivity.	***Mood.*** Natural nervous system relaxant. Inward, calm, introverted. Excess in menopause can cause depression.
Sleep. Excess keeps awake.	***Sleep.*** Helps sleep, prevents insomnia.
Breasts. Excess enlarges breasts and makes them more sensitive.	***Breasts.*** Deficiency causes tenderness, fibrocystic syndrome, lumpiness, swelling.
Thyroid. Excess can increase prolactin hormone which can lower thyroid.	***Thyroid.*** No effect on prolactin, facilitates thyroid action.
Blood clotting. Increases, if estrogen excess.	***Blood clotting.*** Normalizes.
Libido. Increases.	***Libido.*** Decreases.
Energy. Increases, extroverted.	***Energy.*** Decreases, introverted.
Cancer. Excess estrogen increases risk of breast and endometrial (uterine) cancer.	***Cancer.*** Helps prevent estrogen-dependent cancers.
Food cravings. Imbalances, crave chocolate, sweet, fried, salty foods. Ravenous appetite.	***Food cravings.*** No effect.
Microbiome. Maintains the gut microbiome and protects against insulin resistance.	***Microbiome.*** No effect.
Immunity. Increases immunity. Strongest right before ovulation and during pregnancy.	***Immunity.*** No effect.

after miscarriage, and when coming off birth control pills (BCPs). There is *usually* no ovulation while breastfeeding, but that is *not* a guarantee, so breastfeeding is an unreliable birth control method. Anovulation is also common during menarche and menopause.

Hormone Replacement Therapy (HRT) and Bioidentical Hormones

Hormone replacement therapy (HRT) is a controversial subject. Common wisdom always held that estrogen protected women from heart disease. When a woman goes through menopause, her heart disease risk increases. The Women's Health Initiative at the National Institutes of Health (NIH) was a landmark study, carried out between 1993 and 1998 to determine, among many other things, the effect of the synthetic estrogenic drug Premarin (derived from pregnant mare's urine) and progestin (synthetic progesterone like Provera) on women who had not had hysterectomies. However, the study was shut down midstream because it was too dangerous. The hormones were actually *increasing* the risk of stroke, heart disease, breast cancer, and dementia, not the other way around.[10] This finding was a very big deal and caused a media furor.

A debate ensued on whether or not a woman should be taking any artificial hormones at all, including BCPs or intentionally prescribed HRT for various reproductive problems. Some doctors stopped prescribing them; many didn't. The problem with synthetic hormones is that, yes, their structure is similar enough to hook onto receptor sites, but these molecules are not an exact fit. They do the damage described in the Women's Health Initiative study.

This brings us to *bioidentical hormones*, which are specially formulated and custom-made by prescription in a compounding pharmacy. These molecules fit perfectly onto receptor sites and are virtually identical to human-made hormones and are safe and

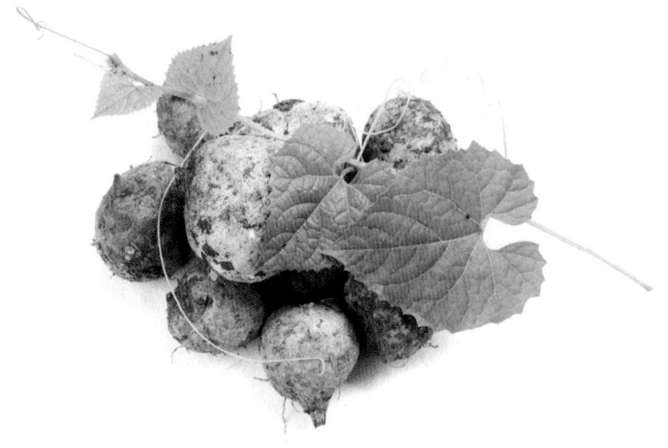

• **Fig. 28.5** *Dioscorea villosa* (Wild Yam root) can be chemically converted into a natural progesterone cream in a laboratory, but the body cannot do this by itself. However, the raw root is mildly phytoestrogenic and can be used for this purpose when made into a tincture or cream by the home herbalist. The root is notably spasmolytic, useful for menstrual and other smooth muscle cramping. (/iStock/Onandter_sean)

effective. When HRT is used, it should always be bioidentical, be it estrogen, progesterone, testosterone, or thyroid hormone.

Natural progesterone must be extracted in a laboratory from Wild Yam root or soybeans (Fig. 28.5). Unfortunately, an herbalist cannot tincture up her own *Dioscorea villosa* (Wild Yam root) and expect it to have the same effect, a popular misconception in herb land. Wild Yam contains a precursor of a steroid hormone called *diosgenin*, a useful phytoestrogen. But diosgenin can only be converted into progesterone in a lab.[11] The body cannot change diosgenin into progesterone by itself. So, homemade Wild Yam cream does *not* contain progesterone, although natural Wild Yam root *does* have a weak phyto-*estrogenic* (not progesteronic) effect, is a lovely smooth muscle relaxant for all kinds of cramping and can lower LDL cholesterol. You will see the hormonal effect of Wild Yam root touted repeatedly in the literature, accurately or not.

Prolactin

The hormone ***prolactin*** is made by the anterior pituitary and is classically known to stimulate milk production after childbirth (*lactation*), hence its name. When there is no pregnancy, levels should be low, but they can become abnormally high from hypothyroidism and a *prolactinoma*, a surprisingly common type of benign pituitary tumor. The most common symptom from high prolactin levels is milk leakage from nipples in women *and* men; the hormone is present in both sexes. It increases water retention, inflammation, stress, and fatigue; shortens the luteal phase; and can stop periods completely. This action leads to anovulation and trouble getting pregnant.

The clinical takeaway is that obtaining a blood prolactin level could shed light on many unsolved reproductive problems, including infertility. Effects of abnormally high blood prolactin levels (*hyperprolactinemia*) are as follows:

- *High prolactin decreases length of luteal phase.* A common result is shorter or cessation of periods. The length of the LH surge and second half of the cycle (luteal phase) decreases.
- *High prolactin can cause infertility.* Because the LH surge and luteal phase are short, there is decreased progesterone produced in the corpus luteum. This results in irregular or infrequent periods with decreased to no ovulation and fewer opportunities to conceive. And with decreased progesterone, the uterine lining is also less conducive to maintaining a pregnancy.[12]
- *High prolactin increases water retention.* Because the luteal phase is shortened, there is less progesterone, a natural diuretic. Water is retained, and there is bloating.
- *High prolactin increases inflammation.* Inflammatory substances, the prostaglandins, are increased, leading to joint aches and pains and breast soreness.
- *High prolactin increases stress and fatigue.* It heightens postpartum depression by preventing hormones from smoothly returning to prepregnancy levels.
- *High prolactin from hypothyroidism.* High estrogen lowers thyroid hormones, and to make matters worse, a low thyroid increases prolactin, spiraling up the problem.
- *High prolactin in men.* High male levels cause erectile dysfunction (ED) and decreased sex drive, along with breast enlargement, tenderness, and breast-milk leakage.
- *Fix for high prolactin.* Lengthen luteal phase progesterone by working on the HPG axis, particularly using Chastetree berry and the essential fatty acids EPA/DHA. Paeonia Bai Shao Yao (White Peony root) and Licorice root are helpful.[12] Decrease stress.

Testosterone and Male Hormone Facts

Testosterone is an ***androgen***, the major male steroid hormone that triggers development of male sexual characteristics at puberty, such as voice changes, enlargement of penis and testes, growth of facial and body hair, and increased muscle mass. Like estrogen, it is triggered by the HPG axis. When levels are low, the hypothalamus releases gonadotropin releasing hormone (GnRH) from the pituitary, which triggers the pituitary to release FSH and LH. These two stimulate the testis to produce testosterone. Testosterone is also responsible for sex drive, sperm, fat, and red blood cell production. In women, testosterone is produced in small amounts in the ovaries and, along with estrogen, helps to maintain sex drive and bone density. Androgen receptors are in all *her* bone cells. It is produced in the adrenals in both sexes. Testosterone facts follow.

- *Testosterone decreases depression.*
- *Testosterone maintains libido and fertility.*
- *Testosterone maintains lean muscle mass.*
- *Testosterone deficiency in men.* Testosterone naturally decreases with age. Very low amounts reduce sex drive and sperm count, and it can lead to erectile dysfunction (ED). It can also cause hot flashes, depression, irritability, and difficulty concentrating. ED calls for yang tonics. If testosterone replacement is prescribed, bioidenticals are best. It is usually given as a topical gel or in pellets that are implanted under the skin by an healthcare provider or a trained nurse practitioner and last for about 6 months.
- *Manopause or andropause.* A man's biological clock ticks, just like a woman's, except more gradually. Consider manopause a transition into becoming a Wise-Man or sage. The term *manopause* was coined at the University of California, Los Angeles (UCLA) and is defined as a slow, steady decline in testosterone levels over many decades; average age is between 40 and 60 years. Common signs and symptoms are similar to female menopause. There is declining sexual function, low

bone density, decreased energy and concentration, loss of body hair, breast tenderness, increased body fat, and heart disease risk. Bioidentical HRT containing testosterone might help but is overrated. Use yang tonics and love. Tribulus fruit and Ashwagandha root are classical yang tonic remedies. Nettle root also helps.

- *Testosterone in women.* It is the most bioactive hormone in women and does not cause masculinity. Female androgen insufficiency (FAIS) is a real thing. It is common for a woman's HRT formula to include a little testosterone.

Chinese Medicine Perspective: Reproduction and Major Syndromes

The Kidney organ system has an enormous influence on reproduction. This list includes some reproduction aspects of Kidney.

- *Reproduction.* The Kidneys store the jing or essence. The vital essence (Kidney yin function) is largely responsible for mental and physical development and forms the basis of our ability to reproduce. Imbalances may include infertility, sexual issues, and physical and/or mental developmental issues.
- *Inheritance.* The Kidneys are the home of the *ancestral chi*, our inherited constitution (DNA), what we came in with. The *Gates of Vitality*, an acupuncture point in the lower back known as *Ming Men* is associated with this energy, ancestral qi, the energy molecule adenosine triphosphate, and Kidney yang. Its location is near the physical kidneys. The Kidneys are the *root of yin and yang* for the entire body.
- *Kidney yin function.* The receptive female principle is Kidney yin. It deals with moisture and coolness. Estrogen and progesterone are the classic female yin hormones. Kidney yin function is the basis for reproduction, growth, and development; formation of the bone marrow; and nourishment of the brain and bones. Kidney yin vacuity, also called *empty heat*, is responsible for hot flashes in menopause. Symptoms include the *five hots*, a feeling of heat of the palms, chest, and soles of feet.
- *Kidney yang function.* The active male principle is Kidney yang. It deals with warmth, fertility, and libido. Testosterone is the archetypal hormone. Kidney Yang Deficiency can be a cause of infertility, decreased libido, and miscarriages.
- *Liver qi and female reproduction.* The Liver is intimately associated with the menstrual cycle and reproduction. Qi moves the blood and the Liver's job is to maintain the free flow of qi. When qi becomes sluggish or stagnant, there is pain and distention, or dull, crampy menstrual pain. If there is long-term stagnation, there can be fixed, stabbing pain. Solid masses such as blood clots, fibroids, or cystic breasts can form.[13]

Chinese Medicine Major Reproductive Syndromes

- *Kidney Yang Deficiency.* This syndrome can occur with women during menses and menopause; and with men, it can involve impotence and infertility. Yang implies heat, dryness, and strength, so yang deficiencies involve the energetics of cool, damp, and/or weakness.
  - *Kidney Yang Deficiency in menses.* Cold limbs, weak back and knees, thin reddish-pink flow, pallor, long irregular cycles. **P** Deep and weak. **T** Pale, scalloped, thin white, moist coat. Use warming, drying, and strengthening herbs.
  - *Kidney Yang Deficiency in menopause.* Menstrual cycles are long, few, and far between; flow can be scanty or heavy; limbs cold; back and knees sore and weak; face and limbs show edema, or loose stools occur. **P** Thready and deep. **T** Body pale and scalloped, thin white coat. Fix is to tonify yang and dry damp.
  - *Kidney Yang Deficiency in male erectile dysfunction or infertility.* There is infertility, low sperm count, and infrequent and weak erections. **P** Deep and weak. **T** Pale. Use Yang tonics like Epimedium Yin Yang Ho (Horny Goat weed) or Eucommia Du Zhong (Eucommia bark).
- *Kidney Yin Deficiency.* Two major female problems come to mind: scanty menstrual flow and the hot flashes of menopause.
  - *Scanty menstrual flow.* Blood looks pinkish or watery red; woman experiences irritability, dizziness, or insomnia. **P** Rapid and thready. **T** Red with less coating than normal. Rehmannia Shu Di Huang (Prepared Rehmannia root) tonifies Kidney and Liver yin.
  - *Empty heat, the hot flashes of menopause.* These occur from burned-out yin and lack of coolant and moisture, both of which Kidney yin should supply. Hot flashes are known as *false* or *empty heat.* The body feels hot and dry because Kidney yin is unable to cool the yang, not like true heat that is caused by a yang excess. Symptoms include night sweats, insomnia, hot flashes, and feelings of heat in the evening; the five hots; incontinence; scant, dark urine; dry throat; restlessness; and headaches. **P** Thready, wiry, and rapid. **T** Red with scant coat. The fix is to add yin and moisture to cool things down and to cause sweating. Use cooling and moisturizing herbs such as Asparagus Tian Men Dong (Shiny Asparagus tuber) or Chickweed herb.
- *Blood Deficiency.* Presents with lots of bleeding, accompanied by anemia, or a pink, scanty, watery flow. Causes include estrogen or thyroid deficiency, malnourishment, excess postpartum bleeding, and intense athletic training. Long cycles. **P** Weak and slow, thin or knotted. **T** Pale and dry. There is weakness, dryness, and cold. Fixes are to restore the blood with Nettle herb, Angelica Dang Gui (Dong Quai root), Codonopsis Dang Shen (Downy Bellflower root), or Zizyphus Da Zao (Jujube berry, Chinese date) and to add phytoestrogens, demulcents, and arterial stimulants.
- *Liver Qi and Blood Stagnation.* Liver Blood Stagnation occurs in the uterus when the blood flow gets sluggish in the vessels and capillaries and starts to pool and clot. There is a feeling of dragging, dull abdominal pain and heaviness, generally in the luteal half of the menstrual cycle. If not addressed, the blood flow gets slower and slower and stagnates, becoming *Liver Qi Stagnation*, the lumps manifesting as uterine fibroids, endometriosis, breast hardenings, cysts, cervical dysplasia, or worst of all, cancer. These hardenings usually indicate estrogen dominance. Menses are irregular and flow can be heavy or scant, with clots that are helped by warmth. There may be breast pain. **P** Slippery or forceful. **T** Body has purple tinge. Therapeutic strategy is to (1) move blood and decongest the Liver with Bupleurum Chai Hu (Asian Buplever root), Lady's Mantle, or Pasqueflower; (2) restore the Spleen with Atractylodes Bai Zhu (White Atractylodes root) and nourish and move qi and blood with Citrus Chen Pi (Ripe tangerine peel); or (3) use the classic formula, Free and Easy Wanderer, Xiao Yao Wan (Fig. 28.6).

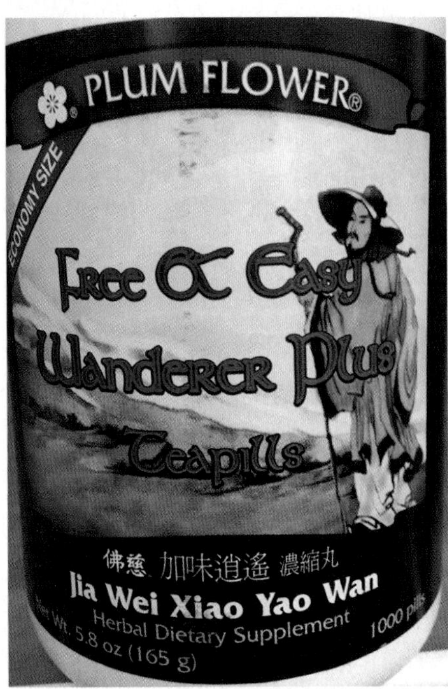

• **Fig. 28.6** Free and Easy Wanderer Teapills, a Chinese patent formula often used for blood clots seen in Liver Qi Stagnation and other menstrual symptoms. The chief herbs are illustrated in Box 28.4.

Reproductive Materia Medica

Reproductive Herbs Worth Honorable Mention

- *Achillea millefolium* (Yarrow herb). Because Yarrow is so complex chemically and has so many qualities, it can be considered a universal regulator of female reproductive functions from prepuberty to postmenopause.[14] Its astringency stops heavy bleeding. Its uterine stimulating effect brings on delayed menses. Its steroidal saponin content makes it estrogenic *and* progesteronic for deficiencies of either hormone. Its spasmolytic effect helps cramping, as does its venous stimulating effect on congestive dysmenorrhea. When you don't have a clue what to use, reach for Yarrow as part of the formula. It is quite bitter and might need some Licorice root to balance the taste.
- *Serenoa serrulata* (Saw Palmetto berry). This trophorestorative heads straight to the reproductive hormones and organs. A yang tonic, it stimulates reproductive qi and blood in men and women, an ally for both sexes, even though its primary reputation is as a man's herb. It is sweet, oily, astringent, and nutritive, promoting sexual organ development, conception, lactation, and stimulating testosterone, progesterone, and prolactin hormones on a pituitary level. It ramps up libido in men *and* women.
  - *For men* it contains the androgenic steroid hormone, sitosterol, so is a *pituitary-gonadal stimulant.* It is famous for shrinking the prostate in benign prostatic hypertrophy (BPH) and normalizing sperm production. For older men especially, it stops urinary leakage and irritation, often caused by pressure on the bladder from an enlarged prostate (Kidney Qi Deficiency).
  - *For women* it normalizes ovulation, menstruation with scanty, delayed periods, irregular cycles, and PMS. It also helps milk production when lactation is insufficient. Later in life, it helps normalize menopausal symptoms.[14]

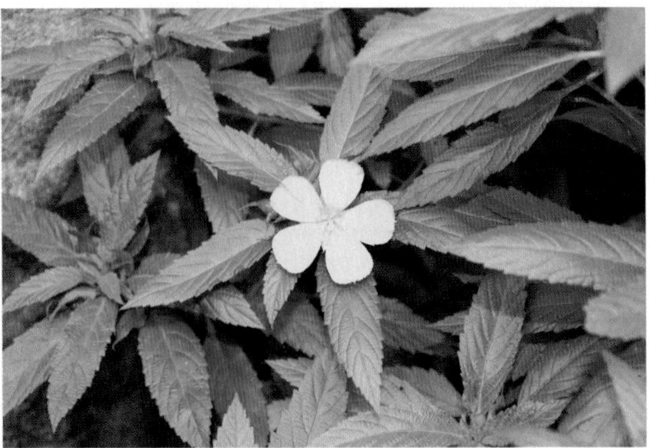

• **Fig. 28.7** *Turnera diffusa* (Damiana leaf) is a warming and drying yang tonic used for Kidney Yang Deficiency. For that reason, it helps libido and decreases frigidity. It is useful for progesterone and testosterone deficiencies. (/iStock/im a photographer and an artist).

- *Turnera diffusa* (Damiana leaf) (Fig. 28.7). This subtropical plant contains essential oils and caffeine-like alkaloids. It is stimulating, restoring and astringing, and it loves the reproductive organs and the pituitary gland. Think of Damiana for Kidney Yang Deficiency, with impotence and ED, lack of sex drive, testosterone deficiency, and urinary incontinence. It strengthens the reproductive organs and increases male testosterone and female progesterone. For women, it regulates late periods and helps PMS caused by progesterone deficiency.
- *Epimedium saggitatum* Yin Yang Huo (Horny Goat Weed leaf). The *horny-ness* refers to the fact that the leaves have sharp prickly tips. It is an important medium-strength Chinese Kidney yang tonic that works on the pituitary level, regulating hormones in men and women. It is both androgenic and estrogenic, notably for impotence, low libido, and irregular menses. It stimulates cerebral circulation, a lot like Ginkgo leaf.

Restoratives and Tonics for Men and Women

This group has a normalizing effect on the reproductive organs and other actions as well. Many of the same tonics are used for men and women (Table 28.3). For instance, Ashwagandha root normalizes mood, energy levels, hormones, and overall immune function. Hawthorn berry supports the heart; Nettle herb builds blood and increases immune function and energy. Maca root keeps libido healthy and promotes energy and natural fertility. Nettle herb builds blood. Its root slows prostate growth, used historically to decrease symptoms of prostate enlargement.

Kidney yin tonics are moisturizing, nutritive, and especially useful in menopause with declining estrogen levels, dryness, and hot flashes. *Kidney yang tonics* help stamina, sex drive, ED, fertility, and energy in men and women. *Blood tonics* are nutrient dense, high in minerals, and improve blood quality. Indications for blood tonics are thin menses with watery, pale-pink blood, heavy flow with blood loss resulting in anemia, and during postpartum after blood has been lost in childbirth. Angelica Dang Gui is used in the follicular phase to enhance fertility caused by blood deficiency and is often combined with Ginger root and Cinnamon bark to protect the stomach.[13]

Tonics and restoratives are used to moderate other types of herbs and are included in most gynecological formulas, especially with uterine involvement, for prolapse, during childbirth, and

TABLE 28.3 Restoratives, Kidney Yin, Kidney Yang, and Blood Tonics

Herb	Notes
Serenoa serrulata Saw Palmetto berry	Trophorestorative for men and women. A yang tonic that helps libido, shrinks prostate in benign prostatic hypertrophy, normalizes menses and menopause.
Avena sativa Milky Oat berry	For neuroendocrine deficiency, tonifies reproductive qi, balances menses, premenstrual syndrome (PMS), and menopause. Helps all reproductive hormones.
Turnera diffusa Damiana leaf	Kidney yang tonic. Reproductive restorative. For low sperm count, erectile dysfunction, low libido, and increases testosterone.
Epimedium saggitatum Yin Yang Huo Horny Goat Weed leaf	Kidney yang tonic. Reproductive restorative for men and women. Androgenic, estrogenic, warm, dry, and astringent. For impotence, infertility. Works at hypothalamus-pituitary level.
Rubus idaeus Red Raspberry leaf	Classic mild and safe uterine-toning tonic during pregnancy.
Nutritive blood tonics. *Medicago sativa* Alfalfa herb *Trifolium pratense* Red Clover flower	Blood tonics for men and women with important nutritives, vitamins, and minerals. Balances estrogen excess and/or deficiency in PMS. For uterine fibroids, fibrocystic breasts, and menopause.[15] Red Clover flower increases fertility.
Angelica sinensis Dang Gui Dong Quai root	Blood tonic, estrogenic, and emmenagogue. For uterus qi and blood deficiency with weakness, pale flow, pallor, dryness, late, absent periods.
Polygonum multiflorum He Shou Wu Flowery Knotweed root, Fo Ti	Yin tonic. Nervous system trophorestorative. For infertility, fatigue, and nervous exhaustion. Said to restore black hair color.
Rehmannia glutinosa Shu Di Huang Prepared Rehmannia root	Yin tonic. Moisturizing for menopause, hot flashes, adrenals, and estrogen deficiency.
Asparagus spp. Tian Men Dong Shatavari in Ayurvedic. Asparagus root in the West.	Yin tonic. Moisturizing for menopausal hot flashes.
Anemarrhena Zhi Mu Know Mother root	Yin tonic that clears heat. Great for hot flashes in menopause.

postpartum. A famous women's gynecology Chinese Medicine tonic is Four Things Soup or Decoction, Si Wu Tang (Box 28.2). If an emmenagogue is used to bring on menses, a tonic moderates this. If a spasmolytic is used for cramping, the restorative retains muscle tone. Tonics are used for men needing assistance with energy, libido, fertility, and testosterone building. If an herb is used to shrink the prostate, tonics balance this action.

Phytoestrogens

Phytoestrogens are plants with estrogen-like activity (Table 28.4). They have structural similarities to human estrogens, allowing them to bind to receptor sites and to block harmful exogenous estrogens in the environment and endogenous ones produced in the body.

Phytoestrogens help women with PMS and menopausal women with hot flashes and vaginal dryness, and phytoestrogens reduce risk of stroke, osteoporosis, and breast cancer. Phytoestrogens can make human estrogen levels rise or fall, depending on need. This balancing action works similarly to a class of drugs called ***selective estrogen receptor modulators (SERMs)***; one example is the breast cancer drug, Tamoxifen.[15] SERMs are selective because they block estrogen from entering breast tissue but leave it alone in the uterus and bone where it is needed.

All sex hormones are derived from cholesterol, variations changing them into specific types. Phytoestrogens contain different active chemicals. *Isoflavones* are commonly found in Red Clover or Kudzu root. *Steroidal saponins* are in Jamaican Sarsaparilla root and Wild Yam root, and *phytosterols* are in Licorice root. In fact, plants with steroidal molecules have traditionally and intuitively been used for women's menstrual functions throughout the Wise-Woman tradition.

Progesteronics

Naturally occurring progesterone is not known to exist in plants in biologically active levels, but certain botanicals seem to calm down overactive estrogen (Table 28.5). Phytoestrogens, like Licorice root and other Pea family plants, have a weak binding capacity for human receptor sites, but progesterone receptor sites are pickier and more selective. Plants containing steroidal saponins (more progesteronic) and phytosterols (more estrogenic) have chemical structures similar to those of many human hormones, but whether their structures are similar to those of progesterone or estrogen is not clear. Whether and why certain plants are actually progesteronic is a debatable topic.

Science aside, certain plants have been successfully used historically for hormonal balance. *Dioscorea villosa* (Wild Yam root), *Trillium grandiflorum* (Birthroot) (Fig. 28.8), and the endangered *Chamaelirium luteum* (Helonias root or False Unicorn root) seem to have an indirect effect, improving the balance of estrogen to

• BOX 28.2 **Four Things Soup or Decoction, Si Wu Tang**
(An exemplary general female blood tonic)

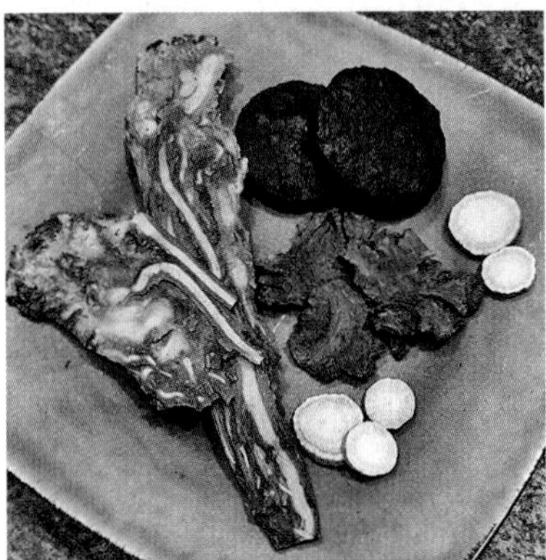

Four Things Soup Si Wu Tang. This popular woman's tonic features four famous roots: (clockwise from left) Angelica Dang Gui, Rehmannia Shu Di Huang, Paeonia Bai Shao and (center) Ligusticum Chuan Xiong.

This is a notable and important Chinese gynecology formula for premenstrual syndrome (PMS), threatened miscarriage, menstrual cramps, or anemia. It builds blood and tonifies the Liver and Kidneys. It is given most typically to women with symptoms of sallow complexion, pale lips and fingernails, dizziness, vertigo, tinnitus, irregular menstruation, decreased blood flow, abdominal pain or amenorrhea. **P** Thin or wiry. **T** Pale.

Equal parts

1. Rehmannia Shu Di Huang (Prepared Rehmannia root). Nourishes blood.
2. Angelica Dang Gui (Dong Quai root). Nourishes blood.
3. Ligusticum Chuan Xiong (Sichuan Lovage root). Moves blood.
4. Paeonia Bai Shao (White Peony root). Nourishes blood.

Directions

Grind herbs and use the mixture of roots listed to prepare remedy of your choice.

- Decoction. (1 tbsp herb mixture per cup, 1–2 times daily.)
- Tincture. 1:4 60% tincture (5 mL 2 times daily.)
- Capsules. (Two 00 capsules 3 times daily.)

progesterone. Another good herbal bet for increasing progesterone is the HPG axis level approach, which stimulates the release of FSH and LH. One of the all-time best HPG influencers is *Vitex agnus-castus* (Chastetree berry).

Bleeding: Hemostatics and Emmenagogues

Some herbs exist to decrease bleeding, and others to increase bleeding (Table 28.6). Reproductive ***hemostatics*** are herbs that discourage abnormally heavy menstrual bleeding by causing capillary constriction or by speeding up blood clotting (*coagulants*). They are usually astringents that tighten tissue with a tropism to the uterus, such as Witch Hazel leaf or Shepherd's Purse herb (Fig. 28.9). A normal amount of bleeding for a girl or woman to expect is 30 to 80 mL a month, or a need to change menstrual pads or regular-sized tampons three to six times a day.[6] Of course this amount varies and tapers off toward the end of the cycle. ***Menorrhagia*** refers to excessive menstrual bleeding beyond reasonable parameters.

For hemostatics to work, ***pulse dosing*** is used, which involves herbs given frequently and close together (Appendix A). A dosing example might be 5 mL (1 teaspoon) every 15 to 30 minutes until bleeding lessens, up to 2 hours maximum. (Note that extremely heavy bleeding that doesn't let up *could* be a medical emergency.) Some important hemostatics are, from strong to weak: Cotton root bark, strongest; Goldenseal root and Shepherd's Purse herb, next strongest; and Red root, Yarrow herb and Birthroot, medium-strength.

Emmenagogues are uterine stimulants. They increase uterine contractions and menstrual flow. Some work through stimulation because of their bitter taste, others through localized irritation.[16] They do not cause miscarriages but could bring on a late period if there is no pregnancy; Ginger root and Mugwort herb are examples. Late periods could be caused by life's occurrences, such as stress, lifestyle disruptions, relationship angst, travel, anovulation, and excessive exercise. The absence of a period for at least three previous menstrual cycle lengths or at least 6 months in a previously menstruating woman is termed ***amenorrhea***.[17] Unless reasons are natural causes such as pregnancy, breastfeeding, going off BCPs, or perimenopause, amenorrhea is generally treated with HRT, and emmenagogues are not used.

Caution: Some emmenagogues are so strong they have been used as abortifacients by ancient Wise-Women and by the Eclectics and should be used only by very experienced herbalists. These include *Hedeoma pulegioides* (Pennyroyal essential oil, which has caused death), *Ruta graveolens* (Rue herb), and *Senecio* spp. (Ragwort herb).[6] They all can have extremely toxic effects (Table 28.6).[18]

Uterine Pain, Part I: Move Blood with Venous Decongestants and Arterial Stimulants

For pain relief, we use herbs that move blood in the veins and arteries (Table 28.7). The uterine muscle is very vascular. Blood can accumulate and get congested there, causing dull, heavy cramping, especially in the luteal phase. This is called *congestive dysmenorrhea*. In Chinese Medicine, it is called *blood congestion*. This type of menstrual cramping is solved by increasing the circulation and moving accumulated venous blood away from the uterus, moving it upward, against gravity, and back to the heart. Herbs that do this are cool, dry, astringent *venous decongestants* that squeeze the blood up and away. Examples are Lady's Mantle herb, Pasqueflower herb, or Shepherd's Purse herb.

In addition to moving venous blood, arterial circulation should be encouraged because of blood becoming engorged in the uterine capillaries. Use warming *arterial stimulants* in small amounts in formula along with the venous decongestants. Examples here are Prickly Ash bark, Ginger root, or Cayenne pepper.

Uterine Pain, Part II: Relax Smooth Uterine Muscles with Spasmolytics

Spasmolytics relax smooth uterine muscles and are used to stop cramps caused from muscle spasms (Table 28.8). It is useful to use them in conjunction with the venous and arterial blood movers just described. The former help congestive dysmenorrhea by moving pooling blood away from the uterus, and the latter relaxes the uterine muscles. Because we don't always know the cause, it is a good idea to use them all.

TABLE 28.4 Estrogenic Herbs

Herb	Description
Glycyrrhiza glabra Gan Cao Licorice root	Contains phytosterols for estrogen deficiency and high blood sugar.
Angelica sinensis Dang Gui Dong Quai root	Moist, estrogenic and progesteronic. Builds blood, emmenagogue in scanty menses. Enhances luteinizing hormone surge, so shortens long cycle. Anticoagulant, so contraindicated in heavy bleeding. Helps vaginal dryness and menopausal hot flashes.
Trifolium pratense Red Clover	Established phytoestrogen for premenstrual syndrome (PMS), menopause, hot flashes. Nutritive yin tonic.
Caulophyllum thalictroides Blue Cohosh root (Note that Blue Cohosh is a totally different genus and species from Black Cohosh.)	Steroidal saponin, spasmolytic, and tones uterus. For estrogen deficiencies, including PMS. Classic obstetrical use in labor and delivery. Loved by the Eclectics.
Smilax officinalis Jamaican sarsaparilla root	Steroidal saponin. For estrogen and progesterone deficiencies and a blood cleanser.
Pueraria lobata Ge Gen Kudzu root	High isoflavone content with high estrogenic activity. Used in Chinese Medicine for hypertension and migraines. Cooling demulcent for hot flashes.
Dioscorea villosa Wild Yam root	Contains *diosgenin*, a steroidal phytoestrogen. It is also an excellent spasmolytic for cramps.
Panax quinquefolius Xi Yang Shen American ginseng root	Works on hypothalamic-pituitary-adrenal and hypothalamic-pituitary-gonadal levels. Classic neuro-endocrine and digestive restorative. Yin, qi, and Spleen tonic; more estrogenic and less stimulating than Asian ginseng.
Humulus lupus Hops flower	Phytoestrogenic with nervous system-relaxing and sleep-inducing actions. Helps hot flashes.
Salvia officinalis Garden Sage leaf	Phytoestrogen, cooling, drying, specifically for menopausal night sweats and mental clarity.
Medicago sativa Alfalfa herb *Urtica dioica* Nettle herb	Estrogenic nutritives. For estrogen deficiency with pale blood and skin. Also, for PMS and menopause.
Foeniculum vulgare Fennel seed	For estrogenic deficiency with scanty, delayed periods, clots and cramps, PMS, and insufficient lactation.
Actaea racemosa Black Cohosh root	Controversial as a phytoestrogen. Research reports the herb is *not* estrogenic, although traditionally used for this with reported success.[19] But it *is* an effective smooth-muscle relaxant for cramping.

Male-Oriented Herbs

Every culture has addressed male reproductive health. Many of these herbs are traditional Chinese Medicine *yang tonics*, warming and energizing (Table 28.9). They address signs of incontinent urination caused by enlarged prostate, premature ejaculation, loss of libido, and low sperm count, and they tend to stimulate the HPG axis.[20] By approaching the problem from that level, they can help both sexes, and *Panax* spp. (Ginseng root) and Epimedium Yin Yang Ho (Horny Goat weed) do just that. Although they are traditionally oriented toward males, they should not be overlooked for women, the yin principle balancing the male yang.

Other herbs that help men's reproductive health include Ayurvedic tonics, Tribulus fruit, or Ashwagandha root. Western examples are Damiana herb and Saw Palmetto berry. Yang tonics tend to contain subgroups of predominantly androgenic/testosterone steroid hormones.

Other Herbal Reproductive Categories

There are many herbal categories discussed elsewhere in this book that are often used in reproductive formulas. *Liver decongestants, tonics, and stimulators* are very important to include in estrogen-dominant conditions. They improve liver function and help metabolize estrogen. Remember the bitters: berberines, the docks, and others like Blue Flag root, Chaparral leaf, Fringe Tree bark, and Dandelion root. Include herbs such as Salvia Dan Shen, Milk Thistle seed, and Poke root. Remember the *lymphatic circulators* in formulas for uterine fibroids, fibrocystic breasts, and other lumps: Cleavers herb, Marigold flower, Echinacea root, Red root, Pau d'arco bark, and Yellow Dock root.

Cooling and/or estrogenic herbs for hot flashes dealing with Chinese Medicine's *empty heat* designation include Anemarrhena Zhi Mu (Know Mother root), Chickweed herb, Elderflower, Garden Sage leaf, Solomon's Seal root, Schisandra Wu Wi Zi (Five Taste berry), and Scrophularia Xuan Shen (Black Figwort root).

TABLE 28.5 **Herbs that Increase Progesteronic Effect**

Vitex agnus-castus Chastetree berry Essential to keep in large quantities in your women's apothecary.	Normalizes cycles by giving good follicle stimulation hormone and luteinizing hormone (LH) surges in the pituitary. Very useful for luteal phase. Must use for 3 to 6 months for results.
Chamaelirium luteum Helonias root, False Unicorn root Endangered species, please find sustainable sources or substitute others.	Steroidal saponin. Normalizes progesterone and estrogen deficiencies. For congestive dysmenorrhea, miscarriage prevention, last trimester prophylaxis, and to harmonize labor.
Trillium erectum Birthroot or Bethroot	Steroidal saponin. For progesterone and estrogen deficiencies, congestive dysmenorrhea, helps childbirth contractions.
Dioscorea villosa Wild Yam root	Steroidal saponin, spasmolytic, and analgesic. Used by Eclectics for progesterone deficiency type problems, although progesterone from Wild Yam requires laboratory extraction.
Achillea millefolium Yarrow herb	Universal hormonal normalizer, more on the progesterone side. Hemostatic and for all kinds of cramping.
Turnera diffusa Damiana bark	Yang tonic that increases libido. Luteal hormone balancer (the half of the cycle where progesterone dominates).
Gossypium spp. Cotton root bark Highly sprayed, so use organic.	Progesteronic, increases LH and ovulation, strong hemostatic.
Smilax officinalis Jamaican Sarsaparilla root	Steroidal saponin, more on progesteronic side. For luteal problems like swollen breasts, and inverted nipples.
Lepidium spp. Maca root	Works on hypothalamic–pituitary level, helping female hormonal balance and adrenal health. On the progesterone side. Helps menopause.

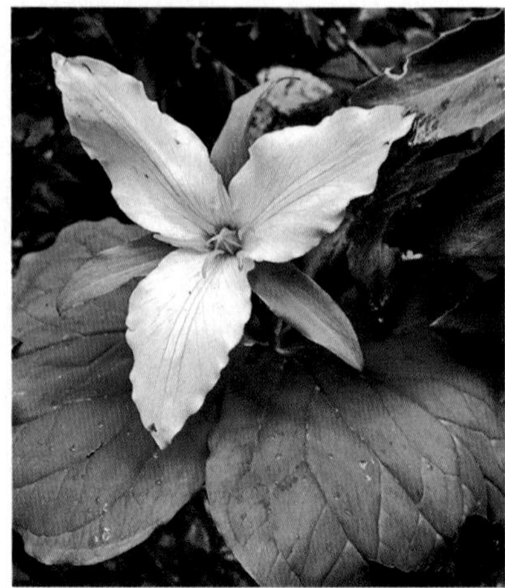

• **Fig. 28.8** *Trillium grandiflorum* (Birthroot, White Trillium). Appropriately named Birthroot, this lovely forest dweller is used to promote contractions in labor and to lessen postpartum bleeding. Trillium root is a uterine restorative, a steroidal saponin that balances hormones (estrogen or progesterone) when one or the other is deficient.

For *fertility enhancers*, use the yang tonics listed earlier. Nutritious Red Clover flower is Susun Weed's go-to fertility choice for women. Use herbs that work on the HPG axis, like Chastetree berry, Saw Palmetto berry, the ginsengs, and other adaptogens. Consider Cotton root bark, Mugwort herb, Damiana leaf, Jamaican sarsaparilla root, and Yarrow herb.

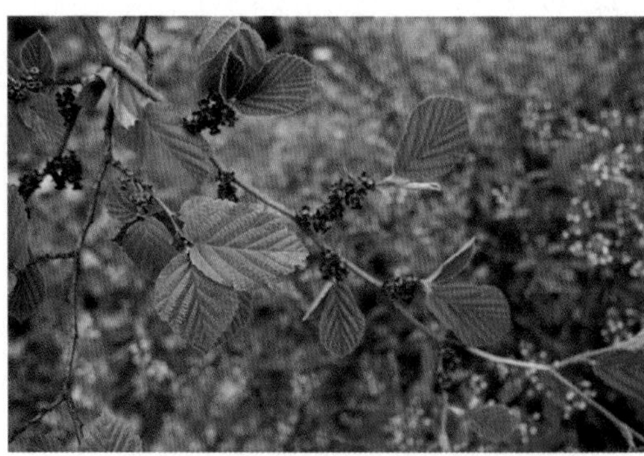

• **Fig. 28.9** *Hamamelis virginiana* (Witch Hazel leaf). Its high tannin content makes it a good astringent, used for menorrhagia and other types of bleeding. It dries damp, stopping other discharges and diarrhea and also restores weak veins present in varicosities and hemorrhoids. (/iStock/seven75)

Common Reproductive Conditions

Phase Dosing

Because of the complexity of female reproduction, sometimes it makes sense to administer different formulas at specific times of the menstrual cycle. ***Phase dosing*** is the dispensing of a separate formula at different phases (halves) of the cycle, depending on a woman's condition, or giving a symptomatic formula during the menstrual phase. Normally the follicular phase is when

TABLE 28.6 Hemostatics and Emmenagogues (*For menorrhagia, pulse dose 5 mL every 15 min for 2 hours*)

HEMOSTATICS *Slows down menstrual flow.*	EMMENAGOGUES *Stimulates menstrual flow.*
Gossypium spp. (Cotton root bark) Constricts and coagulates. Use organic. Very strong hemostatic.	*Zingiber officinale* (Ginger root) For delayed periods, warming, spasmodic dysmenorrhea. Strong emmenagogue.
Capsella bursa-pastoris (Shepherd's purse herb) For any type of bleeding, varicose veins. Strong hemostatic.	*Artemisia* spp. (Mugwort herb and other Artemisias) For delayed periods, amenorrhea, long cycles. Strong emmenagogue.
Trillium spp. (Birthroot or Beth root) Astringent. For bleeding, discharges, diarrhea, prolapse. Often used pre- and postpartum. Medium-strength hemostatic.	*Actaea racemosa* (Black Cohosh root) For delayed periods, spasmodic dysmenorrhea, difficult labor. Moderately strong emmenagogue.
Alchemilla vulgaris (Lady's Mantle herb) General for heavy menses and diarrhea.	*Mitchella repens* (Partridge berry). Moderately strong emmenagogue.
Hamamelis virginiana (Witch Hazel leaf) General hemostatic and astringent for heavy menses, GI bleeding, and hemorrhoids. A capillary restorative and vasoconstrictor.	*Angelica sinensis* Dang Gui (Dong Quai root) For scanty periods, amenorrhea, spasmodic dysmenorrhea, and blood deficiency.
Typha angustifolia Pu Huang (Cattail pollen) General hemostatic for heavy menses, styptic, hematuria. Also, hypotensive, vasodilating, and antilipemic.	*Caulophyllum thalictroides* (Blue Cohosh root) Moderately strong emmenagogue.
Chamaelirium luteum (Helonias root, False Unicorn root) Mildly astringent, so helps heavy bleeding. A steroidal saponin, and progesteronic.	*Salvia officinalis* (Garden Sage herb) For delayed periods, estrogenic, hot flashes especially at night. Mild emmenagogue, but a medium-strength herb.
Achillea millefolium (Yarrow herb) Heavy menses with bright red blood, wounds, hemorrhoids, GI, phlebitis. Mild astringent. (Notice that Yarrow appears in both columns.) Its astringency stops heavy bleeding, but it brings on delayed menses because of its stimulating effect.	*Achillea millefolium* (Yarrow herb) For delayed periods, a mild emmenagogue that can paradoxically stimulate menses when slowed down by exposure to cold.[14] Progesteronic, venous decongesting and antispasmodic, for all kinds of cramps, and menopausal symptoms.
Cinnamomum cassia Cinnamon bark Arrests flow, astringes, dries damp. Add 1 drop essential oil per ounce of tincture to slow bleeding.	*Artemisia vulgaris* Mugwort herb Uterine stimulant and relaxant. Can help stagnant qi and bring on periods.

estrogen dominates, the luteal phase is when progesterone peaks, and bleeding time is the menstrual phase when hormones bottom out. Here are some examples of when phase dosing might be appropriate.

- *If a young woman had menstrual cramps* in the first couple of days during menses, a pain formula with smooth-muscle relaxants begun perhaps 2 days before and all during menses would be logical.
- *If an older perimenopausal woman had severe cramping* and a dull ache before and during menses, it would make sense to give her a formula beginning at ovulation to decongest the uterus, continuing through the second half of the cycle (luteal) and during her period (Case History 28.1).
- *If a woman had estrogen dominance PMS* (too much unopposed estrogen overpowering progesterone in the luteal half), and there was heavy bleeding with bright red clots, then the luteal half would need greater emphasis on progesteronic and Liver qi decongesting botanicals (Case History 28.3). The best herb to increase the progesteronic effect is large amounts of Chastetree berry, working indirectly from the pituitary level. It also helps to supplement with an OTC laboratory-produced topical Wild Yam cream, such as Pro-Gest (Fig. 28.10).
- *If a woman had estrogen deficiency* in the follicular half when estrogen peaks, and her blood was scant and pale, that phase would need a formula higher in phytoestrogenic herbs (Table 28.4). A different hormone normalizing formula could then be administered during the luteal phase.
- *If there were very short periods with difficulty conceiving*, there could be a weak LH surge with skipped ovulations requiring a high dose of Vitex berry to begin before ovulation and to continue throughout the luteal phase.
- *If a woman had PMS with bloating, water retention, breast tenderness and insomnia*, there is a luteal phase defect. An increased progesteronic effect is needed to help diuresis and to relax and calm the nervous system.
- *If using a follicular or luteal formula*, stop them at menses and then resume in the proper phase. Because both estrogen and progesterone are at their lowest ebb during bleeding, it is counterproductive to boost them at that time.

Dysmenorrhea (Menstrual Cramps)

- *Definition*. ***Dysmenorrhea*** means painful menses (Case History 28.1).

TABLE 28.7 Venous Decongestants and Arterial Stimulants
(For congestive dysmenorrhea)

Herb	Notes
Paeonia lactiflora Bai Shao Yao White Peony root	Uterine blood decongestant, astringent, muscle relaxant. For cramps, regardless of cause. Helps hot flashes, too.
Ligusticum wallichii Chuan Xiong Sichuan Lovage root	Uterine decongestant. Capillary stimulant.
Aesculus hippocastanum Horse Chestnut seed	Strong venous decongestant for uterine congestion and stagnation, varicose veins, or hemorrhoids. Anticoagulant.
Collinsonia canadensis Stone root	Venous decongestant for uterine congestion, cramps, and for stagnation with varicosities, leg cramps, hemorrhoids, constipation.
Chamaelirium luteum Helonias root, False Unicorn root	Excellent uterine decongestant. Helps uterine prolapse. Use only nonendangered sources.
Ceanothus americanus Red root	Venous decongestant. Excellent hemostatic.
Trillium grandiflorum or T. erectum Birthroot or Bethroot	Uterine decongestant. Good hemostatic.
Capsella bursa-pastoris Shepherd's Purse herb	Venous decongestant for cramps. Hemostatic.
Alchemilla vulgaris Lady's Mantle herb	Venous decongestant and hemostatic.
Achillea millefolium Yarrow herb	General uterine venous decongestant and mild systemic astringent. Mild hemostatic.
Mitchella repens Partridgeberry herb	Venous uterine decongestant, diuretic.
Cinnamomum cassia Cinnamon bark	Arterial stimulant. Regulates blood glucose. Warming.
Zingiber officinalis Ginger root	Arterial and capillary stimulant. Protects stomach. Warming and pungent.
Zanthoxylum americanum Prickly Ash bark	Arterial stimulant, very dry and warming.

TABLE 28.8 Uterine Spasmolytics

Herb	Notes
Viburnum opulus (Cramp bark) *Viburnum prunifolium* (Black Haw bark)	Both are spasmolytic and interchangeable.
Ligusticum wallichii Chuan Xiong Sichuan Lovage root	Relaxes smooth muscle and also a blood tonic/builder, often used with Dong Quai and Paeonia Bai Shao Yao (White Peony root).
Bupleurum chinensis Chai Hu Asian Buplever root	Spasmolytic and liver restorative, antiinflammatory.
Paeonia lactiflora Bai Shao Yao White Peony root	Famous for any type of menstrual cramping. Can use either Red or White Peony.
Actaea racemosa Black Cohosh root	Antispasmodic, but probably not estrogenic according to latest studies.
Caulophyllum thalictroides Blue Cohosh root.	Spasmolytic, famous Eclectic, Native American remedy. Used in labor and delivery.
Leonurus cardiaca Motherwort herb	Queen of spasmolytics that also supports heart, stops palpitations, calms anxiety in all mothers, tones uterus. For menopause with hot flashes. Emmenagogue potential.
Anemone pulsatilla Pasqueflower herb	Antispasmodic, relaxing. Combines well with Cramp bark, Black Cohosh, White Peony.

TABLE 28.9 Male Oriented Herbs

Herb	Notes
Panax ginseng Ren Shen Asian ginseng root	Works on hypothalamic-pituitary-gonadal (HPG) and hypothalamic-pituitary-adrenal (HPA) levels. Androgenic, aphrodisiac, estrogenic, pituitary-adrenal, fertility stimulant. For deficiencies of qi, blood, and essence. Yang tonic.
Eleutherococcus senticosus Ci Wu Jia Siberian Ginseng root	Works on HPG and HPA axis. Adaptogen, fertility, yang tonic.
Serenoa serrulata Saw Palmetto berry	Works on HPG axis, contains sitosterol. Androgenic hormonal-gonadal stimulant. Shrinks prostate in BPH. Helps fertility, sperm production, and urinary leakage.
Epimedium saggitatum Yin Yang Ho Horny Goat weed	Yang tonic. Stimulates HPG axis. For infertility, impotence, low sperm count. Estrogenic: helps estrogen deficiency, irregular menses, and menopause.
Eucommia ulmoides Du Zhong Eucommia bark	For Kidney Yang Deficiency with damp on board. Helps libido and infertility. Also, classic connective tissue strengthener.
Turnera diffusa Damiana leaf	Kidney yang tonic. Reproductive restorative. For Kidney yang deficiency with impotence, erectile dysfunction, low libido.
Cervus nippon Lu Rong Velvet Deer antler	Tonifies Kidney yang. Endocrine restorative of the HPA axis, nutritive. For impotence, infertility, chronic weight loss.
Schisandra chinensis Wu Wei Zi Schisandra berry, Five Taste berry	For Kidney Yang and qi deficiency. Adaptogen, Liver trophorestorative, works on pituitary level. Helps low libido.
Tribulus terrestris Puncturevine root and fruit, Goathead (Must use large doses to be effective.)	Contains steroidal saponins that improve sperm count and motility; helps erectile dysfunction, and libido.
Lepidium meyenii Maca root	Peruvian herb that works on pituitary level. Androgenic, adaptogenic, increases sperm count, motility, mental clarity; helps thyroid.
Pausinystalia johimbe Yohimbe bark	African herb that increases circulation to penis, helps sustain firm erection. Contraindicated with high blood pressure.
Withania somnifera Ashwagandha root	Ayurvedic adaptogen that increases testosterone, energy, sperm count, motility.
Crataeva nurvala Three-leaved Caper root, root bark and leaf	Ayurvedic herb valued for treatment of renal conditions such as enlarged prostate, stones, cystitis.
Urtica dioica Nettle root	The root is used to decrease nocturia and increase prostate health.

- *Spasmodic primary dysmenorrhea* with muscle cramping lasts for only 2 to 3 days during bleeding, so administer spasmolytics to deal with acute short-term symptoms. *Phase dose* a couple of days before menses and then during bleeding time. Use in high doses. Improves over time. Usually occurs in teenagers and young women.
- *Congestive secondary dysmenorrhea* with blood pooling in the uterus occurs during the luteal phase and during menses, requiring administration during those times using *phase dosing*. Common in older women with liver congestion, not improving over time.[18]

- *Signs and symptoms.* Cramps and menstrual pain.
- *Allopathic treatment.* Tylenol, ibuprofen, and muscle relaxants.
- *General therapeutic principles.* (1) Uterine decongestants like Lady's Mantle or Red Root to get uterine capillary blood moving. (2) Venous systemic decongestants to circulate blood back to the heart: Yarrow or Witch Hazel herb. (3) Arterial stimulants like Ginger root or Prickly Ash bark. (4) Spasmolytic uterine relaxants to calm down smooth-muscle spasms in the uterine wall. (5) Nervines for stress and anxiety.

Dysfunctional Uterine Bleeding

- *Definition.* The designation ***dysfunctional uterine bleeding (DUB)*** covers a lot of territory. It refers to abnormal uterine bleeding and is a symptom, not a disease. Patterns and causes vary. There is a wide range of what's normal, so become familiar with that (Box 28.3). There can be too much or too little bleeding, erratic cycles, and spotting (Case History 28.2). Rule out cancer, abnormal uterine size and shape, endometriosis, and ovarian cysts. If not those, DUB is usually a symptom of hormonal imbalances on the HPG level and a failure to ovulate. There is unopposed (too much) estrogen and deficient or no progesterone. If there is spotting, some parts of the endometrium are probably shedding, and others are not.[12] DUB is common in menarche and perimenopause. Leave it alone if no problems arise.
- *Signs and symptoms.* Many symptoms are possible. *Menorrhagia* is very heavy bleeding (more than seven soaked-through pads per period or a need to change tampons every hour for 2 to 3 days). *Scanty flow* looks pale pink and watery (decreased estrogen).

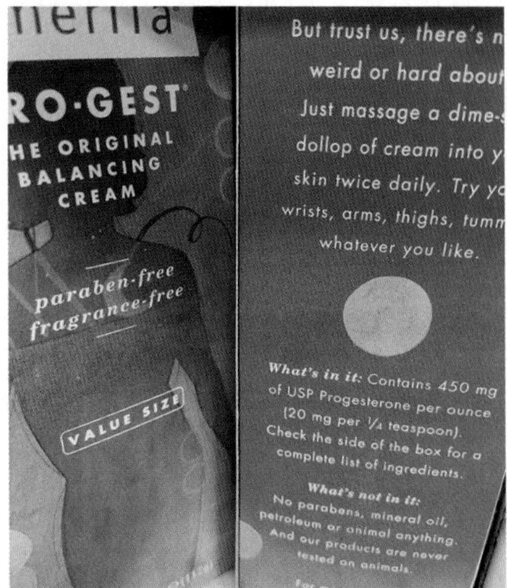

• **Fig. 28.10** Pro-Gest is an over the counter laboratory-produced progesterone cream made from Wild Yam. Use topically for progesterone deficiencies such as menopausal insomnia and hot flashes, or fibrocystic and tender breasts.

Long flow length means lasting over 7 to 10 days (Box 28.3). *Amenorrhea* is lack of a period for more than 6 months. (Rule out pregnancy, menopause, and extreme athletics.)

- *Allopathic treatment.* Varied, depending on cause. HRT and surgery.
- *General therapeutic principles.* (1) Increase the hypothalmic-pituitary pathway with Vitex. (2) Scanty flow is usually estrogen deficiency; in such case, Angelica Dang Gui or Red Clover herb. (3) Use mild uterine tonics to tone muscle. (4) Reduce stress with nervines. (5). Normalize anemia, so if flow is extremely heavy, supplement with iron-rich herbs and foods. (6) Use two formulas, one to correct underlying problem and other to use during period for excess bleeding, as needed.

Premenstrual Syndrome

- *Definition.* The name *premenstrual syndrome* was coined in the 1950s but the syndrome has been recognized since the days of Hippocrates. It involves an extensive variety of physical and behavioral symptoms, usually occurring in the luteal phase of the menstrual cycle (Case History 28.3). Varying subgroups with predominant symptoms have been described by diverse sources. Here is one easy-to-grasp grouping of four types. PMS-A features *anxiety* and has an estrogen excess or progesterone deficiency aspect. PMS-C involves *carbohydrate cravings*. In PMS-D, *depression* predominates. PMS-H refers to *hyperhydration* and bloating.[18]
- *Signs and symptoms.* Most common are depression, anxiety, mood swings, or anger. Women may also experience pelvic pain; abdominal bloating; abnormal appetite with food cravings for sugar, alcohol, or fatty foods; cyclic weight gain; and changes in bowel habits. Also, breast swelling and tenderness, headaches, fatigue, insomnia, and joint pain may occur. There are many others.
- *Allopathic treatment.* Hormone therapy and/or symptomatic drug therapy such as antidepressants, diuretics, and analgesics.
- *General therapeutic principles.* (1) Correct imbalances on HPG level. Vitex throughout cycle long-term. (2) Correct any estrogen

CASE HISTORY 28.1

Case History for Dysmenorrhea (Menstrual Cramps)

S. Caroline complains of cramps and pain 2 weeks before and during her periods. Her blood has clots. She appears quite anxious and stressed out.
O. **P** Wiry and choppy. **T** Purplish.
A. Blood and Qi stagnation. Congestive and spasmodic dysmenorrhea.
P. *Specific therapeutic principles.* (1) Uterine decongestants. (2) Spasmolytics. (3) Venous and arterial stimulants to move blood. (4) Liver decongestants. (5) Nervines for pain and stress.

Herbal Formula and dose.

Phase dosing 5 mL 3 × day after ovulation and during menses

Parts	Herbs	Rationale
3	Paeonia Bai Shao Yao White Peony root	Uterine decongestant, all kinds of cramps.
2	Motherwort herb	Spasmolytic and relaxant for anxiety.
2	Stone root	Venous and uterine decongestant.
2	Passionflower herb	Calming nervine.
2	Dandelion root	Decongest the liver, bitter.
1	Ginger root	Move blood. Arterial stimulant, spasmolytic, protects stomach.

Suggestions

- *Diet.* Antiinflammatory.
- *Supplements.* EPA/DHA, and magnesium to ease strong muscle contractions.
- *Essential oils.* Lavender for relaxation; Clary Sage and Rose for hormone balance.
- *Warm castor oil pack for pain.* The oil from Castor beans (*Ricinus communis*) is a remedy that goes as far back as ancient Egypt, and its use was revived in modern times by medical clairvoyant Edgar Cayce. Soak a cotton or flannel cloth in castor oil and place over crampy area. Castor oil is very thick and sticky. Cover it with a piece of plastic and then a towel. Put heating pad on top of the whole thing. Can reuse the oil-soaked pack for the next few days, by storing it in refrigerator overnight in a plastic bag. The oil increases circulation, is antiinflammatory, moves qi and blood, and relieves pain.

• BOX 28.3 Handy Moon Cycle Facts

- ***Length of periods.*** Three to eight days is normal.
- ***Length of menstrual cycle.*** Refers to time from the start of one period until the day before the next flow; average length is 28 days, but 21 to 35 days is still normal.
- ***Counting cycle length.*** Day 1 begins on the *first* day of bleeding to the next bleed.
- ***Amenorrhea.*** Abnormal absence of menstruation between 3 and 6 months and not from natural causes such as pregnancy, breastfeeding, coming off birth control pills, or menopause.
- ***Ovulation.*** Occurs at midcycle but varies. Average is day 14 of a 28-day cycle.
- ***Fertile time.*** Five days around ovulation. Two days before, 1 day during, and 2 days after the egg leaves its sac.
- ***Dispensary.*** Herbs that work on most female menstrual problems usually take three to four cycles for a normal rhythm to be established. Eventually the body self-corrects, and herbs are no longer needed.[18]

CASE HISTORY 28.2

Case History for Dysfunctional Uterine Bleeding (DUB)

S. Jane is 33 years old and complains of erratic and sometimes excessive menstrual bleeding. She is soaking a tampon every hour in the first three days of her period. There are no clots. She has been to a health care provider and was told it was not serious, but she could go on HRT if she wants. She doesn't. She has been under excessive stress.

O. **P** Weak. **T** Pale with white coating.

A. Kidney and Spleen Qi Deficiency. Metrorrhagia.

P. *Specific therapeutic principles.* (1) Increase progesterone. (2) Nervines for stress. (3) Tone uterus. (4) Iron-rich herbs. (5) Adaptogen for HPA/adrenal support. (6) Spleen tonic to hold blood up. (5) Separate formula for heavy bleeding, as needed.

Formula #1 for DUB and Dose. 5 ml 3 × day between menses.

Part	Herbs	Rationale
3	Chastetree berry	HP axis and increases progesterone and ovulation.
3	St. John's Wort or Motherwort	Nervine and possible hormone regulation.
2	Bethroot	Tones uterus, saponin effect helps regulate blood flow.
2	Eleutherococcus Ci Wu Jia	Adrenal support, adaptogen.
2	Codonopsis Dang Shen	Spleen restorative.
2	Nettle herb	Iron and minerals for anemia.

Formula #2 for Heavy Bleeding and Dose.

Phase and pulse dosing. Begin just before menses and during period.
2–5 ml every 15 minutes up to 2 hours till bleeding stops.[18]

Part	Herb	Rationale
2	Yarrow herb	Hemostatic.
2	Shepherd's Purse herb	Hemostatic.
2	Lady's Mantle herb	Hemostatic.
1	Cinnamon bark	Stops bleeding, Warms up uterus.

Suggestions

- *Diet.* Anti-inflammatory. Green leafy veggies and iron-rich foods.
- *Supplements.* EPA/DHA.
- Stress management.
- Note: For pale pink, scanty flow, it's the *opposite* problem from above. *More* estrogen is needed. Remove Vitex and add estrogenic herbs like Red Clover or Garden Sage leaf.

CASE HISTORY 28.3

Case History for Premenstrual Syndrome

S. Sarah is 43 years old and runs a daycare center. On about day 13 of her generally 21-day cycle, she feels angry, irritable, and impatient with everyone. She reports sharp menstrual cramps, stress, anxiety, irritability, and sweating. She has bloating and has gained weight. On the first 3 days of her period, she changes tampons every hour. There are lots of dark clots.

O. **P** Wiry, thin, and choppy. **T** Red with purple edges.

A. Liver Qi and Blood Stagnation. Estrogen dominant/Premenstrual Syndrome-A with short cycles and clots.

P. *Specific therapeutic principles.* (1) Phase dose with two formulas: one for follicular and other beginning at ovulation and throughout luteal. Discontinue during menses. (2) Balance hypothalamic-pituitary axis with Chasteberry, larger proportion during ovulation and in luteal. (3) Hormonal balance, most in luteal. (4) Decongest the liver to ease stagnation and decrease bloating, more in luteal. (5) Tonify nervous system and give anxiolytics for anxiety throughout follicular and luteal. (6) Strengthen adrenals throughout both halves. (7) Decongest uterus for pain in luteal. (8) Dry damp from bloating, sweating; both halves. (9) Move qi and blood in follicular and luteal.

Formula #1 for Follicular Phase and Dose

Phase dosing. 5 mL or squeezes 3 × day until ovulation (day 14).

Parts	Herbs	Rationale
3	Chasteberry berry	Increase progesterone, balance pituitary, decrease bleeding.
3	Bupleurum Chai Hu	Relax uterus, decongest liver.
2	Schisandra Wu Wei Zi	Hypothalamic-pituitary-adrenal (HPA) axis and Hypothalamic-pituitary-gonadal (HPG) axis, adrenal and liver support.
2	Poria Fu Ling	Dry damp, help bloating, tonify Spleen.
1	Prickly Ash bark	Move qi and blood.
1	Passionflower herb	Decrease anxiety and stress

Formula #2 for Ovulation and Luteal Phase and Dose

Phase dosing, 5 mL or squeezes 3 × day
Begin at ovulation (usually between days 13 and 15) and through luteal phase until first bleeding.

Parts	Herbs	Rationale
4	Chastetree berry	Increase progesterone, balance pituitary, decrease bleeding.
2	Yarrow herb	Hormonal balance, dry damp.
2	Bupleurum Chai Hu	Decongest liver, relax uterus.
2	Schisandra Wu Wei Zi	HPA, gonadal, adrenal, and liver support to metabolize estrogen.
1	Poria Fu Ling	Dry damp, stop sweating, tonify Spleen.
1	Prickly Ash bark	Move qi and blood.
1	Pasqueflower herb	Decrease anxiety and stress, decongest uterus for pain.

Suggestions

- *Diet* Antiinflammatory; be conscientious at least 10 days before menses. Reduce any soy products, alcohol, and junk food Fat organic to decrease xenoestrogens in pesticides. Maca smoothie (Box 27.1).
- *Supplements.* Progesterone cream in luteal phase. Large doses EPA/DHA for antiinflammatory effect. B vitamins: B_6, methyl B_{12}, and B_9 in the form of MTHF folate, a stable and absorbable kind with the long chemical name, methylenetetrahydrofolate (MTHF) to help stress.
- *Go within.* Remind client that the luteal phase is a quiet time of the month, to be peaceful and introspective. Suggest yoga and meditation.
- *Alternative Chinese formula:* Free and Easy Wanderer, Xiao Yao Wan (Box 28.4).

• BOX 28.4 Free and Easy Wanderer for PMS (Xiao Yao Wan "Free Up the Spirit")

For the Childbearing Years

One of the most popular and effective multipurpose Chinese formulas for women. Classic for Liver Qi and Blood Stagnation that presents with estrogen dominance premenstrual syndrome (PMS), irregular periods, abdominal pain, and indigestion.[22] Xiao Yao Wan gets Liver qi flowing to help pain, strengthens the Spleen to help digestion, relieves abdominal pain, nourishes the blood, and calms stress, which makes it perfect for PMS.

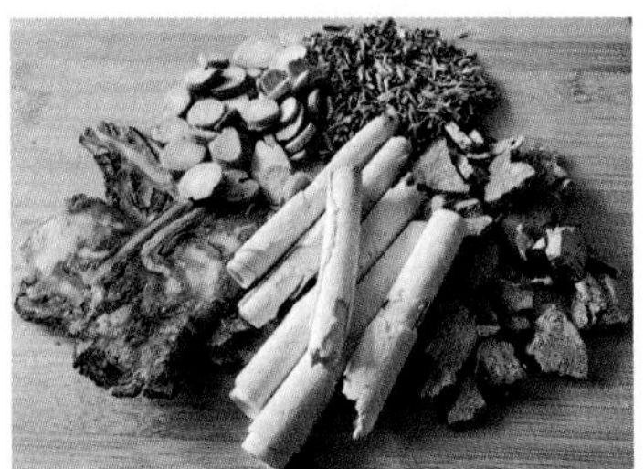

Herbs to free the spirit in patent formula *Free and Easy Wanderer*. Clockwise from top: Bupleurum Chai Hu, Atractylodes Bai Zhu, Poria Fu Ling, Angelica Dang Gui, Paeonia Bai Shao.

Parts	Herb	Rationale
9	Bupleurum Chai Hu (Asian Buplever root)	Moves stuck Liver qi. Improves liver function.
9	Angelica Dang Gui (Dong Quai root)	Tonifies Liver blood. Improves liver function.
9	Paeonia Bai Shao (White Peony root)	Nourishes Liver yin, strengthens blood.
9	Atractylodes Bai Zhu (White Atractylodes root)	Spleen/digestive restorative.
9	Poria Fu Ling (Hoelen fungus)	Strengthens Spleen, drains damp.
6	Glycyrrhiza Gan Cao (Licorice root)	Helps Spleen, harmonizes other herbs.
6	Zingiber Wei Jiang (Ginger root)	Regulates and warms Spleen.
2	Mentha Bo He (Asian Field mint herb)	Reduces Liver heat and wind.

Directions. Purchase this patent in any Chinese pharmacy (4 pills 3 × day); tincture up the formula (5 mL 3 × day); or grind herbs and place in 00 capsules (2 caps 2–3 × day.)

and progesterone imbalances. (3) Treat emotional disturbances for anxiety/depression. (4) Incorporate Liver stimulation to detox. (5) Choose adaptogens for stress. (6) Treat any other symptoms, such as stabilizing blood sugar with bitters for sweet cravings.

Cyclic Breast Changes and Fibrocystic Breasts

- *Definitions.*
  - *Cyclic changes*: Changes in breast size and tenderness, usually in the luteal phase.
  - *Fibrocystic breasts*: Benign fibrous cystic breast lumps are called ***fibrocystic breasts.*** They are fluid-filled sacs that change in size during menses, becoming larger under the influence of estrogen and smaller or disappearing at other times. (Case History 28.4). They are not cancerous, but solid tumors *can* indicate cancer. Fibrous cysts are common in the 40- to 50-year-old age group. The cysts grow when estrogen peaks because estrogen is *proliferative*; it makes tissue larger.

CASE HISTORY 28.4

Case History for Fibrocystic Breasts

S. Livia is 36 years old and complains of large breast lumps, especially just before her period. They are tender. She eats a lot of fast food and coffee and has a high-stress job. She complains of indigestion after fast-food consumption, but that does not stop her.
O. P Wiry and choppy. **T** Purplish body with thin white coat.
A. Liver Qi and Blood Stagnation. Fibrocystic breasts.
P. *Specific therapeutic principles.* (1) Increase progesterone. (2) Use Liver stimulants (decongestants). (3) Use alteratives, especially lymphatic drainers. (4) Use relaxing nervines. (5) Move qi and blood. (6) Help digestion and restore Spleen.

Herbal Formula and Phase dosing.

6 mL 3 × daily from mid-cycle (ovulation) to menses.

Part	Herbs	Rationale
3	Chastetree berry	Increases progesterone, hypothalamic-pituitary-gonadal axis.
2	Poke root	Moves lymph, decongests liver, detoxification, moves qi.
2	Bupleurum Chai Hu	Moves blood, decongests the liver, moves qi.
2	Atractylodes Bai Zhu	Restore Spleen/digestion.
2	Jamaican Sarsaparilla root	Progesteronic, alterative, moves lymph, decongests liver.
2	Lemon balm herb	Decreases stress.

Suggestions

Red Flag. Eighty percent of breast lumps are benign. If not sure, refer out to healthcare provider. Women often seek herbal help *after* they have ruled out cancer.

- *Diet.* Antiinflammatory, more omega-3 fatty acids, fewer omega-6. Cruciferous veggies. Decrease all caffeinated foods. Sometimes decreasing foods high in tyramine helps such as aged cheeses, wine, mushrooms, and processed meats.
- *Prevention.* Diindolylmethanes, referred to as DIMs, from cruciferous veggies, lignins from flaxseeds, soy isoflavones from soy products. Phytoestrogens modify effects of *bad* estrogen.[18] Decrease xenoestrogen exposure. Sort through collection of hygiene products, soaps, plastic containers, and use only pure products.
- *Decrease stress.*

- *Diagnosis*. If a dominant lump does not resolve after menses when estrogen is low, it should be checked out with an ultrasound, mammogram, or biopsy to rule out cancer or a benign fatty tumor called a *lipoma*. Self-breast exam techniques should be taught to clients.
- *Signs and symptoms*. Cyclic changes include pain, ropy and lumpy breasts, warmth, and enlargement, usually in the upper outer quadrant of both breasts.
- *Causes*. Estrogen excess with progesterone deficiency, lots of caffeine and fat in diet, HRT, and subclinical hypothyroidism. Elevated prolactin may increase estrogen and cell growth in breasts.
- *Allopathic treatment*. Drugs, surgery.
- *General therapeutic principles*. (1) Decrease estrogen with HPG and other progesteronic herbs. (2) Choose liver stimulants and

cholagogues to clear estrogen. (3) Move lymph. (4) Use alteratives. (5) Address any hypothyroidism. (6) Restore Spleen with Atractylodes Bai Zhu (White Atractylodes root). (7) Nourish the blood with Angelica Dang Gui (Dong Quai root).

Uterine Fibroids

- *Definition. **Uterine fibroids*** are the most common noncancerous, smooth-muscle uterine tumors affecting women past age 35 years (Case History 28.5). Varies in size and location from pea to watermelon size, and abdomen can get very large and resemble a pregnancy. Fibroids, like fibrocystic breasts, are estrogen driven and go away after menopause. Not serious, and no need to treat unless symptomatic. Other names for fibroids are *myomas* and *leiomyomas*.

CASE HISTORY 28.5

Case History for Uterine Fibroids

S. Ellen is 39 years old and woke up one morning with pain and blood in her bed, and she was not having her period. She felt a walnut-sized lump in her uterine area and had fixed, stabbing uterine pain. She jumped out of bed, very upset.

O. **P** Choppy. **T** Purplish on the sides, perhaps with distended sublingual veins.

A. Blood stagnation. Uterine fibroid.

P. *Specific therapeutic principles.* (1) Decrease estrogen excess. (2) Check bleeding with hemostatics. (3) Shrink fibroid with dissolvents. (4) Decongest liver. (5) Pelvic decongestant for pain. (6) Move lymph. Expect fibroid shrinkage within 3 to 6 months.

Herbal Formula and Dose.
5 mL 3 × day between meals in a little water

Parts	Herbs	Rationale
4	Chastetree berry	Reduces estrogen by increasing luteal phase.
3	Creosote leaf or Poke root	Shrink/dissolve fibroids; liver stimulant.
3	Cotton root bark	Hemostatic for bleeding.
2	Nettle herb	Iron-rich uterine tonic.
2	Cleavers herb	Pelvic decongestant moves lymph.
2	Schisandra Wu Wei Zi (Five Taste berry)	Metabolize estrogen through liver.

Suggestions

Red Flag. Rule out cancer. Soaking two maxi-pads in 30 minutes is a medical emergency.

- *Diet.* Reduce exposure to xenoestrogens. Eat organic food with lots of fiber. Increase lignins and soy foods to prevent binding of 16-hydroxyestrone (16-OHE), the *bad* estrogen metabolite.[9] Diindolylmethanes, referred to as DIMs, such as cruciferous veggies, Green tea.
- *Castor oil packs for pain*, (as explained under suggestions in Case History 28.1).
- *Yucca-Chaparral syrup.* From late herbalist Michael Moore, helps shrink fibroids. Fill crock pot one herb at a time with water. Cook each one on low for 2 to 3 days to make a thick syrup. For Yucca root syrup, add 25% glycerin to preserve. Chaparral (Creosote leaf) syrup is a strong antioxidant that preserves itself. Blend 60% Chaparral with 40% Yucca.[23] Take as a tincture 5 mL 3 × day for a few months. Keep extra syrup in the refrigerator.

CASE HISTORY 28.6

Case History for Perimenopause

S. Leila is "going nutty." She is 53 years old, complains of night sweats that wake her up at night and hot flashes during the day. She can't lose weight, periods are sporadic, and when they come, she has flooding. She is exhausted and worried.

O. **P** Thready, wiry, and rapid. **T** Red with scant coat.

A. Kidney Yin Deficiency with empty heat. Perimenopause.

P. *Specific therapeutic principles.* (1) Cool, moisturizing Kidney yin tonics. (2) Balance hormones on hypothalamic-pituitary-gonadal level. (3) Cooling herbs for hot flashes. (4) Liver restoratives. (5) NS restoratives. (6) Daytime formula and separate sleep and hot flash formula.

Formula #1 Daytime Formula and Dose. 5 mL 3 × day

Parts	Herbs	Rationale
3	Chastetree berry	Hormonal balance on HPG level.
3	Anemarrhena Zhi Mu	Yin tonic, clears heat, balance NS, adrenals, moisturizing.
2	Prepared Rehmannia Shu Di Huang	Yin tonic increases moisture and blood.
2	Hawthorn berry	Heart protective, helps with hot flashes.
1	Milk Thistle seed	Liver restorative, stimulant.
1	Chickweed herb	Cools hot flashes.

Formula #2 Sleep and Hot Flash Formula and Dose

4 squeezes at bedtime, and 4 squeezes every 15 min for 2 hours as needed. Keep bottle by bedside.

Parts	Herb	Rationale
1	Hops flower	Estrogenic and relaxing for sleep.
1	Skullcap herb	Estrogenic and relaxing for sleep.
1	Garden Sage herb	Dry secretions, estrogenic, cooling.
1	Schisandra Wu Wei Zi	Dry secretions, restore nervous system.
1	Lemon balm herb	Cooling, relaxing.

Suggestions

- *Diet.* Antiinflammatory. Increase high fiber foods, reduce sugar, caffeine if symptoms are bad.
- *Supplements.* EPA/DHA, vitamins E, D_3 and B complex (especially vitamins B_6, methyl B_{12}, and B_9 in the form of MTHF folate).
- *Hot flash control.* Avoid tobacco, spicy foods, sugar, hot drinks, hot tubs, hot baths, hot anything, stress. Lavender essential oil tepid bath before bed.
- *Consume less alcohol.* It decreases osteoporosis risk, and hot flashes.
- *Phytoestrogens* such as soy foods for hot flashes may help.
- *Stop smoking.* To decrease risk of heart disease, smoking-related cancers, and osteoporosis.
- *Exercise.* Aerobics for cardiovascular health and weight-bearing for bone density. Yoga for stress.
- *Regular sexual activity.* Use it or lose it. Helps with vaginal dryness and depression. No worries about getting pregnant.
- *Chinese patent formula.* Rehmannia Six, Liu Wei Di Huang Wan (Box 28.5).
- Remind client her Wise-Woman years are approaching.

• BOX 28.5 Rehmannia Six for Menopause (Liu Wei Di Huang Wan)

For Kidney Yin Deficiency in menopause, with intolerable hot flashes

This classic Chinese formula tonifies Kidney and Liver yin, balances hormones, increases bone density, all recommended measures for menopausal symptoms. It can be made up as a tincture or purchased as a patent medicine in teapill form. *Teapills* are small black spherical pills made by cooking ingredients into an herbal tea and then condensing them down into a solid.

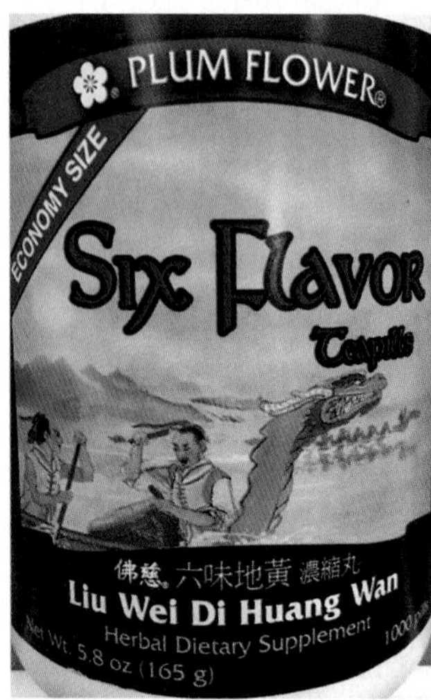

Six Flavor Teapills, Chinese patent for night sweats, afternoon heat, or irregular menses. The chief herb of the big six is prepared Rehmannia Shu Di Huang.

24 g	Prepared Rehmannia Shu Di Huang	Chief herb. Yin, jing, and blood tonic.
12 g	Cornus Shan Zhu Yu (Cornelian Cherry fruit)	Nourishes Liver and Kidney.
12 g	Dioscorea Shan Yao (Chinese Yam root)	Tonifies the Spleen and Kidney.
9 g	Alisma Zi Xie (Water Plantain rhizome)	Sedates the Kidney and dries damp.
9 g	Moutan Mu Dan Pi (Peony root)	Sedates deficiency fire of the Liver.
9 g	Poria Fu Ling (Hoelen fungus)	Strengthens Spleen, dries damp.

Dose. 8–12 teapills 3 times daily. Tincture 5 mL 3 × day.

CASE HISTORY 28.7

Case History for Benign Prostatic Hypertrophy

S. Eric is 40 years old and not able to urinate strongly. He feels an urgent need to urinate, but the stream is hard to start. There is pressure, no pain. He is angry. Prostate-specific antigen tests are slightly elevated.

O. P Wiry. **T** Normal with possible teeth marks.

A. Liver Qi Stagnation. Enlarged prostate.

P. *Specific therapeutic principles.* (1) Shrink prostate. (2) Treat potential urinary tract infection. (3) Soothe urethra with demulcents. (4) Kidney yang restoratives. (5) Bladder tonic.

Herbal Formula and Dose.

5 mL 3 × day between meals in a little water

Parts	Herbs	Rationale
2	Saw Palmetto berry	Shrink prostate, inhibit dihydrotestosterone (DHT).
2	Three-leaved Caper root or Nettle root	Shrink prostate, bladder tonic.
2	Ganoderma Ling Zhi Reishi mushroom	Inhibits DHT.
2	Oregon Grape root	Decrease inflammation and possible UTI.
2	Corn silk	Urinary demulcent.
2	Kava root	Decrease muscle spasms.

Suggestions

Red Flag. Blood in urine, erectile dysfunction, lower back or pelvic pain, and a decrease in ejaculate during sex are warning signs of prostate cancer.

- *Diet.* Antiinflammatory. Pumpkin seeds, cruciferous veggies, the antioxidant lycopene in cooked tomatoes (unsweetened sauce) all inhibit dihydrotestosterone (DHT), the prostate-damaging form of testosterone. Green tea.
- *Supplements.* EPA/DHA, zinc 20 mg. Over the counter Saw Palmetto oil extract standardized to a dose of 320 mg; amino acid L-lysine is a natural DHT inhibitor.

- *Signs and symptoms.* Asymptomatic or heavy bleeding, sometimes low back or dragging pelvic pain. If large, could cause miscarriage or infertility. Could cause urinary frequency and feeling of heaviness or congestion in lower abdomen. Anemia, if heavy blood loss.
- *Allopathic treatment.* Rule out cancer; ultrasound to diagnose. Wait and see; laser or surgical removal.
- *General therapeutic principles.* Try to wait it out. (1) Downgrade estrogen excess. Vitex in large doses has been proven to help.[18] (2) Shrink fibroids with dissolvents. (3) Control bleeding. (4) Use pelvic decongestants. (5) Choose liver stimulants. (6) Move lymph to detoxify. (7) Use uterine tonics. (8) Use iron-rich herbs if anemic.

Menopausal Symptoms

- *Definition.* Medically, ***menopause*** is the cessation of menstruation that has lasted for 12 consecutive months. Ovaries gradually decrease in size and function after age 30 years. The process is a natural event, a metamorphosis (Case History 28.6).
  - *Perimenopause*: Takes about 2 to 8 years before menses stops for good. Irregular cycles with decreased ovulation, elevated FSH and LH as the HPG axis compensates for estrogen and progesterone decline.
  - *Menopause:* Periods have ceased for 1 year.
  - *Post menopause:* The time after menses has stopped. Median worldwide age for menopause is 51 years but ranges from 40 to 58 years.
- *Signs and symptoms*. Most common for herbalists to see.
  - *Perimenopause:* Hot flashes, insomnia, memory problems, fatigue, anxiety, vaginal dryness, heavy bleeding or spotting, and stress incontinence. Flooding and irregular cycles caused by nonovulatory periods. There is no LH surge, so no progesterone is produced in the corpus luteum, and the endometrium lining keeps growing. When menses comes, the lining sheds a lot of blood.

CASE HISTORY 28.8

Case History for Infertility in Women

S. Joline is 30 years old and has been trying to conceive for 2 years. She is exhausted, her complexion is pale, skips a lot of periods, and was told by her healthcare provider that she didn't always ovulate. She is a full-time caregiver for her live-in father, who has Alzheimer's. This caretaking creates plenty of stress for her and her husband, whose sperm and sperm count are normal.

O. **P** Thready and weak. **T** Pale with moist coat.

A. Kidney Yang, Qi and Blood Deficiency. Infertility, probably caused by anovulation.

P. *Specific therapeutic principles.* (1) Increase chances of ovulation by strengthening LH surge. (2) Tone uterus. (3) Nervines for stress. (4) Liver detoxifiers. (5) Build blood. (6) Yang tonic.

Herbal Formula and Dose.

6 mL 3 × day between meals

Parts	Herbs	Rationale
2	Chastetree berry	Helps ovulation.
2	Prepared Rehmannia Shu Di Huang	Builds blood.
2	Saw Palmetto berry	Yang tonic, increases qi and blood.
2	Milk Thistle seed	Liver restorative and detox.
2	Asparagus root	Increases uterine tone.
2	Motherwort herb	Relieves stress.
2	Paeonia Bai Shao Yao White Peony root	Decongests pelvis.

Suggestions

- *Diet.* Antiinflammatory, high nutrition essential. High-zinc foods such as mushrooms, egg yolk, Brewer's yeast, sunflower and pumpkin seeds. Leafy greens for folic acid and blackstrap molasses for iron, citrus, Rosehips tea for vitamin C, cold water fish for omega-3 fatty acids.
- *Supplements.* High-dose vitamin B-complex. EPA/DHA, trace minerals, bioflavonoids.
- *Mind-body approach.* Stress reduction modalities. Take time out for self. Take time alone with her husband and find a substitute caregiver or look into adult day care.

    - *Post menopause.* The time after a woman has not bled for a year, through the rest of her life. Concerns about heart health and osteoporosis. The Wise-Woman years.
- *Chinese medicine perspective.* Kidney Yin Deficiency. Hot, tense, and dry condition.
- *Allopathic treatment.* HRT, but if not bioidentical, there is risk of breast and uterine cancer.
- *General therapeutic principles.* (1) Nourish organs with Kidney yin tonics. (2) Balance hormones. (3) If flooding: increase progesterone and hemostatics. (4) If hot flashes or empty heat occur, use cooling and anhidrotic herbs. (5) Use Liver restoratives. (6) If there is emotional depression: use NS restoratives. For rage: NS tonics and B vitamins. (7) For insomnia: adrenal/NS tonics; fix night sweats, use central nervous system relaxants. (8) For fatigue, use adrenal restorative. (9) Use Spleen tonics.

CASE HISTORY 28.9

Case History for Infertility in Men

S. Jack is 40 years old and complains of decreased energy and sex drive and weaker erections. His wife, who is 10 years younger, would like another child before *her* biological clock runs out. They have been trying for a year. He is discouraged, anxious, and overweight with large abdominal girth and bloating; he is trying to cut out fast food and caffeine. Urine flow is weak. Reported blood pressure 165/90.

O. **P** Deep and weak. **T** Pale. Bloating and apple shape observed. Blood pressure taken by herbalist 170/94.

A. Kidney Yang Deficiency. Low libido, probable low sperm count and benign prostatic hypertrophy, insulin resistance.

P. *Specific therapeutic principles.* Two formulas. One for fertility and other for insulin resistance. (1) Promote fertility and libido with Kidney yang tonics. (2) Improve microcirculation. (3) Shrink probable enlarged prostate. (4) Nervines for anxiety and to bring down BP. (5) Antihypertensives. (6) Bitters formula before meals for insulin resistance.

Formula #1 for Infertility and Dose 5 squeezes 3 × day between meals.

Parts	Herbs	Rationale
3	Ashwagandha root	Kidney yang tonic specific.
3	Saw Palmetto berry	Kidney yang tonic, shrink prostate.
2	Epimedium Yin Yang Huo	Yang tonic.
2	Ginkgo leaf	Increase microcirculation.
2	Ligusticum Chuan Xiong	Hypotensive, antilipemic, nervous sedative.

Formula #2 for Insulin Resistance and Dose 3 × day.

Parts	Herb	Rationale
3	Dandelion root	Bitters for insulin resistance.
2	Bitter melon	Bitters for insulin resistance.
1	Yellow Dock root	Bitters for insulin resistance, elimination.
1	Ginger root	Warmth and digestive aid.
1	Poria Fu Ling	Dry damp, bloating.

Suggestions

- *Diet.* Antiinflammatory, high nutrition. Bitter greens for glucose balance. Help couple implement dietary changes. Lower caffeine by switching from coffee to Green tea. Consider Four-R protocol.
- *Supplements.* Grape seed extract for microcirculation. EPA/DHA. Consider probiotics.
- Maca/Turmeric smoothie daily to increase libido and help gut. Mix herbs with veggies, a little fruit, or make Golden Milk (Box 27.1).

Benign Prostatic Hypertrophy (BPH)

- *Definition.* ***Benign prostatic hypertrophy (BPH)*** refers to a slow growing, non-cancerous enlargement of the prostate gland in men over 40 years old that slowly narrows the urethra (Case History 28.7). This can disrupt normal life. It becomes difficult to empty bladder completely, and residual leads to susceptibility to urinary tract infections (UTIs), bladder stones, and kidney damage. Danger is that it can lead to slow-growing prostate cancer.

- *Signs and symptoms.* Frequency and urgency to urinate, especially at night. Weak stream that is hard to start and dribbling, and there is difficulty emptying bladder completely.
- *Allopathic treatment.* Drugs: Proscar to shrink prostate, antibiotics for UTI. Prostate-specific antigen (PSA) blood test to check for cancer. This test is inconclusive. Surgery.
- *Herbs that inhibit dihydrotestosterone* (DHT*)*. An enzyme called *5-alpha reductase* metabolizes and converts testosterone into prostate-damaging DHT. Presence of the enzyme, combined with decreased testosterone levels in men, leads to prostate enlargement. Research with Saw Palmetto berry, Ganoderma Ling Zhi (Reishi mushroom), and Pumpkin seed showed they block the 5-alpha reductase pathway.[21]
- *General therapeutic principles.*[1] (1) Shrink prostate. (2) Help bladder function with Nettle root, or if obtainable, *Crataeva nurvala* (Three leaved Caper root and herb), an Ayurvedic classic tonic for BPH, UTI, and stones; a Kidney tonic. (3) Decrease inflammation or any UTI. (4) Decrease muscle spasms with spasmolytics.

Infertility in Women and Men

- *Definition.* Inability to have a child for whatever reason creates stress in and out of the bedroom. Herbal therapy can last up to a year. Large doses of love and understanding are necessary.
  - *Women. Infertility* in a woman is an inability to get pregnant (conceive) a child after a year or longer of unprotected sex, provided her partner is fertile. (Case History 28.8). Often caused by poor lifestyle choices: SAD, excessive drugs, alcohol, caffeine, stress, coming off BCPs, and environmental toxins. Common physical causes are anovulation, hormone imbalances, endometriosis, and polycystic ovary disease.
  - *Men. Infertility* in a man is an inability to create a pregnancy in a fertile woman after a year of unprotected sex. (Case History 28.9). Usually from androgen deficiency with decreased sperm count and lower volume of ejaculate. Frequently accompanied by or caused by other chronic health problems.
- *Signs and symptoms.*
  - *Women.* Irregular or long periods; painful and heavier or lighter periods, depending on hormone imbalances; acne; body hair growth; and pain during sex.
  - *Men.* Decrease in libido, energy, strength, and height; weaker erections.
- *Allopathic treatment.* Fertility tests. Hormone therapy. Artificial insemination, *in vitro* fertilization.
- *General therapeutic principles for women.* Treat underlying cause, if known, or attend to general treatment. (1) Use Vitex to insure ovulation. (2) Use nervines for stress. (3) Support liver detoxification to decrease environmental toxins. (4) Use nutritive herbs to build qi and blood. (5) Increase pelvic tone.[16]
- *General therapeutic principles for men.*[1] (1) Use testosterone and fertility promotors with yang tonics. (2) Use adaptogens. (3) Use prostate herbs if BPH in history (it usually is). (4) Increase micro circulation. (5) Treat other underlying health problems. (6) Improve pelvic circulation/decongest. (7) Recommend frequent sex to help libido and fertility in men and women. Use it or lose it.

Summary

Human reproduction is a major topic and we just scratched the surface. An herbalist's clinical practice could be in this area alone. Metaphysically, the second chakra deals with sex and relationships. The menstrual cycle was approached as moon centered, moon driven, and circular. Physically, the female hormones estrogen, representing the outwardly oriented first, follicular half of the menstrual cycle, and progesterone, epitomizing the second half or luteal phase of the cycle, were explained and contrasted. This information, along with the role of FSH and LH, are basics for herbalists to internalize. The role of testosterone in men's reproductive health is a lot easier to grasp.

Pertinent Chinese Medicine reproductive syndromes are usually related to Kidneys and Liver. Classic patent formulas that herbalists might easily use in clinic included (1) Four Things Soup or Decoction, Si Wu Tang, a female tonic to tonify blood and regulate menses. (2) Free and Easy Wanderer, Xiao Yao Wan, a multipurpose formula for PMS. (3) Rehmannia Six, Lu Wei Di Huang Wan, a timeless menopausal remedy. Any of these may be embellished or modified, depending on the situation.

The reproductive Materia Medica included many herbs encountered in other chapters, plus a few more. Black Cohosh root has enjoyed a long reputation for being the go-to phytoestrogenic plant but according to new research may not hook on to receptor sites. Consequently, it has been omitted from most of our case history formulations, usually substituted with herbs like Red Clover flower, Licorice root, or Wild Yam root.

Phase dosing is a women's reproductive strategy to dispense herbs. The conditions chosen for case histories were those most commonly encountered but are by no means a complete collection. Please refer to the bibliography for further related references.

Review

Fill in the Blanks

(Answers in Appendix B.)

1. Menstrual cycle hormones for first half are ___ that trigger ___.
2. Menstrual cycle hormones for the second half are ___ that trigger ___.
3. The major androgen is _____.
4. Name five measures to maintain a healthy reproductive system: ___, ___, ___, ___, ___.
5. Name six places estrogen receptor sites are found: ___, ___, ___, ___, ___, ___.
6. Four foods with isoflavones are ___, ___, ___, ___. Four foods with lignins are ___, ___, ___, ___.
7. Which two problems does Kidney Yang Deficiency lead to in men? ___, ___. P ___ T ___.
8. Which two main problems does Kidney Yin Deficiency lead to in women? ___, ___. P ___, T ___.

9. Herbs for infertility are usually ___ tonics. Herbs for menopause are usually ___ tonics.
10. Answer as to estrogen or progesterone excess or deficiency. Pale, scanty menstrual flow is usually caused by ___. A long cycle and skipped periods are usually caused by ___.

Critical Concept Questions

(Answers for you to decide.)

1. What is the difference between the hypothalamic-pituitary-adrenal (HPA) axis as discussed in Chapter 27, and the hypothalamic-pituitary-gonadal (HPG) axis as discussed throughout this chapter?
2. What is the mind-body relationship between the second chakra, the moon, emotions, and menses?
3. Discuss the Chinese Medicine Kidney's role in the life cycle.
4. What is the role of DIMs in reproductive health?
5. Client asks about HRT. Explain bioidentical hormones. Would you recommend them? Why?
6. Give examples of soy isoflavones and lignins. What are they used for?
7. Why is Liver Qi and Blood Stagnation so important in women's health problems? It leads to what? Pulse and tongue? Herb categories and examples used to fix it?
8. What are xenoestrogens and why are they so problematic?
9. Could you explain the menstrual cycle to a client? Try doing it out loud.
10. Your client has purchased Black Cohosh in hopes of helping her hot flashes. Your response?

References

1. Bone, Kerry and Simon Mills. *Principles and Practice of Phytotherapy* (London, UK: Elsevier, 2013).
2. Myss, Caroline. *Anatomy of the Spirit* (New York, NY: Three Rivers, 1996).
3. Kresser, Chris. "The Gut Hormone Connection: How Gut Microbes Influence Estrogen Levels." Kresser Institute. https://kresserinstitute.com/gut-hormone-connection-gut-microbes-influence-estrogen-levels/ (accessed September 5, 2019).
4. Meyers, Amy. "Nine Causes of Estrogen Dominance and What To Do About It." https://www.amymyersmd.com/2019/03/9-causes-estrogen-dominance/ (accessed September 2, 2019).
5. Gersh, Felice. Notes from Xymogen Seminar, Denver, CO, 2018.
6. Northrup, Christiane. *Women's Body, Women's Wisdom* (New York, NY: Bantam, 2002).
7. Charnow, Jody W. "Low Estrogen Explains Some Hypogonadal Symptoms in Men". Renal and Urology News. https://www.renalandurologynews.com/home/departments/mens-health-update/hypogonadism/low-estrogen-explains-some-hypogonadal-symptoms-in-men/ (accessed October 10, 2019).
8. Zorn, Kaitlyn. "Estrogen Dominance & Excess Estrogen in Naturopathic Practice." Naturopathic Doctor News & Review (ndnr) https://ndnr.com/womens-health/estrogen-dominance-excess-dietary-and-tcm-approaches-to-hormone-balance/ (accessed March 14, 2021).
9. Hall, Sidney et al. "Lignins as a Novel Targeted Therapy for Breast Cancer." Emerging Researchers National Conference. https://emerging-researchers.org/projects/19734/ (accessed September 2, 2019).
10. National Institutes of Health. U.S. Department of Health and Human Services. "WHI Follow up Study Confirms Health Risks of Long-Term Combination Hormone Therapy Outweigh Benefits for Post Menopausal Women". https://www.nih.gov/news-events/news-releases/whi-follow-study-confirms-health-risks-long-term-combination-hormone-therapy-outweigh-benefits-postmenopausal-women (accessed September 5, 2019).
11. Weil, Andrew. "Had Enough Wild Yams?" Andrew Weil, MD. https://www.drweil.com/health-wellness/health-centers/women/had-enough-wild-yams/ (accessed September 5, 2019).
12. Trickey, Ruth. *Women, Hormones & the Menstrual Cycle* (St. Leonard's, Australia: Allen and Unwin, 1998).
13. "Managing Women's Issues with Chinese Medicine." Staff of Pacific College of Oriental Medicine, 2021.
14. Holmes, Peter. *Energetics of Western Herbs* (Boulder CO: Snow Lotus, 2006).
15. Ganora, Lisa. *Herbal Constituents: Foundations of Phytochemistry* (Louisville, CO: Herbalchem, 2009).
16. Hoffman, David. *Medical Herbalism: The Science and Practice of Herbal Medicine* (Rochester, VT: Healing Arts, 2003).
17. Kass-Annese, Barbara and Hal C. Danzer. *The Fertility Awareness Handbook* (Redondo Beach, CA: Patterns, 1981).
18. Romm, Aviva. *Botanical Medicine for Women's Health* (UK: Elsevier, 2010).
19. Brinckmann, Josef, and Thomas Brendler. "Black Cohosh, Herb Profile." HerbalGram: Journal of the American Botanical Council. February-April 2019.
20. Holmes, Peter. *Jade Remedies: A Chinese Herbal Reference for the West* (Boulder, CO: Snow Lotus, 1996).
21. Hartfield, William. "Best Alpha 5 Reductase Inhibitors." Hairguard. https://www.hairguard.com/best-natural-5-alpha-reductase-inhibitors/ (accessed September 5, 2019).
22. Naeser, Margaret. *Outline Guide to Chinese Patent Medicines in Pill Form* (Ann Arbor, MI: Edward Brothers, 1990).
23. Remedy passed down to author from Shelley Torgove, teacher and clinician, obtained from herbalist Michael Moore. This really works to shrink fibroids. It's a project, so make up a large quantity and store extra in fridge.

29 Herbal Legalities

"Health is a state of complete physical, mental and social well-being and not merely the absence of disease or infirmity."

—***World Health Organization***

CHAPTER REVIEW

- Historical aspects of herbalism in the United States: Food and Drug Administration (FDA), the Dietary Supplement Health and Education Act (DSHEA), the standardization issue, standardized herbal extracts, Generally Regarded as Safe (GRAS), Wise-Woman tradition and the Women's Self-Help Movement, and National Center for Complementary and Integrative Health (NCCIH).
- State of herbalism around the world: Kampo and the Japanese Pharmacopeia (JP), World Health Organization (WHO), Pharmacopoeia of the People's Republic of China (PPRC), British Pharmacopeia (BP), Commission E, Therapeutic Goods Act (TGA) of Australia, Canadian Natural and Non-Prescription Health Products Directorate (NNHPD).
- Herbal timeline of legislation and important events.

KEY TERMS

Active component
British Pharmacopeia (BP)
Canadian Natural and Non-Prescription Health Products Directorate (NNHPD)
Commission E
Dietary Supplement and Health Education Act (DSHEA)
Drug
Extract, standardized
Extract, weight-to-volume
Generally Regarded as Safe (GRAS)
Japanese Pharmacopeia (JP)
Kampo
Marker compound
National Center for Complementary and Integrative Health (NCCIH)
National Institutes of Health (NIH)
Pharmacopeia of the People's Republic of China (PPRC)
Phytopharmaceutical
Standardization
Therapeutic Goods Act of Australia (TGA)
World Health Organization (WHO)

The legal practice of herbalism in the United States and around the world is in a state of flux. The United States comes up short with respect to legal recognition of plant medicine in comparison with the United Kingdom (UK), Germany, Australia, China, and others.

Herbal medicine and other complementary modalities are used extensively throughout Europe. Regulation and practice vary, but public demand is strong. Changes are in progress in the Netherlands and the UK. In Africa, a large percentage of the population uses some form of traditional herbal medicine, and the topic enjoys significant attention in global health debates.

Herbalists in the United States must keep their radar tuned to the doings of the Food and Drug Administration (FDA), because legal use of targeted herbs can go under fire and the herbs can be quickly banned. Private herbal organizations such as the American Botanical Council keep its members informed of pertinent impending legislation. It is important to stay knowledgeable, informed, and aware of the politics of the healing arts because it could affect herbal practices and businesses in a blink. To appreciate how we got to this point historically, refer to Chapter 2.

Historical Aspects of Herbalism in the United States

Federal Drug Administration (FDA) Established by Congress in 1928

The sad story of modern herbal regulations in the United States, and the herbal profession's association with the *Federal Drug Administration (FDA)* began with the passage of the Pure Food and

Drugs Act in 1906. The act was passed to ensure food and drug safety and eventually merged into the FDA by 1928. The FDA's responsibilities range from regulating new medicines and herbs to inspecting food processing centers. The organization is powerful, complete with lobbyists and millions of dollars thrown its way in the interests of large pharmaceutical companies, Big Pharma.

The FDA was originally lax about drug laws. Then in 1959, the Thalidomide scare occurred, and the situation changed. Thalidomide was an over-the-counter (OTC) drug used to treat morning sickness in pregnancy, and it caused horrible birth defects. Children were born without limbs, hands, or ears. In response, a Congressional OTC Review Panel was formed, and it directed the FDA to tighten their standards.[1] Drug companies thereafter had to demonstrate safety in elaborate studies at costs of hundreds of millions of dollars. Attempts to recoup their losses caused prescription drug prices to skyrocket. This situation persists today, and research costs are used as an excuse for the exorbitant prices so many pharmaceutical companies charge for lifesaving drugs.

OTC drug producers were required to conduct expensive research not only on drugs, but also on herbs and other products in their resale inventory, products that historically had been used safely for years. As a result of their complaints and pressure, the Congressional Over the Counter Panel wrote reports called *monographs*, which served as the basis for including past approvals of OTC drugs and herbs previously deemed safe and effective. The catch was that the Congressional Panel only reviewed what was submitted by the drug manufacturers. Many drugs were presented, but only a limited number of herbs made it to review, primarily laxatives like Senna bark, Psyllium seed, and Cascara Sagrada herb; a few decongestants such as Peppermint and Eucalyptus essential oil; and two ingredients derived from Chinese Ephedra Ma Huang.

These were only a tiny fraction of the more than 100 herbs that had historically and clinically been deemed safe and effective and that were listed in the United States Pharmacopeia (USP). For instance, Valerian-based sleep aids were available in pharmacies before World War II, but Valerian root was dropped in place of drug sedative antihistamines such as Benadryl. As of 2020, as far as herbalists are concerned, the outcome of this sorry tale is that any drug or herb not grandfathered into the USP after the Thalidomide scare must now undergo the same expensive, time-consuming testing the FDA requires of all new drugs. From the 1920s to the present, the inclusion of healing herbs was rapidly dropped from the USP.[2]

The Important Dietary Supplement Health and Education Act (DSHEA) 1994

The ***Dietary Supplement and Health Education Act (DSHEA)*** was passed by the United States Congress in 1994, and all herbalists need to know its specifications, definitions, and requirements. Herbs are considered *dietary supplements* or *foods*. They are *not* considered drugs. A ***drug*** is legally defined as a substance "intended for use in the diagnosis of, cure, mitigation, treatment, or prevention of disease."[3] The fact that herbs are not considered drugs has pros and cons. Herbs, unlike drugs, cannot have medical claims made about them, even though they have been used as effective medicine for centuries. On the other hand, herbs don't require the same extensive testing as a drug. For example, an herb label cannot claim that Goldenseal root will cure the flu (a medical claim), but it *can* state that it *supports the immune system*. Herbal product labels and internet statements must be extremely vague and unclear about an herb's therapeutic effects and uses. To be designated a *drug*, it must undergo rigorous and expensive testing and be FDA approved, which is about impossible to accomplish without large financial backing.

The DSHEA spells out regulations regarding manufacture and sale of dietary supplements and defines permissible labeling claims. A *dietary supplement* is a product intended to supplement the diet that bears or contains one of more of these dietary ingredients: a vitamin, a mineral, an herb or other botanical, or an amino acid.[4] (Tobacco is excluded from this classification.)

The DSHEA also outlines safety requirements for new dietary ingredients. Still in effect as of early 2020, it allows the FDA to consider petitions that would allow manufacturers of herbs and dietary supplements to make medicinal claims. To date, very few medical claims have been approved. One approved claim was that soy protein helps to lower cholesterol.

Generally, the FDA has declined many requests to reopen the OTC review process to accommodate healing herbs. Thus medicinal herbs are sold as dietary supplements, a designation several rungs down the ladder from a drug, significantly decreasing its status. For now, *herbalists must be very careful not to call an herb a drug.*

The Standardization Issue

Drugs are standardized. Most herbs are not. ***Standardization*** means that one or more components (deemed the *active ingredients*) are present in a specific, guaranteed amount, usually expressed as a percentage. It guarantees that the consumer gets a product in which the chemistry of the product is specific from batch to batch. In a strong, potentially toxic drug, it is critical to know how much is being delivered every time. Nevertheless, there are arguments for and against this specification (Table 29.1).

Plants follow nature's standard, not the drug model. There are many, many constituents in any given plant existing in varying amounts, depending on climate, location, soil, and other factors. Dandelion greens harvested in one location are not exact chemical replicas of those growing elsewhere. In drugs, so-called *active ingredients* are isolated and often artificially synthesized in a lab. An adult-sized tablet of Bayer aspirin *always* contains 325 mg of acetylsalicylic acid. That is a given standardized amount, the bioactive chemical.

Herbs are *synergistic* and many ingredients, perhaps some not yet chemically isolated, play an important role in an herb's action. What may be toxic in isolation is often much safer when combined with other chemicals in the plant, tempering the toxicity. There may be currently unidentified constituents contributing to a plant's healing magic. Once removed, the botanical becomes less effective.

As Big Pharma gets increasingly interested in entering the herbal market, they see the potential to make big bucks. But money cannot be made from natural Dandelion greens growing in the earth. An apple can't be patented. So, the way around this profitability problem is to isolate the *assumed* active ingredient, send it to a lab, and have it synthetically produced. The active ingredient is studied, clinical trials are done to establish safety, and FDA approval for the newly created drug follows. The plant has become a *phytopharmaceutical*, an herbal drug. It is now patentable and with patents come exclusive rights to manufacture, produce, and aggressively market the product, and to rake in the profits. This limits the broad range of traditionally known properties and uses of an herb, in favor of a single-use mentality based on the action of a particular active ingredient. Do herbalists want to give up their power in that way?

TABLE 29.1 Herb Standardization Pros and Cons

	Positives	Negatives
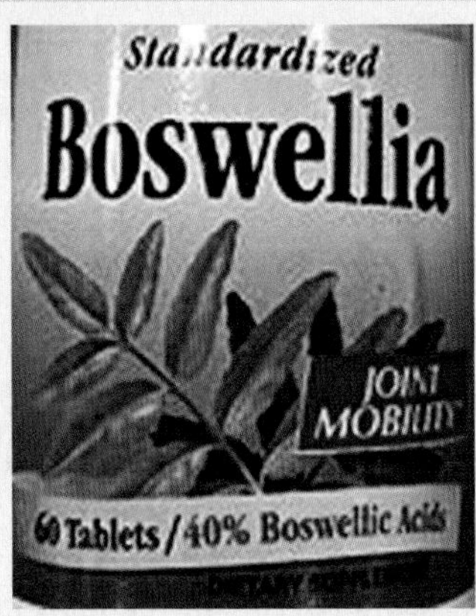 *Boswellia* spp. (Frankincense resin) is standardized in this product to contain 40% boswellic acids, the deemed active ingredients.	• The exact amount of active chemicals or constituents is known in measured amounts. • The stated plant is guaranteed to actually be in the product. • Nothing else is added. • The herbal products are reproducible, batch for batch.	• A plant has synergy. It is more than the sum of its parts. The combination of many constituents, active or not, helps it work in a safe manner. • A whole plant is milder acting than one extracted chemical. Overdose is rare. • The entire chemical makeup of a plant might be unknown. Its so-called active *ingredient* may not be the only therapeutic factor. • Herbs have been safely used for centuries with no institutional interference. • Herbs are considered a food, not a drug under the Dietary Supplement Health and Education Act. • If an herb is standardized, it is being treated like a drug.

Standardized Herbal Extracts

Earlier on (Chapter 7), the strength of an herbal tincture and extract was expressed in terms of its *weight-to-volume* (w/v) concentration. A w/v *tincture* was said to range from a 1:5 (meaning 1-to-5) to a 1:3 concentration of whole herb to menstruum. A ***weight-to-volume extract*** was considered to be a stronger liquid tincture, having a 1:2 to 1:1 concentration of whole herb to menstruum. The lower the second number, the stronger the tincture. The first number is always 1. These tinctures and extracts ensure that one part of whole herb was infused in a specified proportion of liquid menstruum. It gives no information about amounts of any specific chemical constituents contained in the whole herb.

Standardized extracts are different and are approaching the status of drugs. Instead of a w/v ratio, they are expressed as a *weight-to-weight* (w/w) ratio. The numbers are in the *opposite* order from w/v tinctures or extracts. For instance, a 4:1 (meaning 4 to 1) concentration of a standardized extract means that a powdered extract contains the extracted constituents from 4 g of starting material in 1 g of finished extract. Stated another way, 1 part of the extract is equivalent to or derived from 4 parts crude herb.[5] A 10:1 extract means 10 parts of raw plant was used to create 1 part of extract. The higher the first number, the stronger the extract. The second number is always 1 in the ratio.

Advanced analytical methods have taken herbal production one step further toward attaining drug status, a determination of active ingredient (in milligrams or percentage) present in the extract. The plant is manufactured into extremely strong liquid or solid form. Commercial fluid and solid extracts get their strength by distilling off some of the alcohol by processes known as vacuum distillation and countercurrent filtration. To convert a fluid extract into a solid or powder, the liquid solvent must be removed. This removal is done by either method just mentioned, or by thin layer evaporation, a type of drying out procedure.[5] What is left is then ground into a powder, a solid extract. Ordinarily, 4:1 is the typical concentration of a solid extract.

Proceeding down the road toward drug creation, standardized products can be analyzed in a laboratory to ensure that the extract is guaranteed to contain what is considered the ***active component*** at an accepted standardized level in milligrams or to contain a specific percentage of a ***marker compound***, the biochemical constituent characteristic of the plant.[2] A saving grace (distinguishing them from an official drug) is that the entire plant and all its constituents still remain in the extract with its synergistic factors intact. This is a bit better than an isolated ***phytopharmaceutical***, a botanical product reduced to one or several plant substances or active ingredients. The following bulleted list gives examples of herbal standardizations on the market and products based either on active components or characteristic marker compounds.

- *Cucurbita pepo* (Pumpkin seed) standardized to contain 52% linoleic acid, 18% oleic acid, and 12.5% palmitic acid (Fig. 29.1).
- *Vaccinium myrtillus* (Bilberry berry) standardized to contain 40 mg of anthocyanosides. Active component in milligrams.

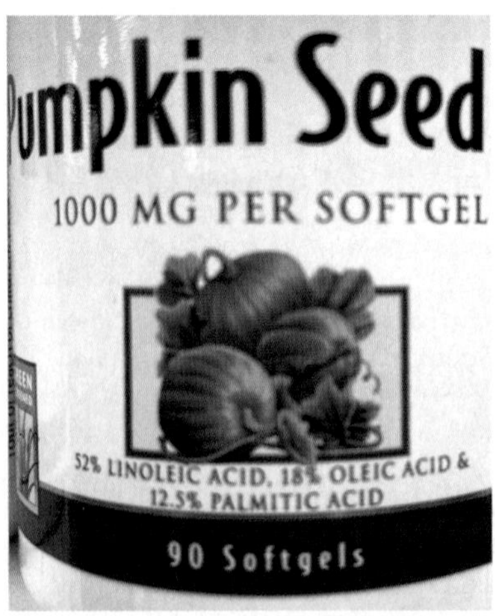

• **Fig. 29.1** *Curcurbita pepo* (Pumpkin seed) is standardized here to contain specific percentages of its marker compounds, the constituents characteristic of the plant.

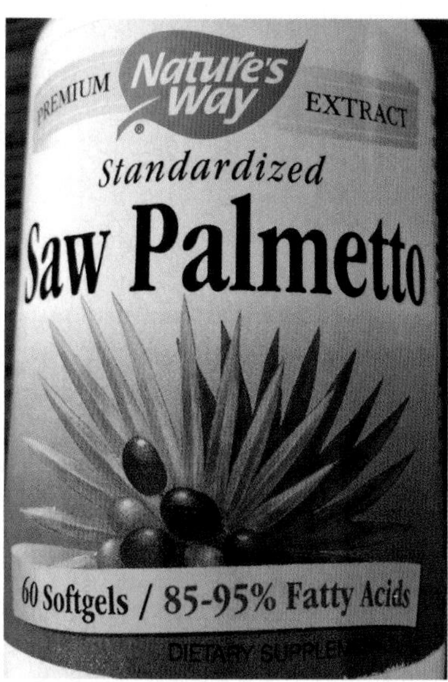

• **Fig. 29.2** *Serenoa repens* (Saw Palmetto berry) is known for its high fat content. This label shows the percentage of that marker compound, guaranteeing a high fatty acid percentage.

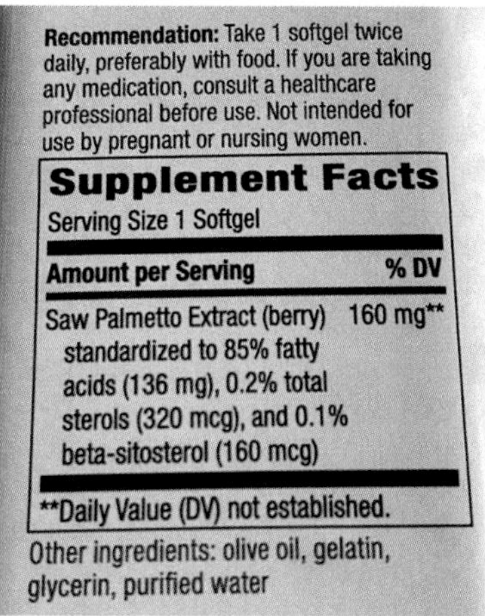
Recommendation: Take 1 softgel twice daily, preferably with food. If you are taking any medication, consult a healthcare professional before use. Not intended for use by pregnant or nursing women.

Supplement Facts

Serving Size 1 Softgel

Amount per Serving	% DV
Saw Palmetto Extract (berry) standardized to 85% fatty acids (136 mg), 0.2% total sterols (320 mcg), and 0.1% beta-sitosterol (160 mcg)	160 mg**

**Daily Value (DV) not established.

Other ingredients: olive oil, gelatin, glycerin, purified water

• **Fig. 29.3** Here is a later, more explicit version of the same company's Saw Palmetto berry label that was shown in Fig. 29.2. The back of the bottle breaks down the types of fatty constituents (sterols and beta-sitosterols) into percentages of the total, plus grams and micro-grams. A little closer on the continuum of drug-style labeling.

- *Silybum marianum* (Milk Thistle seed) standardized to contain 70 mg of silymarin. Active component in milligrams.
- *Curcuma longa* (Turmeric root) standardized to contain 95% curcumin. Marker compound characteristic of the plant expressed as a percentage.
- *Valerian officinalis* (Valerian root) standardized to contain 0.8% to 1% valerenic acid. Marker compound characteristic of the plant expressed as a percentage.
- *Serenoa repens* (Saw Palmetto berry) standardized to contain 85% to 95% fatty acids. Marker compound characteristic of the plant is expressed as a percentage (Fig. 29.2) on this label. Fig. 29.3 shows a more recent label of the same brand providing a breakdown of the total fatty acids in percentages *and* milligrams.

Arriving at a truly standardized extract requires expensive technology that only large companies have at their disposal, almost certainly pushing small businesses and stand-alone herbalists out of the picture. It is far beyond the scope of small apothecaries, folk methods, and kitchen tincture making. The traditional w/v method is no longer sufficient in the eyes of Big Pharma.

Food and Drug Administration (FDA) Introduced Generally Regarded as Safe (GRAS) Status 1958

Generally Regarded as Safe (GRAS) is the designation the FDA gave to food additives in 1958. However, the label has little consistency or clarity and is not as good as it sounds. For a substance to be considered GRAS, it has to meet certain criteria. Substances that were in general use as food additives prior to January 1, 1958, were grandfathered in for this designation, based on common knowledge gained through a history of safe use. No further safety testing was required.[6]

Substances put into use *after* January 1, 1958 are considered GRAS only if their safety is based on scientific procedures and research. GRAS status does not have to be affirmed by the FDA, and it *is* legal for GRAS additives to be based on the research of qualified experts in the food industry, without requiring independent investigation. A conflict of interests, perhaps?

Furthermore, GRAS status is designated for substances considered safe for ingestion as additives in foods taken *orally*. No testing is required for other paths of body entry. Toxicity can vary greatly, depending on route of administration. The fragrance industry and the essential oil industry, which sell products that enter the body through the nose and the skin, both use GRAS status.

Many herbal products fall into a gray area of regulation. About half the herbs sold by the herb industry are not on the GRAS list but are widely imported and sold for food use. Their omission does not imply that they are unsafe. For example, Barley and Arrowroot are not on the GRAS list of food additives, yet these foods have been safely ingested for hundreds of years. Examples of herbs that are included on the GRAS list range alphabetically from Alfalfa herb and Red Algae to Yucca root and Zedoary bark. Listed essential oils range from Alfalfa, Allspice, Almond, and Cherry bark to Ylang Ylang,[7] implying safety in commonly used quantities. The GRAS status list may be found on the FDA website,[8] but the designation does not appear on most product labels.

Wise-Woman Tradition Continues: The Self-Help Movement 1960s to Present

Women's status in healing and herbalism has come full circle or, more accurately, full spiral. The Women's Self-Help Movement that began in the 1960s and 1970s is thriving and stresses the importance of taking charge of one's health without total trust and dependence on the medical establishment. The heart-centered Wise-Woman Tradition is being reinvented with a different name. Of course, this passage of herbal lore and wisdom handed down through generations has always existed. Many Wise-Men have joined, adding and blending their important yang to the yin. Empowering folks to take responsibility for their own healing is the way of the herbalist. We are reclaiming our power.

The Wise-Woman Tradition cites the 12th century mystic, prophet, and herbalist Hildegard von Bingen to be the first acknowledged woman who actually wrote anything down, moving us from an oral to a written tradition. Many courageously followed her example, and countless well-respected herbalists enjoyed a revival in the 1960s and 1970s.

Individuals of the modern herbalist movement are numerous. One such Wise-Woman elder was Juliette de Bairacli Levy, who passed in 2009. She was a breeder of Afghan hounds, a friend of the Romani people, and a pioneer of holistic veterinary medicine. *Juliette of the Herbs* is a classic film about her life.[9] Another beloved grandmother was Hannah Kroeger, at one time owner of the only herb shop in Boulder, Colorado. She dispensed her healing wisdom along with packets of herbs in the 1950s. Hannah's wheat germ and carrot juice were revolutionary items at the time. She was a Boulder institution.

Present-day herbal grandmothers and grandfathers range from folk herbalists to scientists to modern healthcare providers. Many have written books leaving their legacy. A few well-known grandmothers are Rosemary Gladstar, Mindy Green, Feather Jones, Susun Weed, Brigitte Mars, Lisa Ganora, Rosalee de la Forêt, Kiva Rose, and Aviva Romm. The male principle has contributed stars such as Jim Duke, Christopher Hobbs, Michael Tierra, Michael Moore, Matthew Wood, Stephen Buhner, Simon Mills, Kerry Bone, Peter Holmes, and Dr. John R. Christopher. (For those omitted, my deep apologies.)

National Center for Complementary and Integrative Health (NCCIH) 1998

The ***National Center for Complementary and Integrative Health (NCCIH)*** was founded in 1998 under ***National Institutes of Health (NIH)*** in the United States. Its purpose is to conduct scientific research on complementary and integrative health approaches, so it can provide well-informed recommendations to the public. It is interesting that NIH played around with appropriate naming of its center. They went through three names. It was originally called the Office of Alternative Medicine (OAM), then the National Center for Complementary and Alternative Medicine (NCCAM). Now it is known as the National Center for Complimentary and Integrative Medicine (NCCIH). Notice that the word *alternative* was eventually dropped; whereas *complementary* and *integrative* were either added or retained. The implication is that holistic medicines have moved up a notch and are now considered legitimate parts of health care delivery that *merge* into the whole, rather than a last-ditch resort or an *alternative*. Herbalism, chiropractic, massage, reflexology, and many others presently integrate with and complement status quo allopathic medicine.

NCCIH has funding in the millions of dollars. It is used for studies, surveys, and research, including grants and training. One NCCIH 2007 survey conducted on the subject of pain found that American adults who use complementary health approaches to treat or manage pain spent an estimated $14.9 billion out of pocket. The four types of pain with the highest estimated out-of-pocket spending on complementary approaches were back, neck, joint, and arthritic pain. Back pain was the *number-one* pain disorder.[10]

Because the NCCIH funds scientific research on complementary and integrative health, an herbalist can apply for a grant or funding to be trained as a researcher. It is telling and encouraging that the U.S. government finally finds complementary health worth investigating.

State of Herbalism Around the World

Kampo and the Japanese Pharmacopeia (JP) 1886

In Japan, herbal medicine has been used effectively for over 1400 years; the first version of the official ***Japanese Pharmacopeia (JP)*** was published in 1886. Japanese Medicine consists of traditional folk use of raw herbs and ***Kampo***, a Japanese adaptation of traditional Chinese Medicine and the official medicine of Japan. Many Kampo herbal formulations dispensed in granules and powdered forms (designated in Japan as *drugs*) are covered under their national health insurance. Kampo herbals are regulated in a manner similar to the regulation of drugs in the West.

The 14th edition of the JP lists 165 herbal ingredients that were approved for use in Kampo remedies. The most common herb listed is *Glycyrrhiza uralensis* Gan Cao (Licorice root), which appears in 94 of Tsumura formulas, the leading manufacturer of Kampo medicines in Japan.[11]

World Health Organization (WHO) 1948

The ***World Health Organization (WHO)*** directs and coordinates international health within the United Nations' system. It defines traditional use of herbal medicines as having had "long historical use that is well-established and widely acknowledged to be safe and effective and may be accepted by national authorities." The WHO further and reasonably concludes that "a traditional medicine is the sum total of the knowledge, skills, and practices based on the theories, beliefs, and experiences indigenous to different cultures." Their function is to "help mothers and children survive and thrive so they can look forward to a healthy old age." It ensures "the safety of the air people breathe, the food they eat, the water they drink, and the medicines and vaccines they need."[12] The founding date of the WHO was April 7, 1948, and nations celebrate *World Health Day* annually on April 7.

The Pharmacopeia of the People's Republic of China (PPRC) 1953

Herbal medicine is part of Chinese culture. Over the last century, traditional Chinese Medicine has coexisted with allopathic medicine. Hospitals have units for traditional medicine, and most rural doctors are able to provide either modality. Doctors are trained in both, and the two systems are practiced side by side at every level of the health care system. Herbal medicine plays an enormous and respected role.

The ***Pharmacopoeia of the People's Republic of China (PPRC)*** began publication in China in 1953. Tellingly, Volume One is the herbal volume that covers single herbs and fixed herbal formulas, the patents. Volume Two is the Western medicine volume that addresses conventional pharmaceuticals.[13] Additional volumes have been added over the years. In China, the word *drug* applies to plants and plant medicines, and botanicals have equal footing with allopathic remedies.

Monographs in the English edition appear in alphabetical order according to the pharmaceutical name, indicating the plant part used (Glycyrrhiza radix), and then by Latin name (*Glycyrrhiza uralensis*), giving the genus and species. Some of the PPRC features reflecting China's long history of traditional Chinese herbal medicine include thousands of herbal monographs, application of contemporary analytical technologies, emphasis on safety, protection, sustainable development of traditional remedies, and development of green standards.

The United Kingdom and *The British Pharmacopoeia* (BP) 1968

Ever since Henry VIII ordained parliament to pass the *Herbalist's Charter* in 1543, (Chapter 2) to assure himself access to herbal treatment for his painfully gouty ulcers, herbalists in the UK and its present and former territories, such as Australia, have had an amazing amount of freedom to practice and dispense herbal medicine. The first issue of the ***British Pharmacopoeia (BP)*** was published in 1864, although its legal status didn't occur until 1968.[14] The BP is used by individuals and organizations involved in pharmaceutical research, development, manufacture, and testing.

King Henry VIII's ordained freedom to practice herbalism now seems to be under attack and flux, with pressure from some factions to create a licensure requirement for the practice of herbal medicine.[15] With the advent of and subsequent withdrawal of Britain from the European Union (EU), the situation has become more complicated and muddier in terms of an herbalist's access to herbs, herbal products, and formulas. Herb shops and apothecaries that once freely sold herbs to the public had to undergo an expensive and complicated licensing process to comply with EU standards, resulting in many herbs disappearing from the market.

Depending on issues such as claims, presentation, and dosage, a single substance can be designated a food *or* a medicine. *Echinacea* spp., for example, can be marketed as a fully licensed product or as a medicine exempt from licensing. Garlic bulb can be a food or a medicine. Saw Palmetto berry can be a food, a medicine exempt from licensing, or a fully licensed product. The British Herbal Medicine Association tries to keep this all straight and its members informed, as the legal situation of herbals remains in flux.

Germany's Commission E, Established 1978

Germany's ***Commission E*** monographs stand out as the world's most authoritative government-sponsored, expert-developed information on medicinal herbs. An Expert Advisory Panel similar to the FDA's earlier OTC Review Panel, routinely publishes monographs that list uses, dosages, side effects, and any known drug/herb interactions. It also lists herbs deemed unsafe. So far, they have declared more than 300 herbs to be safe and effective.[16] Commission E monographs can be obtained in English translation from the American Botanical Council (ABC).

German herb companies are allowed to make medicinal claims in line with Commission E monographs, which are intended to inform consumers, not provide a scientific basis for safety. Legally, herbals are considered to be medicines in Germany and are distributed through OTC sales in pharmacies and by medical prescription through pharmacies. Herbals are, in principle, reimbursable by the health insurance system, unless special criteria for their exclusion apply, such as substances negatively assessed by Commission E. Herbal medicines are not prescription-bound but can be prescribed by healthcare providers for reimbursement.[17] What an enlightened idea.

Therapeutic Goods Act Regulations of Australia (TGA) 1989

In Australia, medicinal products containing herbs, vitamins, minerals, nutritional supplements, homeopathies, and certain aromatherapy preparations are considered complementary medicines and regulated as medicines under the ***Therapeutic Goods Act (TGA)*** of 1989.[18] It is the national framework for the regulation of herbs to ensure quality, safety, and performance. It is based on a risk management approach designed to ensure public health and safety and at the same time frees industry from any unnecessary regulatory burden. Australian manufacturers of *all medicines* must be licensed, and their manufacturing processes must comply with the principles of Good Manufacturing Practice (Chapter 30). The TGA does not regulate practitioners; it regulates products, which must all be licensed.

Canadian Natural and Non-Prescription Health Products Directorate (NNHPD) 2004

Canada is a country that enjoys free medical care and subsidized medicine. That said, its provisions apply only to orthodox medicine, which also covers supplements prescribed by naturopathic healthcare providers that are tax deductible within certain parameters.

The ***Canadian Natural and Non-Prescription Health Products Directorate (NNHPD)*** is the regulating authority for natural health products for sale in Canada. According to WHO, herbal medicines are regulated as *drugs* in Canada and must therefore conform to labeling and other requirements, as set out in the Food and Drugs Act and Regulations.[19] This proviso means that, in contrast to requirements in the United States, large numbers of herbal medicines with indication claims are legally on the Canadian market.

To be legally sold in Canada, natural health products must have a product and site license. This requirement applies neither to health care practitioners who compound products on an individual basis for their patients nor to retailers. Canada considers traditional usage to be the use of a medicinal ingredient within a cultural belief system or healing paradigm for at least 50 consecutive years. One example is Traditional Chinese Medicine. This 50-year time span was chosen to represent two generations, allowing possible reproductive effects to be identified.

Herbal Timeline

The herbal timeline (Table 29.2) is a continuation of events that have occurred since we left off in Chapter 2 with mention of Rene Caisse's Essiac formula. This timeline proceeds with happenings and landmark legislation in the United States, pharmacopeas, and regulations from around the world, and the founding of notable herbal organizations (Chapter 30).

TABLE 29.2 Herbal Timeline of Legislation and Important Events

1864	National Institute of Medical Herbalists (NIMH) is the United Kingdom's leading professional body and voluntary regulator of herbal practitioners.
1870s	Founding of National Institutes of Health (NIH). U.S. federal agency responsible for biomedical and public health research.
1886	*Japanese Pharmacopeia* (JP). Regulates drugs and Kampo herbs and Japanese adaptations of traditional Chinese herbs.
1906	Pure Food and Drugs Act established by U.S. Congress. Allegedly for consumer protection. Inspects restaurants and food processing facilities.
1928	Alexander Fleming discovers penicillin, ushering in the pharmaceutical craze.
1928	U.S. Federal Drug Administration (FDA) established. Emerged out of the Pure Food and Drugs Act of 1906. Regulates, approves, recalls, classifies medicines, herbs, foods, drugs, and medical devices. Now under Department of Health and Human Services.
1946	Centers for Disease Control (CDC) established. U.S. federal agency founded to monitor public health, communicable diseases, epidemics, and health threats.
1948	World Health Organization (WHO). Role is to "direct and coordinate health within United Nations' system."
1953	U.S. Department of Health and Human Services. Regulates many departments, including all welfare, social security, restaurants, and the FDA.
1953	*Official Pharmacopoeia of the People's Republic of China* (PPRC). Consists of drugs and herbal medicine. English editions available.
1958	Generally Regarded as Safe (GRAS) status introduced by the FDA.
1960s to present	Women's Health and Self-Help Movement. Continuation of the Wise-Woman Tradition with notable male herbalists joining in. Reclaiming the power of herbal medicine and still going strong.
1962	The drug Thalidomide causes deformed babies. FDA cracks down, and their powers in drug approval and monitoring are greatly extended.
1968	*British Pharmacopeia* (BP). The United Kingdom's standard for drugs and herbs.
1970	U.S. Controlled Substances Act includes *Cannabis sativa* as a Schedule I drug, with a "high potential for abuse" and "no currently accepted medical use." This law restricted its access for researchers.
1978	Commission E in Germany. Standard research-based herbal monographs published. These are added to and updated regularly.
1988	American Botanical Council (ABC). Prestigious organization founded by Mark Blumenthal to provide traditional and science-based herbal education to herbalists, health care professionals, public, and the media.
1989	American Herbalist Guild (AHG) founded. A nonprofit, educational organization representing the goals and voices of herbalists.
1989	Therapeutic Goods Act (TGA) regulations of Australia. Sets policy on complementary medicines, herbals, homeopathics, and nutritional supplements.
1994	U.S. Dietary Supplement Health Education Act (DSHEA). Herbs are designated as dietary substances (not drugs) and regulated as such.
1995	American Herbal Pharmacopeia (AHP) founded by herbalist Roy Upton to promote responsible use, safety, and standards of herbal medicine. Publishes herbal monographs and other educational materials.
1997	Eisenberg Survey. Showed that one out of three people used complementary and alternative medicine, paid for mostly out of pocket.
1998	First edition of *Physician's Desk Reference for Herbal Medicine*. Signified understanding that healthcare providers needed information about herbal medicine.

(*Continued*)

TABLE 29.2 Herbal Timeline of Legislation and Important Events—cont'd

1998	National Center for Complementary and Integrative Health (NCCIH) formed as part of the National Institutes of Health.
2000	*Pharmacopeia of the People's Republic of China* (PPRC) published first English edition. Volume One: herbal monographs. Volume Two: Western drugs.
2004	Dietary supplements containing the alkaloid ephedrine banned by the FDA because they were misused in dietary supplements to increase fat loss and energy and to decrease weight. Ephedrine is an active ingredient in the raw Chinese herb, Ephedra Ma Huang, safely used in Chinese Medicine as a bronchodilator for thousands of years. The ban caused most wholesale herbal companies to remove Ma Huang from their shelves.
2004	*Canadian Natural and Non-Prescription Health Products Directorate* (NNHPD) includes herbals.
2018	FDA approval of first *Cannabis*-based prescription drug, Epidolex, an oral solution for severe forms of epilepsy.
2019	U.S. Drug Enforcement Agency takes steps to process 2016 applications to register more qualified growers to produce *Cannabis* spp. for research purposes but retains its Schedule I status.[20]
Present	Herbalists need to be informed, vigilant, and active in influencing favorable botanical medicine legislation. It won't happen by itself.

Summary

It is evident from this historical overview that the United States lags behind many countries in its legal recognition and acceptance of herbal remedies for everyday use. Major reasons are politics, economics, protection of turf, and unwillingness to change. The situation fluctuates, and the herbal community has a responsibility to stay current and aware of impending legislation that might work for or against us. There is strength in numbers and in staying connected.

Regulations imposed by the FDA and the DSHEA tend to represent and favor Big Pharma at the expense of herbalists and the general public, who so frequently turn to complementary remedies. The two sides could ideally make a harmonious pairing in the interests of national health. Regardless of laws and regulations, herbal medicine always was and will be practiced.

As more herbal research is conducted, and new healing plants are discovered worldwide, particularly in our rain forests, undiscovered and wondrous remedies of the future are silently growing. Many drugs were derived from plants in the first place. A renaissance is occurring in herbal medicine, not because of herbalists already part of the chorus, but from public interest and renewed scientific inquiry into healing plants.

Review

Fill in the Blanks

(Answers in Appendix B.)

1. According to the DSHEA, an herb is considered a ___, not a ___.
2. Thalidomide was a ___ used to ___.
3. Thalidomide caused ___. The FDA responded by ___.
4. A NCCIH survey found that the number-one type of pain was ___.
5. Commission E monographs list four major facts about herbs: ___, ___, ___, ___.
6. Kampo is the ___.
7. In China, an herb is considered a ___. Its Pharmacopeia lists more than ___ herbs (state how many).
8. An accepted standardized level of a substance in milligrams is the ___ ___.
9. A biochemical constituent characteristic of the plant is called a ___ ___ and is usually designated by a ___.
10. Name four areas in which the WHO coordinates international health: ___, ___, ___, ___.

Critical Concept Questions

(Answers for you to decide.)

1. What is the difference between a *complementary* and *alternative* medicine?
2. Are you in favor of herbal standardization? Give pros and cons.
3. What is a phytopharmaceutical?
4. What is the difference between a 1:5 extract and a 5:1 extract?
5. How does the regulation of herbals in the United States compare with herbal regulation in other countries? Support your answer.
6. What is Thalidomide? What did it have to do with the FDA?
7. Why are so few herbs listed in the USP today?
8. What is the significance of Commission E?
9. What do you think about the status of herbal medicine in China?
10. What is the status of the Wise-Woman in the modern era?

References

1. "US Regulatory Response to Thalidomide, 1950-2000." Embryo Project Encyclopedia. https://embryo.asu.edu/pages/us-regulatory-response-thalidomide-1950-2000 (accessed September 7. 2019).
2. Tierra, Michael. "Why Standardized Herbal Extracts?" East West School of Planetary Herbology. https://planetherbs.com/research-center/phytotherapy-articles/why-standardized-herbal-extracts/ (accessed September 7. 2019).
3. "Drug Substance Law and Legal Definition." U.S. Legal. https://definitions.uslegal.com/d/drug-substance/ (accessed July 29, 2019).
4. "FDA 101: Dietary Supplements." U.S. Food and Drug Administration. https://www.fda.gov/consumers/consumer-updates/fda-101-dietary-supplements (accessed September 7. 2019).
5. Murray, Michael. *The Healing Power of Herbs* (Rocklin, CA: Prima, 1999).
6. "Generally Recognized as Safe: GRAS." U.S. Food and Drug Administration. https://www.fda.gov/food/food-ingredients-packaging/generally-recognized-safe-gras (accessed September 7, 2019).
7. "Botanicals Generally Recognized as Safe." Herb Research Foundation. https://s10.lite.msu.edu/res/msu/botonl/b_online/library/dr-duke/gras.htm (accessed September 8, 2019).
8. "Food Additive Status List." U.S. Food and Drug Administration. https://www.fda.gov/food/food-additives-petitions/food-additive-status-list (accessed January 26, 2020).
9. "Juliette of the Herbs." IMDB. http://www.imdb.com/title/tt0208242/ (accessed September 7, 2019).
10. "U.S. Adults Spend Billions Out-Of-Pocket on Complementary Approaches for Pain." National Center for Complementary and Integrative Health, National Institutes of Health. https://nccih.nih.gov/research/results/spotlight/082715 (accessed September 7, 2019).
11. "List of Kampo Herbs." Wikipedia. https://en.wikipedia.org/wiki/List_of_kampo_herbs (accessed September 8, 2019).
12. "About WHO." and "What We Do." World Health Organization. https://www.who.int/about and http://www.who.int/about/what-we-do/en/ (accessed September 8, 2019).
13. "The Chinese Pharmacopoeia 2015 English Edition." United States Pharmacopeia. https://www.usp.org/products/chinese-pharmacopoeia (accessed September 8, 2019).
14. "The British Pharmacopoeia." British Pharmacopoeia. https://www.pharmacopoeia.com/the-british-pharmacopoeia (accessed September 8. 2019).
15. Tierra, Michael. "Current Herbal Regulation in the UK." East West School of Planetary Herbology. https://planetherbs.com/blogs/michaels-blogs/current-herbal-regulation-in-the-uk/ (accessed September 8, 2019).
16. "The German Legal and Regulatory Environment and the History and Background of Commission E." American Botanical Council. http://cms.herbalgram.org/commissione/history.html?ts = 1567974260&signature = 3bc59a036f1ead978616f401d5a31b1a (accessed September 8, 2019).
17. Foster, Steven. "Germany's Rich Herbal Traditions: Exploring the Impact of the German Commission E." Mother Earth Living. https://www.motherearthliving.com/mother-earth-living/germanys-rich-herbal-traditions (accessed March 12, 2021).
18. "An Overview of the Regulation of Complementary Medicines in Australia." Australian Government Department of Health. https://www.tga.gov.au/overview-regulation-complementary-medicines-australia (accessed September 8, 2019).
19. "Natural and Non-prescription Health Products Directory." Government of Canada. http://www.hc-sc.gc.ca/ahc-asc/branch-dirgen/hpfb-dgpsa/nhpd-dpsn/index-eng.php (accessed September 8, 2019).
20. Stone, Will. "Researching Medical Marijuana May Soon Get Easier." NPR. https://www.npr.org/sections/health-shots/2019/08/27/754761944/researching-medical-marijuana-may-soon-get-a-lot-easier (accessed January 30, 2020).

30

Business Thoughts for a Modern Herbalist

"Never doubt that a small group of thoughtful, committed citizens can change the world; indeed, it is the only thing that ever has."

—Margaret Mead

CHAPTER REVIEW

- Worldwide popularity of herbalism and other holistic modalities. The Eisenberg National Survey. *HerbalGram* market report.
- Legal status of herbalists in the United States: Licensure and implications, scope of practice, educational requirements, herb schools and certifications, financial aspects, ethics, and self-regulation. Practicing herbalism safely.
- Legal obligations for making and selling herbal products: Good Manufacturing Practice (GMP). Who has to comply and why? Getting down to details of GMP compliance. Recalls.
- Important herbal organizations: American Botanical Council, American Herbalists Guild, American Herbal Pharmacopeia, and National Institute of Medical Herbalists in the United Kingdom.
- Seed banks and maintaining biodiversity.
- What herbalists do.
- Photo gallery of herbalists in action.

KEY TERMS

American Botanical Council (ABC)
American Herbal Pharmacopeia (AHP)
American Herbalists Guild (AHG)
David Eisenberg National Survey
Ethics
Good Manufacturing Practice (GMP)
National Institute of Medical Herbalists (NIMH)
Recalcitrant species
Recalls
Seed banks

Pertinent issues and information are presented for 21st century herbalists hoping to get out into the real world and use their skills. Facts and figures that substantiate the dramatic upswing of herbal usage in the last 30 years or more in the United States are given; not a bad marketing tool.

Arguments for and against herbal licensure are explored, as is the advent of the Good Manufacturing Practice (GMP) requirements of the U.S. Food and Drug Administration (FDA), and how they are bound to affect any herbalist desiring to produce and sell herbal products. Herbalists, as members of a respected profession, have a responsibility to support and to benefit from our professional organizations.

Just as a knowledge of plant medicine is our ultimate health insurance policy, seed banks are vital ways to preserve our plant DNA. The Millennium Seed Bank Partnership coordinated by the Royal Botanic Gardens, Kew, in the United Kingdom, is one such endeavor. A collection of ideas for herbal entrepreneurship and avenues of employment is presented, followed up with a photo gallery showing actual herbalists in action.

Worldwide Popularity of Herbalism and Other Holistic Modalities

In the United States, herbs and herbalists are enjoying an upswing in popularity. We are once again in the midst of a paradigm shift, where many traditional practitioners, doctors, nurses, and pharmacists are beginning to appreciate and embrace our buried lore. Positive attitudes and an openness to herbal medicine can be attributed to people taking responsibility for their own health and self-care, coupled with disillusionment about the medical system. In 2016 herbal supplement sales in the United States increased more than 7% from the year before. The top three best sellers were Horehound herb (*Marrubium vulgare*), Cranberry berry (*Vaccinium macrocarpon*), and *Echinacea* spp.[1]

Prestigious allopathic medical journals such as *The Journal of the American Medical Association* (*JAMA*), *The New England Journal of Medicine* (*NEJM*), and others, publish studies and articles on the benefits of healing herbs. Public interest and demand have played a role in changing the status quo of the medical and herbal fields. For example, it is no accident that the well-used and respected *Physician's Desk Reference* (*PDR*), a collection of all prescription drugs available in the United States, now includes an herbal volume, the *PDR for Herbal Medicines*, though it is a very conservative take on herbal medicine. Nevertheless, it became necessary for allopathic healthcare providers, in self-defense, to understand and learn about botanicals and their possible interactions with the drugs they prescribe and the surgeries they perform.

It is telling that many of the pharmaceutical chemicals currently available to allopathic healthcare providers have a long history of use as herbal remedies. These chemicals include codeine and morphine from the Opium poppy, digitalis present in Foxglove herb, and quinine in the bark of the Cinchona tree. In the over-the-counter (OTC) scenario, we have capsicum in Cayenne pepper used in arthritis creams, menthol from Peppermint herb, and camphor from the Camphor tree featured in Bengay. According to the World Health Organization (WHO) approximately 25% of modern drugs used in the United States have been derived from plants.[2]

About 90% of the population of African countries and 70% in India currently use herbal medicine for some aspect of primary health care. In the United States, $17 billion was spent on alternative and complementary medicine in 1990, and that amount had doubled by 1997. Herbal medicines are common in Europe; France and Germany lead the pack in OTC sales. Herbal medicinal products have been their citizens' first choice in the treatment of minor diseases or disorders, evidenced by the success and prestige of Commission E monographs.[3]

The Eisenberg National Survey

A well-known 1997 study, the ***David Eisenberg National Survey***, showed that one out of three people in the United States used complementary therapies. Most people paid from out-of-pocket sources, declining to share this information with their doctors. Holistic health is rarely covered by health insurance. In 2002 the most significant change revealed a 50% jump in the use of herbal supplements over the past 5 years, and that has been growing. Next up was yoga at 40%. The Eisenberg survey concluded that alternative medicine use and expenditures increased substantially between 1990 and 1997, attributable primarily to an increase in the proportion of the population seeking alternative therapies, rather than increased visits to doctors.[4] These are significant and hopeful findings.

Market Report from HerbalGram States that Herbal Sales are Up

HerbalGram: The Journal of the American Botanical Council reported that "Herbal Dietary Supplement Sales in United States increased 6.8% in 2014, marking the 11th consecutive year of growth ... American consumers spent roughly $6.4 billion on herbal supplements according to aggregated market statistics provided by Nutrition Business Journal." The top supplements in order of expenditures from 2013 to 2014 were Turmeric root, Wheat or Barley Grass, Flaxseed and Flaxseed oil, Spirulina, Milk Thistle seed, Elderberry, Maca root, Echinacea root, and Oregano herb.[1] There is always some herb in vogue, a popular *herb of the year*. Apparently, in 2013 Turmeric root led the pack.

The Legal Status of Herbalists in the United States

Licensure and Implications

Herbalism is *not* regulated in the United States. At this writing (January 2020), there are no herbal licenses awarded in any state. However, state licenses are required for other medical professionals such as doctors, nurses, acupuncturists, chiropractors, massage therapists, and in certain states, naturopaths and reflexologists. No licensure means herbalists practicing clinical herbalism operate in legal shades of gray. The profession is vulnerable to unwarranted legal restrictions, making all professional herbalists more or less work outside the boundaries of the law.

Some herbalists are fine with potential licensure requirements, and others vehemently oppose any regulation whatsoever, preferring to stay off the radar, hoping they can continue to do what they have always done well in peace and quiet. Some might feel outraged or threatened, having always practiced herbalism in their communities and wish to pass on the Wise-Woman/Wise-Men traditions, give sage council, and be allowed to dispense the medicine of our plant allies freely and without fear.

Before you jump to any conclusions for or against, consider the path it takes to even obtain a state licensure requirement. When none exists, a profession usually works at it state by state, provided a group, organization, or individual is motivated to do so. It is a long process that involves lobbying, public speaking, and educating state legislators as to why licensing is even necessary, what an herbalist act (ordinance) would look like, and what the educational standards should be. This last is a sticky topic (see later section). Licensing is a trade-off, where certain liberties are exchanged for greater privileges. The ensuing section lays out some of the arguments.

Scope of Practice

Medical doctors, chiropractors, and licensed naturopaths have the authority to *diagnose*, *treat*, or *prescribe*. Acupuncturists do, provided they adhere to Chinese Medicine diagnoses. Nurses do not. Exactly what a profession's scope of practice entails is enumerated in their Practice Act. With no legal backup, herbalists must be *extremely* careful about being construed as practicing medicine without a license, including not diagnosing, treating, or prescribing. One way to dance around this is to use descriptions such as Chinese syndromes (Kidney Qi Deficiency), and by defining illnesses by their symptoms rather than actually naming a disease. We cannot assign a client a Western diagnosis such as the flu, pneumonia, or Alzheimer's. We can *suggest* a treatment but cannot *prescribe* one. It's all about using careful and correct wording.

Educational Requirements, Herb Schools and Certifications

Licensure assures that the licensee has acquired a minimum amount of knowledge in her field to practice safely and do no harm due to lack of training. Licensure is designed to *protect the public*, and the state gives an examination to verify this. Once passed, the person becomes a state registered *something*. Licensure confirms that the practitioner has received proper training, is not a quack, or in our case (if it existed), would assure no one could claim to be a master herbalist after a paltry 2-week training, and that said herbalist will not endanger anyone's life because of insufficient education.

It is hard to get any group or profession to agree on what an herbal education should include, much less to decide on the number of training hours. What would or should be included on a licensure examination to assure competency? Should an herbalist be required to know all traditions? Or is Western herbalism enough? What about people trained in Ayurvedic but not Western, and so on? Should they be required to study and be tested on a tradition they will never use? (Massage therapists and others have run into this exact bitter debate and dilemma.)

From a legal standpoint, lack of licensure means that titles and certificates awarded by any U.S. herb school have no legal clout, regardless of quality or hours spent in class. With licensure, schools are generally required to follow state-approved curricula. It would be up to the herbal community to make those educational recommendations. Most state licensing agencies do not have a clue what an herbalist is, what s/he does, or what an herbal education would/should look like. Whereas a licensed nurse attended an accredited college, followed a set curriculum preparing her to pass the state Nursing Board Exam, and received a license to perform nursing within a stated scope of practice. Herbalists have no such opportunity, and some would just as soon not upset the status quo.

What about the many competent herbalists who have apprenticed or are self-taught and do not have the proper credentialing *on paper?* They could still be recognized for their knowledge, perhaps by passing an exam to fulfill any licensure requirements. Or as with other newly formed licensures, they could be grandfathered in because they were in practice prior to the law's inception. They would not have to return to school for a certificate and still be allowed to legally practice.

Financial Aspects

Everything has a cost. Even setting up a state exam and oversight board with a paid staff involves funding. So herbalists (as other licensees) would be charged fees to obtain and maintain their license. Then there are continuing education requirements with personnel needed to monitor those. Therefore, it could be argued that licensure is just a state money-making venture, where periodic fees are charged to oversee and regulate the whole shebang.

However, with the expenses of licensure comes legitimacy. And with legal clout, third-party payment from insurance companies is more likely. It is doubtful any insurance company will reimburse a dime for herbal services rendered unless they are delivered by a licensed herbalist or are recognized under the umbrella of an already licensed acupuncturist, naturopath, or chiropractor who is additionally trained in botanical medicine.

With insurance available for herbal clients, more people could afford it, and practices would increase along with incomes. Then the insurance companies would have to be billed; and taking the time and filling out all *that* paperwork is itself a learning curve. Do we want to go down that rabbit hole?

Licensure would supposedly protect the public from malpractice and poorly trained herbalists. But an herbalist would then need to have (and pay for) malpractice insurance. State licensure laws require proof of that. No one wants to be sued, and, yes, herbal medicine has a very good safety record (especially compared with allopathic), but even so, it does open up another can of worms.

Ethics and Self-Regulation

The fact that there is no state regulation or licensure means that herbalists must regulate themselves. This is something all professions do (with or without licensure). We need to be mature enough to adhere to a self-imposed code of conduct, moral principles, values, or ***ethics***, and do the *right thing*, so as not to misrepresent our knowledge or to cause harm through irresponsible practice. Self-regulation is supposed to weed out those who practice dangerous herbal medicine.

For instance, the American Herbalists Guild (AHG) has a code of ethics that lays out how herbalists should conduct themselves, including full disclosure of education, not misrepresenting skills, maintaining confidentiality, exercising professional courtesy, using quality botanicals, avoiding needless therapy, and other items. Should an infringement or complaint occur, AHG has a complaint-resolution procedure to investigate and ultimately revoke membership.[5] Beyond that, there is no recourse, whereas with state licensure, a license could be withdrawn because of malpractice, and that person would no longer be allowed to practice.

Licensure can arguably be good or bad.[6] As far as legalities go, at this point the best an herbalist can do in the United States is to get the very best possible herbal training, similar to the curriculum laid out in this text, and to be very conscious and careful. Lack of licensure has not stopped countless successful herbalists out there with a passion and desire to practice.

Practice Herbalism Safely

To be safe, herbalists can recommend remedies, educate clients, and dispense specific herbs that are mild to medium strength and certainly not very strong or toxic plants without appropriate knowledge and experience. Err on the side of safety and refer onward and outward if unsure. This recommendation means using intuition *and* book learning. If you get a funny feeling, act on it. Refuse to treat and refer out to a qualified practitioner. *When in doubt, refer it out.* Only suggest remedies within your comfort zone. This also means sizing up your client and yourself. Do you have a trusting relationship? If an herbal side effect occurs (and someday, it inevitably will) what will *you* do? What will *they* do? In all my years of practice, I have never been sued. On the other hand, I would never have taken on a cancer patient without a physician on board, nor would I have handled a situation by myself that I felt was beyond my ability. The many reasons, pro and con, for herbal licensure are summarized in Table 30.1.

Legal Obligations for Making and Selling Herbal Products

Good Manufacturing Practice

An important area where transitions are affecting herbalists (and OTC supplement producers) in the United States concerns FDA regulations regarding the manufacture of food supplements, which includes herbal products. It is a system for ensuring that products are consistently produced and controlled according to quality standards. It requires having a method in place so an herb can be tracked from the ground to the consumer. ***Good Manufacturing Practice (GMP)*** was put into effect in the United States by the FDA on June 25, 2007; other countries and the World Health Organization have their own versions.

TABLE 30.1 Positives and Negatives of Herbal Licensure
(As of April 2021, there are no requirements for herbal licensure in the United States.)

Reasons Against	Reasons For
Should not have to give up any freedoms and be able to practice the art of herbalism without government interference.	Would not have to practice in shades of gray and would have legal status and the privileges that entails.
No state fees to pay, and no hassle with paperwork.	Paperwork and fees are worth assurance of recognition as a respected, legitimate, and qualified practitioner.
No certificates needed, and no expense of a formal education.	Proof of education assures the public that an herbalist has adequate training to practice safely.
Apprentices and self-taught herbalists should be recognized for their knowledge without passing any test.	Testing assures competence and ability to practice safely.
Herb schools might have to revise curriculums and pay large fees for approved programs.	Herb schools should meet high standards and award meaningful certifications that are recognized by states, allowing for licensure.
How can we determine what an herbal education should include, and number of required educational hours? There are too many traditions and ways to practice.	Basic educational requirements should be determined by herbal organizations to reflect a minimum knowledge for safe practice.
The medical system and the insurance industry are broken. Herbalists may want no part of that and all the paperwork involved.	Clients could be covered by third-party payment, and herbalists would have a larger practice with increased income.
Herbalists are ethical and can self-regulate.	The herbalist profession, like any other, should self-regulate even *with* licensure and oversight.
The Wise-Woman tradition should be maintained.	Things are going in this direction, and the world is changing.

Herbalists are now being considered healthcare professionals who are more noticeable and accepted than ever. Traditional folk methods of producing herbal remedies for public sale are no longer part of the modern world. Change and transitions are inevitable, and the 2000s are a new age. Setting up an apothecary from the establishment of your practice with a system in place to follow current GMP guidelines will be much easier than playing catch-up later or perhaps having to reinvest in brand new, expensive equipment.

Good Manufacturing Practice, as applied to herbalists, is beginning its baby steps in the United States. Regulators and practitioners are feeling their way, determining how to adapt it into a workable system for herbal remedy production. Acupuncture schools and Chinese Medicine apothecaries are also involved. No clear guidebook exists for herbalists *yet*, but organizations such as the American Herbalists Guild are presenting classes and seminars on the practical aspects of accomplishing GMP compliance. This information will inevitably become part of herb school curricula. As learning tools, their student apothecaries will have to comply.

Naturally, healing botanicals would do better having their *own* stand-alone category, rather than being lumped into the Dietary Supplement Health and Education Act (Chapter 29). Herbs are neither food supplements nor drugs. If they *must* be regulated, it would make more sense to have guidelines structured specifically to herbal medicine, instead of fitting a square peg into an existing round hole.

Who Has to Comply, and Why?

GMP applies to any herbalist turning raw material or herb (dietary supplement) into a product sold directly to the public. If an herbalist is planning on producing and selling ingestible or topical herbal products, such as teas, tinctures, percolations, glycerites, capsules, lip balms, lotions, and so forth, GMP regulations will affect how to set up the business, whether in-house or online. The larger and more visible an enterprise, the more exposed and greater the pressure for compliance. As with licensure and standardization issues, how an herbalist chooses to use this information will be for her to decide. It is a far cry from kitchen folk herbalists who weren't concerned with such details. The point is to be aware and informed.

Once a method is in place, it becomes routine and will just need occasional tweaking, as more efficient and easier procedures are established by trial and error. I am acquainted with two forward-thinking herb shop proprietresses, both complying with GMP, who have shared their logs and record-keeping systems with me. The particulars are uniquely individual with no single template, but both satisfy GMP inspections and requirements. Each herbalist must accomplish GMP compliance as they see fit.

The GMP inspectors themselves are going through a learning curve. It is doubtful if most FDA and health department examiners even understand what herbal medicine and remedy production are about. Some *get* this concept; others have nary a clue, and in such cases we must patiently and kindly *educate* them.

Getting Down to Details of GMP Compliance

The FDA's rationale for GMP is to ensure the supplement industry delivers "safe, accurately labeled products to the consumer." They consider it an important tool to help ensure dietary supplement products' "quality, purity, consistency, and safety."[7]

In plain English, this means that if you purchase a pound of raw Milk Thistle seed from Mountain Rose Herbs, make it into a tincture, and then use it as one of six herbs in a client's formula and she has a bad reaction, there must be a system to trace that herb back to its source, to determine whether, what, and where a mistake was made. Was it the fault of the grower, the harvesters, the herb company, or an error in your production methods of a perfectly fine and correctly identified and labeled herb? Or was it an individual reaction your client had to an uncontaminated, properly labeled and identified herb prepared in your shop?

This process really isn't a bad idea. If practicing due diligence, it is very unlikely an herbalist will be sued when operating in good faith according to regulations, having built up a trusting herbalist-client relationship. Customers and clients can also purchase products with confidence, assured they are getting a pure, unadulterated, high-quality remedy containing what is stated on the label in the specified proportions. It may seem daunting, depending on your penchant for detail, but it is doable. For an herbalist GMP, broadly speaking, breaks down into these elements:

- *Clean and sanitary conditions.* The conditions under which herbal products are produced must be clean and hygienic, as laid out by the state departments of health, not unlike sanitary conditions in a restaurant. This includes proper handwashing, wearing of protective latex or vinyl gloves and an apron, and having hair pulled back or covered by a hat, scarf, or net. Cleaning supplies should be in a separate closed area, in the olden days called a *broom closet.*
  - *Some typical physical requirements.* You will need a three-basin sink to soap and double rinse utensils at the proper water temperature, *even* if there is also a dishwasher. Other considerations are having nonporous stainless-steel surfaces that are easily cleaned and sanitized and equipment for proper sealing, covering, and storage of herbs. A closed-off area for grinding herbs with ventilation of dust to the outside is essential for breathing and cleanliness (Fig. 30.1). Also needed is a refrigerator dedicated to herbs and not food, and a floor drain for mop-bucket waste and dirty water disposal. Items like these are a monetary investment best worked into a business plan before, not after, the fact.
- *Proper record keeping.* Logs and a record-keeping system must be in place so that an herb is traceable all along the line from source to consumer. Details include recording suppliers' lot numbers, shipment dates, your *own* lot numbers, dates, and batch numbers for each product produced from those herbs, and a system to determine which herbs or formulas were dispensed to which client. More specifics to consider:
  - *Arrival of new herbal shipments and samples of each.* Keep invoices and record online or on paper the date, herb company, lot number, botanical and common name, and weight. Then reserve 1 to 2 g of raw sample to stash away in an organized, accessible place. Small zip-lock jewelry (earring) bags obtainable at crafts stores work well.
  - *Verifiable and up-to-date records.* Current records that will pass any periodic health department or FDA inspection must be kept.
  - *Housekeeping check-off lists.* These records provide evidence of posted cleaning schedules for work areas and bathrooms, checked off and initialed.
  - *Physical sample of each apothecary batch.* A tiny vial of each tincture, percolation, etc. must be kept so that it could be chemically analyzed, if that ever became necessary. It should be labeled with Latin name, plant part, date made, type of preparation and proportions, and apothecary lot and unique identification number assigned by herbalist to that product.
- *Adverse reactions.* Should any client or customer report a side effect, bad reaction, or severe allergic response, it must be documented. How was the situation handled? What was done or modified? Medical records should always contain this information. It is not meant to be incriminating or threatening, just safe practice, as long as the information is truthful, and the herbalist responded like any other reasonable herbalist would have. Unexpected client reactions occur in the practices of even well-intentioned, experienced, and skillful herbal clinicians. Be proactive and protect yourself, and your client, because herbal malpractice insurance is not even available. Give yourself and your clients peace of mind.

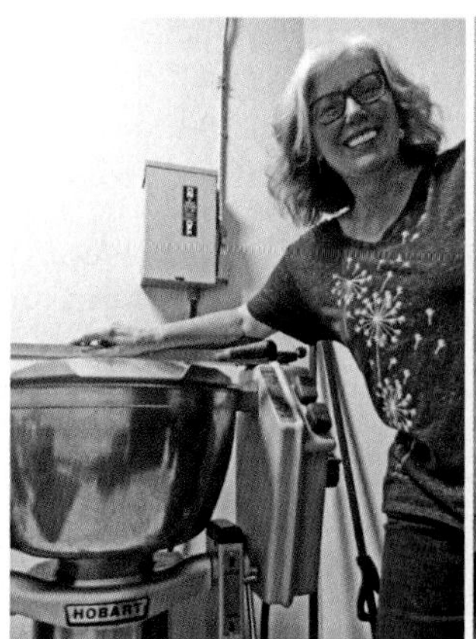

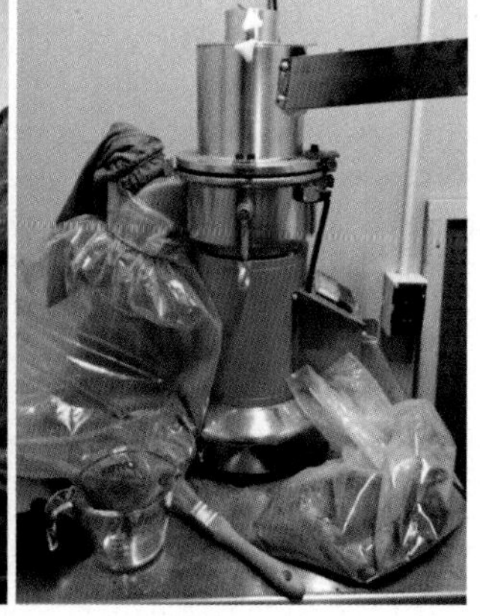

• **Fig. 30.1** An apothecary's dream set-up. A dedicated room containing large herb grinders and a custom ventilation system that removes the finely powdered dust which invariably accumulates. Operated by herbalist Valerie Blankenship, Sage Consulting & Apothecary Colorado Springs, CO.

Recalls

Recalls are actions taken by a firm to remove a faulty product from the market. GMP provides a way to determine exactly what the problem is and where down the line the problem occurred, so that appropriate measures can be taken. It is not a crime to make an honest mistake; but it *is* criminal and unethical if there is not full disclosure or there are no measures taken to rectify the situation.

One of the most notorious drug recalls in history was the so-called "Tylenol murders" in the west side of Chicago in 1982. Drug company Johnson & Johnson recalled 31 million bottles of Tylenol-branded acetaminophen capsules from store shelves. The capsules had been laced with deadly potassium cyanide. Seven people died in the original poisonings and several more from copycat crimes. Before it was over, Johnson & Johnson changed their bottle tops to tamper-proof safer designs and offered replacement products free of charge. This led to massive OTC product packaging reforms and to federal antitampering laws.[8] That's why drugs and OTC medicines are now so impossibly hard to open.

Another recall happened on February 22, 2013, when Herbalife International of America announced the voluntary recall of certain lots of its niche Instant Healthy Meal Nutritional Shake Mix packets because the label identified the product as dairy-free. This was not true, because the drink had trace amounts of milk proteins, causing severe allergic reactions in sensitive individuals. Herbalife publicized and recalled the specific lot numbers involved.[9]

Another example: if a small herbal business owner was found to have contaminated Licorice root tincture on her shelves, she would be able to track which actual bottles and/or formulas contained Licorice with that specific lot number and could then easily remove only that batch from her shelves. She would also have to discard the dried herb that matched that lot number, and the supplier would need to be notified as well.

Important Herbal Organizations

Professional herbal organizations help us stay connected and keep us up to date with the latest resources, classes, gatherings, information, and opportunities we might not have known about otherwise. A professional organization also self-regulates and establishes and disseminates ethical standards for the profession. It keeps us informed of pertinent legislation such as the latest on GMP, provides prospects for networking, and gives us ways to stay linked with the herbal community. They help us promote what we love.

The American Botanical Council

The ***American Botanical Council (ABC)*** is a nonprofit educational and research organization that states as its mission to "Provide education using science-based and traditional information to promote responsible use of herbal medicine—serving the public, researchers, educators, health care professionals, industry, and media."[10] It publishes *HerbalGram: The Journal of the American Botanical Council*, a peer-reviewed quarterly that posts herbal news, legislative issues, and updates on its website, and offers information databases and herbal information for its members. It also has a media education program that responds to inaccuracies and misrepresentations about herbs in the media. The ABC is an organization deserving of an herbalist's membership and support.

The American Herbalists Guild

American Herbalists Guild (AHG) is a professional organization founded in 1989 for herbalists. It encourages herbal educational opportunities, sponsors seminars, publishes a quarterly journal, and offers other member benefits. Its founding members read like a *Who's Who* in American herbal medicine. AHG provides webinars and classes, and it sponsors periodic herbal conferences held in rotating, gorgeous outdoor settings, perfect for herb walks, gatherings, and celebrations. I can testify that these get-togethers will provide herbalists with an overwhelming amount of information, which can take a full year (or more) to absorb and will give opportunities to connect to the local flora and to meet and network with herbal enthusiasts from all over the country. The booths themselves are amazing.

One becomes a professional member by passing a test to become and receive an *AHG Registered Herbalist* membership. As described on its website, "AHG Registered Herbalist Membership exists as a way for herbalists to demonstrate a core level of knowledge and experience in botanical medicine practice that is recognizable as a meaningful standard to themselves, to the general public, and to other health professionals and institutions."[11]

To earn this designation, an herbalist is required to submit three case histories, similar to those used throughout this text. Also required are three letters of recommendation and background information. If U.S. state licensure for herbalists ever comes down the pike, it is quite likely that AHG educational standards will carry a lot of weight. Its *AHG, Registered Herbalist* title is one of the best designations an herbalist can presently attain in the United States.

American Herbal Pharmacopeia

The ***American Herbal Pharmacopeia (AHP)*** is a nonprofit founded by herbalist Roy Upton in 1995. Its mission is to publish critically reviewed herbal monographs, similar to, but more complex than, Germany's Commission E. AHP also stores AHP-verified herbal samples called Botanical Reference Materials (BRMS), which are analyzed and used as a standard or baseline. Other samples may then be submitted, analyzed, and compared with the baseline plant to determine chemical authenticity and quality.

AHP focuses on Ayurvedic, Chinese Medicine, and Western herbs most frequently used in the United States. The monographs represent "the most comprehensive and critically reviewed body of information on herbal medicines in the English language, and serve as a primary reference for academicians, health care providers, manufacturers, and regulators" and provide "the most relevant information needed to comply with cGMPs."[12] The small *c* means *current* GMP and is sometimes used to indicate that GMP standards can change and must remain up to date as technology changes.

The monographs are long, thorough, and complex. A sample 64-page monograph for the aerial parts of *Echinacea purpurea* may be viewed on the website. The monograph contains (among many other features) beautiful color photos of the plant; compares *E. purpurea* to other species on the market; includes images of microscopic characteristics; gives details about cultivation, harvesting, preparation; and provides chemical breakdown charts and the scientific procedures used to isolate ingredients, not to mention the therapeutics, actions, and safety profile of the plant.[13] That's a lot of info.

National Institute of Medical Herbalists in the United Kingdom

The ***National Institute of Medical Herbalists (NIMH)***, established in 1864, is the U.K.'s leading professional body and voluntary regulator of herbal practitioners. Notice that their name is the Institute of *Medical* Herbalists, a lofty designation. It sets high standards for professional education, practice, and conduct. It accredits herbal schools, maintains a member register, establishes a code of ethics and codes of conduct and practice, and self-regulates the profession by taking complaints and using disciplinary procedures. Admission to the institute is only for those who have graduated from an accredited course. It has members from all over the world.[14] It also operates a mandatory malpractice block insurance program.

This organization is a *little* like the American Herbalists Guild in that it is a self-regulating body that sets herbal educational standards, but goes many steps further by limiting admission to qualified herbalists who have met their specifications and by providing malpractice insurance. It is also about 125 years *older* than the baby AHG.

Seed Banks and Maintaining Biodiversity

Seed banks are places where seeds are stored to preserve genetic biodiversity, insurance policies for medicinal plants and food security. Climate change, natural and environmental disasters, nuclear war, extinction, hybridization, and biodiversity loss all threaten our pure plant DNA pool. In fact, the Amazon rain forest, the world's present and future medicine chest is endangered. There are hundreds of seed banks of different sizes around the world that function as backup systems in case of catastrophe. Should the unspeakable occur and an entire crop be wiped out, planters could use seed reserves to start over. One famous seed bank, the Svalbard Global Seed Vault, is located on an island nearly 600 miles north of Norway. It is fortified deep under the permafrost into solid rock, known as the doomsday vault. It is under such tight security that no one person knows all the codes to open any seed package.[15]

The Millennium Seed Bank Partnership is an international conservation mission coordinated by the Royal Botanic Gardens, Kew, outside London, a global resource for conservation, sustainable solutions, and research. It holds the largest concentration of seed-bearing plants on Earth, including the entire plant population of the United Kingdom and many endangered species, which have top priority for collection. The seeds are dried, frozen, and stored in deep-freeze chambers of $-18°$ to $-20°C$. Some seeds do not retain viability when dried, especially those from the hot wet tropics. Therefore they cannot be banked in this manner. They are known as ***recalcitrant species***, and studies are underway to see if they might be preserved by cryogenic storage techniques.[16]

Another approach to preserving biodiversity and food security is not storing seeds in underground or frozen seed banks but to keep them alive and growing cycle after cycle, a *live* seed bank. One such is the Yupaichani Network in Vilcabamba, Ecuador, a consortium of friends and associates working together on various stated initiatives: to protect seed biodiversity, rehydrate and coordinate reforesting, run a land collective and eco-arts school, create organic corridors, and operate an herbal medicine and seed collective. Because of its biodiversity, Ecuador is considered a living seed bank with altitudes that support species from three climate zones: the costal lowlands, the low Amazon tropical rainforests, and the high Andean mountains. The Ecuadorian group coordinates local seed saving hubs throughout their country and much of South America. Their seed saving is on a personal-neighborhood-bioregional level. They also operate the Vilcabamba Organic Market, where the vendors produce what they sell (pictured in photo gallery).[17]

An example of plant conservation and preservation of live plants in North America is United Plant Savers (UpS), based in Rutland, Ohio. It was begun in 1994 by founding president, Rosemary Gladstar, and encourages private cultivation, sustainable practices, and preservation of endangered wild medicinals, such as Slippery Elm, American gingeng, and Goldenseal. The group encourages the creation of *botanical sancturaries* across the country, where at-risk medicinal plants can be preserved and propagated. You could be part of this effort to preserve medicinal plants for generations to come.

For herbalists desiring to grow their own herbs, quality seeds are available from non-GMO heirloom seed companies specializing in organic medicinal seeds from all over the world. One such resource is Horizon Herbs/Strictly Medicinal Seeds in Williams, Oregon. They sell hard-to-find seeds and seedlings, ranging from ancient grains like quinoa and amaranth to medicinal herbs such as Comfrey root, Codonopsis Dang Shen (Downy Bellflower root), Ephedra Ma Huang (Ephedra stem), and many more. Just perusing their catalog is an education and a joy.

What Herbalists Do

There are numerous possibilities for herbal entrepreneurship. Choose clinical herbalism, maintain private practices, or work in established clinics. Teach in or launch a school; become a guest speaker, conduct community classes, or lead herb walks. Establish and run an herb shop, orchestrating an entire business. Become a grower selling high-quality organic herbs. (We need more of those.)

Quite a few herbalists work in health food stores or pharmacies, giving consults and dispensing their wisdom to the public. Others are associated with supplement companies and manage entire herbal departments and customer education. One former student went to work for an herbal product company, helping them devise their own proprietary formulas, and another artistic herbalist is studying botanical illustrating. Herbalists with scientific backgrounds might consider conducting research studies and chemical analysis of botanicals. National Institutes of Health grants are available for botanical research.

Some innovative herbalists who love large-scale medicine making and have the wherewithal and organizational skills to become GMP certified, wholesale *their own* tinctures, proprietary formulas, and other botanical products to established clinics, apothecaries, and shop owners who would rather not be involved in the production process. The service includes individualized labeling and provides creative labels printed with GMP certification designation, customer's name, and logo. This sounds like an up-and-coming business that could be in demand.

Another unique and exciting idea is to convert a camper, van, or bus into a mobile herbal clinic, equipped with on-site consulting, apothecary, and dispensary. This unit might travel around serving ethnic communities, rural neighborhoods, or Indian reservations. Or the mobile clinic could administer herbal first aid at public gatherings, concerts, marches, foot or bike races, and other events. ***The only thing stopping herbal entrepreneurship is lack of imagination and courage.***

Photo Gallery of Herbalists in Action

The following collection (Boxes 30.1 through 30.5) shows some of the many herbal entrepreneurs out there doing their *thing*. As you can see, they conduct botanical walks, run herbal shops, do consultations, teach and own schools, participate in sustainable seed banks and commune with their plant allies. Enjoy perusing the gallery.

• BOX 30.1 Photo Gallery: Brigitte Mars

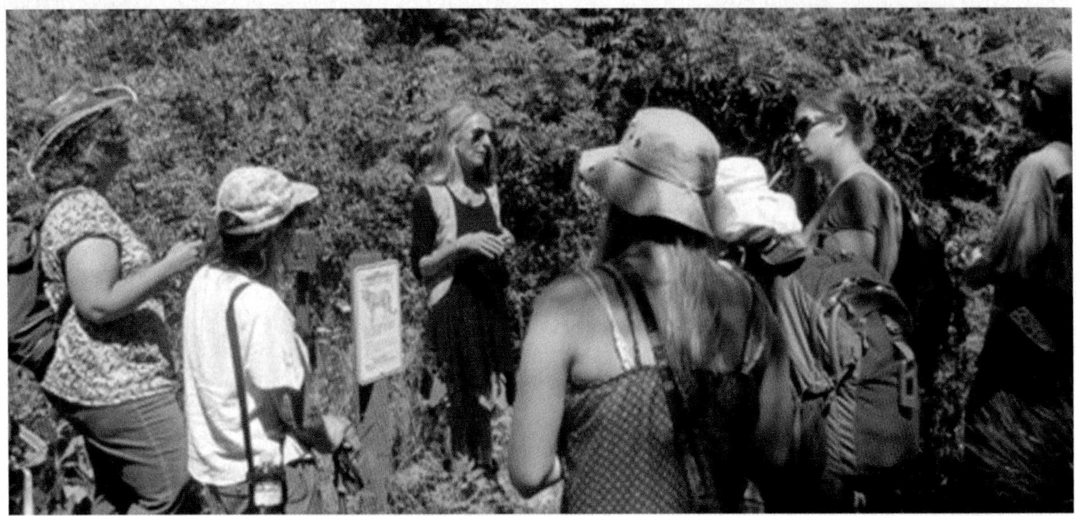

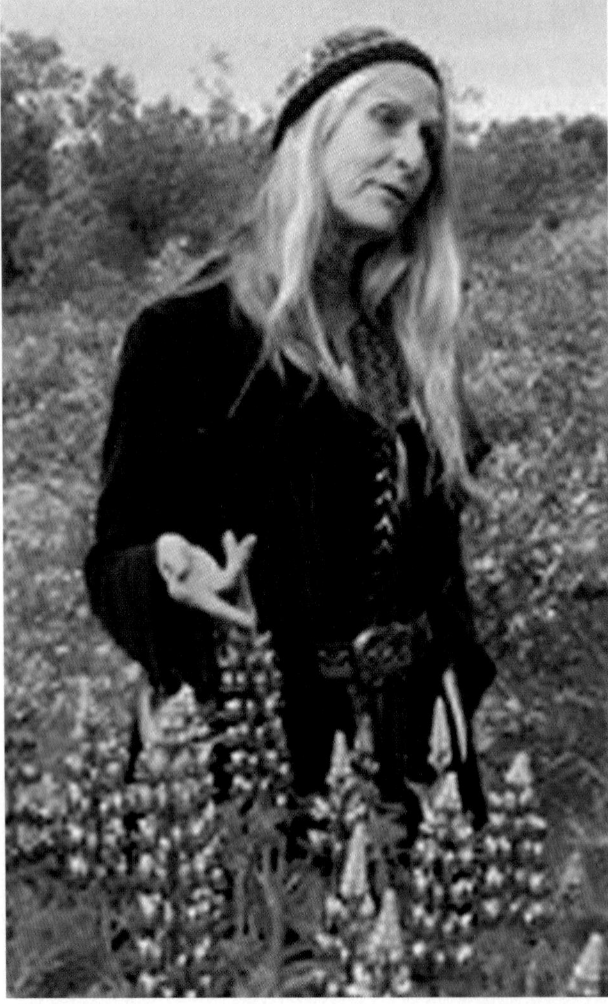

BRIGITTE MARS. Herbalist, author, and university professor, Boulder, CO, leading herb walks (top and left); consulting and selling herbs at Pharmaca Integrative Pharmacy in Boulder (lower right). https://brigittemars.com/about/

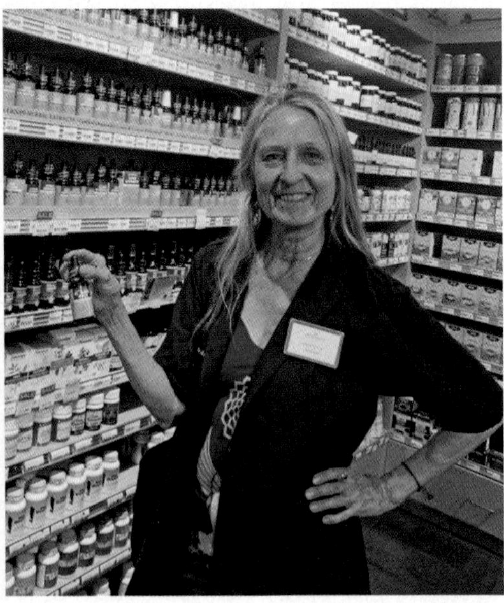

• BOX 30.2 Photo Gallery: Lisa Ganora, Mindy Green, Feather Jones

LISA GANORA, Director, Colorado School of Clinical Herbalism (CSCH) and author of *Herbal Constituents,* teaching at her school (right). https://clinicalherbalism.com and https://herbalconstituents.com

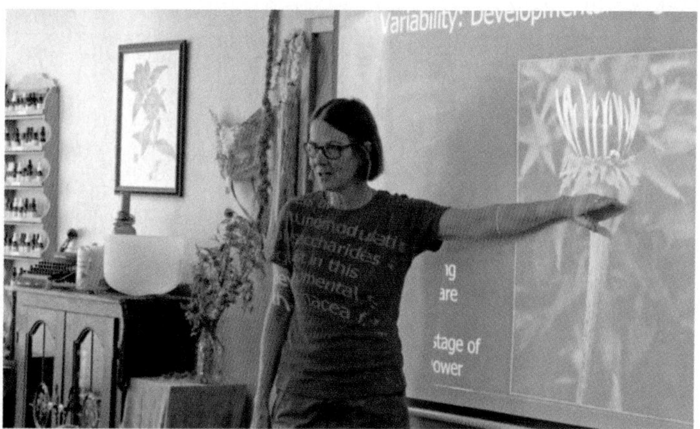

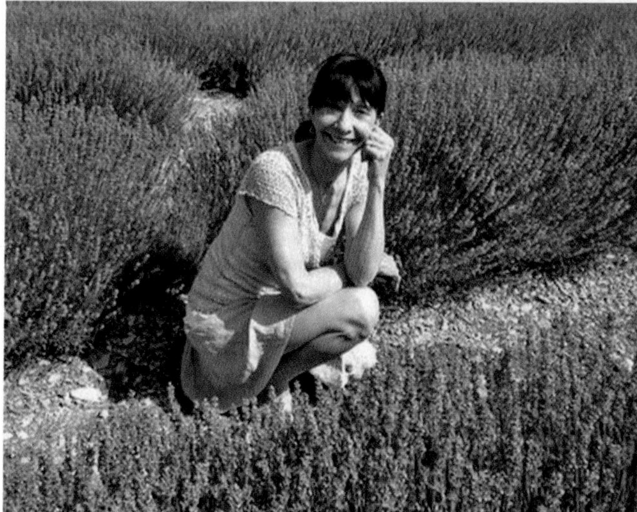

MINDY GREEN in Lavender field (left). She is passionate about the healing powers of plants and their wondrous essential oils. www.greenscentsations.com

FEATHER JONES, RH (AHG) (below) leading an herb walk. feather@sedonateablends.com www.sedonateablendscom www.canyonspiritventures.com

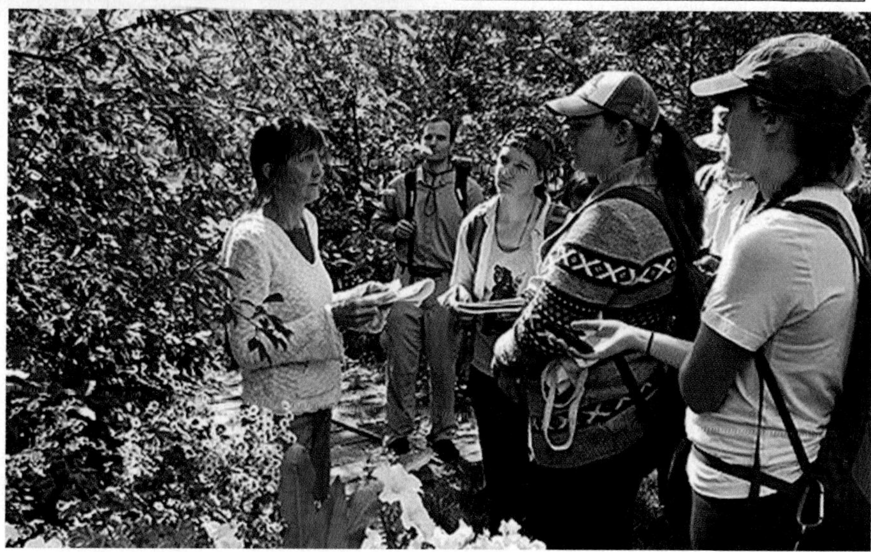

• BOX 30.3 Photo Gallery: Yupaichani Network in Equador, Vilcabamba Organic Market
(A sustainable live seed bank with a mission to preserve seed biodiversity and eco-activism)

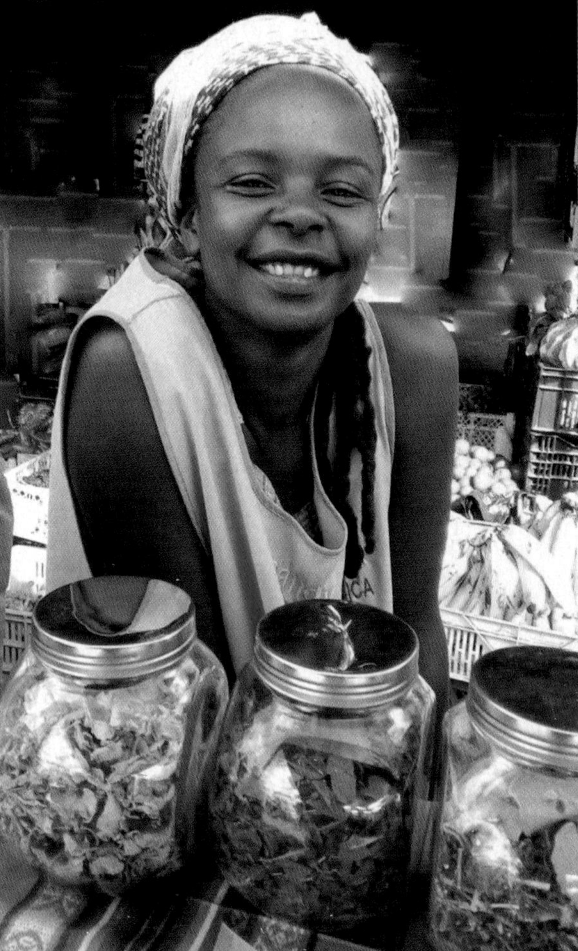

Pictures from ZIA PARKER, founder of the Yupaichani Network in Ecuador that protects seed biodiversity. Scenes from herbalists at their Vilcabamba Organic Market. Top left: Deb selling herbs. Lower left: Zia Parker and friends sorting herbs. Top right: Herb growers and market vendors. Lower right: Valvina laughs.
http://vidaverde.info/yupaichani-

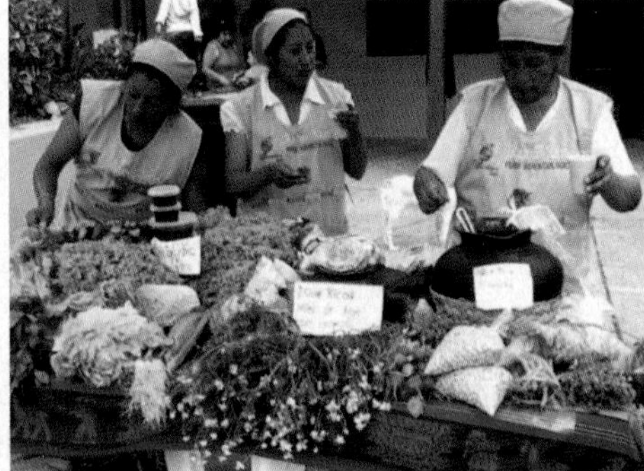

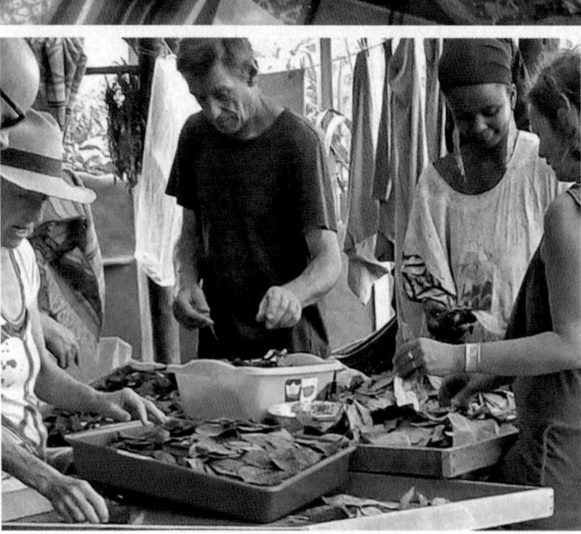

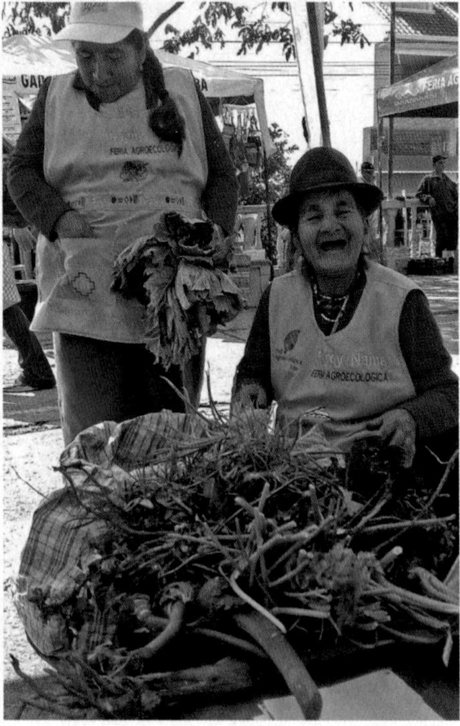

• BOX 30.4 Photo Gallery: Valerie Blankenship, Matthew Berk, Rebecca Luna

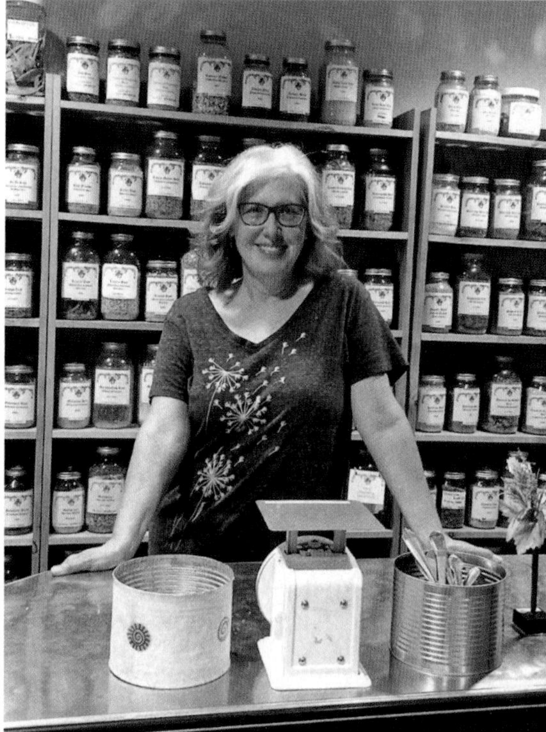

VALERIE BLANKENSHIP (above), owner of Sage Consulting & Apothecary, Colorado Springs, CO. valerie@sagewomanherbs.com https://www.sagewomanherbs.com

MATTHEW BERK, L.Ac. MSTOM (below). Reviewer for Chinese herbal portion of this book, shown consulting and selling herbs at Herbs & Arts, Denver, CO. calmmindacu@gmail.com

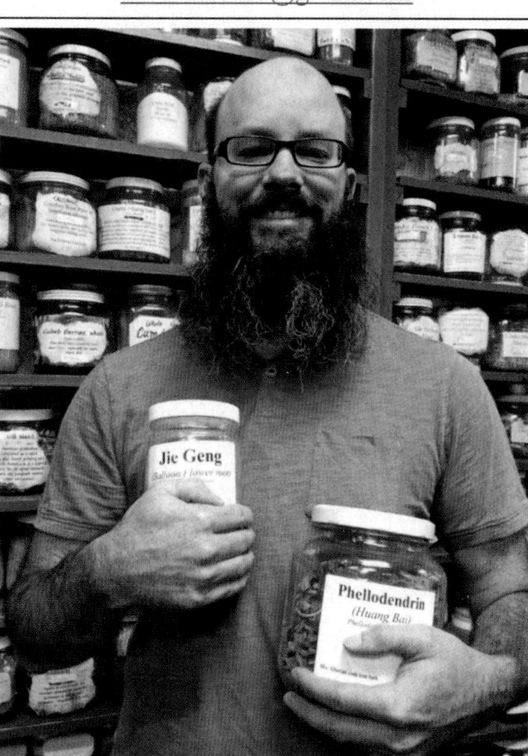

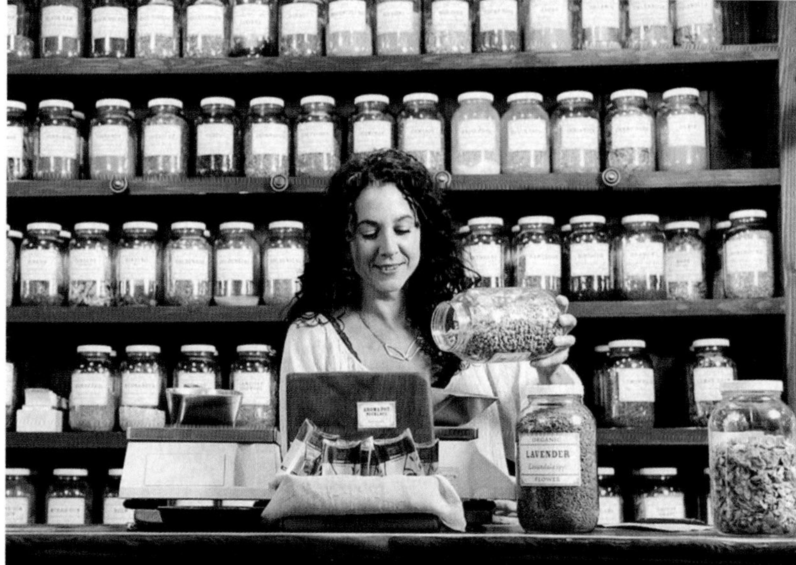

REBECCA LUNA (left), herbalist and shopkeeper of Rebecca's Herbal Apothecary & Supply in Boulder, CO. https://www.rebeccasherbs.com

• BOX 30.5 Photo Gallery: Rachel Lord, Joan Zinn

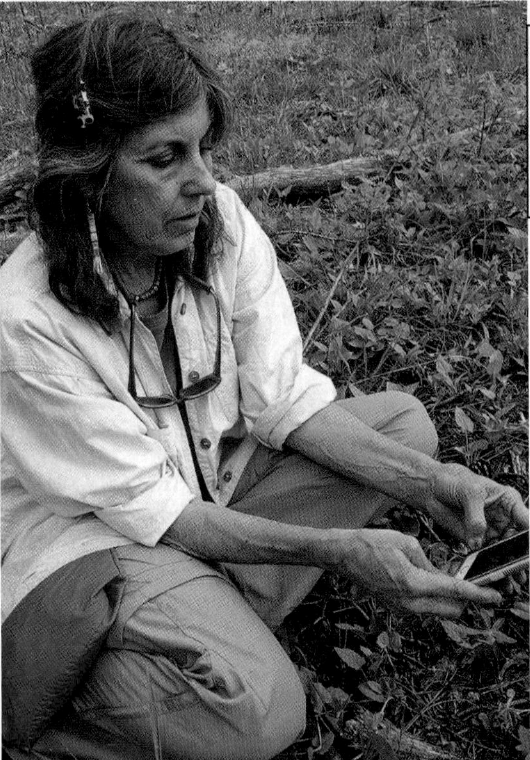

RACHEL LORD, MH, RN, AHG, author of this text. Taking pictures for the book and wildcrafting with Joan Zinn in Colorado mountains (top left).
https://clinicalherbalismwisdom.blogspot.com

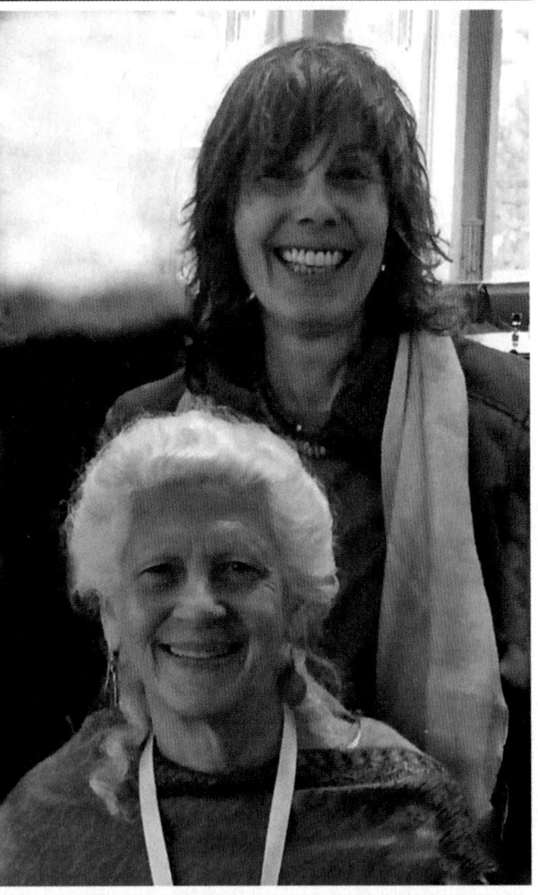

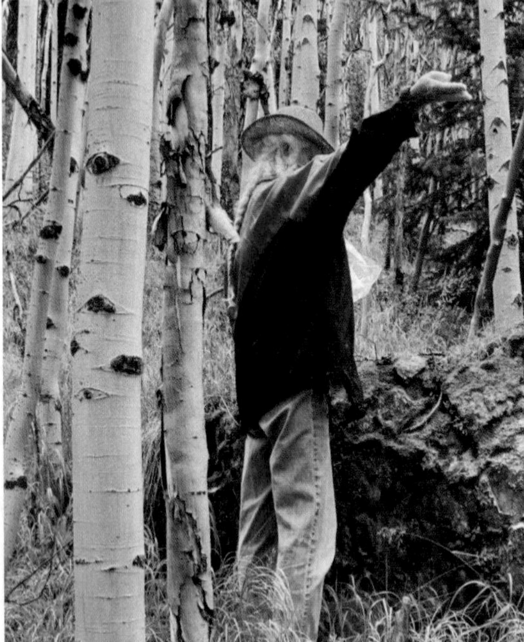

Above right: Rachel Lord, author, and Joan Zinn of Medicine Hill Herbs at the AHG conference in Granby, CO.

Lower left: Ceremony among the aspens on herb walk with JOAN ZINN, AHG, herbalist, teacher, book editor, illustrator, Western herb consultant for this book.
www.medicinehillherbs.com

Summary

Public interest in and use of botanical medicine for healing are on the rise, as are market sales of herbals and other supplements. These increases are creating a growing demand for knowledgeable herbalists. Licensure does not yet exist for us in the United States, but because herbalists are increasingly being accepted as valid health care professionals, it a likely future scenario.

GMP requirements are an FDA regulation. GMP involves two main areas: (1) Having clean and sanitary medicine-making facilities similar to restaurants. (2) Having a system in place that tracks an herb from grower or wildcrafter, to production, to a consumer carrying it out the door. In the event someone gets sick from ingesting or applying a faulty product, a recall can be initiated to quickly remove it from the market in the interests of public safety.

There are many implications for and against licensure. With or without it, herbalists can self-regulate to ensure high standards and safe practice for the public. One way to reach this goal is to belong to and support professional herbal organizations. Self-regulation is the ethical path, as is preservation of our botanical bounty and resources. Conscious and sustainable herbal purchasing, wildcrafting, and seed bank maintenance will ensure there are healing plants for the seventh generation to come.

Chapter Review

Fill in the Blanks

(Answers in Appendix B.)

1. The top three bestselling herbs in 2016 were ___, ___, ___.
2. Name three sanitation requirements of GMP: ___, ___, ___.
3. Name three record-keeping requirements of GMP: ___, ___, ___.
4. What are four professional herbal organizations? ___, ___, ___, ___.

Critical Concept Questions

(Answers for you to decide.)

1. What is the David Eisenberg National Survey?
2. What is the implication of doctors having a *PDR for Herbal Medicine*?
3. What do you think of GMP certification? Would you pursue it?
4. What do you think about requiring licensure for herbalists?
5. Discuss ethical obligations for herbalists.
6. Discuss the importance of seed banks.
7. How do you plan to use your herbal knowledge?

References

1. Smith, Tyler, et al. "Herbal Supplement Sales in US Increase 7.7% in 2016." *HerbalGram: Journal of the American Botanical Council*, 2017 Number 115.
2. Murray, Michael. *The Healing Power of Herbs* (Rockville, CA: Prima, 1999).
3. Wachtel-Galor, Sissi, and Iris F.F. Benzie. "Herbal Medicine: A Growing Field with a Long Tradition." National Center for Biotechnology Information. https://www.ncbi.nlm.nih.gov/books/NBK92773/ (accessed January 27, 2020).
4. Eisenberg, DM, et al. "Trends in Alternative Medicine Use in the United States, 1990–1997: Results of a Follow-Up National Survey." *JAMA*. 280(18) 2011:1569, http://www.ncbi.nlm.nih.gov/pubmed/9820257 (accessed January 27, 2020).
5. "AHG Code of Ethics Policy." American Herbalists Guild. https://www.americanherbalistsguild.com/ethics (accessed February 4, 2020).
6. Buhner, Stephen Harrod. "Some Arguments Against the Standardization of Herbalists." https://www.stephenharrodbuhner.com/wp-content/uploads/2018/11/standardization.art_.pdf (accessed February 7, 2010).
7. "Federal GMPs for Dietary Supplements." Natural Products Association. https://www.npanational.org/regulatory/federal-gmps-dietary-supplements/ (accessed January 28, 2020).
8. Markel, Howard. "How the Tylenol Murders of 1982 Changed the Way We Consume Medication." PBS. https://www.pbs.org/newshour/health/tylenol-murders-1982 (accessed March 15, 2021).
9. "Herbalife Recalls Some Nutritional Shake Mix Due to Milk Allergen." Reuters. http://www.reuters.com/article/us-herbalife-productrecall-idUSBRE91M01420130223 (accessed January 28, 2020).
10. "About the American Botanical Council." http://abc.herbalgram.org/site/PageServer?pagename = About_Us#VisionMission (accessed January 30, 2020).
11. "Becoming an AHG Registered Herbalist." https://www.americanherbalistsguild.com/becoming-ahg-rh-member (accessed January 30, 2020).
12. "About AHP Monographs." https://herbal-ahp.org/about-ahp-monographs/ (accessed January 30, 2020).
13. "Sample AHP Monograph: *Echinacea purpurea* Aerial Parts." https://herbal-ahp.org/sample-ahp-monograph-echinacea/ (accessed January 30. 2020).
14. Stannard, Laura. "National Institute of Medical Herbalists." Laura Stannard Medical Herbalist. http://www.themedicalherbalist.co.uk/national-institute-of-medical-herbalists.html (accessed January 30, 2020).
15. Ronca, Debra. "How Seed Banks Work: Seed Banks Around the World." How Stuff Works. https://science.howstuffworks.com/environmental/green-science/seed-bank4.htm (accessed January 30, 2020).
16. "Seed Collection." Royal Botanic Gardens, Kew. https://www.kew.org/science/collections-and-resources/collections/seed-collection (accessed January 30, 2020).
17. Parker, Zia. "Yupaichani Network." Vida Verde: The Green Life. http://vidaverde.info/yupaichani-network/ (accessed February 3, 2020).

Appendix A

Essential Information

Conversions Frequently Used by Herbalists

• BOX A.1 Absolutely Necessary Equivalents

- ***Weight to volume (w/v) equivalents***. 1 g = 1 mL One cm^3 (cubic centimeter or cc) water weighs 1 g.
- 1 oz = 30 g approximately (Rounded up unless you need to be exact because 1 oz = 28.3495231 g precisely.)
- 1 mL = 1 dropper full (squeeze) = about 25–30 drops (gtt) = 1 g (Most herbalists round this up to 30 gtts for convenience.)
- 30 mL = 1 oz (1 oz Boston round bottle)
- 60 mL = 2 oz (2 oz Boston round bottle)
- 120 mL = 4 oz (4 oz Boston round bottle)
- 240 mL = 8 oz (8 oz Boston round bottle)

• BOX A.2 English to Metric Conversions

- 1 tsp = 5 mL = 5 dropper squeezes = about 180 drops of 60% alcohol tincture
- 3 tsp = 1 tbsp = 15 mL = 15 dropper squeezes
- 8 oz = 1 cup = 250 mL
- 2 cups = 1 pint = 500 mL
- 2 pints = 1 quart = 1000 mL (or approximately 1 liter since 1 liter = 0.946353 of a quart.)
- 4 quarts = 1 gallon = 4000 mL
- 3 tsp = 1 tbsp = 15 mL = 15 dropper squeezes
- 8 oz = 1 cup = 250 mL
- 2 cups = 1 pint = 500 mL
- 2 pints = 1 quart = 1000 mL or approximately 1 liter because 1 liter = 0.946353 of a quart.)
- 4 quarts = 1 gallon = 4000 mL

TABLE A.1 Teaspoons to Droppers to Milliliters *(In case client is using a measuring spoon instead of a dropper.)*

Teaspoon	Squeeze of Dropper and Total Drops	Milliliters
¼	1 squeeze = 30 drops	1.0 mL approximately
½	2.5 squeezes = 75–88 drops	2.5 mL approximately
1	5.0 squeezes = 150–175 drops	5.0 mL approximately

TABLE A.2 Tincture Equivalents to Grams of Dried Herb

Tincture Proportion	Tincture Amount	Equivalent of Dried Herb in Grams
1:3 (33% w/v tincture)	100 mL	33 g
1:4 (25% w/v tincture)	100 mL	25 g
1:5 (20% w/v tincture)	100 mL	20 g
1:10 (10% w/v tincture)	100 mL	10 g

w/v = weight to volume.

Medical Abbreviations

TABLE A.3 Medical Abbreviations *(Accepted by the medical field).*

As needed = prn
Bedtime = H. S.
Before meals = a.c.
By mouth = p.o.
Capsule = cap.
Drop = gtt.
Every = q
Every day or 1 × daily = q day
Four × day = q.i.d.
Hour = h
Minute(s) = min
Ointment = ung.
Suppository = supp.
Tablespoon = tbsp
Teaspoon = tsp
Three × a day = t.i.d.
Tincture = tinc.
Two times a day = b.i.d.
With = c
Without = s

Average Doses for Adults

• BOX A.3 Doses for Adults, Acute Conditions

- **Infusions** ¼-½ cup throughout the day every 2 h up to 3–4 cups
- **Decoctions** ¼-½ cup throughout the day every 2 h up to 3–4 cups
- **Tinctures in formula, infectious onset/acute** 2–4 mL every 2 h when awake, or 1–2.5 mL every 30–60 min (¼-½ tsp every 30–60 min)

• BOX A.4 Doses for Adults, Chronic Conditions

- **Infusions** 1 cup 3 × daily for several weeks
- **Decoctions** 1 cup 3 × daily for several weeks
- **Tinctures in formula** 1–5 mL 3 × a day
- **Fluid extracts in formula** 1.0–2.4 mL 3 × a day (1:1 or 1:2 proportion)

• BOX A.5 Adults, Pulse Dosing Schedule

- **Diarrhea or hemorrhage** ½-2 tsp every 15 min–2 h maximum.
- **Pain** 1 tsp or 3–5 mL every 15–30 min as needed, for 2 h maximum. Then taper down.
- **Stalled labor** ¼-½ tsp every 30 min as needed, up to 3 times maximum.
- **Insomnia** 4 mL at bedtime; then 2 mL every 15 min as needed, up to 2 h, then STOP.

• BOX A.6 Adults, Essential Oil Dosages

Make sure all essential oils (EOs) taken internally are safe to do so. Consult a reliable text. Use high quality, pure oils with no adulterants.

- **Internal dose of EOs in tinctures**. Approximately 1 drop per ounce of tincture.
- **Internal dose of EOs in teas**. 2–4 drops in warm water or mild herbal tea 2–3 × daily.
- **Internal dose of EOs in capsules**. Some EOs are irritating to the mucosa and must be encapsulated with a carrier oil. They are too harsh to swallow and could burn on the way down. Use 1–2 drops topped off with a carrier such as olive or flaxseed. Examples are Oregano, Cinnamon, and Thyme. (Check EO books.)
- **Topical or external dose for skin**. 1 drop neat (if tolerated) or 1–3 drops diluted into ½ tsp vegetable carrier (fixed) oil. Douches, 20 drops-1 pint warm water daily × 1 week.
- **EOs for massage**. Add 10–25 drops per ounce of carrier vegetable oil such as olive, almond, avocado, or grape seed.

• BOX A.7 Adult Doses for Syrups, Glycerites, and Capsules

Syrups

- Typically, 1 tsp as needed.

Glycerites

- 5 dropperfuls (squeezes) 2–3 × daily for a tonic or mild herb.
- 10–25 drops 3 to 4 × daily for more intense herbs.

Capsules

- **Chronic problems**. Average adult dose is 2 double 00 caps 2–3 × daily. Children 1 double 00 cap 2–3 × daily. Take with juice or water, as you would any pill.
- **Acute problems**. Average adult dose is 1 double 00 capsule every hour until symptoms subside and then wean down. Average child's dose is 1 single 0 capsule every hour until symptoms subside and then wean down.

Amount of Dried Herb Related to Capsules

- 2 small 0 size caps = 1 large size 0 cap.
- 1 oz finely ground herb fills about 60 size 0 caps.
- 1 oz finely ground herb fills about 30 size 00 caps.
- One size 00 cap holds about ¼ tsp or 0.5 g of dried finely powdered herb.

Average Doses for Children

• BOX A.8 Formulas for Children's Dosing

CLARK'S RULE[a] (weight-based)

Divide weight of the child in pounds by 150 = fraction of adult dose.
Then multiply fraction by adult dose.
Adult Dose × (Child's weight in pounds ÷ 150) = Child's Dose
Example: Adult dose is 3 mL. Child weighs 35 lb.
35 ÷ 150 = 0.2333 = fraction of adult dose. Then: 0.2333 × 3 mL = 0.699. Round up to 0.7 mL (child's dose)

YOUNG'S RULE (age-based)

Child's age in years divided by age plus 12 = fraction of adult dose.
Then multiply fraction by adult dose.
Adult Dose × Child's age ÷ (Age + 12) = Child's Dose
Example: Adult dose is 3 mL, and child age is 3 y old.
3 ÷ 15 = 0.2 = (fraction of adult dose). Then, 0.2 × 3 mL = 0.6 mL (child's dose)

FRIED'S RULE[b] (Infants up to 24 months)

Age in months divided by 150 = fraction of adult dose.
Then multiply fraction by adult dose to get child's dose.
(Age in months ÷ 150) × adult dose = child's dose
Example: Child is 4 months old. Adult's dose is 5 mL.
4 months ÷ 150 = 0.266 (fraction of adult dose). Then: 0.266 × 5 mL = 0.13 mL (child's dose)

[a]"Clark's Rule and Young's Rule." Pharmacy Tech Study. https://www.pharmacy-tech-study.com/dosecalculation.html (accessed August 12, 2019).
[b]"Pediatric Dosage Rules." Austin Community College. https://www.austincc.edu/rxsucces/ped5.html (accessed August 12, 2019).

Clinic Forms to Copy and Use

- **Herbal Health History**. Fill out together with client. and keep in your records. (Fig A.1)
- **Herbalist's Assessment Form**. Fill out for your records. (Fig A.2)
- **Herbal Consult Suggestions**. Keep a copy for your records and give one to your client. (Fig A.3)

Lab Sheets to Copy and Use

- Dried Plant Tincture Worksheet. (Fig A.4)
- Fresh Plant Tincture Worksheet. (Fig A.5)
- Percolation Worksheet. (Fig A.6)
- Dual Extraction Worksheet (Fig A.7)
- Vegetable Glycerite Worksheet (Fig A.8)
- Wildcrafting Information Sheet (Fig A.9)

HERBAL HEALTH HISTORY

Today's Date______________

Last Name:________________________ First Name: ___________________

Middle_______

Address:________________________________ City: _________ State:_______

Zip________

Phone: Cell: ______________ Home:_________________ Work:

____

Email: ____________________________

Date of Birth: ______________ Age: _____ Place

raised:____________________________

Occupation:____________________________ Employer

____

Referred By: ______________________

Who do you live with? Myself ☐ Other(s) ☐ (Adults and relationship to you)

____

____

____

____

____

Children: Name (s), Age(s), Living with

You?____

____

____

____

Height: _______Weight:______ Happy With Weight?________ Desired weight: _______

Allergies:_________________________ Food Sensitivities

____

____

Do you have a Primary Care Practitioner? ☐ No ☐ Yes Name and Title

__________________ ____ Phone

________________ For what _____

____

Other Current Practitioners

Name/Title:______________________Address:_____________________Phone:____________

Name/Title:______________________Address:_____________________Phone:____________

• **Fig. A.1** Herbal Health History.

HERBAL HEALTH HISTORY

Herbal Treatment Goals: Why did you come in today?

1. ______________________________
2. ______________________________
3. ______________________________

Stressors in your life: (Rate stress level 1-10; 10 is the worst.) Family: ______ Social: ______ Work related: ______ Stress in your body? ______ Other? ______________________________

Where do you hold your tension? ______________________________

How do you relax? ______________________________

Do you exercise? ☐ Yes ☐ No What type? ______________ How often? ______________ How long is each session? ______________ Weight bearing? ______

Energy level and pattern? (least and most productive time of day)

____

Are you pregnant? ____________ Due date: ____________

Serious Past Illnesses?

____

Accidents, Injuries and Dates

____

Hospitalizations and Dates

____

Current prescription medications and what condition is being treated?

____

Current herbs and supplements and why are you taking them?

____

• **Fig. A.1** Herbal Health History (Continued).

HERBAL HEALTH HISTORY

Current Medical Concerns

☐ Asthma	☐ Headaches	☐ Multiple Sclerosis
☐ Blood Clots	☐ Heart Problems	☐ Osteoarthritis
☐ Breast Lumps	☐ Hemophilia	☐ Osteoporosis
☐ Cancer	☐ HIV	☐ Rheumatoid Arthritis
☐ Chronic Fatigue	☐ Infections	☐ Stomach ulcers
☐ Diabetes	☐ Liver Problems	☐ Other: ______________________
☐ Epilepsy	☐ Lupus	____________________________

Family History

☐ Arthritis	☐ Obesity	☐ Ovarian Cancer
☐ Heart Disease	☐ Thyroid	☐ Depression/Anxiety
☐ Diabetes	☐ Epilepsy	☐ Mental Health Disorders
☐ Alcoholism	☐ Breast Cancer	☐ Other ___________
☐ Asthma	☐ Prostate Cancer	

Wellness Continuum (Please mark where you think you fall on this wellness continuum)

Sick -- **Your Optimum health**

| Getting sick | O | Good | Healthy |

Addictions or Frequent Habits			
☐ Sugar	☐ Smoking tobacco/marijuana	☐ Alcohol	☐ Drugs
☐ Caffeine	How many a day? ___	How much? ________	What? ____________
☐ Salt	How long? _________	How long? _________	How Long? ________

Insomnia: ☐ Yes ☐ No ☐ Can't fall asleep ☐ Can't stay asleep What time do you wake up? ______ How often does this happen? ________________ Average hours sleep per night____ _________ Do you feel rested in the am? __________________

Frequent headaches or migraines? ☐ No ☐ Yes Describe type of pain like stabbing, aching.

____

Relationship to Food

Cravings: ☐ Salt ☐ Sweets ☐ Carbs ☐ Fats ☐ Chocolate

How much water do you drink a day? ________________

How much soda do you drink a day? ________________

How many cups of coffee do you drink a day? __________

How many cups of tea do you drink a day and what kind?

• **Fig. A.1** Herbal Health History (Continued).

HERBAL HEALTH HISTORY

____

What are your favorite snacks? ______________________________ How often do you partake?__________ ______________________________

What kind of cooking oil do you use? ______________________

Are you on any specific kind of diet? (gluten-free, vegetarian, vegan)

____

Do you buy organic? _____

How many times a day/week/month do you eat the following? Indicate how often.

Red Meat ____	Syrup ____	All vegetables ____	Miso _____
Poultry ____	Honey ____	Organic? _____	Sauerkraut _____
Fish ____	Refined Sugar ____	Yellow/orange veggies ___	Umeboshi _____
Pork _____	Brown Sugar ____	Green veggies ____	Kimchi ______
Wild Meats ____	Agave ____	White/purple veggies ____	Pickles ______
Quinoa ____	Candy ____	Coconut/rice milk_____	Sprouts _____
Soy Foods ____	Ice Cream ____	Rice white or brown _____	Salads ______
Beans ____	Baked goods ____	Millet ______	Vinegar _____
Eggs ____		Package cereal _____	Crackers _____
Mushrooms ____		Oats _____	Chips _____
Nuts ____		Barley _____	Pretzels _____
Dairy – organic? ____		Bulgur ______	Green smoothies ___
Yogurt _____		Pasta _____	Seaweeds ____
Kefir ____		Bread ________	
Cheese ____		Type? ________	
Nuts _____		White Flour _____	

SYMPTOM SURVEY

General:
- ☐ General fatigue
- ☐ Loss of or excessive gain in weight
- ☐ Motion Sickness

Other: __________

Respiratory
- ☐ Allergies
- ☐ Sinus Problems
- ☐ Difficulty breathing deeply
- ☐ Nosebleeds
- ☐ Frequent coughing
- ☐ Frequent colds/sore throats
- ☐ Asthma

Cardiovascular
- ☐ Rapid or skipped beats
- ☐ Varicose veins
- ☐ Bruise easily
- ☐ Chest pain
- ☐ Cold hands/feet
- ☐ Shortness of breath with activity
- ☐ High blood pressure

Neuromuscular
- ☐ Headaches
- ☐ Muscle pain – Where? ____________
- ☐ Muscle cramping
- ☐ Weakness in arms or legs
- ☐ Swollen joints

Senses
- ☐ Hearing Loss
- ☐ Earaches
- ☐ Ringing in ears
- ☐ Glasses/Contact Lenses
- ☐ Eye Problems ______________________

Digestive
- ☐ Frequent indigestion
- ☐ Heartburn
- ☐ Gas/bloating
- ☐ Nausea/vomiting
- ☐ Abdominal cramps
- ☐ Frequency of bowel movements___________
- ☐ Alternating constipation/diarrhea
- ☐ Consistency of stools: hard, firm, soft , loose
- ☐ Pain/itching in rectum
- ☐ Hemorrhoids
- ☐ Excessive or loss of appetite

Other:_________________________

Endocrine
- ☐ Swollen glands
- ☐ Excessive thirst, hunger, sweating, urination
- ☐ Slow/fast metabolism
- ☐ Blood sugar imbalances
- ☐ Thyroid problem such as low energy

Other: ________________________________

____

• **Fig. A.1** Herbal Health History (Continued).

HERBAL HEALTH HISTORY

☐ Painful joints
☐ Frequent dislocations
☐ Jaw/pain tension (TMJ)
☐ Frequent bone fractures
☐ Memory loss
☐ Absent minded
☐ Numbness/tingling Where?______________
Other:_______________________________

Skin

☐ Skin eruptions
☐ Excessive sweating – Where?___________
☐ Dry or oily skin

☐ Hair loss
Other: _______________________________
____

Urinary

☐ Frequent urination
☐ Involuntary escape of urine
☐ Burning/discharge on urination
☐ Weak urine stream
☐ Difficulty starting urine
☐ Constant urge to urinate
☐ Bedwetting
☐ Flank pain
☐ Number of times awaken in night to urinate_____
☐ Frequent urinary tract infections
Other:_______________________________

For Men:

☐ Burning/discharge on urination
☐ Lumps/swelling of testicles
☐ Pain in prostate or testicles
☐ Sores on penis or scrotum
☐ Hernia
☐ Impotence
☐ Erectile Dysfunction
Other:_________________________
____
____
____
____

For Women:

Menses

Do you have periods? ☐ Yes ☐ No
☐ Frequency and duration
☐ Amount of bleeding: scant, average, heavy, spotting
☐ Color: bright red, dark red, pink
☐ Clots? Color: _______________
☐ Bleeding between periods
Other: _______________________________

PMS

☐ Breast Lumps
☐ Sore breasts
☐ Irritable
☐ Depressed
☐ Emotional swings
☐ Bloating
☐ Other _____________________________

Menopause

☐ Do you think you have started? ☒ Yes ☒ No
☐ Irregular cycle time frame: ______________
☐ Anxiety or Depression? ________________
☐ Spotting
☐ Hot flashes
☐ Vaginal dryness/itching

Childbirth

☐ Number of pregnancies: ___________________
☐ Number of births: _________________________
☐ Miscarriages: ☒ Yes ☒ No
☐ Premature births
☐ Cesareans
☐ Abortions

Other

☐ Vaginal pain/rash/irritation
☐ Vaginal discharge __Color:
____

Muscular-Skeletal

☐ Arthritis
☐ Pain _______
☐ Stiff neck
☐ Mobility limitations
☐ Spinal curvature
☐ Other _______

Cancellation Policy

So that I may better serve my clients, 24 hours'notice is required for cancellation. You will be charged the full session with less than 24 hours' notification.

Disclaimer

1. I understand that this work does not constitute, nor it is a substitute for medical treatment, but rather is a form of health maintenance. I realize that this therapist is not a doctor, and does not diagnose, prescribe, or treat any specific conditions.
2. I understand and agree that I am responsible for keeping my therapist informed of any changes in my physical condition, as this could affect the treatment I receive.

Signature ____ Date __________

• **Fig. A.1** Herbal Health History (Continued).

HERBALIST'S ASSESSMENT FORM

S. Client Name ______________________ Date _______ Sex _____ Age_____

Chief Complaint or status since last visit

Secondary Problem(s) or status since last visit

Body Systems: Initial history or status since last visit.

Respiratory______________________________________

Cardiovascular______________________________________

Nervous______________________________________

Urinary______________________________________

Endocrine______________________________________

Gastrointestinal______________________________________

Urinary______________________________________

Skin______________________________________

Musculoskeletal______________________________________

Reproductive

____

Emotional/ Mental Health

____

____

____

General Questions:

Body pain

____

Headache

____

Digestion

____

Stools ______________________________________

Thirst ______________________________________

Sleep ______________________________________

Energy Level

____

Menses/Menopause

____

EENT/Phlegm

____

Emotions

____

• **Fig. A.2** Herbalist's Assessment Form.

HERBALIST'S ASSESSMENT FORM

Lifestyle

____

Exercise

____

Are they taking the herbs/supplements?

____

Typical diet or dietary progress since last visit

____

____

____

H_2O intake________ Favorite foods __________________________ hot or cold ______

raw_______ cooked______ caffeine_______ dairy______ gluten_______

Breakfast	Lunch	Dinner	Snacks

Overall reported progress since last visit

☐ Much Improved ☐ Slightly Improved ☐ No change ☐ Slightly worse ☐ Much worse

O. Pulse rate________ Blood Pressure ___________

Tongue body/ color/shape ____

Tongue coat/color____

Right Pulses	Left Pulses
Overall Depth Overall Strength Overall Quality	Overall Depth Overall Strength Overall Quality
Lung	Heart
Spleen	Liver
Kidney Yin	Kidney Yang

Other Physical Findings (complexion, heart/lung/gut auscultation, lab results, etc.).

• **Fig. A.2** Herbalist's Assessment Form (Continued).

HERBALIST'S ASSESSMENT FORM

____

____

____

____

____

A. Conditions

Hot /Cold Dry/Damp Tense/Weak Hard/Soft Interior /Exterior Excess/Deficient

Chinese Syndromes

____

Western Syndromes (Signs/symptoms, MD diagnosis)

____

Predisposing Causes/Triggers

____

P. Therapeutic Principles (Herbal, dietary, supplements, lifestyle)

Herbal Formula Name ______________________

Dose ______________________________

Instructions ______________________________________

Part	Herb	Rationale

Supplements, Dietary Changes, Lifestyle Suggestions

Treatment Priorities and Sequence

____

____

____

Return visit/referrals ______________________________

Herbalist Signature and Date ______________________________

• **Fig. A.2** Herbalist's Assessment Form (Continued).

HERBAL CONSULT SUGGESTIONS

Herbalist ________________________ *Phone* ____________ *Email* ______________

Client Name ____ **Date** ______________

Herbs (instructions) ____

____

Dietary ____

____

Supplements ____

____

Lifestyle ____

Aromatherapy ____

Referrals ____

Next Appointment Date/Time ____

• **Fig. A.3** Herbal Consult Suggestions.

DRIED PLANT TINCTURE WORKSHEET

GENERAL INFORMATION
Herb botanical name ____
Common name ____________________________ Pinyin name ____________________
Company or location of collection ____
Date received/wildcrafted _____________ Company lot number _______________
Apothecary production lot number_____________ Batch number __________
Herbalist's name____

W/V = Weight-to-Volume **TM = Total Menstruum**

TOM = Total Original Menstruum **OE = Original Ethanol**

AM = Added Menstruum **AE = Added Ethanol**

ETHANOL/WATER MACERATION
W/V ratio □ 1:2 □ 1:3 □ 1:4 □ 1:5 □ Other _____________
Ethanol % ________
Weight of herb _________ g
W/V ratio ______ g x ________ = TM mL _________
Ethanol needed % Ethanol _______ x TM = _______ = mL of needed ethanol ______
Water needed % Water _________ x TM = _______ = mL of needed water ________
Maceration date ______. Date pressed _____. TM _____ mL. Yield _____mL. Loss _____ mL
Initials _____
Notes (Taste, energy, changes next time):

• **Fig. A.4** Dried Plant Tincture Worksheet.

FRESH PLANT TINCTURE WORKSHEET

GENERAL INFORMATION
Herb botanical name
____
Common name ______________________ Pinyin name
____
Company or location of collection ______________________________
Date received/wildcrafted ___________ Company lot number ___________
Apothecary production lot number___________ Batch number ________
Herbalist's Name______________________________

W/V = Weight to volume **TM = Total menstruum**
TOM = Total original menstruum **OE = Original ethanol**
AM = Added menstruum **AE = Added ethanol**

W/V Ratio ☑ 1:2
Ethanol 95-100 %
Weight of fresh herb ________ grams
W/V Ratio ______ g x 2 = TM ________ mL
Ethanol Needed _______ TM mL
Water Needed None
Maceration date ______. Date pressed _____.TM _____mL. Yield ____ mL. Loss _____mL.
Initials _____
Notes (Taste, energy, changes next time)

• **Fig. A.5** Fresh Plant Tincture Worksheet.

PERCOLATION WORKSHEET

GENERAL INFORMATION
Herb botanical name
____
Common name ______________________ Pinyin name ______________________
Company or location of collection ______________________________
Date received/wildcrafted ___________ Company lot number ___________
Apothecary production lot number___________ Batch number ________
Herbalist's name______________________________
W/V = Weight to volume **TM = Total menstruum**
TOM = Total original menstruum **OE = Original ethanol**
AM = Added menstruum **AE = Added ethanol**

W/V Ratio ☐ 1:2 ☐ 1:3 ☐ 1:4 ☐ 1:5 ☐ Other ___________
Ethanol % ______
Weight of Herb _______ grams
W/V Ratio ______ g x _______ = TOM _______ mL
Add to cone TOM ______x 30% or mL of dry herb pressed in cup =AM ______mL
Total menstruum TOM ______mL + AM _______ mL = TM ________mL
Ethanol Needed % EtOH______ x TM = ______mL = mL of needed ethanol ________
Water Needed % water _______ x TM = _______ = mL of needed water ________
Sandcastle date ________ Initial _______
Perc date _____. Date bottled _____. TM _____mL. Yield _____mL. Loss _____mL
Initials _____
Notes (Taste, energy, adjustment for cone addition, did herb perc well, changes next time)

• **Fig. A.6** Percolation Worksheet.

DUAL EXTRACTION WORKSHEET

GENERAL INFORMATION
Herb Botanical Name
____
Common Name ____________________ Pinyin Name ____________________
Company or Location of Collection
____
Date Received/Wildcrafted ___________ Company Lot Number ______________
Apothecary Production Lot Number___________ Batch Number _________
Herbalist's Name________________________________
W/V ratio ☐ 1:2 ☐ 1:3 ☐ 1:4 ☐ 1:5 ☐ Other __________
Ethanol % _______
Weight of Herb _______ g
Method: Maceration and Decoction
W/V Ratio _____ g x _______ = TM _______ mL
Ethanol Needed % EtOH_______ x TM = _______ = mL of needed ethanol ________
Water Needed % water _______ x TM = _______ = mL of needed water ________
Alcohol to Macerate = _________ mL
Water to Decoct = Needed water mL _____ x 2 = _____mL. Decoct down to ½ = _______mL
Date completed _________ OM ______mL Yield_______ mL Loss _______mL
Initials _______
Notes (Taste, energy, changes next time, did more water need to be added to decoction?)

• **Fig. A.7** Dual Extraction Worksheet.

VEGETABLE GLYCERITE WORKSHEET

GENERAL INFORMATION
Herb Botanical Name ____
Common Name ____________________ Pinyin Name ________________
Company or Location of Collection ________________________________
Date Received/Wildcrafted ___________ Company Lot Number ______________
Apothecary Production Lot Number___________ Batch Number _________
Herbalist's Name________________________________

W/V Ratio ☐ 1:2 ☐ 1:3 ☐ 1:4 ☐ 1:5 ☐ Other __________
Glycerin percentage of menstruum (If only using glycerin, it has to be at least 60% by volume to maintain shelf life/stability, a 60% glycerite.)
Glycerite includes what percent ethanol? ______%. **Glycerin %**______
Glycerite includes what percent vinegar? _____% **Weight of herb** _____ grams
W/V Ratio ______ grams x ________ = TM _______ mL
Glycerin needed % glycerin ______ x TM ____ ___ = _______mL glycerin
Ethanol needed % ethanol ________ x TM = ___ ___ = _______ mL ethanol
Vinegar needed % vinegar _______ x TM = ______ = ______mL vinegar
Water needed Glycerin mL _____ + EtOH mL _____ + Vinegar mL ____ = ______mL
TM _______mL – sum of glycerin + ethanol + vinegar = _____mL water
Date completed ______ TM ______mL Yield_______ mL Loss _______mL
Initials _____
Notes: Taste, energy, changes next time, how did it taste? Need more or less glycerin?

• **Fig. A.8** Vegetable Glycerite Worksheet.

WILDCRAFTING INFORMATION SHEET

Herbalist name ______________________________
Date gathered ___________________ **Time of day gathered** _____________
Botanical name________________________________
Common name(s)______________________________ **Batch number**_______
Type of plant part(s) gathered ________________________
Weather conditions during harvest ________________________
Location of area where gathered (Map, directions as needed.)

Description of area where gathered (Terrain, distance from highway, mountain, prairie, river, open field, back yard.)

Permit information (Whose land? permit-Yes, No From where or whom, date?)

Cleaning Method (shaking, peeling, washing, tools)

Drying method and conditions (Tinctured fresh, racks, dehydrator, basket, temperature, ventilation, indoors or outdoors?)

Assessment of process (Did drying, cleaning, gathering methods work? Suggestions.)

Fresh weight (grams or ounces) _____________ **Dried weight (grams or ounces)** ________

I have gathered these herbs in a manner which is harmonious and respectful to the Earth and in an area which was unpolluted and did not disrupt the eco-system.

Gatherer _____________________________ **Date** ________________

• **Fig. A.9** Wildcrafting Information Sheet.

Appendix B

Answers to Chapter Review Questions, Fill in the Blanks

Part I: The Basics

Chapter 2: The History of Herbalism

(1) Hippocrates. **(2)** Syphilis. **(3)** Physica. **(4)** Bloodletting, mercury, arsenic. **(5)** Caduceus. **(6)** Galen. **(7)** Avicenna (Ibn Sina). **(8)** United States Pharmacopeia. **(9)** John King, John Uri Lloyd, Harvey Felter, John Milton Scudder, and Finley Ellingwood. **(10)** Physiomedicalists, William Cook, *Physio-Medical Dispensary*.

Chapter 3: Philosophical Constructs of Herbalism

(1) Right. **(2)** Traditional, Ayurvedic, Western European, and Chinese Medicine. **(3)** Traditional. **(4)** Thought process in making health care decisions. **(5)** Analytical. **(6)** Breaking and entering. **(7)** Altering energy. **(8)** Doing nothing.

Chapter 4: Taxonomy and Botany for Herbalists

(1) A two-name system of classification for all living things. The first name is the genus, the second name is the specie**s**. **(2)** Division, class, subclass, order, family, genus, species. **(3)** Gymnosperm: vascular, naked seeds in cones. Angiosperm: vascular, seeds fully enclosed and protected in an ovary which grows into a flower. **(4)** Monocot: one seed leaf, parallel veins in the leaves, horizontal rootstalks, floral parts mostly in threes. Dicot: two seed leaves, netted veins in the leaves, generally tap rooted, complex branching, floral parts mostly in fours and fives. **(5)** A stamen consists of pollen, anther, and filament. **(6)** A pistil consists of a stigma, style, ovary, and ovule. **(7)** Lamiaceae, Apiaceae, Brassicaceae, Fabaceae, Liliaceae, Poaceae, Rosaceae, Asteraceae **(8)** Square stalks, opposite leaves, usually aromatic. **(9)** Flowers with banner, wings, and keel. Seeds with pods. Leaves are pinnate. **(10.)** Flower is a compound umbel. Stalk is hollow.

Chapter 5: Wildcrafting, Preparation, Storage and Purchasing

(1) Downward, fall. **(2)** Upwards, aerial, late spring, summer. **(3)** Hori hori, shovel, knife, collecting bag, clippers, water, hat. **(4)** More than two years. **(5)** Nylon screens, drying racks, dehydrators, upside down bunches, flat baskets. **(6)** Heat, light, moisture. **(7)** Circulate all around the plant. **(8)** greens and flowers: 1 year. Roots, seeds, and barks: 2 to 3 years. **(9)** Common name, botanical name, date, place of origin (where wildcrafted or herb company name and lot number). **(10)** Longitudinal cuts, no more than one quarter of the branch circumference or from cut or fallen branch.

Chapter 6: Types of Herbal Remedies

(1) Water, alcohol, glycerin, vinegar, wine, fixed oil. **(2)** Relaxing, restoring, stimulating, sitz, douche, clear heat. **(3)** Gargles, compresses, baths. **(4)** Tinctures: 1 part root or herb to 3 to 5 parts solvent or menstruum. Extracts or concentrates: 1 part herb to 1 to 2 parts menstruum. **(5)** Internal or ingestible, tinctures, ethane. **(6)** External, liniments, propane. **(7)** Oxymel, cordial, medicated syrup. **(8)** Alcohol, glycerin, vinegar, water. **(9)** Salve: oil or fat. Cream: water and oil/fat base and requires emulsification. **(10)** Maceration, menstruum, marc.

Chapter 7: Preparation of Tinctures, Infused oils, Salves, Lotions, Creams and Syrups

(1) One cubic centimeter (cc) of water weighs 1 gram (g). **(2)** Ethanol, isopropyl. **(3)** Tannins, mucilage, some flavonoids and saponins. **(4)** Alkaloids, essential oils, most saponins, and some glycosides. **(5)** Resins and oleoresins, 60% to 90% alcohol. Wormwood, Yarrow, Myrrh. **(6)** Herb weight = 240 g. TM = 960 mL. Total alcohol = 576 mL. Total water = 384 mL. **(7)** OM = 600 mL. AM = 180 mL. TM = 780 mL. Total water = 390 mL. Total alcohol = 390 mL. **(8)** Hot water decoction and ethanol maceration **(9)** Solar oil method 4 to 6 weeks. Double boiler digestion method, a few hours. Accelerated blender version, one-half hour**.** **(10)** Pour oil in slowly. Don't touch the cream because of contamination. Get out all bubbles.

Chapter 8: Chemical Constituents for Herbalists

(1) Pharmacognosy**.** **(2)** Carbohydrates, amino acid derivatives, lipids, phenolic compounds, terpenes, and alkaloids. **(3)** Carbohydrates, fats, and proteins. **(4)** White Willow bark, Meadowsweet, Wintergreen leaf, Sweet Birch bark, Cramp bark, Black Haw bark, and the Poplars, including Aspen bark. **(5)** Allicin. **(6)** Flax seed, Milk Thistle seed, Schisandra Wu Wei Zi. **(7)** Flavonoids, Phenols. **(8)** Angelica Dong Quai, Alfalfa herb, Red and White Clover flower, Hops flower. **(9)** Terpenes. Thymol, limonene, iridoids, menthol, glycyrrhizin. **(10)** Berberines, antimicrobial. Oregon Grape root, Barberry, and Coptis Huang Lian (Goldthread root).

Chapter 9: Basic Concepts of Chinese Medicine

(1) Medical qi gong, massage, nutrition, herbal medicine, acupuncture. **(2)** Internal, damp, cold, and moist. **(3)** The body's immune system. **(4)** Wood, Fire, Earth, Metal, and Water. **(5)** Liver-Gallbladder, Heart-Small Intestine, Spleen-Stomach, Lung-Large Intestine, and Kidney-Bladder. **(6)** Heart. **(7)** Liver. **(8)** **P** Weak and thin. **T** Pale, absent coat. **(9)** **P** slippery. **T** Puddled with moisture, scalloped, and/or a thicker or greasier coat. **(10)** Spleen Damp Heat.

Chapter 10: Energetics and Western Herbology

(1) Taste, warmth, and moisture. **(2)** Sweet, salty, bitter, pungent, sour. **(3)** Stimulate/sedate, restore/relax, moisten/decongest. **(4)** Bee pollen, Shitake mushroom, Oat Straw, Blue-green Algae, Nettle, sea vegetables, wheat grass. **(5)** Ginger, Oregano, Barley, Docks, Goldenseal, Water Hemlock. **(6)** Soften hardened tissue or lumps or stones. Use for kidney and gall stones, cholesterol deposits, hardenings. **(7)** Litholytics, antiatherosclerotics, antilipidemics. **(8)** Cold, hot, weak, tense, dry, damp. **(9)** Licorice root. **(10)** Acute urinary tract infection, urinary retention, congestive heart failure, and face and limb edema.

Part II: Materia Medica

Chapter 11: Basic Materia Medica

(1) Relaxes. **(2)** Astringent/coagulant for bleeding. Astringent for fibroids or diarrhea. Antimicrobial for infection. Progesteronic for premenstrual syndrome or menopause. Diaphoretic for early onset colds/flu. **(3)** Antilipemic, antilithic, anticoagulant. Tonifies heart and blood qi. **(4)** Nervine. Coptis Huang Lian, Goldenseal root, and Oregon Grape root. **(5)** Viral infections such as cold sores, genital herpes, shingles. Damp heat. **(6)** Boils, sores, ulcers, eczema, or psoriatic arthritis. **(7)** Cold, bitter, and dry. **(8)** Red Clover flower. Yarrow herb. Vitex berry. **(9)** Hypertension, increased sodium, aldosterone effect, or hyperglycemia. **(10)** *Crataegus oxyacantha* L. Heart tonic, antilipemic, antilithic, and anticoagulant. **(11)** Ginkgo leaf and Turmeric root.

Chapter 12: Materia Media Groupings

(1) Lobelia herb, Chamomile flower. **(2)** Asparagus root. Comfrey root, allantoin. Vulnerary. **(3)** Ayurvedic adaptogen: Ashwagandha. Chinese Medicine adaptogen: Schisandra Wu Wei Zi or Astragalus Huang Qi. Adaptogenic mushrooms: Ganoderma Ling Zhi (Reishi mushroom) and shitake mushroom. Adaptogen for depression: Rhodiola root. **(4)** Super foods are broccoli, bee pollen, sea veggies. Companion herbs are Ginkgo herb, Nettle herb, Elderberry berry, Hawthorn berry, Saw Palmetto berry, Lycium Gou Qi Zi (Wolfberry), and Bilberry berry. Also, Green and Rooibos tea. **(5)** Burdock root and Celery seed work on kidneys. Cleavers herb for lymph. **(6)** Thyme or Garden Sage leaf for a cool, hacking cough with white sputum. Chrysanthemum Ju Hua or Coltsfoot herb for yellow/green sputum. **(7)** Platycodon Jie Geng and Wild Cherry bark. **(8)** Pregnancy: Raspberry leaf. Menopause: Vitex berry and Rehmannia Shu Di Huang. Dysmenorrhea: Cramp bark, Paeonia Bai Shao Yao (White Peony root) or Pasque flower herb. **(9)** Andrographis Chuan Xin Lian (Heart-thread Lotus leaf) for infection and Xanthium Cang Er Zi (Siberian cocklebur fruit) for secretions. **(10)** Lonicera Jin Yin Hua (Honeysuckle flower) is cold and sweet. Garlic bulb is hot and pungent. Andrographis Chuan Xin Lian is cold and bitter. Osha root is warm and pungent/bitter. Wormwood herb is cold and bitter. Uva Ursi leaf is cold and astringent.

Part III: The Herbalist in Action

Chapter 13: Herbal Safety

(1) Allergic reactions. **(2)** Meadowsweet herb, Sweet Clover herb, Saw Palmetto berry, Willow bark. **(3)** Sweet Birch bark, Willow bark, Wintergreen herb and root, Meadowsweet herb, various Poplars including Aspen bark. **(4)** Increase force of contractions, decrease heart rate. Treat congestive heart failure. Drugs are Digoxin and Lanoxin derived from digitalis. Herbs with cardiac glycosides are Lily of the Valley herb, Squill bulb leaf scales, Dogbane seed, root, and bark, Pleurisy root, Oleander herb, Night Blooming cactus stem, Foxglove herb and root. **(5)** Vasodilators, emmenagogues, uterine stimulants. **(6)** Intestinal cramping, uterine contractions, watery diarrhea. Long-term use leads to dependency, dehydration, and electrolyte imbalance. Examples: *Cascara sagrada* bark, Aloe Vera resin, Senna leaf and fruit, Rhubarb root. **(7)** Adrenal cortex. Tumors can cause hyperaldosteronism. Symptoms are edema, hypertension, low K^+, high Na^+ and cardiac involvement. Licorice root can mimic this. Syndrome is then called pseudoaldosteronism. **(8)** Aconite root, Bloodroot, Ephedra stem, Poke root, Lobelia herb, Yarrow herb, and essential oils of Chamomile, Tansy, Pennyroyal, and Rue. **(9)** Comfrey leaf and root, Coltsfoot herb. PAs can cause liver damage.

Chapter 14: Formulating, Dispensing and Dosing

(1) Therapeutic principle. **(2)** Primary therapeutic action. **(3)** Compliment effect of principle action. **(4)** Address symptoms not yet covered. **(5)** Fine tune formula. **(6)** 60 mL of each herb. **(7)** 1 part = 40 mL. Need 120 mL Dandelion root, 80 mL Bupleurum Chai Hu, 40 mL Milk Thistle seed for an 8-oz bottle. **(8)** 3 to 4 cups daily for several weeks. **(9)** ¼ to ½ cup throughout day up to 3 to 4 cups. **(10)** 1 to 5 mL three × day.

Chapter 15: History, Assessment, and Documentation

(1) Herbal Health History form, Herbalist's Assessment form, Herbal Consult Suggestions form. **(2)** Taste, emotion, sense organ, tissue, voice or sound, environmental factor, element, season. **(3)** Liver 1 a.m. to 3 a.m., Heart 11:00 a.m. to 1:00 p.m., Spleen

9:00 a.m. to 11 a.m., Kidney 5:00 p.m. to 7:00 p.m., Lungs 3:00 a.m. to 5:00 a.m., Pericardium 7:00 p.m. to 9 p.m. **(4)** Subjective, Objective, Assessment, Plan. **(5)** African-American descent, elderly, obese, heavy drinker, insulin and leptin resistance, gout, kidney disease, birth control pills. **(6)** Health Insurance Portability and Accountability Act. **(7)** Suspected cancer, undiagnosed lumps, chest pain, difficulty breathing, uneven pupils, slurred speech, droopy mouth, loss of movement, black, tarry stools. **(8)** Right wrist: Lung, Spleen, Kidney yang. Left wrist: Heart, Liver, Kidney yin. **(9)** Depth, strength, quality. **(10)** Body color, body shape, fur quality, fur color.

Part IV: Case Histories, Therapeutics and Formulations

Chapter 16: Maintaining the Body in Health

(1) Prostaglandins, interleukins, leukotrienes, eicosanoids. **(2)** Intestinal permeability, dysbiosis. Caused by genetically modified organisms (GMOs), refined sugar, high fructose corn syrup, food allergens, artificial hormones, processed foods. **(3)** Antimicrobials, bitters, cholagogues, gut restoratives, herbs to dry mucous damp. **(4)** Premature aging and degenerative diseases, including cancer. **(5)** Liver: Milk Thistle seed. GI: Licorice root or Atractylodes Bai Zu (White Atractylodes root). Adrenals: Nettle herb or Ashwagandha root. Lungs: Sage leaf. Heart: Hawthorn berry. Kidneys: Goldenrod herb. **(6)** Arugula, coffee, dark chocolate, endive. **(7)** Healthy diet, avoiding electric and magnetic fields, connection to friends and family, adequate sleep, stress management, full-spectrum lighting and sunlight, handwashing. **(8)** Normalize stress, balance the hypothalamic-pituitary-adrenal axis. **(9)** Restoratives, adaptogens, tonics. **(10)** Qi, blood, yin, yang tonics.

Chapter 17: Infection and Toxicosis

(1) Cold, bitter, astringent, drying, and sinking. **(2)** *Echinacea angustifolia*, *Ligusticum porterii*, Andrographis Chuan Xin Lian. **(3)** Coptis Huang Lian, Oregon Grape root, Juniper berry, honey, Garlic bulb. **(4)** Antimicrobials, immunostimulants, detoxicants/alteratives, restoratives, synergists. **(5)** Antiparasitic herbs. If external, treat internally also. Treat underlying problem. Flush out helminths. Immunostimulants. **(6)** *Echinacea* spp., Ganoderma Ling Zhi, Lonicera Jin Yin Hua, Forsythia Lian Qiao, Andrographis Chuan Xin Lian. **(7)** Wind cold, wind heat, damp heat, and toxic heat. **(8)** Tumors, cysts, ulcers, boils, skin rashes, eczema. **(9)** Quorum sensing, multiple drug resistant efflux pump, layering of different species within the biofilm, aerobic and anaerobic organisms within same biofilm. **(10)** *Echinacea* spp., *Ligusticum porterii*, *Andrographis paniculata*, *Scutellaria baicalensis* Huang Qin, *Lonicera japonica* Jin Yin Hua, *Glycyrrhiza glabra* or *G. sinensis*.

Chapter 18: The Gastrointestinal System

(1) Digestion. Worry or overthinking. Sweet, dry, warm. **(2)** **P** Weak, slow, deep. **T** Pale, swollen, wet. Diarrhea. **(3)** Food triggers, parasites, bacteria, small intestine bacterial overgrowth (SIBO), yeast, non-steroidal anti-inflammatory drugs (NSAIDs). **(4)** Digestive enzymes, hydrochloric acid, prebiotics. **(5)** Digestive enzymes, stimulate appetite, balance glucose levels, stimulate bile flow, antimicrobial, repair the gut lining. **(6)** Western: Burdock root, Irish Moss, Slippery Elm bark. Chinese Medicine: Codonopsis Dang Shen, White Atractylodes Bai Zhu and Panax Xi Yang Shen (American Ginseng root). **(7)** Tannin and astringent. Calamus root, White Oak bark, Cranesbill root, Yarrow herb. **(8)** Meadowsweet herb, Iceland Moss, Chickweed herb, Calamus root. **(9)** Unsweetened yogurt or kefir, miso, kimchi, fermented veggies. **(10)** Rectal itching and burning, extreme exhaustion, sweet cravings, gas and bloating, food sensitivities, and brain fog.

Chapter 19: The Hepato-biliary System

(1) *Silybum marianum* (Milk Thistle seed), *Taraxacum officinale* (Dandelion root), *Schisandra chinensis* Wu Wei Zi (Five Taste berry), *Bupleurum chinense* Chai Hu (Asian Buplever root), *Cynara scolymus* (Artichoke leaf), *Urtica dioica* (Nettle herb), *Zizyphus* jujube Da Zao (Jujube berry). **(2)** Extreme fatigue, skin outbreaks, environmental sensitivity, chronic headaches, mental confusion, muddled thoughts, bitter taste, and digestive problems. **(3)** Drugs, alcohol, polluted air or water, heavy metals, chemical fertilizers, nonorganic food, food additives, and leaky gut. **(4)** Lead, mercury, cadmium, and inorganic arsenic. **(5)** Many skin problems, fatigue, depressed immunity, neurological symptoms including brain fog, memory loss, gastrointestinal symptoms, and bitter taste in mouth. **(6)** Strong: Wormwood herb, Gentian root, Blue flag root. Mild: Dandelion root, Garden Sage leaf, Artichoke leaf. **(7)** Chinese Medicine: Scutellaria Huang Qi, Rhubarb Da Huang, Bupleurum Chai Hu, Coptis Huang Lian. Western: Gentian root, Wormwood herb, Fringe Tree bark, Celandine herb. **(8)** Gallbladder Damp Heat. **P** Slippery and wiry. **T** Red body with thick, sticky, yellow coating. **(9)** Gardenia Zhi Zi, Rhubarb root, Gentian root, Barberry root, Fringe Tree bark. **(10)** Glutathione. Foods: cruciferous veggies, mushrooms, avocados, onions, spinach. Herbs: Milk Thistle seed, Platycodon Jie Geng, Turmeric root, Astragalus Huang Qi.

Chapter 20: The Respiratory System

(1) Expectorants, demulcent, antitussive, antimicrobial, nervous relaxant, or nervine. **(2)** External Wind Heat, External Wind Cold, External Wind Damp Heat, Lung Yin Deficiency, Lung Qi Deficiency, Lung Phlegm Damp. **(3)** Warming: Angelica root or Osha root. Cool: *Calendula officinalis*, *Echinacea* spp. Very cold: Andrographis Chuan Xin Lian, Goldenseal root or Coptis Huang Lian. **(4)** Stimulating expectorants are warm and dry. Thyme herb, *Angelica archangelica* root, Elecampane root, Hyssop herb, Yerba Santa leaf, Basil herb, Pinellia Ban Xia. Used in cold, damp conditions. **(5)** Bronchodilators, antitussives, demulcents, antiasthmatic remedies. **(6)** Western: Marshmallow root, Slippery Elm bark, Irish Moss, Iceland Moss. Chinese Medicine: Ophiopogon Mai Men Dong, Glycyrrhiza Gan Cao, Codonopsis Dang Shen, Astragalus Huang Qi. **(7)** **T** body red, coat sticky yellow. **P** rapid and slippery. **(8)** Lung Yin tonic for a dry, hacky cough. Use mucogenics and demulcents. **(9)** Lung qi tonic for weak conditions like chronic asthma, seasonal allergies, and chronic bronchitis/sinusitis. Use Lung adaptogens. **(10)** Treat infection, treat pain, lymphatic drainers for detox and draining tonsils, throat gargles.

Chapter 21: Pediatrics

(1) Clark's dose 1.12 mL; Young's Rule 1.0 mL. **(2)** 0.45 mL, Fried's rule. **(3)** Respiratory, gastrointestinal, nervous, integumentary. **(4)** Immunity, building gut flora, no milk allergies. **(5)** Liver matures at age 3, gut matures by ages 10 to 12. **(6)** Chamomile flower, Passionflower, Lemon Balm leaf, California poppy herb, Lavender herb. **(7)** Diaphoretics: Elderberry, Catnip herb, Ginger root, Melissa balm leaf. **(8)** Dehydration; high carb, low fruit and vegetable diet; bed rest; lack of exercise. **(9)** Herbal popsicles, gelatin cubes, licorice root sticks, baths, putting tincture in apple juice. **(10)** Dehydration, persistent cramping, bloody stools, diarrhea lasting more than 2 weeks.

Chapter 22: The Cardiovascular System

(1) Simple sugars/carbohydrates, trans fats. **(2)** Smoking, hypertension, high cholesterol, diabetes, obesity, family history of insulin and leptin resistance, gluten sensitivity, dysbiosis, diet high in saturated and trans fats. **(3)** Lp(a), ApoB/ApoA ratio, and triglyceride/HDL ratio. **(4)** General restoratives, arterial stimulants, venous decongestants, and capillary stimulants. **(5)** Thrombolytics. Chinese Medicine: Ligusticum Chuan Xiong and Salvia Dan Shen. Western: Hawthorn berry, Ginkgo leaf, and Lily of the Valley herb. **(6)** Hypertension. Coleus root, Hawthorn berry, Passionflower, and Olive leaf. **(7)** Astringents to decrease vein diameter. Restoratives to tone and strengthen connective tissue vessels. Antiinflammatories to ease discomfort. Bioflavonoids to strengthen vessels. Circulatory stimulants to stop stasis. **(8)** Congestive heart failure. Heart Qi Deficiency. **(9)** Antilipidemics. Turmeric root, Globe Artichoke leaf, Hawthorn berry, Oregon Grape root, Garlic bulb capsules, and Gotu Kola herb. **(10)** Decrease heart rate and increase force of contractions.

Chapter 23: The Neurological System

(1) Fermented foods, no simple sugars, good quality sleep, sunshine, and eliminate food sensitivities like gluten or lactose. **(2)** Dopamine, serotonin, glutamate, norepinephrine, nitric oxide. **(3)** Cause drowsiness, depress the CNS, can inhibit motor function, and induce a healing state of sleep. **(4)** Herbal hypnotics: Kava root, Passionflower, Wild Lettuce leaf, Jamaican Dogwood root bark, and Valerian root. **(5)** Nervous system restoratives: Basil leaf, Ginkgo leaf, Polygonum He Shou Wu, Garden Sage leaf, Rosemary leaf, Skullcap herb. Relaxants include categories of anxiolytics, spasmolytics, hypnotics, analgesics, and anticonvulsants. **(6)** Western: Jamaican Dogwood root bark. Eastern: Corydalis Yan Hu Suo. **(7)** Panax Xi Yang Shen (American Ginseng root), Ginkgo leaf, Rosemary leaf, Basil leaf, Garden Sage leaf, and Polygonum He Shou Wu (Flowery Knotweed root). **(8)** Shen disturbance of the Heart. **(9)** St. John's Wort. **(10)** Chamomile flower, Hops flower, Melissa Balm leaf, Valerian root, Cramp bark, and Fennel seed.

Chapter 24: The Muscular-Skeletal System

(1) Gout. **(2)** Tendon, ligaments, muscle, bone, cartilage, fascia, blood. **(3)** Red meats, soft drinks, processed foods, excessive amounts of alcohol and caffeine. **(4)** Lupus, rheumatoid arthritis, fibromyalgia, sarcoidosis. **(5)** Bones, sinews (ligaments and tendons). **(6)** Dairy, canned fish with bones such as sardines, sesame seeds, almonds, dark green leafy veggies. **(7)** Siegesbeckia Xi Xian Cao, Angelica Du Ho, Cinnamomum Gui Zhi, Ledebouriella Fang Feng; Prickly Ash bark, Blue Cohosh root, Ginger root, Jamaican Sarsaparilla root. **(8)** Stephania Han Fang Ji, Siegesbeckia Xi Xian Cao, Bupleurum Chai Hu; Black Cohosh root, Celery seed, Devil's Claw root, Cat's Claw root, Meadowsweet herb. **(9)** Eucommia Du Chong, Eleuthero Ci Wu Jia, Panax San Qi; Horsetail, Nettle herb, Walnut hull and leaf. **(10)** Moxibustion, cupping, tui na, and acupuncture.

Chapter 25: The Integumentary System

(1) Protection from sun, heat, cold, first line of defense against the exterior (immune function), endocrine gland, exocrine gland, temperature regulation, sensory organ, and detoxifier. **(2)** Skin and body hair. **(3)** Clubbing is oxygen lack. Pale is anemia or blood deficiency. Pitting indicates psoriasis. Thickening and yellowing indicates poor circulation or fungal infection. **(4)** Endocrine: Vitamin D manufacture. Exocrine: sweat and oil glands. **(5)** **P** Wiry, rapid. **T** Red body, yellow, thick sticky coat. **(6)** Lymphatic: Red Root, Cleavers herb, and Calendula flower. Kidney: Burdock root, Goldenrod herb, and Nettle herb. Liver: Blue Flag root, Yellow Dock root, and Poke root. **(7)** Antimicrobial, antiinflammatory, prevents scarring, controls odor, absorbs moisture, doesn't spoil. **(8)** Lacerations: cut in the skin. Abrasions: superficial scrapes. Hematomas: a bruise. Puncture wounds: splinters, thorns, or foreign objects piercing the skin. **(9)** *Stellaria media* (Chickweed herb), *Hamamelis virginica* (Witch Hazel leaf), *Calendula officinalis* (Marigold flower), *Avena sativa* (Oats in the form of a colloidal Oatmeal bath). **(10)** Wind Damp Heat with dryness. Wind Damp Heat. Toxic Heat.

Chapter 26: The Urinary System

(1) Water balance, electrolyte balance, pH balance, manufacture of urine, detoxification, maintains BP. **(2)** Kidneys open to the ears, govern the bones (marrow) and teeth, manifest in the head hair. Kidney emotion is fear. Element is water. Color is dark blue or black. **(3)** Chinese Medicine: Dianthus Qu Mai (Proud Pink herb), Alisma Zi Xie (Water Plantain root), Akebia Mu Tong. (Akebia stem). Western: *Arctostaphylos uva-ursi*, *Elymus repens* (Couch Grass root), *Vaccinium myrtillus* (Bilberry leaf and fruit), *Piper mysticum* (Kava root). **(4)** Lin, hot, cold. **(5)** Western: *Arctium lappa* (Burdock root), *Collinsonia canadensis* (Stone root), *Eupatorium purpureum* (Gravel root), *Hydrangea arborescens* (Hydrangea root), *Polygonum aviculare* (Knot grass root), *Crataeva nurvala* (Crataeva stem and root bark). **(6)** Stress incontinence or qi deficiency. Weak pelvic-floor muscles. Spastic neurogenic bladder due to muscle spasms when bladder is empty but there is urgency. Atonic neurogenic bladder where there is no muscle tone, so there is leakage. Estrogen deficiency from thinning of tissue and dryness. **(7)** Astringe and tone bladder wall smooth muscles and help flush out residual urine. Chinese Medicine restoratives: Cuscuta Tu Si Zi (Asian Dodder seed) and Coix Yi Yi Ren (Job's Tears seed). Western restoratives: *Solidago virgaurea* (Goldenrod herb), *Piper methysticum* (Kava root), *Equisetum arvense* (Horsetail herb). **(8)** Western antimicrobial diuretics: Fresh Yarrow herb, Uva ursi leaf, Couch Grass root. Chinese Medicine antimicrobial diuretics: Dianthus Qu Mai, Alisma Zi Xie (Water Plantain root). **(9)** Multiple pregnancies and childbirths, menopause, overweight, and prostatitis. **(10)** Re Lin damp heat, acute urinary tract infection. Xue Lin, passing blood. Shi Lin, stones. Gao Lin, greasy urine. Lao Lin, kidney spleen deficiency, dribbling, and incontinence.

Chapter 27: The Endocrine System

(1) Adrenal cortex, adrenal medulla, stress hormones. **(2)** Insulin resistance, syndrome X, type 2 diabetes. **(3)** Broccoli, cauliflower, and kale. **(4)** Blood test marker that reflects average glucose levels over a 2- to 3-month period, providing a long-term risk factor in diabetes. **(5)** *Spirulina* spp. and *Chlorella* spp. **(6)** Kidney Qi Deficiency. **P** Slow, soft and deep. **T** Pale with a white coat. **(7)** *Gymnema sylvestre* (Gymnema leaf), *Momordica charantia* (Bitter Melon), *Curcuma longa* (Turmeric root), *Olea europea* (Olive leaf), *Trigonella foenum-graecum* (Fenugreek seed), and all the berberines. **(8)** Maca root, Rooibos tea, blue-green algae, sea vegetables, Bee Pollen, blue and red berries. **(9)** Fluorine, chlorine, bromine, iodine. Sources are chlorinated water, fluoridated toothpaste, brominated flour. **(10)** Yin tonics*:* *Rehmannia glutinosa* Shu Di Huang (Prepared Rehmannia root), *Glycyrrhiza uralensis* Gan Cao (Licorice root), *Eleutherococcus senticosus* Ci Wu Jia (Siberian ginseng root). Yang tonics: *Cervus nippon* Lu Rong (Velvet Deer Antler), *Dioscorea opposita* Shan Yao (Mountain Yam root), *Schisandra chinensis* Wu Wei Zi (Five Taste berry). Qi tonics: *Ganoderma lucidum* Ling Zhi (Reishi mushroom), *Panax quinquefolius* Xi Yang Shen (American Ginseng root,) *Eleutherococcus senticosus* Ci Wu Jia (Siberian Ginseng root).

Chapter 28: The Reproductive System

(1) Follicle Stimulating Hormone (FSH), estrogen. **(2)** Luteinizing Hormone (LH), progesterone. **(3)** Testosterone. **(4)** Balance microbiome, minimize xenoestrogens, maintain liver health, eat cruciferous veggies, balance immune system, manage stress, supplementation. **(5)** Cells of ovaries, fat, gut, breasts, skin, muscles, lungs, mitochondrial liver cells. **(6)** Soy isoflavones: edamame, soybeans, miso, tempeh, soymilk. Lignins: golden flax seed, whole grains, legumes, sesame seeds. **(7)** Male erectile dysfunction and infertility. **P** Deep and weak. **T** Pale. **(8)** Scanty, pale menstrual flow and menopausal hot flashes. **P** Thready, wiry and rapid. **T** Red with scant coat. **(9)** Yang, yin. **(10)** Estrogen deficiency, progesterone deficiency.

Part V: Getting Out There

Chapter 29: Herbal Legalities

(1) Food supplement, not a drug. **(2)** Over-the-counter drug used to treat morning sickness in pregnancy. **(3)** Birth defects, tightening up regulations. **(4)** Back pain. **(5)** Uses, dosages, side effects, and any known drug/herb interactions. **(6)** Japanese study and adaptation of traditional Chinese Medicine. **(7)** Drug, more than 4000 herbs. **(8)** Active ingredient. **(9)** Marker compound, percentage. **(10)** World Health Organization ensures safety of air, food, water, medicines, and vaccines.

Chapter 30: Building Your Practice

(1) Horehound herb, Cranberry, and *Echinacea* spp. **(2)** Three basin sink, floor waste drains, proper covering of herbs, hair coverings, and gloves. **(3)** Recording manufacturer's and apothecary lot numbers, dates, supplier, and proper labeling. **(4)** American Herbalists Guild, American Botanical Council, American Herbal Pharmacopeia, and National Institute of Medical Herbalists.

Glossary

A

Abortifacients Herbs that can terminate pregnancy.

Abrasion A superficial tearing away of the skin, no deeper than the epidermis. A scrape or road rash.

Acne Vulgaris Inflammatory skin condition involving over-secretion of sebum (oil) from the sebaceous glands into the hair follicles.

Active Component Constituent considered to be the active ingredient in an herb. Example: Curcumin in *Curcuma longa* (Turmeric root). Does not account for all the other chemicals contained in the plant, nor their synergy.

Acupuncture Chinese practice of inserting fine needles through the skin at meridian points to cure disease or relieve pain.

Acute Otitis Media (AOM) Painful middle ear inflammation and bacterial infection with pus behind the eardrum, common in children.

Acute New, unexpected sudden outbreak of a condition or disease.

Adaptogens Herbs that stimulate the HPA axis, restore, nourish, and help the body balance stress. Examples: Eleuthero Ci Wu Jia (Siberian Ginseng root), Rhodiola root, and Ashwagandha root.

Adrenal Burnout or Fatigue Collection of symptoms, such as body aches, fatigue, nervousness, sleep disturbances, digestive problems, and hormonal imbalances occurring when cortisol production runs out of steam and becomes chronically low.

Adrenaline Stress hormone secreted by the adrenal medulla that initiates sudden stress, fight, or flight reactions.

Aerial The parts of a plant above ground: flowers, seeds, stems, and leaves. Referred to as the *herb*.

Alchemy The forerunner of modern chemistry. A philosophy practiced in the Middle Ages, Renaissance, and by some today. Some alchemist's goals were to discover methods for transmuting baser metals into gold and for finding a universal solvent and elixir of life.

Alkaloids The most potent group of herbal constituents with at least one nitrogen atom in a heterocyclic ring. Classification is based on the type of ring system present. Alkaloids have a wide range of uses and many are synthesized and used in the drug industry. Examples of herbs that contain alkaloids: Comfrey root, Lobelia herb, and Coptis Huang Lian (Goldthread root).

Alkamides A class of lipophilic (fat soluble) polyunsaturated fatty acid molecules. Herbal examples: Echinacea root, Prickly Ash bark, and several peppers including Black Pepper and Long Pepper.

Allicin The active ingredient in Garlic bulb derived from the amino acid, cysteine.

Allopathic Medicine Refers broadly to medical practice that is also termed Western medicine or evidence-based medicine. Adheres to drugs, surgery, and the scientific method.

Alteratives Herbs that improve cellular nutrition and lymphatic drainage through detoxification, sometimes called *depuratives*. Eclectics called them *blood purifiers*. Examples: Burdock root, Yellow Dock root, and Red Clover flower.

Amenorrhea A period stopped for at least three previous menstrual cycles or at least 6 months in a previously menstruating woman, and not from normal causes such as pregnancy, menopause, or breastfeeding.

American Botanical Council (ABC) Founded in 1988 by Mark Blumenthal. Prestigious herbal organization that provides traditional and science based herbal education to herbalists, healthcare professionals, the public, and the media.

American Herbal Pharmacopeia (AHP) Founded in 1995 by herbalist Roy Upton. Publishes herbal monographs and other educational materials, the closest the United States has to Commission E.

American Herbalist Guild (AHG) A non-profit, educational organization founded in 1989 that represents the goals and voices of herbalists. Mission is to support access to herbal medicine for all and excellence in herbal education.

Amino Acids The building blocks of plant and animal proteins, a macronutrient. Contains various numbers of amine and carboxylic acid functional groups.

Anabolism Form of metabolism where the body builds up substances needed in growth and repair. The process requires energy. Example: the creation of bone mass (protein).

Analgesics Herbs that remove symptoms of pain.

Analytic Approach The scientific method. An approach to healing that sees the body as a machine made up of parts and chemicals. If those aspects are addressed, the person is healed.

Anaphylactic Shock Type I immediate sensitivity allergic reaction manifested by hives, face swelling, swollen tongue, and difficulty breathing. A medical emergency.

Androgen The major male steroid hormone that triggers development of male sexual characteristics at puberty.

Angina Pectoris Temporary chest pain on exertion and/or stress when the heart muscle is not getting enough oxygen. It abates with rest and is caused by a partial blockage in the coronary arteries due to fatty plaque or a blood clot.

Angiosperms All flowering plants with seeds enclosed in an ovary, the most recent and numerous plants on Earth.

Angiotensin Converting Enzyme (ACE2) An enzyme (protein) triggered by the kidney's renin from the juxtaglomerular (JG) apparatus. ACE2 triggers conversion of angiotensin I into the powerful vasoconstrictor, angiotensin II. The resultant vessel narrowing helps maintain blood pressure. ACE2 is also present in the heart, lungs, and other tissues.

Anhidrotics Herbs that decrease sweating by astringing, tightening and tonifying tissues. Examples: Garden Sage or Witch Hazel leaf.

Anthelmintics: Herbs that eliminate or destroy internal parasites. They kill helminths (parasitic worms). Examples: Wormwood herb, Black Walnut leaf and hull, Oregano and Clove essential oils.

Antiasthmatics Herbs that open and increase the diameter of the bronchioles. Examples: Lobelia herb and Ephedra Ma Huang.

Anticoagulants Herbs that increase clotting time and decrease blood clots. Examples: Garlic bulb, Ginkgo leaf, and Ginseng root.

Anticonvulsants Herbs that help stop seizures, Liver wind. Examples: Uncaria Gou Teng, Gastrodia Tian Ma, and Lobelia herb.

Antidiarrheals Herbs that eliminate/stop/decrease diarrhea by astringing and tightening tissue. Examples: Raspberry leaf, Blackberry leaf and root, and Cranesbill herb.

Antiemetics Herbs that stop nausea and vomiting. Examples: Ginger root and Fennel seed.

Antihistamines Herbs that block histamine. Examples: Xanthium Cang Er Zi (Siberian Cocklebur), Goldenrod herb, and Nettle herb.

Antihyperlipidemics Herbs that reduce abnormally high lipid levels in the blood. Examples: Green Tea leaf, artichoke leaf, and Hawthorn berry.

Antilithics Herbs that break down mineral deposits, particularly in gall stones and kidney stones. Examples: Gravel root, Horsetail herb, Cleavers herb, and Celery seed or root.

Antimicrobials Herbs that can help the body destroy or resist pathogenic microorganisms. Usually used internally. Examples: Calendula flower, Isatis Ban Lan Gen (Isatis root), and Chaparral/Creosote leaf.

Antineoplastic Inhibits tumors. Possible herbal examples: Oldenlandia Bai Hua She She Cao and Pau D'Arco bark.

Antioxidants A substance that inhibits oxidation and donates electrons to neutralize free radicals. Examples: vitamins C and E, selenium, and flavonoids, all of which are found in plants.

Antipruritics Herbs that inhibit itching associated with sunburns, allergic reactions, eczema, and insect bites. Examples: Peppermint leaf or Witch Hazel leaf.

Antipyretics Herbs that reduce fever. Examples: Elderberry berry, Linden flower, Catnip herb, or Boneset herb.

Antiseptics Herbs used for local application to skin or mucous membranes to destroy or resist infection. Examples: Calendula flower or Chamomile flower.

Antispasmodics (Alternately called spasmolytics.) Herbs that decrease muscle spasms. Examples:

Cramp bark, Valerian root, Corydalis Yan Hu Suo (Asian Corydalis corm), and Black Cohosh root.

Antitussives Herbs that suppress the cough reflex due to presence of cyanogenic glycosides and saponins. Examples: Wild Cherry bark, Coltsfoot herb, White Horehound herb, and Licorice root.

Anxiety A state of excessive uneasiness and apprehension, sometimes with compulsive behavior or panic attacks.

Anxiolytics Herbs that reduce anxiety, sometimes called nervines. Examples: California poppy, Catnip herb, and Chamomile flower.

Apiaceae The Parsley or Carrot family with compound umbels and usually hollow flower stalks.

Apoptosis Normal programmed cell death that kills off unhealthy, old, or malfunctioning cells within a predictable time span.

Apothecary In the Middle Ages, a medical professional who formulated and dispensed herbs and medical remedies to physicians, patients, and surgeons. Today an apothecary is an herb shop with a collection of herbs.

Aromatherapy Use of aromatic plant oils, including essential oils for improving psychological or physical well-being.

Arterial Stimulants Class of herbal diaphoretics that are warm and pungent and encourage sweating by warming up the exterior. Used for external wind cold conditions. Examples: Peppermint herb, Angelica root, and Ledebouriella Fang Feng (Wind Protector root).

Arthritis Inflammation of the joints. A category of diseases within the large connective tissue rheumatology specialty. Examples: autoimmune rheumatoid arthritis and fibromyalgia, wear and tear osteoarthritis, and uric acid forming gout.

Asteraceae The Sunflower family with composite flowerheads (ray and disk flowers).

Asthma A respiratory condition marked by spasms in the bronchi causing narrowing of the airway and difficulty breathing.

Astringents Herbs that tighten tissue and help resolve damp discharges, bleeding, and loose tissues. Examples: White Oak bark and Garden Sage leaf.

Atherosclerosis Fatty plaques on the vessel linings of the coronary arteries.

Athlete's Foot Common fungal infection occurring between the toes and on soles of the feet caused from *Tinea* spp.

Attention Deficit Hyperactivity Disorder (ADHD) Chronic condition marked by persistent inattention, hyperactivity, and sometimes impulsivity.

Autoimmune Response When the body attacks its own healthy cells, building up antibodies against them.

Ayurveda A 5000-year-old system of traditional Hindu medicine native to India. Recognizes three body types or doshas: Vata, Pitta, Kapha. If these become out of balance, illness occurs.

B

Bacteria One celled organisms that have cell walls but lack organelles and an organized nucleus.

Bath, Therapeutic The emersion of the body or a body part into hot, warm, tepid, or cold water with or without the addition of herbs.

Benign Prostatic Hypertrophy/Hyperplasia (BPH) A slow growing, non-cancerous enlargement of the prostate gland, common in men over 40 years, that slowly narrows the urethra leading to difficulty urinating a good stream.

Bi syndromes (Chinese Medicine) Painful obstructions of the muscular skeletal system associated with pain, arthritis, trauma, swelling, spasms, stiffness, and decreased range of motion.

Bile A yellow-dark green fluid made by the liver, stored in the gallbladder, and released into the duodenum on demand where it helps digest fat. The bilirubin pigment gives the stool its brown color.

Bilirubin Pigment formed in the liver by the breakdown of hemoglobin in red blood cells and excreted in the bile. Can cause jaundice in newborns with immature livers, in metabolic overload, and in liver disease.

Binomial System of Nomenclature The two-part system of classification for all living things originated by Carolus Linnaeus. The first name is the *genus* and second name, *species*. Yarrow's two names are *Achillea millefolium*. Considered the botanical or Latin name.

Biofilms Communities of multiple bacteria species that live together within a protective slimy coating. Biofilms are resistant to antibiotics and responsible for many chronic diseases.

Bioidentical Hormone Replacement Therapy (HRT) Specially formulated hormone therapy made by prescription in a compounding pharmacy. These hormone molecules fit perfectly onto receptor sites and are virtually identical to human-made hormones.

Bitters Herbs with a predominantly bitter taste. Examples: Gentian root, *Artemisia* spp., and Dandelion leaf.

Bland A description of the absence of taste. Examples: Slippery elm bark, Poria Fu Ling (Hoelen fungus), or medicinal mushrooms such as Ganoderma Ling Zhi (Reishi mushroom).

Blood (Chinese Medicine) A yin liquid/substance that travels through the vessels and also through the energy meridians. Its function is to nourish, maintain and repair the entire body.

Blood–Brain Barrier A highly selective semipermeable membranous barrier formed by endothelial cells lining the blood vessels of the brain. This *wall* protects the brain and blocks many toxins and bacteria from entering.

Blood Pressure (BP) The force in the arteries when the heart beats. *Systolic* is the highest pressure and *diastolic*, the lowest pressure when the heart is at rest. BP is measured in millimeters of mercury (mmHg).

Blood Tonics (Chinese Medicine) Herbs that nourish the blood. Examples: Angelica Dang Gui (Angelica root), Burdock root, and Red Clover flower.

Bone The hardest connective tissue in the body that forms the skeleton, gives support, and protects internal organs.

Botanical Medicine, Herbal Medicine, Herbalism A medical model or system that uses natural plants or plant extracts that are taken internally, inhaled, or applied to the skin.

Botanical Name The binomial name written in Latin. Includes the genus followed by the species. Examples: *Taraxacum officinalis*, *Serenoa repens*, *Schisandra chinensis*.

Botany The science of plants and the branch of biology that deals with plant life and their structure.

Bowel Transit Time Refers to length of time it takes for food to move from the mouth to the end of the intestine (anus). Ideal is 18 hours.

Brassicaceae The Mustard family with four petals and six stamens, four tall and two short.

British Pharmacopoeia (BP) An annual published collection of quality standards for United Kingdom on herbs and medicinal substances. Established in 1968.

Broad-Spectrum Referring to antibiotics, effective against a large variety of organisms.

Bronchitis Inflammation of the bronchial tubes.

Bronchodilator Herbs that stop airway constriction in the bronchi by relaxing smooth muscles. Examples: *Grindelia squarrosa* (Gumweed flower) and Ephedra Ma Huang.

Bruise A discoloration caused when blunt force causes capillaries to tear and bleed, leaving a purplish discoloration under the skin.

C

Canadian Natural and Non-Prescription Health Products Directory (NNHPD) Canadian Directory that regulates herbs as drugs and lists large numbers of herbal medicines with indications. Established in 2004.

Cannabinoid (CB) Receptors Receptor sites on cell membranes that receive cannabinoids (naturally occurring bioactive constituents). The endocannabinoid system is found throughout the body and controls appetite, mood, and memory.

Capsules Clear soft or hard containers used for filling and administration of dry, powdered herbs and essential oils. Some are cellulose based (vegetarian), and others are animal gelatin based (usually bovine).

Carbohydrates Any type of sugar, a major class of phyto-molecules. Made from carbon, hydrogen, and oxygen. Subclasses are monosaccharides, disaccharides, oligosaccharides, and polysaccharides.

Cardiac Glycosides A class of drugs that strengthen the function of the heart muscle and decrease heart rate, used to treat congestive heart failure. Examples: Digoxin and Lanoxin, originally derived from the highly toxic Foxglove herb. Safer herbal examples are medium strength plants: *Convallaria majalis* (Lily of the Valley herb) and *Scilla maritima* (Squill bulb).

Carminatives Herbs that help digestion and stomach aches. Examples: Fennel seed, Peppermint leaf, and Aniseed.

Cartilage Flexible connective tissue on the articulating surface of joints.

Catabolism Form of metabolism where the body breaks down substances into simpler parts. Examples: digestion, where food is broken down into simpler molecules; and cellular respiration, where glucose is broken apart to release the energy molecule, adenosine triphosphate.

Catarrh Excessive build-up of respiratory mucus associated with inflammation of the mucous membranes.

Cathartics Violent purging herbs that accelerate defecation. Can cause electrolyte imbalance and dehydration. Popular historically. Examples: May Apple root, Turkey Rhubarb root, and Cascara sagrada bark.

Celiac Disease Genetic, autoimmune inflammatory disorder where the ingestion of gluten protein triggers antibodies that damage the villi in the small intestine lining, leading to severe malabsorption. Caused by gluten-containing grains. Examples: wheat, rye, and barley.

Chakra Sanskrit word meaning *wheel*. They are energy centers or spinning wheels of light, ascending from the base of the spine to the crown or top of the head.

Chelation A form of heavy metal detoxification, where heavy metal ions are chemically bound to ions of another substance. Herbal chelators: Kelp and other seaweeds; Spirulina and other microalgae.

Chemists British designation for professionals who dispense drugs.

Chief Complaint When taking a health history, the client's most pressing problem, the reason for the visit.

Cholagogues Herbs that promote discharge of bile from the gallbladder. Examples: Turmeric rhizome, Blue Flag rhizome, and Dandelion root.

Cholecystitis Inflammation of the gallbladder with possible infection, usually caused by gallstones.

Cholelithiasis Formation of gallstones.

Cholesterol A sterol made by the liver found in most body tissues, especially the blood. Necessary precursor of sex hormones and important component of cell membranes. Implicated in heart decease.

Chronic A disease that comes with time: persistent or otherwise long-lasting in its effects.

Chronic Otitis Media with Effusion (OME) Chronic bacterial ear infection with pus, liquid, and pressure building up in middle ear. Often caused by allergies.

Cirrhosis A widespread death of liver cells that perform no function. There is inflammation and fibrous thickening of tissue, often a result of chronic alcohol abuse or all types of viral hepatitis.

Clades Refers to monocots.

Clark's Rule Formula for children's dosage using weight. Divide the weight of the child by 150 to give the approximate fraction of the adult dose.

CNS (Central Nervous System) Depressants A drug classification that slows down the central nervous system. Examples: Valium, Benadryl, and Dilantin.

Cold Sores Tiny, fluid-filled blisters on and around the lips, caused by *Herpes simplex* virus.

Colic Long periods of vigorous crying that persists despite all efforts at consolation.

Commission E Established in Germany, 1978. Publishes herbal monographs that list uses, dosages, side effects, and any known drug/herb interactions. German herb companies are allowed to make medicinal claims in line with the Commission E monographs and herbs are legally considered as medicines.

Common Cold Viral infection and inflammation of the upper respiratory tract caused by many types of viruses.

Common Name A plant's nickname based on common usage; what it is called in a certain location or region. Example: Purple Coneflower or Comb flower for *Echinacea purpurea*.

Compress Hot or cold water and herbs applied externally with a wrung-out cloth. Also called a *fomentation*.

Congestive Heart Failure (CHF) Condition where the heart cannot supply enough blood to the body because of weak, inadequate pumping action. Fluid eventually backs up to the lungs causing shortness of breath, coughing, fatigue, fluid retention and edema in feet/ankles with buildup of fluid and sodium.

Conjunctiva Thin transparent layer of tissue lining the inner surface of the eyelid and sclera.

Conjunctivitis Pinkeye. Inflammation of the conjunctiva manifesting as a red, watery, itchy, yellow-green discharge.

Constipation Bowel frequency of less than three times a week, with the need to strain more than 25% of the time.

Contusion A bruise, an injured capillary or blood vessel that leaks blood into the surrounding area, often under the skin, causing a black-and-blue mark.

Conversion Changing medical measurements back and forth from English to metric. Finding equivalents.

Cordial A syrup with 1 part tincture to 3 parts simple syrup.

Corolla The sum of all the petals, sometimes called the inflorescence.

Coronary Artery Disease (CAD) A full or partial blockage of one or more of the coronary arteries that supply blood to the heart.

Corpus Luteum The term means *yellow body*, and it is a hormone-secreting structure that develops in an ovary after an egg has been discharged (ovulation) but degenerates after a few days unless pregnancy has begun. It produces high amounts of progesterone.

Correspondences (Chinese Medicine) The relationship or correspondence of each organ with the natural world. These include aspects such as taste, color, season, emotion, direction, sense organ, and associated body parts.

Cortisol Antiinflammatory steroid hormone secreted by the adrenal cortex. When stress becomes continual, cortisol blood levels rise, creating many health problems including adrenal fatigue.

Cotyledon The first leaf or leaves that sprout from the seed.

Cough Sudden expelling of air, a reflex in response to irritation of the larynx or tracheobronchial tree. Involuntary mechanism to expel foreign bronchial irritants and excess mucus.

Coumarin Phenolic compound found in legumes of the Pea family (Clovers) and in the Grass family. If it spoils or ferments, it turns into dicoumarol, which can cause blood thinning. However, unspoiled coumarin is *not* anticoagulant.

Counterirritants Organic substance that raises body temperature, causes sweating, and creates a mild irritation to the skin to reduce hot inflammation deeper in the body. Examples: Cayenne fruit, Horseradish root, and menthol in Peppermint herb.

Cream Topical application that is a combination of fat and water. These ingredients will separate, so must be stabilized (emulsified). A *lotion* is a more liquefied cream.

Cupping (Chinese Medicine) Pain therapy where glass cups are applied to the skin along the meridians. They create suction, a way of stimulating the flow of qi.

Cyanogenic Glycosides Sugar compounds that yield cyanide on hydrolysis in the digestive tract. Commonly found in the Rose, Pea, and Daisy families. Occur in many seeds of stone fruits. Examples: apples, cherries, apricots, and peaches.

Cystitis Condition where the urinary bladder, urethra, or both become infected with bacteria.

Cytochrome P450 Enzyme System Liver detoxification system. Consists of 14 enzyme families inside liver cells that metabolize (break down fat-soluble substances such as drugs, foods, alcohol, and herbs) into water-soluble chemicals that can be excreted via the bile and urine.

D

Decoction Standard method for preparing hard plant parts such as dried roots, barks, twigs, and some seeds, using prolonged simmering for 10 to 20 minutes.

Decongestants Herbs that break up mucus and treat or resolve damp conditions where excessive fluid has built up in the body. Examples: Goldenrod herb or Thyme herb.

Deconjugation Metabolic liver pathway that breaks down a substance into simple parts that can be excreted through the bile or urine. A detoxification function.

Demulcents Herbs that when used internally moisten tissues and are cooling, harmonizing, and sometimes nourishing. Examples: Mullein leaf, Marshmallow root, and Platycodon Jie Geng (Balloonflower root).

Depuratives Herbs with a detoxifying/alterative effect that work through the kidneys and lymph to break down and eliminate toxic waste. Examples: Celery seed, Burdock root, and Echinacea root.

Diabetes Mellitus Type 1 (DM1) An autoimmune, often inherited disease where the body attacks its own beta cells. The pancreas produces very little or no insulin at all.

Diabetes Mellitus Type 2 (DM2) Nonautoimmune, noninsulin-dependent diabetes, alternately known as insulin resistance or metabolic syndrome. In early stages, it is reversable with diet, herbs, supplements, and lifestyle changes.

Diagnosis Identifying a disease by an assessment of a patient's signs and symptoms.

Diaphoretics Herbs that cause sweating. Examples: Cinnamon bark and fresh Ginger root.

Diarrhea Frequent liquid bowel movements that can be acute or chronic.

Diastolic Pressure Arterial pressure when the ventricular valve muscles relax. The blood pressure is at its lowest.

Dicots Flowering plants with two seed leaves, netted leaf veins, tap roots, complex branching, floral parts mostly in fours and fives. Also called dicotyledons.

Die-off Negative reaction from killing off parasites, worms, and yeast from the body. The pathogens can release toxins that overwhelm the body's abilities to clear them out. Can cause fever, muscle aches, headaches, or skin rash.

Dietary Supplement Health and Education Act (DSHEA) A law passed in 1994 in the United States classifying herbs as dietary supplements or foods and not drugs.

Dispensary Dedicated space where herbs are prepared, combined (formulated), and provided to a client. Sometimes called an apothecary.

Dissolvents Herbs that soften hardened deposits or tissue, such as gallstones, kidney stones, and plaque on arterial walls. Examples: Artichoke leaf as an antihyperlipidemic that reduces fatty deposits and Hydrangea root bark, a litholytic that dissolves kidney stones.

Diuretics Herbs that increase the elimination of fluids through urination. Examples: Goldenrod herb or Dandelion leaf.

Doctrine of Signatures Belief that a plant's overall shape, smell, or characteristic can reveal its healing abilities. Originated in 1621 based on a book by German mystic Jacob Boehme called *The Signature of All Things*.

Douche A vaginal wash using herbal tea preparations, diluted tinctures, or essential oils in water.

Draining Diuretics Herbs with a stronger designation than *diuretic*. Indicated in generalized edema anywhere in the body, including ankles and lower legs (congestive heart failure and renal failure). Examples: Alisma Zi Xie (Water Plantain root) or Couch Grass root.

Drug A substance legally defined as "intended for use in the diagnosis of, cure, mitigation, treatment or prevention of disease" and standardized to a specific amount of active ingredient.

Dual Extraction or Double Extraction A tincture-making method where an alcohol maceration and a hot-water decoction of the same plant are combined. This combination allows for extraction of most of the water- and alcohol-soluble plant constituents.

Dysbiosis Imbalance of the gut microorganisms (*flora*).

Dysfunctional Uterine Bleeding (DUB) A broad term describing irregularities in the menstrual cycle involving frequency, regularity, duration, and volume of flow outside of pregnancy.

Dysplasia Abnormal cell growth.

Dysuria Pain, burning, or discomfort on urination, often caused by a urinary tract infection.

Dysmenorrhea Menstrual pain or cramps.

E

Eclectics Health movement in late 19th century America founded by John King, M.D. Borrowed herbal knowledge from many cultures and established medical schools. The movement included notables such as Harvey Felter, M.D., John Scudder, M.D., and pharmacist John Lloyd.

Eczema Superficial skin inflammation that comes and goes, caused by direct contact with solvents, soaps, etc., or by internal sources. Caused by food allergies and sensitivities, stress, and toxicity, often with an allergic component.

Eight Principle Patterns of Assessment (Chinese Medicine) The four sets of opposites that help interpret data collected during examination: cold and heat, deficiency and excess, interior and exterior, and yin and yang.

Eisenberg National Survey National health survey of 1997 showing that one out of three people in the United States used complementary therapies.

Electrolytes Compounds that separate into ions in solution and conduct an electrical charge. They are important parts of body fluids. Examples: Sodium (Na^+), Potassium (K^+), Calcium (Ca^+), and Magnesium (Mg^+) have positive charges. Chloride (Cl^-), Phosphate ($PO3^-$), and Bicarbonate ($HCO3^-$) have negative charges.

Electuary An herbal confection or preserve.

Elimination Diet A short-term eating plan that removes certain foods that may be causing food sensitivities or autoimmune reactions. It then reintroduces the food categories one at a time to determine how and which foods are tolerated.

Emmenagogues Herbal uterine stimulants that increase or start menses. Examples: Wild Ginger root or Blue Cohosh root.

Emollients Herbs having the quality of softening, soothing, and keeping the skin moist. Includes creams, salves, and ointments. Examples: Aloe Vera gel, Slippery Elm bark, and Calendula flower.

Endocannabinoid System (ECS) Neurotransmitter signaling system that helps pain and other functions. Endocannabinoids are made in the body and stimulate receptor sites. Some plants also make substances that stimulate human cannabinoid receptors. Examples: *Cannabis* spp., *Echinacea* spp., and Peppercorns.

Endocrine System A system of glands that secrete hormones (chemical messengers) or other products directly into the blood.

Endogenous Originating inside the body. Often refers to the normal toxic end products of metabolism (chemical processes) that occur in the body, as with endogenous waste.

Energetics In herbalism refers to categories or qualities of herbs such as taste, warmth, and moisture.

Enteric Nervous System (ENS) Mesh-like system of neurons that governs the function of the gastrointestinal tract.

Enuresis Involuntary urination especially at night; bedwetting.

Environmental Toxicosis Environmental factors such as pollutants, chemicals, drugs, organisms, hormones, heavy metals, or contaminated drinking water that overwhelm liver detoxification pathways, resulting in toxic overload in the body.

Epidemic Disease outbreak that spreads quickly and affects many individuals at the same time in the same area or community.

Epinephrine Hormone secreted by the adrenal medulla, the fight-or-flight hormone that activates the sympathetic nervous system. Originally called adrenaline, the gland's namesake.

Essential Amino Acids The nine proteins that cannot be made by the body. As a result, they must come from food sources and are *essential* to the diet.

Essential Oils Extremely strong steam or water distillations of aromatic plants. Examples: Peppermint, Lemon, and Bergamot essential oils.

Estrogen Dominance Too much unopposed estrogen, usually a result of not enough progesterone to counteract or balance it out.

Estrogen Major female hormone. Primary functions are to stimulate development of female characteristics and to regulate the menstrual cycle.

Ethics Moral principles that govern behavior for the good of a profession or society. A value, not a law.

Ethyl Alcohol Ethanol, grain alcohol or EtOH refers to pure ingestible medicinal-grade alcohol that is used in tincture making. It is the only type of alcohol that is safe to use internally.

Exogenous Coming from the environment, external, outside the body. Example: a flu virus carried through the air and entering the body through the nose and mouth.

Expectorants Herbs that move mucus up and out of lungs. Examples: Pleurisy root or Osha root.

External Pernicious Influences (Chinese Medicine) Refers to the *six evils* that come from outside the body and can cause illness: external wind, cold, heat, damp, dry, and summer heat.

Extract, Standardized A strong herbal extract based on standardization. Guarantees that a certain weight of a finished extract is derived from a certain weight of crude herb. A 4:1 powdered extract contains the extracted constituents from four grams of starting material in one gram of finished extract. May be in liquid or solid form. The higher the first number, the stronger the extract.

Extract, Weight-to-Volume A strong and highly concentrated herbal tincture based on a weight-to-volume ratio with either 1-part herb in grams to 1-part liquid menstruum in milliliters (1:1); or 1-part herb in grams to 2 parts liquid menstruum in milliliters (1:2). The lower the second number, the stronger the extract.

F

Fabaceae The Pea family with banner, wings, and keel flowers, pealike pods, and often pinnate leaves.

Family Taxonomical classification for plants with similar flowers, fruit, and seed structures. Examples: Mint, Pea, and Rose families.

Fascia Thin fibrous sheets of connective tissue that enclose and separate muscles and organs.

Fatty Acid (FA) Building blocks of fat in the body and foods. They have hydrocarbon tails that terminate with a carboxylic acid group.

Federal Drug Administration (FDA) U.S. federal agency that evolved out of the Pure Food and Drugs Act of 1906. Ensures safety and regulates new medicines and herbs, medical appliances, food inspection, and processing centers. Mandates that any newly added drug or herb requires extensive research.

Fibrocystic Breasts Fluid-filled sacs inside the breast that get larger under influence of estrogen and smaller at other times. Sacs usually disappear after menopause.

Fibromyalgia Autoimmune rheumatic disease with a large group of symptoms such as widespread musculoskeletal pain with trigger points, sleep disturbances and gastrointestinal and emotional problems.

Fire Toxins (Chinese Medicine) Material with pus and oozing that can be internal or external. Takes form of abscesses, tumors, cysts, ulcers, boils, skin rashes, and eczema. Herbs that clear fire toxins, cool heat, drain pus, and kill microorganisms. Examples: Coptis Huang Lian (Goldthread root), Andrographis Chuan Xin Lian (Heart-Thread Lotus leaf), and Isatis Ban Lan Gen (Woad root).

Five Alpha Reductase (5-AR) Enzyme that converts testosterone to the more potent dihydrotestosterone (DHT). Mechanism of action of Saw Palmetto berry in treating benign prostatic hypertrophy (BPH).

Five Element Cycles (Chinese Medicine) These show how the five yin organs with their corresponding element interact and work with each other and/or against each other, resulting in health or disease. Concept shown as a circular chart.

Five Element Theory (Chinese Medicine) World view that includes our relationship with the earth and its natural cycles. Incorporates the five yin-yang organ pairs and their association with the five seasons, five elements, five tastes, five colors, five emotions, and the five sense organs. These encompass the correspondences.

Five Hots (Chinese Medicine) Heat in yin surfaces of the body: such as the palms, soles of the feet, and the chest. Indicates a yin deficiency condition where the body needs moisture. Often seen in night sweats and hot flashes of menopause.

Five Organ Network (Chinese Medicine) Refers to the five paired yin-yang organs: Liver and Gall Bladder, Heart and Small Intestine, Spleen and Stomach, Lung and Large Intestine, and Kidney and Urinary Bladder.

Fixed Oils Nonvolatile true fats found in plants and animals. Examples: olive, almond, sesame, or fish oil. They do not evaporate.

Flavonoids Large subclass of polyphenols that occur in plants as flavonoid glycosides responsible for yellow, red, blue, and purple coloring. Many are antioxidant and antiinflammatory.

Flexner Report U.S. federal government report in 1920 that exposed the alleged shortcomings of the Eclectics in America and that was responsible for removing herbalism from medical school curriculums.

Fluids (Chinese Medicine) All bodily fluids other than blood. Includes semen, urine, lymph, sweat, gastric juices, and mucous membrane linings.

Folk Method Tincture making process done without measuring out ingredients.

Follicle Stimulating Hormone (FSH) A gonadotrophic hormone produced in the anterior pituitary gland that stimulates the growth of the ovarian follicle, the sac where the egg grows in the ovary and that produces estrogen.

Formulating The art of making up or composing an herbal blend, formula, or formulation.

Four Humors Hippocrates' four body types or humors: sanguine, yellow bile, black bile, and white phlegm.

Four-R Program Developed by Jeffrey Bland, Ph. D., of the Functional Medicine Institute. A clinical tool or method to normalize dysbiosis and heal damage to cells of intestine lining. The Four-R's are Remove, Replace, Reinoculate, and Repair.

Fractionated or Advanced Lipid Panel Advanced blood test that is highly predictive of cardiac risk. It tests for cholesterol markers such as the dangerous Lp(a), the ApoB/ApoA ratio and a triglyceride/HDL ratio.

Free Radicals Unstable oxygen molecules that have an unpaired electron. Causes damage to cellular DNA and cell membranes. Sometimes called *reactive oxygen species* (ROS). Implicated as a cause of aging and cancer.

Fried's Rule Dosage calculation for infants up to 24 months. Age in months divided by 150 equals fraction of adult dose. Multiply fraction by adult dose to get child's dose.

Functional Foods Foods that are used as medicine.

Functional Medicine Healing style that addresses the underlying causes of disease, using a systems-oriented approach and engaging both patient and practitioner in a therapeutic partnership. It addresses the root causes of illness and uses functional foods, herbs, supplements, and lifestyle approaches.

Fundamental Substances (Chinese Medicine) Refers to qi, blood, jing, shen, and fluids.

Fungi Mushrooms, yeasts, molds, mildews, smuts, and rusts that live by breaking down and absorbing dead or live organic matter. Some are parasitic and cause athlete's foot and ringworm.

G

Galactagogues Herb or food that stimulates oxytocin, which causes milk ejection. Examples: Hops flower, Blessed Thistle, Fenugreek seed, or Fennel seed.

Gallstones Hardened bile sediments or calculi in the gallbladder.

GAPS Diet Stands for *Gut and Psychology Syndrome* diet. Comprehensive six-stage healing practice developed by Dr. Natasha Campbell-McBride. Used in the treatment of stubborn autoimmune diseases, dysbiosis, inflammatory bowel disease, autism, and attention deficit hyperactivity disorder.

Garbling Sorting out and sifting through a dried plant to remove unwanted material such as twigs, dirt, and pieces of grass.

Gastritis Inflammation of the stomach lining. A stomachache.

Gastroesophageal Reflux Disease (GERD) Condition that results when the cardiac sphincter muscle at the lower end of the esophagus relaxes at the wrong time and hydrochloric acid from the stomach backs up into the esophagus. This can cause heartburn and esophageal cancer.

Gastrointestinal (GI) Pertains to the disgestive system, the stomach, and intestines specifically.

Gastrointestinal (GI) Ulcer Open sores on the inside lining of the stomach (peptic or gastric) and the upper portion of the small intestine (duodenal).

Generally Regarded as Safe (GRAS) The U. S. Food and Drug Administration status given to food additives, including herbs, that were in general use prior to January 1, 1958, and considered safe based on common knowledge gained through a history of safe use. Any herbs coming into use after that date must undergo scientific procedures and research to attain GRAS status.

Genus A group of plants within a family that has more traits in common with each other than with any other plants in that family.

Germ Theory Developed in the 1800s by Louis Pasteur and Robert Koch, this theory states that specific microorganisms cause specific diseases.

Ghrelin Fast-acting hormone secreted in the stomach that increases appetite, hunger, and weight gain.

Gingivitis Inflammation of the gums, usually with infection. Can loosen teeth and cause teeth to fall out. A Myrrh resin rinse is indicated.

Gliadin Protein present in wheat and other grains that can trigger a severe autoimmune inflammatory response producing antibodies that damage villi in the small intestine, eventually leading to severe malabsorption.

Glucagon Pancreatic hormone that turns off insulin, thereby raising blood sugar. The second half of the negative feedback system in the pancreas, the other hormone being insulin.

Gluconeogenesis Liver's transformation of stored glycogen into glucose with release into the blood.

Glutathione Compound containing three amino acids: glutamate, cysteine, and glycine. It is the master antioxidant liver detoxifier. Herbal examples: Milk Thistle seed, Platycodon Jie Geng (Balloonflower root), and Turmeric root.

Gluten Sensitivity A continuum that ranges from mild indigestion and food intolerances when gluten is consumed to flat-out celiac disease where gluten cannot be eaten under any circumstances.

Gluten Proteins responsible for the elastic texture in dough, especially wheat products, barley, and rye, triticale, and oats. Can cause autoimmune response leading to food sensitivities and celiac disease.

Glycerin The sweet faction of a fixed oil found in fats of plants and animals. A *glycerite* is an herbal extraction using mainly vegetable glycerin as the menstruum.

Goitrogens Substances that disrupt the production of thyroid hormones by interfering with iodine uptake in the thyroid gland. Examples: raw cruciferous veggies in some situations.

Good Manufacturing Practice (GMP) Protocol laid out by the U.S. Food and Drug Administration to assure that products are of high quality and do not pose any risk to the consumer or public. Herbalists are beginning to use this system.

Gonads The primary reproductive organs, the female ovaries and the male testes. The ovaries produce and contain the ova/egg cells, and the testes/testicles produce sperm cells.

Gout Very painful form of arthritis caused by uric acid crystals building up in the joints and kidneys.

Gram Stain The Gram stain test is named for bacteriologist Hans Gram. Method of identifying bacteria by applying a crystal violet stain to bacterial slides. If the cells stain purple, they're gram-positive. If the stain takes on the color of a red counterstain, they're gram-negative.

Gripe An old-fashioned term for sharp, gripping, bowel pains or cramps.

Gum A water-soluble polysaccharide secretion produced by algae and plants in response to trauma, insect, damage, or infection. Example: *Acacia senegal* (Gum Arabic).

Gut-Associated Lymphoid Tissue (GALT) Part of the immune system, a mucosal barrier in the lining of the colon that activates immune cells to guard against penetration of microbes from outside sources. It also excretes mucus and traps and expels harmful bacteria.

Gut-Brain Axis/Connection Refers to the physical connections (nerves) and the chemical connections (neurotransmitters) running between the gut and the brain and how they affect health and emotions.

Gut-Liver Axis Relationship between the gut and the liver. Intestinal permeability (leaky gut) can lead to liver disease and failure by overtaxing its detoxification pathways.

Gymnosperm Plants with naked seeds not enclosed in an ovary. Their egg cells are exposed to the air and fertilized when pollen lands directly on them. Example: a pinecone.

H

Half-life Period of time required for the concentration or amount of a drug in the body to be reduced by one-half in the blood plasma.

Halogens A group of elements on the periodic table that include fluorine, chlorine, bromine, and iodine. Being chemically similar, they compete with iodine for binding sites. They appear in drinking water and countless foods and products.

Hashimoto's Thyroiditis An autoimmune disease where the immune system attacks the thyroid gland with a resultant decrease of thyroid hormones.

Hay Fever Common and annoying seasonal allergy caused by pollens that trigger IgG antigen reactions that are not life threatening.

Headache A symptom characterized by continuous pain over various parts of the head.

Health Insurance Portability and Accountability Act (HIPAA) U.S. law that protects and ensures right to privacy for a patient's written and electronic medical records and health information.

Helminths Parasitic worms such as flukes, tapeworms, or nematodes that feed on living hosts. Many live in the human digestive tract and are known as intestinal parasites. They interfere with nutrient absorption and cause disease.

Hematoma A bruise. Localized swelling of clotted or partially clotted blood caused by a break in the wall of a blood vessel. The blood seeps out into surrounding tissue, causing a black-and-blue mark.

Hematuria Blood in the urine.

Hemoglobin A1c (HgA1c) Test for risk of diabetes that averages blood sugar levels over a 2- to 3-month period.

Hemostatics Herbs that lessen internal or external bleeding by causing capillary constriction or by speeding up blood clotting (coagulants). Examples: Beth root and Oak bark.

Hepatocyte A liver cell.

Herb A plant used for medicinal purposes.

Herbalism The study or practice of the medicinal and therapeutic use of plants.

Herbalist/Herbologist One who uses and studies plant parts for medicine.

Herbology The study of plants.

Herpes Simplex Virus 1 (HSV) Virus that causes cold sores. Once in the body, it remains dormant in the nervous system and can mutate into other *Herpes* family viruses later.

Histamine Substance produced by mast cells as part of a local immune response to an allergen.

The *histamine response* causes inflammation and typical immediate allergy symptoms.

Hives A rash of pale or red welts on the skin that itch intensely, sometimes with dangerous swelling, caused by an allergic reaction, typically, to specific foods.

Hormones Chemical substances produced in the body that control and regulate the activity of certain cells or organs. Many are secreted by the ductless glands of the endocrine system.

Hydrosol An aromatic water and volatile oil combination. The process of distillation is used to separate the liquid parts (water and volatile oils) from the solid parts of a plant. May be used alone or as a water base for making creams, lotions, syrups, and fomentations.

Hydrotherapy The therapeutic use of water in various forms and temperatures.

Hyperhidrosis Abnormal, profuse sweating when body does not need cooling down.

Hyperlipidemia Elevated fat levels in the blood (cholesterol, triglycerides), which can lead to blood clots and fatty plaques in the coronary arteries, causing heart attack and stroke.

Hypnotics Herbal remedies that cause drowsiness, depress the central nervous system (CNS), and may inhibit motor function. They induce a deep and healing state of sleep. They are *not* related to hypnotism or to the sedative-hypnotic classification of Western drugs. Examples: Hops flower, Passionflower herb, and Valerian root.

Hypoglycemics Herbs that lower blood sugar. Examples: Fenugreek seed or Bitter Melon.

Hypohidrosis Decreased ability to sweat when body is too hot. *Anhidrosis*, inability to sweat at all.

Hypotensives Herbs that help bring down blood pressure. Examples: Ziziphus Suan Zao Ren (Sour Jujube seed), Hawthorn berry, and Hops flower.

Hypothalamic-Pituitary-Adrenal Axis (HPA axis) Interactive endocrine pattern where the hypothalamus in the brain relays hormonal or electrical messages to the pituitary, which then relays chemical hormonal message to the adrenal glands.

Hypothalamic-Pituitary-Gonadal Axis (HPG axis) Interactive endocrine pattern/pathway/axis where the hypothalamus in the brain relays hormonal and/or electrical messages to the pituitary, which then relays chemical hormonal messages to the gonads (ovaries and testes).

Hypothalamic-Pituitary-Thyroid Axis (HPT axis) Interactive endocrine pattern where the hypothalamus in the brain relays hormonal or electrical messages to the pituitary, which then relays a chemical hormonal message to the thyroid gland.

I

Immunomodulatory Polysaccharides (IPs) Phytochemically complex carbohydrates present in most adaptogenic herbs, including medicinal mushrooms.

Incontinence Lack of voluntary control over urination. Major types are stress incontinence, neurogenic bladder, and estrogen deficiency.

Inducing Agent Enzyme or substance in the CYP450 system that increases rate of metabolism, shortens half-life, and decreases blood levels of the *substrate* (the therapeutic drug that is acted on by the enzyme or inducing agent).

Infection An invasion and multiplication of microorganisms such as bacteria, viruses, or parasites that are not normally present within the body.

Inflammation, Acute and Pathological *Acute inflammation* is the body's normal response to injury and infection. The inflammatory cascade is manifested by redness, edema, heat, and pain. It facilitates healing. *Pathological* (chronic) *inflammation* is a prolonged immune response that remains long after an infection, injury, or toxic exposure is gone, acting as if it is still there. It is a set-up for chronic disease and pain.

Inflammatory Bowel Disease (IBD) Autoimmune bowel inflammation that causes serious illnesses involving bleeding. Examples: ulcerative colitis and Crohn's disease.

Influenza A highly contagious respiratory infection caused by enveloped viruses called influenza A and B.

Infused Oils Macerations of fresh or dried herbs in a fixed oil menstruum. May be used alone for skin care or added to creams and lotions.

Infusion Standard method for preparing dried leaves, seeds, flowers, stems, and other light plant parts in hot or cold water.

Inhibiting Agent Substance or enzyme in the CYP450 system that reduces rate of metabolism, prolongs half-life, and raises blood levels of the substrate (the therapeutic drug that is acted upon by the inhibiting agent).

Insulin Hormone produced in pancreatic beta cells that drives glucose-rich carbohydrates from digested food in the bloodstream into the cells, so that glucose can then be used as a raw material in the manufacture of the energy molecule, adenosine triphosphate (ATP).

Insulin Resistance Condition where the pancreatic islet cells become resistant to insulin hooking on to their receptor sites, requiring more and more insulin to do the job of forcing glucose into the cells in order to maintain normal blood glucose levels. Leads to type 2 diabetes. Also called metabolic syndrome.

Integument The skin, the tough outer layer. The human integumentary system includes the hair, nails, skin glands, and nerves.

Intermittent Fasting Restricting daily eating to 14 to 16 hours a day, allowing the gut time to empty and shift from burning sugar to burning fat as its primary fuel. Regimen includes no late-night eating before bedtime.

International Code of Binomial Nomenclature (ICBN) Set of rules for the scientific Latin/Greek naming of plants. The International Botanical Congress (IBC) meets every few years to establish the guidelines for the naming of plants, their additions, and their revisions.

Intestinal Permeability (IP) Spaces that form between the cell walls of the intestinal lining due to dysbiosis. Condition is called intestinal permeability or *leaky gut*.

Inulin Indigestible oligosaccharide prebiotic. It is not insulin. It is a prebiotic that feeds the intestinal flora and lowers serum triglycerides, among other things. Herbs with inulin: Garlic bulb, Chicory root, Dandelion root, and Elecampane root.

Irritable Bowel Syndrome (IBS) Common syndrome caused from leaky gut resulting in indigestion with crampy pain, bloating, diarrhea, or constipation.

Ischemia Inadequate blood supply to an organ or part of the body, especially the heart muscle.

Isopropol Alcohol Non-ingestible rubbing alcohol that contains propane and may only be used externally. It is highly poisonous but safe in external liniments.

J

Japanese Pharmacopeia (JP) Founded in 1886. Regulates drugs and Kampo herbs (Japanese adaptation of Chinese herbs).

Jaundice Yellowish discoloration under the skin and whites of the eyes from buildup of bilirubin when the liver doesn't break it down.

Jing (Chinese Medicine) The substance that underlies life from birth to death. Jing is the basis of reproduction and development, part of our DNA.

K

Kampo Japanese study and adaptation of Chinese Medicine.

Keying Out System for identifying a plant in the wild using the process of elimination. Found in some field guides.

L

Laceration A cut or tear in the skin where none of the skin is missing, just separated.

Lactose A sugar present in milk and dairy.

Lamiaceae The Mint family with square stalks, opposite leaves, irregular flowers, and usually aromatic scent.

Larynx The voice box or vocal cords.

Latin name Specific plant name written in Latin that includes its genus and species. Sometimes called the botanical name and/or scientific name. Examples: *Iris versicolor*, *Sticta pulmonaria*.

Laudanum A whole opium preparation containing all the opium alkaloids. Used in the Victorian era as a pain killer and available at any apothecary at that time without a prescription. Many people became addicted without realizing the drug's danger.

Laxatives (Purgatives, Aperients) Herbs that loosen stools and increase bowel movements. Examples: Senna pod or Cascara bark.

Leaky Brain or Blood-Brain Barrier Hyperpermeability Syndrome Condition where cell junctions around the capillaries of the blood brain barrier become too large, allowing harmful bacteria and toxins to leak into the brain, causing chronic inflammation. This can result in neurological diseases such as Alzheimer's, Parkinson's, dementia, multiple sclerosis, amyotrophic lateral sclerosis, autism, and seizures. Leaky gut often results in leaky brain.

Leaky Gut or Intestinal Permeability (IP) Both are names for condition where undigested large protein food particles (macromolecules) leak out between enlarged cell wall junctions into the blood, acting as environmental antigens, causing inflammation and autoimmune responses.

Lectins Toxic glycoproteins found in seeds of some Bean family and Spurge family plants. Causes cell agglutination (clotting). Examples: Castor bean, Mistletoe herb, and Poke root.

Leptin Hormone secreted by fat cells, stomach, and other places that signals a decrease of hunger and induces weight loss.

Leptin Resistance Condition often causing weight gain. Occurs through negative feedback. Excessive circulating leptin hormone decreases the brain's sensitivity to it. Results in decrease of leptin's appetite-regulating effect by not getting signal of satiety (being full).

Ligament Tough fibrous connective tissue that connects one bone to another.

Lignins High fiber class of polyphenols. Various kinds are part of the active constituents in adaptogens, phytoestrogens, anticarcinogenics, and hepatoprotective herbs. Examples: Flax seeds, Milk Thistle seed, and Schisandra Wu Wei Zi (Five Taste berry).

Liliaceae The Lily family with monocot flowers and parts in threes. The three sepals and three petals are usually identical and hard to differentiate; leaves have parallel veins.

Lin Syndromes (Chinese Medicine) Term for a group of physical urinary disorders involving frequency, dribbling, painful issues. They involve infection, hematuria, stones, chronic Kidney and Spleen deficiencies.

Liniment An external thin medicated tincture that is rubbed onto the skin.

Lipids Fatty, oily substances that are usually not water soluble. The properties of fats and fatty acids depend on their degree of hydrogen saturation and the length of their molecules, or chain length.

Local An herb (or drug) that acts locally, or directly on a tissue or organ. The substance must make direct contact with the cells to be effective. Examples: Oregon Grape root and Juniper berry.

Lotion Moisturizing combinations of fat and water requiring emulsification to stabilize them. Examples: Creams and lotions (a thinner cream).

Luteinizing Hormone (LH) A gonadotropic hormone produced in the anterior pituitary that stimulates ovulation and the growth of the empty egg sac, the corpus luteum, which produces progesterone.

Lymphatic Drainers Herbs that help lymphatic circulation, used to drain toxins and excess fluids. Examples: Red root, Ocotillo bark, and Cleavers herb.

M

Maceration Slow steeping of an herb in any type of liquid menstruum.

Marc The insoluble residue that remains after extracting the soluble components of an herb in a menstruum.

Marker Compound A biochemical constituent characteristic of a plant. Examples: curcumin in Turmeric root or polyphenols in Grape seed extract.

Materia Medica An herbal list of medicinal plants. Literally means the *materials of medicine*.

Mediterranean Diet Traditional diet in Mediterranean countries (Italy and Greece) characterized by a high consumption of vegetables and olive oil and moderate intake of protein.

Menarche Onset of menstruation at puberty, usually around 11 to 12 years old.

Menopause Cessation of menstruation that has lasted for 12 consecutive months.

Menorrhagia Abnormally heavy menstrual bleeding.

Menstrual Cycle The hormonal process women go through each month to prepare for a possible pregnancy. The cycle begins from the start of one period until the day before the next vaginal blood flow (*menstruation*). Average cycle lasts 28 days.

Menstruation The process where blood and other materials are discharged through the vagina as the uterine lining sheds. Happens in intervals of about one lunar month from puberty until menopause, except during pregnancy.

Menstruum Solvent used for extraction of plant constituents resulting in a tincture or extract. May be water, alcohol, vinegar, wine, brandy, glycerin, or combinations thereof. Note: Plural of menstruum can be menstruums or menstrua.

Metabolism Chemical processes in the body needed to sustain life. Happens either by breaking down organic substances (*catabolism*) or by combining molecules to create new substances (*anabolism*) with the use of energy.

Microbiome Collection or community of microbes or microorganisms in the gut.

Mind-Body Connection Theory that refers to how thoughts, feelings, beliefs, and attitudes can positively or negatively affect biological functioning.

Monoamine Oxidase Inhibitors (MAOIs) Class of antidepressant drugs that block breakdown of the enzyme monamine oxidase. Examples: Nardil and Parnate. Saint John's Wort (hypothesized to be a weak MAO inhibitor) has been contraindicated for use with MAOIs and other antidepressant drug categories.

Monocots Flowering plants with one seed leaf, parallel leaf veins, horizontal rootstalks, simple branching, and floral parts mostly in threes. Also called *monocotyledons*.

Monograph Herbal compendium that lists uses, dosages, side effects, and any known drug/herb interactions. Example: German Commission E Monographs.

Monounsaturated Fats Lipids that have one double bond in the molecular chain with all of the remainder carbon atoms being single-bonded. Examples: olives, almonds, peanuts, macadamia nuts, hazelnuts, pecans, cashews, and avocados.

Moxibustion (Chinese Medicine) Pain therapy using a smoking stick of moxa, *Artemisia vulgaris* (Mugwort herb), near the skin to warm the blood, stimulate circulation, and relieve stagnation.

Mucilage Polysaccharides that form viscous, slimy solutions with water, known as demulcents. They coat mucous membranes. Examples: Slippery Elm bark, Comfrey root and leaf.

Mucogenic Stimulates production of mucus. Herbal Example: Marshmallow root.

Mucolytic Expectorants Herbs that break up thick, respiratory mucus (*mucolytics*) and help induce coughing (*expectorants*). Examples: Mullein leaf, Coltsfoot herb, and White Horehound herb.

Mucostatics or Mucus Decongestants Herbs that break up mucus in the body, either by astringing (Goldenrod herb, Thyme, and Sage herb) or by action of essential oil glycosides (Cayenne fruit and Yerba Mansa herb).

Muscle Type of connective tissue that contracts and relaxes. Skeletal muscle moves joints, smooth muscle supports blood vessels and hollow organs, and cardiac muscle pumps blood.

Myalgia Pain in a muscle or muscle group.

Myocardial Infarction (MI) Heart attack. Refers to reduced blood flow to one or more of the coronary arteries (*infarction*) resulting in lack of oxygen (*ischemia*) and ultimate cell death (*necrosis*) to the portion of the heart muscle supplied by that artery.

N

National Center for Complementary and Integrative Health (NCCIH) Founded in 1998 under National Institutes of Health in the United States. Its purpose is to "conduct scientific research on complementary and integrative health approaches" and to provide well-informed recommendations to the public.

National Institute of Medical Herbalists (NIMH) The United Kingdom's leading professional body and voluntary regulator of herbal practitioners, established 1864.

National Institutes of Health (NIH) Founded in the 1870s. U.S. federal agency responsible for biomedical and public health research. Funds scientific research on complementary health, including herbal medicine.

Neat Application of an essential oil that is undiluted.

Negative Feedback Loop In the endocrine system or any other, a self-regulating inhibitory system that maintains the correct amount of hormones or other substances to create balance. When a level gets too high, production is turned off; when a level gets too low, production is turned back on. Examples: blood pressure, thyroid hormone, and blood sugar regulation.

Nervines Western classification of herbs that affect the nervous system in various ways: relaxing, cooling it down, warming it up, strengthening, and harmonizing. Examples: Passionflower herb, Hops flower, and Pasqueflower root and herb.

Neuralgia Intense burning or stabbing pain caused by irritation, compression, or damage to a nerve.

Neuroendocrine System The interaction between the nervous and the endocrine system. The hypothalamus of the brain and an assortment of endocrine glands working together to regulate body functions, such as stress, reproduction, glucose, and energy metabolism.

Neurogastroenterology The study of the brain, the gut, and their interactions. Encompasses the understanding and management of gastrointestinal motility, mental health, gastrointestinal disorders, and mind-body connection.

Neuropathy Damaged or diseased nerves. *Peripheral neuropathy* refers to diseased or damaged nerves that carry messages to and from the brain and spinal cord, to the extremities.

Neurotransmitters Chemical messengers causing the transfer of a nerve impulse to another nerve fiber, muscle fiber, or some other structure. Examples: Acetylcholine, serotonin, and dopamine.

Nonsteroidal Antiinflammatory Drugs (NSAIDs) A class of drugs that stop pain and inflammation by blocking cyclo-oxygenase (COX) enzymes, which in turn inhibit production of prostaglandins, part of the inflammatory cascade. They are the most commonly used painkillers on the market. Examples: aspirin, ibuprofen, Advil, Motrin.

Nutrigenomics Interaction of nutrition and genes, especially when used to prevent disease.`

O

Organic Acids Plant acids derived from monosaccharides. There are many types. Examples: fruit acids of citric, malic, and tartaric and others, such as formic acid, oxalic acid, and ascorbic acid (Vitamin C).

Organoleptics Using the senses. Judging the potency, quality, and phytochemical composition of an herb or herbal preparation by using sense of taste, smell, temperature, vision, and body effects.

Osteoarthritis Damage of weight-bearing joints due to mechanical stress on a joint that progresses to wearing down of articular cartilage, joint fusion, and immobility. Common on knees, hips, fingers, and back.

Osteoporosis Porous bone, where calcium is lost more quickly than it is replaced.

Otitis Media with Effusion (OME) Chronic bacterial ear infection with pus, liquid, and pressure building up in middle ear with an allergic component. Common in children.

Ovulation When a mature egg is released from the ovary, usually day 14 of the menstrual cycle.

Oxalates Substance that can be toxic to kidneys in people with calcium oxalate kidney stones and fat malabsorption problems. Present in many foods. Examples: Spinach, rhubarb, and beets.

Oxidative Stress Imbalance in free radical production in the liver with inability to detoxify their harmful effects. Oxidative stress damages cell DNA and leads to inflammation.

Oxymel A specialized sweet and sour herbal honey.

Oxytocics Herbs hastening or facilitating childbirth, especially by stimulating contractions of the uterus. Examples: Blue Cohosh and Cotton root bark.

P

Paleo Diet The hunter-gatherer diet featuring whole, unprocessed foods such as grass-fed meat, free-range poultry, wild fish, vegetables (including root vegetables), fruit, berries, some nuts, and some seeds. It includes avoidance of grains, legumes, refined sugars, and dairy. Good for insulin resistance and weight loss.

Palpate An assessment technique done by feeling. Example: feeling a pulse.

Pandemic Outbreak of an infectious disease that has spread quickly through human populations across the world or in a very large region.

Papules Raised, red, solid, inflamed pimples.

Paradoxical Effect A substance that causes the opposite effect of what would normally be expected. Example: Valerian root when used for full heat conditions instead of empty heat. In some instances, occurs with narcotic drugs.

Parasites Organisms that live on other organisms and get their nutrients from their host, such as helminths (worms) or protozoa.

Parasiticides Herbs that treat parasites. Examples: Aloe vera gel and Lemon essential oil.

Pectins Water-trapping colloidal polysaccharides found in the primary walls of most plant cells. It has a pulling action in the gut that helps with detoxification. Examples: apples and the white inside rind of citrus fruits.

Percolation Preparation where the soluble constituents of an herb are extracted by slow passage of the solvent through a column or cone of dried, powdered plant that has been packed in a percolator.

pH Potential of hydrogen (acid-base balance). The pH is a number expressing the acidity or alkalinity of a solution on a logarithmic scale on which 7 is neutral, lower values are more acid, and higher values more alkaline.

Pharmacognosy Study of plants as a potential source of drugs and science of plant chemistry.

Pharmacokinetics Study of what happens to a constituent from the time it enters the body to when it exits.

Pharmacology Study of the interaction of biologically active agents within a living system, the key chemical constituents in a plant.

Pharmacopoeia of the People's Republic of China (PPRC) Official Chinese compendium of drugs and herbal medicine, established in 1953. English editions are available.

Pharynx The throat tube extending from the back of the nasal passages and mouth to the esophagus.

Phase Dosing Type of dosing administration. Dispensing a separate formula for different phases (halves) of the menstrual cycle.

Phase I Liver Detoxification First stage of liver detoxification involving oxidation, reduction, and hydrolysis. Cytochrome P450 enzymes break down fat-soluble toxins and produce free radicals that can damage liver cells if excessive.

Phase II Liver Detoxification Second stage of liver detoxification utilizing methylation and sulfation. Harmful free radicals formed in Phase I are converted in Phase II into water-soluble form, which are then easily excreted through the kidneys and liver.

Phenolic Compounds Phytochemical classification containing coumarins, salicylic acids, flavonoids, lignins, and phytoestrogens.

Photosensitizing Herbal side effect caused by ingestion of certain substances combined with sunlight exposure. Example: St. John's Wort and many Apiaceae family members such as *Angelica* spp.

Photosynthesis Process where plants use light to convert carbon dioxide and water into glucose and oxygen for their food. The light absorbing pigment is green chlorophyll.

Phylogeny Classifying plants based on their genetic and evolutionary relationships, rather than by form (morphology) or by chemical constituents.

***Physician's Desk Reference* (PDR)** A collection of all the prescription drugs available in the United States. The information is the same as the leaflet in the drug package, also known as the package insert. Drug companies pay to have their drugs included, so many generic medicines do not appear.

Physiomedicalists Offshoot of Thomsonian Movement of 19th century America led by William Cook M.D., who wrote *The Physio-Medical Dispensatory*, still in use today.

Phytocannabinoids Plant substances that stimulate cannabinoid receptors. Were initially discovered in *Cannabis* spp. but later identified in *Echinacea* spp., among other plants including Hops.

Phytochemistry Branch of chemistry concerned with major substances found in plants and the therapeutic properties that result.

Phytoestrogens Plants with estrogen-like activity that bind to human estrogen receptor sites and block harmful estrogens. They are not identical to human estrogens but have structural similarities. Examples: Red Clover flower and Soy.

Phytopharmaceutical Herbal product that is standardized to contain a given amount of a particular ingredient, has received a patent, and is now a standardized drug.

Pinyin Official phonetic system for transcribing Mandarin pronunciations of Chinese characters into the Latin alphabet. Examples: *Huang Qi* for Astragalus root and *Shu Di Huang* for prepared Rehmannia root.

Pistil (Stigma, Style, Ovary, Carpel) The female part of a flower. Consists of the top *stigma*, the middle *style*, and the bottom *ovary*. The ovary contains the *ovules*. A single ovary is a *carpel*. After fertilization, an ovule develops into a seed.

Plaque Waxy substance that builds up inside the coronary arteries causing atherosclerosis. Can eventually block an artery, causing a heart attack.

Plaster A long-lasting oil or wax-based medication applied topically.

Poaceae The Grass family, with hollow stems and kneelike joints or nodes.

Polarity A molecule with an uneven distribution of electrical charges. There are areas of partial positive charge and areas of partial negative charge. Substances of similar polarities will dissolve within one another, and those of dissimilar polarities will not. Important when considering proportions of alcohol, water, or glycerin relative to a plant's constituents.

Polyunsaturated Fats Lipids in which the hydrocarbon chain possesses two or more carbon double bonds. They are unsaturated because the molecule contains less than the maximum amount of hydrogen. Examples: nuts, seeds, fish, algae, leafy greens, and krill.

Portal System The liver's private circulatory system that receives raw nutrients from digestion to be processed or stored before being passed on to the heart.

Potentiation Interaction between two or more drugs or herbs resulting in a pharmacologic response greater than the sum of individual responses to each single drug or herb. Example: Jamaican Dogwood bark combined with the narcotic alkaloid morphine.

Poultice A soft, mushy external application of herbs made into a paste.

Prebiotics Fibers acting as food sources for probiotics. Consist of fructooligosaccharides, inulin, and beta-glucans. Examples: cooked onions, raw garlic, leeks, and asparagus.

Precipitate Falling out of solution and settling at the bottom of a liquid.

Premenstrual Syndrome (PMS) Large variety of physical and behavioral symptoms, usually occurring in the luteal phase of the menstrual cycle. Examples: depression, anxiety, mood swings, food cravings, and/or weight gain.

Primary Qualities Taste, warmth, and moisture are the primary qualities in herbal energetics.

Probiotics Live, friendly bacteria making up the microbiome of a healthy digestive track. Examples: *lactobacillus bulgaricus*, *lactobacillus acidophilus*, and *bifidobacteria*.

Progesterone Female hormone released by the corpus luteum in the second half of the menstrual cycle.

Prolactin Anterior pituitary hormone that stimulates lactation. When not breastfeeding, high levels can cause short luteal phases, hypothyroidism, and infertility; it can cause erectile dysfunction in men.

Proof Twice the percentage of the alcohol content. Example: 95% alcohol is 190 proof.

Property of an Herb The effect an herb has on the body. An herb's potential for achieving a particular outcome. Examples: herbal actions that stimulate, sedate, restore, relax, astringe, or eliminate.

Proportion or Part The amount (usually in milliliters) of one herb in relation to another herb in formula. A constant. Example: a formula with 1 part Calendula flower, 2 parts Lavender herb, and 3 parts Lemon balm leaf.

Proteinuria Protein in the urine.

Pruritis Severe itching of the skin.

Pseudoaldosteronism Adverse herb effect caused from very high doses of Licorice root in susceptible individuals. Mimics hyperaldosteronism (too much aldosterone). The effect causes high sodium, low potassium, edema, hypertension, and cardiac problems. Reversible when the herb is discontinued.

Psoriasis Noncontagious raised skin plaques caused by abnormally fast turnover of skin cells that do not shed, which is caused by autoimmune factors.

Psychoneuroimmunology The study of the interaction between the brain, nervous system, and immune system, and how they affect each other.

Pulse Dosing Frequent herbal doses given every 15 minutes to 30 minutes to 1 hour. Often used for pain, insomnia, acute infection, or bleeding.

Pulse (Chinese Medicine) A reflection of the blood and qi circulating through the vessels that tell about the condition of each organ.

Puncture Wound Sharp penetrating wound caused from splinters, thorns, or foreign objects that pierce the skin.

Purgatives Very strong, forceful stimulating anthraquinone laxatives that can be habit forming. Examples: *Rhamnus purshiana* (Cascara Sagrada bark), *Rheum officinale* (Rhubarb root), and *Cassia acutifolia* (Senna leaf/pod).

Purulence Condition of containing or secreting pus.

Pyelonephritis Inflammation of the kidney as a result of bacterial infection.

Pyrrolizidine Alkaloids (PAs) Alkaloids that might/can cause liver toxicity in large amounts. Examples: Comfrey leaf and root, and in lesser quantity Coltsfoot herb.

Q

Qi (Chinese Medicine) The body's natural life force or energy that flows through pathways called meridians.

Qi Tonics (Chinese Medicine) Herbs that increase physiological energy production in the body. Example: Astragalus Huang Qi (Astragalus root), Panax Ren Shen (Asian Ginseng root), and Codonopsis Dang Shen (Downy Bellflower root).

Qigong (Chinese Medicine) A mind-body practice and an energetic form of movement used to enhance the flow of qi through the body. Uses body movements, breathing, and focused intention to improve mental and physical health.

Quality An herb's nature or sensory description. How it acts upon contact with the mouth, skin, stomach, and sense organs. Refers to taste, heat, and moisture.

R

Rainbow Diet Healthy dietary concept embracing a multicolored plate of food, guaranteeing intake of a full selection of vitamins, minerals, and antioxidants.

Rancidity Spoilage of oils or fats due to oxidation (combining with oxygen in the atmosphere). To prevent this, store oils away from heat, light, air, and moisture.

Recalcitrant Species Seeds that cannot be dried and frozen and still retain viability. Therefore, seed bank storage is ineffective.

Recalls Actions taken by a firm to remove a faulty product from the market.

Relaxants Herbs that treat tense, restrained conditions in the body. Examples: antispasmodics (stop spasms), anticonvulsants (stop seizures), and muscle relaxants.

Renal Calculi Hardened stone formation anywhere in in urinary tract. Made from calcium oxalate, calcium phosphate, or uric acid.

Renin-Angiotensin-Aldosterone (RAA) Pathway Complex system in the kidneys that maintains normal blood pressure and assures proper heart function. Pathway involves release of the enzyme renin, and the conversion of angiotensin I, (under the stimulus of ACE2 enzyme), into the strong vasopressor, angiotensin II. Aldosterone is also released from the adrenals which brings sodium and more water into the blood.

Restoratives Herbs that build and nourish tissues. In Chinese medicine terms they support the body's vital energy or qi and treat weak, deficient conditions. Examples: Red Clover flower, Codonopsis Dang Shen (Downy Bellflower root), and Milky Oat berry.

Rheumatoid Arthritis Chronic systemic autoimmune inflammatory disease that attacks peripheral joints and surrounding muscles, tendons, and ligaments, especially the hands, feet, ankles, and knees.

RICE Acronym for Rest, Ice, Compression, and Elevation, a first aid protocol for sprains and strains and trauma injury.

Rosaceae The Rose family with five sepals, five petals, numerous stamens, and oval serrated leaves.

Rubefacients Herbs used topically in analgesic liniments, sometimes called *counterirritants.* Cause varying degrees of skin redness by dilating the capillaries and increasing blood circulation. Examples: Cayenne fruit, Mustard seed, Garlic bulb, Camphor resin, and Nettle herb.

S

Salicylates and Salicylic Acid A phenolic acid derived from the naturally occurring salicylic glycosides found in plants. Examples: White Willow bark, Meadowsweet herb, and Aspen bark. The drug version is acetylsalicylic acid (ASA) or aspirin.

Saluretics Diuretic herbs that increase renal excretion of sodium chloride. Examples: Dandelion leaf and Goldenrod herb.

Salves A semisolid fatty herbal mixture prepared for external use made from a wax and oil base. Other names: *ointments* and *unguents.*

Saturated Fatty Acids (SFAs) Molecules with hydrogen atoms filling up the tail making them solid at room temperature. Examples: animal fats and the tropical plant oils of palm and coconut.

Sebum A light yellow, oily substance secreted by the sebaceous (oil) glands that help keep the skin and hair moisturized.

Secondary Qualities In herbal energetics, herbs possessing a specific therapeutic action. They can be stimulating, sedating, restoring, relaxing, or moistening. Each quality treats the opposite condition. Example: a warm stimulating, moving herb such as Prickly Ash bark could be used for cold sluggish blood circulation.

Sedating Herb quality that treats excess hot conditions or hyperactivity. It reduces heat of infection and is cool, dry, and bitter. It cools the nervous system in a hyperactive person. Examples: Hops flower, Passionflower herb, California Poppy herb.

Seed Bank A place where seeds are stored to preserve genetic diversity.

Selective Estrogen Receptor Modulators (SERMs) Drug classification used for prevention of osteoporosis and breast cancer. SERMs allow estrogen to enter the uterine and bone tissue but block it from entering breast tissue. Example: Tamoxifen.

Serotonin Syndrome Adverse side effect from use of antidepressive selective serotonin reuptake inhibitor (SSRI) drugs like Prozac and Zoloft. Serotonin syndrome can cause diarrhea, sweating, shaking, and possible life-threatening seizures. Herbal implication: St John's Wort has been cited in potentiating this if combined with SSRIs in treating depression. Opinions are mixed about the truth of this drug/herb interaction.

Shen (Chinese Medicine) The spirit or essence that is stored in the Heart associated with the human personality and the ability to live life fully and happily. Shen disharmonies lead to mental illnesses.

Shingles A viral infection causing a painful rash that follows a nerve ganglion on one side of the body. St. John's Wort is a key antiviral herb for shingles.

Sialagogues Herbs that increase the flow of saliva. Example: Prickly Ash bark.

Signs Objective information about a client's condition that can be observed or measured, such as external bleeding, blood pressure, pulse rate, or lab results.

Simple The use of a single herb in a remedy.

Sinews (Chinese Medicine) Refers to tendons and ligaments. The Liver rules the sinews.

Sinusitis Inflammation and infection in the paranasal sinuses. Condition may be acute or become chronic and linger for years.

Sitz bath Specialized bath taken by sitting in hot or cold water to cover the pelvis. Herbs may be included. Used for gynecological, urinary, and lower gastrointestinal problems.

Small Intestinal Bacterial Overgrowth (SIBO) The presence of excessive bad/toxic bacteria in the small intestine.

Smokes The therapeutic smoking of dried, relaxing herbs.

S.O.A.P. Acronym for subjective, objective, assessment, and plan. An organizational method of charting.

Solubility The ability of a given substance to dissolve in a particular solvent such as water, alcohol, or vinegar.

Spasm Abnormal and involuntary contraction of a skeletal muscle that can cause a great deal of pain.

Spasmolytics (Alternately called antispasmodics.) Herbs that decrease smooth muscle spasms. Examples: Cramp bark, Valerian root, Corydalis Yan Hu Suo (Asian Corydalis corm), and Black Cohosh root.

Species A group of organisms that resemble each other more closely than those of any other group and are capable of reproducing with one another to produce fertile offspring.

Sphygmomanometer Instrument used to measure blood pressure, an inflatable cuff with a gauge attached that is wrapped around a limb above a radial pulse.

Spirits Combinations of ethanol and essential oils used for flavoring or added to tinctures, syrups, honeys, and elixirs.

Spleen Tonics (Chinese Medicine) Herbs that restore and heal the Spleen (digestion), such as Codonopsis Dang Shen (Downy Bellflower root) and Atractylodes Bai Zhu (White Atractylodes root.

Sprain A torn or twisted ligament.

Stagnation (Chinese Medicine) A slowing of the circulation of body fluids (blood or lymph) or energy in the body. The slower something circulates, the more solid it gets, eventually becoming a mass. The action of an organ or muscle may also slow from stagnation.

Stamen (Pollen, Anther, Filament) The male part of a flower consisting of the *pollen* on the tip, the *anther* on which the pollen sits, and the *filament* or stalk. Stamen is pronounced *stay men.*

Standardization Implies that one or more components, usually that deemed active ingredient(s), are present in a specific, guaranteed amount, often expressed as a metric measurement or a percentage. It guarantees that the consumer gets a product in which the chemistry of the product is specific from batch to batch.

Standardized Dose Refers to an herbal extract or pill guaranteed to have a set number of active constituents per dose, determined by laboratory analysis.

Steam Breathing in the vapors of an herbal infusion high in essential oils.

Sterols A group of antiinflammatory saponins naturally occurring in plants. Some lower cholesterol, some are adrenal tonics, and some act as steroids in muscular skeletal pain.

Stimulants Herbs that help to create movement or increase an action in the body caused by cold conditions. They are warming. Stimulants can move blood in the limbs or internal organs, move lymphatic flow, release muscle spasms. Examples: Cayenne pepper, Ephedra Ma Huang (Ephedra stem), and Cardamom pod.

Strain A stretching or tearing of a muscle or its tendon.

Stye A bacterial infected, pus-filled oil gland present at the eyelash base. Not contagious but irritating, itchy, and painful.

Styptics Herbs that stop external bleeding, often used in compresses or poultices. Examples: Plantain leaf, Oak bark, Cayenne pepper, and Yarrow herb.

Subfamily Taxonomical classification directly under family, with smaller botanical differences. Example: Faboideae, with flowers having a banner, wings, and keel structure in the Pea family.

Substrate The therapeutic drug, herb, or food that is acted upon by an enzyme in the cytochrome P450 system.

Suppository (Bolus) A single-dosed preparation inserted into the rectum or vagina for local or systemic healing.

Symbiotic Relationship Mutually beneficial relationships such as with fungi and algae.

Symptoms Subjective evidence of disease, such as pain, anxiety, or depression.

Syndrome or Disharmony (Chinese Medicine) Phrase for functional disturbances or illnesses, such as Wind Damp Heat, or Liver Yang Rising.

Synergy Two or more chemicals potentiating the effect of the herb and/or decreasing its toxicity. Concept that the effect of the whole herb is greater than its parts.

Syrup A thick, sweet herbal preparation. A saturated solution of sugar in pure water or other aqueous liquid.

Systemic Affecting the whole body by traveling through the blood stream.

Systolic Pressure The highest blood pressure number. Occurs when the right ventricular valve in the heart contracts, pushing the blood out into circulation.

T

Tannins A class of water-soluble astringent polyphenols, biomolecules in roots, seeds, bark, and leaves. Have a drying astringent taste. Examples: Oak bark, Green tea, or Coffee.

Taxonomy Classification of organisms, both plant and animal, based on their structural characteristics and evolutionary history.

Tendon Tough band of fibrous connective tissue that connects a muscle to a bone. A sinew.

Teratogenesis Relating to or causing malformations of an embryo or fetus. Any agent that can do this is referred to as *teratogenic.*

Terpenes The largest group of secondary plant metabolites. Their basic structure is a 5-carbon precursor isoprene. These units can be assembled chemically in many different ways, accounting for their diversity. Types include essential oils, resins, saponins, steroids, carotenoid pigment, and rubber.

Testosterone An androgen, the major male sex hormone.

Therapeutic Bath Emersion of the body or a body part into hot, warm, tepid, or cold water where herbs have been added.

Therapeutic Goods Act of Australia (TGA) The Australian standard for regulation of herbs, vitamins, minerals, nutritional supplements, and homeopathics, established in 1989. They are referred to as *complementary medicines* based on a risk management approach designed to ensure public health and safety.

Therapeutic Principles Main intentions in a formula. A list of what the herbalist intends to accomplish.

Thomsonian Movement American health movement of the 1800s started by Samuel Thomson. Supported the body's inclination to heal itself and championed gentle herbs over dramatic dangerous practices of the time.

Thrombus A blood clot in the vascular system that blocks or impedes blood flow.

Tincture Alcohol or alcohol and water preparation suitable for roots, seeds, fruits, or herbs, usually in a 1:5 to 1:3 concentration of crude plant material to menstruum.

Tonics (Chinese Medicine) Herbs that nourish, strengthen, and build up tissues and vitality, and treat deficiencies. They build yin, yang, qi or blood, or combinations thereof. Examples: *Panax* spp. (the Ginsengs), Astragalus Huang Qi (Astragalus root), Ganoderma Ling Zhi (Reishi mushroom), Schisandra Wu Wei Zi (Five Taste berry).

Toxicosis Build-up of poisons in the body from environmental (exogenous) factors or from factors that originate in the body (endogenous).

Trans Fatty Acid (FA) Fatty acid that is chemically altered by overheating, oxidation, and partial hydrogenation because of the forced addition of hydrogen into Omega-6 polyunsaturated oils to make it semihard at room temperatures. Examples: Margarine and most junk foods.

Transit Time Number of hours for food to move from the mouth to the end of the intestine or anus.

Tribe Taxonomical classification directly under subfamily, only with smaller botanical differences. Example: Trifolieae, Clover tribe with three-parted leaves in the Pea family.

Tridosha In Ayurveda, the three fundamental energies or principles governing the function of our bodies on a physical and emotional level. The three doshas are Vata, Pitta, and Kapha.

Triglycerides The main constituents of natural fats and oils. Consist of three molecules of fatty acid combined with a molecule of the alcohol glycerol. Elevated levels are a risk factor for heart disease and stroke.

Tropho-Restoratives Nutritive restoratives that have an affinity or tropism to particular organs and tissues and that improve structure and function. Examples: Burdock root or Horsetail herb (skin), or Dandelion root and Milk thistle seed (liver).

Tuina (Chinese Medicine) Therapeutic bodywork combining massage, acupressure, and other forms of body manipulation. Opens the body's blockages and stimulates movement in the meridians and muscles.

Twenty-Four-Hour Organ Clock (Chinese Medicine) A representation of the yin/yang organ pairs showing the time of day when each is dominant and having the most vital energy. Each organ cycles through a two-hour period and the complete cycle takes 24 hours.

U

Unani-Tibb Also called Unani Medicine, a form of traditional medicine practiced in the Middle East and South Asia. It is based on the teachings of Hippocrates and Galen who were influenced by Islamic theories.

United States Pharmacopeia (USP) Formed in 1820, a science-based, nonprofit public health organization. It is the official public standard-setting authority for all dietary supplements (including herbs), prescription and over-the-counter medicines, and other health care products manufactured and sold in the United States.

Unsaturated Fatty Acid (UFA) A fat that has at least one double bond, and the hydrogens do not fill up the tail, making it liquid at room temperature. Examples: Vegetable oils of olive, avocado, and canola.

Urea The end product of protein metabolism, from which *urine* is named.

Urethritis Inflammation of the ureters.

Urinary Tract Infection (UTI) An infection in any part of the urinary system. Usually ascends from the outside and up the tract. Terms for infection in: the urethra (*urethritis*), the bladder (*cystitis*), the ureter (*urethritis*), to kidney level (*pyelonephritis*).

Urticaria Hives. An allergic skin rash with raised, itchy bumps or raised flat wheals.

Uterine Fibroid Most common noncancerous uterine tumor affecting women past age 35. Varies in size and location. They are driven by hormones and shrink after menopause.

V

Vaccine Substance that stimulates the production of antibodies and provides immunity against one or several diseases, often viral.

Vagus The 10th cranial nerve, longest of the 12 paired cranial nerves that physically connect the gut to the brain, carrying chemical messages back and forth.

Varicose Veins A weakening and widening of the venous walls in the lower legs, a type of peripheral vascular disease (PVD).

Vasoconstriction Narrowing or constricting of the muscular walls of the blood vessels. Can cause blood pressure to increase.

Vasodilation Dilation or widening of the muscular walls of the blood vessels that allows blood to flow more easily. Can lower blood pressure.

Vasodilators Class of herbs and medications that are cooling and relaxing. They can lower blood pressure and encourage diaphoresis by relaxing and dilating the capillaries near the skin. In Chinese Medicine, used for External Wind Heat. Examples: Elderflower blossoms and Chrysanthemum Ju Hua.

Vasopressor Drug classification that causes blood vessels to constrict and increases blood pressure. Example: Epinephrine.

Vegetarian Diet There are three main types. None allow meat, fish, or fowl. *Ovo-lactovegetarians* eat plants, eggs, and dairy. *Lactovegetarians* eat plants and dairy but not eggs. *Vegans* eat plants but no animal products at all, including eggs and dairy.

Vermifuges Herbs that expel helminths or worms, also known as *anthelmintics*. Examples: Areca Bing Lang (Betel Nut), Eugenia Ding Xiang (Clove bud), Rue herb, and Garlic bulb. Technically, *vermicides* kill the worms, and *vermifuges* flush them out.

Vinegar A sour-tasting liquid containing acetic acid, obtained by fermenting dilute alcoholic liquids used as menstruums, such as wine, cider, or beer.

Virus Tiny infective microorganism consisting of a nucleic acid molecule (RNA or DNA) in a protein coat. A virus is too small to be seen by light microscopy and is able to multiply only in the living cells of a host.

Vitalism Holistic approach aimed at preventing and treating disease through supporting a person's vital force. Sees the body as a whole unit working together and more than the sum of its parts. The use of energetics in herbalism.

Volatile Oil An oil having the odor or flavor of the plant from which it comes. A tendency to vaporize. Example: Peppermint and Hyssop essential oils.

Vulneraries Herbs that heal tissues or cuts, bruises, and lacerations. Examples: Comfrey root, Goldenseal root, and Marigold herb.

W

Warmth One of the primary qualities, along with moisture and taste. The entire spectrum of gradations from hot to warm to neutral to cool to cold.

Weight-to-Volume (W/V) Method of tincture production that assumes 1 gram of herb (weight) is equal to 1 cubic centimeter of water or menstruum (volume). Precise weights of herbs and menstruum volumes are calculated and measured to produce a specific tincture strength.

Whitehead Whitish elevations of sebum in blocked skin pores.

Wildcrafting The gathering or harvesting of wild plants in a conscious manner.

Wind (Chinese Medicine) One of the Six Pernicious Influences. Wind denotes movement. *External Wind* brings cold, damp, and pathogens into the body from the external environment. *Internal Wind* originates in the liver and implies involuntary movements such as seizures, spasms, and dizziness.

Wise-Woman Tradition Oldest type of healing known, where oral information about the healing attributes of local plants is passed down by women from generation to generation.

World Health Organization (WHO) Established in 1948, the World Health Organization defines the traditional use of herbal medicines as having had long history that is well established and widely acknowledged to be safe and effective and may be accepted by national authorities.

X

Xenoestrogens Industrial compounds found in the environment that mimic human estrogen molecules and hook on to estrogen receptor sites in the body, displacing human estrogen.

Y

Yang Deficiency (Chinese Medicine) Condition of coldness due to deficiency of warming yang. Symptoms are lethargy, poor digestion, and lower back pain.

Yang Tonics (Chinese Medicine) Herbs that are warm and circulating and help deficient, weak conditions and therefore strengthen yang. Examples: Cervus Lu Rong (Velvet Deer Antler) that tonifies Kidney yang and Eucommia Du Zhong (Eucommia bark) that builds up bone and sinews.

Yin Deficiency (Chinese Medicine) Condition of warmth and dryness due to lack of cooling yin. Symptoms are night sweats and the five hots: burning sensations in the palms, soles of the feet, and the chest.

Yin Tonics (Chinese Medicine) Herbs that are moist and nourishing and strengthen yin. Examples: Asparagus Tien Men Dong (Shiny Asparagus tuber) or Anemarrhena Zhi Mu (Know Mother root).

Young's Rule Formula for calculating children's dosage using age. Child's age divided by 12 plus the age.

Z

Zoology Study of the behavior, structure, physiology, classification, and distribution of animals.

Cross Index: Herbs by Botanical Name

Latin Binomial	Common Name	Pinyin Name (Cantonese)
A		
Achillea millefolium	Yarrow herb and essential oil	None
Aconitum carmichaelii	Prepared Sichuan Aconite root	Fu Zi
Acorus calamus	Calamus root	Bai/Shui Chang Pu
Actaea racemosa	Black Cohosh root	None
Adenophora stricta	Upright Ladybell root	Nan Sha Shen
Aesculus chinensis	Chinese Horse Chestnut	Suo Luo Zi
Aesculus hippocastanum	Horse Chestnut	None
Agastache rugosa	Rugose Giant Hyssop herb	Huo Xiang
Agathosma betulina and spp.	Buchu leaf	None
Agrimonia eupatoria	Agrimony herb	None
Akebia quinata	Akebia stem	Bai Mu Tong
Alchemilla arvensis	Parsley piert herb	None
Alchemilla vulgaris	Lady's Mantle herb	None
Aletris farinose	Unicorn root	None
Alisma orientalis	Water plantain root	Ze Xie
Allium sativum	Garlic bulb	Da Suan
Allium spp.	Wild Onion bulb	None
Alnus serrulata	Alder bark	None
Aloe vera and spp.	Aloe resin and gel	Lu Hui
Althea officinalis	Marshmallow root	None
Ambrosia artemisiifolia	Ragweed herb	None
Amomum villosum	Wild Cardamom pod	Sha Ren
Andrographis paniculata	Heart-thread Lotus leaf	Chuan Xin Lian
Anemarrhena asphodeloides	Know Mother root	Zhi Mu
Anemone pulsatilla/patens	Pasqueflower herb	None
Anemopsis californica	Yerba Mansa herb	None
Anethum graveolens	Dill seed and essential oil	None
Angelica archangelica	Angelica root and essential oil	None
Angelica pubescens	Hairy Angelica root	Du Ho
Angelica sinensis	Angelica root, Dong Quai	Dang Gui
Anticlea elegans	Mountain Death Camus plant	None
Apium graveolens	Celery seed and root	None
Arctium lappa	Burdock root	Niu Bang Zi (seed)
Arctostaphylos uva-ursi	Uva ursi leaf, Bearberry, Kinnikinnick	None
Areca catechu	Betel nut	Bing Lang
Arnica montana and spp.	Arnica flower	None
Artemisia absinthium	Wormwood herb	None
Artemisia annua	Sweet Annie herb	Huang Hua Hao
Artemisia argyi	Asian Mugwort leaf	Ai Ye
Artemisia dracunculus	Tarragon herb and essential oil	None
Artemisia tridentata and spp.	Sagebrush herb	None
Artemisia vulgaris	Mugwort herb and essential oil	None
Asarum canadensis	Wild Ginger root	None
Asarum spp.	Asian Wild Ginger root and herb	Xi Xin
Asclepias speciosa	Milkweed	None
Asclepias tuberosa	Pleurisy root	None
Asparagus cochinchinensis	Shiny Asparagus root	Tian Men Dong
Asparagus officinalis	Asparagus root	None
Asparagus racemosus	Shatavari root	None
Astragalus membranaceus	Astragalus root	Huang Qi
Astragalus spp.	Astragalus seed	Sha Yuan Zi
Atractylodes lancea	Black Atractylodes root	Cang Zhu
Atractylodes macrocephala	White Atractylodes root	Bai Zhu
Avena sativa	Milky Oat tops, berry, and straw	None
B		
Bacopa monnieri	Water Hyssop, Bacopa, whole plant	None
Baptisia tinctoria	Wild Indigo root	None
Barosma betulina	Buchu leaf	None

Latin Binomial	Common Name	Pinyin Name (Cantonese)
Berberis vulgaris	Barberry root bark	None
Betonica officinalis	Wood betony herb	None
Betula alba and spp.	Birch leaf, bark, and essential oil	Hua Mu Pi (bark)
Borago officinalis	Borage leaf	None
Boswellia carterii and serrata	Frankincense resin and essential oil	Ru Xiang
Brassica spp.	Mustard seed	None
Brucea javanica	Java berry	Ya Dan Zi
Bupleurum chinense	Asian Buplever root	Chai Hu

C

Latin Binomial	Common Name	Pinyin Name (Cantonese)
Calendula officinalis	Calendula, Marigold, Pot Marigold flower	None
Camellia sinensis	Tea leaf	Cha Ye
Cannabis sativa and *C. indica*	Marijuana bud/ Grass/Pot	None
Capsella bursa-pastoris	Shepherd's Purse herb	Jia Cai
Capsicum annuum	Cayenne Pepper fruit	None
Carduus benedictus	Blessed Thistle herb	None
Carthamus tinctorius	Safflower	Hong Hua
Cassia acutifolia	Senna leaf	None
Cassia obtusifolia	Sickle Senna seed	Jue Ming Zi
Caulophyllum thalictroides	Blue Cohosh root	None
Ceanothus spp.	Red Root	None
Centella asiatica	Gotu Kola leaf	Ji Xue Cao
Cereus grandiflorus, syn. *Selenicereus grandiflorus*	Night Blooming Cactus flower and stem	None
Cervus nippon and spp.	Mature Deer antler	Hua Lu Gen
Cetraria islandica	Iceland Moss thallus	None
Chamaelirium luteum	Helonias, False Unicorn root	None
Chelidonium majus and spp.	Celandine herb	Bai Qu Cai
Chimaphila umbellata	Pipsissewa herb and root	None
Chionanthus virginicus	Fringe Tree root bark	None
Chlorella spp	Microalgae	None
Chondrus crispus	Irish Moss thallus	None
Chrysanthemum parthenium	Feverfew herb	None
Chrysanthemum x *morifolium*	Chrysanthemum flower	Ju Hua
Cichorium intybus	Chicory root	None
Cicuta maculata	Spotted Water Hemlock plant	None
Cinchona spp.	Cinchona bark	None
Cinnamomum spp.	Cinnamon bark, twig, and essential oil	Rou Gui (bark), Gui Zhi (twig)
Citrus aurantium	Bitter Orange fruit, Neroli essential oil (flower)	Zhi Shi (unripe), Zhi Ke (ripe)
Citrus limonum	Lemon rind and essential oil	None
Citrus reticulata and spp.	Tangerine peel and essential oil	Qing Pi (unripe), Chen Pi (ripe)
Citrus x *aurantium var. sinensis*	Sweet Orange fruit	Tian Chen
Cochlearia armoracia	Horseradish root	None
Codonopsis pilosula	Downy Bellflower root	Dang Shen
Coffea arabica	Coffee bean	None
Coix lachryma	Job's Tears seed	Yi Yi Ren
Coleus forskohlii	Coleus root	None
Collinsonia canadensis	Stoneroot	None
Commiphora myrrha	Myrrh resin and essential oil	Mo Yao
Conium maculatum	Poison Hemlock plant	None
Convallaria majalis	Lily of the Valley herb	None
Coptis chinensis	Coptis root	Huang Lian
Cordyceps sinensis	Chinese Caterpillar mushroom	Dong Chong Xia Cao
Coriandrum sativum	Cilantro herb and seed	Hu Sui (herb), Hu Shi Zi (seed)
Cornus officinalis	Japanese Dogwood berry	Shan Zhu Yu
Corydalis spp.	Prepared Asian Corydalis corm	Yan Hu Suo
Crataegus spp.	Hawthorn berry	None
Crataegus spp.	Asian Hawthorn berry	Shan Zha
Crataeva nurvala	Crataeva stem and root bark	None
Crocus sativus	Saffron flower styles, stigmas	Xi Hong Hua
Cucurbita spp.	Pumpkin seed	None
Cupressus sempervirens	Cypress tip	None
Curcuma longa	Turmeric root	Yu Jin
Cuscuta chinensis	Asian Dodder seed	Tu Si Zi
Cynara scolymus	Artichoke leaf	None
Cytisus scoparius syn. *Sarothamnus scoparius*	Broom, Scotch Broom tops	None

D

Latin Binomial	Common Name	Pinyin Name (Cantonese)
Datura stramonium and *D. alba* and spp.	Jimsonweed, Angel's Trumpet plant	Yang Jin Hua (flower)
Daucus carota	Wild Carrot seed	Nan He Zao
Dendrobium nobile	Stonebushel stem	Shi Hu
Desmodium styracifolium	Coin-Leaf Desmodium herb	Guang Jin Qian Cao
Dianthus superbus	Proud Pink herb	Qu Mai

Latin Binomial	Common Name	Pinyin Name (Cantonese)
Dioscorea spp.	Mountain Yam root	Shan Yao
Dioscorea villosa	Wild Yam rhizome	None

E

Latin Binomial	Common Name	Pinyin Name (Cantonese)
Echinacea angustifolia, E. purpurea	Echinacea root, flower cone	None
Elettaria cardamomum	Cardamom pod and essential oil	None
Eleutherococcus senticosus	Siberian/Eleuthero ginseng root	Ci Wu Jia
Emblica officinalis	Amla, Indian Gooseberry	None
Ephedra sinica	Ephedra twig	Ma Huang
Epimedium saggitatum	Horney Goat Weed leaf	Yin Yang Huo
Equisetum arvense and spp.	Horsetail herb	Mu Zei
Eriobotrya japonica	Loquat leaf	Pi Pa Ye
Eriodictyon spp.	Yerba Santa leaf	None
Eryngium maritimum	Sea Holly root	None
Eschscholzia californica	California Poppy root and herb	None
Eucalyptus globulus	Eucalyptus leaf and essential oil	An Ye
Eucommia ulmoides	Eucommia bark	Du Zhong
Eugenia caryophyllata and syn. *Syzygium aromaticum*	Clove bud and essential oil	Ding Xiang
Eupatorium perfoliatum	Boneset herb	None
Eupatorium purpureum	Gravel root	None
Euphoria longan	Longan berry and fruit	Long Yan Rou
Euphrasia spp.	Eyebright herb	None

F

Latin Binomial	Common Name	Pinyin Name (Cantonese)
Filipendula ulmaria	Meadowsweet herb	None
Foeniculum vulgare	Fennel seed and essential oil	None
Forsythia suspensa	Forsythia valve	Lian Qiao
Fouquieria splendens	Ocotillo bark	None
Fragaria vesca	Strawberry leaf	None
Fritillaria thunbergii	Zhejiang Fritillaria bulb	Zhe Bei Mu
Fucus vesiculosus	Bladderwrack thallus	None

G

Latin Binomial	Common Name	Pinyin Name (Cantonese)
Galium aparine	Cleavers herb	Ba Xian Cao
Ganoderma lucidum	Reishi mushroom	Ling Zhi
Gardenia jasminoides	Gardenia pod	Zhi Zi
Gastrodia elata	Celestial Hemp corm	Tian Ma
Gaultheria procumbens	Wintergreen herb (Eastern N. America)	None
Gentiana lutea and spp.	Gentian root	None
Gentiana scabra	Scabrous Gentian root	Long Dan Cao
Geranium maculatum	Cranesbill root	Lao Guan Cao
Ginkgo biloba	Ginkgo leaf	Yin Xing Ye
Glycyrrhiza glabra and *G. lepidota*	Licorice root	None
Glycyrrhiza uralensis	Licorice root	Gan Cao, Zhi Gan Cao (honey fried)
Gossypium spp.	Cotton root bark	Mian Hua Gen
Granum floris pollinis	Flower pollen	None
Grifola frondosa	Maitake mushroom, Hen of the Woods	Hui Shu Hua
Grindelia robusta	Gum Weed flower	None
Gymnema sylvestre	Gymnema herb	Wu Xue Teng

H

Latin Binomial	Common Name	Pinyin Name (Cantonese)
Hamamelis virginiana	Witch Hazel leaf	None
Harpagophytum procumbens	Devil's Claw root	None
Heracleum spp.	Cow Parsnip leaf and seed	None
Houttuynia cordata	Fishwort herb	Yu Xing Cao
Humulus lupulus	Hops flower	None
Hydrangea arborescens	Hydrangea root	None
Hydrastis canadensis	Goldenseal root	None
Hypericum perforatum	St. John's Wort	Guan Ye Lian Qiao
Hyssopus officinalis	Hyssop herb and essential oil	None

I

Latin Binomial	Common Name	Pinyin Name (Cantonese)
Ilex paraguariensis	Yerba Maté leaf and twig	None
Inula helenium	Elecampane root	Tu Mu Xiang
Iris versicolor	Blue Flag rhizome	None
Isatis tinctoria, I. indigotica	Isatis, Woad root	Ban Lang Gen
Isatis tinctoria, I. indigotica	Isatis, Woad leaf	Da Qing Ye

J

Latin Binomial	Common Name	Pinyin Name (Cantonese)
Juglans regia and *J. nigra*	Walnut leaf and hull, Black Walnut seed, leaf, and hull	Hu Tao Ren (meat), Ye (leaf), Zhi (twig)
Juniperus communis and spp.	Juniper berry and essential oil	None

L

Latin Binomial	Common Name	Pinyin Name (Cantonese)
Lactuca serriola	Prickly Lettuce	None
Lactuca virosa	Wild Lettuce leaf	None
Laminaria spp.	Kelp thallus	Kun Bu
Larrea divaricata	Creosote, Chaparral leaf	None
Lavandula angustifolia	Lavender flower and essential oil	None
Ledebouriella divaricata	Wind Protector root	Fang Feng
Lentinula edodes	Shitake mushroom (Japanese)	Xiang Gu
Leonurus cardiaca	Motherwort herb	None
Leonurus spp.	Asian Motherwort herb	Yi Mu Cao
Lepidium meyenii	Maca root	None
Ligusticum levisticum	Lovage root and essential oil	Ou Dang Gui
Ligusticum porteri	Osha root	None
Ligusticum sinense	Chinese Lovage root	Gao Ben
Ligusticum wallichii	Sichuan Lovage root	Chuan Xiong
Ligustrum lucidum	Glossy Privet berry	Nu Zhen Zi
Linum usitatissimum	Flax seed	Ya Ma Zi
Lobelia chinensis	Lobelia herb	Ban Bian Lian
Lobelia inflata	Lobelia herb	None
Lonicera japonica and spp.	Japanese Honeysuckle flower	Jin Yin Hua
Lycium chinense and spp.	Goji berry, Wolfberry, Lycii	Gou Qi Zi
Lycopus virginicus	Bugleweed herb	None

M

Latin Binomial	Common Name	Pinyin Name (Cantonese)
Macuna pruriens	Velvet bean	None
Magnolia liliiflora	Magnolia bud	Xin Yi Hua
Magnolia officinalis	Magnolia bark	Hou Po
Mahonia repens	Oregon Grape root	None
Malpighia glabra	Acerola or Barbados cherry	None
Marrubium vulgare	White Horehound leaf	None
Matricaria recutita	German Chamomile flower and essential oil	None
Medicago sativa	Alfalfa herb	None
Melaleuca alternifolia	Tea Tree leaf and essential oil	None
Melia toosendan	Sichuan Bead Tree berry	Chuan Lian Zi
Melilotus officinalis	Melilot, Sweet Yellow Clover herb	None
Melissa officinalis	Lemon Balm leaf and essential oil	None
Mentha arvensis	Mint herb, Asian field mint, field mint, Poléo mint	Bo He
Mentha pulegium	Pennyroyal herb	None
Mentha spicata	Spearmint leaf and essential oil	Xiang Hua Cai
Mentha x *piperita*	Peppermint leaf and essential oil	None
Menyanthes trifoliata	Bogbean leaf and herb	Shui Cai Ye
Mitchella repens	Partridgeberry herb	None
Mitragyna speciosa	Kratom leaf	None
Momordica charantia	Bitter Melon fruit	Ku Gua (Gan)
Monarda fistulosa	Wild Oregano, Beebalm herb	None
Myristica fragrans	Nutmeg seed and essential oil	Rou Dou Kou

N

Latin Binomial	Common Name	Pinyin Name (Cantonese)
Nardostachys jatamansi, N. chinensis	Indian Spikenard root and essential oil	Gan Song
Nasturtium officinale	Watercress herb	None
Nepeta cataria	Catnip leaf	None
Notopterygium incisum	Notopterygium root	Qiang Huo

O

Latin Binomial	Common Name	Pinyin Name (Cantonese)
Ocimum basilicum	Basil herb and essential oil	Jiu Ceng Ta
Ocimum tenuiflorum, O. sanctum	Holy Basil herb, Tulsi	None
Oldenlandia diffusa	Snake-tongue grass herb	Bai Hua She
Olea europaea	Olive leaf	None
Ophiopogon japonicus	Dwarf Lilyturf root	Mai Men Dong
Oplopanax horridus	Devil's Club root	None
Opuntia spp.	Prickly Pear cactus, whole plant	Xian Ren (root)
Origanum majorana	Marjoram herb and essential oil	None
Origanum vulgare	Oregano herb and essential oil	Tu Yin Chen
Oxalis acetosella	Wood Sorrel herb	None

P

Latin Binomial	Common Name	Pinyin Name (Cantonese)
Paeonia lactiflora	White Peony root	Bai Shao Yao
Paeonia lactiflora, P. obovata	Red Peony root	Chi Shao Yao
Paeonia suffruticosa	Tree Peony root bark	Mu Dan Pi
Palmaria palmata	Dulse seaweed	None
Panax ginseng	Asian ginseng root	Ren Shen
Panax notoginseng	Pseudoginseng root, Tienchi	San Qi/ Tian Qi
Panax quinquefolius	American ginseng root	Xi Yang Shen
Parietaria officinalis	Pellitory of the Wall herb	None
Passiflora incarnata	Passionflower herb	None
Pausinystalia johimbe	Yohimbe bark	None
Pedicularis spp.	Lousewort, Elephant head, Betony	None

Latin Binomial	Common Name	Pinyin Name (Cantonese)
Pelargonium graveolens	Geranium herb and essential oil	Xiang Ye
Perilla frutescens	Perilla seed	Zi Su Zi
Petroselinum crispum	Parsley leaf, root, seed	None
Peumus boldus	Boldo leaf	None
Pfaffia paniculata	Suma root, Brazilian ginseng	None
Phellodendron amurense	Siberian Cork tree bark	Huang Bai
Phytolacca decandra and spp.	Poke root	Shang Lu
Pimpinella anisum	Aniseed and essential oil	None
Pinellia ternata	Prepared Pinellia corm	Ban Xia
Pinus pinaster	Maritime Pine bark	None
Pinus sylvestris	Scotch Pine needle and essential oil	None
Piper methysticum	Kava root	None
Piper nigrum	Black Peppercorn and essential oil	Hu Jiao
Piscidia erythrina	Jamaican Dogwood root bark	None
Plantago psyllium	Psyllium fiber	None
Plantago spp.	Plantain leaf and seed	Che Qian Cao
Platycodon grandiflorum	Balloonflower root	Jie Geng
Podophyllum peltatum	Mayapple root	None
Polygonatum multiflorum and spp.	Solomon's Seal root	Huang Jing
Polygonum aviculare	Common Knotgrass herb	Bian Xu
Polygonum multiflorum	Flowery Knotweed root	He Shou Wu
Populus tremuloides, P. tremula	Quaking Aspen bark	None
Poria cocos	Hoelen fungus	Fu Ling
Porphyra spp.	Nori seaweed	Zi Cai
Portulaca oleracea	Purslane herb	Ma Chi Xian
Potentilla erecta	Tormentil root	None
Potentilla spp.	Cinquefoil herb	Wei Ling Cai
Prunella vulgaris	Selfheal Spike	Xia Ku Cao
Prunus armeniaca	Apricot kernel	Tian Xing Ren (sweet)
Prunus domestica	Plum kernel	None
Prunus persica	Peach kernel	Tao Ren
Prunus serotina	Wild Cherry bark	None
Pueraria lobata	Kudzu root	Ge Gen
Pulmonaria officinalis	Lungwort lichen	None
Pygeum africanum	Pygeum bark	None
Pyrola rotundifolia and spp.	Wintergreen, round-leafed	Lu Xian Cao
Q		
Quercus alba and spp.	White Oak bark, Oak bark	None

Latin Binomial	Common Name	Pinyin Name (Cantonese)
R		
Raphanus sativus niger	Black Radish root	None
Ravensara aromatica	Ravensara essential oil	None
Rehmannia glutinosa	Rehmannia root	Shu Di Huang (prepared), Sheng Di Huang (raw)
Rhamnus catharticus	Buckthorn bark	None
Rhamnus purshiana	Cascara sagrada bark	None
Rheum officinale, R. palmatum	Rhubarb root	Da Huang
Rhodiola rosea	Rhodiola root	None
Rhus glabra	Sumac root bark and berry	None
Ricinus communis	Castor bean seed pods and leaf	None
Rosa woodsii and spp.	Wild Rose flower and hips and essential oil	Mei Gui Hua (flower), Jin Ying Zi (hip)
Rosmarinus officinalis	Rosemary leaf and essential oil	Mai Die Xiang
Rubia tinctorum	Madder root	None
Rubus idaeus	Raspberry leaf	Tai Bing Mei
Rubus villosus	Blackberry	None
Rumex acetosella	Sheep Sorrel herb and root	None
Rumex crispus	Yellow Dock root	Niu Er Da
Ruscus aculeatus	Butcher's Broom root	None
Ruta graveolens	Rue herb	Chou Cao
S		
Salix alba	White Willow bark	None
Salvia miltiorrhiza	Cinnabar Sage root	Dan Shen
Salvia officinalis	Garden Sage leaf and essential oil	Shu Wei Cao
Salvia sclarea	Clary Sage essential oil	None
Sambucus nigra	Black Elderberry	None
Sanguinaria canadensis	Bloodroot	None
Santalum album	Sandalwood and essential oil	Tan Xiang
Sargassum fusiforme and spp.	Sargassum seaweed	Hai Zao
Sarothamnus scoparius and syn. *Cytisus scoparius*	Broom, Scotch Broom tops	None
Schisandra chinensis	Five Taste berry, Schisandra	Wu Wei Zi
Schizonepeta tenuifolia	Japanese Catnip herb	Jing Jie
Scilla maritima	Squill bulb	None
Scrophularia ningpoensis	Black Figwort root	Xuan Shen
Scrophularia nodosa	Figwort root and herb	None
Scutellaria baicalensis	Baikal Skullcap root	Huang Qin

Latin Binomial	Common Name	Pinyin Name (Cantonese)
Scutellaria lateriflora	Skullcap herb	None
Senecio aureas	Life root, Groundsel, Golden Ragwort	None
Senna acutifolia	Senna leaf	Fan Xie Ye
Serenoa serrulata	Saw Palmetto berry	None
Sesamum indicum	Black sesame seed	Hei Zhi Ma
Siegesbeckia pubescens	Hairy Siegesbeckia herb	Xi Xian Cao
Silybum marianum	Milk Thistle seed	Shui Fei Ji
Smilax officinalis	Jamaican Sarsaparilla root	None
Solidago virgaurea and spp.	Goldenrod herb and essential oil	None
Spirulina spp.	Microalgae	None
Stellaria media	Chickweed herb	None
Stephania tetrandra	Stephania root	Han Fang Ji
Stricta pulmonaria	Lungwort lichen	None
Strychnos pierriana	Prepared Vomit nut	Ma Qian Zi
Symphytum officinale	Comfrey root and leaf	None

T

Latin Binomial	Common Name	Pinyin Name (Cantonese)
Tabebuia avellanedae	Pau d'arco bark	None
Tamarindus indica	Tamarind pulp	None
Tanacetum parthenium	Feverfew herb	None
Taraxacum mongolicum	Dandelion root	Pu Gong Ying
Taraxacum officinale	Dandelion root and leaf	None
Theobroma cacao	Cocoa bean/ Chocolate	None
Thymus vulgaris and spp.	Thyme herb and essential oil	Di Jiao
Tilia cordata	Linden flower	Duan Shu Hua
Toxicodendron diversilobum	Poison Oak plant, Western	None
Toxicodendron radicans, syn. *Rhus radicans*	Poison Ivy plant, Eastern	None
Toxicodendron rydbergii	Poison Ivy plant, Western	None
Toxicoscordion venenosum	Meadow Death Camus plant	None
Tribulus terrestris	Caltrop fruit. Puncture vine, Goathead	Bai Ji Li
Trichosanthes kirilowii	Snake Gourd seed	Gua Lou Ren
Trifolium pratense	Red Clover flower	None
Trigonella foenum-graecum	Fenugreek seed	Hu Lu Ba
Trillium pendulum, T. erectum	Bethroot, Birthroot	None
Tripterygium wilfordii	Yellow Vine root	Lei Gong Teng
Triticum repens	Couch Grass root	None
Turnera diffusa	Damiana leaf	None
Tussilago farfara	Coltsfoot herb	Kuan Dong Hua (flower)

U

Latin Binomial	Common Name	Pinyin Name (Cantonese)
Ulmus fulva	Slippery Elm bark	None
Uncaria rhynchophylla	Gambir Vine twig	Gou Teng
Urtica dioica	Nettle herb, seed, and root	None
Usnea diffracta and spp.	Usnea thallus, Old Man's Beard	None

V

Latin Binomial	Common Name	Pinyin Name (Cantonese)
Vaccinium macrocarpon	Cranberry	None
Vaccinium myrtillus	Bilberry leaf and fruit	None
Valerian officinalis	Valerian root and essential oil	Xie Cao
Veratrum californicum and spp.	False Hellebore plant	Li Lu (root)
Verbascum thapsus	Mullein leaf, flower, root	None
Verbena officinalis and spp.	Vervain herb, Blue Vervain	None
Viburnum opulus	Cramp bark	None
Viola tricolor	Heartsease herb	None
Viola yedoensis	Asian Violet root and herb	Zi Hua Di Ding
Viscum album	Mistletoe herb	Hu Ji Sheng
Vitex agnus-castus and spp.	Chastetree berry	Man Jing Zi
Vitis vinifera	Grapevine	None

W

Latin Binomial	Common Name	Pinyin Name (Cantonese)
Withania somnifera	Ashwagandha root	None

X

Latin Binomial	Common Name	Pinyin Name (Cantonese)
Xanthium sibiricum	Siberian Cocklebur	Cang Er Zi

Y

Latin Binomial	Common Name	Pinyin Name (Cantonese)
Yucca spp.	Yucca root	None

Z

Latin Binomial	Common Name	Pinyin Name (Cantonese)
Zanthoxylum americanum	Prickly Ash bark	None
Zea mays	Corn Silk style	None
Zingiber officinalis	Ginger root and essential oil	Jiang Gan (dried), Sheng (fresh), Pi (skin)
Ziziphus jujuba	Black or Red Chinese date, berry	Da Zao (black) Hong Zao (red)
Zizyphus spinosa	Sour Jujube seed	Suan Zao Ren

Cross Index: Herbs by Common Name

Common Name	Latin Binomial	Pinyin Name (Cantonese)
A		
Acerola or Barbados cherry	*Malpighia glabra*	None
Agrimony herb	*Agrimonia eupatoria*	None
Akebia stem	*Akebia quinata*	Bai Mu Tong
Alder bark	*Alnus serrulata*	None
Alfalfa herb	*Medicago sativa*	None
Aloe resin and gel	*Aloe vera* and spp.	Lu Hui
American ginseng root	*Panax quinquefolius*	Xi Yang Shen
Amla, Indian Gooseberry	*Emblica officinalis*	None
Angelica root and essential oil	*Angelica archangelica*	None
Angelica root, Dong Quai	*Angelica sinensis*	Dang Gui
Aniseed and essential oil	*Pimpinella anisum*	None
Apricot kernel	*Prunus armeniaca*	Tian Xing Ren (sweet)
Arnica flower	*Arnica montana* and spp.	None
Artichoke leaf	*Cynara scolymus*	None
Ashwagandha root	*Withania somnifera*	None
Asian Buplever root	*Bupleurum chinense*	Chai Hu
Asian Dodder seed	*Cuscuta chinensis*	Tu Si Zi
Asian ginseng root	*Panax ginseng*	Ren Shen
Asian Hawthorn berry	*Crataegus* spp.	Shan Zha
Asian Motherwort herb	*Leonurus* spp.	Yi Mu Cao
Asian Mugwort leaf	*Artemisia argyi*	Ai Ye
Asian Violet root and herb	*Viola yedoensis*	Zi Hua Di Ding
Asian Wild Ginger root and herb	*Asarum* spp.	Xi Xin
Asparagus root	*Asparagus officinalis*	None
Astragalus root	*Astragalus membranaceus*	Huang Qi
Astragalus seed	*Astragalus* spp.	Sha Yuan Zi
B		
Baikal Skullcap root	*Scutellaria baicalensis*	Huang Qin
Balloonflower root	*Platycodon grandiflorum*	Jie Geng
Barberry root bark	*Berberis vulgaris*	None
Basil herb and essential oil	*Ocimum basilicum*	Jiu Ceng Ta
Betel nut	*Areca catechu*	Bing Lang
Bethroot, Birthroot	*Trillium pendulum, T. erectum*	None
Bilberry leaf and fruit	*Vaccinium myrtillus*	None
Birch leaf, bark, and essential oil	*Betula alba* and spp.	Hua Mu Pi (bark)
Bitter Melon fruit	*Momordica charantia*	Ku Gua (Gan)
Bitter Orange fruit, Neroli essential oil (flower)	*Citrus aurantium*	Zhi Shi (unripe), Zhi Ke (ripe)
Black Atractylodes root	*Atractylodes lancea*	Cang Zhu
Black Cohosh root	*Actaea racemosa*	None
Black Elderberry	*Sambucus nigra*	None
Black Figwort root	*Scrophularia ningpoensis*	Xuan Shen
Black or Red Chinese date, berry	*Ziziphus jujuba*	Da Zao (black) Hong Zao (red)
Black Peppercorn and essential oil	*Piper nigrum*	Hu Jiao
Black Radish root	*Raphanus sativus niger*	None
Black sesame seed	*Sesamum indicum*	Hei Zhi Ma
Blackberry	*Rubus villosus*	None
Bladderwrack thallus	*Fucus vesiculosus*	None
Blessed Thistle herb	*Carduus benedictus*	None
Bloodroot	*Sanguinaria canadensis*	None
Blue Cohosh root	*Caulophyllum thalictroides*	None
Blue Flag rhizome	*Iris versicolor*	None
Bogbean leaf and herb	*Menyanthes trifoliata*	Shui Cai Ye
Boldo leaf	*Peumus boldus*	None
Boneset herb	*Eupatorium perfoliatum*	None
Borage leaf	*Borago officinalis*	None
Broom, Scotch Broom tops	*Sarothamnus scoparius* and syn. *Cytisus scoparius*	None
Buchu leaf	*Agathosma betulina* and spp.	None
Buchu leaf	*Barosma betulina*	None
Buckthorn bark	*Rhamnus catharticus*	None
Bugleweed herb	*Lycopus virginicus*	None
Burdock root	*Arctium lappa*	Niu Bang Zi (seed)
Butcher's Broom root	*Ruscus aculeatus*	None

Common Name	Latin Binomial	Pinyin Name (Cantonese)
C		
Calamus root	*Acorus calamus*	Bai/Shui Chang Pu
Calendula, Marigold, Pot Marigold flower	*Calendula officinalis*	None
California Poppy root and herb	*Eschscholzia californica*	None
Caltrop fruit. Puncture vine, Goathead	*Tribulus terrestris*	Bai Ji Li
Cardamom pod and essential oil	*Elettaria cardamomum*	None
Cascara sagrada bark	*Rhamnus purshiana*	None
Castor bean seed pods and leaf	*Ricinus communis*	None
Catnip leaf	*Nepeta cataria*	None
Cayenne Pepper fruit	*Capsicum annuum*	None
Celandine herb	*Chelidonium majus* and spp.	Bai Qu Cai
Celery seed and root	*Apium graveolens*	None
Celestial Hemp corm	*Gastrodia elata*	Tian Ma
Chastetree berry	*Vitex agnus-castus* and spp.	Man Jing Zi
Chickweed herb	*Stellaria media*	None
Chicory root	*Cichorium intybus*	None
Chinese Caterpillar mushroom	*Cordyceps sinensis*	Dong Chong Xia Cao
Chinese Horse Chestnut	*Aesculus chinensis*	Suo Luo Zi
Chinese Lovage root	*Ligusticum sinense*	Gao Ben
Chrysanthemum flower	*Chrysanthemum* x *morifolium*	Ju Hua
Cilantro herb and seed	*Coriandrum sativum*	Hu Sui (herb), Hu Shi Zi (seed)
Cinchona bark	*Cinchona* spp.	None
Cinnabar Sage root	*Salvia miltiorrhiza*	Dan Shen
Cinnamon bark, twig, and essential oil	*Cinnamomum* spp.	Rou Gui (bark), Gui Zhi (twig)
Cinquefoil herb	*Potentilla* spp.	Wei Ling Cai
Clary Sage essential oil	*Salvia sclarea*	None
Cleavers herb	*Galium aparine*	Ba Xian Cao
Clove bud and essential oil	*Eugenia caryophyllata* and syn. *Syzygium aromaticum*	Ding Xiang
Cocoa bean/Chocolate	*Theobroma cacao*	None
Coffee bean	*Coffea arabica*	None
Coin-Leaf Desmodium herb	*Desmodium styracifolium*	Guang Jin Qian Cao
Coleus root	*Coleus forskohlii*	None
Coltsfoot herb	*Tussilago farfara*	Kuan Dong Hua (flower)
Comfrey root and leaf	*Symphytum officinale*	None
Common Knotgrass herb	*Polygonum aviculare*	Bian Xu
Coptis root	*Coptis chinensis*	Huang Lian
Corn Silk style	*Zea mays*	None
Cotton root bark	*Gossypium* spp.	Mian Hua Gen
Couch Grass root	*Triticum repens*	None
Cow Parsnip leaf and seed	*Heracleum* spp.	None
Cramp bark	*Viburnum opulus*	None
Cranberry	*Vaccinium macrocarpon*	None
Cranesbill root	*Geranium maculatum*	Lao Guan Cao
Crataeva stem and root bark	*Crataeva nurvala*	None
Creosote, Chaparral leaf	*Larrea divaricata*	None
Cypress tip	*Cupressus sempervirens*	None
D		
Damiana leaf	*Turnera diffusa*	None
Dandelion root	*Taraxacum mongolicum*	Pu Gong Ying
Dandelion root and leaf	*Taraxacum officinale*	None
Devil's Claw root	*Harpagophytum procumbens*	None
Devil's Club root	*Oplopanax horridus*	None
Dill seed and essential oil	*Anethum graveolens*	None
Downy Bellflower root	*Codonopsis pilosula*	Dang Shen
Dulse seaweed	*Palmaria palmata*	None
Dwarf Lilyturf root	*Ophiopogon japonicus*	Mai Men Dong
E		
Echinacea root, flower cone	*Echinacea angustifolia, E. purpurea*	None
Elecampane root	*Inula helenium*	Tu Mu Xiang
Ephedra twig	*Ephedra sinica*	Ma Huang
Eucalyptus leaf and essential oil	*Eucalyptus globulus*	An Ye
Eucommia bark	*Eucommia ulmoides*	Du Zhong
Eyebright herb	*Euphrasia* spp.	None
F		
False Hellebore plant	*Veratrum californicum* and spp.	Li Lu (root)
Fennel seed and essential oil	*Foeniculum vulgare*	None
Fenugreek seed	*Trigonella foenum-graecum*	Hu Lu Ba
Feverfew herb	*Chrysanthemum parthenium*	None
Feverfew herb	*Tanacetum parthenium*	None
Figwort root and herb	*Scrophularia nodosa*	None
Fishwort herb	*Houttuynia cordata*	Yu Xing Cao
Five Taste berry, Schisandra	*Schisandra chinensis*	Wu Wei Zi
Flax seed	*Linum usitatissimum*	Ya Ma Zi
Flower pollen	*Granum floris pollinis*	None

Common Name	Latin Binomial	Pinyin Name (Cantonese)
Flowery Knotweed root	*Polygonum multiflorum*	He Shou Wu
Forsythia valve	*Forsythia suspensa*	Lian Qiao
Frankincense resin and essential oil	*Boswellia carterii* and *B. serrata*	Ru Xiang
Fringe Tree root bark	*Chionanthus virginicus*	None

G

Common Name	Latin Binomial	Pinyin Name (Cantonese)
Gambir Vine twig	*Uncaria rhynchophylla*	Gou Teng
Garden Sage leaf and essential oil	*Salvia officinalis*	Shu Wei Cao
Gardenia pod	*Gardenia jasminoides*	Zhi Zi
Garlic bulb	*Allium sativum*	Da Suan
Gentian root	*Gentiana lutea* and spp.	None
Geranium herb and essential oil	*Pelargonium graveolens*	Xiang Ye
German Chamomile flower and essential oil	*Matricaria recutita*	None
Ginger root and essential oil	*Zingiber officinalis*	Jiang Gan (dried), Sheng (fresh), Pi (skin)
Ginkgo leaf	*Ginkgo biloba*	Yin Xing Ye
Glossy Privet berry	*Ligustrum lucidum*	Nu Zhen Zi
Goji berry, Wolfberry, Lycii	*Lycium chinense* and spp.	Gou Qi Zi
Goldenrod herb and essential oil	*Solidago virgaurea* and spp.	None
Goldenseal root	*Hydrastis canadensis*	None
Gotu Kola leaf	*Centella asiatica*	Ji Xue Cao
Grapevine	*Vitis vinifera*	None
Gravel root	*Eupatorium purpureum*	None
Gum Weed flower	*Grindelia robusta*	None
Gymnema herb	*Gymnema sylvestre*	Wu Xue Teng

H

Common Name	Latin Binomial	Pinyin Name (Cantonese)
Hairy Angelica root	*Angelica pubescens*	Du Ho
Hairy Siegesbeckia herb	*Siegesbeckia pubescens*	Xi Xian Cao
Hawthorn berry	*Crataegus* spp.	None
Heart-thread Lotus leaf	*Andrographis paniculata*	Chuan Xin Lian
Heartsease herb	*Viola tricolor*	None
Helonias, False Unicorn root	*Chamaelirium luteum*	None
Hoelen fungus	*Poria cocos*	Fu Ling
Holy Basil herb, Tulsi	*Ocimum tenuiflorum, O. sanctum*	None
Hops flower	*Humulus lupulus*	None
Horney Goat Weed leaf	*Epimedium saggitatum*	Yin Yang Huo
Horse Chestnut	*Aesculus hippocastanum*	None
Horseradish root	*Cochlearia armoracia*	None
Horsetail herb	*Equisetum arvense* and spp.	Mu Zei
Hydrangea root	*Hydrangea arborescens*	None
Hyssop herb and essential oil	*Hyssopus officinalis*	None

I

Common Name	Latin Binomial	Pinyin Name (Cantonese)
Iceland Moss thallus	*Cetraria islandica*	None
Indian Spikenard root and essential oil	*Nardostachys jatamansi, N. chinensis*	Gan Song
Irish Moss thallus	*Chondrus crispus*	None
Isatis, Woad leaf	*Isatis tinctoria, I. indigotica*	Da Qing Ye
Isatis, Woad root	*Isatis tinctoria, I. indigotica*	Ban Lang Gen

J

Common Name	Latin Binomial	Pinyin Name (Cantonese)
Jamaican Dogwood root bark	*Piscidia erythrina*	None
Jamaican Sarsaparilla root	*Smilax officinalis*	None
Japanese Catnip herb	*Schizonepeta tenuifolia*	Jing Jie
Japanese Dogwood berry	*Cornus officinalis*	Shan Zhu Yu
Japanese Honeysuckle flower	*Lonicera japonica* and spp.	Jin Yin Hua
Java berry	*Brucea javanica*	Ya Dan Zi
Jimsonweed, Angel's Trumpet plant	*Datura stramonium* and *D. alba* and spp.	Yang Jin Hua (flower)
Job's Tears seed	*Coix lachryma*	Yi Yi Ren
Juniper berry and essential oil	*Juniperus communis* and spp.	None

K

Common Name	Latin Binomial	Pinyin Name (Cantonese)
Kava root	*Piper methysticum*	None
Kelp thallus	*Laminaria* spp.	Kun Bu
Know Mother root	*Anemarrhena asphodeloides*	Zhi Mu
Kratom leaf	*Mitragyna speciosa*	None
Kudzu root	*Pueraria lobata*	Ge Gen

L

Common Name	Latin Binomial	Pinyin Name (Cantonese)
Lady's Mantle herb	*Alchemilla vulgaris*	None
Lavender flower and essential oil	*Lavandula angustifolia*	None
Lemon Balm leaf and essential oil	*Melissa officinalis*	None
Lemon rind and essential oil	*Citrus limonum*	None
Licorice root	*Glycyrrhiza glabra* and *G. lepidota*	None

Common Name	Latin Binomial	Pinyin Name (Cantonese)
Licorice root	*Glycyrrhiza uralensis*	Gan Cao, Zhi Gan Cao (honey fried)
Life root, Groundsel, Golden Ragwort	*Senecio aureas*	None
Lily of the Valley herb	*Convallaria majalis*	None
Linden flower	*Tilia cordata*	Duan Shu Hua
Lobelia herb	*Lobelia chinensis*	Ban Bian Lian
Lobelia herb	*Lobelia inflata*	None
Longan berry and fruit	*Euphoria longan*	Long Yan Rou
Loquat leaf	*Eriobotrya japonica*	Pi Pa Ye
Lousewort, Elephant head, Betony	*Pedicularis* spp.	None
Lovage root and essential oil	*Ligusticum levisticum*	Ou Dang Gui
Lungwort lichen	*Pulmonaria officinalis*	None
Lungwort lichen	*Stricta pulmonaria*	None

M

Common Name	Latin Binomial	Pinyin Name (Cantonese)
Maca root	*Lepidium meyenii*	None
Madder root	*Rubia tinctorum*	None
Magnolia bark	*Magnolia officinalis*	Hou Po
Magnolia bud	*Magnolia liliiflora*	Xin Yi Hua
Maitake mushroom, Hen of the Woods	*Grifola frondosa*	Hui Shu Hua
Marijuana bud/Grass/Pot	*Cannabis sativa* and *C. indica*	None
Maritime Pine bark	*Pinus pinaster*	None
Marjoram herb and essential oil	*Origanum majorana*	None
Marshmallow root	*Althea officinalis*	None
Mature Deer antler	*Cervus nippon* and spp.	Hua Lu Gen
Mayapple root	*Podophyllum peltatum*	None
Meadow Death Camus plant	*Toxicoscordion venenosum*	None
Meadowsweet herb	*Filipendula ulmaria*	None
Melilot, Sweet Yellow Clover herb	*Melilotus officinalis*	None
Microalgae	*Chlorella* spp	None
Microalgae	*Spirulina* spp.	None
Milk Thistle seed	*Silybum marianum*	Shui Fei Ji
Milkweed	*Asclepias speciosa*	None
Milky Oat tops, berry, and straw	*Avena sativa*	None
Mint herb, Asian field mint, field mint, Poléo mint	*Mentha arvensis*	Bo He
Mistletoe herb	*Viscum album*	Hu Ji Sheng
Motherwort herb	*Leonurus cardiaca*	None
Mountain Death Camus plant	*Anticlea elegans*	None
Mountain Yam root	*Dioscorea* spp.	Shan Yao
Mugwort herb and essential oil	*Artemisia vulgaris*	None
Mullein leaf, flower, root	*Verbascum thapsus*	None
Mustard seed	*Brassica* spp.	None
Myrrh resin and essential oil	*Commiphora myrrha*	Mo Yao

N

Common Name	Latin Binomial	Pinyin Name (Cantonese)
Nettle herb, seed, and root	*Urtica dioica*	None
Night Blooming Cactus flower and stem	*Cereus grandiflorus*, syn. *Selenicereus grandiflorus*	None
Nori seaweed	*Porphyra* spp.	Zi Cai
Notopterygium root	*Notopterygium incisum*	Qiang Huo
Nutmeg seed and essential oil	*Myristica fragrans*	Rou Dou Kou

O

Common Name	Latin Binomial	Pinyin Name (Cantonese)
Ocotillo bark	*Fouquieria splendens*	None
Olive leaf	*Olea europaea*	None
Oregano herb and essential oil	*Origanum vulgare*	Tu Yin Chen
Oregon Grape root	*Mahonia repens*	None
Osha root	*Ligusticum porteri*	None

P

Common Name	Latin Binomial	Pinyin Name (Cantonese)
Parsley leaf, root, seed	*Petroselinum crispum*	None
Parsley piert herb	*Alchemilla arvensis*	None
Partridgeberry herb	*Mitchella repens*	None
Pasqueflower herb	*Anemone pulsatilla/patens*	None
Passionflower herb	*Passiflora incarnata*	None
Pau d'arco bark	*Tabebuia avellanedae*	None
Peach kernel	*Prunus persica*	Tao Ren
Pellitory of the Wall herb	*Parietaria officinalis*	None
Pennyroyal herb	*Mentha pulegium*	None
Peppermint leaf and essential oil	*Mentha* x *piperita*	None
Perilla seed	*Perilla frutescens*	Zi Su Zi
Pipsissewa herb and root	*Chimaphila umbellata*	None
Plantain leaf and seed	*Plantago* spp.	Che Qian Cao
Pleurisy root	*Asclepias tuberosa*	None
Plum kernel	*Prunus domestica*	None
Poison Hemlock plant	*Conium maculatum*	None
Poison Ivy plant, Eastern	*Toxicodendron radicans*, syn. *Rhus radicans*	None
Poison Ivy plant, Western	*Toxicodendron rydbergii*	None
Poison Oak plant, Western	*Toxicodendron diversilobum*	None
Poke root	*Phytolacca decandra* and spp.	Shang Lu
Prepared Asian Corydalis corm	*Corydalis* spp.	Yan Hu Suo

Common Name	Latin Binomial	Pinyin Name (Cantonese)
Prepared Pinellia corm	*Pinellia ternata*	Ban Xia
Prepared Sichuan Aconite root	*Aconitum carmichaelii*	Fu Zi
Prepared Vomit nut	*Strychnos pierriana*	Ma Qian Zi
Prickly Ash bark	*Zanthoxylum americanum*	None
Prickly Lettuce	*Lactuca serriola*	None
Prickly Pear cactus, whole plant	*Opuntia* spp.	Xian Ren (root)
Proud Pink herb	*Dianthus superbus*	Qu Mai
Pseudoginseng root, Tienchi	*Panax notoginseng*	San Qi/Tian Qi
Psyllium fiber	*Plantago psyllium*	None
Pumpkin seed	*Cucurbita* spp.	None
Purslane herb	*Portulaca oleracea*	Ma Chi Xian
Pygeum bark	*Pygeum africanum*	None
Q		
Quaking Aspen bark	*Populus tremuloides, P. tremula*	None
R		
Ragweed herb	*Ambrosia artemisiifolia*	None
Raspberry leaf	*Rubus idaeus*	Tai Bing Mei
Ravensara essential oil	*Ravensara aromatica*	None
Red Clover flower	*Trifolium pratense*	None
Red Peony root	*Paeonia lactiflora, P. obovata*	Chi Shao Yao
Red root	*Ceanothus* spp.	None
Rehmannia root	*Rehmannia glutinosa*	Shu Di Huang (prepared), Sheng Di Huang (raw)
Reishi mushroom	*Ganoderma lucidum*	Ling Zhi
Rhodiola root	*Rhodiola rosea*	None
Rhubarb root	*Rheum officinale, R. palmatum*	Da Huang
Rosemary leaf and essential oil	*Rosmarinus officinalis*	Mai Die Xiang
Rue herb	*Ruta graveolens*	Chou Cao
Rugose Giant Hyssop herb	*Agastache rugosa*	Huo Xiang
S		
Safflower	*Carthamus tinctorius*	Hong Hua
Saffron flower styles, stigmas	*Crocus sativus*	Xi Hong Hua
Sagebrush herb	*Artemisia tridentata* and spp.	None
Sandalwood and essential oil	*Santalum album*	Tan Xiang
Sargassum seaweed	*Sargassum fusiforme* and spp.	Hai Zao
Saw Palmetto berry	*Serenoa serrulata*	None
Scabrous Gentian root	*Gentiana scabra*	Long Dan Cao
Scotch Pine needle and essential oil	*Pinus sylvestris*	None
Sea Holly root	*Eryngium maritimum*	None
Selfheal Spike	*Prunella vulgaris*	Xia Ku Cao
Senna leaf	*Cassia acutifolia*	None
Senna leaf	*Senna acutifolia*	Fan Xie Ye
Shatavari root	*Asparagus racemosus*	None
Sheep Sorrel herb and root	*Rumex acetosella*	None
Shepherd's Purse herb	*Capsella bursa-pastoris*	Jia Cai
Shiny Asparagus root	*Asparagus cochinchinensis*	Tian Men Dong
Shitake mushroom (Japanese)	*Lentinula edodes*	Xiang Gu
Siberian Cocklebur	*Xanthium sibiricum*	Cang Er Zi
Siberian Cork tree bark	*Phellodendron amurense*	Huang Bai
Siberian/Eleuthero ginseng root	*Eleutherococcus senticosus*	Ci Wu Jia
Sichuan Bead Tree berry	*Melia toosendan*	Chuan Lian Zi
Sichuan Lovage root	*Ligusticum wallichii*	Chuan Xiong
Sickle Senna seed	*Cassia obtusifolia*	Jue Ming Zi
Skullcap herb	*Scutellaria lateriflora*	None
Slippery Elm bark	*Ulmus fulva*	None
Snake Gourd seed	*Trichosanthes kirilowii*	Gua Lou Ren
Snake-tongue grass herb	*Oldenlandia diffusa*	Bai Hua She
Solomon's Seal root	*Polygonatum multiflorum* and spp.	Huang Jing
Sour Jujube seed	*Zizyphus spinosa*	Suan Zao Ren
Spearmint leaf and essential oil	*Mentha spicata*	Xiang Hua Cai
Spotted Water Hemlock plant	*Cicuta maculata*	None
Squill bulb	*Scilla maritima*	None
St. John's Wort	*Hypericum perforatum*	Guan Ye Lian Qiao
Stephania root	*Stephania tetrandra*	Han Fang Ji
Stonebushel stem	*Dendrobium nobile*	Shi Hu
Stoneroot	*Collinsonia canadensis*	None
Strawberry leaf	*Fragaria vesca*	None
Suma root, Brazilian ginseng	*Pfaffia paniculata*	None
Sumac root bark and berry	*Rhus glabra*	None
Sweet Annie herb	*Artemisia annua*	Huang Hua Hao
Sweet Orange fruit	*Citrus* x *aurantium* var. *sinensis*	Tian Chen
T		
Tamarind pulp	*Tamarindus indica*	None
Tangerine peel and essential oil	*Citrus reticulata* and spp.	Qing Pi (unripe), Chen Pi (ripe)

Common Name	Latin Binomial	Pinyin Name (Cantonese)
Tarragon herb and essential oil	*Artemisia dracunculus*	None
Tea leaf	*Camellia sinensis*	Cha Ye
Tea Tree leaf and essential oil	*Melaleuca alternifolia*	None
Thyme herb and essential oil	*Thymus vulgaris* and spp.	Di Jiao
Tormentil root	*Potentilla erecta*	None
Tree Peony root bark	*Paeonia suffruticosa*	Mu Dan Pi
Turmeric root	*Curcuma longa*	Yu Jin

U

Common Name	Latin Binomial	Pinyin Name (Cantonese)
Unicorn root	*Aletris farinose*	None
Upright Ladybell root	*Adenophora stricta*	Nan Sha Shen
Usnea thallus, Old Man's Beard	*Usnea diffracta* and spp.	None
Uva ursi leaf, Bearberry, Kinnikinnick	*Arctostaphylos uva-ursi*	None

V

Common Name	Latin Binomial	Pinyin Name (Cantonese)
Valerian root and essential oil	*Valerian officinalis*	Xie Cao
Velvet bean	*Macuna pruriens*	None
Vervain herb, Blue Vervain	*Verbena officinalis* and spp.	None

W

Common Name	Latin Binomial	Pinyin Name (Cantonese)
Walnut leaf and hull, Black Walnut seed, leaf, and hull	*Juglans regia* and *J. nigra*	Hu Tao Ren (meat), Ye (leaf), Zhi (twig)
Water Hyssop, Bacopa whole plant	*Bacopa monnieri*	None
Water plantain root	*Alisma orientalis*	Ze Xie
Watercress herb	*Nasturtium officinale*	None
White Atractylodes root	*Atractylodes macrocephala*	Bai Zhu
White Horehound leaf	*Marrubium vulgare*	None
White Oak bark, Oak bark	*Quercus alba* and spp.	None
White Peony root	*Paeonia lactiflora*	Bai Shao Yao
White Willow bark	*Salix alba*	None
Wild Cardamom pod	*Amomum villosum*	Sha Ren
Wild Carrot seed	*Daucus carota*	Nan He Zao
Wild Cherry bark	*Prunus serotina*	None
Wild Ginger root	*Asarum canadensis*	None
Wild Indigo root	*Baptisia tinctoria*	None
Wild Lettuce leaf	*Lactuca virosa*	None
Wild Onion bulb	*Allium* spp.	None
Wild Oregano, Beebalm herb	*Monarda fistulosa*	None
Wild Rose flower and hips and essential oil	*Rosa woodsii* and spp.	Mei Gui Hua (flower), Jin Ying Zi (hip)
Wild Yam rhizome	*Dioscorea villosa*	None
Wind Protector root	*Ledebouriella divaricata*	Fang Feng
Wintergreen herb (Eastern N. America)	*Gaultheria procumbens*	None
Wintergreen, round-leafed	*Pyrola rotundifolia* and spp.	Lu Xian Cao
Witch Hazel leaf	*Hamamelis virginiana*	None
Wood betony herb	*Betonica officinalis*	None
Wood Sorrel herb	*Oxalis acetosella*	None
Wormwood herb	*Artemisia absinthium*	None

Y

Common Name	Latin Binomial	Pinyin Name (Cantonese)
Yarrow herb and essential oil	*Achillea millefolium*	None
Yellow Dock root	*Rumex crispus*	Niu Er Da
Yellow Vine root	*Tripterygium wilfordii*	Lei Gong Teng
Yerba Mansa herb	*Anemopsis californica*	None
Yerba Maté leaf and twig	*Ilex paraguariensis*	None
Yerba Santa leaf	*Eriodictyon* spp.	None
Yohimbe bark	*Pausinystalia johimbe*	None
Yucca root	*Yucca* spp.	None
Zhejiang Fritillaria bulb	*Fritillaria thunbergii*	Zhe Bei Mu

Bibliography

Achterberg, Jeanne. *Woman as Healer* (Boston, MA: Shambhala Press, 1990).

Alfs, Matthew. *300 Herbs: Their Indications & Contraindications* (New Brighton, MN: Old Theology Book House, 2003).

Battaglia, Salvatore. *The Complete Guide to Aromatherapy,* 3rd ed. (Australia: Black Pepper Creative, 2018).

Beinfield, Harriet and Efrem Korngold. *Between Heaven and Earth: A Guide to Chinese Medicine* (New York: Ballantine Books, 1991).

Bensky Dan, et al., editors. *Materia Medica: Chinese Herbal Medicine,* 3rd ed. (Seattle, WA: Eastland Press, Inc., 2004).

Blumenthal M, et al., editors. *The Complete German Commission E Monographs: Therapeutic Guide to Herbal Medicines.* (Austin, TX: American Botanical Council published in cooperation with Integrative Medicine Communications, 1998).

Bone, Kerry and Simon Mills. *Principles and Practice of Phytotherapy* (London, UK: Elsevier, 2013).

Bone, Kerry. *The Ultimate Herbal Compendium* (Warwick, Queensland, Australia: Phytotherapy Press, 2007).

Brinker, Francis. *Herb Contraindications and Drug Interactions,* 2nd ed. (Sandy, OR: Eclectic Medical, 1998).

Buhner, Stephen Harrod. *Herbal Antibiotics,* 2nd ed. (North Adams, MA: Storey, 2012).

Buhner, Stephen Harrod. *Herbal Antivirals* (North Adams, MA: Storey, 2013).

Buhner, Stephen Harrod. *The Lost Language of Plants* (Chelsea, VT: Chelsea Green, 2002).

Coffman, Sam. *The Herbal Medic,* vol I. (San Antonio, TX: The Human Path, 2014).

Cook, William. *The Physio-Medical Dispensatory: A Treatise on Therapeutics, Materia Medica, and Pharmacy in Accordance with the Principles of Physiological Medication* (Cincinnati, OH: William Cook, 1869).

Corrado, Monica. *The Complete Cooking Techniques for the GAPS™ Diet* (Fort Collins, CO: Selene River Press, 2019).

Craighead, John J, et al. (Peterson Field Guides) *A Field Guide to Rocky Mountain Wildflowers* (New York: Houghton Mifflin, 1963).

De La Forêt, Rosalee. *Alchemy of Herbs* (Carlsbad, CA: Hay House Lifestyles, 2017).

Eisler, Riane. *The Chalice and the Blade, Our History, Our Future* (New York: Harper Collins, 1995).

Elpel, Thomas J. *Botany in A Day,* 6th ed. (Pony, MT: HOPS Press, 2013).

Essential Science Publishing, compilers. *PDR: People's Desk Reference for Essential Oils* (Essential Science Publishing, 1999).

Flanagan, Sabina. *Hildegard of Bingen, a Visionary Life* (London, UK: Routledge, 1989).

Flint, Margi. *The Practicing Herbalist: Meeting with Clients, Reading the Body,* 3rd ed. (Marblehead, ME: Earth Song, 2013).

Ganora, Lisa. *Herbal Constituents: Foundations of Phytochemistry* (Louisville, CO: Herbalchem, 2009).

Gladstar, Rosemary. *Herbal Healing for Women* (New York: Fireside, Simon & Schuster, 1993).

Gladstar, Rosemary. *Rosemary Gladstar's Herbal Recipes for Vibrant Health* (North Adams, MA: Storey, 2008).

Govinda, Kalashatra. *A Handbook of Chakra Healing: Spiritual Practice for Health, Harmony, and Inner Peace* (Old Saybrook, CT: Konecky and Konecky, 2002).

Green, James. *The Herbal Medicine-Maker's Handbook* (New York: Crossing Press, 2002).

Griggs, Barbara. *Green Pharmacy: The History and Evolution of Western Herbal Medicine* (Rochester, VT: Healing Arts, 1991).

Hofmann, Albert, et al. *Plants of the Gods: Origins of Hallucinogenic Use* (New York: Van der Marck, 1987).

Hoffman, David. *Medical Herbalism: The Science and Practice of Herbal Medicine* (Rochester, VT: Healing Arts, 2003).

Holmes, Peter. *Energetics of Western Herbs: A Materia Medica Integrating Western & Chinese Herbal Therapeutics.* vols. I and II. 4th ed. (Boulder, CO: Snow Lotus, 2006).

Holmes, Peter. *Jade Remedies: A Chinese Herbal Reference for the West,* vols. I and II. (Boulder, CO: Snow Lotus, 1996).

Kane, Charles W. *Medicinal Plants of the American Southwest* (Lincoln Town Press, 2011).

Kaptchuk, Ted J. *The Web That Has No Weaver* (New York: Congdon and Weed, 1983).

Kass-Annese and Hal Danzer. *The Fertility Awareness Handbook* (Redondo Beach, CA: Patterns Publishing, 1981).

Kershaw, Linda. *Edible and Medicinal Plants of the Rockies* (Auburn, WA: Lone Pine, 2000).

Kizior, Robert J and Barbara B. Hodgson. *Saunders Nursing Drug Handbook 2017* (Salt Lake City, UT: Elsevier, 2017).

Lieberman, Daniel E. *The Story of the Human Body* (New York: Vintage, 2014).

Mars, Brigitte. *The Desktop Guide to Herbal Medicine,* 2nd ed. (Columbus, OH: Basic Health, 2016).

McGuffin Michael, et al., editors. *American Herbal Products Association's Botanical Safety Handbook.* (New York: CRC Press, 1997).

Meyers, Amy. *The Autoimmune Solution: Prevent and Reverse the Full Spectrum of Inflammatory Symptoms and Diseases* (New York: Harper Collins, 2017).

Mills, Simon Y and Kerry Bone. *Essential Guide to Herbal Safety* (London, UK: Elsevier, 2005).

Mills, Simon Y. *The Essential Book of Herbal Medicine* (Middlesex, UK: Penguin, 1991).

Moore, Michael. *Medicinal Plants of the Desert and Canyon West* (Santa Fe, NM: Museum of New Mexico Press, 1989).

Moore, Michael. *Medicinal Plants of the Mountain West* revised and expanded ed. (Santa Fe, NM: Museum of New Mexico Press, 2003).

Murray, Michael and Joseph Pizzorno. *Encyclopedia of Natural Medicine* (Rocklin, CA: Prima, 1991).

Murray, Michael. *Encyclopedia of Nutritional Supplements* (Rocklin, CA: Prima, 1996).

Murray, Michael. *The Healing Power of Herbs,* 2nd ed. (Rocklin, CA: Prima, 1999).

Myss, Caroline. *Anatomy of the Spirit* (New York: Three Rivers, 1996).

Naeser, Margaret A. *Outline Guide to Chinese Herbal Patent Medicines in Pill Form* (Ann Arbor, MI: Edwards Brothers, 1990).

Northrup, Christiane. *The Wisdom of Menopause* (New York: Bantam Books, 2001).

Northrup, Christiane. *Women's Body, Women's Wisdom* (New York: Bantam Books, 2002).

Nozedar, Adele. *The Illustrated Signs and Symbols Sourcebook* (New York: Metro Books, 2008).

O'Brien, Mary and Karen Vail. *Edible and Medicinal Plants of the Southern Rockies* (Steamboat Springs, CO: Leaning Tree Tales, 2015).

Romm, Aviva. *Naturally Healthy Babies and Children* (Berkeley, CA: Celestial Arts, 2000).

Romm, Aviva. *Adrenal Thyroid Revolution* (New York: Harper Collins, 2017).

Romm, Aviva. *Botanical Medicine for Women's Health* (London, UK: Elsevier, 2010).

Santich, Rob and Kerry Bone. *Phytotherapy Essentials: Healthy Children, Optimizing Children's Health with Herbs* (Warwick, Queensland, Australia: Phytotherapy Press, 2008).

Skidmore-Roth, Linda. *Mosby's Nursing Drug Reference 2017,* 30th ed. (Salt Lake City, UT: Elsevier, 2017).

Strehlow, Wighard and Gottfried Hertzka. *Hildegard of Bingen's Medicine* (Santa Fe, NM: Bear and Company, 1988).

Taylor, James and Barbara Cohen. *Memmler's Structure and Function of the Human Body,* 10th ed. (Philadelphia, PA: Lippincott, 2013).

Teeguarden, Ron. *Chinese Herbal Tonics* (Venice, CA: Cha Yuan Press, 1991).

Tierra, Michael. *The Way of Chinese Herbs* (New York: Pocket Books, 1998).

Tilford, Gregory L. *Edible and Medicinal Plants of the West* (Missoula, MT: Mountain Press, 1997).

Trickey, Ruth. *Women, Hormones & the Menstrual Cycle* (St. Leonards, NSW, Australia: Allen and Unwin, 1998).

Weed, Susun S. *Down There: Sexual and Reproductive Health* (Woodstock, NY: Ash Tree, 2011).

Weil, Andrew. *Eight Weeks to Optimum Health* (New York: Random House, 2003).

Wentz, Izabella. *Hashimoto's Protocol* (New York: Harper Collins, 2017).

Wolfson, Jack. *The Paleo Cardiologist* (New York: Morgan James, 2015).

Yance, Donald R. *Adaptogens in Medical Herbalism* (Rochester, VT: Healing Arts, 2013).

Zand, Janet, et al. *Smart Medline for a Healthier Child: A Practical A-Z Reference to Natural and Conventional Treatments for Infants and Children* (Garden City, NY: Avery, 1994).

Index

Page numbers followed by *b* indicates boxes, *f* indicates figures and *t* indicates tables.

H

M

Q

R

S

T

U

V

W